MECHANISMS IN PARKINSON'S DISEASE – MODELS AND TREATMENTS

Edited by **Juliana Dushanova**

Mechanisms in Parkinson's Disease – Models and Treatments
Edited by Juliana Dushanova

Published by InTech

Janeza Trdine 9, 51000 Rijeka, Croatia

Publishing Process Manager Silvia Vlase

Technical Editor Teodora Smiljanic

Cover Designer InTech Design Team

Additional hard copies can be obtained from orders@intechopen.com

Mechanisms in Parkinson's Disease – Models and Treatments, Edited by Juliana Dushanova
p. cm.
ISBN 978-953-307-876-2

For EU product safety concerns:
IN TECH d.o.o., Prolaz Marije Krucifikse Kozulić 3, 51000 Rijeka, Croatia,
info@intechopen.com or visit our website at intechopen.com.

Meet the editor

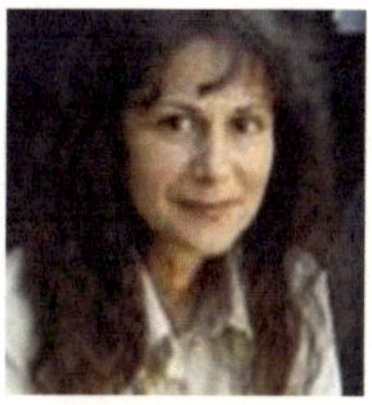

Dr Dushanova's research interests are in motor neurophysiology, pathophysiology of Parkinson's disease, and in the development of approaches for diagnostics. Her works span human and non-human primate research, computational modeling, and simulations. She received her MS degree from Sofia University, Bulgaria and her pre-doctoral fellowship from Professor Pfurtscheller at the Department of Medical Informatics at the Ludwig Boltzmann Institute for Medical Informatics and Neuroinformatics, Technical University Graz, Austria. Her PhD was received from the Institute of Neurobiology, Bulgarian Academy of Sciences, and she studied neurophysiology under the supervision of Professor J.P. Donoghue in the Neuroscience Department of Brown University, Rhode Island, USA. Associate Professor Dushanova's research is in the field of movement disorders, and she has been involved in electroencephalography research and practice since 1994.

Contents

Preface

Parkinson's disease (PD) is the second most common neurodegenerative disorder that affects one to two per cent of the world's population over the age of 65. Continued research into the pathogenesis of PD is essential as it mainly affects the elderly population.

PD is characterized by a loss of dopaminergic neurons from the substantia nigra pars compacta (SNc). The SNc is part of the substantia nigra, which belongs to the group of nuclei in the midbrain, called the basal ganglia. The function of the basal ganglia requires signaling of both excitatory and inhibitory neurotransmitters to balance the two main signaling pathways, the direct and indirect pathways. These pathways remain balanced by the nigrostriatal pathway or the dopaminergic projections from the SNc to the striatum (caudate nucleus and putamen) with a basal level of striatal dopaminergic DA integral for proper function of the basal ganglia. A basal ganglia structure performs neurotransmitter-mediated operations through somatotopically organized projections to GABAergic medium spiny projection neurons (MSNs). These striatal cells are innervated by excitatory glutamatergic fibers from cortex and thalamus, and modulatory dopaminergic fibers from the midbrain and transmit neural information to the basal ganglia output structures. Neural transmission at the level of MSNs has been associated with the regulation of voluntary movement and cognitive functions. Knowledge of the new transmitter mechanisms by which such interactions take place can provide new insight into the basal ganglia physiopathology and new clues for therapy of severe motor disorders, such as Parkinson's disease. Thus, in PD, the loss of dopamine neurons causes the subsequent loss of striatal dopamine, and the presentation of motor symptoms, such as bradykinesia, akinesia, rigidity and postural instability. The movement disorders are often associated with abnormalities in electrical activity within the substantia nigra pars reticulata. Parkinson's is a complex disorder involving alterations in brain chemistry, morphology and activity. An enhanced understanding of the interdependence of these processes will increase our understanding of this devastating disease.

Accordingly, current treatment of PD involves increasing striatal dopamine content, by either direct replacement or reduction of its breakdown. Unfortunately, these treatments only provide symptomatic relief and the efficacy is somewhat limited. For example, the current "gold-standard" treatment for PD, L-DOPA, the precursor to dopamine, only alleviates symptoms for five to 10 years before debilitating side effects such as dyskinesia appears. The underlying pathogenesis of degenerating DA neurons still remains unknown. Importantly for potential PD therapeutics, the loss of neurons occurs slowly over many years, suggesting that there is a window of opportunity within which a neuroprotective therapy could be administered to slow or halt the progression of the disease. However, to date, no neuroprotective therapies are in clinical use. As this is the case, new avenues of research into the pathogenesis of PD and the discovery of possible neuroprotective agents are critical.

Evidence from both clinical and experimental models of PD have elucidated a number of mechanisms that are attributed to the continuing loss of DA neurons, such as oxidative stress, mitochondrial dysfunction, and glutamate excitotoxicity. More recently, inflammatory processes, particularly the chronic activation of microglia, and blood brain barrier (BBB) dysfunction have gained much attention for their potential role in the pathogenesis of PD. There is evidence that oxidative stress participates in the neurodegeneration. Neutrophils express a primary alteration of nitric oxide release in PD patients, where reactive oxygen species and oxidative stress parameters are more probably related to the evolution of PD. Peripheral markers of oxidative stress in red blood cells of neurological patients could be a reflection of the brain condition and suggests that oxygen-free radicals are partially responsible for the damage observed in PD living patients. Other reports suggest that mitochondrial dysfunction and impairment of the respiratory complexes are associated with the neuronal loss. Substantial evidence suggests diet, in particular iron intake, and environmental risk factors, such as pesticides and heavy metals as causative of PD. However, the way genetic and environmental factors are related to the nutritional status of PD patients is still unknown. Moreover, how the nutritional status of PD patients might contribute to the development of the disorder is not yet established. Drosophila melanogaster is used as a valid model in PD research to investigate the effect of paraquat and iron alone or in combination, and polyphenols upon two different glucose feeding regimens on the life span and locomotor activity of the fly. The concept of oxidative stress is defined as an imbalance with increased oxidants or decreased antioxidants. The situations of oxidative stress, evaluated by the peripheral markers of oxidative stress in the blood of neurological patients, seem to afford a reflection of the brain condition. Brain oxidative stress, with oxygen free radicals being responsible for brain damage, provides signals to peripheral blood, at least, through the diffusible products of lipid peroxidation.

The neuropeptide, substance P (SP), is widely distributed throughout both the central and peripheral nervous systems. Generally in PD, it is considered that SP expression within the SN is decreased, with such loss of SP also being attributed to symptom presentation. However, most studies have used post-mortem PD cases or experimental models of PD with maximal dopaminergic degeneration, which replicate the late stages of the disease. In these final stages, the reduction in striatal DA input has resulted in a loss of the SP/DA positive feedback mechanism and consequently the reduction in nigral SP. Indeed, it has been shown that SP content within the SN is not reduced until greater than 90 per cent of striatal DA has been depleted. SP content within the SN has yet to be directly measured in early clinical PD.

A prevalent etiologic hypothesis is that PD may result from a complex interaction between environmental toxic factors, genetic susceptibility traits, and aging. In the initial stages of disease, levodopa therapy is the most effective for improving motor symptoms in individuals with PD. However, long-term treatment with levodopa is accompanied by fluctuations in motor performance, dyskinesias, and neuropsychiatric complications. A disease-modifying therapy is the most important unmet medical need in the treatment of PD. New information has become available on the mechanism responsible for levodopa-induced motor complications and the potential value of therapies that provide more continuous dopaminergic stimulation.

Little mathematical modeling has been offered for Parkinson's disease. Drosophila research into PD has focused on the transgenic expression of human alpha–synuclein in fly neurons and on the comprehensive investigation of two genes responsible for recessive PD, parkin and PINK1. Finally, the advantages of Drosophila as a model will continue to advance our understanding of the mechanisms that contribute to PD, and to aid in the design of therapeutic treatments with implications for other degenerative diseases and aging processes.

Many drugs used to treat PD are effective in many patients, but do not retard the degeneration of the brain regions affected by the disease. Their effectiveness diminishes over time and their adverse effects become increasingly more troublesome. Therefore, new therapeutic approaches are required. Clinical and biochemical evidences suggest that PD involves multifactorial oxidative neurodegeneration, and that levodopa therapy aggravates the oxidative burden. It is demonstrated that PD is primarily an oxidative disease and can be induced by endogenous and exogenous environmental oxidant stressors. Several lines of evidences indicate also that mitochondrial dysfunctions play an important role in the pathophysiology of PD contributing to the development and progression of the disease. Recent studies show that two of the four major genes (DJI and PINK1) involved in familial Parkinson's disease are of mitochondrial origin. Mutations of these genes increase cell susceptibility to stressful conditions inducing mitochondrial dysfunction and apoptosis. Mitochondrial antioxidants/nutrients can improve mitochondrial functions and protect mitochondria against oxidative damage. It has been shown that they have neuroprotective effects against PD in cellular and animal models as well as in clinical trials. The mitochondrial antioxidant/nutrient acetyl-L-carnitine (ALC), with its well-known antioxidant energizing protective activities and with its trophic effects, at optimal doses can be an effective and safe prevention strategy for PD.

Idiopathic Parkinson's disease is thought to represent a complex interaction between the inherent vulnerability of the nigrostriatal dopaminergic system, a possible genetic predisposition, and exposure to environmental toxins, including inflammatory triggers. Accumulating evidence now suggests that chronic neuroinflammation is consistently associated with the pathophysiology of PD. Activation of microglia, the resident immune cells of the brain have been reported after post-mortem analysis of the substantia nigra pars compacta in brains from PD patients. Equally, increased levels of pro-inflammatory mediators, reactive oxygen species and eicosanoids have been repeatedly reported in the brain of PD patients. It is hypothesized that chronically activated microglia secrete high levels of pro-inflammatory mediators, which damage neurons and further activate microglia, resulting in a feed forward cycle, promoting further inflammation and neurodegeneration. Moreover, nigrostriatal dopaminergic neurons are more vulnerable to pro-inflammatory and oxidative mediators than other cell types because of their low intracellular glutathione concentration. Systemic inflammation has also been suggested to contribute to neuroinflammation and, consequently, neurodegeneration in PD, as lymphocyte infiltration has been observed in brains of PD patients. Epidemiological reports of reduced susceptibility to PD among chronic users of anti-inflammatory drugs have also provided evidence of a link between inflammation and PD. Intriguing new evidence now suggests that exposure to systemic inflammation pre-birth or in early life, and the consequent induction of neuroinflammation throughout the lifespan of an individual, contributes to the evolution of neurodegenerative disorders like PD. Sustained microglial activation, elevated pro-inflammatory mediators and lymphocyte infiltration have also all been observed in animal models of PD, substantiating the current belief of a fundamental role of inflammation in neurodegeneration.

The molecular pathways underlying the pathogenesis of the disease remain poorly understood. Interestingly, recent studies suggest that cyclin-dependent kinase 5 (Cdk5), a serine/threonine kinase that is predominantly active in neurons, plays a pivotal role in neuronal loss in models of Parkinson's disease. Cdk5 is typically activated by its activator p35 and p39, and is implicated in a plethora of neuronal functions including neuronal migration, neuronal survival and differentiation, and the regulation of synaptic functions. Cleavage of p35 into a p25 fragment during pathological condition results in prolonged and aberrant activation of Cdk5. Importantly, p25-mediated activation of Cdk5 has been associated with neuronal loss in MPTP-toxicity model of Parkinson's disease. MPTP-induced neuronal loss is markedly attenuated in p35-deficient mice. Subsequent studies have identified several substrates of Cdk5 that may be the underlying critical role of Cdk5 in MPTP toxicity. For example, phosphorylation of survival factor MEF2 by Cdk5 was found to inactivate MEF2, in addition to promoting its degradation. In addition, Cdk5-mediated phosphorylation of antioxidant enzyme Prx2 and an enzyme crucial for repair of DNA damage, Ape1, have both been demonstrated to contribute to MPTP-induced neuronal loss.

The tridecapeptide neurotensin (NT), widely distributed both in the peripheral and in the central nervous system (CNS) of mammals, including humans, acts as a primary neurotransmitter or neuromodulator of classical neurotransmitters. NT is synthesized in neurons and released by sodium and calcium-dependent mechanisms and three major subtypes of NT receptors named NTS1, NTS2, and NTS3, are largely distributed in different discrete areas in the brain, as well as in the periphery. NT has been shown to be closely associated with the dopaminergic system, implicated in Parkinson's disease. The functional evidence that NT modulates dopaminergic transmission, especially the nigrostriatal and mesocorticolimbic DA pathways, has suggested that the NT regulation of this system may have important implications for the pathophysiology and development of treatments of these disorders. The NT receptor antagonists could be used as a treatment strategy for Parkinson's disease. In addition, NT also plays a crucial role in the regulation of the glutamatergic transmission. Evidence has accumulated that glutamate is an important mediator of neuronal injury. In view of the enhancing effects of NT on glutamate transmission, this peptide may play a relevant role in reinforcing the glutamate-mediated excitotoxicity, as demonstrated in primary cultures of mesencephalic DA and cortical neurons.

The majority of cases of Parkinson's disease are idiopathic, and with the exception of isolated toxin induced cases such as MPTP (1-methyl-4-phenyl-1,2,3,6-tetrahydropyridine), underlying environmental causes remain to be discovered. However, approximately 15 per cent of individuals with Parkinson's disease have a first-degree relative who also has the disease, and five to10 per cent of Parkinson's disease sufferers are known to have monogenic forms of the disease. Furthermore, a number of the genes identified in familial Parkinson's disease have been implicated in, and as risk factors for, sporadic disease. Currently, without a defined aetiology of the sporadic disease, studying the molecular mechanisms by which the genetic and toxic forms progress in animal models offers a valuable resource to gain insight into the sporadic disease.

The loss of nigrostriatal dopaminergic neurons (predominately in the substantia nigra pars compacta) as well as noradrenergic neurons of the locus coeruleus with the concomitant of intracytoplasmic protein aggregates termed Lewy bodies in surviving neurons, is considered the defining pathological feature of Parkinson's disease. Based on Lewy body deposition, it has been suggested that Parkinson's disease first affects the olfactory bulbs and caudal brainstem nuclei and then progresses rostrally to the substantia nigra, which does not become involved until the disease is moderately advanced. However, dopamine supplementation to reverse depleted dopamine output from the substantia nigra pars compacta is the mainstay pharmacological intervention for Parkinson's disease. Drugs, such as levodopa, alleviate the symptomatic motor decline of Parkinson's disease only; they do not address the nonmotor features related to degeneration of nondopaminergic systems. As the disease progresses, dopamine supplementation becomes less efficient, and dyskinesia and behavioral abnormalities may develop. Interestingly, a recent study has reported that the neural loss in PD in locus coeruleus is greater than that in substantia nigra. The influence of noradrenergic neurotransmission on dopamine-mediated behavior has been the focus of several studies over the last four decades, and has confirmed the importance of the relationship between dopaminergic and noradrenergic pathways in the control of locomotor activity. It has been suggested that progressive neurodegeneration of the main noradrenergic nucleus – the locus coeruleus – might influence not only the progression of Parkinson's disease but also the response to dopaminergic replacement. Furthermore, additional evidence supports the notion that noradrenaline deficit might be relevant to the pathogenesis of long-term complications of L-DOPA treatment, such as the wearing-off phenomenon and dyskinesias.

In spite of the bulk of data on the influence of an alteration of noradrenergic transmission on locomotor behavior, much of this data is conflicting and not conclusive. Therefore, definitive conclusions as to the specific role of the noradrenergic system in the generation of symptoms of Parkinson's disease and L-DOPA-induced dyskinesia LID, cannot yet be drawn. Based on a number of behavioral studies demonstrating the alleviation of dyskinesia by α_2 adrenergic receptor antagonists, in addition to other biochemical studies, some studies hypothesized that the noradrenergic system also plays a role in the neural mechanisms underlying Parkinson's disease and L-DOPA-induced dyskinesia.

New intervention strategies focused on modifying the disease process, as opposed to the current symptom-alleviating management of the disease, are considered necessary for Parkinson's disease. Since direct regeneration of brain tissues is difficult to achieve, an alternative supply of neural cells is required in order to attain any therapeutic goal. Recent progress in stem cell biology has led to new approaches to the generation of neurons.

Animal models provide a platform to delineate the pathogenic mechanisms of Parkinson's disease, and studies involving primates, rodents (rat and mouse), zebrafish, nematodes and fruit flies have been instrumental in further understanding of PD. Models of neurotoxins, such as MPTP, can mimic the loss of dopaminergic neurons and are useful as models of characteristic motor symptoms of PD. However, they lack age-dependent progressive neuronal loss, presence of Lewy bodies, and extensive non-motor symptoms that are found in PD. These models are valuable in advancing the understanding of dopaminergic neuronal death and concomitant physiological consequences, but there are limits to what can be accomplished with neurotoxin models, as they are not founded on mechanisms known to cause human Parkinson's disease. On the contrary, genes linked to rare forms of PD, or the processes which they regulate, are potential therapeutic targets. Studies using genetically modified animal models have implicated abnormal handling of misfolded proteins by the ubiquitin-proteasome and autophagy-lysosomal systems, increased oxidative stress, and mitochondrial and lysosomal dysfunctions as key processes perturbed in the neurodegenerative process of PD. Apart from the obvious preference for vertebrate (rodents and primates) models to investigate PD, an increasing number of studies have also shown a number of advantages and the utility of invertebrate (flies and nematodes) models. The central nervous system of invertebrate animals have a rather small number of neuron and glia as compared to vertebrates. However, essential functional features such as neurotransmitter system of vertebrates and invertebrates are conserved. A concern of current animal models is the ability of models to reproduce some, but not all, characteristic pathological features of the human Parkinson's disease.

Glutathione GSH is the most abundant and the main antioxidant agent in the central nervous system. Early post-mortem studies revealed decreased levels of GSH in degenerating substantia nigra of PD patients. Although diminished GSH levels could be secondary to increased oxidative stress, it has been postulated as an early event in PD-associated neuronal death, in which the decrease in GSH content results in a direct inhibition of complex I. Decreased activity of mitochondrial complex I, found in post-mortem tissue of PD patients, is probably a founding event in neuronal death. Interestingly, this phenotype is replicated in experimental PD induced by 1-methyl-4-phenyl-l,2,3,6-tetrahydropyridine (MPTP) intoxication, which induces parkinsonian symptoms in mice, primates, and humans. Inhibition of complex I leads to impaired mitochondrial ATP production and an accelerated production ROS. The increased ROS could generate a positive loop between complex I inhibition and oxidative stress. Iron accumulation is another element relevant to neuronal death in PD. In particular, iron accumulation has been demonstrated in the dopaminergic neurons of the substantia nigra pars compacta. The iron dyshomeostasis takes place in the late stages of the disease as part of a vicious cycle resulting in uncontrolled oxidative damage. Over the years, many chemical compounds and toxins have been identified as causative agents of PD. 1-Methyl-4-phenyl-1,2,3,6-tetrahydropyridine (MPTP) is a representative strong neurotoxin that has been recognized from several young drug addicts who developed severe parkinsonism. In addition, epidemiologically, environmental neurotoxins such as agricultural chemicals (pesticides, herbicides, and fungicides) are promising candidates for causative factors of PD. Rotenone and paraquat could promote and accelerate the development of PD. Oxidative stress and mitochondrial dysfunction induced by these toxins could contribute to the progression of PD. While most cases of PD are sporadic, specific mutations in genes that cause familial forms of PD have led to provide new insights into its pathogenesis. Analysis of these gene products may provide vital clues to our understanding of the molecular pathogenesis of dopaminergic neuronal death in PD. Over 10 causative genes for autosomal-dominant (a-synuclein, UCHL1, and LRRK2) or autosomal-recessive (parkin, PINK1, and DJ-1) inheritance PD have been identified and classified for PARK loci.

Oxytocin and vasopressin are important modulators of diverse social and anxiety-related behaviors. The enzyme that regulates the function of both peptides, called oxitocinase (OX) or vasopressinase, is also involved in cognitive functions. These results may reflect changes in the levels of oxytocin and vasopressin in the medial prefrontal cortex (mPFC) and, consequently, in the functions in which they are involved and might account, in part, for the cognitive abnormalities observed in hemi-parkinsonism.

6-Hydroxydopamine (6-OHDA) is a specific dopaminergic neurotoxin and has been commonly used to produce experimental animal models of PD. The stereotaxic injection of 6-OHDA into the substantia nigra and striatum of the brain injures dopaminergic neurons. Gynostemma pentaphyllum (Cucurbitaceae, GP) is usually used as an herbal tea and is widely believed to have various protective and/or improving functions for diabetes, depression, anxiety, fatigue and hyperlipidemia. GP has been also found to have an anti-stress function and immunomodulatory activity in mice. Recently, it is reported that an oral administration of GP extracts amelioration and reduction of tyrosine hydroxylase (TH)-immunopositive cells induced by 6-OHDA-lesioning in the dopaminergic neurons of substantia nigra of rat brain.

Human leucine-rich-repeat kinase 2 (LRRK2) has been found to be thus far the most frequent cause of late-onset and idiopathic PD. The mutations are found in five to six per cent of patients with familial PD and, importantly, also have been implicated with sporadic PD with unprecedented one to two per cent prevalence.

The pathogenic role and associated biochemical pathways responsible for LRRK2-linked disease remain unknown, however the described disease-linked mutations represent a unique opportunity to biochemically explore the pathogenicity of LRRK2 and identify therapeutic targets for related neurodegenerative disorders. Since LRRK2 kinase activity is critically linked to toxicity, it presents a viable target for therapeutic modulation.

Two of the cardinal characteristics of PD are the death of dopaminergic neurons in the substantia nigra pars compacta and the presence of intracellular inclusions in surviving neurons. Although a direct link between the two events is unclear, it is generally thought that these inclusions, referred to as Lewy bodies, are either causal or predictive of the oncoming neuronal death cascade. It is the loss of these dopaminergic neurons that leads to the disruptions in basal ganglia circuitry and causes the gross motor dysfunction seen in those afflicted with PD. As such, a better understanding of the components of Lewy bodies and how they may contribute to PD pathology is important. The main component of Lewy bodies is a protein known as a-nucleic. Aside from its prominence in Lewy bodies, a-nucleic is of particular interest because genetic mutations such as gene multiplication and amino-acid substitutions cause autosomal-dominant inherited forms of the disease. Manipulation of a-nucleicα-synuclein gene expression is the basis for many experimental transgenic PD models and a target for therapeutic intervention in humans. There is also evidence to suggest that the smaller, oligomeric aggregates of a-nucleicα-synuclein may be more cytotoxic than bona fide Lewy bodies. However, there is still much left to be uncovered about how a-nucleicα-synuclein contributes to the progression of PD or even regarding the normal function of the protein. A clue to the answers to both of these questions may lie in the ability of a-nucleicα-synuclein to switch between a membrane-bound and a cytosolic form. Pathologically, the balance between the populations of membrane-bound and cytosolic forms is thought to be important in the development of oligomeric species and/or Lewy bodies.

Current symptomatic treatment methods based on administration of L-3, 4-dihydroxyphenylalanine (L-DOPA) and other drugs that stimulate dopaminergic neurotransmission result in dyskinesia and psychiatric complications. As such, there are no effective neuroprotective or neurorestorative therapies. Recently, a novel class of compounds called neuroimmunophilin (NIL) ligands derived from the natural product FK506 (tacrolimus) have shown efficacy in treatment in a number of neurodegenerative disease models. The tyrosine hydroxylase TH protein and its regulation by phosphorylation is emerging as a promising molecular target to combat the locomotor deficits seen not only in PD but in aging as well.

Chapter 1 is designed to be a comprehensive review of all aspects of clinical, pathophysiological, and therapeutic aspects concerning PD, as well as an update on the innovative aspects of the disease primarily focused on identifying new pathophysiological factors and new outlook therapeutics. The next chapter examines research that points to timing deficits in upper limb repetitive and coordinated movements in PD, when required to integrate a timing cue. Further, to evaluate how attention and processing of sensory feedback may contribute to timing control, it has taken a close look at new methodologies to investigate timing control during gait in PD. The results of these studies are discussed in terms of how timing deficits may be an important underlying factor contributing to many of the motor symptoms seen in PD. The hypotheses described in chapter 3 are that brain oxidative stress and damage are involved in the pathogenesis of neurodegenerative diseases such as Alzheimer's and Parkinson's diseases, and non-neurodegenerative vascular dementia. The peripheral markers could be a useful tool in determining the evolution of brain oxidative stress in neurological patients. The subject of C

chapter 4 is the pathognomonic signs of dopaminergic neuron death observed in PD including inhibition of mitochondrial complex I, iron accumulation and decreased glutathione (GSH) content, and the interplay between the three factors. The results in chapter 5 suggest that filterable nocardiae are likely to multiply within astrocytes, through which they may invade neurons, and play a significant role in both neuronal loss and Lewy body formation.

The aim of chapter 6 is to ascertain that inflammation in both the periphery, as well as the brain, may be a major factor in the progression of PD. This chapter identifies the latest results on the identification of inflammatory markers in the blood of PD patients, and the possibility that these may be able to traverse the blood brain barrier to initiate and propagate inflammation in the brain. A range of anti-inflammatory agents are discussed which have been shown in animal studies as well as PD patients to have a beneficial effect. Chapter 7 introduces the cellular functions of cyclin-dependent kinase 5 (Cdk5) and summarizes existing knowledge on the involvement of Cdk5 in various aspects of PD pathology. Chapter 8 suggests that the factors involved in regulating a-nucleica-synuclein membrane dissociation are likely to provide new insight into a-nucleica-synuclein function and its role in PD. The review in chapter 9 provides a mechanistic framework to our current understanding of the structural and molecular basis of FKBP function in neuronal cells in relation to PD. In summary, a deeper understanding of FKBP function in PD will not only open up new targets for treatment but will also aid the design of new NILs for more effective therapeutic intervention. Chapter 10 summarizes that enhancement of tyrosine hydroxylase TH activity is a central feature of growth factor related increases in locomotor activity and nigral DA may be critical for specific aspects of locomotor activity.

Several models are offered in chapter 11, considering the relationships within the striata nigra: a model for dendritic spine density as a function of dopamine levels, a model of temperature-dependent neuronal firing patterns, and a model of dopamine-dependent mitochondrial damage and calcium release. The aim of chapter 12 is to describe the investigations into PD genes in Drosophila. These studies provide great insights into the underlying mechanisms that contribute to the progressive neurodegeneration caused by the disease and the future importance of Drosophila as a model organism to understanding the disease. Chapter 13 reviews the genetic PD animal models including those available in rodent, zebrafish, nematodes and fruit fly, and other animal models such as primate. The aim of this review is to assess the current models and the design of experiments to resolve the limitations of the animal models of PD. Chapter 14 aims to analyze OX in the left and right medial prefrontal cortex of spontaneously hypertensive rats with left or right hemi-parkinsonism, induced by intrastriatal injections of 6-hydroxydopamine (6-OHDA), and compared with sham controls. The next studies (Chapter 15) are focused on Dictyostelium discoideum Roco proteins which have similar domain architecture and very similar characteristics to LRRK2. The social amoeba Dictyostelium discoideum provides a well-established model in the study of the basic aspects of directed cell movement and development. This chapter tries to answer key questions for the intramolecular regulation of LRRK2 and gives insight in the function of the LRR, the mechanism by which the Roc domain regulates kinase activity, the role that COR plays in this process and, importantly, how the PD-linked mutations alter the interactions between the different domains. Chapter 16 shows that striatal depletion of dopamine DA-depletion generates an abnormal circuit dynamics in the rodent striatum - basically, abnormal synchronized oscillatory activity at multiple levels of the cortico-basal ganglia loops, and that dopamine receptor agonists dissolve the dominant state and open the way to create a bioassay for the testing of drugs with potential therapeutic value. The next review (chapter 17) focuses on animal models of both toxin-induced and genetically determined PD that have provided significant insight for understanding this disease. It also discusses the validity, benefits, and limitations of representative models.

Chapter 18 further investigates the protective effects of herbal butanol extracts from GP (GT-BX) on stressful exposure and L-DOPA treatment in 6-OHDA-lesioned rat model of PD. In this chapter, the results suggest that BP-BX develops the neuroprotective activity on stress- and L-DOPA-induced toxic reaction in the 6-OHDA-lesioned rat models of PD. The protection provided by acetyl-L-carnitine (ALC) offered the possibility of new therapeutic strategies for neurodegenerative diseases which can share the same final neurotoxic pathway in mitochondria (chapter 19). A novel striatum-specific transcript encoding an orphan G protein coupled receptor, the Gpr88, has been identified in rodent and human brains (chapter 20). Gpr88 protein is highly concentrated throughout the striatum of rodents and primates with membrane/cytoplasmic expression in MSNs. Ultrastructural immunolabelling revealed concentration of Gpr88 at post-synaptic sites, preferentially contacted by asymmetrical excitatory axodendric synapses. Moreover, dopaminergic and cortico-striatal lesions, followed by administration of dopaminergic ligands in rats, reveals that Gpr88 expression is modulated by dopamine- and glutamate-regulated mechanisms, providing anatomical basis for potential therapeutic strategies for striatum-related motor disorders. Chapter 21 proposes that a combined therapy with antioxidant and high energetic agents should be provided to individuals at risk of suffering from PD to delay or to prevent motor symptoms and/or frank PD. This data may contribute to a better understanding of the inherent nutritional status, genetic predisposition and environmental agents as causative factors of PD. Chapter 22 examines the current evidence in the literature which offers insight into the premise that inflammation may either cause or be a consequence of neurodegeneration in PD and presents the immunomodulatory therapeutic strategies that are now under investigation and in clinical trials as potential neuroprotective drugs for PD. Chapter 23 suggests that NTS1 activation may be involved in the etiology or progression of neurodegenerative pathologies and the treatment with selective NTS1 receptor antagonists in combination with conventional drug treatments could provide a novel therapeutic approach, especially for the treatment of PD. Chapter 24 offers one interesting approach using embryonic stem cells. ESCs could be an excellent source for cell replacement therapy of neurodegenerative medicine such as PD. Chapter 25 hypothesizes that due to the compensatory additional release of striatal DA by remaining DA neurons early during dopaminergic degeneration, SP through this positive feedback mechanism may also be locally increased within the SN. Here, SP may subsequently contribute to the activation of microglia and the dysfunction of the BBB, and thus perpetuate the ongoing degeneration of DA neurons. Thus, treatment with a NK1 receptor antagonist may represent a novel neuroprotective therapy for PD that may slow disease progression.

The behavioral and biochemical studies presented in Chapter 26 suggest that the noradrenaline system exerts a compensatory mechanism in PD, whereas the enhanced activation of α_{2a} adrenoceptors following repeated L-DOPA treatment may contribute to the development of L-DOPA-induced dyskinesia. Chapter 27 describes an analysis method which can predict a person's mitochondrial single nucleotide polymorphism (mtSNP) constitution and probabilities of becoming a PD patient, centenarian, Alzheimer's disease patient, or type 2 diabetes patient. It may be useful in the initial diagnosis of various diseases. In addition, a slight decrease in cardiac uptake of 123i-metaiodobenzylguanidine (MIBG) has been reported in some patients with multiple system atrophy (MSA). Taking these careful considerations together, ^{123}I-MIBG myocardial scintigraphy may not be regarded as the first and best choice of diagnostic aid for Lewy body disease, especially in the early stages (chapter 28).

We would like to thank all the people who supported the preparation of this book, who contributed to the book and, in particular, all who made the book possible by their positive evaluations of its proposal.

Dr. Juliana Dushanova
Institute of Neurobiology,
Bulgarian Academy of Sciences,
Sofia,
Bulgaria

1

Update in Parkinson's Disease

Fátima Carrillo and Pablo Mir
Unidad de Trastornos del Movimiento. Servicio de Neurología. Instituto de Biomedicina de Sevilla (IBiS). Hospital Universitario Virgen del Rocío/CSIC/Universidad de Sevilla, Spain

1. Introduction

Parkinson's disease (PD) was first described in 1817 by James Parkinson, who described in his monograph entitled "*An Essay on the Shaking Palsy*" the description of the clinical features of this disease (Parkinson, 1817). The cardinal clinical manifestations of PD are resting tremor, rigidity, bradykinesia, and gait dysfunction. It is now appreciated that PD is also associated with many nonmotor features, including autonomic dysfunction, pain and sensory disturbances, mood disorders, sleep impairment, and dementia (Olanow et al, 2009). PD is the second most common neurodegenerative disorder, with an average age at onset of about 60 years and the mean duration of the disease from diagnosis to death is 15 years, with a mortality ratio of 2 to 1 (Katzenschlager et al, 2008). The incidence of the disease rises steeply with age, from 17 - 4 in 100 000 person years between 50 and 59 years of age to 93 - 1 in 100 000 person years between 70 and 79 years, with a lifetime risk of developing the disease of 1 - 5% (De Rijk et al, 1995). With the aging of the population and the substantial increase in the number of at-risk individuals older than 60 years, it is anticipated that the prevalence of PD will increase dramatically in the coming decades (De Lau and Breteler, 2006).
The etiology remains obscure but important genetic and pathological clues have recently been found. This monograph is designed to make a comprehensive review of all aspects of both clinical as pathophysiological and therapeutic concerning PD, as well as an update on the innovative aspects of the disease primarily focused on identifying new genetic factors and new outlook therapeutics.

2. Neuropathology

Pathologically, PD is characterized by degeneration of dopaminergic neurons in the substantia nigra pars compacta (SNc). However, cell loss in the locus coeruleus, dorsal nuclei of the vagus, raphe nuclei, nucleus basalis of Meynert, and some other catecholaminergic brain stem structures including the ventrotegmental area also exists (Damier et al, 1999). This nerve-cell loss is accompanied by three distinctive intraneuronal inclusions: the Lewy body, the pale body, and the Lewy neurite. A constant proportion of nigral neurons (3–4%) contain Lewy bodies, irrespective of disease duration. This finding is consistent with the notion that Lewy bodies are continuously forming and disappearing in the diseased substantia nigra (Greffard et al, 2010). The brain-stem shape is a spherical structure measuring 8–30μm with a hyaline core surrounded by a peripheral pale-staining halo, and is composed ultrastructurally of 7–20-nm wide filaments with dense granular material and vesicular structures. Pale bodies are large rounded eosinophilic structures that often displace neuromelanin and are the predecessor of the Lewy body.

Aggregated α-synuclein is the main component of Lewy bodies in dopaminergic neurons of all PD patients, including those in whom PD occurred sporadically. Aggregated α-synuclein in the cytosol of cells does not only occur in the Substantia nigra but already earlier, pre-symptomatically in the motor part of the Nucleus vagus, in the olfactory bulb and in the Locus coeruleus. In later stages cortical areas of the brain are also frequently involved (Braak and Tredici, 2010). In fact, these bodies are present in small numbers in almost all cases of PD (Halliday et al, 2008). Neocortical Lewy bodies are not necessarily the pathological correlate of dementia in PD (Colosimo et al, 2003; Parkkinen et al, 2005). The amount of associated cortical β-amyloid seems to be the key factor for the cognitive decline in PD (Holton et al, 2008; Halliday et al, 2008). The hypothesis that the aggregation of α-synuclein and the build up of Lewy bodies results in toxicity has been challenged.

Currently, most evidence indicates that oligomers but not the fibrils of α-synuclein that are deposited in the Lewy bodies, are the toxic species. This would also imply that the rapid conversion of α-synuclein from an oligomeric to an aggregated state, deposited in Lewy bodies, may help to detoxify the oligomeric form of α-synuclein (Goldberg and Lansbury, 2000). Fetal mesencephalic neurons implanted in patients with PD to restore dopaminergic transmission may develop Lewy bodies. The existence of different striatal level factors present in the striatal microenvironment of the host probably triggers the propagation of alpha- α-synuclein pathology. Inflammation, oxidative stress, excitotoxicity, and loss of neurotrophic support of the grafted neurons could all be important factors (Li et al, 2008, 2010). A prion hypothesis implicating permissive templating has also been proposed (Hardy 2005).

The few patients with PD of genetic origin (α-synuclein, *LRRK-2*, and *GBA* mutations) who have had autopsy have all shown changes indistinguishable from those found in patients with PD (Lees et al, 2008). Some families with *LRRK-2* mutations also have tangle pathology and non-specific neuronal loss (Gilks et al, 2005). In contrast, parkin mutations lead to nigral loss, restricted brain-stem neuronal loss, and absence of associated Lewy bodies or neurofibrillary degeneration. Heterozygous parkin carriers, however, have been associated with both Lewy body and neurofibrillary tangle pathology (Van de Warrenburg et al, 2001; Pramstaller et al, 2005).

3. Genetic of Parkinson's disease

The PD is mostly idiopathic. However, at present, genetics has taken a very important role in clinical diagnosis. The first genetic contribution to PD was made by William Richard Gowers, in 1902, with the observation of familial aggregation in some patients with PD, but it was not until 1997 that discovered the first gene mutation associated with it (*SNCA*/α-synuclein).

Today there are two kinds of Mendelian PD: autosomal dominant and autosomal recessive PD. Generally, the recessive autosomal forms are associated with PD onset age of juvenile (age of onset <40 years) and an unknown condition. Parkin (*PRKN*) is the most frequently mutated gene in early-onset PD. Dominant autosomal PD is later onset, usually appears between 50-60 years of age, and pathologically with Lewy bodies. *LRRK2* is the most frequently mutated gene in dominant PD (Lees et al, 2009).

Mutations in the glucocerebrosidase gene (*GBA*) are associated with Gaucher's disease, the most common lysosomal storage disorder. Parkinsonism is an established feature of Gaucher's disease and an increased frequency of mutations in *GBA* has been reported in several different ethnic series with sporadic PD. Heterozygous mutations in the *GBA* gene significantly increased (five times) the risk of PD (Sidransky et al, 2009). In addition, patients with heterozygous mutations in the *GBA* gene also have pathology similar to idiopathic PD, with the presence of Lewy bodies and α-synuclein aggregate. *GBA* mutations represent a significant risk factor for the development of PD and suggest that to date, this is the most common genetic factor identified for the disease (Neumann et al, 2009).

3.1 Autosomal dominant forms of Parkinson's disease

To date, there are two genes associated with dominant autosomal dominant PD: *SNCA*/α-synuclein (PARK1) and leucine rich repeat kinase 2 (*LRRK2*, PARK8).

3.1.1 *SNCA*/α-synuclein (PARK1)

SNCA located on chromosome 4q21 (PARK1) was the first gene associated with PD. First, mutations in this gene were identified in families of Greek and Italian origin in 1997 (Polymeropoulos et al, 1997). This discovery was very important, because the identification of mutations in this gene was the first evidence that PD could be due to a genetic cause. After the discovery of the first pathogenic mutation, p.Ala53Thr (Polymeropoulos et al, 1997), two mutations were identified in the *SNCA* gene: mutation in a German family p.Ala30Pro (Kruger et al, 1998) and p.Glu46Lys mutation in a Spanish family (Zarranz et al, 2004). Years later, in 2003, was discovered the first affecting the genomic triplication of *SNCA* locus in a large family with PD (known as the 'Iowa kindred') (Singleton et al, 2003). After identification of the *SNCA* triplication, duplication *SNCA* genomic locus have also been identified in familial and sporadic forms of PD (Chartier-Harlin et al, 2004).

The *SNCA* gene encodes a protein called α-synuclein. This protein consists of 140 amino acids and is highly expressed in the central nervous system. α-Synuclein is the major fibrillar component of the Lewy body (Spillantini et al, 1997). Although its function is still unknown, appears to be involved in synaptic plasticity, neuronal differentiation, and axonal transport and synaptic vesicles (Biskup et al, 2008).

Symptoms caused by mutations in the *SNCA* gene are variable, but usually comes with age at onset around 50 years and phenotypic characteristics common to Lewy body dementia, with deposits of α-synuclein fibril and / or protein Tau, where Lewy bodies are more distributed throughout the brain of what we usually see in the PD. Some patients have dementia, visual hallucinations, parkinsonism and fluctuating cognition and attention (for example, patients with the mutation p.Glu46Lys and *SNCA* locus triplication). In contrast, the families described with duplication of the *SNCA* locus appear to have a slower progression of the disease, age of onset is usually late and not have dementia (Hardy et al, 2009). These latter observations led to suggest that the evolution of the disease may be associated with a dose-related effect of the *SNCA* locus (Singleton et al, 2003).

3.1.2 *LRRK2*/Dardarin (PARK 8)

Another locus for a dominant form of PD was first mapped in a Japanese family on chromosome 12 and named PARK8 (Funayama et al, 2002). Missense mutations in the gene for *LRRK2* were found to be disease causing in 2004 (Paisan-Ruiz et al, 2004; Zimprich et al,

2004). The most common mutation is the p.Gly2019Ser, which also constitutes the most common mutation of both mendelian and sporadic PD (Healy et al, 2008). Although there are over 50 different mutations described in the gene for confirmation dardarin pathogenicity in some of these mutations are difficult (Paisán-Ruiz 2009).

LRRK2 contains 51 coding exons and encodes a protein of 2,257 amino acids called dardarin. Endogenous LRRK2 is ubiquitiously expressed within neurons and associates with membranes and lipid rafts. The protein is found in presynaptic terminals where it associates with vesicles and endosomes (Biskup et al, 2008). Its function remains unknown, although functional studies have found that certain mutants alter *LRRK2* kinase activity and this activity is crucial for the toxic effect of the protein. It has also been seen that certain *LRRK2* gene mutations cause neuronal death (Biskup et al, 2008). It is also believed that dardarin could be involved in vesicular traffic system (Shin et al, 2008).

Mutations in the *LRRK2* gene vary greatly depending on the patient's geographical origin. There is some ethnic influence in the changes associated with the gene *LRRK2*. p.Arg1628Pro and p.Gly2385Arg as mutations, which, being absent in the Caucasian population, significantly increase the risk of PD in Asian populations. Both mutations are present in the normal population with a frequency of 2.65% (p.Arg1628Pro) and 1.8% (p.Gly2385Arg), but its prevalence is significantly higher in patients with PD. In addition, the mutation p.Gly2019Ser, common in the Caucasian population, is rarely identified in the Asian population (<0.1%), however, two mutations adjacent to amino p.Gly2019, p.Ile2012Thr and p.Ile2020Thr, occur more frequently in Asians than in Caucasians (Paisán-Ruiz 2009).

The clinical presentation closely resembles sporadicPD, but patients tend to have a slightly more benign course and are less likely to develop dementia and a favorable response to treatment with levodopa. Unilateral tremor is usually the first symptom of the disease, progressing slowly and benign. Patients with mutations in the LRRK2 gene are prone to develop dystonia (Healy et al, 2008). The age of onset is very variable (from 28 to 90 years old), but with an average age approaching 60 years. A person who inherits the Gly2019Ser mutation has only 28% risk of developing parkinsonism when younger than 60 years of age, but the risk rises to 74% at 79 years of age (Paisán-Ruiz 2009). p.Gly2019Ser mutation carriers have been described with no parkinsonian symptoms, suggesting the existence of incomplete penetrance associated with this mutation, and homozygous carriers without additional clinical effect caused by gene dosage (Paisán-Ruiz 2009).

3.2 Autosomal recessive forms of Parkinson's disease

Loss-of-function mutations in four genes (*PRKN, DJ-1, PINK1*, and *ATP13A2*) cause early onset recessive parkinsonism (age of onset <40 years). Parkin mutations are the second most common genetic cause of L-dopa-responsive parkinsonism, whereas mutations in the other three genes are rare.

3.2.1 *PRKN*/parkin (PARK2)

The PARK2 locus was cloned by extensive linkage analysis conducted in 13 consanguineous families from Japan in 1997. Today, mutations (> 100 different mutations) in the *PRKN* gene are the most common genetic cause of early-onset parkinsonism (onset age <40 years). The clinical picture associated with mutations in this gene is also similar to idiopathic PD, with a slow disease progression and response generally appropiate to treatment with levodopa.

Patients often develop dyskinesias at low doses of levodopa and generally develop dystonia. Lewy bodies are usually not a common pathology (Khan et al, 2003).
Parkin protein localizes, although not predominantly, to the synapse and associates with membranes. In general parkin is a cytoplasmic protein and functions in the cellular ubiquitination/ protein degradation pathway as an ubiquitin ligase (Kubo et al, 2001).

3.2.2 *PINK1*/PTEN-induced putative kinase 1(PARK6)

Initially, the PARK6 locus was cloned in a large Sicilian family in 2001. Three years later, pathogenic mutations in a gene called *PINK1* were identified in several Italian families (Valente et al, 2004). Symptoms caused by this gene are very similar to that described in patients with mutations in the *PRKN* gene. However, the age of onset may be more variable, reaching present even at 68 years of age, but typically has a juvenile onset (Kumazawa et al, 2008).
PINK1 encodes a primarily mitochondrial protein kinase. Mutations in the PINK1-gene are much less common than parkin mutations, and probably account for only 1 to 4 % of early-onset cases (Valente et al, 2004; Kumazawa et al, 2008; Rogaeva et al, 2004).

3.2.3 *DJ-1* (PARK7)

Mutations in the *DJ-1* gene (PARK7) are another rare cause of recessive autosomal parkinsonism (Bonifati et al, 2003; Hedrich et al, 2004). The clinical picture with early-onset and slow progression is similar to other recessive autosomal forms of PD. The normal function of DJ-1 and its role in dopamine cell degeneration is unknown, but there is evidence linking DJ-1 to oxidative stress response and mitochondrial function (Hardy et al, 2009).

3.2.4 ATP13A2-5P-type ATPase (PARK9)

The locus PARK9, *ATP13A2* was first identified in families of Chilean and Jordanian origin who had a syndrome known as Kufor-Rakeb. This disease is rare and presents with a rigid and akinetic parkinsonism and juvenile onset. Spasticity, Babinski signs, supranuclear gaze palsy and cognitive impairment are some of the clinical symptoms that often occur in this disease (Paisán-Ruiz et al, 2010). The gene encodes a protein lysosomal of 1,180 amino acids that are abundantly expressed in the brain and might act in the proteolytic degradation carried out in the lysosomes (Ramirez et al, 2006).

3.2.5 Other autosomal recessive forms of parkinsonism

Recently, mutations in the gene *PLA2G6* (phospholipaseA2 calcium-independent)(PARK 14) were also found present in individuals who had an akinetic and progressive parkinsonism. Cognitive impairment is a clinical symptom that often accompanies these patients. *PLA2G6* encodes a phospholipase enzyme of 752 amino acids. In general, the phospholipases induce changes in the composition of the membrane, activate the inflammatory cascade and alter cell signaling pathways of unknown function (Paisán-Ruiz et al, 2010).
Several familial cases with a complex parkinsonism and dystonia have been identified with mutations in the gene FBX07 (PARK15). The clinical features resembling parkinsonism caused by mutations in the *PRKN* gene. In fact, FBXO7 gene encodes a protein of 522 amino acids, which seems to be also involved in the system of ubiquitin-proteasome protein degradation (Di Fonzo et al, 2009; Paisán-Ruiz et al, 2010).

Recently, it has been shown that patients with mutations in the gene spatacsin (*SPG11*) (Non PARK locus) develop a juvenile parkinsonism similar to that caused by genes *ATP13A2*, *PLA2G6* and *FBX07*. These patients show a thinning of the corpus callosum, very characteristic signs of spastic paraplegia. The presenting symptoms of the disease are often both spasticity and parkinsonism (Paisán-Ruiz et al, 2010).

4. Clinical features

PD commonly presents with impairment of dexterity or, less commonly, with a slight dragging of one foot. The onset is gradual and the earliest symptoms might be unnoticed or misinterpreted for a long time. Fatigue and stiffness are common but non-specific complaints. Other initial symptoms are lugubrious stiff face, a hangdog appearance, a flexion of one arm with lack of swing, a monotonous quality to the speech, and an extreme slowing down. The early physical signs are often erroneously and a lag of 2 - 3 years from the first symptoms to diagnosis is not unusual. A change in a patient's writing can be present for several years before diagnosis, with a tendency to slope usually in an upward direction and for the writing to get progressively smaller and more cramped after a line or two (Lee et al, 2009).

Complaints within the first 2 years of the disease of falls (especially backwards), fainting, urinary incontinence, prominent speech, disturbed swallowing, amnesia, or delirium should raise the possibility of an alternative diagnosis.

In the late stages of PD, the face of patients is masked and expressionless, the speech is monotonous, festinant, and slightly slurred, and posture is flexed simian with a severe pill rolling tremor of the hands. Freezing of gait for several seconds can happen when attempting to enter the consulting room and, when starting to move again, the patient tends to move all in one piece with a rapid propulsive shuffle. These motor blocks lead to falls. All dextrous movements are done slowly and awkwardly, and assistance might be needed for dressing, feeding, bathing, getting out of chairs, and turning in bed. Constipation, chewing and swallowing difficulties, drooling of saliva, and urge incontinence of urine are common complaints.

Although PD has long been considered primarily a motor disorder Nonmotor symptoms (NMS) in PD are common and were recognized by James Parkinson himself. Thus, in his Essay on the Shaking Palsy in 1817, he referred to sleep disturbance, constipation, urinary incontinence and delirium (Parkinson, 1817). Numerous studies have now indicated that NMS is an integral symptom complex of PD, affecting memory, bladder and bowel, and sleep among others (Table 1) (Chaudhuri et al, 2006). It is commonly thought that NMS occur only in late or advanced PD but NMS can indeed present at any stage of the disease including early and pre-motor phase of PD. Several NMS of PD such as olfactory problems, constipation, depression and erectile dysfunction may predate the motor signs, symptoms and diagnosis of PD by a number of years (Chaudhuri et al, 2006; Tolosa et al, 2007).

Patients with PD are prone to have sleep disturbances that result in excessive daytime somnolence (EDS) and require proper identification and treatment (Comella, 2007). Sleep dysfunction in PD is usually manifest by difficulty in initiating sleep, fragmented sleep, REM behavior disorder (RBD), reversal of the sleep cycle, and EDS (Porter et al, 2008). It is possible that RBD might be early features of PD that antecede the onset of the classic motor features of the disease. In fact, in one study, RBD was found to have preceded the onset of PD symptoms in 52% of patients (Postuma et al, 2006). RBD in patients with PD is frequently seen in association with visual hallucinations (Meral et al, 2007). The presence of RBD in patients with PD is also frequently associated with neuropsychiatric problems and cognitive impairment. Even the presence of RBD in a patient with PD without dementia predicts the subsequent development of cognitive impairment (Vendette et al, 2007).

Although, troublesome dysautonomia is recognized in advanced PD, cardiac (123)I-metaiodobenzylguanidine (MIBG) imaging demonstrates early cardiac sympathetic denervation in PD (low cardiac uptake) and not multiple system atrophy (MSA) where the heart is usually visualized (Goldstein et al, 2000). Cardiac sympathetic denervation has also been found in genetic forms of PD with alpha synuclein mutation (Singleton et al, 2004).

Neuropsychiatric problems such as dementia, delirium, anxiety, and depression occur at one time or another in most patients, and can potentially be more disabling than motor dysfunction.

Risk of dementia exists, particularly in those patients who present with prominent gait and speech disorders, depression, and a poor response to L-dopa. The greatest risk factor for dementia, however, is the age of the patient and not the duration of the disease (Levy, 2007). Visuospatial difficulties, disturbances of attention and vigilance, delirium, and executive dysfunction are more common in PD than in Alzheimer's disease (Noe et al, 2004). Visual hallucinations are commonly associated with PD dementia.

Depression is pervasive in PD and affects approximately 40% of patients at least once during the course of their disease (Starkstein et al, 1992). Studies have suggested that symptoms of depression may precede the development of PD.

5. Pharmacologic treatment

5.1 Neuroprotection

Several putative neuroprotective agents have been tested in placebo-controlled clinical trials. Some clinical trials had negative outcomes despite promising theoretical or preclinical evidence. These include the antioxidant vitamin E (Parkinson Study Group, 1993), the glutamate release inhibitor riluzole (Jankovic and Hunter, 2002) , coenzyme Q10 (Shults et al, 2002), glial cell line-derived neurotrophic factor (GDNF) (Nutt et al, 2003), the antiapoptotic agents TCH346 (Olanow et al, 2006), CEP-1437 (Parkinson Study Group, 2007), and the neuroimmunophilins (Gold and Nutt, 2002) which are thought to act via a possible trophic mechanism. Conversely, some putative neuroprotective agents have demonstrated significant benefits compared with controls, but still could not be unequivocally deemed to be neuroprotective because of the possibility of confounding symptomatic or pharmacologic effects. Although it is not possible to claim with certainty that any of these drugs are neuroprotective, many are routinely used by physicians based on the hope that they might slow disease progression. These agents are considered below.

5.1.1 Selegiline

Selegiline is a selective, irreversible inhibitor of monoamine oxidase-B (MAO-B). Selegiline was the first drug to be tested as a putative neuroprotective therapy in patients with PD based on its capacity to protect dopamine neurons by inhibiting the MAO-B oxidation of MPTP and blocking the formation of free radicals derived from the oxidative metabolism of dopamine (Olanow 1996). The initial advantages shown by selegiline have not been maintained. Furthermore, evidence is insufficient to make a conclusion on the neuroprotective, as opposed to the symptomatic effect of selegiline in PD (Parkinson Study Group, 1996).

Neuropsychiatric symptoms
Depression, apathy, anxiety
Anhedonia
Attention deficit
Hallucinations, illusion, delusions
Dementia
Obsessional and repetitive behaviour (usually drug induced)
Confusion
Delirium (could be drug induced)
Panic attacks
Sleep disorders
Restless legs and periodic limb movements
REM behaviour disorder and REM loss of atonia
Non-REM sleep related movement disorders
Excessive daytime somnolence
Vivid dreaming
Insomnia
Sleep disordered breathing
Autonomic symptoms
Bladder disturbances
Urgency
Nocturia
Frequency
Sweating
Orthostatic hypotension
Coat hanger pain
Sexual dysfunction
Hypersexuality (likely to be drug induced)
Erectile impotence
Dry eyes (xerostomia)
Gastrointestinal symptoms
Dribbling of saliva
Ageusia
Dysphagia/ choking
Reflux, vomiting
Nausea
Constipation
Unsatisfactory voiding of bowel
Fecal incontinence
Sensory symptoms
Pain
Paraesthesia
Olfactory disturbance
Other symptoms
Fatigue

Diplopia
Blurred vision
Seborrhoea
Weight loss
Weight gain (possibly drug induced)

Table 1. Nonmotor features of PD

5.1.2 Rasagiline

Rasagiline is another selective, irreversible MAO-B inhibitor. There are data from studies in vitro and in animal models have shown neuroprotective capacity by rasagiline (Sagi et al, 2007; Zhu et al, 2008).

To test for a possible neuroprotective effect in patients with PD, rasagilina had been shown to have a symptomatic effect in the TEMPO study (The Rasagiline Mesylate in Early Monotherapy for PD Outpatients) (Parkinson Study Group, 2002). ADAGIO (the Effect of Rasagiline Mesylate in Early PD patients) study was designed to verify these results. It demonstrated that early treatment with rasagiline 1 mg daily provided a benefit that was not obtained with the delayed introduction of the drug. These results are consistent with rasagiline having a possible neuroprotective effect (Olanow et al, 2009).

5.1.3 Dopamine agonist

Dopamine agonists have been studied for putative neuroprotective effects in PD, based on their capacity to protect dopamine neurons from a variety of toxins (Schapira, 2002). Indeed, the dopamine agonist pramipexole has been reported to protect dopamine neurons in MPTP-lesioned primates (Iravani et al, 2006).

Clinical trials have attempted to test the capacity of dopamine agonists to provide disease-modifying effects in PD. However, Class I randomized, controlled trials with bromocriptine (Olanow et al, 1995), pramipexol (Parkinson Study Group, 2000; Parkinson Study Group, 2002), and ropinirole (Rakshi et al, 2002; Whone et al, 2003) produced no convincing evidence of neuroprotection in early PD.

5.1.4 Levodopa

The only available placebo-controlled study of levodopa in relation to neuroprotection is inconclusive about any Neuroprotective, as opposed to symptomatic effect (Fahn et al, 2004). Mortality studies suggest improved survival with levodopa therapy (Rajput 2001).

5.2 Motor symptoms treatment of PD

5.2.1 Levodopa

Levodopa is the most effective drug for the symptomatic treatment of PD and the gold standard against which new therapies must be measured. Benefits are usually seen in all stages of the disease and can be particularly noteworthy in patients with early PD, in whom the drug can control virtually all of the classic motor features. Although prediction of the therapeutic response in an individual is not possible, motor symptoms initially improve by 20 - 70%. Speech, swallowing, and postural instability can improve initially, but axial symptoms are generally less responsive and seem to escape more readily from long-term control (Fahn et al, 2004).

Levodopa exerts its symptomatic benefits through conversion to dopamine, and is routinely administered in combination with a decarboxylase inhibitor (carbidopa, benserazide) to prevent its peripheral conversion to dopamine and the resultant nausea, vomiting and orthostatic hypotension. A combination of carbidopa/levodopa and the COMT inhibitor entacapone is available. There are also sustained-release formulations of levodopa although sustained-release formulations of levodopa are not as well absorbed as regular formulations, and doses 20% to 30% higher may be necessary to achieve the same clinical effect. A gel preparation of levodopa (Duodopa) has been used for intraintestinal infusion of the agent and is used in more advanced stages of disease.

Levodopa is absorbed in the small bowel by active transport through the large neutral amino acid (LNAA) pathway, and can be impaired by alterations in gastrointestinal motility and by dietary LNAAs, such as phenylalanine, leucine, and valine, which compete with levodopa for absorption through the LNAA (Nutt et al, 1984).

Acute side effects associated with levodopa include nausea, vomiting, and hypotension, but levodopa is generally well tolerated when it is gradually increased. Levodopa is generally started at a low dose to minimize these risks. Most people can be maintained over the first 5 years of the disease on 300 - 600 mg/day levodopa. Levodopa maintain a similar level of control in de novo PD after 5 years (Koller et al, 1999), and also in more advanced PD with a duration of about 10 years and without motor fluctuations(Goetz et al, 1988).

Chronic levodopa therapy is associated with motor complications, such as dyskinesias and motor fluctuations, in the majority of patients. Motor fluctuations include delayed onset of levodopa's therapeutic effect or its wearing off between doses. Dyskinesias are involuntary choreiform movements that can involve any part of the body and sometimes impose disabling or painful postures. A meta-analysis found 40% likelihood of motor fluctuations and dyskinesias after 4–6 years of levodopa therapy (Ahlskog and Muenter, 2001). Risk factors are younger age, longer disease duration, and levodopa (Denny AP and Behari M, 1999; Fahn et al, 2004). In individual studies, the percentage of fluctuations and dyskinesia may range from 10% to 60% of patients at 5 years on disease duration, and up to 80–90% in later years (Olanow et al, 2001). Patients with PD can also experience fluctuations in such nonmotor symptoms as mood, cognition, autonomic disturbances, pain, and sensory function (Witjas et al, 2002). Levodopa may also be associated with neuropsychiatric side effects, including cognitive impairment, confusion and psychosis. Importantly, many PD features are not satisfactorily controlled by, or do not respond to, levodopa. These include freezing episodes, postural instability with falling, autonomic dysfunction, mood disorders, pain and sensory disturbances, and dementia. Levodopa treatment can also be associated with a dopamine dysregulation syndrome in which patients compulsively take extra doses of levodopa in an addictive fashion. Although levodopa has been associated with impulse control disorders (ICDs) such as hypersexuality and pathologic gambling, these behaviors have primarily been reported to be associated with dopamine agonists (Ceravolo et al, 2010). In addition, chronic levodopa treatment has been associated with punding, which is a series of repetitive and purposeless behaviors, such as collecting or assembling and disassembling objects for no apparent reason (Evans et al, 2004).

There has long been a theoretical concern that levodopa might accelerate neuronal degeneration in PD because of the potential of the drug to generate free radicals through its oxidative metabolism (Olanow et al, 2004). However, most studies in animal models and humans do not show an accelerated loss of dopaminergic neurons to long-term levodopa therapy in usual clinical doses (Olanow et al, 2004). The Earlier vs Later Levodopa Therapy in PD (ELLDOPA) study was the first double-blind, placebo-controlled trial to assess the safety and efficacy of different doses of levodopa and address the potential toxicity of levodopa in patients with PD (Fahn et al, 2004). The clinical results of this study certainly do not provide any evidence to suggest that levodopa is toxic or accelerates the development of disability in patients with PD and do not demonstrate any adverse effect of levodopa on PD progression.

5.2.2 Dopamine agonist

Dopamine agonists are a class of drugs with diverse physical and chemical properties. They share the capacity to directly stimulate dopamine receptors, presumably because they incorporate a dopamine-like moiety within their molecular configuration. Dopamine agonists have drawn particular interest as a treatment for PD because of their potential to provide antiparkinsonian effects with a reduction in the motor complications associated with levodopa. Today, dopamine agonists are also used as early symptomatic therapy to reduce the risk of developing the motor complications associated with levodopa therapy.

It is generally accepted that the shared D2-like receptor agonistic activity produces the symptomatic antiparkinsonian effect. This D2 effect also explains peripheral (gastrointestinal nausea and vomiting), cardiovascular (orthostatic hypotension) and neuropsychiatric (somnolence, psychosis, and hallucinations) side effects.

The first group of dopamine agonists used in the treatment of PD were ergot derivatives (bromocriptine, cabergoline, lisuride, pergolide, dihidroergocriptine). Numerous studies have demonstrated the effectiveness of these agents in PD as adjuncts to levodopa and shown that as monotherapy they are associated with a reduced risk of inducing dyskinesia compared with levodopa (Montastruc et al, 1994; Bracco et al, 2004; Oertel et al, 2006). However, their use has markedly declined due to the risk of valvular fibrosis and the introduction of nonergot dopamine agonists (apomorfine, pramipexole, ropinirole, rotigotine, piribedil). Although rare, cardiac dysfunction with valvular thickening and fibrosis has been reported with pergolide and cabergoline, presumably because they activate the 5HT2b receptor (Morgan and Sethi 2006; Zanettini et al, 2007; Roth BL 2007). In the nineties, nonergot dopamine agonists have largely supplanted the ergot agonists as the dopamine agonists of choice for the treatment of PD. Apomorphine is a short-acting dopamine agonist that is available in injectable form as a rescue drug for the management of "off" periods, and in some countries as an subcutaneous infusion therapy for the management of patients with advanced motor complications.

Levodopa is more efficacious than any orally active dopamine agonist monotherapy. The proportion of patients able to remain on agonist monotherapy falls progressively over time to <20% after 5 years of treatment. For this reason, after a few years of treatment, most patients who start on an agonist will receive levodopa as a replacement or adjunct treatment to keep control of motor parkinsonian signs. Over the last decade, a commonly tested strategy has been to start with an agonist and to add levodopa later if worsening of symptoms cannot be controlled with the agonist alone (Rinne et al, 1998; Parkinson Study Group 2000; Rascol et al, 2000).

From the limited data available (bromocriptine versus ropinirole, bromocriptine versus pergolide), the clinical relevance of the reported difference between agonists, if any, remains questionable (Mizuno Y et al, 1995; Korczyn et al, 1999).

Class I randomized, controlled trials demonstrate how early use of an agonist can reduce the incidence of motor complications versus levodopa (cabergoline (Bracco et al, 2004), pramipexole (Parkinson Study Group, 2000), and ropinirole (Rascol et al, 2000; Whone et al 2003). Similar conclusions were reported with bromocriptine (Montastruc et al, 1994), and pergolide (Oertel et al, 2006) in several class II studies. There is no evidence to suggest that an agonist is more effective than another in preventing or delaying the time to onset of motor complications. Dopamine agonists serve to delay the onset of motor complications by delaying the time until levodopa is required, but do not prevent motor complications once levodopa is introduced. Indeed, two studies have now shown that the time to onset of motor complications from when levodopa is introduced is the same whether levodopa is used as initial therapy or as an adjunct to the dopamine agonist (Rascol et al, 2000; Constantinescu et al, 2007).

Regarding the treatment of non-motor symptoms in PD pramipexole has shown to have an antidepressant effect in several randomized, double-blind controlled studies (Corrigan et al, 2000; Lemke et al, 2006; Bxarone et al, 2010). A recent study with transdermal rotigotine 24 hours monotherapy vs placebo has shown an improvement in nocturnal sleep disturbance (assessed by the "Modified Parkinson's Disease Sleep Scale) and early-morning motor dysfunction (Trenkwalder et al, 2011).

There are long-acting preparation of pramipexole and ropinirole with 24-hour prolonged release. Also rotigotine by transdermal administration has been shown to have constant levels of drug with a single patch daily. This allows for less fluctuation in plasma drug levels and permits drug levels to be maintained during the waking day and to drop off during the night. This may lead to better compliance and more consistent symptom response throughout the day and perhaps better nighttime symptom control. In adjunct studies, ropinirole (Pahwa et al, 2007) and pramipexol (Hauser et al, 2010) 24 hours provided improvement in UPDRS motor and quality-of-life scores comparable with the immediate release form of the drug and was well tolerated.

Dopamine agonists and all other active dopamine-mimetic medications share a common safety profile. Accordingly, side effects such as nausea, vomiting, orthostatic hypotension, confusion and psychosis, may occur with administration of any of these agents. Hallucinations and somnolence are more frequent with some agonists than with levodopa and are particularly common in elderly people or patients with cognitive impairment (Etminan et al, 2001). The ergot-derived dopamine agonists can be associated with a Raynaud's-like phenomena, erythromelalgia, and pulmonary or retroperitoneal fibrosis (Andersohn and Garbe, 2009). These events are relatively uncommon and are not seen with the nonergot dopamine agonists. Valvular fibrosis may occur in as many as 30% of patients receiving ergot-based dopamine agonists and can lead to valvular dysfunction with the need for surgical repair in extreme cases. This has resulted in withdrawal of pergolide from the market, and a marked reduction in the use of the other ergot agonists (Zanettini et al, 2007; Roth 2007). When these agents are used, it is essential that patients be periodically monitored with echocardiography to detect valvular alterations.

Sedation with EDS and possible unwanted sleep episodes has been associated with the use of dopamine agonists. Dopaminergic medications and dopamine agonists in particular, are known to have dose-related sedative side effects (Frucht et al, 1999; Ferreira et al, 2000; Paus et al, 2003).

Other problems related to the use of dopamine agonists include weight gain (possibly related to overeating) (Nireberg and Waters, 2006), edema (especially in the lower extremities) (Kleiner-Fisman G and Fisman, 2007) and a variety of ICDs, such as pathologic gambling, hypersexuality, and compulsive eating and shopping (Weintraub et al, 2006). Risk factors for ICDs include current use of dopamine agonists, particularly in high doses, young age of PD onset, and a premorbid or family history of ICDs or depression (Voon et al, 2006). ICDs were first identified in association with pramipexole, but have now been described with ropinirole and pergolide. Interestingly, they occur much less frequently with levodopa, although punding is primarily associated with chronic levodopa treatment. The precise mechanism whereby dopamine agonists might induce these ICDs is not known. It remains to be determined if dopamine agonists are directly responsible for inducing an ICD through a particular pattern of receptor stimulation, or if there is an underlying personality disorder that becomes clinically manifest with restoration of striatal dopaminergic tone.

5.2.3 Catechol-O-methyltransferase (COMT) inhibitors

Catechol-O-methyltransferase (COMT) inhibitors reduce the metabolism of levodopa, extending its plasma half-life and prolonging the action of each levodopa dose. Administration of levodopa with a COMT inhibitor increases its elimination half-life (from about 90 minutes to about 3 hours).

Two COMT inhibitors have been approved as adjuncts to levodopa for the treatment of PD; tolcapone and entacapone. Tolcapone inhibits COMT at peripheral level and to a lesser extent at the central level whereas entacapone acts only in the periphery.

COMT inhibitors are effective when administered in conjunction with levodopa and increase interdose, trough, and mean levodopa concentrations. Administration of levodopa plus a COMT inhibitor results in smoother plasma levodopa levels and more continuous brain availability compared with levodopa alone (Muller et al, 2006). Thus, administering levodopa with a COMT inhibitor has the potential to deliver levodopa to the brain in a more predictable and stable fashion, thus decreasing the fluctuations in levodopa concentrations seen when standard levodopa is administered intermittently.

Double-blind, placebo-controlled trials have demonstrated that both tolcapone and entacapone increase "on" time, decrease "off" time, and improve motor scores for patients with PD who experience motor fluctuations. Moreover, this benefit was associated with a reduction in the mean daily dose of levodopa (Kurth et al, 1997; Parkinson Study Group, 1997). Benefits have been shown to persist for 3 years or longer (Larsen et al, 2003). In general, superior clinical benefits have been achieved with tolcapone, reflecting the increased level of COMT inhibition.

Benefits with COMT inhibitors have also been observed in stable patients PD who have not yet begun to experience motor fluctuations (Waters et al, 1997; Olanow et al, 2004).

There has also been interest in the potential of COMT inhibitors to reduce the risk for motor complications associated with standard doses of levodopa (Olanow and Stocchi, 2004). This is based on the concept that intermittent doses of short-acting levodopa leads to pulsatile stimulation of dopamine receptors and motor complications. COMT inhibitors extend the elimination half-life of levodopa and thus, if administered frequently enough, might provide continuous levodopa to the brain. Although studies in monkeys showed that administration of levodopa plus the COMT inhibitor entacapone reduced dyskinesias compared with treatment with levodopa alone (Smith et al, 2005), these results have not been observed in patients. Specifically, in a recent clinical trial, Stalevo Reduction in Dyskinesia Evaluation (STRIDE-PD), which compared the time to onset and frequency of dyskinesia in levodopa-naïve PD patients who were randomized to initiate levodopa therapy with carbidopa/levodopa compared with carbidopa/levodopa/entacapone (Stalevo), was demonstrated that patients randomized to Stalevo had an increased frequency and a shorter time to dyskinesia than did those on standard levodopa (Stocchi et al, 2010).

COMT inhibitors increase levodopa bioavailability, and hence they increase the incidence of dopaminergic adverse reactions, including nausea, and cardiovascular and neuropsychiatric complications. Diarrhoea and urine discoloration are the most frequently reported non-dopaminergic adverse reactions. Tolcapone can elevate liver transaminases, and fatal cases of liver injury are reported (Assal et al, 1998). Currently, the drug has been reintroduced to the market in many countries, but has been imposed strict safety restrictions.

5.2.4 MAO-B inhibitors

Selegiline and rasagiline inhibit the action MAO-B. MAO-B prevents the breakdown of dopamine, leading to greater dopamine availability. Mechanisms besides MAO-B inhibition may also contribute to the clinical effects (Olanow, 1996). Unlike selegiline, rasagiline is not metabolized to amphetamine, and has no sympathomimetic activity.

Selegiline was initially approved as an adjunct to levodopa in patients with motor fluctuations. However, selegiline is primarily used in early disease, based on its putative neuroprotective effects (see section on Neuroprotection) and its capacity to provide mild symptomatic benefits (Parkinson Study Group 1993). When combined with levodopa, it can enhance dopaminergic side effects and lead to increased dyskinesia and neuropsychiatric problems, particularly in the elderly.

Rasagiline has been approved for use in patients with both early and advanced PD. Rasagiline is an irreversible inhibitor of MAO-B. It is more potent and more selective than selegiline, and does not generate amphetamine or methamphetamine metabolites. TEMPO study, a class I study with rasagiline, showed improvement of both the total UPDRS and the motor subscale of the UPDRS in patients treated with rasagiline versus placebo (Parkinson Study Group 2002). Recently published data on long-term efficacy of rasagiline in patients who participated in the TEMPO study, showing maintenance of rasagiline as monotherapy in about half of patients after two years of follow-up (Lew et al, 2010). In ADAGIO study early vs delayed start rasagiline 1 or 2 mg/day were compared. The results of this study suggest that early treatment with rasagiline 1 mg/ day provides benefits that cannot be attained with later initiation of the drug, and argues for starting symptomatic treatment at an earlier time point than has conventionally been used (Olanow et al, 2009). The PRESTO (Parkinson Study Group, 2005) and LARGO (Rascol et al, 2005) study have demonstrated the benefit of rasagiline in patients with motor fluctuationes.

Safinamide is a new MAO-B inhibitor that is currently being studied as a treatment for early and advanced PD. In addition to its MAO-B inhibitor properties, it also inhibits dopamine uptake, and blocks sodium channels and glutamate release. A randomized, placebo-controlled trial of safinamide in early to midstage PD demonstrated modest antiparkinsonian effects, with benefits specifically noted in patients who were already receiving a dopamine agonist (Stocchi et al, 2004).

MAO inhibitors are generally well tolerated. Amphetamine metabolites of selegiline may induce insomnia. At the daily doses currently recommended, the risk of tyramine-induced hypertension (the cheese effect) is low. Also this reaction has not been reported with selective inhibitors of MAO-B (Heinonen EH and Myllylä, 1998). Concerns that the selegiline/levodopa combination increased mortality rates (Ben-Shlomo et al, 1998) have been allayed (Olanow et al, 1998). MAO inhibitors may also interfere with serotonin metabolism and induce a serotoninergic syndrome, although this reaction is rarely presented (Ritter and Alexander, 1997).

5.2.5 Other antiparkinsonian drugs

5.2.5.1 Anticholinergics

The precise mechanism of action of anticholinergic drugs in PD is not known although are believed to act by correcting the disequilibrium between striatal dopamine and acetyl choline activity. Some anticholinergics, e.g. benzotropine, can also block dopamine uptake in central dopaminergic neurons. The anticholinergics used to treat PD specifically block muscarinic receptors.

The use of anticholinergics has dramatically declined in the era of levodopa and dopamine agonists, but these agents are still occasionally used. Anticholinergic drugs are typically used in younger patients with PD in whom resting tremor is the dominant clinical feature and where cognitive function is preserved. Anticholinergic drugs are of little value in the treatment of other parkinsonian features such as rigidity, akinesia, gait dysfunction, or impaired postural reflexes (Cantello et al, 1986). Currently trihexyphenidyl is the most widely used of the anticholinergic drugs.

The most commonly reported side effects are blurred vision, urinary retention, nausea, constipation (rarely leading to paralytic ileus), and dry mouth. The incidence of reduced sweating, particularly in those patients on neuroleptics, can lead to fatal heat stroke. Anticholinergics are contraindicated in patients with narrow-angle glaucoma, tachycardia, hypertrophy of the prostate, gastrointestinal obstruction, and megacolon. Impaired mental function (mainly immediate memory and memory acquisition) is a well-documented central side effect that resolves after drug withdrawal. Therefore, if dementia is present, the use of anticholinergics is contraindicated (Van Herwaardenet al, 1993).

5.2.5.2 Amantadine

Amantadine's mechanism of action remains unclear. A blockade of N-methyl-D-aspartate (NMDA) glutamate receptors and an anticholinergic effect are proposed, whereas other evidence suggests an amphetamine-like action to release presynaptic dopamine stores (Kornhuber et al, 1994).

Amantadine has been shown to improve akinesia, rigidity, and tremor in placebo-controlled trials when used as monotherapy or in combination with levodopa. Early studies suggested that benefit with amantadine is transient, but some patients enjoy more sustained benefits (Butzer et al, 1975; Timberlake and Vance, 1978).

Amantadine is the only currently available agent that is capable of blocking dyskinesia without interfering with the parkinsonian response and has proven to be of considerable benefit for some patients. The utilization of amantadine, however, may be limited by its propensity to cause cognitive impairment, particularly in patients with advanced PD (Verhagen Metman et al, 1998; Metman et al, 1999).

Side effects include confusion, hallucinations, insomnia, and nightmares. These are more common in older patients, but can be seen in patients of any age. Peripheral side effects include livedo reticularis and ankle edema, although these are rarely severe enough to limit treatment. Dry mouth and blurred vision can occur and are presumed related to its peripheral anticholinergic effects.

5.3 Nonmotor symptoms treatment of Parkinson's disease (Table 2)

NMS in PD include neuropsychiatric symptoms, sleep disturbances, autonomic dysfunction, and pain or sensory problems. Such symptoms are a frequent accompaniment to the motor disability with continuing disease progression (Chaudhuri et al, 2006). Although several nondopaminergic systems within the brainstem and cortex are involved in PD, specific clinicopathological correlation for such features remains uncertain, and despite the increasing recognition of these problems, specific pharmacological therapies that target the relevant nondopaminergic neurotransmitter system are limited.

The management of dementia in PD is a pressing problem because cognitive impairment is a common and important source of disability. As dementia in PD is associated with a cholinergic deficit, trials of the cholinesterase inhibitors donepezil and rivastigmine have been carried out in patients with dementia. In these studies, both rivastigmine (Emre et al, 2004) and donepezil (Ravina et al, 2005) showed a modest but significant improvement compared with controls without worsening of parkinsonism.

The cause of psychotic symptoms in PD is probably multifactorial, involving interplay between pathological processes and dopaminergic medications. The management of hallucinations and delirium in the patient with PD must begin with a pretreatment setting eliminating those drugs that can cause hallucinations or delusions and adjusting the dose of levodopa. When the adjustments fail to eliminate or sufficiently alleviate hallucinations and/or cannot be accomplished without inducing a meaningful deterioration in PD features, neuroleptic therapy should be considered. Haloperidol, perphenazine, or chlorpromazine are effective antipsychotics, but are not recommended for patients with PD because of their capacity to block striatal dopamine D2 receptors and exacerbate parkinsonian features. The "atypical" neuroleptics are the preferred agents to use (especially clozapine (Parkinson Study Group, 1999) and quetiapine (Fernandez et al, 2003)), and can often effectively treat hallucinations and psychosis induced by dopaminergic medications. They are called "atypical" because among other factors they preferentially block limbic and cortical dopamine receptors, but are relatively devoid of D1 and D2 receptor-blocking properties (Friedman and Factor, 2000).

Anxiety and depression are extremely common in PD and frequently coexist. Both might respond to dopaminergic therapies, and anxiety in particular can be experienced when the motor effects of levodopa have worn off (ie, during an "off period). However, successful management of these mood disorders often requires treatments in addition to dopaminergic agents, which suggests that non-dopaminergic neurotransmitters are involved. The current management of depression and anxiety in PD involves the use of conventional treatments that enhance serotonergic neurotransmission, such as selective serotonin reuptake inhibitors (SSRIs) or tricyclic antidepressants. Although in clinical practice many patients with PD do experience a significant improvement in mood symptoms with these agents (whatever the exact mechanism of action), the true effectiveness in PD has not been established owing to the limited numbers of available randomised controlled trials (Weintraub et al, 2005; Chung et al, 2003). Some antidepressants, which are undergoing investigation for depression and anxiety in PD, are also selective noradrenergic reuptake inhibitors (eg, duloxetine, venlafaxine, and desipramine).

Patients with PD can experience various behavioural problems as a consequence of dopaminergic medications, including impulse control disorders, such as pathological gambling, shopping, eating, and hypersexuality,(Voon et al, 2011) and abnormal excessive motor behaviours ranging from purposeless fiddling to complex stereotypic activities, known as "punding" (Evans et al, 2004). These problems have been particularly associated with dopamine agonists, but also with levodopa. The precise mechanism whereby dopamine agonists might induce these ICDs is not known. Treatment of each patient should be individualized based on the magnitude of the ICD problem and the need for dopaminergic drugs to control PD features. The symptoms might resolve on reducing or discontinuing the dopamine agonists, although they can persist in some patients (Mamikonyan et al, 2008). Other approaches could include trials of various psychoactive agents and psychosocial interventions and referring patients for appropriate counseling services.

Sleep dysfunction in PD is usually manifest by difficulty in initiating sleep, fragmented sleep, reversal of the sleep cycle, and EDS. Sleep disturbances in PD are multifactorial and may be related to aging, parkinsonian motor dysfunction, dyskinesia, pain, nocturia, nightmares, dopaminergic and nondopaminergic medications, cognitive impairment, and a variety of specific sleep disorders, including restless legs syndrome (RLS), periodic limb movements of sleep (PLMS), RBD, and sleep apnea. Collectively, they contribute to the increase in daytime sleepiness that is so frequently found in patients with PD (Tandberg et al, 1999; Comella, 2007). Dopaminergic medications and particularly dopamine agonists can have a complex effect on sleep. Sometimes these medications cause insomnia or sleepiness. In other situations they may improve nocturnal immobility, and in this way improve the quality of sleep (Montastruc et al, 2001; Brodsky et al, 2003). Thus, dopaminergic medications can either improve or worsen sleep in patients with PD. RBD in patients with PD may be effectively treated with low-dose clonazepam (0.25 to 1.0 mg nightly). The wake-promoting drug modafinil, which possibly affects histamine release in the hypothalamus, is currently used as an option to treat excessive daytime sleepiness in patients with PD (Morgenthaler et al, 2007). Is currently being assessed two other drugs (the BF 2.649 a selective histamine H3 inverse agonist and the caffeine, a non-selective adenosine antagonist) in the treatment of EDS in PD patients.

Drugs currently used to treat orthostatic hypotension in PD include midodrine, a sympathomimetic, and fludrocortisone, a mineralocorticoid. Supine hypertension is a potential side-effect of both of these approaches. The acetylcholinesterase inhibitor pyridostigmine bromide has been suggested to reduce orthostatic hypotension with less effect on supine hypertension, although evidence is limited (Low and Singer, 2008). L-threo-3, 4- dihydroxyphenylserine is a synthetic amino acid precursor of noradrenaline that is available for freezing of gait in PD and orthostatic hypotension in autonomic failure (Mathias et al, 2001). However, few randomised controlled trials few randomised controlled trials (RCTs) of treatment for orthostatic hypotension have been undertaken specifically in PD, but rather have involved mixed populations of patients including multiple system atrophy, in which the pathophysiology of orthostatic hypotension is different. Thus, the true efficacy of treatments for orthostatic hypotension in PD remains unclear.

Urinary symptoms can be troublesome in advanced PD. Current treatments are drugs for overactive bladder symptoms, such as the muscarinic antagonists oxybutynin and tolterodine. However, such drugs are typically poorly tolerated in patients with advanced PD due to central and peripheral anticholinergic side-effects. Another muscarinic antagonist, trospium chloride, has potentially fewer central side-effects due to poor penetration of the blood - brain barrier, and is effective for treating overactive bladder symptoms (Staskin, 2006).

Postural instability is a late complication of PD which can lead to a mounting fear of falls with increasing immobilisation and dependency. Most falls in patients with PD occur in a forward or sideways direction and are due to turning difficulties, gait and postural asymmetries, problems with sensorimotor integration, difficulties with multitasking, failure of compensatory stepping, and orthostatic myoclonus (Bloem et al, 2004). Skilled physical therapy with cueing to improve gait, cognitive therapy to improve transfers, exercises to improve balance, and training to build up muscle power and increase joint mobility, is efficacious (Keus et al, 2007). Regular physical and mental exercise should be encouraged at all stages of the disease. Benzodiazepines should be avoided wherever possible because they increase the risk of falling.

Insomnia
Adjust dopaminergic drugs, sleep hygiene techniques or clonazepam
Depression
Serotonin and noradrenergic reuptake inhibitors or tricyclic antidepressants
Rapid eye movement behaviour disorders
Adjust Parkinson's disease drugs or clonazepam
Fatigue
Amantidine or selegiline
Day time sleepiness
Modafinil
Psychosis and hallucinations
Adjust Parkinson's disease drugs or antipsychotic (clozapine, quetiapine)
Constipation
Osmotic laxatives (macrogol)
Urinary urgency
Check drugs, anticholinergic bladder stabilisers, and desmopressin for nocturia
Impotence
Sildenafil, tadalafil, and vardenafil
Pain
Adjust Parkinson's disease drugs and muscle relaxants
Restless legs
Dopamine agonists
Orthostatic hypotension
Adjust Parkinson's disease drugs; increase water and salt intake; fludrocortisone, ephedrine, or midodrine
Drooling
0-5% atropine eye drops sublingually, scopoderm patch, or botulinum toxin injections into salivary glands
Excessive sweating
Adjust Parkinson's disease drugs, propantheline, propranolol, or topical aluminium creams

Table 2. Treatment of Non motor symptoms of PD

6. Surgical procedure for the treatment of Parkinson's disease

The capacity of surgical therapies to provide benefit for patients with PD who can no longer be satisfactorily controlled with medical therapies due to motor complications has been a major advance in the modern treatment of PD (Hallett and Litvan, 2000). Surgical therapies have historically used ablative procedures (e.g., chemical, radiofrequency, or thermal lesions) to make a destructive lesion in overactive or abnormally firing brain targets. However, ablative procedures are associated with the risk of inducing damage to neighboring structures with consequent neurologic dysfunction. The introduction in 1987 of high-frequency deep brain stimulation (DBS) procedures in PD has resolved many of these issues. High frequency stimulation of specific brain targets induces functional benefits that simulate the effects of a destructive lesion, but without the need for making a destructive brain lesion. DBS is performed by implanting an electrode with four contacts into a target site within the brain and connecting it to a pulse generator placed subcutaneously over the chest or abdomen wall. Stimulator settings can be adjusted periodically with respect to electrode configuration, voltage, frequency, and pulse width (Bergman et al, 1990; Olanow et al, 2000).

The mechanism of action of high-frequency DBS is still not clear, even more than 21 years after its introduction. The mechanism is believed to be independent of the target, because DBS mimics the effects of ablation in all targets used to date, but its effects depend on stimulation rather than on the creation of a lesion.

Patients who are thought to benefit from DBS are those affected by clinically diagnosed idiopathic PD, in whom the cardinal symptoms of the disease— bradykinesia, rigidity, and tremor— are likely to be significantly improved (Krack et al, 2003; Deuschl et al, 2006). Those who show improvement with the optimum adjustment of anti-PD drugs or suprathreshold levodopa dose (300 mg per dose) are highly likely to show a similar improvement after optimum placement of the electrodes (Charles et al, 2002). Higher baseline scores on section III (motor) of the unified PD rating scale (UPDRS) and higher baseline levodopa responsiveness are independent predictors of greater change in motor score after surgery. Midline symptoms, dysautonomic symptoms, and gait disturbance unresponsive to levodopa (ie, freezing) are only slightly improved, if at all (Xie et al, 2001).

The different surgical targets exist in the treatment of PDare as follows: - Ventral intermediate (VIM) nucleus of the thalamus: stimulation procedures in this target provide potent antitremor (Narabayashi, 1989) and antidyskinesia (Narabayashi et al, 1984) effect in PD. However, the thalamus is rarely selected as a target site today because similar benefits can be obtained with other targets that are associated with more widespread antiparkinsonian effects. Subthalamic nucleus (STN) or internal segment of the globus pallidus (GPi)—physiologic and metabolic studies indicate that neurons in both the STN and GPi are overactive in PD (Crossman et al, 1985; Mitchell et al, 1989), and that lesions of these structures provide antiparkinsonian benefits in animal models of PD (Bergman et al, 1990; Brotchie et al, 1991; Guridi et al, 1994;). Both ablation and high frequency stimulation of these targets have been shown to provide antiparkinsonian benefits as well as a profound reduction in dyskinesia (especially GPi) in patients with PD. Although the STN is currently the preferred surgical target in most centers, there is no conclusive data indicating that comparable results cannot be obtained with stimulation of the GPi (Follet et al, 2010). Patients undergoing subthalamic stimulation required a lower dose of dopaminergic agents

than did those undergoing pallidal stimulation.- Pedunculopontine nucleus (PPN)—the PPN is a diffuse nucleus that extends throughout the upper brainstem. Stimulation and lesions in the PPN influence locomotion, and for this reason it has been referred to as the mesencephalic locomotor center (Pahapill and Lozano, 2000). Preliminary studies suggest that stimulation of the PPN may provide locomotor benefits for patients with PD (Stefani et al, 2007). DBS of the PPN is being actively investigated.
Side effects of DBS can be related to the surgical procedure, the device, or to the stimulation. There is a risk of hemorrhage and damage to neighboring brain structures, although risks are less than are seen with ablative procedures, particularly when performed bilaterally (Hallett and Litvan, 2000). Complications associated with the device can be related to infection or mechanical problems (e.g., lead fracture, movement of the electrode, skin erosion), and may require lead removal or reimplantation. Side effects related to stimulation are generally transient and may be controlled by adjusting the stimulation variables. The battery must be periodically replaced.

7. Recommendations for the management of Parkinson's disease

The optimal time frame for onset of therapy has not been clearly defined. Once parkinsonian signs start to have an impact on the patient's life, initiation of treatment is recommended. For each patient, the choice between the numerous effective drugs available is based in several factors. These factors include considerations related to the drug (efficacy for symptomatic control of parkinsonism/prevention of motor complications, safety, practicality, costs, etc.), and the patient (symptoms, age, needs, expectations, experience, co-morbidity, socioeconomic level, etc.).
Currently, there is no uniform proposal on initiating symptomatic medication for PD. In the past, levodopa was traditionally used to initiate therapy for PD because it was the most effective symptomatic agent, and levodopa is still commonly used as initial therapy by some physicians. Today, many movement disorder neurologists have elected to initiate symptomatic therapy with a dopamine agonist in appropriate patients, and to supplement with levodopa when satisfactory control cannot be attained with dopamine agonist monotherapy. This treatment philosophy is based on the body of laboratory and clinical information indicating that dopamine agonists are associated with a reduced risk of inducing motor complications compared with levodopa. Dopamine agonist use as as initial therapy because they delay the time until levodopa is required and permit use of lower doses of levodopa. To begin with levodopa is the preferred treatment for patients with PD with cognitive impairment, the elderly who have a reduced propensity to develop motor complications, and patients suspected of having an atypical parkinsonism who are undergoing a trial of dopaminergic therapy.
MAO-B inhibitors such as selegiline and rasagiline provide another therapeutic option in early disease. MAO-B inhibitors have been shown to provide modest antiparkinsonian effects when used as monotherapy and also delay the need for levodopa. The symptomatic effect is more modest than that of levodopa and (probably) dopamine agonists, but they are easy to administer (one dose, once daily, no titration). Furthermore the TEMPO and the ADAGIO studies suggest that early treatment with rasagiline provides benefits that cannot be attained with later introduction of the same medication (Parkinson Study Group, 2002;

Olanow et al, 2009). Although this does not establish neuroprotection and long-term studies are required to determine the effect of the drug on cumulative disability in the long run, it does indicate that earlier treatment with rasagiline may provide a better outcome, at least at the 18-month time point. For these reasons, many physicians now choose to initiate therapy in patients with early PD with an MAO-B inhibitor.

There may be advantages to initiating therapy in patients with early PD with both an MAO-B inhibitor and a dopamine agonist (not at the same time) to enhance clinical benefits and further delay the need for levodopa. However, there have been no studies as yet examining the effects of combining an MAO-B inhibitor with a dopamine agonist on the need for levodopa and the risk of inducing dyskinesia. However, subset analyses in studies testing rasagiline in advanced patients (Parkinson Study Group, 2005; Rascol et al, 2005) and preliminary studies with a new MAO-B inhibitor safinamide, (Stocchi et al, 2004) suggest that adding an MAO-B inhibitor to a dopamine agonist improves UPDRS scores.

Amantadine or anticholinergics are not routinely prescribed in patients with early PD, although some movement disorder specialists might use anticholinergics if tremor is the predominant feature in young patient with PD.

There are a variety of ways to enhance motor response in patients who experience suboptimal motor control with dopamine agonist or levodopa monotherapy. The simplest approach is to gradually raise the dose of the dopaminergic agent. However, high doses of dopamine agonists can be associated with neuropsychiatric side effects, sedation and ICDs. If patients cannot be satisfactorily controlled on an agonist, then levodopa should be added. If the patient is receiving levodopa monotherapy, increased doses might be effective. Higher doses are associated with an increased risk of motor complications, but may be justified if required to provide a satisfactory clinical response. The addition of a dopamine agonist may enhance benefit without increasing the risk of motor complications. COMT and/or MAO-B inhibitors may also be useful in managing patients with a suboptimal clinical response. The use of a subcutaneous apomorphine penject as a rescue device for unpredictable refractory off periods can also be helpful in some instances, and its fast action helps to restore confidence in patients becoming insecure about leaving home (Ostergaard et al, 1995).

Despite adjustments of the timing and dose frequency of levodopa, motor fluctuations and dyskinesias can mark the long-term therapeutic benefit. Amantadine is an effective anti-dyskinetic agent in some patients. Subcutaneous waking day apomorphine pump is a highly effective treatment for refractory motor fluctuations. Orally administered anti-parkinsonian medication should be adjusted obtain thebest results for dyskinesia reduction and off periods. Enteric administration of a soluble formulation of levodopa (Duodopa) through gastro-jejunostomy is another highly effective medical option for patients who failed to, or are reluctant to, try the apomorphine pump. Infusion therapies is based on the principle that continuous infusion of a dopaminergic agent provides more constant and physiologic activation of striatal dopamine receptors than is accomplished with intermittent administration of the same drug, and thereby reduces the risk of motor complications. Continuous infusion of either levodopa or apomorphine has been tested in patients with advanced PD and consistently been reported to reduce the frequency of motor complications (Manson et al, 2002; Antonini et al, 2007). Sustained improvement in motor performance with a great reduction in drug-induced involuntary movements can also be achieved by functional neurosurgery with bilateral deep brain stimulation of the STN or GPi.

8. Experimental approaches

Cell-based therapies have been studied based on the notion that transplantation of dopaminergic cells could replace dopamine neurons, which degenerate in PD, and restore dopaminergic function in a more physiologic manner than can be achieved with oral therapies (Lindvall and Bjo¨rklund, 2004). Fetal nigral transplantation has been the best studied of these approaches to date. Numerous laboratory studies have demonstrated that embryonic dopaminergic neurons implanted into the denervated striatum can survive, extend axons, provide organotypic innervations of the striatum, produce dopamine, and provide behavioral benefits in the 6-OHDA rodent and MPTP-monkey (Olanow et al, 1996). These studies have served as the basis for initiating clinical trials in patients with PD. To date, there is no universal agreement on the optimal transplant protocol. Open-label clinical trials using a variety of different transplant regimens produced variable clinical results. Various types of cells have been used (adrenal gland, mesencephalic fetal grafts, and more recently, epithelial retinal cells). Stem cells are also being investigated, which might be better tolerated immunologically, but raise their own (oncological) problems. Despite the elegance of this approach, it is still experimental and is not currently available to patients (Morizane et al, 2008). Intrastriatal carotid body (CB) transplants have been assayed in animal models of PD to test whether they increase the striatal dopamine levels and/or exert a neuroprotective action on the nigrostriatal pathway. Currently it being studied the in vitro formation of new CB tissue derived from adult CB stem cells, given the limitations of previous studies have been presented with autotransplantation of CB in patients with PD (López-Barneo et al, 2009).

Gene delivery approaches are also being actively investigated as a possible treatment for PD. In this technology, viruses are used as vectors to introduce the DNA of a desired protein into the genome of cells within a specific brain target. Furthermore, promoters can ensure that the virus vector infects specific brain cells (e.g., TH promoter targets dopamine cells). This sequence can thus potentially result in continuous production of the desired therapeutic protein in the desired target region of the brain (Dass et al, 2006). Most human studies have used the adeno-associated virus serotype 2 (AAV-2) as the vector, as AAV-2 does not induce an immune response and permits long-term expression of the transgene. No clinically significant or unanticipated adverse events have been encountered in any of the gene therapy studies performed to date (Svendsen, 2007). Different gene therapy approaches are currently being tested in PD, e.g trophic factors such as glial-derived nerve factor (Lang et al, 2006) or neurturin (Marks et al, 2010).

9. Conclusions

The current knowledge of the disease continues to evolve and be challenged by scientific discovery. Further research on the function of the proteins identified by the susceptibility genes, the interplay of the disease process with normal ageing, and the nature of environmental triggers that unmask the disease process will be needed if we are to develop reliable biomarkers and a cure for this disabling movement disorder. Although it is producing significant progress in new therapeutic options important unmet medical needs remain, and even more effective therapeutic interventions are required for the successful management of the patient with PD. Many such agents are now in development. However, future strategies need to focus on more selective targeting of subtypes of neurotransmitter receptors to reduce side effects and optimise benefit. Finally, the development of neuroprotective agents in PD has to date focused on preventing dopamine cell loss. However, to be optimally effective, such therapies will also need to target nondopamine cells involved in the multisystem disease process.

10. References

[1] Ahlskog JE and Muenter MD(2001). Frequency of levodopa related dyskinesias and motor fluctuations as estimated from the cumulative literature. *Movement Disorders* 16, 3 (May 2001): 448–458, 0885-3185.

[2] Andersohn F, Garbe E (2009). Cardiac and noncardiac fibrotic reactions caused by ergot- and nonergot-derived dopamine agonists. *Mov Disord* 24, 1(Jan 2009):129-33, 1531-8257.

[3] Antonini A, Isaias IU, Canesi M, Zibetti M, Mancini F, Manfredi L, Dal Fante M, Lopiano L and Pezzoli G. (2007). Duodenal levodopa infusion for advanced Parkinson's disease: 12- month treatment outcome. *Mov Disord* 22, 8 (Jun 2008):1145-1149, 0885-3185.

[4] Assal F, Spahr L, Hadengue A, Rubbia-Brandt L and Burkhard PR (1998). Tolcapone and fulminant hepatitis. *Lancet* 352, 9132 (Sep 1998):958, 0140-6736.

[5] Ben-Shlomo Y, Churchyard A, Head J, Hurwitz B, Overstall P, Ockelford J and Lees AJ (1998). Investigation by Parkinson's Disease Research Group of United Kingdom into excess mortality seen with combined levodopa and selegiline treatment in patients with early, mild Parkinson's disease: further results of randomized trial and confidential inquiry. *British Medical Journal* 316, 7139 (Apr 1998): 1191–1196.

[6] Bergman H, Wichmann T and DeLong MR (1990). Reversal of experimental parkinsonism by lesions of the subthalamic nucleus. *Science* 249, 4975 (Sep 1990): 1436 - 38, 0036-8075.

[7] Biskup S, Gerlach M, Kupsch A, Reichmann H, Riederer P, Vieregge P, Wüllner U and Gasser T. (2008). Genes associated with Parkinson syndrome. *J Neuro*, 255, 5 (Sep 2008), 8-17, 0340-5354.

[8] Bloem BR, Hausdoroff JM, Visser JE and Giladi N (2004). Falls and freezing of gait in Parkinson 's disease: a review of two interconnected, episodic phenomena. *Mov Disord* 19, 8 (Aug 2004): 871-84, 0885-3185.

[9] Bonifati V, Rizzu P, van Baren MJ, Schaap O, Breedveld GJ, Krieger E, Dekker MC, Squitieri F, Ibanez P, Joosse M, van Dongen JW, Vanacore N, van Swieten JC, Brice A, Meco G, van Duijn CM, Oostra BA and Heutink P (2003). Mutations in the DJ-1 gene associated with autosomal recessive early-onset parkinsonism. *Science* 299, 5604 (Jan 2003) :256–259, 1095-9203.

[10] Braak H and Del Tredici K. (2010). Pathophysiology of sporadic Parkinson's disease. *Fortschr Neurol Psychiatr*, 78, Suppl 1 (Mar 2010), S2-4, 1439-3522.

[11] Bracco F, Battaglia A, Chouza C, , Dupont E, Gershanik O, Marti Masso JF and Montastruc JL (2004); PKDS009 Study Group. The long-acting dopamine receptor agonist cabergoline in early Parkinson's disease: final results of a 5-year, double-blind, levodopa-controlled study. *CNS Drugs* 18, 11 (Aug 2004):733–746, 1172-7047.

[12] Brotchie JM, Mitchell IJ, Sambrook MA and Crossman AR (1991). Alleviation of parkinsonism by antagonist of excitatory amino acid transmission in the medial

segment of the globus pallidus in rat and primate. *Mov Disord* 6, 2 (Jan 1991): 133–138, 0885-3185.

[13] Brodsky MA, Godbold J, Roth T and Olanow CW (2003). Sleepiness in Parkinson's disease: a controlled study. *Mov Disord* 18, 6 (June 2003):668–672, 0885-3185.

[14] Butzer JF, Silver DE and Sahs AL (1975). Amantadine in Parkinson's disease. A double-blind, placebo-controlled, crossover study with long-term follow-up. Neurology 25, 7 (Jul 1975): 603-6, 0028-3878.

[15] Bxarone P, Poewe W, Albrecht S, Debieuvre C, Massey D, Rascol O, Tolosa E, Weintraub D (2010). Pramipexole for the treatment of depressive symptoms in patients with Parkinson's disease: a randomised, double-blind, placebo-controlled trial. *Lancet Neurol* 9, 6 (Jun 2010): 573-80, 1474-4465.

[16] Cantello R, Riccio A, Gilli M, Delsedime M, Scarzella L, Aguggia M and Bergamasco B. (1986). Bornaprine vs placebo in Parkinson disease: double-blind controlled cross-over trial in 30 patients. *Ital J Neurol Sci* 7, 1 (Feb 1986): 139-43, 0392-0461.

[17] Ceravolo R, Frosini D, Rossi C and Bonuccelli U (2010). Spectrum of addictions in Parkinson's disease: from dopamine dysregulation syndrome to impulse control disorders. *J Neurol* 257(Suppl 2)(Nov 2010):S276-83, 1432-1459.

[18] Charles PD, Van Blercom N, Krack P, Lee SL, Xie J, Besson G, Benabid AL, Pollak P (2002). Predictors of effective bilateral subthalamic nucleus stimulation for PD. *Neurology* 59, 6 (Sep 2002): 932-34, 0028-3878.

[19] Chartier-Harlin MC, Kachergus J, Roumier C, Mouroux V, Douay X, Lincoln S, Levecque C, Larvor L, Andrieux J, Hulihan M, Waucquier N, Defebvre L, Amouyel P, Farrer M and Destée A. (2004). Alpha-synuclein locus duplication as a cause of familial Parkinson's disease. *Lancet* 364, 9440 (Sep 2004),1167-9, 1474-547X.

[20] Chaudhuri KR, Healy DG and Schapira AH (2006). National Institute for Clinical Excellence. Non-motor symptoms of Parkinson' s disease: diagnosis and management. *Lancet Neurol* 5, 3 (Mar 2006): 235 - 45, 1474-4422.

[21] Chung TH, Deane KH, Ghazi-Noori S, Rickards H and Clarke CE (2003). Systematic review of antidepressant therapies in Parkinson' s disease. *Parkinsonism Relat Disord* 10, 2 (Dec 2003): 59 - 65, 1353-8020.

[22] Colosimo C, Hughes AJ, Kilford L and Lees AJ. (2003). Lewy body cortical involvement may not always predict dementia in Parkinson' s disease. *J Neurol Neurosurg Psychiatry* 74, 7 (Jul 2003), 852 - 56, 0022-3050.

[23] Comella CL (2007). Sleep disorders in Parkinson' s disease: an overview. *Mov Disord* 22 (suppl 17)(Sep 2007): S367 - 73, 0885-3185.

[24] Constantinescu R, Romer M, McDermott MP, Kamp C and Kieburtz K; CALM-PD Investigators of the Parkinson Study Group (2007). Impact of pramipexole on the onset of levodopa-related dyskinesias. *Mov Disord* 22, 9 (Jul 2007):1317– 1319, 1531-8257.

[25] Corrigan MH, Denahan AQ, Wright CE, Ragual RJ and Evans DL (2000). Comparison of pramipexole, fluoxetine, and placebo in patients with major depression. *Depress Anxiety* 11, 2 (May 2000): 58-65, 1091-4269.

[26] Crossman AR, Mitchell IJ and Sambrook MA (1985). Regional brain uptake of 2-deoxyglucose in *N*-methyl-4-phenyl-1,2,3,6- tetrahydropyridine (MPTP)-induced

parkinsonism in the macaque monkey. *Neuropharmacology* 24, 6 (Jun 1985):587-591, 0028-3908.

[27] Dass B, Olanow CW and Kordower J (2006). Gene transfer of trophic factors and stem cell grafting as treatments for Parkinson's disease. *Neurology* 66, 10 suppl 4 (May 2006):S89- S103, 1526-632X.

[28] De Lau LM and Breteler MM. (2006). Epidemiology of Parkinson's disease. *Lancet Neurol* , 5, 6(june 2006), 525-535, 1474-4422.

[29] Damier P, Hirsch EC, Agid Y and Graybiel AM. (1999). The substantia nigra of the human brain. II. Patterns of loss of dopamine-containing neurons in Parkinson 's disease. *Brain* 122, 8 (Aug 1999), 1437-48, 0006-8950.

[30] Denny AP and Behari M (1999). Motor fluctuations in Parkinson's disease. *Journal of the Neurological Sciences* 165, 1(May 1999): 18-23, 0022-510X.

[31] De Rijk MC, Breteler MM, Graveland GA, Grobbee DE, van der Meché FG and Hofman A. (1995). Prevalence of Parkinson's disease in the elderly: the Rotterdam Study. *Neurology,* 45, 12 (Dec 1995), 2143-46, 0028-3878.Di Fonzo A, Dekker MC, Montagna P, Baruzzi A, Yonova EH, Correia Guedes L, Szczerbinska A, Zhao T, Dubbel-Hulsman LO, Wouters CH, de Graaff E, Oyen WJ, Simons EJ, Breedveld GJ, Oostra BA, Horstink MW and Bonifati V (2009). FBXO7 mutations cause autosomal recessive, early-onset parkinsonian-pyramidal syndrome. *Neurology* 72, 3 (Jan 2009):240-5, 1526-632X.

[32] Deuschl G, Schade-Brittinger C, Krack P, Volkmann J, Schäfer H, Bötzel K, Daniels C, Deutschländer A, Dillmann U, Eisner W, Gruber D, Hamel W, Herzog J, Hilker R, Klebe S, Kloss M, Koy J, Krause M, Kupsch A, Lorenz D, Lorenzl S, Mehdorn HM, Moringlane JR, Oertel W, Pinsker MO, Reichmann H, Reuss A, Schneider GH, Schnitzler A, Steude U, Sturm V, Timmermann L, Tronnier V, Trottenberg T, Wojtecki L, Wolf E, Poewe W and Voges J; German Parkinson Study Group, Neurostimulation Section (2006). A randomized trial of deep-brain stimulation for Parkinson's disease [published erratum in *N Engl J Med* 355, 9 (Aug 2006): 896-908, 1533-4406.

[33] Emre M, Aarsland D, Albanese A, Byrne EJ, Deuschl G, De Deyn PP, Durif F, Kulisevsky J, van Laar T, Lees A, Poewe W, Robillard A, Rosa MM, Wolters E, Quarg P, Tekin S and Lane R (2004). Rivastigmine for dementia associated with Parkinson's disease. *N Engl J Med* 351, 24 (Dec 2004):2509-18, 1533-4406.

[34] Etminan M, Samii A, Takkouche B and Rochon P (2001). Increased risk of somnolence with the new dopamine agonists in patients with Parkinson's disease. A metaanalysis of randomised controlled trials. *Drug Safety* 24, 11 (Oct 2001): 863-868, 0114-5916.

[35] Evans AH, Katzenschlager R, Paviour D, O'Sullivan JD, Appel S, Lawrence AD and Lees AJ (2004). Punding in Parkinson's disease: its relation to the dopamine dysregulation syndrome. *Mov Disord* 19, 4 (Apr 2004):397-405, 0885-3185.

[36] Fahn S, Oakes D, Shoulson I, Kieburtz K, Rudolph A, Lang A, Olanow CW, Tanner C and Marek K; Parkinson Study Group (2004). Levodopa and the progression of Parkinson´s disease. *N Engl J Med* 351, 24 (Dec 2004): 2498-508, 1533-4406.

[37] Fernandez HH, Trieschmann ME, Burke MA, Jacques C and Friedman JH (2003). Long-term outcome of quetiapine use for psychosis among Parkinsonian patients. *Mov Disord* 18; 5 (May 2003):510-4, 0885-3185.

[38] Ferreira JJ, Galitzky M, Montastruc JL and Rascol O (2000). Sleep attacks and Parkinson's disease treatment. *Lancet* 355, 9212 (Apr 2000):1333-4, 0140-6736.

[39] Follett KA, Weaver FM, Stern M, Hur K, Harris CL, Luo P, Marks WJ Jr, Rothlind J, Sagher O, Moy C, Pahwa R, Burchiel K, Hogarth P, Lai EC, Duda JE, Holloway K, Samii A, Horn S, Bronstein JM, Stoner G, Starr PA, Simpson R, Baltuch G, De Salles A, Huang GD and Reda DJ; CSP 468 Study Group (2010). Pallidal versus subthalamic deep-brain stimulation for Parkinson's disease. *N Engl J Med* 362, 22 (Jun 2010):2077-91, 1533-4406.

[40] Friedman JH and Factor SA (2000). Atypical antipsychotics in the treatment of drug-induced psychosis in Parkinson's disease. *Mov Disord* 15, 2 (Mar 2000):201–211, 0885-3185.

[41] Frucht S, Rogers JD, Greene PE, Gordon MF and Fahn S (1999). Falling asleep at the wheel: motor vehicle mishaps in persons taking pramipexole and ropinirole. *Neurology* 52, 9 (Jun 1999): 1908-10, 0028-3878.

[42] Funayama M, Hasegawa K, Kowa H, Saito M, Tsuji S and Obata F (2002). A new locus for Parkinson's disease (PARK8) maps to chromosome 12p11.2–q13.1. *Ann Neurol* 51, 3 (Mar 2002), 296–301, 0364-5134.

[43] Gilks WP, Abou-Sleiman PM, Gandhi S, Jain S, Singleton A, Lees AJ, Shaw K, Bhatia KP, Bonifati V, Quinn NP, Lynch J, Healy DG, Holton JL, Revesz T and Wood NW. (2005). A common LRRK2 mutation in idiopathic Parkinson' s disease. *Lancet* 365, 9457(Jan 2005), 415-16, 1474-547X.

[44] Goetz CG, Tanner CM, Shannon KM, Shannon KM and Carroll VS (1988). Controlled release carbidopa/levodopa (CR4-Sinemet) in Parkinson's disease patients with and without motor fluctuations. *Neurology* 38, 5(May): 1143–1146, 0028-3878.

[45] Gold BG, Nutt JG (2002). Neuroimmunophilin ligands in the treatment of Parkinson's disease. *Curr Opin Pharmacol* 2, 1 (Feb 2002):82- 86, 1471-4892.

[46] Goldberg MS and Lansbury PT. (2000). Is there a cause-and-effect relationship between alpha-synuclein fibrillization and Parkinson's disease?. *Nat Cell Biol* 2, 7 (Jul 2000), E115–E119, 1465-7392.

[47] Goldstein DS, Holmes C, Li ST, Bruce S, Metman LV and Cannon RO 3rd (2000). Cardiac sympathetic denervation in Parkinson disease. *Ann Intern Med* 133, 5 (Sep 2000):338–347, 0003-4819.

[48] Greffard S, Verny M, Bonnet AM, Seilhean D, Hauw JJ and Duyckaerts C. (2010). A stable proportion of Lewy body bearing neurons in the substantia nigra suggests a model in which the Lewy body causes neuronal death. *Neurobiol Aging* 31, 1(Jan 2010), 99-103, 1558-1497.

[49] Guridi J, Herrero MT, Luquin R, Guillen J and Obeso JA (1994). Subthalamotomy improves MPTP-induced parkinsonism in monkeys. *Stereotact Funct Neurosurg* 62, 1-4 (Jan 1994): 98–102, 1011-6125.

[50] Hallett M and Litvan I; Members of the Task Force on Surgery for Parkinson's Disease of the American Academy of Neurology Therapeutic and Technology Assessment Committee (2000). Scientific position paper of the Movement Disorder Society

evaluation of surgery for Parkinson's disease. *Mov Disord* 15, 3 (May 2000):436–438, 0885-3185.

[51] Halliday G, Hely M, Reid W and Morris J. (2008). The progression of pathology in longitudinally followed patients with Parkinson' s disease. *Acta Neuropathol,* 115, 4 (Apr 2008), 409-15, 0001-6322.

[52] Hardy J. (2005). Expression of normal sequence pathogenic proteins for neurodegenerative disease contributes to disease risk: permissive templating as a general mechanism underlying neurodegeneration. *Biochem Soc Trans* 33; 4 (Aug 2005), 578-81, 0300-5127.

[53] Hardy J, Lewis P, Revesz T, Lees A and Paisán-Ruiz. (2009). Genetics of Parkinson's syndromes: a critical review. *Curr Opin Genet Dev* 19, 3 (Jun 2009), 254-65, 1879-0380.

[54] Hauser RA, Schapira AH, Rascol O, Barone P, Mizuno Y, Salin L, Haaksma M, Juhel N and Poewe W (2010). Randomized, double-blind, multicenter evaluation of pramipexole extended release once daily in early Parkinson's disease. *Mov Disord* 25, 15 (Nov 2010):2542-9, 1531-8257.

[55] Healy DG, Falchi M, O'Sullivan SS, Bonifati V, Durr A, Bressman S, Brice A, Aasly J, Zabetian CP, Goldwurm S, Ferreira JJ, Tolosa E, Kay DM, Klein C, Williams DR, Marras C, Lang AE, Wszolek ZK, Berciano J, Schapira AH, Lynch T, Bhatia KP, Gasser T, Lees AJ and Wood NW (2008). Phenotype, genotype, and worldwide genetic penetrance of LRRK2-associated Parkinson's disease: a case-control study. *Lancet Neurol* 7, 7 (Jul 2008), 583–590, 1474-4422.

[56] Hedrich K, Djarmati A, Schafer N, Hering R, Wellenbrock C, Weiss PH, Hilker R, Vieregge P, Ozelius LJ, Heutink P, Bonifati V, Schwinger E, Lang AE, Noth J, Bressman SB, Pramstaller PP, Riess O and Klein C (2004). DJ-1 (PARK7) mutations are less frequent than Parkin (PARK2) mutations in early-onset Parkinson disease. *Neurology* 62, 3 (Feb 2004):389–394, 1526-632X.

[57] Heinonen EH and Myllylä V (1998). Safety of selegiline (deprenyl) in the treatment of Parkinson's disease. *Drug Saf* 19, 1 (Jul 1998): 11-22, 0114-5916.

[58] Iravani MM, Haddon CO, Cooper JM, Jenner P and Schapira AH (2006). Pramipexole protects against MPTP toxicity in nonhuman primates. *J Neurochem* 96, 5 (Mar 2006):1315–1321, 0022-3042.

[59] Jankovic J, Hunter C (2002). A double-blind, placebo-controlled and longitudinal study of riluzole in early Parkinson's disease. *Parkinsonism Relat Disord* 8, 4 (Marz 2002): 271-6, 1353-8020.

[60] Katzenschlager R and Lees AJ (2002). Treatment of Parkinson's disease: levodopa as the first choice. *Journal of Neurology* 249(Suppl. 2)(Sep 2002): II19-II24, 0340-5354.

[61] Katzenschlager R, Head J, Schraq A, Ben-Shlomo Y, Evans A and Lees AJ. Fourteen-year final report of the randomized PDRG-UK trial comparing three initial treatments in PD. *Neurology* , 71, 7 (Aug 2008), 474–80, 1526-632X.Lashley T, Holton JL, Gray E, Kirkham K, O'Sullivan SS, Hilbig A, Wood NW, Lees AJ and Revesz T. (2008). Cortical alpha-synuclein load is associated with amyloid-beta plaque burden in a subset of Parkinson' s disease patients. *Acta Neuropathol,* 115, 4 (Apr 2008), 417-25, 0001-6322.

[62] Keus SH, Bloem BR, Hendriks EJ, Bredero-Cohen AB and Munneke M; Practice Recommendations Development Group (2007). Evidence-based analysis of physical therapy in Parkinson' s disease with recommendations for practice and research. *Mov Disord* 22, 4 (Mar 2007): 451-60, 0885-3185.

[63] Khan NL, Graham E, Critchley P, Schrag AE, Wood NW, Lees AJ, Bhatia KP and Quinn N (2003). Parkin disease: a phenotypic study of a large case series. *Brain* 126, 6 (June 2003), :1279-92, 0006-8950.

[64] Kitada T, Asakawa S, Hattori N, Matsumine H, Yamamura Y, Minoshima S, Yokochi M, Mizuno Y and Shimizu N (1998). Mutations in the parkin gene cause autosomal recessive juvenile parkinsonism. *Nature* 392, 6676 (Apr 1998):605-8, 0028-0836.

[65] Kleiner-Fisman G and Fisman DN (2007). Risk factors for the development of pedal edema in patients using pramipexole. *Arch Neurol* 64, 6 (Jun 2007): 820-4, 0003-9942.

[66] Koller WC, Hutton JT, Tolosa E and Capilldeo R (1999). Immediate-release and controlled-release carbidopa/levodopa in PD: a 5-year randomized multicenter study. Carbidopa/Levodopa Study Group. *Neurology* 53, 5(Sep 1999): 1012–1019, 0028-3878.

[67] Korczyn AD, Brunt ER, Larsen JP, Nagy Z, Poewe WH and Ruggieri S (1999). A 3-year randomized trial of ropinirole and bromocriptine in early Parkinson's disease. The 053 Study Group. *Neurology* 53, 2 (Jul 1999): 364-70, 0028-3878.

[68] Kornhuber J, Weller M, Schoppmeyer K and Riederer P (1994). Amantadine and memantine are NMDA receptor antagonists with neuroprotective properties. *J Neural Transm* 43: 91–104, 0303-6995.

[69] Krack P, Batir A, Van Blercom N, Chabardes S, Fraix V, Ardouin C, Koudsie A, Limousin PD, Benazzouz A, LeBas JF, Benabid AL and Pollak P. (2003). Five-year follow-up of bilateral stimulation of the subthalamic nucleus in advanced Parkinson' s disease. *N Engl J Med* 349, 20 (Nov 2003): 1925-34, 1533-4406.

[70] Kruger R, Kuhn W, Muller T, Woitalla D, Graeber M, Kosel S, Przuntek H, Epplen JT, Schols L and Riess O. (1998). Ala30Pro mutation in the gene encoding alpha-synuclein in Parkinson's disease. *Nat Genet* 18, 2 (Feb 1998), 106–108, 1061-4036.

[71] Kubo SI, Kitami T, Noda S, Shimura H, Uchiyama Y, Asakawa S, Minoshima S, Shimizu N, Mizuno Y and Hattori N (2001). Parkin is associated with cellular vesicles. *J Neurochem* 78, 1 (Jul 2001):42–54, 0022-3042.

[72] Kumazawa R, Tomiyama H, Li Y, Imamichi Y, Funayama M, Yoshino H, Yokochi F, Fukusako T, Takehisa Y, Kashihara K, Kondo T, Elibol B, Bostantjopoulou S, Toda T, Takahashi H, Yoshii F, Mizuno Y and Hattori N (2008) Mutation analysis of the PINK1 gene in 391 patients with Parkinson disease. *Arch Neurol* 65, 6 (Jun 2008):802–808, 1538-3687.

[73] Kurth MC, Adler CH, Hilaire MS, Singer C, Waters C, LeWitt P, Chernik DA, Dorflinger EE and Yoo K (1997). Tolcapone improves motor function and reduces levodopa requirement in patients with Parkinson's disease experiencing motor fluctuations: a multicenter, double-blind, randomized, placebo-controlled trial. *Neurology* 48, 1 (Jan 1997):81– 87, 0028-3878.

[74] Lang AE, Gill S, Patel NK, Lozano A, Nutt JG, Penn R, Brooks DJ, Hotton G, Moro E, Heywood P, Brodsky MA, Burchiel K, Kelly P, Dalvi A, Scott B, Stacy M, Turner D,

Wooten VG, Elias WJ, Laws ER, Dhawan V, Stoessl AJ, Matcham J, Coffey RJ and Traub M (2006). Randomized controlled trial of intraputamenal glial cell line-derived neurotrophic factor infusion in Parkinson disease. *Ann Neurol* 59, 3 (Mar 2006):459-466, 0364-5134.

[75] Larsen JP, Worm-Petersen J, Siden A, Gordin A, Reinikainen K and Leinonen M (2003). The tolerability and efficacy of entacapone over 3 years in patients with Parkinson's disease. *Eur J Neurol* 10, 2 (Mar 2003):137-146,1351-5101.

[76] Lees AJ, Hardy J and Revesz T. (2009). Parkinson's disease. *Lancet* 373, 9680 (Jun 2009), 2055-2066, 1474-547X.

[77] Li JY, Englund E, Holton JL, Soulet D, Hagell P, Lees AJ, Lashley T, Quinn NP, Rehncrona S, Björklund A, Widner H, Revesz T, Lindvall O and Brundin P. (2008). Lewy bodies in grafted neurons in subjects with Parkinson' s disease suggest host-to-graft disease propagation. *Nat Med* 14, 5 (May 2008), 501-03, 1546-170X.

[78] Lemke MR, Brecht HM, Koester J and Reichmann H (2006). Effects of the dopamine agonist pramipexole on depression, anhedonia and motor functioning in Parkinson's disease. *J Neurol Sci* 248, 1-2 (Oct 2006): 266-70, 0022-510X.

[79] Levy G (2007). The relationship of Parkinson disease with aging. *Arch Neurol* 64, 9 (Sep 2007): 1242-46, 0003-9942.

[80] Lew MF, Hauser RA, Hurtig HI, Ondo WG, Wojcieszek J, Goren T and Fitzer-Attas CJ. (2010). Long-term efficacy of rasagiline in early Parkinson's disease. *Int J Neurosci* 120, 6 (Jun 2010): 404-8, 1563-5279.

[81] Li JY, Englund E, Widner H, Rehncrona S, Björklund A, Lindvall O and Brundin P. (2010). Characterization of Lewy body pathology in 12- and 16-year-old intrastriatal mesencephalic grafts surviving in a patient with Parkinson's disease. *Mov Disord* 25, 8, 1091-06, 1531-8257.

[82] Lindvall O and Bjo¨rklund A (2004). Cell therapy in Parkinson's disease. *NeuroRx* 1, 4 (Oct 2004):382-393, 1545-5343.

[83] Low PA and Singer W (2008). Management of neurogenic orthostatic hypotension: an update. *Lancet Neurol* 7, 5 (May 2008): 451-58, 1474-4422.

[84] López-Barneo J, Pardal R, Ortega-Sáenz P, Durán R, Villadiego J and Toledo-Aral JJ (2009). The neurogenic niche in the carotid body and its applicability to antiparkinsonian cell therapy. *J Neural Transm* 116, 8 (Aug 2009):975-82, 1435-1463.

[85] Mamikonyan E, Siderowf AD, Duda JE, Potenza MN, Horn S, Stern MB and Weintraub D (2008). Long-term follow-up of impulse control disorders in Parkinson' s disease. *Mov Disord* 23, 1 (Jan 2008): 75-80, 1531-8257 .

[86] Manson AJ, Turner K and Lees AJ (2002). Apomorphine monotherapy in the treatment of refractory motor complications of Parkinson's disease: long-term follow-up study of 64 patients. *Mov Disord* 17, 6:1235-41, 0885-3185.

[87] Marks WJ Jr, Bartus RT, Siffert J, Davis CS, Lozano A, Boulis N, Vitek J, Stacy M, Turner D, Verhagen L, Bakay R, Watts R, Guthrie B, Jankovic J, Simpson R, Tagliati M, Alterman R, Stern M, Baltuch G, Starr PA, Larson PS, Ostrem JL, Nutt J, Kieburtz K, Kordower JH and Olanow CW (2010). Gene delivery of AAV2-neurturin for Parkinson's disease: a double-blind, randomised, controlled trial. *Lancet Neurol* 9, 12 (Dec 2010):1164-72, 1474-4465.

[88] Mathias CJ, Senard JM, Braune S, Watson L, Aragishi A, Keeling JE and Taylor MD. (2001). L-threodihydroxyphenylserine (L-threo-DOPS; droxidopa) in the management of neurogenic orthostatic hypotension: a multinational, multi-center, dose-ranging study in multiple system atrophy and pure autonomic failure. *Clin Auton Res* 2001; 11, 4 (Aug 2001): 235-42, 0959-9851.

[89] etman LV, Del Dotto P, LePoole K, Konitsiotis S, Fang J and Chase TN (1999). Amantadine for levodopa-induced dyskinesias: a 1-year follow-up study. *Arch Neurol* 56, 1 (Nov 1999):1383–1386, 0003-9942.

[90] Meral H, Aydemir T, Ozer F, Ozturk O, Ozben S, Erol C, Cetin S, Hanoglu L, Ozkayran T and Yilsen M. (2007). Relationship between visual hallucinations and REM sleep behavior disorder in patients with Parkinson's disease. *Clin Neurol Neurosurg* 109, 10 (Dec 2007):862- 867, 0303-8467.

[91] Mitchell IJ, Clarke CE and Boyce S, Robertson RG, Peggs D, Sambrook MA and Crossman AR (1989). Neural mechanisms underlying parkinsonian symptoms based upon regional uptake of 2-deoxyglucose in monkeys exposed to 1-methyl-4-phenyl-1,2,3,6-tetrahydropyridine. *Neuroscience* 32, 1 (Jan 1989):213–226, 0306-4522.

[92] Mizuno Y, Kondo T and Narabayashi H (1995). Pergolide in the treatment of Parkinson's disease. *Neurology* 45, 3(Suppl. 31)(Mar 1995): S13–S21, 0028-3878.

[93] Montastruc JL, Rascol O, Senard JM and Rascol A (1994). A randomized controlled study comparing bromocriptine to which levodopa was later added, with levodopa alone in previously untreated patients with Parkinson's disease: a five year follow up. *J Neurol Neurosurg Psychiatry* 57, 9 (Sep 1994):1034 –1038, 0022-3050.

[94] Montastruc JL, Brefel-Courbon C, Senard JM, Bagheri H, Ferreira J, Rascol O and Lapeyre-Mestre M. (2001) . Sleep attacks and antiparkinsonian drugs: a pilot prospective pharmacoepidemiologic study. *Clin Neuropharmacol* 24, 3 (May-June 2001):181–183, 0362-5664 .

[95] Morgan JC and Sethi KD (2006). Pergolide-induced ergotism. *Neurology* 67, 1 (Jul 2006):104, 1526-632X.

[96] Morgenthaler TI, Kapur VK, Brown T, Swick TJ, Alessi C, Aurora RN, Boehlecke B, Chesson AL Jr, Friedman L, Maganti R, Owens J, Pancer J and Zak R; Standards of Practice Committee of the American Academy of Sleep Medicine. (2007). Practice parameters for the treatment of narcolepsy and other hypersomnias of central origin [published erratum in Sleep 2008; 31: TOC]. *Sleep* 30, 12 (Dec 2007): 1705-11, 0161-8105.

[97] Morizane A, Li JY and Brundin P (2008). From bench to bed: the potential of stem cells for the treatment of Parkinson' s disease. *Cell Tissue Res* 331, 1 (Jan 2008): 323-36, 1432-0878.

[98] Muller T, Erdmann C, Muhlack S, Bremen D, Przuntek H and Woitalla D (2006). Inhibition of catechol-*O*-methyltransferase contributes to more stable levodopa plasma levels. *Mov Disord* 21, 3 (Mar 2006):332–336, 0885-3185.

[99] Neumann J, Bras J, Deas E, O'Sullivan SS, Parkkinen L, Lachmann RH, Li A, Holton J, Guerreiro R, Paudel R, Segarane B, Singleton A, Lees A, Hardy J, Houlden H, Revesz T and Wood NW (2009). Glucocerebrosidase mutations in clinical and

pathologically proven Parkinson's disease. *Brain* 132, Pt 7 (Jul 2009):1783-94, 1460-2156.

[100] Narabayashi H, Yokochi F and Nakajima Y (1984). Levodopainduced dyskinesia and thalamotomy. *J Neurol Neurosurg Psychiatry* 47, 8 (Aug 1984):831- 839, 0022-3050.

[101] Narabayashi H (1989). Stereotaxic vim thalamotomy for treatment of tremor. *Eur Neurol* 29, (suppl 1)(Jan 1989):29 -32, 0014-3022.

[102] Nirenberg MJ and Waters C (2006). Compulsive eating and weight gain related to dopamine agonist use. *Mov Disord* 21, 4 (Apr 2006): 524-9, 0885-3185.

[103] Noe E, Marder K, Bell KL, Jacobs DM, Manly JJ and Stern Y (2004). Comparison of dementia with Lewy bodies to Alzheimer's disease and Parkinson's disease with dementia. *Mov Disord* 19, 1 (Jan 2004):60–67, 0885-3185.

[104] Nutt JG, Woodward WR, Hammerstad JP, Carter JH and Anderson JL (1984). The "on-off " phenomenon in Parkinson's disease. Relation to levodopa absorption and transport. *N Engl J Med* 310, 8 (Feb 1984):483- 488, 0028-4793.

[105] Nutt JG, Burchiel KJ, Comella CL, Jankovic J, Lang AE, Laws ER Jr, Lozano AM, Penn RD, Simpson RK Jr, Stacy M and Wooten GF; ICV GDNF Study Group. Implanted intracerebroventricular. Glial cell line-derived neurotrophic factor. (2003). Randomized, double-blind trial of glial cell line-derived neurotrophic factor (GDNF) in PD. *Neurology* 60, 1 (Jan 2003): 69-73, 1526-632X.

[106] Nyholm D, Nilsson Remahl AI, Dizdar N, Constantinescu R, Holmberg B, Jansson R, Aquilonius SM and Askmark H (2005). Duodenal levodopa infusion monotherapy vs oral polypharmacy in advanced Parkinson disease. *Neurology* 64, 2 (Jan 2005):216–223, 1526-632X.

[107] Oertel WH, Wolters E, Sampaio C, Gimenez-Roldan S, Bergamasco B, Dujardin M, Grosset DG, Arnold G, Leenders KL, Hundemer HP, Lledó A, Wood A, Frewer P and Schwarz J (2006). Pergolide versus levodopa monotherapy in early Parkinson's disease patients: the PELMOPET study. *Mov Disord* 21, 3 (Mar 2006): 343–353, 0885-3185.

[108] Olanow CW, Hauser RA, Gauger L, Malapira T, Koller W, Hubble J, Bushenbark K, Lilienfeld D and Esterlitz J (1995). The effect of deprenyl and levodopa on the progression of Parkinson's disease. *Ann Neurol* 38, 5 (Nov 1995): 771-7, 0364-5134.

[109] Olanow CW. Selegiline: current perspectives on issues related to neuroprotection and mortality (1996). *Neurology* 47, (6 suppl 3)(Dec 1996):S210 -S216, 0028-3878.

[110] Olanow CW, Kordower JH and Freeman TB (1996). Fetal nigral transplantation as a therapy for Parkinson's disease. Trends *Neurosci* 19, 3 (Mar 1996):102–109, 0166-2236.

[111] Olanow CW, Myllyla VV, Sotaniemi KA, Larsen JP, Pålhagen S, Przuntek H, Heinonen EH, Kilkku O, Lammintausta R, Mäki-Ikola O and Rinne UK (1998). Effect of selegiline on mortality in patients with Parkinson's disease: a meta-analysis. *Neurology* 51, 3 (Sep 1998): 825–830, 0028-3878.

[112] Olanow CW, Brin M and Obeso JA (2000). The role of deep brain stimulation as a surgical treatment for Parkinson's disease. *Neurology* 55, 12(suppl 6)(Feb 2000):60–66, 0028-3878.

[113] Olanow CW, Watts RL and Koller WC (2001). An algorithm (decision tree) for the management of Parkinson's disease: treatment guidelines. *Neurology* 56, 11 Suppl. 5 (Jun 2001): S1–S88, 0028-3878.

[114] Olanow CW and Stocchi F (2004). COMT inhibitors in Parkinson's disease: can they prevent and/or reverse levodopa induced motor complications? *Neurology* 62, 1 suppl 1 (Jan 2004):S72–S81, 1526-632X.

[115] Olanow CW, Agid Y, Mizuno Y, Albanese A, Bonuccelli U, Damier P, De Yebenes J, Gershanik O, Guttman M, Grandas F, Hallett M, Hornykiewicz O, Jenner P, Katzenschlager R, Langston WJ, LeWitt P, Melamed E, Mena MA, Michel PP, Mytilineou C, Obeso JA, Poewe W, Quinn N, Raisman-Vozari R, Rajput AH, Rascol O, Sampaio C and Stocchi F(2004). Levodopa in the treatment of Parkinson's disease: current controversies. *Movement Disorders* 19, 9 (Sep 2004): 997-1005, 0885-3185.

[116] Olanow CW, Kieburtz K, Stern M, Watts R, Langston JW, Guarnieri M and Hubble J; US01 Study Team (2004). Double-blind, placebo-controlled study of entacapone in levodopa-treated patients with stable Parkinson disease. *Arch Neurol* 61, 10 (Oct 2004):1563–1568, 0003-9942.

[117] Olanow CW, Schapira AHV, LeWitt PA, Kieburtz K, Sauer D, Olivieri G, Pohlmann H and Hubble J(2006). TCH346 as a neuroprotective drug in Parkinson's disease: a double-blind, randomised, controlled trial. *Lancet Neurol* 5, 12 (Dec 2006):1013–1020, 1474-4422.

[118] Olanow CW, Rascol O, Hauser R, Feigin PD, Jankovic J, Lang ALangston W, Melamed E, Poewe W, Stocchi F and Tolosa E; ADAGIO Study Investigators (2009) . A double-blind, delayed-start trial of rasagiline in Parkinson's disease. *N Engl J Med* 361, 13 (Sep 2009): 1268-78, 1533-4406.

[119] Olanow CW, Stern MB and Sethi K. (2009). The scientific and clinical basis for the treatment of Parkinson disease. *Neurology,* 26, 72(21 Suppl 4)(Dec 2009), S1-136, 0028-3878.

[120] Ostergaard L, Werdelin L, Odin P, Lindvall O, Dupont E, Christensen PB, Boisen E, Jensen NB, Ingwersen S and, Schmiegelow M (1995). *J Neurol Neurosurg Psychiatry* 58, 6 (Jun 1995):681-7, 0022-3050.

[121] Pahwa R, Stacy MA, Factor SA, Lyons KE, Stocchi F, Hersh BP, Elmer LW, Truong DD and Earl NL; EASE-PD Adjunct Study Investigators. (2007). Ropinirole 24-hour prolonged release: randomized, controlled study in advanced Parkinson disease. *Neurology* 68, 14 (Apr 2007): 1108-15, 1526-632X.

[122] Pahapill PA and Lozano AM (2000). The pedunculopontine nucleus and Parkinson's disease. *Brain* 123, 9 (Sep 2000):1767–1783, 0006-8950.

[123] Paisan-Ruiz C, Jain S, Evans EW, Gilks WP, Simon J, van der Brug M, Lopez de Munain A, Aparicio S, Gil AM, Khan N, Johnson J, Martinez JR, Nicholl D, Carrera IM, Pena AS, de Silva R, Lees A, Marti-Masso JF, Perez-Tur J, Wood NW and Singleton AB (2004) Cloning of the gene containing mutations that cause PARK8-linked Parkinson's disease. *Neuron* 44, 18 (Nov 2004), 595–600, 0896-6273.

[124] Paisán-Ruiz (2009). LRRK2 gene variation and its contribution to Parkinson disease. *Hum Mutat* 30, 8 (Aug 2009): 1153-60, 1098-1004.

[125] Paisán-Ruiz C, Guevara R, Federoff M, Hanagasi H, Sina F, Elahi E, Schneider SA, Schwingenschuh P, Bajaj N, Emre M, Singleton AB, Hardy J, Bhatia KP, Brandner S, Lees AJ, and Houlden H (2010). Early-onset L-dopa-responsive parkinsonism with pyramidal signs due to ATP13A2, PLA2G6, FBXO7 and spatacsin mutations. *Mov Disord* 25, 12 (Sep 2010): 1791-800, 1531-8257.

[126] Parkinson J. *An Essay on the Shaking Palsy*. London: Whittingham and Rowland for Sherwood, Neely and Jones; 1817.

[127] Parkkinen L, Kauppinen T, Pirttila T, Autere JM and Alafuzoff I (2005). Alpha-synuclein pathology does not predict extrapyramidal symptoms or dementia. *Ann Neurol* 57, 1 (Jan 2005), 82 - 91, 0364-5134.

[128] Parkinson Study Group (1993). Effects of tocopherol and deprenyl on the progression of disability in early Parkinson's disease. *N Engl J Med* 328, 21 (Jan 1993:176 -183, 0028-4793.

[129] Parkinson Study Group (1996). Impact of deprenyl and tocopherol treatment on Parkinson's disease in DATATOP subjects not requiring levodopa. *Ann Neurol* 39, 1 (Jan 1996): 29-36, 0364-5134.

[130] Parkinson Study Group (1997). Entacapone improved motor fluctuations in levodopa-treated Parkinson's disease patients. *Ann Neurol* 42, 5(Nov 1997):747–755, 0364-5134.

[131] Parkinson Study Group (1999). Low dose clozapine for the treatment of drug-induced psychosis in Parkinson's disease. *N Engl J Med* 340, 10 (Mar 1999):757–763, 0028-4793.

[132] Parkinson Study Group (2000). Pramipexole vs levodopa as initial treatment for Parkinson disease: a randomized controlled trial. Parkinson Study Group. JAMA 284, 15 (Oct 2000): 1931-8, 0098-7484.

[133] Parkinson Study Group (2002). Dopamine transporter brain imaging to assess the effects of pramipexole vs levodopa on Parkinson disease progression. JAMA 287, 13 (Jul 2002): 1653-61, 0098-7484.

[134] Parkinson Study Group (2002). A controlled trial of rasagiline in early Parkinson disease: the TEMPO Study. *Arch Neurol* 59, 12 (Dec 2002): 1937-43, 0003-9942.

[135] Parkinson Study Group (2005). A randomized placebo-controlled trial of rasagiline in levodopa-treated patients with Parkinson disease and motor fluctuations: the PRESTO study. *Arch Neurol* 62, 2 (Feb 2005):241–248, 0003-9942.

[136] Parkinson Study Group PRECEPT Investigators (2007). Mixed lineage kinase inhibitor CEP-1347 fails to delay disability in early Parkinson disease. *Neurology* 2007;69, 15 (Oct 2007):1480– 1490, 1526-632X.

[137] Paus S, Brecht HM, Köster J, Seeger G, Klockgether T and Wüllner U (2003). Sleep attacks, daytime sleepiness, and dopamine agonists in Parkinson's disease. *Mov Disord* 18, 6(Jun 2003):659-67, 0885-3185.

[138] Polymeropoulos MH, Lavedan C, Leroy E, Ide SE, Dehejia A, Dutra A, Pike B, Root H, Rubenstein J, Boyer R, Stenroos ES, Chandrasekharappa S, Athanassiadou A, Papapetropoulos T, Johnson WG, Lazzarini AM, Duvoisin RC, Di Iorio G and Nussbaum RL. (1997). α- Synuclein gene identified in families with Parkinson's disease. Science 276, 5321 (June 1997), 2045–2047, 0036-8075.

[139] Porter B, Macfarlane R and Walker R (2008). The frequency and nature of sleep disorders in a community-based population of patients with Parkinson's disease. *Eur J Neurol* 15, 1 (Jan 2008):50 -54, 1468-1331.

[140] Postuma RB, Lang AE, Massicotte-Marquez J and MontplaisirJ (2006). Potential early markers of Parkinson disease in idiopathic REM sleep behavior disorder. *Neurology* 66, 6 (Mar 2006):845- 851, 1526-632X.

[141] Pramstaller PP, Schlossmacher MG, Jacques TS, Scaravilli F, Eskelson C, Pepivani I, Hedrich K, Adel S, Gonzales-McNeal M, Hilker R, Kramer PL and Klein C . (2005). Lewy body Parkinson' s disease in a large pedigree with 77 Parkin mutation carriers. *Ann Neurol* 58: 3 (Sep 2005), 411-22, 0364-5134.

[142] Rajput AH (2001). Levodopa prolongs life expectancy and is non-toxic to substantia nigra. *Parkinsonism Relat Disord* 8, 2 (Oct 2001): 95-100, 1353-8020.

[143] Rakshi JS, Pavese N, Uema T, Ito K, Morrish PK, Bailey DL and Brooks DJ. (2002). A comparison of the progression of early Parkinson's disease in patients started on ropinirole or L-dopa: an 18F-dopa PET study. *J Neural Transm*; 109, 12 (Dec 2002): 1433-43, 0300-9564.

[144] amirez A, Heimbach A, Grundemann J, Stiller B, Hampshire D, Cid LP, Goebel I, Mubaidin AF, Wriekat AL, Roeper J, Al-Din A, Hillmer AM, Karsak M, Liss B, Woods CG, Behrens MI, Kubisch C (2006) Hereditary parkinsonism with dementia is caused by mutations in ATP13A2, encoding a lysosomal type 5 P-type ATPase. *Nat Genet* 38, 10 (Oct 2008):1184–1191, 1061-4036.

[145] Rascol O, Brooks DJ, Korczyn AD, De Deyn PP, Clarke CE and Lang AE (2000). A five-year study of the incidence of dyskinesia in patients with early Parkinson's disease who were treated with ropinirole or levodopa. 056 Study Group. *N Engl J Med* 342, 20 (May 2000): 1484–91, 0028-4793.

[146] Rascol O, Brooks DJ, Melamad E, Oertel W, Poewe W, Stocchi F and Tolosa E: LARGO study group. (2005). Rasagiline as an adjunct to levodopa in patients with Parkinson's disease and motor fluctuations (LARGO, Lasting effect in Adjunct therapy with Rasagiline Given Once daily, study): a randomised, double-blind, parallel-group trial. *Lancet* 2005;365, 9463 (Mar 2005):947–954, 1474-547X.

[147] Ravina B, Putt M, Siderowf A, Farrar JT, Gillespie M, Crawley A, Fernandez HH, Trieschmann MM, Reichwein S and Simuni T (2005). Donazepil for dementia in Parkinson's disease: a randomized, double blind, crossover study. J Neurol *Neurosurg Psychiatry* 76, 7 (Jul 2005):934 -939, 0022-3050.

[148] Renkwalder C, Kies B, Rudzinsca M, Fine J, Nikl J, Honczarenco K, et al. Rotigotine effects on early morning motor function and sleep in Parkinson's disease: a doble-blind, randomized, placebo-controlled study (RECOVER). Mov Disord 2010. [Epub ahead of print]

[149] Rinne UK, Bracco F, Chouza C, Dupont E, Gershanik O, Marti Masso JF, Montastruc JL and Marsden CD (1998). Early treatment of Parkinson's disease with cabergoline delays the onset of motor complications. The PKDS009 Study Group. *Drugs* 1998; 55(Suppl. 1)(Mar 1998): 23-30, 0012-6667.

[150] Ritter JL and Alexander B (1997). Retrospective study of selegiline antidepressant drug interactions and a review of the literature. *Ann Clin Psychiatry* 9, 1 (Mar 1997): 7–13, 1040-1237.

[151] Rogaeva E, Johnson J, Lang AE, Gulick C, Gwinn-Hardy K, Kawarai T, Sato C, Morgan A, Werner J, Nussbaum R, Petit A, Okun MS, McInerney A, Mandel R, Groen JL, Fernandez HH, Postuma R, Foote KD, Salehi-Rad S, Liang Y, Reimsnider S, Tandon A, Hardy J, St George- Hyslop P and Singleton AB (2004). Analysis of the PINK1 gene in a large cohort of cases with Parkinson disease. *Arch Neurol* 61, 12(Dec 2004):1898–1904, 0003-9942.

[152] Roth BL (2007). Drugs and valvular heart disease. *N Engl J Med* 356, 1 (Jan 2007):6 –9, 1533-4406.

[153] Shin N, Jeong H, Kwon J, Heo HY, Kwon JJ, Yun HJ, Kim CH, Han BS, Tong Y, Shen J, Hatano T, Hattori N, Kim KS,Chang S, Seol W (2008). LRRK2 regulates synaptic vesicle endocytosis. *Exp Cell Res* 314, 10 (Jun 2008),2055–2065, 1090-2422.

[154] Sagi Y, Mandel S, Amit T and Youdim MB (2007). Activation of tyrosine kinase receptor signaling pathway by rasagiline facilitates neurorescue and restoration of nigrostriatal dopamine neurons in post-MPTP-induced parkinsonism. *Neurobiol Dis* 25, 1 (Jan 2007): 35-44, 0969-9961.

[155] Schapira AH (2002). Dopamine agonists and neuroprotection in Parkinson's disease. *Eur J Neurol* 9(suppl 3)(Nov 2002):7–14, 1351-5101.

[156] Shults CW, Oakes D, Kieburtz K, Beal MF, Haas R, Plumb S, Juncos JL, Nutt J, Shoulson I, Carter J, Kompoliti K, Perlmutter JS, Reich S, Stern M, Watts RL, Kurlan R, Molho E, Harrison M and Lew M; Parkinson Study Group (2002). Effects of coenzyme Q10 in early Parkinson disease: evidence of slowing of the functional decline. *Arch Neurol* 59, 10 (Oct 2002): 1541-50, 0003-9942.

[157] Sidransky E, Nalls MA, Aasly JO, Aharon-Peretz J, Annesi G, Barbosa ER, Bar-Shira A, Berg D, Bras J, Brice A, Chen CM, Clark LN, Condroyer C, De Marco EV, Dürr A, Eblan MJ, Fahn S, Farrer MJ, Fung HC, Gan-Or Z, Gasser T, Gershoni-Baruch R, Giladi N, Griffith A, Gurevich T, Januario C, Kropp P, Lang AE, Lee-Chen GJ, Lesage S, Marder K, Mata IF, Mirelman A, Mitsui J, Mizuta I, Nicoletti G, Oliveira C, Ottman R, Orr-Urtreger A, Pereira LV, Quattrone A, Rogaeva E, Rolfs A, Rosenbaum H, Rozenberg R, Samii A, Samaddar T, Schulte C, Sharma M, Singleton A, Spitz M, Tan EK, Tayebi N, Toda T, Troiano AR, Tsuji S, Wittstock M, Wolfsberg TG, Wu YR, Zabetian CP, Zhao Y and Ziegler SG (2009). Multicenter analysis of glucocerebrosidase mutations in Parkinson's disease. *N Engl J Med* 361, 17 (Oct 2009):1651-61. 1533-4406.

[158] Singleton AB, Farrer M, Johnson J, Singleton A, Hague S, Kachergus J, Hulihan M, Peuralinna T, Dutra A, Nussbaum R, Lincoln S, Crawley A, Hanson M, Maraganore D, Adler C, Cookson MR, Muenter M, Baptista M, Miller D, Blancato J, Hardy J and Gwinn- Hardy K. (2003). Alpha-Synuclein locus triplication causes Parkinson's disease. *Science* 302, 5646 (Oct 2003), 841, 1095-9203.

[159] Singleton A, Gwinn-Hardy K, Sharabi Y, Li ST, Holmes C, Dendi R, Hardy J, Singleton A, Crawley A and Goldstein DS. (2004). Association between cardiac denervation and parkinsonism caused by alpha-synuclein gene triplication. *Brain* 127(Pt 4):768–772, 0006-8950.

[160] Smith LA, Jackson MJ, Al-Barghouthy G, Rose S, Kuoppamaki M, Olanow W and Jenner P (2005). Multiple small doses of levodopa plus entacapone produces continuous dopaminergic stimulation and reduces dyskinesia induction in MPTP-treated drug naïve primates. *Mov Disord* 20, 3(Mar 2005): 306-14, 0885-3185.

[161] Spillantini MG, Schmidt ML, Lee VM, Trojanowski JQ, Jakes R and Goedert M. (1997). Alpha-synuclein in Lewy bodies. *Nature,* 388, 6645 (Aug 1997), 839–840, 0028-0836.

[162] Starkstein SE, Mayberg HS, Leiguarda R, Preziosi TJ and Robinson RG (1992). A prospective longitudinal study of depression, cognitive decline, and physical impairments in patients with Parkinson's disease. *J Neurol Neurosurg Psychiatry* 55, 5 (May 1992):377-82, 0022-3050.

[163] Staskin DR (2006). Trospium chloride: distinct among other anticholinergic agents available for the treatment of overactive bladder. *Urol Clin North Am* 33, 4 (Nov 2006): 465 - 73, 0094-0143.

[164] Stefani A, Lozano AM, Peppe A, , Stanzione P, Galati S, Tropepi D, Pierantozzi M, Brusa L, Scarnati E and Mazzone P. (2007). Bilateral deep brain stimulation of the pedunculopontine and subthalamic nuclei in severe Parkinson's disease. *Brain* 130, 6 (Jun 2007):1596 –1607, 1460-2156.

[165] Stocchi F, Arnold G, Onofrj M, Kwiecinski H, Szczudlik A, Thomas A, Bonuccelli U, Van Dijk A, Cattaneo C, Sala P, Fariello RG; Safinamide Parkinson's Study Group (2004). Improvement of motor function in early Parkinson disease by safinamide. *Neurology* 63, 4 (Aug 2004):746 –748, 1526-632X.

[166] Stocchi F, Rascol O, Kieburtz K, Poewe W, Jankovic J, Tolosa E, Barone P, Lang AE and Olanow CW (2010). Initiating levodopa/carbidopa therapy with and without entacapone in early Parkinson disease: the STRIDE-PD study. *Ann Neurol* 68, 1 (Jul 2010): 18-2, 1531-8249.

[167] Svendsen C (2007). The first steps towards gene therapy for Parkinson's disease. *Lancet Neurol* 6, 9 (Sep 2007):754 –756, 1474-4422.

[168] Tandberg E, Larsen MD and Karlsen MD (1999). Excessive daytime sleepiness and sleep benefit in Parkinson's disease: a community-based study. *Mov Dis* 14, 6 (Nov 1999):922–927, 0885-3185.

[169] Timberlake WH and Vance MA (1978). Four-year treatment of patients with parkinsonism using amantadine alone or with levodopa. *Ann Neurol* 3, 2 (Feb 1978): 119-28, 0364-5134.

[170] Tolosa E, Gaig C, Santamaría J, Compta Y (2009). Diagnosis and the premotor phase of Parkinson disease. *Neurology* 72(7 Suppl)(Feb 2009):S12-20, 1526-632X.

[171] Trenkwalder C, Kies B, Rudzinsca M, Fine J, Nikl J, Honczarenco K, Dioszeghy P, Hill D, Anderson T, Myllyla V, Kassubek J, Steiger M, Zucconi M, Tolosa E, Poewe W, Surmann E, Whitesides J, Boroojerdi B and Chaudhuri KR; Recover Study Group. (2010). Rotigotine effects on early morning motor function and sleep in Parkinson's disease: a doble-blind, randomized, placebo-controlled study (RECOVER). *Mov Disord* 26, 1 (Jan 2011):90-9, 1531-8257.

[172] Valente EM, Abou-Sleiman PM, Caputo V, Muqit MM, Harvey K, Gispert S, Ali Z, Del Turco D, Bentivoglio AR, Healy DG, Albanese A, Nussbaum R, González-Maldonado R, Deller T, Salvi S, Cortelli P, Gilks WP, Latchman DS, Harvey RJ,

Dallapiccola B, Auburger G and Wood NW (2004). Hereditary early-onset Parkinson's disease caused by mutations in PINK1. *Science* 304, 5674 (May 2004):1158-60, 1095-9203.

[173] Van de Warrenburg BP, Lammens M, Lucking CB, Denèfle P, Wesseling P, Booij J, Praamstra P, Quinn N, Brice A and Horstink MW. (2001). Clinical and pathologic abnormalities in a family with parkinsonism and parkin gene mutations. *Neurology* 56, 4 (Feb 2001), 555-57, 0028-3878.

[174] Van Herwaarden G, Berger HJ and Horstink MW (1993). Short-term memory in Parkinson's disease after withdrawal of long-term anticholinergic therapy. *Clin Neuropharmacol* 16, 5 (Oct 1993): 438-43, 0362-5664.

[175] Vendette M, Gagnon JF, De´cary A, Massicotte-Marquez J, Postuma RB, Doyon J, Panisset M and Montplaisir J (2007). REM sleep behavior disorder predicts cognitive impairment in Parkinson disease without dementia. *Neurology* 69, 19 (Nov 2007):1843–1849, 1526-632X.

[176] Verhagen Metman L, Del Dotto P, van den Munckhof P, Fang J, Mouradian MM and Chase TN (1998). Amantadine as treatment for dyskinesias and motor fluctuations in Parkinson's disease. *Neurology* 50, 5 (May 1998):1323-26, 0028-3878.

[177] Voon V, Hassan K, Zurowski M, Duff-Canning S, de Souza M, Fox S, Lang AE and Miyasaki J (2006). Prospective prevalence of pathological gambling and medication association in Parkinson disease. *Neurology* 66, 11(Jun 2006):1750-52, 1526-632X.

[178] Voon V, Sohr M, Lang AE, Potenza MN, Siderowf AD, Whetteckey J, Weintraub D, Wunderlich GR and Stacy M (2011). Impulse control disorders in parkinson disease: A multicenter case-control study. *Ann Neurol* [Epub ahead of print].

[179] Waters CH, Kurth M, Bailey P, Shulman LM, LeWitt P, Dorflinger E, Deptula D and Pedder S. (1997). Tolcapone in stable Parkinson's disease: efficacy and safety of long term treatment. The Tolcapone Stable Study Group. *Neurology* 49, 3 (Sep 1997):665- 671, 0028-3878.

[180] Weintraub D, Morales KH, Moberg PJ, Bilker WB, Balderston C, Duda JE, Katz IR and Stern MB (2005). Antidepressant studies in Parkinson' s disease: a review and meta-analysis. *Mov Disord* 20, 9 (Sep 2005): 1161-69, 0885-3185.

[181] Weintraub D, Siderowf AD, Potenza MN, Goveas J, Morales KH, Duda JE, Moberg PJ and Stern MB (2006). Association of dopamine agonist use with impulse control disorders in Parkinson disease. *Arch Neurol* 63, 7(Jul 2006): 969-73, 0003-9942.

[182] Whone AL, Watts RL, Stoessl AJ, Davis M, Reske S, Nahmias C, Lang AE, Rascol O, Ribeiro MJ, Remy P, Poewe WH, Hauser RA and Brooks DJ (2003). Slower progression of Parkinson'sdisease with ropinirole versus levodopa: The REAL-PET study. *Ann Neurol* 54, 1 (Jul 2003): 93-101, 0364-5134.

[183] Witjas T, Kaphan E, Azulay JP, Blin O, Ceccaldi M, Pouget J, Poncet M and Chérif AA (2002). Nonmotor fluctuations in Parkinson's disease: frequent and disabling. *Neurology* 59, 3 (Aug 2002):408–413, 0028-3878.

[184] Xie J, Krack P, Benabid AL and Pollak P (2001). Effect of bilateral subthalamic nucleus stimulation on parkinsonian gait. *J Neurol* 248, 12 (Dec 2001): 1068-72, 0340-5354.

[185] Zanettini R, Antonini A, Gatto G, Gentile R, Tesei S and Pezzoli G (2007). Valvular heart disease and the use of dopamine agonists for Parkinson's disease. *N Engl J Med* 356, 1 (Jan 2007):39–46, 1533-4406.

[186] Zarranz JJ, Alegre J, Gomez-Esteban JC, Lezcano E, Ros R, Ampuero I, Vidal L, Hoenicka J, Rodriguez O, Atares B, Llorens V, Gomez Tortosa E, del Ser T, Munoz DG and de Yebenes JG. (2004). The new mutation, E46K, of alpha-synuclein causes Parkinson and Lewy body dementia. *Ann Neurol* 55, 2 (Feb 2004), 164–173, 0364-5134.

[187] Zimprich A, Biskup S, Leitner P, Lichtner P, Farrer M, Lincoln S, Kachergus J, Hulihan M, Uitti RJ, Calne DB, Stoessl AJ, Pfeiffer RF, Patenge N, Carbajal IC, Vieregge P, Asmus F, Muller-Myhsok B, Dickson DW, Meitinger T, Strom TM, Wszolek ZK and Gasser T (2004) Mutations in LRRK2 cause autosomal-dominant parkinsonism with pleomorphic pathology. *Neuron* 44, 4 (Nov 2004), 601–607, 0896-6273.

[188] Zhu W, Xie W, Pan T, Jankovic J, Li J, Youdim MB, Le W (2008). Comparison of neuroprotective and neurorestorative capabilities of rasagiline and selegiline against lactacystin-induced nigrostriatal dopaminergic degeneration. *J Neurochem* 2008; 105, 5 (Jun 2008): 1970-8, 1471-4159.

2

Timing Control in Parkinson's Disease

Quincy J. Almeida
*Sun Life Financial Movement Disorders Research & Rehabilitation Centre,
Wilfrid Laurier University
Canada*

1. Introduction

Internal generation and modulation of timing may be an important underlying yet unrecognized mechanism of many symptoms in Parkinson's disease. It has been recently debated whether the basal ganglia or cerebellum might contribute to overall timing control during movement execution. As seen in basal ganglia disorders such as Parkinson's disease (PD) and Huntington's disease (HD), timing dysfunction is present and contributes to the ability to control everyday movements. In some cases, timing deficits may be associated with very debilitating movement impairments such as speech festination, balance control (falling) and freezing of gait.

One interesting example is how the 'shuffling gait' that is typical of PD can be improved with visual step cues spaced appropriately apart, even when dopaminergic medications are withdrawn. While this is a well known fact, it is important to consider whether the observed improvements in stride length may be the result of a spatiotemporal trade-off (Morris et al., 2001; 1994b). That is, while a larger stride length can be achieved with the use of visual step cues, a subsequent timing deficit (i.e. gait rhythmicity becoming even slower) may also result. However, unlike spatial parameters of movement like step length, timing dysfunction is resistant to the typical dopaminergic treatments used in Parkinson's disease (Blin et al., 1991). Thus, research has argued that spatiotemporal trade-off may be the result of a shift of focus to specific spatial components of movement (Georgiou et al., 1993; Zijlstra et al., 1998), while temporal control is simultaneously sacrificed. Alternatively, the inability to modulate timing during movement may be part of an underlying deficit in the ability to process interoceptive sources of feedback that guide the control of movement. If this were the case, then internal timing would be an important direction for therapeutic interventions which might have the potential to improve motor symptoms in PD.

Within this chapter we will examine timing deficits in upper limb repetitive and coordinated movements and also timing during gait in PD. Further, to evaluate how attention and processing of sensory feedback may contribute to timing control, we will take a close look at new methodologies to investigate timing control during gait in Parkinson's disease. Specifically we will evaluate the ability of individuals with PD (while "On" and "Off" their dopaminergic medication) to modulate spatial and temporal components of gait in self-paced, and temporally-cued conditions using an auditory stimulus, and further to determine whether this modulation is dependent on the dopaminergic system. The concept of evaluating timing error will also be introduced as a potential way to better understand the motor symptoms of PD. The results of these studies will be discussed with respect to how the timing deficits might be an important underlying factor that contributes to the typical motor symptoms seen in Parkinson's disease.

2. Timing during upper limb movements

Control of upper limb movements is essential for many activities of daily living, and represents an area of concern for individuals with Parkinson's disease (PD). Many of the well known motor symptoms including tremor, rigidity and bradykinesia have an associated timing control deficit that has the potential to influence the execution of upper limb movements. For example, the dysfunctional motor output that leads to co-contraction of agonist and antagonistic muscles and hence the symptom of rigidity, has the potential to influence any sort of rhythmic movement behaviour that requires timing. Functionally, timing deficits could be reflected in upper limb tasks like typing or handwriting, where it has been commonly reported that 'hastening' (i.e. increased temporal frequency of tapping) is necessary to synchronize rhythmic hand movements requiring a frequency greater than 2Hz with tremor frequency of the hands (Freund, 1989).

It is also notable that many of the standard upper limb clinical tests, rate slowness as the low end of the severity spectrum while greater timing variability (in finger tapping, opening and closing hands, and wrist pronation-supination) represents an increased severity of motor symptoms. In these sorts of tests, the more the timing variability, the greater the severity of motor symptoms is rated.

As early as 1954, Schwab, Chafetz and Walker demonstrated that individuals with PD lacked the ability to maintain two concurrent voluntary motor activities. These observations were made during a rhythmic ergogram-squeezing task with one hand while connecting points on a triangle with the other. Results of this study indicated that the PD participants could do each task very well in isolation, but were unable to maintain both tasks at the same time. They concluded that individuals with PD have difficulty internally regulating continuous rhythmic movements, although the possibility that cognitive resource limitations associated with dual tasking needs to be considered. Since then, internal timing deficits have been commonly reported during upper limb movements in PD (Freeman et al., 1993; Nakamura et al., 1978; OBoyle et al., 1996; Pastor et al., 1992; Yahalom et al., 2004; Ziv et al., 1999).

2.1 Timing during upper limb tapping movements

One of the simplest movements to evaluate clinical timing deficits is tapping. Due to its continuous rhythmical nature, timing deficits would be easily identified. It also the ideal type of clinical test for identifying unilateral deficits, since slowing of tapping frequency and increased in tapping variability are easy to recognize. O'Boyle *et al.* (1996) examined self-paced finger tapping in PD and found that relative to control participants, patients were unable to maintain their own self-selected frequency. Although, PD is typically associated with bradykinesia, they demonstrated that PD participants tapped faster during the self-paced tapping task when compared to healthy control participants. Additionally, they demonstrated that PD had a higher timing variability during the tapping task, which is interesting in itself, since self-paced timing might be considered the optimal state for the motor system to internally generate movement. Similarly, Pastor *et al.* (1992) examined rhythmic flexion-extension movements of the wrist and identified less accurate timing during movements at 2 and 2.5 Hz (but not slower required frequencies) in PD relative to healthy control participants.

In addition, they demonstrated that individuals who had moderate or severe PD were less accurate at all frequencies. The authors suggested that deficits were related to impairment in an internal timekeeper, and it could be argued that progressive neurodegeneration continues to further degrade timing control. This has been supported by other rhythmic unimanual tapping research in PD (Nakamura et al., 1978; Ziv et al., 1999).

Perhaps one of the most thorough evaluations of internal versus external timing control during upper limb tapping was published by Yahalom *et al.* (2004). Their group investigated a number of controlled frequencies that were both internally and externally generated. In this set of studies, self-paced tapping would have been considered as a baseline, and internally-generated tapping would have been considered the 'as fast as possible' frequency of tapping. External timing would have been evaluated by modifying the frequency required by an external auditory metronome. Results revealed that PD had difficulty with internally generated fast rhythmical movements (i.e. slowed tapping) but externally or self-paced tapping was preserved. In contrast to other studies, these findings might be difficult to interpret since self-paced movements might also be argued to be internally driven movements, whereas the deficits identified during fast rhythmical tapping movements might simply be the influence of the cardinal symptom of bradykinesia. One potentially interesting method of evaluating these sorts of deficits further, would be to externally pace movement at a pace that is faster than the internally-generated fast pace. If participants are still unable to match the fast required frequencies, it might be concluded that attempting to distinguish between externally and internally driven movements would be pointless. The other potential method to evaluate timing control would be to evaluate timing error (or timing accuracy) during the tapping, relative to the timing of the metronome. This alternative might be argued to be a better indicator of control, and will be discussed in the upcoming section on timing control during gait.

The other benefit of evaluating timing control in a motor skill as simplistic as tapping, is that unimanual tapping can easily be combined with other tasks. For example, unimanual tapping can easily be combined with the contralateral limb to evaluate bimanual finger tapping, or in some cases, lip tapping in internally and externally-paced situations in PD (Konczak et al., 1997a). In these experiments, results indicated that PD performed all tasks with reduced tapping amplitude and an increased variability. And that this performance was largely influenced by hastening. Their overall conclusion was essentially a replication other researchers who argue that deficits in PD are associated with an internal cueing deficit. Oddly, since external cueing did not improve these impairments, the authors concluded that external cueing may have further negative effects of repetitive movements (Konczak et al., 1997a), although it might be important to evaluate how dopaminergic treatment response influences timing control during both internally and externally driven rhythmic movements, in order to make stronger conclusions on whether or not the basal ganglia are associated with internal versus external timing.

2.2 Timing during sequential upper limb movements

Generally research suggests that movement execution deficits observed with PD become even more pronounced when they involve coordination of multiple sequences of limb actions (Benecke et al, 1987). In a study involving a two-segmented movement, while individuals with PD displayed a marked delay between movement segments, the movement kinematics were similar to those of healthy control participants (Weiss et al.,

1997). One interpretation of these results is that individuals with PD have difficulty timing a switch between the sequential steps of a motor program, while others might argue that online integration of upcoming movement might represent a deficit in the ability to utilize sensory information in a closed-loop fashion to control movement. In a similar study Roy et al., (1993), observed a marked deficit during movement when participants with PD were required to produce different sequences of movements, as opposed to repeating the same sequence of movement repetitively. This finding would suggest that the difficulty making transitions between motor steps are accentuated in situations where different actions must be planned to complete the movement sequence (Brown & Almeida, 2011).

In contrast, Curra et al.,(1997) argue that individuals with PD may encounter a delay in the timing of movement execution when required to process a greater quantity of information per unit of time. In their sequential line drawing task, Parkinson's patients encountered more difficulty than healthy control participants in completing a full drawing sequence. However, when it was required to produce each segment with a step-wise cueing of the drawing sequence, PD patients were able to improve their performance. The results of these studies support the notion that individuals with PD may suffer from an attentional overload when selecting and preparing appropriate motor steps required for executing a movement sequence (Brown et al., 1993; Jones et al., 1994; Robertson & Flowers, 1990), while timing control itself is not impaired.

Sequencing difficulties of individuals with PD have also been documented in bimanual situations. Horstink (1990) noted that individuals with PD were unable to coordinate two separate plans of action for the upper limbs. While this perspective supports the idea of attentional overload, it may be of further interest since other studies of interlimb coordination have demonstrated that coordination deficits are not apparent when the movement tasks for each upper limb are related to a common goal. For example, Stelmach used a discrete bimanual targeting task in in-phase and anti-phase conditions of varying distances (Stelmach & Worringham, 1988). Unlike the findings of studies with different motor tasks for each limb, their results indicated that individuals with PD were able to coordinate movements as a single unit, and that deficits beyond typical bradykinesia were only present for asymmetrical movements. A detailed review of timing deficits that have been identified during bimanually coordinated movements is discussed further in the next section.

A number of studies have since confirmed that interlimb coordinated movements that involve a common goal between the limbs are less impaired in PD. This would suggest that strategies that help create a single movement goal for coordinated actions between two limbs may have important benefits in working toward improved coordination of timing between limbs. This may have even more important implications for basal ganglia disorders that are primarily or initially unilateral in nature, such as hemi-Parkinsonism, hemiballismus and even unilateral stroke of the basal ganglia. In therapeutic settings, important benefits might be achieved if interventions take into consideration coordinated movements that require both limbs to work together toward a common goal.

2.3 Timing during coordinated upper limb movements

A wide variety of deficits have been found in individuals with PD during bimanual coordination. The most common measures used to describe coordination impairment are the accuracy and variability of the relative phase relationship between the upper limbs. Coordination accuracy and variability were found to be worse in PD during both symmetrically performed (in-phase) movements while greater impairments were identified during non-symmetrical, unidirectional (anti-phase) movements (Serrien et al., 2000). PD were also found to have poorer coordination accuracy and greater variability during anti-phase (but not in-phase) during a medial-lateral sliding task (see Figure 1) and a pronation-supination task of the forearms (Almeida et al., 2002; Byblow et al., 2000).

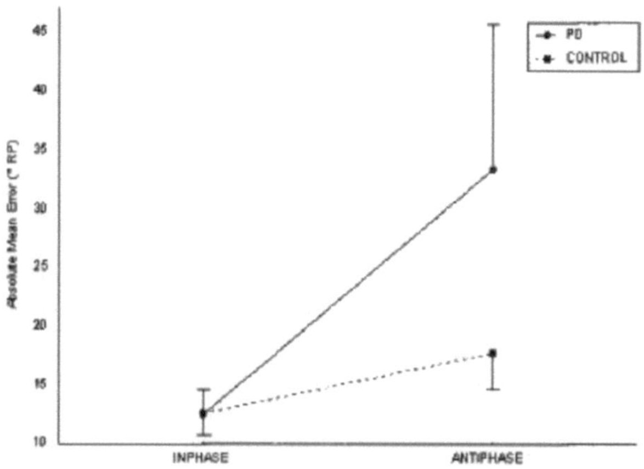

Fig. 1. Coordination accuracy as represented by absolute mean error in PD and healthy age-matched control participants *(Almeida et al., Movement Disorders, 2002)*

It is interesting to note however, that these results may be dependent on temporal parameters and requirements of the task. Some researchers would argue that timing demands might impose movement coordination to be dynamically self-organized. For example, Byblow and colleagues failed to identify coordination deficits in PD (Byblow et al., 2002), but it was proposed that this was a result of individuals with PD selecting a preferred frequencies of 1.02 Hz compared to a self-selected1.56 Hz in healthy controls during a pronation-supination task. Similarly, no differences in relative phase were seen using a frequency of 0.6 Hz with wrist flexion-extension movements (Byblow et al., 2003). Together these experiments suggest that an externally-driven demand imposed by a fast paced metronome is critical to establish coordination deficits. Coordination performance has also been investigated using the number of successful trials. Individuals with PD were shown to have more unsuccessful trials during in-phase at high frequencies and anti-phase at low frequencies than healthy age-matched controls during bimanual circular drawing (Ponsen et al., 2006).

Coordination (i.e. accuracy and stability) involves the temporal and spatial coupling of the limbs (Swinnen, 2002). However (as previously mentioned), the individual assessment of amplitude and frequency are important to consider in bimanual coordination in PD due to the possible contributions of motor symptoms including bradykinesia (slowness of movement) and hypometria (reduced size of movement) (see section 2) to voluntary movement. In addition to coordination deficits, impairments in amplitude and frequency have been documented in individuals with PD while performing bimanual tasks. Smaller amplitudes were seen during both in-phase and anti-phase at a frequency of 1 Hz (Swinnen et al., 1997). During symmetrical (in-phase) triangle drawing, smaller amplitudes were seen but only symmetrical patterns were used (Swinnen et al., 2000). Smaller amplitudes of movements were found predominantly with increasing the frequency from below to above the spontaneous transition frequency (Byblow et al., 2002). More variable amplitude was seen across all conditions for individuals with PD (Serrien et al., 2000). Amplitudes were found to be more variable in symmetrical triangle drawing (Swinnen et al., 2000). However, conflicting evidence has also found that amplitudes were not more variable during a cyclical flexion-extension task (Swinnen et al., 1997). The reason for this finding is unclear but it was suggested that the novel task used in this experiment could have resulted in variability of amplitude to be high across all participants.

Timing deficits as represented by a failure to follow a required frequency of movement has been even more commonly found in individuals with PD during bimanual coordination tasks. The frequency of movements in PD participants was found to be slower than healthy controls (see Fig. 2) only at a frequency of 1.75 Hz but not at 0.75 or 1.25 Hz (Almeida et al., 2002). Longer cycle durations were found in PD participants either when both arms moved 80 degrees or when one moved 80 while the other moved 40 degrees but not during movements of 40 degrees (Serrien et al., 2000). Longer cycle durations were also seen during both in-phase and anti-phase at 1 Hz (Swinnen et al., 1997). During symmetrical triangle drawing, longer cycle durations were seen with a goal of 1.5 seconds per cycle (Swinnen et al., 2000). As such, there may be value to evaluating error in ability to follow a required frequency. This notion will be considered during gait in more detail below.

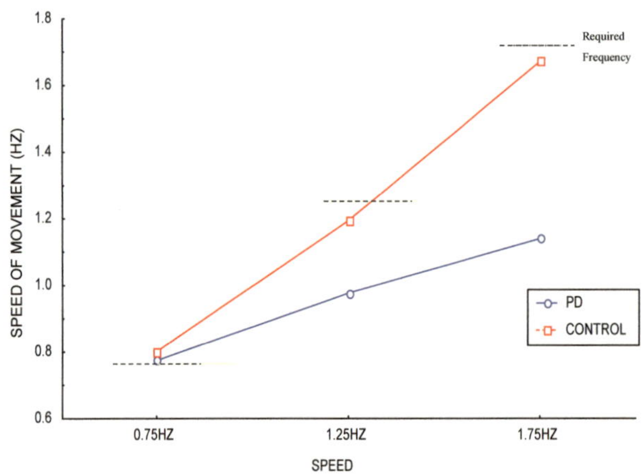

Fig. 2. Timing relative to required frequency during upper limb coordinated movements *(adapted from Almeida et al., Movement Disorders, 2002)*

In order to better appreciate timing deficits during coordinated limb actions, it may be valuable to consider what temporal demands might produce greater variability. For example, coordinated movements were found to be more variable at 1.0 Hz regardless of the complexity of required movement phase (Johnson et al., 1998). A slower and longer time to reach peak velocity as well as a longer time to reach peak negative and positive acceleration was seen in PD (Lazarus & Stelmach, 1992). A more variable frequency was seen at higher speeds and to a greater extent during anti-phase (Ponsen et al., 2006). More variability was seen in cycle durations during a cyclical flexion-extension task (Swinnen et al., 1997) and during in-phase triangle drawing (Swinnen et al., 2000). Thus, the use of auditory feedback to augment movement timing and performance has been controversial during upper limb bimanually coordinated movements in PD. Pacing was provided from a metronome for half of the 20-second trials during an bimanual coordination task, and no difference in coordination, speed or size of movements was seen with the metronome (Almeida et al., 2002). Similarly, no effects of auditory cueing were seen on temporal, spatial, pattern switching or coordination in a bimanual coordination task (Byblow et al., 2000). Furthermore, no differences were seen in temporally regulating symmetrical bimanual triangle drawing with or without a metronome (Swinnen et al., 2000). Based on this evidence, it appears that auditory cueing does not negatively influence coordination performance in PD. However, research demonstrated that external cues from a metronome improved accuracy and stability of bimanual coordination during in-phase coordination but caused individuals with PD to switch from anti-phase to in-phase during anti-phase trials (Johnson et al., 1998). They suggested that this may have increased the complexity of the task. However, this may also have been the contribution of increased attentional demand as proposed by Almeida *et al.* (2003). Thus, it remains unclear whether timing devices such as an external auditory metronome might negatively affect coordination performance in PD. It is suggested that externally pacing devices may increase attentional demands or affect coordination through sensorimotor integration deficits.

3. Gait and timing control in Parkinson's

In comparison to upper limb pointing movements where eye-hand coordination is critical to our normal experience of executing a goal-directed movement, gait may be of particular interest when considering movement deficits because the lower limbs likely require greater integration of a variety of sensory inputs that are not as visually-based. To be explicit, while vision may be important in identifying the goal of a locomotor task or to evaluate how locomotion through the environment progresses, each lower limb can be efficiently controlled by spinal circuitry without a specific dependence on the visual system to monitor the trajectory and progression of each individual step throughout gait. In fact, while the upper limb motor system develops from childhood with a heavy dependence on visual guidance for reaching, pointing and grasping movements, would revert back to a greater dependence on vision in any neurologically-impaired state. Thus, it is important to consider how timing control might be differentially influenced in lower limb (in contrast to upper limb) systems.

3.1 Typical gait deficits associated with Parkinson's

Although the control of gait may be one of the motor system's most useful and versatile capabilities, the contribution of the different sensory systems in a purposeful gait task is not often considered in PD or other basal ganglia disorders. That is, while upper limb pointing studies have been used to evaluate sensory guidance of goal-directed movement (as described above), investigations of gait in PD have spent more time attempting to quantify the unusual characteristics of PD gait rather than examining similar issues during goal-directed locomotion.

Traditionally, research into the gait deficits of PD has focused on differences between PD patients "On" and "Off" their dopaminergic medications, in self-paced walking tasks. Research has well documented the responsiveness of certain gait parameters to dopaminergic therapy in PD. The most typical finding is that both velocity and step length improve with dopaminergic treatment during conditions of self-paced locomotion in PD (O'Sullivan et al., 1998). As such, these studies have been interpreted as evidence that only spatial impairments (e.g. decreased stride length) improve with dopaminergic treatment while temporal characteristics remain unchanged (Blin et al., 1991; Morris et al., 2001), thus concluding that the basal ganglia are involved in scaling movement amplitude (Morris, et al., 1998). The assumption would be that scaling of movement amplitude may be processed through the basal ganglia/supplementary motor-premotor cortex loop, while movement rhythmicity must be controlled by other neural structures such as the brainstem, spinal cord and cerebellum. This conclusion however may be premature, since these types of experiments do not specifically evaluate how individuals with PD are able to incorporate timing cues into an on-going locomotor behaviour.

In contrast, temporal characteristics such as cadence have been demonstrated to show no specific response to medications during self-paced locomotion (Blin et al., 1991; Morris et al., 1994a; O'Sullivan et al., 1998). Since step length and gait velocity both increase in response to drug therapy, while timing (which according to physics, is the only other factor that can contribute to gait slowness) is thought to remain constant, it is not surprising that researchers have been quick to assert that the underlying mechanism responsible for gait disturbance in PD involves the scaling and regulation of stride length.

Interestingly, many of the latest studies examining individuals with PD have determined that stride length regulation may not be the only contributing factor to gait disturbance. Hausdorff and colleagues have proposed that temporal measures, and specifically their stride-to-stride variability may be critical to evaluate since they have been demonstrated to be significantly associated with an increased fate of falling in PD (Hausdorff et al., 1998; Schaafsma et al., 2003). In both of these studies, stride-to-stride variability was investigated during self-paced gait over a large sampling period (80m). Although this variability was responsive to dopaminergic medication, individuals with PD in the "On" state were still considerably more variable than healthy control participants. Increased step-to-step timing variability has also been identified more frequently in those patients who experience episodes of freezing during gait (Hausdorff et al., 2003). This may have important implications for understanding the role of the basal ganglia in the control of timing, in light of recent research that has demonstrated dysfunctional cadence in the three steps proceeding an episode of freezing (Nieuwboer et al., 2001). As suggested by Morris and colleagues, hypokinesia and freezing are aggravated by a number of different ambulatory tasks (Morris et al., 2001) and so it is important to examine other gait tasks that involve a variety of goals rather than step length modulation, in response to visual cues.

However, there are a number of research groups that have argued that gait in PD can be improved through the use of timing cues (Earhart, 2009). Thaut and colleagues (Thaut et al., 1999) have acknowledged that important differences between timing associated-rhythm and auditory stimulation through music exist, but the argument that music might lead to auditory priming of timing control is an interesting one. Researchers have pointed about the suggested benefits of dance therapies such as tango (Hackney et al., 2007) and non-partnered dance (Hackney & Earhart) in PD. Thus, the potential for timing therapy to improve motor control in PD requires further consideration.

3.2 Freezing of gait and timing mechanisms in Parkinson's

Interestingly, severe gait impairments during the on-going execution of movement may also be clinically evident as freezing and are most commonly identified in the gait of individuals with PD. Clinical evaluations have revealed that 14% of impairments associated with freezing phenomena occur during movement execution rather than more common initiation problems (Giladi et al., 1992). Each example described in the study involves a shift in the sensory feedback experience, which may have resulted in an interruption in the on-going movement pattern. Examples include difficulty changing between a climbing and normal gait when reaching the last step of a staircase; continuing gait into an elevator before the door suddenly closes; maintenance of a consistent gait pattern over a change in floor texture and, difficulty switching between forward and side-ways step patterns. Common to these cases of severe movement impairment is the requirement for coordination between the lower limbs with feedback from the visual and proprioceptive senses, which provides a rationale for an examination into gait control in individuals with PD, and it may be important to consider how timing demands might contribute to these sorts of severe gait deficits.

Recent research has identified increases in timing variability as a marker that occurs prior to a freezing of gait episode (Hausdorff et al., 2003), and this has been used to predictably identify situations in which freezing of gait might most commonly occur. For example, our own research has identified an increase in timing variability prior to an unusually narrow doorway (Almeida & Lebold, 2010), and this can be identified in only those patients with PD who experience freezing of gait. Although more research is needed on this topic, anecdotal reports from patients who experience freezing of gait, suggest that if they focus on a single goal (such as timing there steps to dance through a doorway), that freezing episodes can be overcome. And so, in order to fully appreciate the potential underlying mechanisms for gait disturbance, it is important to decipher how gait parameters are modified while attempting to achieve a locomotor goal. As we will discuss later, modulating timing relative to an external rhythm might be such a locomotor goal.

3.3 External cueing and gait in Parkinson's

The most common goal-oriented locomotor task employed to evaluate gait characteristics is the ability to follow or match gait characteristics to an external stimulus. Borrowed from the practice of physical therapy, external cueing has been argued to be a useful tool to bypass deficits associated with basal ganglia dysfunction (Rubinstein et al., 2002). The most universally known example is the improvement in step length that can be seen when visuospatial cues are provided in the form of parallel line in the path of a walk (Azulay et al., 1999; Azulay et al., 1996), compared to the typical shuffling and short-stepped gait of PD. Other sensory cues have also been studied and demonstrate improvements to the cadence (rate of stepping) and overall gait velocity, as a result of auditory cueing (Howe et al., 2003; McIntosh et al., 1997; Thaut et al., 2001), in spite of the fact that cadence control has been suggested to be intact in PD (Iansek & Morris, 1997; Morris et al., 1994b). Large clinical trials are now underway that are more thoroughly investigating the use of auditory cues as a therapeutic intervention for PD (Rochester et al., 2009). In many cases, when the instructions are specific to focusing on the timing of the task, PD performance can be improved with auditory cueing (Ringenbach et al., 2009).

4. Neural correlates of timing control in Parkinson's

Imaging research has implicated the basal ganglia, and specifically the putamen in the neural network involved in timing control during movement (Harrington, Haaland, & Knight, 1998; Rao et al., 1997). Interestingly, the nigrostriatal projections to the putamen are believed to be involved in the loop producing motor dysfunction in PD. These projections are part of a feedback loop between motor cortex, striatum, pallidum, thalamus and supplementary motor cortex (SMA) (Alexander et al.,1986), and are likely involved in the internal regulation of well-practiced, repetitive movements (Almeida et al., 2003). This parallel circuit may play a vital role in the sensorimotor integration of proprioceptive feedback from the limbs with other external stimuli. Integration of proprioceptive feedback and other sensory cues may be a critical aspect of internal guidance of movement that is rarely considered. Bearing this perspective in mind, a sample PD population with a dysfunctional timing neural network might be expected to demonstrate measurable deficits in temporal variability of gait such as cadence, step time and support time when integrating an auditory timing metronome, but not in tasks involving a self-selection of pace.

4.1 An integrated approach toward understanding timing control in gait

As previously mentioned, one of the most important ways to decipher the contribution of the basal ganglia system to movement control is to evaluate motor performance in a neurodegenerative population such as PD, when the patients are in the On and Off medication states. This allows us to make inferences about how movement control changes when the dopaminergic system has an opportunity to contribute to performance. And so, while we know that spatial parameters such as movement amplitude are strongly influenced by dopaminergic status, there would be a reasonably strong rationale to evaluate how timing control might also be influenced by dopamine. Thus, some of our own research has been focused on utilizing tasks that focus on the locomotor goal of modulating or maintaining timing in a movement task.

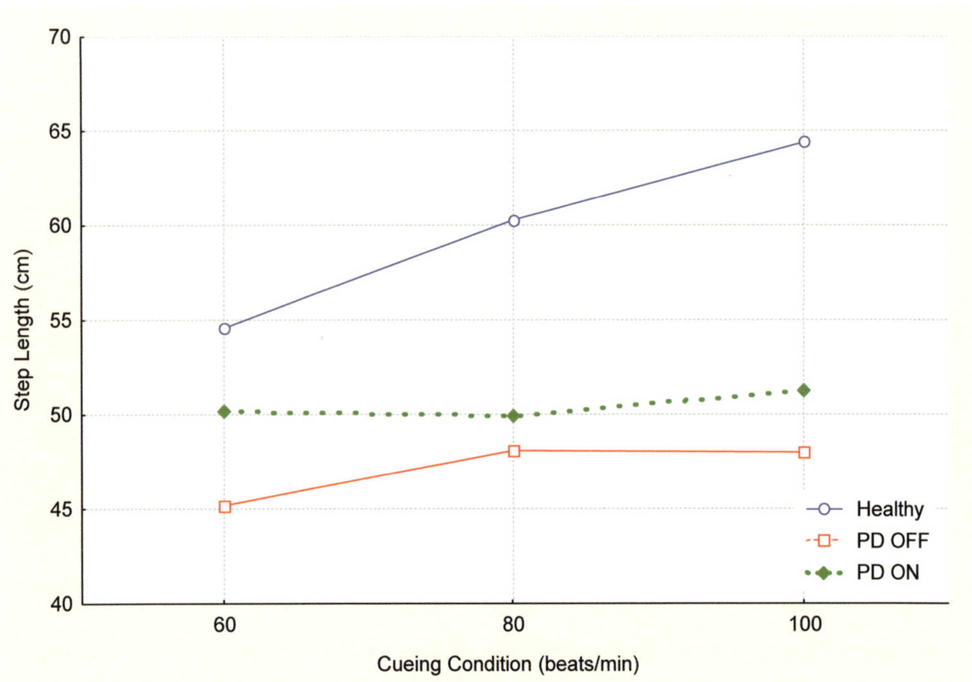

Fig. 3. Externally-paced step length for healthy participants, PD "Off " and "On".
(adapted from Almeida et al., Movement Disorders, 2007)

Since some of our previous research has suggested that auditory timing cues may not be beneficial to upper limb repetitive and coordinated movements in PD (Almeida et al., 2002), we have been attempting to specifically evaluate the ability of individuals with PD (while "On" and "Off" their dopaminergic medication) to integrate an auditory timing cue to modulate the rhythmicity of gait. By manipulating dopaminergic status, we were able to acquire an important glimpse into whether this modulation might be dependent on dopaminergic system involvement (Almeida et al., 2007). As can be seen in Figure 3, only healthy control participants have a resulting increase in step length, when an increase in stepping frequency is prompted by an external timing device. In contrast, while PD participants show the expected step length increase (in response to dopaminergic medication), the same modulation of step length that occurs in healthy participants (when required to increase stepping frequency) does not occur.

This was the first study to demonstrate that while temporal characteristics were unaffected in the self-paced gait of PD patients (regardless of dopaminergic status and in comparison to healthy), PD patients "On" their regular dopaminergic therapy were more variable than both PD "Off" medication and healthy participants when required to integrate an external cue into the regular gait cycle. In fact, none of the timing measures (cadence, step time, double support time) yielded significant between-group differences during self-paced gait, although significant differences were apparent with the provision of external cue.

One of the most intriguing findings of this study (see figure 4a,b) was that temporal measures such as cadence, step time, and double support time identified that only the PD "Off" group now behaved similar to healthy participants, while PD "On" had greater difficulty maintaining appropriate timing in the two slowest cueing conditions (i.e. the PD "On" group performed least like the healthy age-matched participants). At 100 steps per minute, one might have expected that the behavioral response might become more automatically driven, implying less opportunity for supraspinal control. Thus, it might be expected that temporal differences between groups would be minimized. For example researchers have shown that galvanic vestibular stimulation has less of an effect at faster speeds of locomotion than during slower speeds (Jahn et al., 2000) arguing that the gain of this sensory regulation is down regulated at the higher speeds.

4.2 A novel proposal for evaluating timing control in gait

Given that timing modulation differences can be identified between the PD "On" and "Off" states, it seems important to determine whether these dopa-responsive changes are a specific issue of voluntary *control* over timing. One very common method identified for evaluating control and performance during upper limb tasks (described above) is to evaluate accuracy or error of performance. However, there have been very few applications to timing control during gait.

Thus, in order to apply measures of error to timing control during, the goal of our most recent research has been aimed at evaluating the influence of dopaminergic status on timing error (Almeida & Lebold, 2010). This can be achieved by comparing the specific goal of timing a heel strike on the ground relative to the auditory-paced signal from an external auditory metronome. Hence, a timing error could be calculated, with the prediction that if the basal ganglia truly contribute to temporal control, there should be identifiable differences in timing error that are specifically dependent on dopaminergic status.

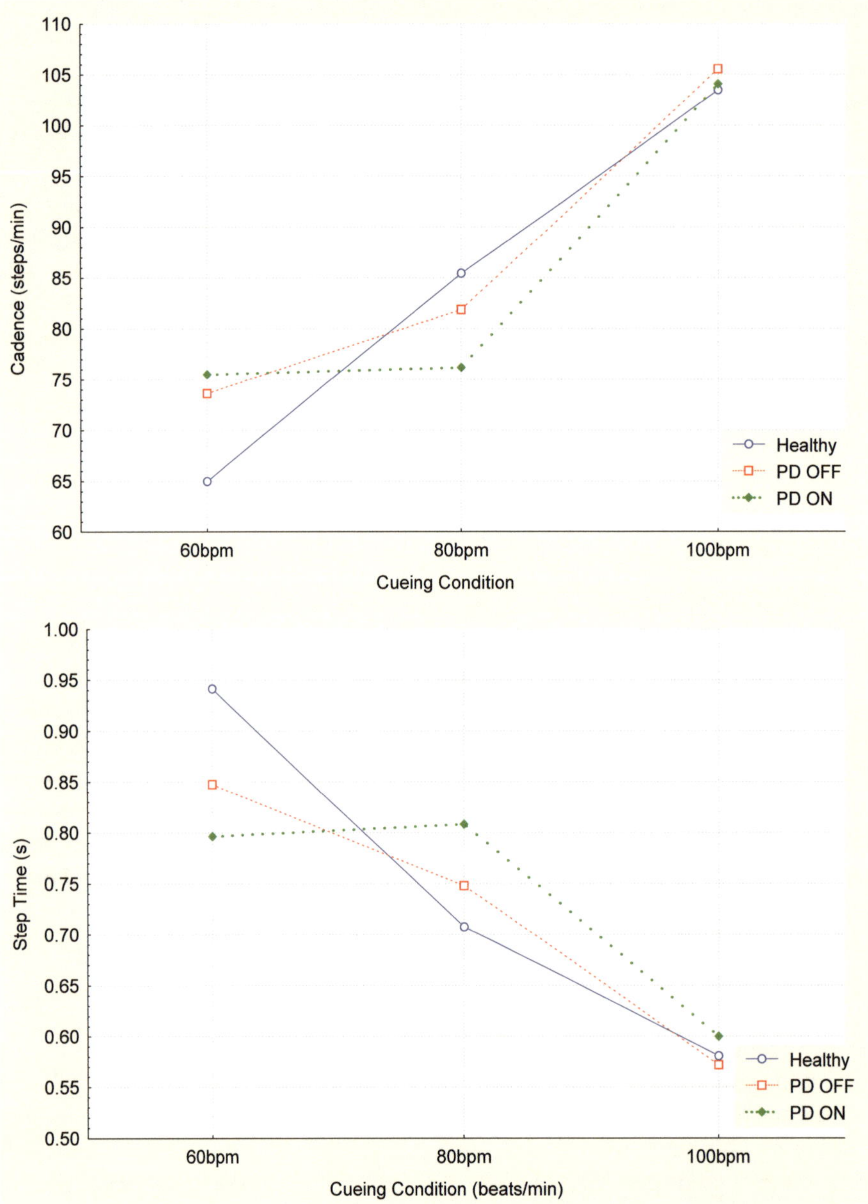

Fig. 4. a) Cadence of gait for the healthy participants, PD "Off " and "On" in the externally-cued conditions, b) Step time for the healthy participants, PD "Off " and "On" in the externally-cued conditions. *(adapted from Almeida et al., Movement Disorders, 2007)*

To test this hypothesis, eighteen PD participants were tested "On" and "Off" dopaminergic medication (consistent with our previous protocols), as well as a group of ten healthy, age-matched control participants. We required all participants to walk in 4 conditions paced by an auditory metronome (5 blocked trials per condition) over a computerized data-collecting and pressure-sensitive carpet (GAITRite®, CIR Systems, Inc., Clifton, New Jersey).

Conditions included self-paced Gait (SP), 30% slower than self-paced gait (-30% SP), 10% slower than self-paced gait (-10% SP) and 10% faster than self-paced gait (+10% SP), and timing error was calculated by comparing the onset of heel strike to the onset of the auditory cue, and averaged over the course of the trial. The error calculating software was created by CIR Systems, Inc., in collaboration with the researchers with the potential aim of creating a new clinical measure to evaluate neurological populations.

Perhaps more interestingly, the primary outcome measure, timing error identified a significant interaction ($F(4,56)=4.87$; $p<.0019$) between medication state and trial. Post hoc analysis revealed that while healthy control participants had a consistently lower timing error than PD, PD "Off" dopaminergic medication were initially less errorful (and behaved more like healthy control participants than PD "On"), but that with practice PD "On" gradually improved timing error while PD "Off" did not (Figure 6).

In addition, PD "Off" were identified to walk with overall greater step-to-step timing variability than PD "On". This difference in variability was specifically identified in the slowest paced condition. Together, the overall interpretation of these findings is that timing variability (which has been linked to falls) and timing error measures reveal an interaction with medication state, suggesting that the basal ganglia may play a role in incorporating sensory timing cues into online control of gait in individuals with PD. Evaluating timing error may be in an important clinical indicator of motor control in PD and other neurological populations.

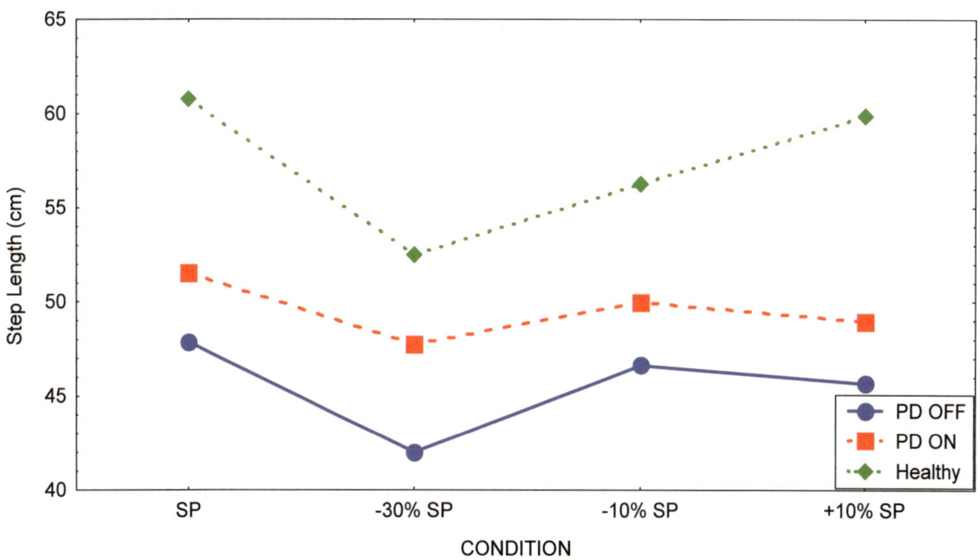

Fig. 5. Regardless of dopaminergic status, PD do not scale step length to the same extent as healthy control participants.

5. Conclusion

Deficits in timing control are evident in both unimanual and bimanual movements, across both the upper and lower limbs. Several methods of identifying timing deficits have been identified, with the important of error and variability being highlighted as important factors that reflect motor control deficits in PD. Although it is clear that amplitude is influenced by basal ganglia dysfunction, it is important to consider how timing may be sacrificed in tasks where amplitude cues are the focus of the task. Similarly, the results of our own research suggest that amplitude (and specifically step length control) appears to be sacrificed when attention must be focused on the goal of modulating timing relative to an external auditory cue. Thus, consideration of sensory-related timing issues in PD may be an important approach in exercise rehabilitation interventions for PD and other basal ganglia-disordered populations.

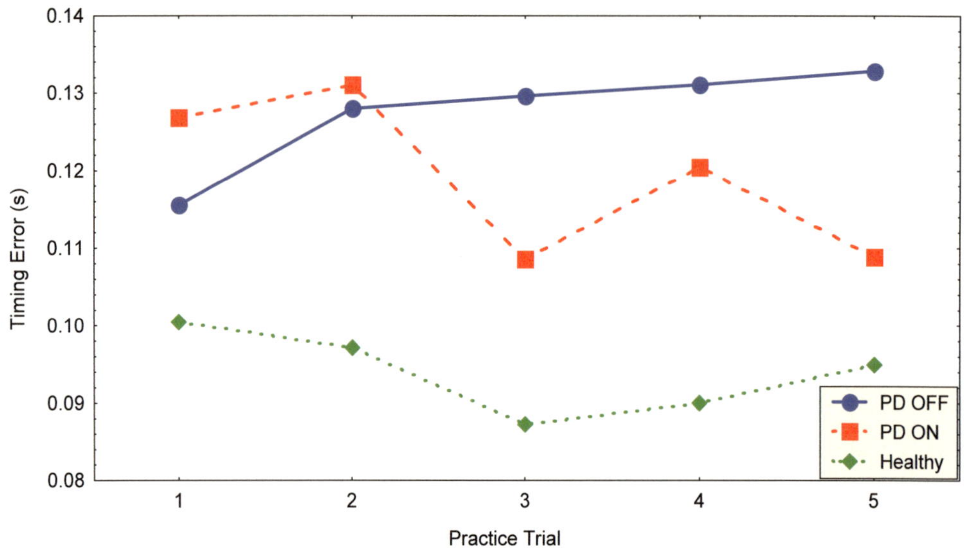

Fig. 6. A significant interaction between medication and trial revealed that with experience utilizing the metronome patients in the OFF state significantly increase their timing error, whereas PD ON improve timing error with practice.

The findings of our own studies on temporal characteristics of gait are consistent with the view that the basal ganglia may be involved in the neural network for precise modulation of timing of repetitive movement relative to external stimuli (Harrington et al., 1998; Rao et al., 1997) and are suggestive of an underlying mechanism for basal ganglia involvement in sensorimotor processing during movement.

In PD, where projections to specific basal ganglia nuclei (such as the putamen) that are implicated in the neural timing system are known to be affected, studies of repetitive finger tapping and lip movements have quantified a basic timing deficit (Freeman et al., 1993; Harrington et al., 1998; Konczak et al., 1997b; O'Boyle et al., 1996). Yet, external cues are heralded to be a potential method of overcoming basal ganglia-related movement impairments (Rubinstein et al., 2002) and a means of enhancing motor performance (Howe et al., 2003; McIntosh et al., 1997; Thaut et al., 2001). As seen in our studies, although provision of external auditory cues may improve certain characteristics of hypokinetic gait such as velocity and cadence, it may also contribute to greater step-to-step variability in PD which can lead to increased risk of falls, lack of stability and may lead to further impairments such as freezing of gait (Hausdorff et al., 1998; Hausdorff et al., 2003).

It is this within-trial variability that may provide insight into the sensorimotor mechanism underlying timing deficits in PD. Perhaps most interesting is the finding that group differences in variability (related to external cueing) are observable in measures of step time and double support time. This may be critically important to consider, in light of recent research that has identified the relationship between step time variability and falls (Schaafsma et al., 2003) and freezing (Hausdorff et al., 2003) in PD. Double support time has been considered an important indicator of abnormal balance control in healthy, older adults and those with cerebellar dysfunction, as well as those with basal ganglia disease (Hausdorff et al., 1998). Increased double support time in medicated PD patients, in light of increased temporal variability may be representative of additional proprioceptive sampling that is required to verify that external cues are being used appropriately. Bearing in mind that the greatest increase in timing variability can be identified in PD "On", this may reflect an increased dependency on proprioceptive feedback for sensorimotor integration with the external stimuli in order to improve timing, with a faulty yet functioning basal ganglia providing input into the neural network for timing. It may be that the basal ganglia are specifically involved in interpreting and integrating proprioception during repetitive and automated movements such as gait. Therefore in timing modulation tasks, where the importance of proprioceptive integration is critical, differences between participants "On" and "Off" their dopaminergic medications can be identified.

Further in support of our view, it should be pointed out that all three groups experienced the most variability in timing at the slowest cueing condition, when there is the greatest opportunity to sample and integrate proprioceptive information with the auditory cues while maintaining balance. In the PD "Off" medication group, performance across temporal measures may approach that of healthy individuals because the basal ganglia loop is not centrally involved when medications are withdrawn. Under these circumstances, a mode of control similar to that for visual cues may be employed.

Finally, timing error was introduced as a novel and potentially interesting method of identifying timing control deficits. Although future research is necessary, evaluating timing error may be an important clinical indicator of disruptions to normal timing control in PD and other neurological disorders.

6. Acknowledgment

Some of this research has been supported by the research grants from the Natural Science and Engineering Research Council of Canada, the Parkinson's Society of Canada, and the Canadian Foundation for Innovation. The author would also like to acknowledge the support of Sun Life Financial to complete research at the Movement Disorders Research & Rehabilitation Centre at Wilfrid Laurier University, Canada.

7. References

Alexander, G. E., DeLong, M. R., & Strick, P. L. (1986). Parallel organization of functionally segregated circuits linking basal ganglia and cortex. *Annu Rev Neurosci, 9*, 357-381.

Almeida, Q. J., Frank, J. S., Roy, E. A., Patla, A. E., & Jog, M. S. (2007). Dopaminergic modulation of timing control and variability in the gait of Parkinson's disease. *Mov Disord, 22*(12), 1735-1742.

Almeida, Q. J., & Lebold, C. A. (2010). Freezing of gait in Parkinson's disease: a perceptual cause for a motor impairment? *J Neurol Neurosurg Psychiatry, 81*(5), 513-518.

Almeida, Q. J., Lebold, C.A. . (2010). *Basal Ganglia Contributions to Timing Control in Parkinson's: Attentional vs. Motor Mechanisms* Paper presented at the 3rd International Congress on Gait and Mental Function, Washington, United States.

Almeida, Q. J., Wishart, L. R., & Lee, T. D. (2002). Bimanual coordination deficits with Parkinson's disease: the influence of movement speed and external cueing. *Mov Disord, 17*(1), 30-37.

Almeida, Q. J., Wishart, L. R., & Lee, T. D. (2003). Disruptive influences of a cued voluntary shift on coordinated movement in Parkinson's disease. *Neuropsychologia, 41*(4), 442-452.

Azulay, J. P., Mesure, S., Amblard, B., Blin, O., Sangla, I., & Pouget, J. (1999). Visual control of locomotion in Parkinson's disease. *Brain, 122 (Pt 1)*, 111-120.

Azulay, J. P., Van Den Brand, C., Mestre, D., Blin, O., Sangla, I., Pouget, J., & Serratrice, G. (1996). [Automatic motion analysis of gait in patients with Parkinson disease: effects of levodopa and visual stimulations]. *Rev Neurol (Paris), 152*(2), 128-134.

Blin, O., Ferrandez, A. M., Pailhous, J., & Serratrice, G. (1991). Dopa-sensitive and dopa-resistant gait parameters in Parkinson's disease. *J Neurol Sci, 103*(1), 51-54.

Brown, M. J., & Almeida, Q. J. (2011). Evaluating dopaminergic system contributions to cued pattern switching during bimanual coordination. *Eur J Neurosci, 34*(4), 632-640.

Byblow, W. D., Lewis, G. N., & Stinear, J. W. (2003). Effector-specific visual information influences kinesthesis and reaction time performance in Parkinson's disease. *J Mot Behav, 35*(2), 99-107.

Byblow, W. D., Summers, J. J., Lewis, G. N., & Thomas, J. (2002). Bimanual coordination in Parkinson's disease: Deficits in movement frequency, amplitude, and pattern switching. *Movement Disorders, 17*(1), 20-29.

Byblow, W. D., Summers, J. J., & Thomas, J. (2000). Spontaneous and intentional dynamics of bimanual coordination in Parkinson's disease. *Human Movement Science, 19*(2), 223-249.

Earhart, G. M. (2009). Dance as therapy for individuals with Parkinson disease. *Eur J Phys Rehabil Med, 45*(2), 231-238.

Freeman, J. S., Cody, F. W., & Schady, W. (1993). The influence of external timing cues upon the rhythm of voluntary movements in Parkinson's disease. *J Neurol Neurosurg Psychiatry, 56*(10), 1078-1084.

Freund, H. J. (1989). Motor dysfunctions in Parkinson's disease and premotor lesions. *Eur Neurol, 29 Suppl 1*, 33-37.

Georgiou, N., Iansek, R., Bradshaw, J. L., Phillips, J. G., Mattingley, J. B., & Bradshaw, J. A. (1993). An evaluation of the role of internal cues in the pathogenesis of Parkinsonian hypokinesia. *Brain, 116*, 1175-1587.

Giladi, N., McMahon, D., Przedborski, S., Flaster, E., Guillory, S., Kostic, V., & Fahn, S. (1992). Motor blocks in Parkinson's disease. *Neurology, 42*(2), 333-339.

Hackney, M. E., & Earhart, G. M. Effects of dance on gait and balance in Parkinson's disease: a comparison of partnered and nonpartnered dance movement. *Neurorehabil Neural Repair, 24*(4), 384-392.

Hackney, M. E., Kantorovich, S., Levin, R., & Earhart, G. M. (2007). Effects of tango on functional mobility in Parkinson's disease: a preliminary study. *J Neurol Phys Ther, 31*(4), 173-179.

Harrington, D. L., Haaland, K. Y., & Hermanowicz, N. (1998). Temporal processing in the basal ganglia. *Neuropsychology, 12*(1), 3-12.

Harrington, D. L., Haaland, K. Y., & Knight, R. T. (1998). Cortical Networks Underlying Mechanisms of Time Perception. *J. Neurosci., 18*(3), 1085-1095.

Hausdorff, J. M., Cudkowicz, M. E., Firtion, R., Wei, J. Y., & Goldberger, A. L. (1998). Gait variability and basal ganglia disorders: stride-to-stride variations of gait cycle timing in Parkinson's disease and Huntington's disease. *Mov Disord, 13*(3), 428-437.

Hausdorff, J. M., Schaafsma, J. D., Balash, Y., Bartels, A. L., Gurevich, T., & Giladi, N. (2003). Impaired regulation of stride variability in Parkinson's disease subjects with freezing of gait. *Exp Brain Res, 149*(2), 187-194.

Howe, T. E., Lovgreen, B., Cody, F. W., Ashton, V. J., & Oldham, J. A. (2003). Auditory cues can modify the gait of persons with early-stage Parkinson's disease: a method for enhancing parkinsonian walking performance? *Clin Rehabil, 17*(4), 363-367.

Iansek, R. T., & Morris, M. (1997). Rehabilitation of gait in Parkinson's disease. *J Neurol Neurosurg Psychiatry, 63*(4), 556-557.

Jahn, K., Strupp, M., Schneider, E., Dieterich, M., & Brandt, T. (2000). Differential effects of vestibular stimulation on walking and running. *Neuroreport, 11*(8), 1745-1748.

Johnson, K. A., Cunnington, R., Bradshaw, J. L., Phillips, J. G., Iansek, R., & Rogers, M. A. (1998). Bimanual co-ordination in Parkinson's disease. *Brain, 121*, 743-753.

Konczak, J., Ackermann, H., Hertrich, I., Spieker, S., & Dichgans, J. (1997a). Control of repetitive lip and finger movements in Parkinson's disease: Influence of external timing signals and simultaneous execution on motor performance. *Movement Disorders, 12*(5), 665-676.

Konczak, J., Ackermann, H., Hertrich, I., Spieker, S., & Dichgans, J. (1997b). Control of repetitive lip and finger movements in Parkinson's disease: influence of external timing signals and simultaneous execution on motor performance. *Mov Disord, 12*(5), 665-676.

Lazarus, J. A. C., & Stelmach, G. E. (1992). Interlimb Coordination in Parkinsons-Disease. *Movement Disorders, 7*(2), 159-170.

McIntosh, G. C., Brown, S. H., Rice, R. R., & Thaut, M. H. (1997). Rhythmic auditory-motor facilitation of gait patterns in patients with Parkinson's disease. *J Neurol Neurosurg Psychiatry, 62*(1), 22-26.

Morris, M., Iansek, R., Matyas, T., & Summers, J. (1998). Abnormalities in the stride length-cadence relation in parkinsonian gait. *Mov Disord, 13*(1), 61-69.

Morris, M. E., Huxham, F., McGinley, J., & Iansek, R. (2001). Gait disorders and gait rehabilitation in Parkinson's disease. *Adv Neurol*, 347-361.

Morris, M. E., Iansek, R., Matyas, T. A., & Summers, J. J. (1994a). Ability to modulate walking cadence remains intact in Parkinson's disease. *J Neurol Neurosurg Psychiatry, 57*(12), 1532-1534.

Morris, M. E., Iansek, R., Matyas, T. A., & Summers, J. J. (1994b). The pathogenesis of gait hypokinesia in Parkinson's disease. *Brain, 117 (Pt 5)*, 1169-1181.

Morris, M. E., Iansek, R., Matyas, T. A., & Summers, J. J. (1996). Stride length regulation in Parkinson's disease. Normalization strategies and underlying mechanisms. *Brain, 119 (Pt 2)*, 551-568.

Nakamura, R., Nagasaki, H., & Narabayashi, H. (1978). Disturbances of Rhythm Formation in Patients with Parkinsons-Disease .1. Characteristics of Tapping Response to Periodic Signals. *Perceptual and Motor Skills, 46*(1), 63-75.

Nieuwboer, A., Dom, R., De Weerdt, W., Desloovere, K., Fieuws, S., & Broens-Kaucsik, E. (2001). Abnormalities of the spatiotemporal characteristics of gait at the onset of freezing in Parkinson's disease. *Mov Disord, 16*(6), 1066-1075.

O'Boyle, D. J., Freeman, J. S., & Cody, F. W. (1996). The accuracy and precision of timing of self-paced, repetitive movements in subjects with Parkinson's disease. *Brain, 119 (Pt 1)*, 51-70.

O'Sullivan, J. D., Said, C. M., Dillon, L. C., Hoffman, M., & Hughes, A. J. (1998). Gait analysis in patients with Parkinson's disease and motor fluctuations: influence of levodopa and comparison with other measures of motor function. *Mov Disord, 13*(6), 900-906.

OBoyle, D. J., Freeman, J. S., & Cody, F. W. J. (1996). The accuracy and precision of timing of self-paced, repetitive movements in subjects with Parkinson's disease. *Brain, 119*, 51-70.

Pastor, M. A., Jahanshahi, M., Artieda, J., & Obeso, J. A. (1992). Performance of Repetitive Wrist Movements in Parkinsons-Disease. *Brain, 115*, 875-891.

Ponsen, M. M., Daffertshofer, A., van den Heuvel, E., Wolters, E., Beek, P. J., & Berendse, H. W. (2006). Bimanual coordination dysfunction in early, untreated Parkinson's disease. *Parkinsonism Relat Disord, 12*(4), 246-252.

Rao, S. M., Harrington, D. L., Haaland, K. Y., Bobholz, J. A., Cox, R. W., & Binder, J. R. (1997). Distributed Neural Systems Underlying the Timing of Movements. *J. Neurosci., 17*(14), 5528-5535.

Ringenbach, S. D., van Gemmert, A. W., Shill, H. A., & Stelmach, G. E. Auditory instructional cues benefit unimanual and bimanual drawing in Parkinson's disease patients. *Hum Mov Sci.*

Rochester, L., Burn, D. J., Woods, G., Godwin, J., & Nieuwboer, A. (2009). Does auditory rhythmical cueing improve gait in people with Parkinson's disease and cognitive impairment? A feasibility study. *Mov Disord, 24*(6), 839-845.

Rubinstein, T. C., Giladi, N., & Hausdorff, J. M. (2002). The power of cueing to circumvent dopamine deficits: a review of physical therapy treatment of gait disturbances in Parkinson's disease. *Mov Disord, 17*(6), 1148-1160.

Schaafsma, J. D., Giladi, N., Balash, Y., Bartels, A. L., Gurevich, T., & Hausdorff, J. M. (2003). Gait dynamics in Parkinson's disease: relationship to Parkinsonian features, falls and response to levodopa. *J Neurol Sci, 212*(1-2), 47-53.

Serrien, D. J., Steyvers, M., Debaere, F., Stelmach, G. E., & Swinnen, S. P. (2000). Bimanual coordination and limb-specific parameterization in patients with Parkinson's disease. *Neuropsychologia, 38*(13), 1714-1722.

Stelmach, G. E., & Worringham, C. J. (1988). The control of bimanual aiming movements in Parkinson's disease. *J Neurol Neurosurg Psychiatry, 51*(2), 223-231.

Swinnen, S. P. (2002). Intermanual coordination: from behavioural principles to neural-network interactions. *Nat Rev Neurosci, 3*(5), 348-359.

Swinnen, S. P., Steyvers, M., Van Den Bergh, L., & Stelmach, G. E. (2000). Motor learning and Parkinson's disease: refinement of within-limb and between-limb coordination as a result of practice. *Behav Brain Res, 111*(1-2), 45-59.

Swinnen, S. P., Van Langendonk, L., Verschueren, S., Peeters, G., Dom, R., & De Weerdt, W. (1997). Interlimb coordination deficits in patients with Parkinson's disease during the production of two-joint oscillations in the sagittal plane. *Mov Disord, 12*(6), 958-968.

Thaut, M. H., Kenyon, G. P., Schauer, M. L., & McIntosh, G. C. (1999). The connection between rhythmicity and brain function. *IEEE Eng Med Biol Mag, 18*(2), 101-108.

Thaut, M. H., McIntosh, K. W., McIntosh, G. C., & Hoemberg, V. (2001). Auditory rhythmicity enhances movement and speech motor control in patients with Parkinson's disease. *Funct Neurol, 16*(2), 163-172.

Yahalom, G., Simon, E. S., Thorne, R., Peretz, C., & Giladi, N. (2004). Hand rhythmic tapping and timing in Parkinson's disease. *Parkinsonism & Related Disorders, 10*(3), 143-148.

Zijlstra, W., Rutgers, A. W., & Van Weerden, T. W. (1998). Voluntary and involuntary adaptation of gait in Parkinson's disease. *Gait Posture, 7*(1), 53-63.

Ziv, I., Avraham, M., Dabby, R., Zoldan, J., Djaldetti, R., & Melamed, E. (1999). Early-occurrence of manual motor blocks in Parkinson's disease: a quantitative assessment. *Acta Neurologica Scandinavica, 99*(2), 106-111.

3

Free Radicals, Oxidative Stress and Oxidative Damage in Parkinson's Disease

Marisa G. Repetto, Raúl O. Domínguez,
Enrique R. Marschoff and Jorge A. Serra
School of Pharmacy and Biochemistry,
University of Buenos Aires (UBA) / PRALIB – CONICET
Argentina

1. Introduction

Parkinson's disease (PD) is an adult-onset disease of unknown etiology, with a prevalence of 0.3% in the entire population, affecting more than 1% of humans over 60 years of age. Primary degeneration occurs in pigmented dopamine-containing neurons in the *pars compacta* of the *substantia nigra*, with projections to the striatum and typical motor signs that appear with a loss of 60% of the dopaminergic neurons of the brain area. While 90-95% of PD cases have no known genetic basis, approximately 5-10% arises from inherited mutations (Farooqui & Farooqui, 2011). While the actual physiopathology of PD remains uncertain, it is currently suggested that the molecular mechanism of the vulnerability of dopaminergic neurons in the *substantia nigra* involves monoamine oxidase-mediated abnormal dopamine metabolism, hydrogen peroxide generation, and abnormal mitochondrial and proteosomal dysfunctions along with microglia cell activation which may be closely associated with neurodegenerative process. The loss of dopaminergic neurons in the *substantia nigra* may be related to resting tremor, rigidity, bradykinesia, postural instability, and gait disturbance in PD patients. Also associated with PD neuropathology are disrupted iron homeostasis, intracellular deposition of proteins in Lewy bodies, and oxidative stress and neuronal damage.

PD is considered the paradigm of α-synucleinopathies within the spectrum of neurodegenerative diseases that exhibit α-synuclein in cytosolic protein aggregates (Navarro et al., 2009).

There is evidence that oxidative stress participates in the neurodegeneration (Lustig et al., 1993; Famulari et al., 1996; Repetto et al., 1999; Fiszman et al., 2003; Domínguez et al., 2008); neutrophils express a primary alteration of nitric oxide release in PD patients, where reactive oxygen species and oxidative stress parameters are more probably related to the evolution of PD (Gatto et al., 1996; Gatto et al., 1997; Repetto & Llesuy, 2004). Peripheral markers of oxidative stress in red blood cells of neurological patients could be a reflection of the brain condition and suggests that oxygen free radicals are partially responsible for the damage observed in PD living patients (Serra et al., 2001; Repetto, 2008). Other reports suggest that mitochondrial dysfunction and impairment of the respiratory complexes are associated with the neuronal loss (Boveris & Navarro, 2008). Moreover, increased mDNA deletions were recognized in nigral neurons in PD (Bender et al., 2006).

1.1 Clinical criteria diagnosis in idiopathic Parkinson's disease

The differential diagnosis of parkinsonian syndromes is considered one of the most challenging in clinical neurology. Despite published consensus operational standards for the diagnosis of idiopathic Parkinson's disease (PD) and the various parkinsonian disorders, such as secondary Parkinson's disease, progressive supranuclear palsy, multiple system atrophy and corticobasal degeneration, the clinical separation of PD requires the application of strict diagnostic criteria.

The diagnosis of the specific secondary Parkinsonism was based on the constellation of clinical features suggestive of a secondary etiology (Gibb et al., 1988; Quinn, 1989; Dalakas et al., 2000; Schrag et al., 2002), namely: Manifestations and suspected etiologies of non PD, Vascular Parkinsonism, Drug-induced Parkinsonism, Multiple System Atrophy, Lewy body dementia, Toxin exposure (carbon-monoxide poisoning), Progressive supranuclear palsy, Hemiparkinsonism - hemiatrophy, Juvenile Parkinsonism with dystonia and hemiatrophy, Walking apraxia-ataxia frontal lobe, Action or postural tremor prominent (essential tremor) and the Stiff person syndrome.

While the clinical characteristics of the Parkinson syndrome facilitate the diagnosis, which is easy in the advanced stages in the paucisymptomatic forms or at the early stages the diagnosis becomes more difficult.

In the absence of a biological marker diagnosis in life can only be performed by clinical criteria. In recent decades the criteria used were not universally recognized, and the PD could be over diagnosed. In a study carried out between 1999 and 2000 (Serra et al., 2001) patients were recruited if they had, at least, two cardinal symptoms of PD according to clinical criteria (Hughes et al., 1992) and, additionally, Hoehn and Yahr stage 1 to 3 (Hoehn & Yahr, 1967), to assess the severity at presentation and progression. Patients also required a history of positive response to levodopa therapy.

Currently, the diagnosis of PD follows the United Kingdom Brain Bank Criteria, which demands bradykinesia and one additional symptom, *i.e.*, rigidity, resting tremor or postural instability. The latter is not a useful sign for the early diagnosis of PD, because it does not appear before Hoehn and Yahr stage 3. Other symptoms of PD which precede the onset of motor disturbances are hyposmia, REM sleep behavioral disorder, constipation and depression. The clinical diagnosis of PD can be supported by levodopa or apomorphine tests. Imaging studies such as cranial CT or MRI are helpful to distinguish PD from atypical or secondary Parkinson's disease.

In the last decade the Unified Parkinson's Disease Rating Scale (UPDRS) is the most widely used clinical rating scale for PD. Authors unanimously considered the concept of a single clinical rating scale to be an important tool for clear and consistent communication among movement disorder colleagues (Fahn et al., 1987; Movement Disorder Society Task Force, 2003).

1.2 Biochemical mechanisms associated to Parkinson's disease

The degradation processes of macromolecules, such as serotonin, norepinephrine, dopamine, and other neurotransmitters of dopaminergic neurons in *substantia nigra*, catalyzed by monoamine oxidase are critically important not only for the regulation of emotional behavior, but also for other neural functions. As a consequence, the brains of PD patients are subject to high levels of oxidative stress. The dopaminergic cell loss and disease progression are accompanied by the accumulation of high iron levels, associated with aggregation of α-synuclein (especially in the mutated form found in familial Parkinson's disease). Increasing evidence indicates that multiple biochemical and cellular factors are involved in neuronal death in PD, some of them involve protein dyshomeostasis, mitochondrial impaired function and metal-induced toxicity. These processes contribute to the oxidative stress and damage and inflammatory response in brain of PD patients (Farooqui & Farooqui, 2011). The current views on PD consider that this disease is not only characterized by *substantia nigra* dysfunction but that it also involves the frontal cortex with a cognitive decline at the early stages of Parkinsonism (McNamara et al., 2007). Oxidative damage and mitochondrial dysfunction in the human frontal cortex are considered factors that lead to impaired cognition in PD patients.

1.2.1 Protein dyshomeostasis

The neuropathological hallmarks of PD include the presence of Lewy bodies mostly composed of α-synuclein, a presynaptic protein that not only plays an important role in neuropathology of PD, but is also known to bind divalent metals as iron (Fe) and copper (Cu), which accelerates the aggregation of α-synuclein to form various toxic aggregates *in vitro*. Although the normal biological function of this protein remains to be elucidated, it is clear that regulation of its expression is essential for healthy neuronal function. Even a 1.5 fold elevation in its expression is sufficient to produce Lewy body disease (Sigletton et al., 2003). Membrane-bound α-synuclein may play a role in fibril formation. Overexpression of α-synuclein impairs mitochondrial function and increases oxidative stress. This prion protein has a neuroprotective function by acting as antiapoptotic factor that inhibits the mitochondria-mediated apoptosis by preventing the formation of the permeability pore of the inner mitochondrial membrane (Opazo et al., 2003; Kozlowski et al., 2009).

These effects are associated to mitochondrial dysfunction due to decreased activity of cytochrome c oxidase and to the increased production of reactive oxygen species, which in turn triggers mitochondria-mediated apoptotic neurodegeneration (Rossi et al., 2004; Spencer et al., 2009).

1.2.2 Mitochondrial impaired function

Neurochemically, PD is characterized by mitochondrial dysfunction and brain mitochondrial oxidative damage. There are also consistent observations of the impaired functioning of mitochondrial respiratory transport chain at the site of complex I (NADH CoQ10 reductase), from PD brain, particularly in the *substantia nigra,* with consequent aggregation and accumulation of α-synuclein (Opazo et al., 2003; Friedlich et al., 2009) and in frontal cortex in PD patients (Boveris & Navarro, 2008). The inhibition of complex I observed in PD has an etiological impact. The question then arises as to the origin of the complex I-deficiency in PD. It could result from an environmental toxin or an acquired or inherited mtDNA mutation(s) (Petrozzi et al., 2007).

The molecular mechanism involved in the inactivation of complex I is likely accounted by the sum of peroxinitrite mediated reactions, reactions with free radical intermediates of the lipid peroxidation process and amine-aldehyde adduction reactions. The inhibitory effects on complex I lead synergistically to denaturation of the protein structure and to further increases of superoxide anion (O_2^-) y peroxinitrite production at the vicinity of complex I (Navarro et al., 2009; Navarro & Boveris, 2009).

Inhibition of complex I creates an environment of oxidative stress that ultimately leads to the aggregation of α-synuclein with the consequent neuronal death. Complex I dysfunction, also called "complex I syndrome" results in complex I inactivation, reduced oxygen (O_2) uptake and ATP formation, increased O_2^- formation, oxidative stress and lipid peroxidation, events that lead to neuronal depolarization and contribute to excitotoxic neuronal injury (Opazo et al., 2003; Kozlowski et al., 2009; Navarro & Boveris, 2009). Mitochondrial dysfunction in the human frontal cortex is to be considered a factor contributing to impaired cognition in PD in comparison to age-matched healthy controls. The mitochondrial impairment observed in frontal cortex in PD patients is properly described as a reduced frontal cortex respiration, with marked decrease in complex I activity, associated with oxidative damage, the latter determined by the increased content of phospholipids and protein oxidation products (Navarro et al., 2009).

Deficient complex I function would likely increase production of superoxide anion by impairing electron flow from NADH to ubiquinone, promoting oxidative stress through subsequent superoxide dismutase and Fenton chemistry. Similar deficits in respiratory transport chain complex I have also been reported in peripheral cells (myocytes and platelets).

Mitochondrial metabolic abnormalities, DNA mutations and oxidative stress contribute to ageing, the greatest risk factor for neurodegenerative diseases. Somatic mitochondrial DNA mutations have been reported in PD brain. These findings are important because the mitochondrial DNA encodes components of the respiratory transport chain complexes, and such mutations may impair efficient electron flow from NADH to molecular oxygen (Friedlich et al., 2009). Further, mitochondrial abnormalities occur early in most of the neurodegenerative disorders, and the evidence of specific interactions of disease-related proteins with mitochondria represents ultimate proof of mitochondrial involvement in neurodegeneration.

Mitochondria are targets of metal toxicity, and in many cases a close link between metal-induced oxidative stress, and damage and mitochondrial dysfunction has been established (Navarro & Boveris, 2004, Navarro & Boveris, 2009; Navarro et al., 2009, Navarro et al., 2010).

1.2.3 Transition metals toxicity

Increasing evidence indicates that metal-induced toxicity is associated with the etiology of neurodegenerative diseases. Two main mechanisms are currently considered likely to be the mechanism for redox active metals: a Haber-Weiss reaction and a depletion of major sulfhydryls, reduced glutathione and protein -SH groups (Repetto & Boveris, 2011).

The cellular and tisular levels of transition metals are apparently determined by regulatory proteins and metallochaperons that control metal capture, transport and storage. The major consequences of metal dyshomeostasis are mitochondrial dysfunction, oxidative stress and mitochondrial genomic damage which enhanced activation of the apoptotic machinery (Kozlowski et al., 2009).

Transition metals including iron (Fe) mediated oxidative damage to cellular components through the one-electron transfer called the Fenton reaction ($Fe^{2+} + H_2O_2 \longrightarrow Fe^{3+} + OH\cdot + OH^-$), which leads to production of the unstable hydroxyl radical (OH.) that will oxidize nucleic acid, protein, carbohydrate and lipid, whichever is proximate (Halliwell & Gutteridge, 1984). Disrupted iron metabolism is implicated in PD, iron levels are increased in the PD *substantia nigra*, associated with α-synuclein pathology, substantial iron deposits are associated with neuronal loss, gliosis and Lewy body pathology. Iron sequestered in

Lewy bodies and other pathobiologic pools of iron in PD brains has the potential to promote Fenton chemistry and oxidative damage to macromolecules. Evidence of oxidative damage to macromolecules is abundant in post-mortem PD tissue, with proteins, nucleic acids, lipids and sugars, all showing evidence of oxidative modification.

The mitochondria of Fe-treated rats show lower respiratory control in association with higher resting (state 4) respiration. This mitochondrial uncoupling elicited by Fe-treatment does not affect the phosphorylation efficiency or the ATP levels, indicating a mild degree of uncoupling in Fe overload (Pardo Andreau et al., 2009).

The Fe accumulation in *substantia nigra* (with up to 255% increases) results in oxidative stress; oxidative damage, decreased reduced glutathione levels and increased dopamine neuronal toxicity (Kozlowski et al., 2009). The Fe-induced oxidative damage to mitochondria contributes to the cellular death mechanisms, arising from a diminished respiratory chain activity and ATP production. The significant reduction in transferrin levels, observed in patients with Parkinson's diseases, is a factor contributing to increase Fe concentrations (Kozlowski et al., 2009; Spencer et al., 2011).

Fe and Cu are prevalent in human tissues, including the brain, and altered levels of these essential metals have been found in brain tissues of patients with neurodegenerative diseases (Repetto & Boveris, 2011). Because approximately 20% of the total Cu is stored in the nucleus, DNA is the major target for copper-catalyzed oxidations. Accumulation of oxidative DNA base modifications, produced by dopamine and other catecholamine neurotransmitters and neurotoxins, is associated with elevated copper (Cu) levels in the presence of O_2^- and H_2O_2 and potentially results from one-electron oxidation and/or the site-attack of hydroxyl radicals via a DNA-Cu(I)OOH complex. Because accumulation of oxidative DNA has been reported as a major contributing factor to genomic instability and mitochondrial dysfunction in aging and neurodegenerative disorders as Alzheimer and PD, it probably contributes to neuronal death associated with these degenerative processes (Spencer et al., 2011).

1.2.4 Oxidative stress and oxidative damage

The concept of oxidative stress is defined as an imbalance with increased oxidants or decreased antioxidants (Sies, 1991). As an imbalance situation, it implies that in the normal physiological condition there is a balance, or a controlled situation of quasi-equilibrium between oxidants and antioxidants. Oxidants are continually produced as secondary products of respiration and oxidative metabolism and antioxidants are continually reacting with oxidant molecules. In the oxidative stress condition, oxidants increase or antioxidants decrease in a progressive and continuous form, sometimes including adaptive responses that involve the synthesis of antioxidants and antioxidant enzymes and that confer elasticity and reversibility to the biological situation of oxidative stress (Boveris et al., 2008). They defined the intracellular oxidative stress as a situation where increases of the steady-state concentrations of any intermediate produces an increase in oxidant intermediates, an increase in the chain reaction rate and a decrease in intracellular antioxidants.

The brain is particularly susceptible to oxidative stress due to its high-energy demand and the specialized redox activities of neurons. Although the brain only constitutes 2 to 3% of total body mass, it utilizes 20% of basal oxygen supplied to the body. Low level of oxidants are needed for normal cellular functions, including, but not restricted to the regulation of neuronal excitability via redox-sensitive ion channels, synaptic plasticity, gene transcription, and the activity of enzymes controlling protein phosphorylation. At higher concentrations, oxidants cause neuronal membrane damage. The biological targets of oxidants include membrane proteins, unsaturated lipids and DNA.

Oxidative stress promotes aggregation and accumulation of α-synuclein, characteristic of Parkinson's disease (Kozlowski et al., 2009; Opazo et al., 2003). The series of observed changes include glycation protein oxidation, lipid peroxidation, depletion of antioxidants and nucleic acid oxidation (Famulari et al., 1996; Gatto et al., 1996; Gatto et al., 1997; Repetto et al., 1999; Fiszman et al., 2003; Boveris et al., 2008; Repetto, 2008). It has been proposed that oxidative damage favors the aggregation of α-synuclein in sporadic PD.

According to a now classical definition, antioxidants are molecules which, when present in small concentrations compared to the biomolecules that are supposed to protect, can prevent or reduce the extent of oxidative destruction of biomolecules. They can prevent initiation or intercept the lipid peroxyl radical involved in the propagation phase. In human plasma there are transition metal binding proteins in order to prevent metal catalysis; on the other side, cell membranes and lipoproteins contain lipophilic antioxidants, which are able to react with lipid peroxyl radicals, eventually terminating the chain reaction of lipid peroxidation. The implication of free radicals in various pathological processes has been detected in an increasing number of human diseases. The assay of oxidative stress parameters has brought substantial insights into the pathogenesis of many diseases in humans, by demonstrating the involvement of free radicals and/or the decrease of antioxidants.

1.2.5 Lipid peroxidation

Lipid peroxidation is a chain reaction initiated by the hydrogen substraction or addition of an oxygen radical, resulting in the oxidative damage of polyunsaturated fatty acids (PUFA). Since polyunsaturated fatty acids are more sensitive than saturated ones, it is obvious that the activated methylene (RH) bridge represents a critical target site. Molecular oxygen rapidly adds to the carbon-centered radical (R·) formed in this process, yielding to lipid peroxyl radical (ROO·). The formation of peroxyl radicals leads to the production of organic hydroperoxides, which, in turn, can subtract hydrogen from another PUFA. This reaction is termed propagation, implying that one initiating hit can result in the conversion of numerous PUFA to lipid hydroperoxides. In sequence of their appearance, alkyl, peroxyl and alkoxyl radicals are involved. The resulting fatty acid radical is stabilized by rearrangement into a conjugated diene that retains the more stable products including hydroperoxides, alcohols, aldehydes and alkanes. Lipid hydroperoxide (ROOH) is the first, comparatively stable, product of the lipid peroxidation reaction. In conditions in which lipid peroxidation is continuously initiated it gives non-radical products (PNR), destroying two radicals at a time. In the presence of transition metal ions, ROOH can give rise to the generation of radicals capable of re-initiating lipid peroxidation by redox-cycling of these metal ions (Halliwell & Gutteridge, 1984).

Lipid peroxidation can have significant downstream effects and possibly play a major role in cell signaling pathways. For example, the mitochondrion lipid cardiolipin makes up to 18% of the total phospholipids and 90% of the fatty acyl chains are unsaturated. Oxidation of cardiolipin may be one of the critical factors initiating apoptosis by liberating cytochrome c from the mitochondrial inner membrane and facilitating permeabilization of the outer membrane. The release of cytochrome c activates a proteolytic cascade that culminates in apoptotic cell death (Navarro & Boveris, 2009).

Many of these products can be found in biological fluids, as well as addition-derivatives of these very reactive end-products. As a result of lipid peroxidation a great variety of aldehydes can be produced, including hexanal, malondialdehyde (MDA) and 5-hydroxynonenal (Repetto, 2008). Oxidation of an endogenous antioxidant reflects an oxidative stress that is evaluated by measuring the decrease in the total level of the antioxidant or the increase in the oxidative form. The only way not to be influenced by nutritional status is to measure the ratio between oxidized and reduced antioxidants present in blood. The published literature provides compelling evidence that MDA represents a side product of enzymatic PUFA-oxygenation and a secondary end product of non enzymatic (autoxidative) fatty peroxide formation and decomposition. Conceptually, these two facts indicate that MDA is an excellent index of lipid peroxidation. With biological materials, it appears prudent to consider the TBARS test more than an empirical indicator of the potential occurrence of peroxidative lipid damage and not as a measure of lipid peroxidation (Repetto, 2008).

1.2.6 Inflammation

Among neural cells, neurons are particularly vulnerable to oxidative damage, not only as a consequence of mitochondrial dysfunction (Boveris & Navarro, 2008), but also due to inactivation of glutamine synthetase, which reduces the uptake of glutamate by glial cells and increases glutamate availability at the synapse producing excitotoxicity. Oxidative damage to lipids and protein of neuronal membrane affects activities of membrane-bound enzymes, ion channels and receptors. Glial cell´s response to oxidative stress-mediated neurodegenerative process is extremely complex. Astrocytes may play a dual function, either protecting neurons from excitotoxicity through glutamate uptake system, or contributing to the extracellular glutamate via reversed glutamate transporter. They may contribute to the inflammatory response by transforming themselves into activated microglia and also release matrix metalloproteinase's, oxidants, prostaglandin E_2 and proinflammatory cytokines such as TNF-α and IL-β1 (Farooqui & Farooqui, 2011). In addition, at the site of neurodegenerative process, neural and non-neural cells express and secrete cytokines, chemokine and complement proteins, which also play important roles in induction, propagation and maintenance of inflammatory response. Cytokines are major effectors of the inflammatory response; they produce their effects by interacting with specific membrane associated receptors. Although physiological levels of cytokines are necessary for normal neuronal function and survival, the increased secretion of cytokines during neurodegenerative process may be detrimental to neurons.

Nitric oxide (NO) is a free radical and potent biological effectors regulating blood vessel dilatation and immune function and serve as a neuronal messenger in the nervous system. Most of the effects of NO are mediated by glutamate, although in high concentrations, may act as a neurotoxin. NO can react with superoxide anion to produce peroxinitrite, an even more potent oxidant associated with lipid peroxidation and cytotoxic effects, in part through the oxidizing of tissue sulfhydrils. Metabolic alterations in circulating blood cells are widely accepted as representative of similar central nervous system changes in human PD. Increased NO release of neutrophils and decreased catalase activity in erythrocytes were observed at the beginning of PD; H_2O_2 release by neutrophils and mitochondrial impaired function may be later signs in PD (Gatto et al., 1996).

1.3 Clinical evidence of oxidative stress and damage in Parkinson's disease

Human neurodegenerative diseases are characterized by cumulative neuronal damage that leads to neurological deficits when neuronal loss reaches a critical level. Actually, the clinical evolution of patients with neurological diseases is based on psychological tests. The current hypotheses are that brain oxidative stress and damage are involved in the pathogenesis of neurodegenerative diseases such as Alzheimer's and Parkinson's diseases and non-neurodegenerative vascular dementia. Involvement of oxidative stress in the pathogenesis of PD is supported both, by postmortem studies and by studies showing the increased level of oxidative stress in the *substantia nigra pars compacta* (Boveris & Navarro, 2008). Under normal conditions, the continuous generation of oxidants is compensated by the powerful action of protective enzymes: superoxide dismutase (SOD), catalase and glutathione peroxidase. Oxidative stress may be a consequence of reduced efficiency of these endogenous antioxidants that may render PD patients more susceptible to oxidative stress. Increases of pro-oxidants, as H_2O_2 and nitric oxide (NO), and decreases of antioxidants, either enzymatic or non enzymatic compounds, are considered an indication of oxidative stress. Oxidative damage is characterized by increases in the levels of the oxidation products of macromolecules, such as thiobarbituric acid reactive substances (TBARS), and protein carbonyls.

Oxidative stress, to which neurons are highly susceptible, is also known to induce oxidative changes in human red blood cells (RBCs), *in vivo* and *in vitro* (Gatto et al., 1996; Repetto & Llesuy, 2004, Repetto, 2008). Based on the hypothesis that oxidative changes are not organ specific, their activities may be evaluated in peripheral and red blood cells.

The situation of oxidative stress evaluated by the peripheral markers of oxidative stress in the blood of neurological patients, seem to provide a reflection of the brain condition. Brain oxidative stress, with oxygen free radicals being responsible for brain damage, signals to peripheral blood, at least, through the diffusible products of lipid peroxidation. The peripheral markers provide a useful tool to determine the evolution of brain oxidative stress in neurological patients (Repetto, 2008).

2. Materials and methods

2.1 Patients

The clinic diagnostic of PD is realized in accordance with the "United Kingdom Parkinson Disease Brain Bank Criteria". Patients (n = 15, age = 66 ± 4 years) were evaluated according to the Hoehn and Yahr's scale in stages 1 to 3, and required a history of positive response to levodopa therapy. No patient presented vascular lesions on CT scanning. The controls groups (Table 1 and Table 2) consisted of 75 and 80 healthy people of 58 ± 2 years and 71 ± 10 years, respectively.

2.2 Peripheral markers of oxidative stress

Blood was obtained by venipuncture and placed into glass tubes with heparinised syringes for separation of erythrocytes or mononuclear cells.

To determine tert-butyl hydroperoxide-initiated chemiluminescence (BOOH-CL), heparinised blood samples were centrifuged at 300 g for 10 min. The plasma fraction (supernatant) was separated for evaluation of the total reactive antioxidant potential (TRAP). Mononuclear cells were discarded by aspiration. Erythrocytes were suspended in saline solution 0.9 % P/V NaCl and were washed three times by centrifugation at 300 g with the same saline solution at 25 °C, and then diluted 1/10 in 1 mM acetic acid and 4 mM

magnesium sulfate. The protein concentration was determines with the Folin reagent, using bovine serum albumin (grade III) as the standard.
The peripheral markers of oxidative stress assayed were:

2.2.1 Tert-butyl hydroperoxide initiated chemiluminescence (BOOH-CL)

The increased values of BOOH-CL indicate the occurrence of oxidative stress in the membrane of the erythrocytes due to consume of the endogenous antioxidants. The chemiluminescence associated to lipid peroxidation (BOOH-CL) was measured with a Packard Tricarb model 3355 liquid scintillation counter in the out-of-coincidence mode. This assay estimates indirectly and with high sensitivity the tissue levels of α-tocopherol by inhibition of the propagation step of lipid peroxidation, as discussed by González Flecha et al. (1991). Red blood cells were suspended in 4 mL of 120 mM KCl, 30 mM phosphate buffer, pH 7.40 at 0.1-0.2 mg protein/mL. Low-potassium glass vials of 25 mm diameter and 50 mm height filled with the sample suspension were used. Instrument background, in the absence of vials, was 2400 ± 60 counts per minutes (cpm) and the emission from the empty vials was 3000 ± 60 cpm. Chemiluminescence measurements were started by the addition of 3 mM tert-butyl hydroperoxide and the counting continued until a maximal level of emission was reached, usually after 20 minutes. Determinations were carried out at 30°C. The results are expressed as cpm/mg protein (González Flecha et al., 1991).

2.2.2 Plasma antioxidant capacity (TRAP)

The decreased values of TRAP in plasma indicate a reduction in the level of plasmatic hydrosoluble antioxidants (*i.e.*, GSH, uric acid, ascorbic acid and bilirubin). The total reactive antioxidant potential of plasma was measured by chemiluminescence. This assay determines total endogenous water soluble antioxidants, mainly glutathione, ascorbic acid, bilirubin and albumin uric acid in plasma. The addition of 10 µL of sample to 20 mM 2,2-azobis (2- amidinopropane) (ABAP) in 100 mM phosphate buffer, pH 7.40 and 40 µM luminol decreased the chemiluminescence to basal levels and prevented the spike of light emission for a period proportional to the amount of antioxidants present in the sample (induction time, δ). The system was calibrated with Trolox (a hydrosoluble vitamin E analogue). The results are expressed as µmoL Trolox per g of organ, or µM Trolox considering 1 g of tissue as 1 mL of water (Lissi et al., 1992).

2.2.3 Thiobarbituric acid reactive substances (TBARS)

The increase in TBARS results from augmented levels of systemic and neuronal hydroperoxides that lead to an increment in lipid peroxidation. TBARS was assayed by the spectrophotometric determination as described by Fraga et al. (1988). Thiobarbituric acid reacts with malondialdehyde, a product of lipid peroxidation, showing maximal absorbance at 535 nm. The reaction mixture consists of 1 mL of plasma, 1 mL of 120 mM KCl, 1 mL of 30 mM phosphate buffer, pH 7.40, 0.05 mL of buthylhydroxytoluene 4 % w/v in ethanol, 1 ml of thrichloroacetic acid 20 % w/v and 1 mL thiobarbituric acid 0.7 % w/v. The deproteinized mixture was heated at 100 °C for 20 minutes. Results (E = 156 $mM^{-1}cm^{-1}$) are expressed as nmol/L plasma (Fraga et al., 1988).

2.2.4 Cu–Zn superoxide dismutase (SOD)

An increase in the activity of the antioxidant enzyme SOD has been regarded as a marker of systemic oxidative stress, since the up-regulation of the antioxidant enzyme expression was considered as an adaptive response to the oxidative stress situation. SOD activity was determined by measuring the ability of red blood cells to inhibit the autoxidation of epinephrine at pH 10.2. The increase in absorbance at 480 nm was 0.025 U-min with no added SOD, and 50% inhibition was achieved by 46 ng/mL of bovine SOD. One unit of SOD activity was defined as the inhibition of the epinephrine oxidation rate by 50%. The inhibition was determined comparing the regression lines of autoxidation of epinephrine standard solutions against varying amounts of sample. Activity is expressed in U SOD/mg protein (Misra & Fridovich, 1972; Serra et al., 2000).

3. Results

The data given in Table 1 show the association of PD with oxidative stress. BOOH-CL was increased by 86% and TRAP values showed a decrease of 33% in PD, together with increases of 19% in TBARS and 55% in SOD, by comparison with the healthy controls (Serra et al., 2001; Repetto, 2008).

Variables	BOOH-CL (cpm/mg Hb) x 10^2	TRAP (μM Trolox)	TBARS (nmol MDA/mL)	SOD (U_{SOD}/mg prot.)
Parkinson's Disease	202 ± 10 $p < 0.001$ n = 12	242 ± 25 $p < 0.001$ n = 12	3.46 ± 0.18 $p < 0.05$ n = 15	15.83 ± 0.57 $p < 0.001$ n = 15

Table 1. BOOH-CL and TRAP in erythrocytes and plasma of patients with Parkinson's disease; TBARS in plasma and SOD in erythrocytes. Probabilities as compared against pooled healthy controls (n = 75) of comparable ages.

The concentration of non-enzymatic antioxidants decreases during oxidative damage. A lower level of antioxidants as a consequence of a previous situation of oxidative damage will correspond to a higher BOOH-CL, TBARS and SOD. These three increases are indicative of the occurrence of systemic oxidative stress.

Present results demonstrate that the BOOH-CL, TBARS, TRAP and SOD variables for determining oxidative stress and antioxidant status would be a useful tool for the biochemical and clinical evaluation of patients during the progression of the disease and clinical treatment (Repetto, 2008; Serra et al., 2009).

Chemiluminescence methods allow evaluating and quantifying the toxic oxygen species and antioxidant defenses in blood samples of the patients. They are: tert-butyl hydroperoxide initiated chemiluminescence (BOOH-CL) and total reactive antioxidant potential (TRAP).

Chemiluminescence occurs when a chemical reaction produces an electronically excited species which emits light on its return to the ground state. Singlet oxygen and triplet carbonyl compounds are the most important chemiluminescent species in lipid peroxidation of biological systems (Figure 1).

The experimental conditions defined here for BOOH-CL (Figure 1) and TRAP (Figure 2) may be used to evaluate oxidative stress in blood of patients in PD patients. The two assays appear as useful to evaluate the overall level of the non-enzymatic antioxidant defenses in the sample. The substances that constitute the non-enzymatic antioxidant defenses (α-tocopherol, ascorbic acid, retinal, uric acid, albumin, ceruloplasmin, glutathione, etc) decrease their concentration during oxidative stress due to their reaction with reactive oxygen or nitrogen species and, in consequence, their elimination.

The levels of methaemoglobin (Met-Hb) are regarded as an index of intracellular damage to the red cell, increased when α-tocopherol is consumed and the rate of lipid peroxidation is increased. Scavenging of free radicals by α-tocopherol is the first and the most critical step in defending against oxidative damage to the red cells. When α-tocopherol is adequate, GSH and ascorbic acid may complement the antioxidant functions of α-tocopherol by providing the reducing equivalents necessary for its recycling/regeneration.

On the other hand, when α-tocopherol is absent, GSH and ascorbic acid may release transitional metals from the bound forms and/or maintain metal ions in a catalytic state. Free radical generation catalyzed by transition metal ions can in turn initiate oxidative damage to cell membranes. Membrane damage leads to the release of heme compounds of the erythrocytes. The heme compounds released may further promote oxidative damage especially when reducing compounds are present.

The lower level of antioxidants as a consequence of the occurrence of oxidative stress is also sustained by higher values of chemiluminescence (Figures 1 and 2). The increase of BOOH-CL is indicative that α-tocopherol is the antioxidant consumed in erythrocytes and suggest that reactive oxygen species and lipid peroxidation catalyzed by reduced transition metals may be responsible for the onset of oxidative damage and the occurrence of systemic oxidative stress in patients suffering PD (Table 1).

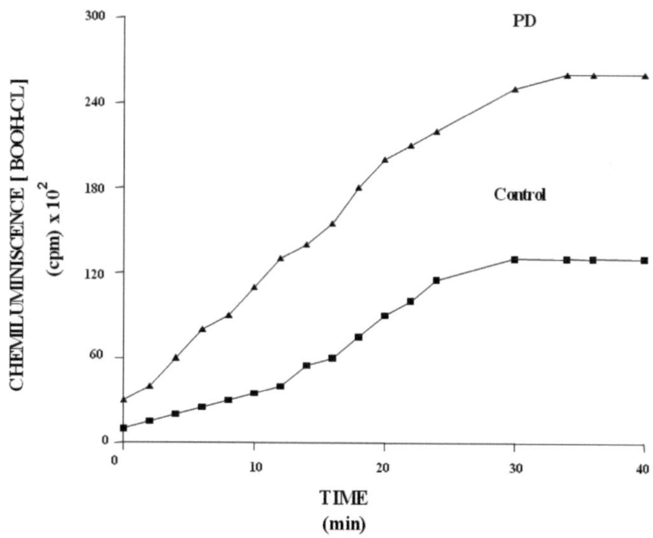

Fig. 1. Photoemission kinetics of chemiluminescence (BOOH-CL) in erythrocytes of a control subject and a PD patient.

The evolution of chemiluminescence shows that at 30 min of the beginning of the lipid peroxidation propagation step, the erythrocyte's BOOH-CL of PD patients were 3 fold greater than those observed in the control subject (control value: 100 x 10^2 cpm) (Figure 1). These results are in agreement with the consumption time of the endogenous hydrosoluble antioxidants in plasma, showing a 50% of decrease in the induction time in PD patients compared with control subject (control value: 4 min) (Figure 2).

As cell membranes and lipoproteins contain lipophilic antioxidants and plasma contains hydrophilic antioxidants, that are able to react with lipid peroxyl radicals, eventually terminating the chain reaction the chemiluminescence technique may be applied to study the antioxidant effect of many compounds or the presence of antioxidant molecules in a biological tissue. The reaction between a lipid and hydroperoxyl radicals with a molecule of antioxidant prevent the emission of light (González Flecha et al., 1991; Repetto, 2008).

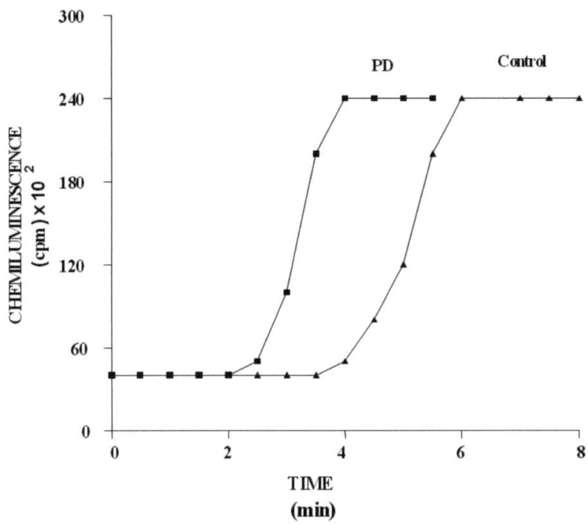

Fig. 2. Time profiles of luminol luminescence with plasma from a PD patient and a control subject.

The biological effects induced by free radicals are neutralized in vivo by antioxidative defense mechanisms, which include ascorbic acid, uric acid, α-tocopherol, carotenoids, glutathione and antioxidant enzymes. However, the extensive generation of oxygen reactive species in some pathological conditions appears to overwhelm natural defense mechanisms, thereby reducing dramatically the levels of endogenous antioxidants.

The non-enzymatic antioxidants decrease their concentration during oxidative damage. A lower level of antioxidants as a consequence of a previous situation of oxidative damage will correspond to a higher chemiluminescence. The increase of BOOH-CL is indicative of the occurrence of systemic oxidative stress.

Accordingly, there is a statistically significant decrease in the measured TRAP, suggesting that an enhanced susceptibility of erythrocytes to the oxidative stress correlates with a decrease in its antioxidant defenses (Figures 3 and 4).

Chemiluminescence is a simple method to providing tools to evaluate the clinical situation of patients, allowing quantification of the plasma antioxidant content, the correlation with the advance of the pathology, the effects of pharmacological treatments and the relative contribution of total endogenous antioxidants to the plasma.

Chemiluminescence is a collective term, which includes the emission of light by molecules which have been excited to a higher energy level as a result of a chemical reaction. Singlet oxygen or triplet carbonyl compounds are likely to be the most important chemiluminescent species in lipid peroxidation of biological systems; both of them can originate from recombination of two peroxyl radicals to a non-radical product according to Russell's mechanism by a number of chemical pathways.

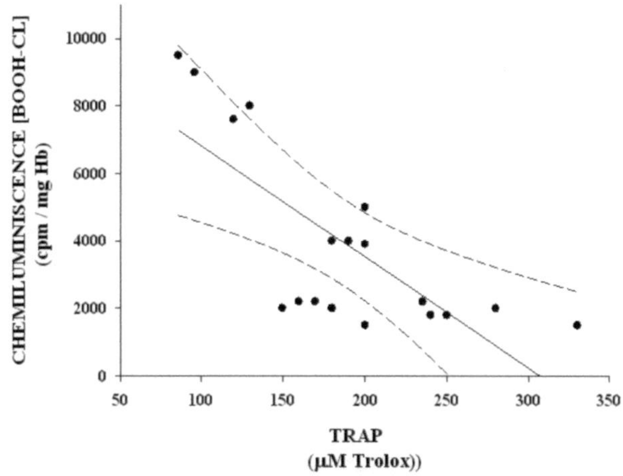

Fig. 3. Correlation between BOOH-CL in erythrocytes and TRAP in plasma of PD patients. Pearson's correlation coefficient was 0.790 ($p < 0.001$). The solid line is the linear regression ($r = -0.752$), dotted lines the 99% confidence intervals.

Although lipids in the cell are protected from autoxidation by a protein coat and/or by the presence of high concentration of antioxidants, it seems evident that some autoxidation of PUFA in cells must occur. Antioxidant status in biological samples is regarded as an indicator of oxidative stress, and in many cases low antioxidant capacity of tissue and body fluids is a consequence of increased oxidative processes (Halliwell & Gutteridge, 1984).

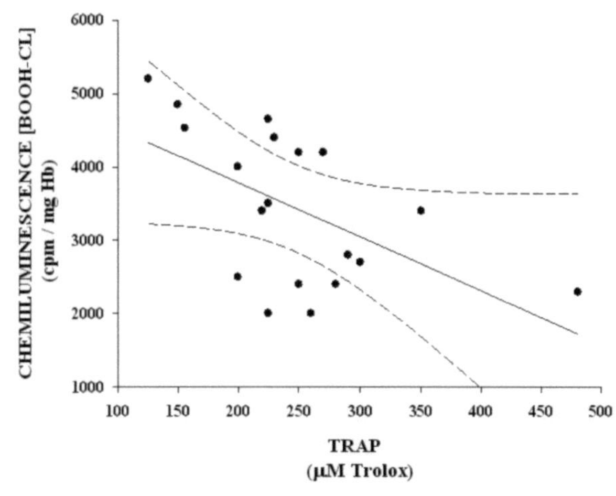

Fig. 4. Correlation between BOOH-CL in erythrocytes and TRAP in plasma of control group. Pearson's correlation coefficient was 0.600 ($p < 0.01$). The solid line is the linear regression ($r = -0.554$), dotted lines the 99% confidence intervals.

Close quantitative correspondences were found when TRAP and BOOH-CL were plotted against the Hoehn and Yahr's scale in Parkinson's patients (Figures 5 and 6).
The evidence linking neurodegenerative diseases with oxidative stress suggested that different substances might be involved in Parkinson´s, Alzheimer´s and Vascular diseases.

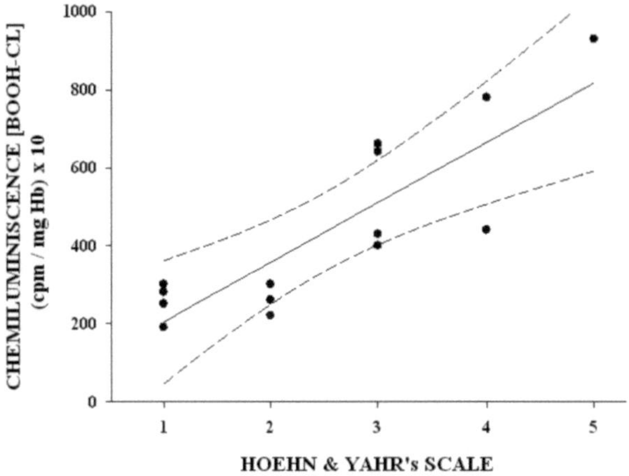

Fig. 5. Correlation between erythrocyte BOOH-CL and Hoehn and Yahr's clinical scale of PD patients (Pearson's correlation coefficient, $r = 0.842$, $p < 0.001$). The solid line is the linear regression ($r = 0.857$), dotted lines the 99% confidence intervals.

This hypothesis was tested using Discriminant Analysis in order to find if it is possible to separate PD, Alzheimer's disease patients (AD), Vascular dementia patients (VD) and healthy controls (C) based on the measured biochemical variables (Serra et al., 2001).
The first Discriminant Function (DF) obtained was: DF 1 = - 18.47 SOD - 1.21 CAT - 0.99 GSH - 3.42 TBARS + 2.42 TRAP - 1.12 Age + 30.23, where CAT and GSH are the values of the antioxidant enzyme catalase and the glutathione system respectively which, albeit not yielding significant differences *per se*, proved useful when included in the discriminant function.
The values assigned by this function to each observation resulted in the correct identification of 100% of PD, 94% of AD and 100% of VD as diseased subjects and 93% of the C group as healthy. It was also possible to discriminate between DAT and VD using the second DF:
DF 2 = - 1.16 SOD + 0.86 CAT + 1.34 GSH + 2.26 TBARS - 1.35 TRAP + 3.58 Age - 5.59, which correctly identified 88.9% of DAT and 73.3% of VD.

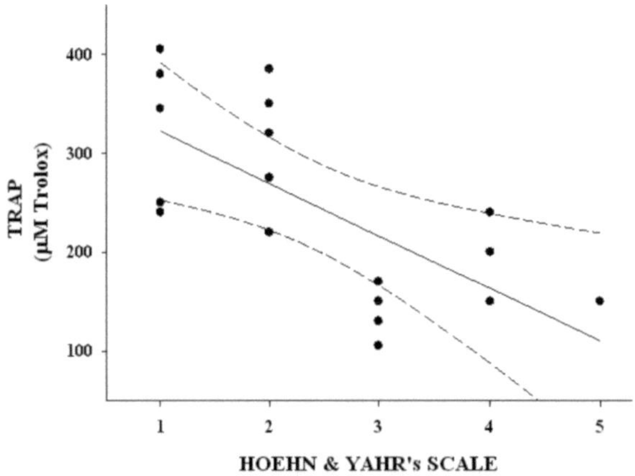

Fig. 6. Correlation between TRAP and Hoehn and Yahr's clinical scale of PD (Pearson's correlation coefficient, $r = 0.890$, $p < 0.003$). Solid line is the linear regression ($r = -0.684$), dotted lines the 99% confidence intervals.

The discriminant functions define four quadrants (Figure 7) with the healthy controls lying in the negative X (first Discriminant Function) region and all the diseased subjects in the positive X. The AD patients fall in the positive X and positive Y (second Discriminant Function) and the VD in the positive X and negative Y. The PD patients were not associated with any of the other groups of patients (9 were classified as AD and 6 as VD).

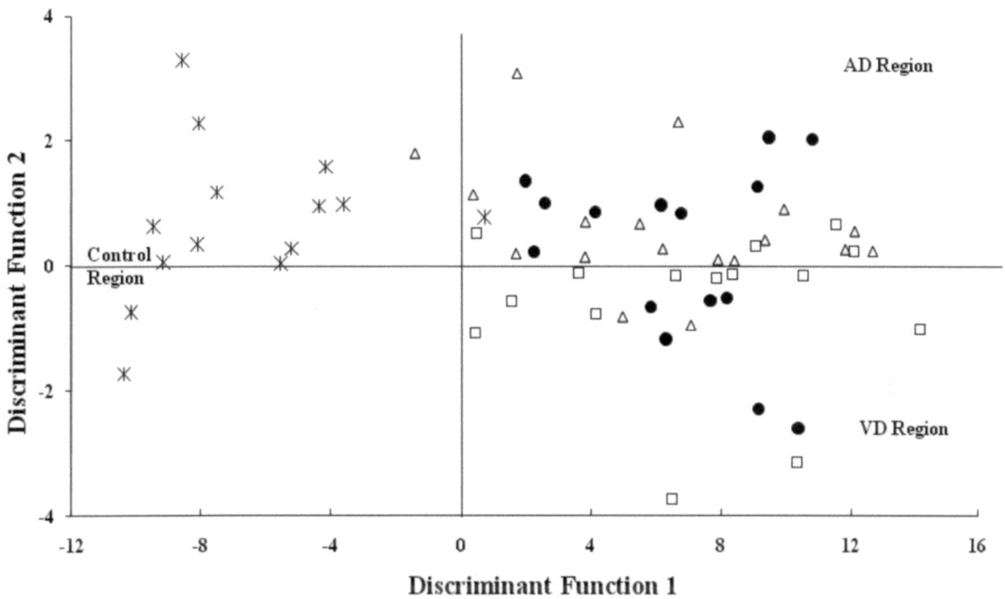

Fig. 7. Plot of pathological and control subjects on the two axes derived from Discriminant Functions. Clinical conditions are: PD patients (n = 15): Filled circles; AD Patients (n = 18): Empty triangles; VD Patients (n = 15): Empty squares; Healthy Controls (n = 14): Asterisks.

The Discriminant Function 2 correctly recognizes AD and VD, showing that these two groups might be considered as separate oxidative disorders (measured by biochemical variables of the peripheral oxidant/antioxidant system). The control and diseased regions are clearly separated, as well as AD and VD regions. PD patients are evenly distributed overlapping AD and VD, suggesting biochemical similarities with both diseases.

The peripheral antioxidant profile of PD shows a degree of overlap (already shown in Figure 7) with those of AD and VD. While dementias can be readily distinguished from each other, the PD profile might be described as intermediate between AD and VD. This might be explained noting that the main neuronal populations affected are different in each disease. Their identity (dopaminergic, noradrenergic, serotoninergic and cholinergic) is well established: mainly dopaminergic neurons die in PD and cholinergic neurons in AD patients; while VD doesn't present neuronal selectivity. The three diseases are associated with oxidative disorders predominating in different anatomical areas of the brain. An intermediate mechanism might be hypothesized for the PD patients (Serra et al., 2001).

Table 2 presents the values of the oxidant and antioxidant variables in the three neurological diseases and healthy controls studied obtained in a different protocol (Serra et al., 2009).

Group	TBARS nmol MDA/ml plasma	TRAP µM Trolox	SOD U_{SOD}/mg protein	CAT k'/ml RBC	GPx µM GPx/ml RBC
Parkinson's Disease n = 15	3.46 ± 0.18 p < 0.05	295 ± 26 p < 0.01	15.83 ± 0.57 p < 0.001	49.5 ± 3.4 N.S.	2.1 ± 0.3 N.S.
Alzheimer's Disease n = 112	3.61 ± 0.13 p < 0.001	277 ± 12 p < 0.001	17.75 ± 0.47 p < 0.001	43.9 ± 3.0 N.S.	1.8 ± 0.1 N.S.
Vascular Dementia n = 57	3.50 ± 0.12 p < 0.01	309 ± 18 p < 0.001	16.69 ± 0.61 p < 0.001	39.4 ± 3.8 N.S.	2.1 ± 0.2 N.S.
Healthy Controls n = 80	2.91 ± 0.08	410 ± 19	10.24 ± 0.28	45.8 ± 3.9	1.9 ± 0.2

Table 2. TBARS, TRAP measured in plasma, the enzymes SOD, CAT and GPx (glutathione peroxidase) measured in erythrocytes of patients with Parkinson's disease, Alzheimer's disease and Vascular dementia. Probabilities as compared against pooled healthy controls of comparable ages. RBC: Red blood cells; N.S.: non-significant differences.

As free radical stress results from an imbalance between free radical production and antioxidant system, it may be possible to measure the antioxidant levels separately or as a total global antioxidant capacity of a biological tissue. The reactive oxygen and nitrogen species are generated in living systems and oxidize a number of cellular constituents like lipids, proteins and DNA. As a consequence of this, antioxidants come into play and act as free radical scavengers, inhibit lipid peroxidation and other free radical mediated processes; they are able to protect the human body from several diseases attributed to the reaction of radicals.

Moreover, the present results show linearity between pairs of oxidative stress variables and the ordering of the neurological patients' diseases along the different regression lines pointing to the existence of an overall balance between oxidative insult, damage and protection (Table 2 and Figures 8 and 9) (Serra et al., 2009).

The linear correlations described between the three variables also include a significant negative linear correlation between plasma TRAP and erythrocyte SOD ($r = -0.980$, $p < 0.001$, not shown), which is implied by the other two relationships.

4. Conclusions

PD is a common neurodegenerative movement disorder, which affects increasing numbers of the elderly population. The disorder is characterized by a selective degeneration of dopaminergic neurons in the *substantia nigra*. Although the molecular mechanism associated with neurodegeneration in PD is not known, it is becoming increasingly evident that neuronal death in this disease is a multifactorial process that may involve monoamino oxidase-mediated abnormal dopamine metabolism, increase of iron levels, hydrogen peroxide generation, transition metal and α-synuclein dyshomeostasis, abnormal mitochondrial function and oxidative stress and damage. Free radicals have been postulated as involved

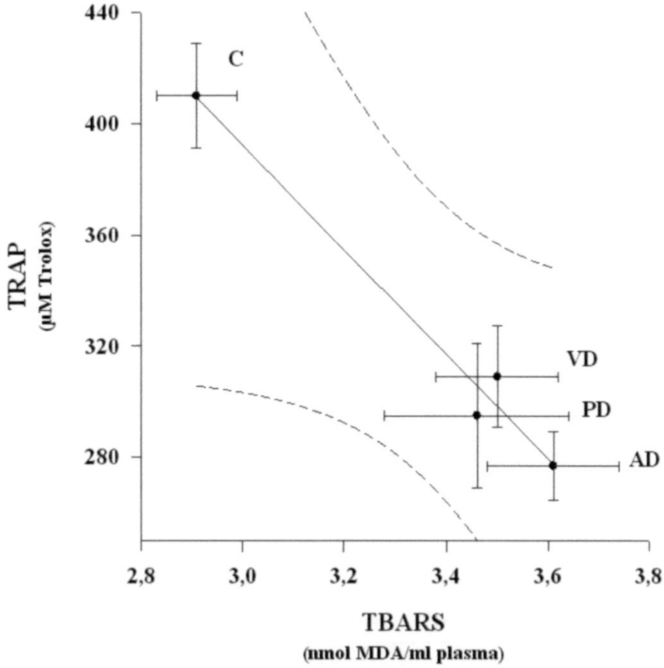

Fig. 8. Correlation between plasma TBARS and plasma TRAP values. Mean values (*points*) and standard error (*bars*), solid line is the linear regression (r = -0.989), dotted lines the 99% confidence intervals. C: healthy controls (n = 80); PD: Parkinson's disease patients (n = 15); AD: Alzheimer's disease patients (n = 112); VD: Vascular Dementia patients (n = 57) (Data from Serra et al., 2009).

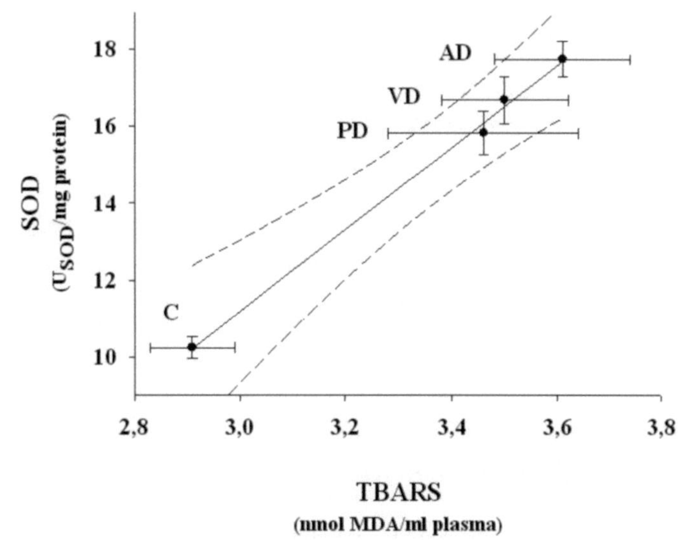

Fig. 9. Correlation between plasma TBARS and erythrocyte SOD values (r = 0.998). Statistics and abbreviations as in Figure 8 (Serra et al., 2009).

in PD disease. The concept of free radical involvement is supported by enhanced basal lipid peroxidation in *substantia nigra* (Navarro & Boveris, 2009) and plasma of PD patients, demonstrated by increased levels of TBARS and lipid peroxidation. The assay of oxidative stress parameters in plasma and red blood cells in humans is usually attempted through the determination of: a decreased in the level of antioxidants, and an increase in the by-products of free radical reactions. The increase of BOOH-CL and TBARS are indicative that α-tocopherol is the antioxidant consumed in erythrocytes and suggest that reactive oxygen species and lipid peroxidation catalyzed by reduced transition metals may be responsible for the onset of oxidative damage and the occurrence of systemic oxidative stress in PD. The levels of intracellular (GSH) and plasma antioxidants are reduced in PD patients, suggesting that changes in GSH homeostasis and metabolism are early component of the pathological process of PD. SOD increases point to the existence of oxidative insult and systemic oxidative stress, alongside with the differences indicated by markers representing conditions that change in a few days period, through a marker representing the homeostatic long term response of the bone marrow in the order of 60–80 days.

It is also interesting to note the coincidence resulting from the linear ordering of the responses in relation with the complexity of the pathologies (Figures 8 and 9), accordingly with the simple Sies scale model. *The steady-state formation of prooxidants in cells and organs is balanced by a similar rate of their consumption by antioxidants that are enzymatic and/or non-enzymatic. Oxidative stress results from imbalance in this prooxidant/antioxidant equilibrium in favor of the prooxidants* (Sies, 1991).

In pathological situations the reactive oxygen species are generated as a consequence of lipid peroxidation and may occur with α-tocopherol deficiency. In addition to containing high concentrations of polyunsaturated fatty acids and transitional metals, red blood cells are constantly being subject to various types of oxidative stress. However, red blood cells are protected by a variety of antioxidant systems, capable of preventing most of the adverse effects under normal conditions. Among the antioxidant systems, in the red cells, α-tocopherol possesses an important and unique role. α-tocopherol may protect the red cells from oxidative damage via a free radical scavenging mechanism or as a structural component of the cell membranes (Repetto, 2008).

Cellular oxidative stress and peroxidation of membrane lipids play a role in the pathogenesis of PD. A condition of systemic oxidative stress, determined in red blood cells by BOOH-CL and SOD activity, and in plasma by TBARS and TRAP, was identified in PD patients. Accordingly, there is a statistically significant decrease in the measured TRAP, suggesting that an enhanced susceptibility of erythrocytes to the oxidative stress correlates with a decrease in its antioxidant defenses. These results indicate that peripheral markers, likely reflecting neuronal conditions in red blood cells and plasma, BOOH-CL, TRAP, TBARS and SOD evaluated by the present procedures, could be a useful complementary measurement when assessing the oxidative stress condition in different clinical pathological situations. Oxidative stress is one of the risk factors, which can initiate and/or promote neurodegeneration in PD, and correlates with the severity of the disease. The concept that free radicals, lipid peroxidation and oxidative stress were involved in the neuronal abnormalities of PD was simultaneous with the recognition of complex I dysfunction in PD. The original idea of oxidative stress has been extended to oxidative and nitrative stress for the protein damage and loss of dopaminergic neurons in Parkinson's disease (Navarro et al., 2009).

5. Acknowledgment

This work was supported by grants from the University of Buenos Aires (B056) and from the PRALIB, CONICET (PIP 6320) from Argentina.

6. References

Bender, A.; Krishnan, K.J.; Morris, C.M.; Taylor, G.A.; Reeve, A.K. & Perry, R.H. (2006). High levels of mitochondrial DNA deletions in *substantia nigra* neurons in aging and Parkinson´s disease. *Nature Genetic,* Vol. 38, pp. 515-517, ISSN: 1061-4036, EISSN: 1546-1718

Boveris, A. & Navarro, A. (2008) Brain mitochondrial dysfunction in aging. *Life,* Vol. 60, No.5, pp. 308-314, ISSN: 1521-6543, EISNN: 1521-6551

Boveris, A.; Repetto, M.G.; Bustamante, J.; Boveris, A.D. & Valdez, L.B. (2008). The concept of oxidative stress in pathology. In: Álvarez, S.; Evelson, P. (ed.), *Free Radical Pathophysiology,* pp. 1-17, Transworld Research Network: Kerala, India, ISBN: 978-81-7895-311-3

Dalakas, M.C.; Fujii, M.; Li, M. & McElroy, B. (2000). The clinical spectrum of anti-GAD antibody-positive patients with stiff-person syndrome. *Neurology,* Vol. 55, pp. 1531-1535, ISSN: 1080-2371; EISSN: 1538-6899

Domínguez, R.O.; Marschoff, E.R.; Guareschi, E.M.; Repetto, M.G.; Famulari, A.L.; Pagano, M.A. & Serra, J.A. (2008). Insulin, glucose and glycated haemoglobin in Alzheimer´s and vascular dementia with and without superimposed Type II diabetes mellitus condition. *Journal of Neural Transmission,* Vol. 115, pp. 77-84, ISSN: 0300-9564, EISSN: 1435-1463

Fahn, S.; Elton, R.L. & UPDRS program members (1987). Unified Parkinson's disease Rating Scale. In: Fahn, S.; Marsden, C.D.; Goldstein, M.; Calne, D.B. (ed.). *Recent developments in Parkinson's disease.* Macmillan Healthcare Information: Florham Park, NJ, USA; Vol. 2, pp. 153–163

Famulari, A.; Marschoff, E.; Llesuy, S.; Kohan, S.; Serra, J.; Domínguez, R.; Repetto, M.G.; Reides, C. & Lustig, E.S. de (1996). Antioxidant enzymatic blood profiles associated with risk factors in Alzheimer's and vascular diseases. A predictive assay to differentiate demented subjects and controls. *Journal of the Neurological Sciences,* Vol. 141, pp. 69-78, ISSN: 0022-510X

Farooqui, T. & Farooqui, A. (2011) Lipid-mediated oxidative stress and inflammation in the pathogenesis of Parkinson´s disease. *Parkinson's disease.* DOI: 10.4061/2011/247467

Fiszman, M.; D´Eigidio, M.; Ricart, K.; Repetto, M.G.; Llesuy, S.; Borodinsky, L.; Trigo, R.; Riedstra, S.; Costa, P.; Saizar, R.; Villa, A. & Sica, R. (2003). Evidences of oxidative stress in Familial Amyloidotic Polyneuropathy Type 1. *Archives of Neurology,* Vol. 60, pp. 593-597, ISSN 0003-9942, EISSN 0375-8540

Fraga, C.; Leibovitz, B. & Tappel, A. (1988). Lipid peroxidation measured as thiobarbituric acid-reactive substances in tissue slices: characterization and comparison with homogenates and microsomes. *Free Radicals in Biology and Medicine,* Vol. 4, pp. 155-161, ISSN: 0891-5849

Friedlich, A.L.; Smith, M.A.; Zhu, X.; Takeda, A.; Nunomura, A.; Moreira, P. & Perry, G. (2009). Oxidative stress in Parkinson´s disease. *The Open Patholology Journal,* Vol. 3, pp. 38-42, ISSN: 1874-3757

Gatto, E.; Carreras, M.C.; Pargament, G.; Reides, C.; Repetto, M.G.; Llesuy, S.; Fernández Pardal, M. & Poderoso, J. (1996). Neutrophil function nitric oxide and blood oxidative stress in Parkinson's disease. *Movement Disorders*, Vol. 11, pp. 261-267, ISSN: 0885-3185

Gatto, E.; Carreras, C.; Pargament, G.; Riobó, N.; Reides, C.; Repetto, M.; Fernández Pardal, N.; Llesuy, S. & Poderoso, J. (1997). Neutrophyl function nitric oxide and blood oxidative stress in Parkinson´s Disease. *Focus Parkinson´s Disease*, Vol. 9, pp. 12-14

Gibb, W.R. & Lees, A.J. (1988). The relevance of the Lewy body to the pathogenesis of idiopathic Parkinson's disease. *Journal Neurology Neurosurgery Psychiatry*, Vol. 51, pp. 745-752, ISSN: 00223050. EISSN: 1468330X

González Flecha, B.; Llesuy, S. & Boveris, A. (1991). Hydroperoxide-initiated chemiluminescence: assay for oxidative stress in biopsies of heart, liver and muscle. *Free Radicals in Biology and Medicine*, Vol. 10, pp. 93-100, ISSN: 0891-5849

Halliwell, B. & Gutteridge, J.M.C. (1984). Oxygen toxicity, oxygen radicals, transition metals and disease. *Biochemical Journal*, Vol. 218, pp. 1-14, ISSN: 0264-6021

Hoehn, M.M. & Yahr, M.D. (1967). Parkinsonism: onset, progression and mortality. *Neurology*, Vol. 17, pp. 427–442, ISSN: 1080-2371; EISSN: 1538-6899

Hughes, A.J.; Ben-Shlomo, S.E.; Daniel, S.E. & Lees, A.J. (1992). What features improve the accuracy of clinical diagnosis in Parkinson's disease: a clinicopathological study? *Neurology*, Vol. 2, pp. 1142–1146, ISSN: 1080-2371; EISSN: 1538-6899

Kozlowski, H.; Janck-Klos, A.; Brasun, J.; Gaggelli, E.; Valensin D. & Valensin, G. (2009). Copper, iron, and Zinc ions homeostasis and their role in neurodegenerative disorders (metal uptake, transport, distribution and regulation). *Coordination Chemistry Review*, Vol. 253, pp. 2665-2685, ISSN: 0010- 8545

Lissi, E.; Pascual, C. & Del Castillo, M. (1992). Luminol luminescence induced by 2, 2'-Azo-bis (2-amidinopropane) thermolysis. *Free Radical Research Communications*, Vol. 17, pp. 299- 311, 1992, ISSN: 8755-0199

Lustig, E.S. de; Serra, J.A.; Kohan, S.; Canziani, G.A.; Famulari, A.L. & Domínguez, R.O. (1993). Copper zinc superoxide dismutase activity in red blood cells and serum in demented patients and in aging. *Journal of the Neurological Sciences*, Vol. 115, pp. 18-25, ISSN: 0022-510X

McNamara, P.; Durso, R. & Harris, E. (2007). "Machiavellianism" and frontal dysfunction: evidence from Parkinson's disease. *Cognitive neuropsychiatry*, Vol. 12, pp. 285-300, ISSN: 0264-3294, EISSN: 1464-0627

Misra, H. & Fridovich, I. (1972). The role of superoxide anion in the autooxidation of epinephrine and a simple assay for superoxide dismutase. *The Journal of Biological Chemistry*, Vol. 247, pp. 3170-3175, ISSN: ISSN 0021-9258, EISSN 1083-351X

Movement Disorder Society Task Force on Rating Scales for Parkinson's disease: The Unified Parkinson's Disease Rating Scale (UPDRS): status and recommendations (2003). *Movement Disorders*, Vol. 18, pp. 738-50, ISSN: 0885-3185

Navarro, A. & Boveris, A. (2004). Rat brain and liver mitochondria develop oxidative stress and lose enzymatic activities on aging. *American Journal of Physiology - Regulatory, Integrative and Comparative Physiology*, Vol. 287, pp. 1244-1249, ISSN: 0363-6119, EISSN: 1522-1490

Navarro, A.; Boveris, A.; Bández, M.J.; Sánchez-Pino, M.J.; Gómez, C.; Muntane, G. & Ferrer, I. (2009). Human brain cortex: mitochondrial oxidative damage and adaptive response in Parkinson's disease and in dementia with Lewy bodies. *Free Radicals in Biology and Medicine*, Vol. 46, pp. 1574-1580, ISSN: 0891-5849

Navarro, A. & Boveris, A. (2009). Brain mitochondrial dysfunction and oxidative damage in Parkinson's disease. *Journal of Bioenergetics and Biomembranes*, Vol. 41, pp. 517-521. ISSN: 0145-479X. EISSN: 1573-6881

Navarro, A.; Bández, M.; Gómez, C.; Sánchez-Pino, M.; Repetto, M.G. & Boveris, A. (2010). Effects of rotenone and pyridaben on complex I electron transfer and on mitochondrial nitric oxide synthase functional activity. *Journal of Bioenergetics and Biomembranes*, Vol. 42, pp. 405-412, ISSN: 0145-479X. EISSN: 1573-6881

Opazo, C.; Barría, M.I.; Ruiz, F.H. & Inestrosa, N.C. (2003). Copper reduction by copper binding proteins and its relation to neurodegenerative diseases. *Biometals*, Vol. 16, pp. 91-98, ISSN: 0966-0844, EISSN: 1572-8773

Pardo Andreu, G.L; Inada, N.M.; Vercesi, A.E. & Curti, C. (2009). Uncoupling and oxidative stress in liver mitochondrial isolated from rats with acute iron overload. *Archives Toxicology*, Vol. 83, pp. 47-53, ISSN: 0340-5761, EISSN: 1432-0738

Petrozzi, L.; Ricci, G.; Giglioli, N.J.; Siciliano, G. & Mancuso, M. (2007). Mitochondria and neurodegeneration. *Bioscience Reports*, Vol. 27, pp. 87-104, ISSN: 0144-8463, EISSN: 1573-4935

Quinn N. (1989). Multiple system atrophy-the nature of the beast. *Journal Neurology Neurosurgery Psychiatry*, Vol. 52, pp. 78-89, ISSN: 00223050. EISSN: 1468330X

Repetto, M.G.; Reides, C.; Evelson, P.; Kohan, S.; Lustig, E.S. de & Llesuy, S. (1999). Peripheral markers of oxidative stress in probable Alzheimer patients. *European Journal of Clinical Investigation*, Vol. 29, pp. 643-649, ISSN: 0014-2972, EISSN: 1365-2362

Repetto, M.G. & Llesuy, S.F. (2004). Peripheral markers of oxidative stress in neurological patients. Reprinted from XIII Bienal Meeting of the Society for Free Radical Research International (SFRR). In: Boveris, A. (ed.), *Proceedings of the Society for Experimental Biology and Medicine*, John Wiley & Sons Inc Publisher: NJ, USA, pp. 251-255, ISSN: 0037-9727, EISSN: 1525-1373

Repetto, M.G. (2008). Clinical use of chemiluminescence assays for the determination of systemic oxidative stress. In: Álvarez, S.; Evelson P. (ed.), *Handbook of chemiluminescent methods in oxidative stress assessment*. Transworld Research Network: Kerala, India; pp. 163-194, ISBN: 978-81-7895-334-2

Repetto, M.G. & Boveris A. (2011). Transition metals: bioinorganic and redox reactions in biological systems. In: *Transition metals: uses and characteristics*. Nova Science Publishers Inc (ed.): New York, USA. In press, ISBN: 978-1-61761-110-0

Rossi, L.; Lombardo, M.; Ciriolo, M. & Rotilio, G. (2004). Mitochondrial dysfunction in neurodegenerative diseases associated with copper imbalance. *Neurochemical Research*, Vol. 29, pp. 493-504, ISSN: 0364-3190, EISSN: 1573-6903

Schrag, A.; Ben-Shlomo, Y. & Quinn, N. (2002). How valid is the clinical diagnosis of Parkinson's disease in the community? *Journal Neurology Neurosurgery Psychiatry*, Vol. 73, pp. 529-534, ISSN: 00223050. EISSN: 1468330X

Serra, J.A.; Marschoff, E.R.; Domínguez, R.O.; Lustig, E.S. de; Famulari, A.L.; Bartolomé, E.L. & Guareschi, E.M. (2000). Comparison of the determination of superoxide dismutase and antioxidant capacity in neurological patients using two different procedures. *Clinica Chimica Acta*, Vol. 301, pp. 87–102, ISSN: 0009-8981

Serra, J.A.; Domínguez, R.O.; Lustig, E.S. de; Guareschi, E.M.; Famulari, A.L.; Bartolomé, E.L. & Marschoff, E.R. (2001). Parkinson's disease is associated with oxidative stress: comparison of peripheral antioxidant profiles in living Parkinson's, Alzheimer's and vascular dementia patients. *Journal of Neural Transmission*, Vol. 108, pp. 1135–1148, ISSN/ISBN: 03009564

Serra, J.A.; Domínguez, R.O.; Marschoff, E.R.; Guareschi E.M.; Famulari, A.L. & Boveris, A. (2009) Systemic oxidative stress associated with the neurological diseases of aging. *Neurochemical Research*, Vol. 34, pp. 2122–2132, ISSN/ISBN: 03643190

Sies, H. (1991). Role of reactive oxygen species in biological processes. *Wiener Klinische Wochenschrift*, Vol. 69, pp. 965–968, ISSN: 1613-7671

Sigleton, A.B.; Farrer, M.; Johnson, J.; Singleton, A.; Hague, S.; Kachergus, J.; Hulihan, M.; Peuralinna, T.; Dutra, A.; Nussbaum, R.; Lincoln, S.; Crawley, A.; Hanson, M.; Maraganore, D.; Adler, C.; Cookson, M.R.; Muenter, M.; Baptista, M.; Miller, D.; Blancato, J.; Hardy, J. & Gwinn-Hardy, K. (2003). Alpha-synuclein locus triplication causes Parkinson´s disease. *Science*, Vol. 302, pp. 841, ISSN: 0036-8075, EISSN 1095-9203

Spencer, W.; Jeyabalan, J.; Kichambre, S. & Gupta, R. (2011). Oxidatively generated DNA damage after Cu (II) catalysis of dopamine and related catecholamine neurotransmitters and neurotoxins: Role of reactive oxygen species. *Free Radicals in Biology and Medicine*, Vol. 50, pp. 139-147, ISSN: 0891-5849

4

The Execution Step in Parkinson's Disease – On the Vicious Cycle of Mitochondrial Complex I Inhibition, Iron Dishomeostasis and Oxidative Stress

Marco T. Núñez, Pamela Urrutia,
Natalia Mena and Pabla Aguirre
University of Chile
Chile

1. Introduction

The evidence for the participation of redox-active iron and reactive oxygen species (ROS) in a number of neurodegenerative diseases, including, Huntington's disease, Alzheimer's disease, Friedreich's ataxia, Amyotrophic lateral sclerosis (ALS) and Parkinson's disease is by now unquestionable.

In particular, in the case of Parkinson's disease (PD) iron accumulation has been demonstrated in the dopaminergic neurons of the substantia nigra pars compacta and neuronal death in this area is prevented by pharmacological agents with iron chelating capacity. Other pathognomonic signs of PD include inhibition of mitochondrial complex I and decreased glutathione (GSH) content. In this chapter we will discuss the effects of complex I inhibition on Fe-S cluster synthesis and iron homeostasis, and the positive feedback loop between iron, glutathione and ROS that ends in cell death. We will also discuss the possible role of hepcidin as a mediator of inflammatory stimuli that trigger iron dishomeostasis.

2. Iron homeostasis and dishomeostasis - the role of iron transporters on iron accumulation

2.1 Iron homeostasis

The components of neuronal iron homeostasis are shown in Figure 1. The scheme includes transferrin and transferrin receptor (TfR), inflow (DMT1; SLC11A2) and efflux (ferroportin 1, FPN1) iron transporters, the iron storage protein ferritin, the ferrireductase Dcytb, responsible for the reduction of extracellular Fe^{3+} to Fe^{2+} prior to transport by DMT1, and the ferroxidase ceruloplasmin, responsible for the oxidation of Fe^{2+} after transport by FPN1 and prior to the binding by apoTf. Transferrin-bound iron uptake starts with the binding of transferrin to surface receptors, followed by internalization into the endosomal system, release of iron mediated by the acidification of the endosome, reduction possibly mediated by Steap3, and transport into the cytosol by endosomal DMT1. Once in the cytoplasm, Fe^{2+}

becomes part of the labile or reactive iron pool where it distributes to mitochondria, neuromelanin and ferritin or engages in electron exchange reactions (Kakhlon & Cabantchik, 2002; Kruszewski, 2003). All the components described in Figure 1 have been detected in the brain (Haeger et al., 2010; Moos et al., 2007; Rouault et al., 2009), with the exception of Steap3, described in erythroid precursor cells (Ohgami et al., 2005).

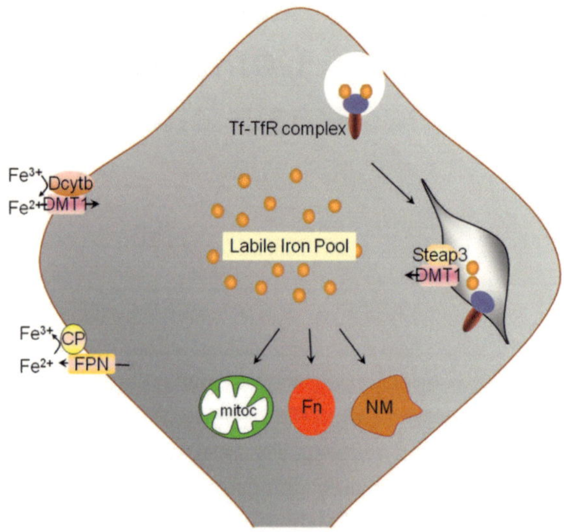

Fig. 1. **Components of neural iron homeostasis.** The molecular components comprise the transferrin-transferrin receptor complex, inflow (DMT1) and efflux (ferroportin, FPN1) iron transporters, the iron storage protein ferritin, the ferrireductase Dcytb, responsible for the reduction of Fe^{3+} prior to transport by DMT1 and the ferroxidase ceruloplasmin, responsible for the oxidation of Fe^{2+} after transport by FPN1 and prior to Fe^{3+} binding to apoTf.

The mammalian DMT1 gene undergoes alternative splicing. The 1A and 1B mRNA DMT1 variants originate from alternative splicing at the 5' end (exons 1A and 1B), while the +IRE or -IRE variants originate from splicing on the 3' end (exons 16/16A and 17) (Hubert & Hentze, 2002). These variants give raise to four DMT1 protein isoforms, all of them active in Fe^{2+} transport (Ludwiczek et al., 2007).

It is generally accepted that the two +IRE isoforms are post-transcriptionally regulated by the IRE/IRP system, which regulates translation of iron homeostasis proteins, which include the TfR, DMT1 and ferritin, in response to the concentration of reactive iron in the cytoplasm (Garrick & Garrick, 2009). Knowledge of differential transcriptional regulation of DMT1 expression is emerging. Both the inflammatory cytokine nuclear factor kappa B (NFκB) and the nuclear factor Y regulate DMT1(1B) expression in embryonic carcinoma cells (Paradkar & Roth, 2006). In contrast, hypoxia up regulates expression of the DMT1(1A) isoform, presumably through activation of hypoxia inducible factor 1b (HIF1b) (Lis et al., 2005; Wang et al., 2010a).

2.2 Iron essentiality in the brain

Iron is an essential element for the development of early cognitive functions. Late fetal and early postnatal iron deficiency causes learning and memory disabilities in humans that persist following iron repletion (Lozoff et al., 1996; Grantham-McGregor & Ani, 2001; Beard & Connor, 2003; Felt et al., 2006). In animal models, nutritional iron deficiency interferes with hippocampus-depending learning (McEchron & Paronish, 2005; Ranade et al., 2008) and synaptic plasticity (Jorgenson et al., 2005). These functional failings have been ascribed to the iron requirements of metabolic pathways involved in neurotransmitter synthesis and myelin formation. Enzymes involved in neurotransmitter synthesis that contain iron as a prosthetic group are recognized targets of iron deficiency (Kwik-Uribe et al., 2000; Taneja et al., 1986; Youdim et al., 1980). Tryptophan hydroxylase, required for serotonin synthesis, tyrosine hydroxylase, required for dopamine and norepinephrine synthesis, monoamine oxidases A and B involved in dopamine catabolism, glutamate decarboxylase , involved in gamma-aminobutyric acid synthesis and glutamate transaminase, involved in L-glutamate synthesis, belong to this group.

Current understanding of the molecular mechanisms underlying the essential role of iron in neuronal function is in large part unknown. Just of late, a role for iron in synaptic plasticity and the associated postsynaptic Ca^{2+} signals has begun to emerge (Hidalgo et al., 2007; Hidalgo & Núñez, 2007). Recent work has shown that in hippocampal neurons, iron chelation with desferrioxamine blocks NMDA-induced calcium signals and the ensuing ERK1/2 activation (Muñoz et al., 2011). Moreover, iron chelation decreases basal synaptic transmission and inhibits iron-induced synaptic stimulation in hippocampal slices, and also impairs sustained long-term potentiation (LTP) induced by strong stimulation. Together, these results suggest that upon NMDA receptor stimulation, iron is required for the generation of calcium signals which in turn promote ERK1/2 activation, an essential step of sustained LTP.

Iron concentration in cerebrospinal fluid (CSF) ranges between 0.2 and 1.1 μM whereas transferrin concentration is around 0.24 μM (Symons & Gutteridge, 1998; Moos & Morgan, 1998). Thus, CSF iron often exceeds the binding capacity of transferrin, and non transferrin bound iron (NTBI) uptake is expected to occur in neurons that express DMT1.

In the brain, DMT1 is expressed in hippocampal pyramidal and granule cells, cerebellar granule cells, pyramidal cells of the piriform cortex, substantia nigra and the ventral portion of the anterior olfactory nucleus, striatum, cerebellum, hippocampus and thalamus, as well as in vascular cells throughout the brain and ependymal cells in the third ventricle (Gunshin et al., 1997; Williams et al., 2000; Burdo et al., 2001).

The pervasive presence of DMT1 in neurons suggests that this transporter is necessary for their regular function (Hidalgo & Núñez, 2007; Wright & Baccarelli, 2007; Pelizzoni et al., 2011; Muñoz et al., 2011). Hippocampal neurons express the 1B, but not the 1A, isoform (Haeger et al., 2010). Since expression of the IB isoform responds to NFkB, regulation of neuronal DMT1 levels by inflammatory stimuli is possible.

2.3 Iron toxicity

Iron is an intrinsic ROS producer. When one or more of its six ligand binding sites is not tightly bound iron becomes redox-active and capable to engage in one-electron exchange reactions producing free radicals (Graf et al., 1984). This is due to the occurrence of the Haber-Weiss and Fenton reactions. The thermodynamic balance of these reactions indicates that in the reductive environment of the cell, iron, in the presence of oxygen, catalyzes the consumption of GSH and the production of the hydroxyl radical (Halliwell, 2006b; Bórquez et al., 2008). In dopaminergic cells, another source of free radicals derives from the non-enzymatic oxidation of dopamine mediated by redox-active iron, resulting in semiquinones and H_2O_2 production (Zoccarato et al., 2005). Thus, iron, both through the Fenton reaction or by dopamine oxidation, is a dangerous pro-oxidant agent.

Overwhelming evidence indicates that iron accumulation is a common feature of a number of neurodegenerative disorders of the central nervous system that include Huntington's disease, Alzheimer's disease, Friedreich's ataxia, Amyotrophic lateral sclerosis (ALS) and Parkinson's disease (Jellinger, 1999; Sayre et al., 2000; Bartzokis et al., 2000; Perry et al., 2003; Zecca et al., 2004; Berg & Youdim, 2006; Wilson, 2006; Weinreb et al., 2011).

Iron accumulation has been demonstrated in the dopaminergic neurons of the substantia nigra pars compacta (Youdim et al., 1989; Hirsch et al., 1991; Gorell et al., 1995; Vymazal et al., 1999). Interestingly, 1-methyl-4-phenyl-1,2,3,6-tetrahydropyridine (MPTP), a drug that causes experimental Parkinson's disease up regulates DMT1(+IRE) protein expression in mice ventral mesencephalon, where it increases neuronal death presumably through abnormal increases in cellular iron content (Salazar et al., 2008; Jiang et al., 2010). Additionally, DMT1(-IRE) mediates L-DOPA neurotoxicity in primary cortical neurons (Du et al., 2009).

The position of iron dishomeostasis in the progression of events leading to neuronal death is unknown, since iron accumulation has been detected in tissue from patients who have died after the final steps of the pathology. Nevertheless, since neuronal death caused by MPTP or 6-hydroxydopamine intoxication is blocked by pharmacologic or genetic chelation of iron (Kaur et al., 2003; Shachar et al., 2004; Youdim et al., 2004; Youdim & Buccafusco, 2005; Zheng et al., 2010) or by dysfunction of the iron transporter DMT1 (Salazar et al., 2008), it is possible that iron dishomeostasis takes place in the late stages of the disease as part of a vicious cycle resulting in uncontrolled oxidative damage and cell death. A recent study in mecencephalic dopaminergic neurons shows that low (0.25-0.5 μM) concentrations of MPP+, the active metabolite of MPTP and a potent mitochondrial complex I inhibitor, induces neuritic tree collapse without loss of cell viability (Gómez et al., 2010). This collapse was effectively prevented by decreasing iron supply or by the addition of antioxidants. Thus, it seems plausible that increased intracellular iron is involved in the early steps of dopaminergic neuron dysfunction.

Iron toxicity is not restricted to dopaminergic neurons. Neurotoxic concentrations of NMDA induces iron-induced the NO-Dexras1-PAP7 signaling cascade in glutamatergic PC12 cells. Upon activation, PAP7 binds to intracellular DMT1 and relocates it to the plasma membrane. Increased intracellular iron, the physiological function of DMT1, increases the production of hydroxyl radicals. Thus, the DMT1-iron uptake-hydroxyl radical signaling pathway appears to mediate NMDA neurotoxicity (Cheah et al., 2006).

3. Decreased mitochondrial Fe-S cluster synthesis as a consequence of complex I dysfunction

3.1 Mitochondrial complex I inhibition in PD

Decreased activity of mitochondrial complex I, found in post-mortem tissue of PD patients (Schapira et al., 1990; Tretter et al., 2004; Banerjee et al., 2009; Hattingen et al., 2009), is probably a founding event in neuronal death. Interestingly, this phenotype is replicated in experimental PD induced by MPTP intoxication, which induces parkinsonian symptoms in mice, primates and humans. Inhibition of complex I leads to impaired mitochondrial ATP production and an accelerated production ROS (Langston et al., 1983; Singer & Ramsay, 1990; Scotcher et al., 1990; Noll et al., 1992).

The association between complex I inhibition and PD is further supported by the observation that rats intoxicated with the selective inhibitor of complex I rotenone, develop a syndrome similar to PD, characterized by neuronal degeneration and the formation of inclusion bodies rich in alpha-synuclein (Betarbet et al., 2000). Likewise, inhibition of glutaredoxin 2, an enzyme involved in Fe-S synthesis, produced an alteration in iron metabolism in a model of Parkinson's disease (Lee et al., 2009). Additionally, mutations in mitochondrial proteins PINK-1 and DJ-1 result in a genetic form of PD, leading further support for an important role of mitochondria in PD neurodegeneration (Bonifati et al., 2003; Valente et al., 2004; Blackinton et al., 2005).

ROS seem to have a negative effect on complex I activity. Experiments with isolated synaptosomal mitochondria revealed that low concentrations of H_2O_2 decrease complex I activity by 10%. This relatively minor effect of H_2O_2 was additive to partial inhibition of complex I induced by low (5 nM-1 μM) concentrations of rotenone (Chinopoulos & Adam-Vizi, 2001). Similarly, sub-mitochondrial particles exposed to $O_2^{\cdot-}$, H_2O_2, or $\cdot OH$ presented decreased activity of NADH dehydrogenase, a marker of complex I activity (Zhang et al., 1990). Thus, an initial inhibition of complex I could generate a positive loop between ROS generation and further complex I inhibition.

3.2 Mitochondrial iron-sulfur cluster synthesis

By being the locus of heme and iron-sulfur (Fe-S) clusters synthesis, the mitochondria is an essential organelle for cell iron homeostasis (Rouault & Tong, 2005). Fe-S clusters, formed by the tetrahedral coordination of sulfur groups with Fe atoms, are small inorganic cofactors believed to be the first catalysts in the evolution of macromolecules. In eukaryotes the most common species of Fe-S clusters are the 2Fe-2S and 4Fe-4S forms (Rouault & Tong, 2005; Lill & Muhlenhoff, 2008; Ye & Rouault, 2010). Today, Fe-S clusters are found as prostetic groups of a wide range of proteins. In mitochondria, proteins such as NADH dehydrogenase (complex I), succinate dehydrogenase (complex II), cytochrome c reductase (complex III) and aconitase contain Fe-S clusters. Fe-S clusters are also exported to cytosol for incorporation into cytoplasmic proteins that require them, such as aconitase, xanthine oxidase, glutamine phosphoribosyl pyrophosphate amidotransferase and nuclear proteins involved in DNA repair (Martelli et al., 2007). For a compendium of Fe-S clusters see The Prosthetic Groups and Metal Ions in Protein Active Sites (PROMISE) http://metallo.scripps.edu/promise/MAIN.html).

The biogenesis of Fe-S clusters in mitochondria has been proposed as a sensor of the cellular Fe status, being high Fe-S cluster levels indicative of high intracellular iron concentrations and vice versa (Rouault & Tong, 2005). Additionally, the loss of function of proteins involved in mitochondrial biogenesis of the clusters or in cluster export to the cytoplasm, has been associated with deregulation of cytoplasmic Fe metabolism, mitochondrial accumulation of Fe and clinical manifestations such as sideroblastic microcytic anemia, myopathy and ataxia (Rouault & Tong, 2008). Recent data from our laboratory indicate that inhibition of complex I by rotenone results in decreased synthesis of Fe-S clusters, as shown by the decreased activity of the Fe-S cluster-containing enzymes cytosolic aconitase, mitochondrial aconitase, xanthine oxidase and glutamyl phosphoribosyltransferase as well as the activation of cytosolic Iron Regulatory Protein 1 (IRP1) (Mena et al., 2011). We think that as a consequence of decrease synthesis of Fe-S complexes, and the consequent activation of IRP1, a decreased activity of complex I results in a false "low iron" signal that activates the iron uptake system.

In consequence, diminished Fe-S cluster synthesis could play a fundamental role in promoting the accumulation of iron observed in PD. Future research is needed to evaluate its participation in neurodegenerative diseases in which iron accumulation is observed.

4. Cell death in PD: necrosis, apoptosis or necroptosis?

The two main pathways of cell death in neurodegenerative and other ROS-related disorders are apoptosis and necrosis. Apoptosis, also termed "programmed cell death" is understood as a regulated process consisting in the activation of caspases by endogenous or external stress signals. Necrosis, morphologically characterized by a gain in cell volume, plasma membrane rupture and subsequent loss of intracellular contents, is considered as an uncontrolled form of cell death. Lately, evidence is accumulating indicating that necrotic death may be also regulated by a set of signal transduction pathways (Kroemer et al., 2009). A third cell death pathway is "necroptosis" or programmed necrosis. Necroptosis death begins by activation of death receptors and its execution involves the active disintegration of mitochondrial, lysosome and plasma membranes. Necroptosis participates in the pathogenesis of several diseases, including ischemic injury, neurodegeneration and viral infection (Vandenabeele et al., 2010). The execution step of necroptosis includes mitochondrial dysfunction, decreased ATP levels, increased oxidative stress and increased labile iron pool mediated by increased ferritin degradation (Vandenabeele et al., 2010).

While the evidence that iron overload in the brain causes necrotic death is scanty (Lobner & Ali, 2002; Maharaj et al., 2006), overwhelming evidence points to apoptosis as the most common pathway of death (Wang et al., 1998; Zaman et al., 1999; Barzilai et al., 2000; Kuperstein & Yavin, 2003; Liu et al., 2003; Zheng et al., 2005; Kooncumchoo et al., 2006; Xu et al., 2008; Kupershmidt et al., 2009; Shi et al., 2010; Ziv et al., 1997). The possible participation of necroptosis in neurodegenerative processes has not been explored but the common characteristics of redox-active iron, oxidative stress and mitochondrial dysfunction, all of which contribute to the execution of necroptosis, make possible that necroptosis may be involved in iron-associated neuronal death.

5. Inflammation and hepcidin – a nexus to iron dishomeostasis

In addition to iron accumulation, other event strongly associated with neuronal death in PD and other neurodegenerative disorders is the presence of inflammatory processes characterized by the occurrence of reactive microglia and the massive production of proinflammatory cytokines. Although both phenomena have been studied as independent events leading to the progression of disease, the recent identification in central nervous system of hepcidin, a hormone that mediates the relationship between systemic iron homeostasis and inflammation, might change our views.

5.1 Hepcidin, the master regulator of iron homeostasis

Hepcidin is a cationic peptide of 25 amino acids secreted into blood circulation by the liver. The mature peptide derives from a precursor of 84 amino acids that after two successive proteolytic cleavages generates the mature peptide. Hepcidin was initially described as a peptide with antimicrobial activity (Krause et al., 2000), however further studies revealed that it also acts as a major regulator of circulating iron levels (Nicolas et al., 2001; Pigeon et al., 2001).

Two processes contribute to the levels of circulating iron, the recycling of senescent red blood cells (RBC) and intestinal iron absorption. The recycling by spleen macrophages of heme iron from senescent RBC is the main contributor of iron to the circulation, providing about 95% of daily turnover. The recycling of RBC iron comprise the phagocytosis of senescent RBC, the release of the iron in the heme moiety of hemoglobin by heme oxygenase-1 and the subsequent release of this iron into the plasma mediated by FPN1 (De Domenico et al., 2008; Kovtunovych et al., 2010).

The physiological function of hepcidin is to down-regulate the levels of circulating iron. It does so by down-regulation of the iron exotransporter FPN1 in macrophages. The binding of hepcidin to FPN1 present in the plasma membrane of splenic macrophages induces the endocytosis of the complex and the subsequent degradation of FPN1 in the lysosome (Nemeth et al., 2004). The decreased levels of FPN1 lead to the accumulation of iron in macrophages and the decrease of circulating iron (Ganz, 2006).

Hepcidin synthesis is regulated by multiple stimuli that have an effect in the regulation of circulating iron levels: (i) increased iron levels induce an increase in hepcidin synthesis in the liver through a mechanism that depends on transferrin receptor 1 and 2, the hemochromatosis protein (HFE) and hemojuvelin/BMP (De Domenico et al., 2007; Gao et al., 2010); (ii) erythropoietin, a hormone that stimulates red blood cell production. Erythropoietin blocks hepcidin synthesis in order to increase circulating levels of iron necessary for hemoglobin synthesis (Wrighting & Andrew, 2006; Pinto et al., 2008); (iii) inflammatory stimuli, mainly the cytokine IL-6, that through stimulation of hepcidin synthesis reduces circulating levels of iron, preventing its use for the proliferation of pathogens (Wrighting & Andrews, 2006) and (iv) hypoxia, that through activation of the hypoxia inducible factor I down-regulates the synthesis of hepcidin in order to increase blood iron levels required for the synthesis of heme in new red blood cells, to counteract oxygen deprivation (Peyssonnaux et al., 2007).

The interaction of hepcidin with FPN1 generates an antiinflammatory response. Binding of hepcidin to FPN1 induces the recruitment and activation of the tyrosine kinase Janus kinase 2 (JAK-2) (De Domenico et al., 2009), which phosphorylates FPN1 in 2 adjacent tyrosines present in a cytosolic loop. Activation of JAK-2 allows for the phosphorylation and translocation to the nucleus of signal transducer and activator of transcription 3 (STAT-3), which induces the expression of genes that encode for proteins whose role is to suppress the inflammatory response (De Domenico et al., 2010a). Within them are the receptor for interleukin 17, a cytokine with antiinflammatory properties and the suppressor of cytokine signaling 3 (SOCS-3) (De Domenico et al., 2010b), a modulator that inhibits the transduction pathways associated with receptors for proinflammatory cytokines IL-6 and tumor necrosis factor-alpha (Croker et al., 2008).

5.2 Hepcidin expression in the CNS

Hepcidin shows a wide distribution in the CNS, most notably in the midbrain, with a clear presence in the superior colliculus, the geniculate nucleus, some fiber bundles of the substantia nigra pars reticulata and the substantia nigra pars compacta (Zechel et al., 2006) and the striatum (Wang et al., 2010b). Hepcidin is expressed mainly in glial cells, as well as in neurons and endothelial cells of choroid plexus (Zechel et al., 2006; Marques et al., 2009).

Hepcidin expression changes with age: increased mRNA levels of hepcidin in cortex, striatum and hippocampus have been observed with aging (Wang et al., 2010b).

As stated above, hepcidin synthesis is induced by inflammatory stimuli. Bacterial lipopolisaccharide (LPS), a potent inflammatory agent, induces liver hepcidin expression. LPS also increases hepcidin expression in the brain. After an intraperitoneal injection of LPS, a transient transcription of the gene for hepcidin ensues in the choroid plexus, which correlates with increased levels of pro-hepcidin in the cerebrospinal fluid (Marques et al., 2009). The highest hepcidin expression was observed at 3 hours returning to baseline levels 24 hours after the injection. Interestingly, LPS treatment induces a 10-fold increase in hepcidin expression in the substantia nigra (Wang et al., 2008), which correlates with a marked increase in iron levels observed in this region in PD.

5.3 FPN1 expression in the CNS

As described above, the iron transporter FPN1 is the receptor for hepcidin. The expression of this transporter-receptor in mouse brain is quite ubiquitous; it is present in oligodendrocytes, microglia, astrocytes and neurons (Song et al., 2010). Space-temporal expression of FPN1 in neurons is variable (Moos & Rosengren Nielsen, 2006). In young brain a high immunoreactivity is found in the neurons of the hippocampus and striatum (cell bodies and in projection fibers), a mild expression in the substantia nigra pars compacta and the superior colliculus and low expression in the substantia nigra pars reticulata (Boserup et al., 2011). In the adult brain, FPN1 immunoreactivity is lower in the projections of the striatum, but no differences have been found in neuronal cell bodies (Moos & Rosengren Nielsen, 2006).

An interesting fact is that the spatial distribution of FPN1 and hepcidin are similar. Although the effects of hepcidin on FPN1 levels can differ according to cell type (Chaston et al., 2008), the injection of hepcidin in mice lateral cerebral ventricle, causes a decrease in the levels of FPN1 in the cerebral cortex, hippocampus and striatum (Wang et al., 2010b), suggesting that their cellular targets in the brain generate the same response than that observed in macrophages, that is, iron retention inside the cells. This conclusion is strengthened by the fact that high doses of hepcidin produce an increase in the iron storage protein ferritin, thus indicating increased cellular iron concentration in these brain areas.

Unexpected for a high cell iron situation, in the hippocampus and cortex of rats treatment with hepcidin induces the decrease of both FPN1 protein and mRNA and an increase in total DMT1 (Li et al., 2011), a situation that should drive further iron accumulation.

Hippocampal neurons in culture treated with hepcidin also show a decrease in the expression of FPN1, which is reflected in a reduction of the iron released from these cells (Wang et al., 2010b). There are no studies in other cell types, however, and it is possible that the response in glial cells should be similar to neurons and macrophages, particularly since microglia cells derive from the same precursor cells that give rise to macrophages (Ginhoux et al., 2010).

5.4 Hepcidin - a nexus between inflammation and iron accumulation in PD

Reports of some cases of PD associated with head trauma (Lees, 1997) and encephalitis (Jang et al., 2009) strongly suggest that inflammation can promote this neurodegenerative disease. Currently, there is a growing array of evidences describing inflammatory properties in the parkinsonian brain. Indeed, many cases of PD are accompanied by general inflammation of the brain, with a dramatic proliferation of reactive amoeboid macrophages and microglia HLA-DR+ in the substantia nigra (McGeer et al., 1988). In the striatum, macrophage proliferation is accompanied by high expression of pro-inflammatory cytokines such as TNF-α, IL-1β, IFN-γ and IL-6 (Mogi et al., 1994; Muller et al., 1998), which are expressed by glial cells (Hirsch et al., 1998). Particularly, the presence of IL-1β, IL-6 and TNF-α has been observed in cerebrospinal fluid and the basal ganglia of patients with PD (Nagatsu, 2002). In addition to increased expression of inflammatory cytokines by activated microglia, factors released by dead dopaminergic cells appear to increase the neuroinflammatory and immune response, leading to irreversible destruction of these cells (Orr et al., 2002).

In general, pro-inflammatory cytokines such as TNF-α and IL-1 have neurotoxic effects, while anti-inflammatory molecules are neuroprotective (Allan & Rothwell, 2001). Intriguingly, IL-6, a classical proinflammatory cytokine, has a dual effect, at low concentrations it protects for neuronal death while at larger concentrations it is highly toxic (Li et al., 2009).

It is not completely understood how the inflammatory response is generated in PD. It has been proposed that the inflammatory response is a product of the oxidative load induced by the metabolism of dopamine (DA). Deamination of DA by monoamine oxidase generates hydrogen peroxide (Gotz et al., 1994), whereas the not enzymatic auto-oxidation produces additionally DA quinones and semiquinones (Stokes et al., 1999). These metabolites, in conjunction with the highly toxic hydroxyl radical generated through the Fenton reaction, are likely to alter protein structure and decrease glutathione levels by generating increased oxidative stress (Halliwell, 2006a), which could lead to activation of an inflammatory response (Park et al., 1999; Di Loreto et al., 2004). In fact, antioxidants such as green tea polyphenols are strong inhibitors of the inflammatory response (Conner and Grisham, 1996; Singh et al., 2010), and may reduce the incidence of dementia, AD, and PD (Mandel et al., 2011).

An inflammatory component has also been observed in several animal models of PD: the injection of 6-hydroxydopamine, MPTP and rotenone generates microglial activation, astrogliogenesis and secretion of inflammatory cytokines (Barnum & Tansey, 2010). The injection of LPS, a potent inducer of inflammation, has also been used as a model of PD. Stereotaxic injection of LPS in the nigro-striatal pathway induced a strong macrophage/microglial reaction in substantia nigra, being the substantia nigra more responsive than the striatum to the inflammatory stimulus (Herrera et al., 2000). Furthermore, no detectable damage to either the GABAergic or the serotoninergic neurons was observed, a demonstration of the particular sensitivity sustantia nigra pars compacta neurons to inflammatory stimuli.

The abundant evidence for the existence of inflammatory processes in PD, and the induction of hepcidin synthesis by cytoquines such as IL-6, suggest that brain hepcidin levels should be higher in inflammatory processes. Hepcidin should induce differential iron accumulation in the diverse cell types present in the brain, based in the different levels of expression of its receptor, FPN1. In the adult brain, the expression of FPN1 is lower in neurons than in glia, thus hepcidin would induce a redistribution of iron, accumulating it mainly in the glial cells, which would act as an "iron sponge". Additionally, the activation of the signal transduction pathway associated with the binding of hepcidin to FPN1, could reduce the inflammatory response generated during neurodegeneration. Alternatively, the decrease in FPN1 induced by hepcidin binding in neurons could result in increased iron accumulation and oxidative stress, which could accelerate the death of these cells.

Future studies on the participation of hepcidin on the disregulation of iron homeostasis in glia and neurons as a response to inflammation, will provide valuable information about its protective or deleterious role in the progress of neurodegenerative diseases.

6. Glutathione metabolism in PD – a cause or a consequence of increased ROS and increased iron content?

The tripeptide glutathione (γ-L-glutamyl-L-cysteinylglycine) is the most abundant and the main antioxidant agent in the central nervous system, where it reaches mM concentrations (Meister & Anderson, 1983; Dringen et al., 2000). In its redox cycling, glutathione is present either in its reduced (GSH) form or its oxidized disulfide (GSSG) form, the ratio GSH/GSSG being faithful reflection of the redox state of the cell (Schafer & Buettner, 2001).

Early post-mortem studies revealed decreased levels of GSH in degenerating substantia nigra of PD patients (Perry et al., 1982; Sofic et al., 1988; Sian et al., 1994), the observation implicating that GSH depletion may play a major role in the neurodegenerative process. The question arises whether GSH depletion is an early event during the progression of the disease or a reflection of increased oxidative stress resulting, for example, from mitochondrial complex I inhibition or from iron accumulation.

Chronic sub-maximal inhibition of GSH synthesis in N27 dopaminergic cells results in about 50% inhibition of mitochondrial electron transport chain complex I without ensuing cell death, inhibition that was reversed upon removal of the inhibitor (Chinta & Andersen, 2006). Thus, increased oxidative stress generated by complex I inhibition should result in decreased GHS levels and further inhibition of complex I. Conversely, a decrease in GSH levels, provoked by unknown causes, could result in inhibition of complex I activity.

Iron induces the consumption of GSH. After exposure to increasing concentrations of iron, SH-SY5Y dopaminergic cells undergo sustained iron accumulation and a biphasic change in intracellular GSH levels, increasing at low (1-5 μM) Fe and decreasing thereafter. Indeed, cell exposure to high iron concentrations (20-80 μM) markedly decreases the GSH / GSSG molar ratio and the GSH half-cell reduction potential, which associated with loss of cell viability (Núñez et al., 2004).

It is therefore possible that a decrease in GSH levels is a consequence of the increased oxidative load produced by the increase in intracellular Fe. Nevertheless, increased iron and decreased GSH may be intertwined in a positive feedback loop, since in dopaminergic neurons the pharmacological reduction of GSH levels results in increased levels of TfR and an increased labile iron pool (Kaur et al., 2009). Thus, the question remains as to which of the three processes initiates the oxidative spiral, but a reasonable assumption is that if one of them ensues the others will follow.

7. A positive feedback loop in the death of neurons

We propose that inhibition of mitochondrial complex I by endogenous and/or exogenous toxins, and inflammatory processes produced by trauma or other causes, result in a vicious cycle of increased oxidative stress, increased iron accumulation and decreased GSH content (Figure 2). In this scheme, neuronal death linked to complex I dysfunction is brought about by a positive feedback loop in which complex I inhibition results in decreased Fe-S cluster synthesis, IRP1 activation, increased DMT1 and TfR expression and iron accumulation. Complex I dysfunction and increased cellular iron result in decreased GSH levels. Both increased oxidative stress and low GSH levels further inhibit complex I activity. Central to this scheme is the deregulation of iron homeostasis since iron chelators effectively block cell death and prevent early events in neurodegeneration such as neuritic tree shortening. Another input to this cycle is brought about by inflammatory cytoquines that induce hepcidin synthesis which, by inducing FPN1 degradation, results in increased cellular iron.

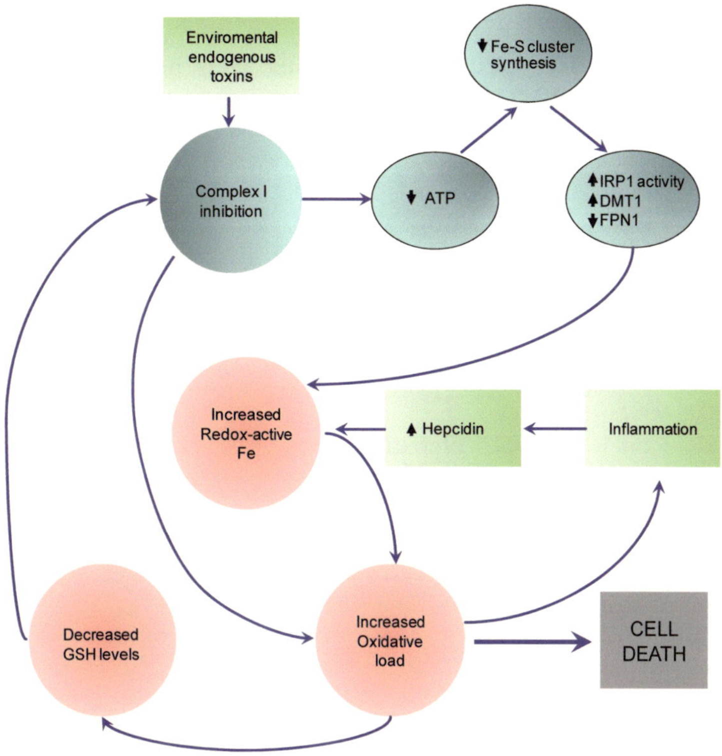

Fig. 2. **A positive feedback loop resulting in uncontrolled oxidative load.** Complex I inhibition results in decreased levels of ATP and decreased Fe-S synthesis (see text). Decreased Fe-S cluster synthesis results in activation of IRP1 that needs a 4Fe-4S cluster to acquire its inactive state. Increased IRP1 activity results in increased DMT1 and transferrin receptor and decreased FPN1 synthesis, which results in increased iron accumulation. Increased iron induces increased oxidative stress and GSH consumption. Both increased oxidative stress and decreased GSH produce further complex I inhibition.

8. Conclusion

Diminished activity of mitochondrial complex I, iron accumulation, oxidative stress and inflammation are common pathognomonic signs of sporadic PD. It is possible that the initiation of any one of these processes will initiate or enhance the others, through the generation of positive feedback loops that will produce apoptotic neuronal death. Intervention of these positive loops should result in prolonged life of the affected neurons. Still unanswered is the question of why substantia nigra pars compacta neurons are so particular prone to this disregulation.

9. Acknowledgment

This work was financed by grant 1100599 from Fondo Nacional de Ciencia y Tecnología Chile, (FONDECYT) and by project ICM-P05-001-F from the Millennium Scientific Initiative, Ministerio de Economía, Chile.

10. References

Allan, S. M. & Rothwell, N. J. (2001). Cytokines and acute neurodegeneration. *Nat Rev Neurosci*, Vol. 2, No. 10, (October 2001), pp. 734-744, ISSN 1471-003X

Banerjee, R., Starkov, A. A., Beal, M. F. & Thomas, B. (2009). Mitochondrial dysfunction in the limelight of Parkinson's disease pathogenesis. *Biochim Biophys Acta*, Vol. 1792, No. 7, (Decembre 2008), pp. 651-663, ISSN 0006-3002

Barnum, C. J. & Tansey, M. G. (2010). Modeling neuroinflammatory pathogenesis of Parkinson's disease. *Prog Brain Res*, Vol. 184, (October 2010), pp. 113-132, ISSN 1875-7855

Bartzokis, G., Sultzer, D., Cummings, J., Holt, L. E., Hance, D. B., Henderson, V. W. & Mintz, J. (2000). In vivo evaluation of brain iron in Alzheimer disease using magnetic resonance imaging. *Arch Gen Psychiatry*, Vol. 57, No. 1, (January 2000), pp. 47-53, ISSN 0003-990X.

Barzilai, A., Zilkha-Falb, R., Daily, D., Stern, N., Offen, D., Ziv, I., Melamed, E. & Shirvan, A. (2000). The molecular mechanism of dopamine-induced apoptosis: identification and characterization of genes that mediate dopamine toxicity. *J Neural Transm Suppl*, Vol. 60, (February 2001), pp. 59-76, ISSN 0303-6995

Beard, J. L. & Connor, J. R. (2003). Iron status and neural functioning. *Annu Rev Nutr*, Vol. 23, (April 2003), pp. 41-58, ISSN 0199-9885

Berg, D. & Youdim, M. B. (2006). Role of iron in neurodegenerative disorders. *Top Magn Reson Imaging*, Vol. 17, No. 1, (December 2006), pp. 5-17, ISSN 0899-3459

Betarbet, R., Sherer, T. B., MacKenzie, G., Garcia-Osuna, M., Panov, A. V. &Greenamyre, J. T. (2000). Chronic systemic pesticide exposure reproduces features of Parkinson's disease. *Nat Neurosci*, Vol. 3, No. 12, (December 2000), pp. 1301-1306, ISSN 1097-6256.

Blackinton, J., Ahmad, R., Miller, D. W., van der Brug, M. P., Canet-Aviles, R. M., Hague, S. M., Kaleem, M. & Cookson, M. R. (2005). Effects of DJ-1 mutations and polymorphisms on protein stability and subcellular localization. *Brain Res Mol Brain Res*, Vol. 134, No. 1, (March 2005), pp. 76-83, ISSN 0169-328X.

Bonifati, V., Rizzu, P., van Baren, M. J., Schaap, O., Breedveld, G. J., Krieger, E., Dekker, M. C., Squitieri, F., Ibanez, P., Joosse, M., van Dongen, J. W., Vanacore, N., van Swieten, J. C., Brice, A., Meco, G., van Duijn, C. M., Oostra, B. A. & Heutink, P. (2003). Mutations in the DJ-1 gene associated with autosomal recessive early-onset parkinsonism. *Science*, Vol. 299, No. 5604, (November 2002), pp. 256-259, ISSN 1095-9203.

Bórquez, D., Valdés, P. & Nuñéz, M.T. (2008). Iron Toxicity: A critical Review on its Role in Parkinson´s Disease, In: *Neurodegenerative Diseases: From Molecular Concepts to Therapeutic Targets*, Von Bernhardi, R. & Inestrosa, N., pp. 189-204, Nova Science Publishers, ISBN 978-160-4561-67-8, New York, USA.

Boserup, M. W., Lichota, J., Haile, D. & Moos, T. (2011). Heterogenous distribution of ferroportin-containing neurons in mouse brain. *Biometals*, (January 2011), ISSN 1572-8773.

Burdo, J. R., Menzies, S. L., Simpson, I. A., Garrick, L. M., Garrick, M. D., Dolan, K. G., Haile, D. J., Beard, J. L. & Connor, J. R. (2001). Distribution of divalent metal transporter 1 and metal transport protein 1 in the normal and Belgrade rat. *J Neurosci Res*, Vol. 66, No. 6, (December 2002), pp. 1198-1207, ISSN 0360-4012.

Chaston, T., Chung, B., Mascarenhas, M., Marks, J., Patel, B., Srai, S. K. & Sharp, P. (2008). Evidence for differential effects of hepcidin in macrophages and intestinal epithelial cells. *Gut*, Vol. 57, No. 3, (October 2007), pp. 374-382, ISSN 1468-3288.

Cheah, J. H., Kim, S. F., Hester, L. D., Clancy, K. W., Patterson, S. E., 3rd, Papadopoulos, V. & Snyder, S. H. (2006). NMDA receptor-nitric oxide transmission mediates neuronal iron homeostasis via the GTPase Dexras1. *Neuron*, Vol. 51, No. 4, (August 2006), pp. 431-440, ISSN 0896-6273.

Chinopoulos, C. & Adam-Vizi, V. (2001). Mitochondria deficient in complex I activity are depolarized by hydrogen peroxide in nerve terminals: relevance to Parkinson's disease. *J Neurochem*, Vol. 76, No. 1, (January 2001), pp. 302-306, ISSN 0022-3042.

Chinta, S. J. & Andersen, J. K. (2006). Reversible inhibition of mitochondrial complex I activity following chronic dopaminergic glutathione depletion in vitro: implications for Parkinson's disease. *Free Radic Biol Med*, Vol. 41, No. 9, (October 2006), pp. 1442-1448, ISSN 0891-5849.

Conner, E. M. &Grisham, M. B. (1996). Inflammation, free radicals, and antioxidants. *Nutrition*, Vol. 12, No. 4, (April 1996), pp. 274-277, ISSN 0899-9007.

Croker, B. A., Kiu, H. & Nicholson, S. E. (2008). SOCS regulation of the JAK/STAT signalling pathway. *Semin Cell Dev Biol*, Vol. 19, No. 4, (August 2008), pp. 414-422, ISSN 1084-9521.

De Domenico, I., Lo, E., Ward, D. M. & Kaplan, J. (2009). Hepcidin-induced internalization of ferroportin requires binding and cooperative interaction with Jak2. *Proc Natl Acad Sci U S A*, Vol. 106, No. 10, (February 2009), pp. 3800-3805, ISSN 1091-6490.

De Domenico, I., Lo, E., Ward, D. M. & Kaplan, J. (2010a). Human mutation D157G in ferroportin leads to hepcidin-independent binding of Jak2 and ferroportin down-regulation. *Blood*, Vol. 115, No. 14, (February 2010), pp. 2956-2959, ISSN 1528-0020.

De Domenico, I., McVey Ward, D. & Kaplan, J. (2008). Regulation of iron acquisition and storage: consequences for iron-linked disorders. *Nat Rev Mol Cell Biol*, Vol. 9, No. 1, (November 2007), pp. 72-81, ISSN 1471-0080.

De Domenico, I., Ward, D. M. & Kaplan, J. (2007). Hepcidin regulation: ironing out the details. *J Clin Invest*, Vol. 117, No. 7, (July 2007), pp. 1755-1758, ISSN 0021-9738.

De Domenico, I., Zhang, T. Y., Koening, C. L., Branch, R. W., London, N., Lo, E., Daynes, R. A., Kushner, J. P., Li, D., Ward, D. M. & Kaplan, J. (2010b). Hepcidin mediates transcriptional changes that modulate acute cytokine-induced inflammatory responses in mice. *J Clin Invest*, Vol. 120, No. 7, (June 2010), pp. 2395-2405, ISSN 1558-8238.

Di Loreto, S., Caracciolo, V., Colafarina, S., Sebastiani, P., Gasbarri, A. & Amicarelli, F. (2004). Methylglyoxal induces oxidative stress-dependent cell injury and up-regulation of interleukin-1beta and nerve growth factor in cultured hippocampal neuronal cells. *Brain Res*, Vol. 1006, No. 2, (March 2004), pp. 157-167, ISSN 0006-8993.

Dringen, R., Gutterer, J. M. & Hirrlinger, J. (2000). Glutathione metabolism in brain metabolic interaction between astrocytes and neurons in the defense against reactive oxygen species. *Eur J Biochem*, Vol. 267, No. 16, (August 2000), pp. 4912-4916, ISSN 0014-2956.

Du, F., Qian, Z. M., Zhu, L., Wu, X. M., Yung, W. H., Tsim, T. Y. & Ke, Y. (2009). L-DOPA neurotoxicity is mediated by up-regulation of DMT1-IRE expression. *PLoS One*, Vol. 4, No. 2, (February 2009), pp. e4593, ISSN 1932-6203.

Felt, B. T., Beard, J. L., Schallert, T., Shao, J., Aldridge, J. W., Connor, J. R., Georgieff, M. K. & Lozoff, B. (2006). Persistent neurochemical and behavioral abnormalities in adulthood despite early iron supplementation for perinatal iron deficiency anemia in rats. *Behav Brain Res*, Vol. 171, No. 2, (May 2006), pp. 261-270, ISSN 0166-4328.

Ganz, T. (2006). Hepcidin and its role in regulating systemic iron metabolism. *Hematology Am Soc Hematol Educ Program*, (November 2006), pp. 29-35, 507, ISSN 1520-4391.

Gao, J., Chen, J., De Domenico, I., Koeller, D. M., Harding, C. O., Fleming, R. E., Koeberl, D. D. & Enns, C. A. (2010). Hepatocyte-targeted HFE and TFR2 control hepcidin expression in mice. *Blood*, Vol. 115, No. 16, (February 2010), pp. 3374-3381, ISSN 1528-0020.

Garrick, M. D. & Garrick, L. M. (2009). Cellular iron transport. *Biochim Biophys Acta*, Vol. 1790, No. 5, (April 2009), pp. 309-325, ISSN 0006-3002.

Ginhoux, F., Greter, M., Leboeuf, M., Nandi, S., See, P., Gokhan, S., Mehler, M. F., Conway, S. J., Ng, L. G., Stanley, E. R., Samokhvalov, I. M. & Merad, M. (2010). Fate mapping analysis reveals that adult microglia derive from primitive macrophages. *Science*, Vol. 330, No. 6005, (October 2010), pp. 841-845, ISSN 1095-9203.

Gomez, F. J., Aguirre, P., Gonzalez-Billault, C. & Núñez, M. T. (2010). Iron mediates neuritic tree collapse in mesencephalic neurons treated with 1-methyl-4-phenylpyridinium (MPP+). *J Neural Transm*, (October 2) [Epub ahead of print], ISSN 1435-1463.

Gorell, J. M., Ordidge, R. J., Brown, G. G., Deniau, J. C., Buderer, N. M. & Helpern, J. A. (1995). Increased iron-related MRI contrast in the substantia nigra in Parkinson's disease. *Neurology*, Vol. 45, No. 6, (June 1995), pp. 1138-1143, ISSN 0028-3878.

Gotz, M. E., Kunig, G., Riederer, P. & Youdim, M. B. (1994). Oxidative stress: free radical production in neural degeneration. *Pharmacol Ther*, Vol. 63, No. 1, (January 1994), pp. 37-122, ISSN 0163-7258.

Graf, E., Mahoney, J. R., Bryant, R. G. & Eaton, J. W. (1984). Iron-catalyzed hydroxyl radical formation. Stringent requirement for free iron coordination site. *J Biol Chem*, Vol. 259, No 6, (March 1984), pp. 3620-3624, ISSN 0021-9258.

Grantham-McGregor, S. & Ani, C. (2001). A review of studies on the effect of iron deficiency on cognitive development in children. *J Nutr*, Vol. 131, No. 2S-2, (February 2001), pp. 649S-666S; discussion 666S-668S, ISSN 0022-3166.

Gunshin, H., Mackenzie, B., Berger, U. V., Gunshin, Y., Romero, M. F., Boron, W. F., Nussberger, S., Gollan, J. L. & Hediger, M. A. (1997). Cloning and characterization of a mammalian proton-coupled metal-ion transporter. *Nature*, Vol. 388, No. 6641, (July 1997), pp. 482-488, ISSN 0028-0836.

Haeger, P., Alvarez, A., Leal, N., Adasme, T., Núñez, M. T. & Hidalgo, C. (2010). Increased hippocampal expression of the divalent metal transporter 1 (DMT1) mRNA variants 1B and +IRE and DMT1 protein after NMDA-receptor stimulation or spatial memory training. *Neurotox Res*, Vol. 17, No. 3, (August 2009), pp. 238-247, ISSN 1476-3524.

Halliwell, B. (2006a). Oxidative stress and neurodegeneration: where are we now? *J Neurochem*, Vol. 97, No. 6, (June 2006), pp. 1634-1658, ISSN 0022-3042.

Halliwell, B. (2006b). Reactive species and antioxidants. Redox biology is a fundamental theme of aerobic life. *Plant Physiol*, Vol. 141, No. 2, (June 2006), pp. 312-322, ISSN 0032-0889.

Hattingen, E., Magerkurth, J., Pilatus, U., Mozer, A., Seifried, C., Steinmetz, H., Zanella, F. & Hilker, R. (2009). Phosphorus and proton magnetic resonance spectroscopy demonstrates mitochondrial dysfunction in early and advanced Parkinson's disease. *Brain*, Vol. 132, No. Pt 12, (December 2009), pp. 3285-3297, ISSN 1460-2156).

Herrera, A. J., Castano, A., Venero, J. L., Cano, J. & Machado, A. (2000). The single intranigral injection of LPS as a new model for studying the selective effects of inflammatory reactions on dopaminergic system. *Neurobiol Dis*, Vol. 7, No. 4, (August 2000), pp. 429-447, ISSN 0969-9961.

Hidalgo, C., Carrasco, M. A., Muñoz, P. & Núñez, M. T. (2007). A role for reactive oxygen/nitrogen species and iron on neuronal synaptic plasticity. *Antioxid Redox Signal*, Vol. 9, No 2, (November 2006), pp. 245-255, ISSN 1523-0864.

Hidalgo, C. & Núñez, M. T. (2007). Calcium, iron and neuronal function. *IUBMB Life*, Vol. 59, No. 4-5, (May 2007), pp. 280-285, ISSN 1521-6543.

Hirsch, E. C., Brandel, J. P., Galle, P., Javoy-Agid, F. & Agid, Y. (1991). Iron and aluminum increase in the substantia nigra of patients with Parkinson's disease: an X-ray microanalysis. *J Neurochem*, Vol. 56, No. 2, (February 1991), pp. 446-451, ISSN 0022-3042.

Hirsch, E. C., Hunot, S., Damier, P. & Faucheux, B. (1998). Glial cells and inflammation in Parkinson's disease: a role in neurodegeneration? *Ann Neurol*, Vol. 44, No. 3 Suppl 1, (September 1998), pp. S115-120, ISSN 0364-5134.

Hubert, N. & Hentze, M. W. (2002). Previously uncharacterized isoforms of divalent metal transporter (DMT)-1: implications for regulation and cellular function. *Proc Natl Acad Sci U S A*, Vol. 99, No. 19, (September 2002), pp 12345-12350, ISSN 0027-8424.

Jang, H., Boltz, D. A., Webster, R. G. & Smeyne, R. J. (2009). Viral parkinsonism. *Biochim Biophys Acta*, Vol. 1792, No. 7, (September 2008), pp. 714-721, ISSN 0006-3002.

Jellinger, K. A. (1999). The role of iron in neurodegeneration: prospects for pharmacotherapy of Parkinson's disease. *Drugs Aging*, Vol. 14, No. 2, (March 1999), pp. 115-140, ISSN 1170-229X.

Jiang, H., Song, N., Xu, H., Zhang, S., Wang, J. & Xie, J. (2010). Up-regulation of divalent metal transporter 1 in 6-hydroxydopamine intoxication is IRE/IRP dependent. *Cell Res*, Vol. 20, No. 3, (February 2010), pp. 345-356, ISSN 1748-7838.

Jorgenson, L. A., Sun, M., O'Connor, M. & Georgieff, M. K. (2005). Fetal iron deficiency disrupts the maturation of synaptic function and efficacy in area CA1 of the developing rat hippocampus. *Hippocampus*, Vol. 15, No. 8, (September 2005), pp. 1094-1102, ISSN 1050-9631.

Kakhlon, O. & Cabantchik, Z. I. (2002). The labile iron pool: characterization, measurement, and participation in cellular processes(1). *Free Radic Biol Med*, Vol. 33, No. 8, (October 2002), pp. 1037-1046, ISSN 0891-5849.

Kaur, D., Lee, D., Ragapolan, S. & Andersen, J. K. (2009). Glutathione depletion in immortalized midbrain-derived dopaminergic neurons results in increases in the labile iron pool: implications for Parkinson's disease. *Free Radic Biol Med*, Vol. 46, No. 5, (January 2009), pp. 593-598, ISSN 1873-4596.

Kaur, D., Yantiri, F., Rajagopalan, S., Kumar, J., Mo, J. Q., Boonplueang, R., Viswanath, V., Jacobs, R., Yang, L., Beal, M. F., DiMonte, D., Volitaskis, I., Ellerby, L., Cherny, R. A., Bush, A. I. & Andersen, J. K. (2003). Genetic or pharmacological iron chelation prevents MPTP-induced neurotoxicity in vivo: a novel therapy for Parkinson's disease. *Neuron*, Vol. 37, No. 6, (April 2003), pp. 899-909, ISSN 0896-6273.

Kooncumchoo, P., Sharma, S., Porter, J., Govitrapong, P. & Ebadi, M. (2006). Coenzyme Q(10) provides neuroprotection in iron-induced apoptosis in dopaminergic neurons. *J Mol Neurosci*, Vol. 28, No. 2, (May 2006), pp. 125-141, ISSN 0895-8696.

Kovtunovych, G., Eckhaus, M. A., Ghosh, M. C., Ollivierre-Wilson, H. & Rouault, T. A. (2010). Dysfunction of the heme recycling system in heme oxygenase 1-deficient mice: effects on macrophage viability and tissue iron distribution. *Blood*, Vol. 116, No. 26, (September 2010), pp. 6054-6062, ISSN 1528-0020.

Krause, A., Neitz, S., Magert, H. J., Schulz, A., Forssmann, W. G., Schulz-Knappe, P. & Adermann, K. (2000). LEAP-1, a novel highly disulfide-bonded human peptide, exhibits antimicrobial activity. *FEBS Lett*, Vol. 480, No. 2-3, (October 2000), pp. 147-150, ISSN 0014-5793.

Kroemer, G., Galluzzi, L., Vandenabeele, P., Abrams, J., Alnemri, E. S., Baehrecke, E. H., Blagosklonny, M. V., El-Deiry, W. S., Golstein, P., Green, D. R., Hengartner, M., Knight, R. A., Kumar, S., Lipton, S. A., Malorni, W., Núñez, G., Peter, M. E., Tschopp, J., Yuan, J., Piacentini, M., Zhivotovsky, B., Melino, G. & Nomenclature Committee on Cell, D. (2009). Classification of cell death: recommendations of the Nomenclature Committee on Cell Death 2009. *Cell Death Differ*, Vol. 16, No. 1, (October 2008), pp. 3-11, ISSN 1476-5403.

Kruszewski, M. (2003). Labile iron pool: the main determinant of cellular response to oxidative stress. *Mutat Res*, Vol. 531, No. 1-2, (November 2003), pp. 81-92, ISSN 0027-5107.

Kupershmidt, L., Weinreb, O., Amit, T., Mandel, S., Carri, M. T. & Youdim, M. B. (2009). Neuroprotective and neuritogenic activities of novel multimodal iron-chelating drugs in motor-neuron-like NSC-34 cells and transgenic mouse model of amyotrophic lateral sclerosis. *FASEB J*, Vol. 23, No. 11, (July 2009), pp. 3766-3779, ISSN 1530-6860.

Kuperstein, F. & Yavin, E. (2003). Pro-apoptotic signaling in neuronal cells following iron and amyloid beta peptide neurotoxicity. *J Neurochem*, Vol. 86, No. 1, (June 2003), pp. 114-125, ISSN 0022-3042.

Kwik-Uribe, C. L., Gietzen, D., German, J. B., Golub, M. S. & Keen, C. L. (2000). Chronic marginal iron intakes during early development in mice result in persistent changes in dopamine metabolism and myelin composition. *J Nutr*, Vol. 130, No. 11, (October 2000), pp. 2821-2830, ISSN 0022-3166.

Langston, J. W., Ballard, P., Tetrud, J. W. & Irwin, I. (1983). Chronic Parkinsonism in humans due to a product of meperidine-analog synthesis. *Science*, Vol. 219, No. 4587, (February 1983), pp. 979-980, ISSN 0036-8075.

Lee, D. W., Kaur, D., Chinta, S. J., Rajagopalan, S. & Andersen, J. K. (2009). A disruption in iron-sulfur center biogenesis via inhibition of mitochondrial dithiol glutaredoxin 2 may contribute to mitochondrial and cellular iron dysregulation in mammalian glutathione-depleted dopaminergic cells: implications for Parkinson's disease. *Antioxid Redox Signal*, Vol. 11, No. 9, (March 2009), pp. 2083-2094, ISSN 1557-7716.

Lees, A. J. (1997). Trauma and Parkinson disease. *Rev Neurol (Paris)*, Vol. 153, No. 10, (July 1998), pp. 541-546, ISSN 0035-3787.

Li, L., Holscher, C., Chen, B. B., Zhang, Z. F. & Liu, Y. Z. (2011). Hepcidin Treatment Modulates the Expression of Divalent Metal Transporter-1, Ceruloplasmin, and Ferroportin-1 in the Rat Cerebral Cortex and Hippocampus. *Biol Trace Elem Res*, (January 2011), ISSN 1559-0720.

Li, X. Z., Bai, L. M., Yang, Y. P., Luo, W. F., Hu, W. D., Chen, J. P., Mao, C. J. & Liu, C. F. (2009). Effects of IL-6 secreted from astrocytes on the survival of dopaminergic neurons in lipopolysaccharide-induced inflammation. *Neurosci Res*, Vol. 65, No. 3, (August 2009), pp. 252-258, ISSN 1872-8111.

Lill, R. & Muhlenhoff, U. (2008). Maturation of iron-sulfur proteins in eukaryotes: mechanisms, connected processes, and diseases. *Annu Rev Biochem*, Vol. 77, (March 2008), pp. 669-700, ISSN 0066-4154.

Lis, A., Paradkar, P. N., Singleton, S., Kuo, H. C., Garrick, M. D. & Roth, J. A. (2005). Hypoxia induces changes in expression of isoforms of the divalent metal transporter (DMT1) in rat pheochromocytoma (PC12) cells. *Biochem Pharmacol*, Vol. 69, No. 11, (May 2005), pp. 1647-1655, ISSN 0006-2952.

Liu, R., Liu, W., Doctrow, S. R. & Baudry, M. (2003). Iron toxicity in organotypic cultures of hippocampal slices: role of reactive oxygen species. *J Neurochem*, Vol. 85, No. 2, (April 2003), pp. 492-502, ISSN 0022-3042.

Lobner, D. & Ali, C. (2002). Mechanisms of bFGF and NT-4 potentiation of necrotic neuronal death. *Brain Res*, Vol. 954, No. 1, (October 2002), pp. 42-50, ISSN 0006-8993.

Lozoff, B., Wolf, A. W. & Jimenez, E. (1996). Iron-deficiency anemia and infant development: effects of extended oral iron therapy. *J Pediatr*, Vol. 129, No. 3, (September 1996), pp. 382-389, ISSN 0022-3476.

Ludwiczek, S., Theurl, I., Muckenthaler, M. U., Jakab, M., Mair, S. M., Theurl, M., Kiss, J., Paulmichl, M., Hentze, M. W., Ritter, M. & Weiss, G. (2007). Ca2+ channel blockers reverse iron overload by a new mechanism via divalent metal transporter-1. *Nat Med*, Vol. 13, No 4, (February 2007), pp. 448-454, ISSN 1078-8956.

Maharaj, D. S., Maharaj, H., Daya, S. & Glass, B. D. (2006). Melatonin and 6-hydroxymelatonin protect against iron-induced neurotoxicity. *J Neurochem*, Vol. 96, No. 1, (November 2005), pp. 78-81, ISSN 0022-3042.

Mandel SA, Amit T, Weinreb O, Youdim MB. (2011). Understanding the Broad-Spectrum Neuroprotective Action Profile of Green Tea Polyphenols in Aging and Neurodegenerative Diseases. *J Alzheimers Dis.* Mar 2. [Epub ahead of print], ISSN ISSN:1387-2877.

Marques, F., Falcao, A. M., Sousa, J. C., Coppola, G., Geschwind, D., Sousa, N., Correia-Neves, M. & Palha, J. A. (2009). Altered iron metabolism is part of the choroid plexus response to peripheral inflammation. *Endocrinology*, Vol. 150, No. 6, (February 2009), pp. 2822-2828, ISSN 1945-7170.

Martelli, A., Wattenhofer-Donze, M., Schmucker, S., Bouvet, S., Reutenauer, L. & Puccio, H. (2007). Frataxin is essential for extramitochondrial Fe-S cluster proteins in mammalian tissues. *Hum Mol Genet*, Vol. 16, No. 22, (June 2007), pp. 2651-2658, ISSN 0964-6906.

McEchron, M. D. & Paronish, M. D. (2005). Perinatal nutritional iron deficiency reduces hippocampal synaptic transmission but does not impair short- or long-term synaptic plasticity. *Nutr Neurosci*, Vol. 8, No. 5-6, (May 2006), pp. 277-285, ISSN 1028-415X.

McGeer, P. L., Itagaki, S., Boyes, B. E. & McGeer, E. G. (1988). Reactive microglia are positive for HLA-DR in the substantia nigra of Parkinson's and Alzheimer's disease brains. *Neurology*, Vol. 38, No. 8, (August 1988), pp. 1285-1291, ISSN 0028-3878.

Meister, A. & Anderson, M. E. (1983). Glutathione. *Annu Rev Biochem*, Vol. 52, (January 1983), pp. 711-760, ISSN 0066-4154.

Mena, N., Hirsch, E. & Núñez, M.T. (2011). Inhibition of mitochondrial complez I results in decreased synthesis of iron-sulfur clusters. In revision, *Biochim Biophys Res Comm.*

Mogi, M., Harada, M., Kondo, T., Riederer, P., Inagaki, H., Minami, M. &Nagatsu, T. (1994). Interleukin-1 beta, interleukin-6, epidermal growth factor and transforming growth factor-alpha are elevated in the brain from parkinsonian patients. *Neurosci Lett*, Vol. 180, No. 2, (October 1995), pp. 147-150, ISSN 0304-3940.

Moos, T. & Morgan, E. H. (1998). Evidence for low molecular weight, non-transferrin-bound iron in rat brain and cerebrospinal fluid. *J Neurosci Res*, Vol. 54, No. 4, (November 1998), pp. 486-494, ISSN 0360-4012.

Moos, T. & Rosengren Nielsen, T. (2006). Ferroportin in the postnatal rat brain: implications for axonal transport and neuronal export of iron. *Semin Pediatr Neurol*, Vol. 13, No. 3, (November 2006), pp. 149-157, ISSN 1071-9091.

Moos, T., Rosengren Nielsen, T., Skjorringe, T. & Morgan, E. H. (2007). Iron trafficking inside the brain. *J Neurochem*, Vol. 103, No. 5, (October 2007), pp. 1730-1740, ISSN 1471-4159.

Muller, T., Blum-Degen, D., Przuntek, H. & Kuhn, W. (1998). Interleukin-6 levels in cerebrospinal fluid inversely correlate to severity of Parkinson's disease. *Acta Neurol Scand*, Vol. 98, No. 2, (September 1998), pp. 142-144, ISSN 0001-6314.

Muñoz, P., Humeres, A., Elgueta, C., Kirkwood, A., Hidalgo, C. & Núñez, M. T. (2011). Iron mediates N-methyl-D-aspartate receptor-dependent stimulation of calcium-induced pathways and hippocampal synaptic plasticity. *J Biol Chem*, (February 2011), ISSN 1083-351X.

Nagatsu, T. (2002). Parkinson's disease: changes in apoptosis-related factors suggesting possible gene therapy. *J Neural Transm*, Vol. 109, No. 5-6, (July 2002), pp. 731-745, ISSN 0300-9564.

Nemeth, E., Tuttle, M. S., Powelson, J., Vaughn, M. B., Donovan, A., Ward, D. M., Ganz, T. & Kaplan, J. (2004). Hepcidin regulates cellular iron efflux by binding to ferroportin and inducing its internalization. *Science*, Vol. 306, No. 5704, (October 2004), pp. 2090-2093, ISSN 1095-9203.

Nicolas, G., Bennoun, M., Devaux, I., Beaumont, C., Grandchamp, B., Kahn, A. & Vaulont, S. (2001). Lack of hepcidin gene expression and severe tissue iron overload in upstream stimulatory factor 2 (USF2) knockout mice. *Proc Natl Acad Sci U S A*, Vol. 98, No. 15, (July 2001), pp. 8780-8785, ISSN 0027-8424.

Noll, T., Koop, A. & Piper, H. M. (1992). Mitochondrial ATP-synthase activity in cardiomyocytes after aerobic-anaerobic metabolic transition. *Am J Physiol*, Vol. 262, No. 5 Pt 1, (May 1992), pp. C1297-1303, ISSN 0002-9513.

Núñez, M. T., Gallardo, V., Muñoz, P., Tapia, V., Esparza, A., Salazar, J. & Speisky, H. (2004). Progressive iron accumulation induces a biphasic change in the glutathione content of neuroblastoma cells. *Free Radic Biol Med*, Vol. 37, No. 7, (September 2004), pp. 953-960, ISSN 0891-5849.

Ohgami, R. S., Campagna, D. R., Greer, E. L., Antiochos, B., McDonald, A., Chen, J., Sharp, J. J., Fujiwara, Y., Barker, J. E. & Fleming, M. D. (2005). Identification of a ferrireductase required for efficient transferrin-dependent iron uptake in erythroid cells. *Nat Genet*, Vol. 37, No. 11, (October 2005), pp. 1264-1269, ISSN 1061-4036.

Orr, C. F., Rowe, D. B. & Halliday, G. M. (2002). An inflammatory review of Parkinson's disease. *Prog Neurobiol*, Vol. 68, No. 5, (January 2003), pp. 325-340, ISSN 0301-0082.

Paradkar, P. N. & Roth, J. A. (2006). Nitric oxide transcriptionally down-regulates specific isoforms of divalent metal transporter (DMT1) via NF-kappaB. *J Neurochem*, Vol. 96, No. 6, (March 2006), pp. 1768-1777, ISSN 0022-3042.

Park, L. C., Zhang, H., Sheu, K. F., Calingasan, N. Y., Kristal, B. S., Lindsay, J. G. &Gibson, G. E. (1999). Metabolic impairment induces oxidative stress, compromises inflammatory responses, and inactivates a key mitochondrial enzyme in microglia. *J Neurochem*, Vol. 72, No. 5, (April 1999), pp. 1948-1958, ISSN 0022-3042.

Pelizzoni, I., Macco, R., Morini, M. F., Zacchetti, D., Grohovaz, F. & Codazzi, F. (2011). Iron handling in hippocampal neurons: activity-dependent iron entry and mitochondria-mediated neurotoxicity. *Aging Cell*, Vol. 10, No. 1, (November 2010), pp. 172-183, ISSN 1474-9726.

Perry, G., Taddeo, M. A., Petersen, R. B., Castellani, R. J., Harris, P. L., Siedlak, S. L., Cash, A. D., Liu, Q., Nunomura, A., Atwood, C. S. & Smith, M. A. (2003). Adventiously-bound redox active iron and copper are at the center of oxidative damage in Alzheimer disease. *Biometals*, Vol. 16, No. 1, (February 2003), pp. 77-81, ISSN 0966-0844.

Perry, T. L., Godin, D. V. & Hansen, S. (1982). Parkinson's disease: a disorder due to nigral glutathione deficiency? *Neurosci Lett*, Vol. 33, No. 3, (December 1982), pp. 305-310, ISSN 0304-3940.

Peyssonnaux, C., Zinkernagel, A. S., Schuepbach, R. A., Rankin, E., Vaulont, S., Haase, V. H., Nizet, V. & Johnson, R. S. (2007). Regulation of iron homeostasis by the hypoxia-inducible transcription factors (HIFs). *J Clin Invest*, Vol. 117, No. 7, (June 2007), pp. 1926-1932, ISSN 0021-9738.

Pigeon, C., Ilyin, G., Courselaud, B., Leroyer, P., Turlin, B., Brissot, P. & Loreal, O. (2001). A new mouse liver-specific gene, encoding a protein homologous to human antimicrobial peptide hepcidin, is overexpressed during iron overload. *J Biol Chem*, Vol. 276, No. 11, (December 2000), pp. 7811-7819, ISSN 0021-9258.

Pinto, J. P., Ribeiro, S., Pontes, H., Thowfeequ, S., Tosh, D., Carvalho, F. & Porto, G. (2008). Erythropoietin mediates hepcidin expression in hepatocytes through EPOR signaling and regulation of C/EBPalpha. *Blood*, Vol. 111, No. 12, (March 2008), pp. 5727-5733, ISSN 1528-0020.

Ranade, S. C., Rose, A., Rao, M., Gallego, J., Gressens, P. & Mani, S. (2008). Different types of nutritional deficiencies affect different domains of spatial memory function checked in a radial arm maze. *Neuroscience*, Vol. 152, No. 4, (March 2008), pp. 859-866, ISSN 0306-4522.

Rouault, T. A. & Tong, W. H. (2005). Iron-sulphur cluster biogenesis and mitochondrial iron homeostasis. *Nat Rev Mol Cell Biol*, Vol. 6, No. 4, (April 2005), pp. 345-351, ISSN 1471-0072.

Rouault, T. A. & Tong, W. H. (2008). Iron-sulfur cluster biogenesis and human disease. *Trends Genet*, Vol. 24, No. 8, (July 2008), pp 398-407, ISSN 0168-9525.

Rouault, T. A., Zhang, D. L. & Jeong, S. Y. (2009). Brain iron homeostasis, the choroid plexus, and localization of iron transport proteins. *Metab Brain Dis*, Vol. 24, No. 4, (October 2009), pp. 673-684, ISSN 1573-7365.

Salazar, J., Mena, N., Hunot, S., Prigent, A., Alvarez-Fischer, D., Arredondo, M., Duyckaerts, C., Sazdovitch, V., Zhao, L., Garrick, L. M., Núñez, M. T., Garrick, M. D., Raisman-Vozari, R. & Hirsch, E. C. (2008). Divalent metal transporter 1 (DMT1) contributes to neurodegeneration in animal models of Parkinson's disease. *Proc Natl Acad Sci U S A*, Vol. 105, No. 47, (November 2008), pp. 18578-18583, ISSN 1091-6490.

Salazar, J., Mena, N. & Núñez, M. T. (2006). Iron dyshomeostasis in Parkinson's disease. *J Neural Transm Suppl*, No. 71, (April 2007), pp. 205-213, ISSN 0303-6995.

Sayre, L. M., Perry, G., Atwood, C. S. & Smith, M. A. (2000). The role of metals in neurodegenerative diseases. *Cell Mol Biol (Noisy-le-grand)*, Vol. 46, No. 4, (June 2000), pp. 731-741, ISSN 0145-5680.

Schafer, F. Q. & Buettner, G. R. (2001). Redox environment of the cell as viewed through the redox state of the glutathione disulfide/glutathione couple. *Free Radic Biol Med*, Vol. 30, No. 11, (May 2005), pp. 1191-1212, ISSN 0891-5849.

Schapira, A. H., Cooper, J. M., Dexter, D., Clark, J. B., Jenner, P. & Marsden, C. D. (1990). Mitochondrial complex I deficiency in Parkinson's disease. *J Neurochem*, Vol. 54, No. 3, (March 1990), pp. 823-827, ISSN 0022-3042.

Scotcher, K. P., Irwin, I., DeLanney, L. E., Langston, J. W. & Di Monte, D. (1990). Effects of 1-methyl-4-phenyl-1,2,3,6-tetrahydropyridine and 1-methyl-4-phenylpyridinium ion on ATP levels of mouse brain synaptosomes. *J Neurochem*, Vol. 54, No. 4, (April 1990), pp. 1295-1301, ISSN 0022-3042.

Shachar, D. B., Kahana, N., Kampel, V., Warshawsky, A. & Youdim, M. B. (2004). Neuroprotection by a novel brain permeable iron chelator, VK-28, against 6-hydroxydopamine lession in rats. *Neuropharmacology*, Vol. 46, No. 2, (December 2003), pp. 254-263, ISSN 0028-3908.

Shi, Z. H., Nie, G., Duan, X. L., Rouault, T., Wu, W. S., Ning, B., Zhang, N., Chang, Y. Z. & Zhao, B. L. (2010). Neuroprotective mechanism of mitochondrial ferritin on 6-hydroxydopamine-induced dopaminergic cell damage: implication for neuroprotection in Parkinson's disease. *Antioxid Redox Signal*, Vol. 13, No. 6, (February 2010), pp. 783-796, ISSN 1557-7716.

Sian, J., Dexter, D. T., Lees, A. J., Daniel, S., Agid, Y., Javoy-Agid, F., Jenner, P. & Marsden, C. D. (1994). Alterations in glutathione levels in Parkinson's disease and other neurodegenerative disorders affecting basal ganglia. *Ann Neurol*, Vol. 36, No. 3, (September 1994), pp. 348-355, ISSN 0364-5134.

Singer, T. P. & Ramsay, R. R. (1990). Mechanism of the neurotoxicity of MPTP. An update. *FEBS Lett*, Vol. 274, No. 1-2, (November 1990), pp. 1-8, ISSN 0014-5793.

Singh, R., Akhtar, N. & Haqqi, T. M. (2010). Green tea polyphenol epigallocatechin-3-gallate: inflammation and arthritis. *Life Sci*, Vol. 86, No. 25-26, (May 2010), pp. 907-918, ISSN 1879-0631.

Sofic, E., Riederer, P., Heinsen, H., Beckmann, H., Reynolds, G. P., Hebenstreit, G. & Youdim, M. B. (1988). Increased iron (III) and total iron content in post mortem substantia nigra of parkinsonian brain. *J Neural Transm*, Vol. 74, No. 3, (January 1988), pp. 199-205, ISSN 0300-9564.

Song, N., Wang, J., Jiang, H. & Xie, J. (2010). Ferroportin 1 but not hephaestin contributes to iron accumulation in a cell model of Parkinson's disease. *Free Radic Biol Med*, Vol. 48, No. 2, (November 2009), pp. 332-341, ISSN 1873-4596.

Stokes, A. H., Hastings, T. G. & Vrana, K. E. (1999). Cytotoxic and genotoxic potential of dopamine. *J Neurosci Res*, Vol. 55, No. 6, (April 1999), pp. 659-665, ISSN 0360-4012.

Symons, M.C.R & Gutteridge, J.M.C. (1998). *Free Radicals And Iron: Chemistry, Biology And Medicine*. Oxford University Press, ISBN 019-8558-92-9, New York, USA.

Taneja, V., Mishra, K. & Agarwal, K. N. (1986). Effect of early iron deficiency in rat on the gamma-aminobutyric acid shunt in brain. *J Neurochem*, Vol. 46, No. 6, (June 1986), pp. 1670-1674, ISSN 0022-3042.

Tretter, L., Sipos, I. & Adam-Vizi, V. (2004). Initiation of neuronal damage by complex I deficiency and oxidative stress in Parkinson's disease. *Neurochem Res*, Vol. 29, No. 3, (March 2004), pp. 569-577, ISSN 0364-3190.

Valente, E. M., Abou-Sleiman, P. M., Caputo, V., Muqit, M. M., Harvey, K., Gispert, S., Ali, Z., Del Turco, D., Bentivoglio, A. R., Healy, D. G., Albanese, A., Nussbaum, R.,

Gonzalez-Maldonado, R., Deller, T., Salvi, S., Cortelli, P., Gilks, W. P., Latchman, D. S., Harvey, R. J., Dallapiccola, B., Auburger, G. & Wood, N. W. (2004). Hereditary early-onset Parkinson's disease caused by mutations in PINK1. *Science*, Vol. 304, No. 5674, (April 2004), pp. 1158-1160, ISSN 1095-9203.

Vandenabeele, P., Galluzzi, L., Vanden Berghe, T. & Kroemer, G. (2010). Molecular mechanisms of necroptosis: an ordered cellular explosion. *Nat Rev Mol Cell Biol*, Vol. 11, No. 10, (October 2010), pp. 700-714, ISSN 1471-0080.

Vymazal, J., Righini, A., Brooks, R. A., Canesi, M., Mariani, C., Leonardi, M. & Pezzoli, G. (1999). T1 and T2 in the brain of healthy subjects, patients with Parkinson disease, and patients with multiple system atrophy: relation to iron content. *Radiology*, Vol. 211, No. 2, (May 1999), pp. 489-495, ISSN 0033-8419.

Wang, D., Wang, L. H., Zhao, Y., Lu, Y. P. & Zhu, L. (2010a). Hypoxia regulates the ferrous iron uptake and reactive oxygen species level via divalent metal transporter 1 (DMT1) Exon1B by hypoxia-inducible factor-1. *IUBMB Life*, Vol. 62, No. 8, (August 2010), pp. 629-636, ISSN 1521-6551.

Wang, Q., Du, F., Qian, Z. M., Ge, X. H., Zhu, L., Yung, W. H., Yang, L. & Ke, Y. (2008). Lipopolysaccharide induces a significant increase in expression of iron regulatory hormone hepcidin in the cortex and substantia nigra in rat brain. *Endocrinology*, Vol. 149, No. 8, (May 2008), pp. 3920-3925, ISSN 0013-7227.

Wang, S. M., Fu, L. J., Duan, X. L., Crooks, D. R., Yu, P., Qian, Z. M., Di, X. J., Li, J., Rouault, T. A. & Chang, Y. Z. (2010b). Role of hepcidin in murine brain iron metabolism. *Cell Mol Life Sci*, Vol. 67, No. 1, (November 2009), pp. 123-133, ISSN 1420-9071.

Wang, Z. J., Lam, K. W., Lam, T. T. & Tso, M. O. (1998). Iron-induced apoptosis in the photoreceptor cells of rats. *Invest Ophthalmol Vis Sci*, Vol. 39, No. 3, (March 1998), pp. 631-633, ISSN 0146-0404.

Weinreb, O., Mandel, S., Bar-Am, O. & Amit, T. (2011). Iron-chelating backbone coupled with monoamine oxidase inhibitory moiety as novel pluripotential therapeutic agents for Alzheimer's disease: a tribute to Moussa Youdim. *J Neural Transm*, (March 2011), ISSN 1435-1463.

Williams, K., Wilson, M. A. & Bressler, J. (2000). Regulation and developmental expression of the divalent metal-ion transporter in the rat brain. *Cell Mol Biol (Noisy-le-grand)*, Vol. 46, No. 3, (July 2000), pp. 563-571, ISSN 0145-5680.

Wilson, R. B. (2006). Iron dysregulation in Friedreich ataxia. *Semin Pediatr Neurol*, Vol. 13, No. 3, (November 2006), pp. 166-175, ISSN 1071-9091.

Wright, R. O. & Baccarelli, A. (2007). Metals and neurotoxicology. *J Nutr* Vol. 137, No. 12, (November 2007), pp. 2809-2813, ISSN 1541-6100.

Wrighting, D. M. & Andrews, N. C. (2006). Interleukin-6 induces hepcidin expression through STAT3. *Blood*, Vol. 108, No. 9, (July 2006), pp. 3204-3209, ISSN 0006-4971.

Xu, Q., Kanthasamy, A. G. & Reddy, M. B. (2008). Neuroprotective effect of the natural iron chelator, phytic acid in a cell culture model of Parkinson's disease. *Toxicology*, Vol. 245, No. 1-2, (February 2008), pp. 101-108, ISSN 0300-483X.

Ye, H. & Rouault, T. A. (2010). Erythropoiesis and iron sulfur cluster biogenesis. *Adv Hematol* 2010, (September 2010), ISSN 1687-9112.

Youdim, M. B., Ben-Shachar, D. & Riederer, P. (1989). Is Parkinson's disease a progressive siderosis of substantia nigra resulting in iron and melanin induced neurodegeneration? *Acta Neurol Scand Suppl*, Vol. 126, (January 1989), pp. 47-54, ISSN 0065-1427.

Youdim, M. B. & Buccafusco, J. J. (2005). Multi-functional drugs for various CNS targets in the treatment of neurodegenerative disorders. *Trends Pharmacol Sci*, Vol. 26, No. 1, (January 2005), pp. 27-35, ISSN 0165-6147.

Youdim, M. B., Green, A. R., Bloomfield, M. R., Mitchell, B. D., Heal, D. J. & Grahame-Smith, D. G. (1980). The effects of iron deficiency on brain biogenic monoamine biochemistry and function in rats. *Neuropharmacology*, Vol. 19, No. 3, (March 1980), pp. 259-267, ISSN 0028-3908.

Youdim, M. B., Stephenson, G. & Ben Shachar, D. (2004). Ironing iron out in Parkinson's disease and other neurodegenerative diseases with iron chelators: a lesson from 6-hydroxydopamine and iron chelators, desferal and VK-28. *Ann N Y Acad Sci*, Vol. 1012, (April 2004), pp. 306-325, ISSN 0077-8923.

Zaman, K., Ryu, H., Hall, D., O'Donovan, K., Lin, K. I., Miller, M. P., Marquis, J. C., Baraban, J. M., Semenza, G. L. & Ratan, R. R. (1999). Protection from oxidative stress-induced apoptosis in cortical neuronal cultures by iron chelators is associated with enhanced DNA binding of hypoxia-inducible factor-1 and ATF-1/CREB and increased expression of glycolytic enzymes, p21(waf1/cip1), and erythropoietin. *J Neurosci*, Vol. 19, No. 22, (November 1999), pp. 9821-9830, ISSN 1529-2401.

Zecca, L., Youdim, M. B., Riederer, P., Connor, J. R. & Crichton, R. R. (2004). Iron, brain ageing and neurodegenerative disorders. *Nat Rev Neurosci*, Vol. 5, No. 11, (October 2004), pp. 863-873, ISSN 1471-003X.

Zechel, S., Huber-Wittmer, K. & von Bohlen und Halbach, O. (2006). Distribution of the iron-regulating protein hepcidin in the murine central nervous system. *J Neurosci Res*, Vol. 84, No. 4, (August 2006), pp. 790-800, ISSN 0360-4012.

Zhang, Y., Marcillat, O., Giulivi, C., Ernster, L. & Davies, K. J. (1990). The oxidative inactivation of mitochondrial electron transport chain components and ATPase. *J Biol Chem*, Vol. 265, No. 27, (September 1990), pp. 16330-16336, ISSN 0021-9258.

Zheng, H., Youdim, M. B. & Fridkin, M. (2010). Site-activated chelators targeting acetylcholinesterase and monoamine oxidase for Alzheimer's therapy. *ACS Chem Biol*, Vol. 5, No. 6, (May 1990), pp. 603-610, ISSN 1554-8937.

Zheng, H., Youdim, M. B., Weiner, L. M. & Fridkin, M. (2005). Novel potential neuroprotective agents with both iron chelating and amino acid-based derivatives targeting central nervous system neurons. *Biochem Pharmacol*, Vol. 70, No. 11, (October 2005), pp. 1642-1652, ISSN 0006-2952.

Ziv, I., Barzilai, A., Offen, D., Nardi, N. & Melamed, E. (1997). Nigrostriatal neuronal death in Parkinson's disease--a passive or an active genetically-controlled process? *J Neural Transm Suppl*, Vol. 49, (January 1997), pp. 69-76, ISSN 0303-6995.

Zoccarato, F., Toscano, P. & Alexandre, A. (2005). Dopamine-derived dopaminochrome promotes H(2)O(2) release at mitochondrial complex I: stimulation by rotenone, control by Ca(2+), and relevance to Parkinson disease. *J Biol Chem*, Vol. 280, No. 16, (February 2005), pp. 15587-15594, ISSN 0021-9258.

5

Filterable Forms of *Nocardia*: An Infectious Focus in the Parkinsonian Midbrains

Shunro Kohbata[1], Ryoichi Hayashi[2], Tomokazu Tamura[3] and Chitoshi Kadoya[4]
[1]*Gifu University,*
[2]*Shinshu University,*
[3]*Fuji National Hospital,*
[4]*Kamisone Hospital*
Japan

1. Introduction

Nocardia is a strictly aerobic gram-positive, partially acid-fast mycelial bacterium that superficially resembles the fungus (Beaman & Beaman, 1994). The bacterium causes L-dopa-responsive movement disorder accompanied by neuronal inclusions resembling Lewy bodies, suggesting a possible link between *Nocardia* and Parkinson's disease (PD) (Kohbata & Beaman, 1991). PD is a slowly progressive, acute monophasic neurological disorder with a lengthy prodromal phase before the onset and with longer duration of disease (Fearnley & Lees, 1991; Hawkes, 2008). It is characterized pathologically by neuronal loss, reactive gliosis, and Lewy bodies in the remaining neurons in the midbrain substantia nigra (Greenfield & Bosanquet, 1953). Spread of Lewy bodies occurs from the brainstem through midbrain and basal forebrain to the cerebral cortex (Braak et al., 2003). Furthermore, the transfer of the nigral lesion to fetal grafts in PD patients with fetal nigral transplantation happens (Braak & Tredici, 2008; Li, et al., 2008). The transfer experiment of the nigral lesion to experimental animals did not attain satisfactory results by using antibiotic-containing homogenizing buffer (Bethlem & Jager, 1960). PD is probably caused by an environmental agent rather than a hereditary factor. The environmental agent may be parasitic to midbrain nigral tissues and bacterial in nature. Heredity might play a role in predisposing certain individuals to PD cause.

Antibody to *Nocardia* is found in the serum of PD patients (Kohbata & Shimokawa, 1993). The 125 human brain specimen (including PD, Dementia with Lewy bodies, and other patients) is not positive for filamentous gram-positive nocardiae by Gram staining (Lu et al., 2005), though *Nocardia*-like beaded cells were present in the midbrain nigral lesions of two patients suffered from encephalitis with a parkinsonian syndrome (Bojinov, 1971 ; Kohbata & Beaman, 1991). On the other hand, an accumulation of acid-fast lipochrome bodies, morphologically identical to filterable forms of *Nocardia* (i.e., filterable nocardiae), within the neuroglia of midbrain nigral lesion is dense in the early stage of PD (Kohbata et al., 1998).

Filterable nocardiae are gram-negative, acid-fast, and PAS-positive granular cells. They are, in vitro & in vivo, morphologically characterized by gelatinous masses containing yellow-fluoresced granules under ultraviolet light when stained with acridine orange and grow to be cylindrical tubules such as that of mycelial bacterium in the presence of erythrocyte lysates. An experimental infection causes a late-onset movement disorder after a long incubation period. Filterable nocardiae, degeneratively generated from *Nocardia,* have a high predilection for erythrocytes and spread through neuroglia to neurons in the mouse brain as intracellular parasites (Kohbata et al., 2009). We attempted to investigate their isolation from the nigral tissues of patients with PD and to detect their presence in the midbrain.

2. Subjects and methods

2.1 Subjects

Six PD patients (aged 65 to 82 years; median age, 72 years) and four patients without neurological disorder (aged 60 to 70 years; median age, 65 years), serving as age-matched controls, were selected from the archives of the Department of Pathology, Chubu National

Subject	Age (yr)	Gender[a]	Duration[b] (yr)	Cause of death	Hoehn & Yahr[c]	Reference
Parkinson's disease						
PD1	65	m	2	Pneumonia	II	Kohbata et al., 1998
PD2	68	m	9	Suicidal attack	III	Kohbata et al., 1998
PD3	75	m	5	Pneumonia	V	This study
PD4	82	f	10	Leukemia	V	This study
PD5	68	f	19	Pneumonia	V	Kohbata et al., 1998
PD6	73	m	26	Choking	V	This study
Control						
C1	60	m	-	Pulmonary cancer	-	Kohbata et al., 1998
C2	61	m	-	Pulmonary cancer	-	Kohbata et al., 1998
C3	70	m	-	Pulmonary cancer	-	Kohbata et al., 1998
C4	70	m	-	Sepsis	-	This study

Table 1. Clinical characteristics in PD and control patients examined.
a, Gender; f = female, m = male.
b, Duration indicates the time from clinical diagnosis of PD to death. c, Hoehn & Yahr 1967.

Hospital (Aichi, Japan), Nagano Red-Cross Hospital (Nagano, Japan), Shinshu University (Nagano, Japan), and Fuji National Hospital (Shizuoka, Japan). Details concerning PD and control patients were shown in the Table. Two suspected PD patients (sPD; female, 78 years old, sPD2 male; 75 years old), in addition to that of PD patients 1 and 4 as shown in Table, were picked up to obtain several frozen midbrain samples of the nigral tissue. Informed consent was obtained from the patients and their family members. The privacy rights of all subjects were always observed. PD was diagnosed by neurologists on the basis of the results of neurological examinations (Kohbata et al., 1998). Paraffin-embedded tissues, serially sectioned into 5-µm sections, and then placed on glass slides according to an atlas (Haines, 1987). The sections at the level of the caudal substantia nigra were examined. The sections were stained with hematoxylin and eosin (H&E). All procedures were performed in compliance with relevant laws and institutional guidelines. The protocol was approved by the appropriate institutional committees.

2.2 Culturing of brain samples

Frozen midbrain samples, ca. one cubic cm in volume, were dissected into small pieces and inoculated into 50 ml of brain heart infusion supplemented with 0.4% (w/v) yeast extract (BYE). After one-day incubation at 37 °C with shaking (130 strokes per minute), the culture was centrifuged for 10 min at 5000 rpm. Supernatant was filtrated through a 0.45 µm and then through a 0.22 µm filter. Filtrate samples were transferred into equal volumes of BYE broth medium and incubated at 37 °C with shaking for two days. One hundred microliters of filtrate samples was inoculated into 50 ml of BYE broth medium with or without 1% (v/v) erythrocyte lysates to be incubated. Erythrocyte lysates were prepared as described previously (Kohbata et al., 2009). Culture samples at various incubation periods were applied to glass slides with a loop and fixed by heat. Samples were histochemically and immunohistochemically examined as described in 2.5. Light microscopy.

2.3 Detection of DNA in the culture samples

DNA was prepared as described previously (Kohbata, 1998; Kohbata et al., 2009). Briefly, five milliliters of extraction buffer (100 mM Tris-HCl, pH 9.0, 40 mM EDTA), 1 ml of 10% SDS, 3 ml of benzyl chloride were added to 10 ml of the culture samples or to 1 wet gram of filamentous gram-positive nocardiae within sterile tubes. For collection of filamentous gram-positive nocardiae, one milliliter of stock culture was transferred into 50 ml of BHI broth and incubated at 37 °C with rotational agitation (150 rpm) as described previously (Kohbata & Beaman, 1991). At 16 h after inoculation, the bacterial pellets were harvested by centrifugation for 15 min at 3000 rpm. The bacterial pellets were washed three times with sterile DW. The tube was vortexed and incubated at 50 °C for 30 min with shaking, ensure the two phases remained thoroughly mixed. Three milliliter of 3 M of sodium acetate, pH 5.0, was then added, and the tube was kept on ice for 15 min. After centrifugation at 5000 rpm at 4 °C for 30 min, the supernatant was collected, and DNA was precipitated with isopropanol. The samples were applied to the wells of a 0.8% gel run in TAE buffer (40 mM Tris, 20 mM acetate, 2 mM EDTA, pH 8.0). Bands were visualized by staining with ethidium bromide (1 µg/ml), destained with distilled water, and photographed. The procedure employed was as follows: A) PCR amplification. B) Restrictive digestion analysis of genome DNA. C) Subcloning of DNA. Amplification of gene fragments and polymerase chain reaction-mediated synthesis were performed as described previously (Kohbata et al., 2009). Genome

DNA was incubated for 1 hr at 37 °C in the presence of 5 U of *Eco*R1 or *Hind* III (Nippon gene, Tokyo, Japan) according to the manufacture's instructions. The fragments produced were separated on a 0.8% gel run in TAE buffer. Several fragments were produced by complete *Hind* III digestion. Eight fragments, each composed of nearly 1000 bases, were selected and inserted into a pUC118 (Takara, Tokyo, Japan) plasmid vector system. Purified plasmids were sequenced as described previously (Kohbata et al., 2009). Sequence analysis was performed through queries of GenBank using the Basic Local Alignment Search Tool (BLAST).

2.4 Light microscopy

Smear samples of broth cultures were Gram-stained. Via a PAS, smear samples or midbrain sections were stained. For immunostaining, smear samples or midbrain sections were stained with antiserum, the specificity of which has been already confirmed (Kohbata et al., 2009). Processing was performed according to conventional peroxidase-antiperoxidase complex or avidin-biotin complex protocols. 3, 3'-diaminobenzine was used as the chromogen. Midbrain sections of PD patients 1, 2, and 5 were stained with 0.1% acridine orange (AO, Polyscience Inc., PA., USA) in McIlvaine's buffer for 4 min. Several sections were stained with 10 µg/ml of 4, 6-diamidino-2-phenylindole (DAPI, Polyscience, PA, USA) and observed with an epifluorescence microscope (Fluorophoto VFR, Nikon, Japan) as described previously (Kohbata, 1998; Kohbata et al., 2009).

3. Results

3.1 Morphological and immunological features of filterable isolates

Several clusters composed of numerous gram-negative granules were observed in one-day cultures of PD patient 1 culture filtrates (Fig. 1A). In two-day cultures, the same granular cells were also seen. Many immunoreactive brilliant granules were present in the clusters (Fig. 1B). PAS-stained clusters were observed (Fig. 1C). Large globules composed of small red PAS-positive granules were seen in the smears from the one-day culture supplemented with erythrocyte lysates (Fig. 1D). Several clusters of gram-negative granules were also seen in one-day culture of PD patient 4 culture filtrates (Fig. 1E). In two-day cultures, similar gram-negative granules were observed. Numerous brilliant immunoreactive granules were present in brown clusters (Fig. 1F). Large globules composed of gram-negative granules were seen when supplemented with erythrocyte lysates. PAS-positive clusters were not seen. In one-day cultures from patient sPD1, many clusters of numerous gram-negative granules were observed (Fig. 1G). They were not reactive to the antiserum (Fig. 1H). Any gram-negative or gram-positive granules were not observed in one-day and two-day cultures of sPD patient 2 filtrates.

3.2 DNA genomic features of filterable isolates

Genomic DNA was detected in broth cultures PD4 (3 & 4 on Fig. 2A), but not in broth cultures PD1 (1 & 2 on Fig. 2A). PCR-mediated synthesis failed to amplify the 16S rDNA of filterable organisms. Genomic DNA digested with *Eco*R1 or *Hind* III revealed a profile (4 & 5 on Fig. 2B) different from that of *Nocardia*. Eight fragment sequences were analyzed. The 4295-base genome was AT-rich, with a G+C content of 41%. G+C content in each fragment varied from 39 to 48%. Most fragments contained several A/T homopolymers. One of these fragments revealed that the genome was AT-rich with a G+C content of 40%; it contained six

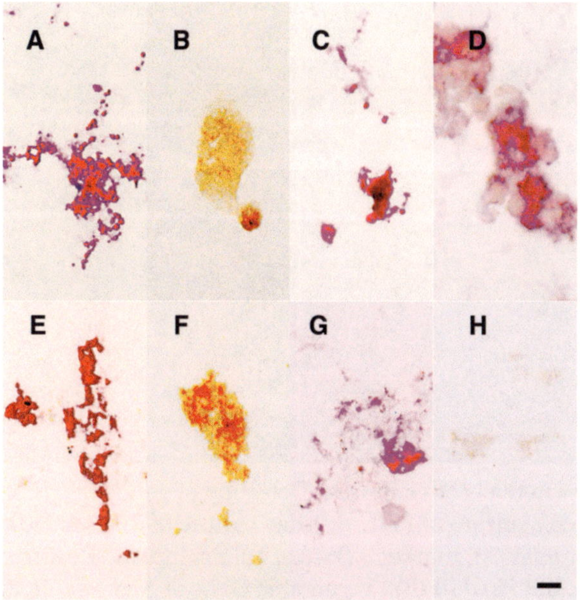

Fig. 1. Light micrographs of broth cultures. Gram-stained (A), immunostained (B), and PAS-stained (C) smears of BYE broth cultures at one day after inoculation of PD1 culture filtrates. PAS-stained smears of BYE broth medium inoculated with PD1 filtrates when supplemented with erythrocyte lysates (D). Gram-stained (E) and immunostained (F) smears of BYE broth cultures at one day after inoculation of PD4 culture filtrates. Gram-stained (G) and immunostained (H) smears of BYE broth cultures at one day after inoculation of suspected PD1 culture filtrates. Panel A through H are the same magnification (bar = 10 µm).

tetramers and three pentamers of adenine or thymine within its 679-base sequence. BLAST analysis indicated that each fragment sequence bore no similarity to genes found in any other sequenced organisms.

3.3 Eosinophilic and immunoreactive inclusion-bearing midbrain neurons of the VL pars compacta and central gray area of PD patient 1

Neurons harbored eosinophilic inclusions such as a peripheral halo with eosinophilic body (Fig. 3A), with small eosinophilic body (Fig. 3B), with eosinophilic body containing a dense center (Fig. 3C), and with double eosinophilic dense bodies (Fig. 3D). Each of next immunostained sections revealed reactive inclusion bodies (Fig. 3E), reactive granular inclusions (Fig. 3F), inclusion bodies with reactive peripheries (Fig. 3G), and tubule-like bodies with reactive peripheries (Fig. 3H). Inclusion bodies within midbrain neurons were negative on several sections stained with PAS.

3.4 Neurons harboring immunoreactive, PAS-positive inclusions and degenerative neurons in the pars compacta of PD patient 2

Immunoreactive and PAS-positive inclusions occupied one half of the neuronal cytoplasm (Figs. 4A & 4B). Immunoreactive corpora were composed of a deformed portion (arrowheads on Fig. 4A). Red inclusions within shrunken pigmented neurons and partially

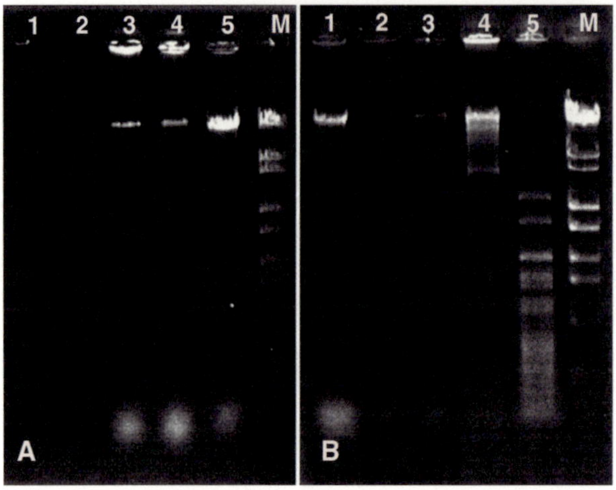

Fig. 2. Genome DNAs in the broth cultures. Detection of genomic DNA (A). 1; 1-day culture of PD1. 2; 2-day culture of PD1. 3; 1-day culture of PD4. 4; 2-day culture of PD4. 5; genomic DNA of *Nocardia*. M; marker 6 (Wako, Tokyo, Japan). Restrictive digestion analysis using *Eco*R1 and *Hind* III (B). 1; genomic DNA of *Nocardia*. 2; digested genomic DNA of *Nocardia* with *Eco*R1. 3; digested genomic DNA of *Nocardia* with *Hind* III. 4; digested genomic DNA of filterable organisms collected from patient PD4 with *Eco*R1. 5; digested genomic DNA of filterable organisms collected from patient PD4 with *Hind* III. M; marker 6. The preparation method is described in the text.

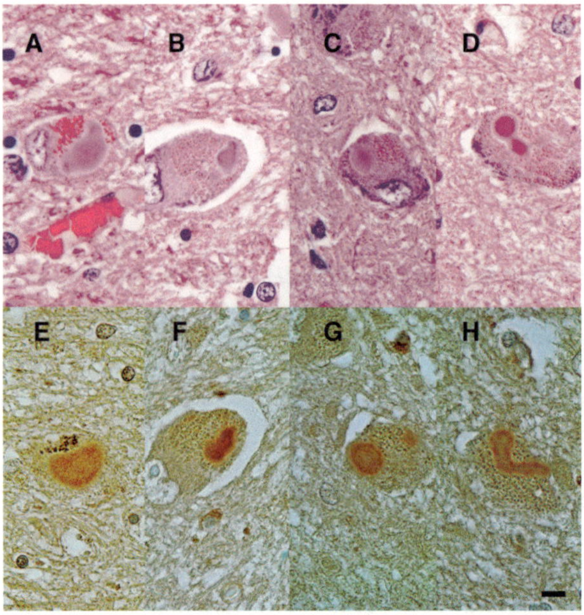

Fig. 3. Light micrograph of the VL pars compacta and the central gray area neurons of patient PD1. H&E-stained sections of the VL pars compacta (A) and of the central gray area (B, C, and D). Immunostained sections of the VL pars compacta (E) and of the central gray area (F, G, and H). Magnification of panels a through h is the same (bar = 10 μm).

red-colored ring-like inclusions within pigmented neurons were observed (Figs. 4C & 4D). The cytoplasm was filled with numerous brilliant brown granules. The same granules were deposited in neuroglia (Fig. 4E). Numerous brown granules were localized within the neuronal cytoplasm (Fig. 4F). One half of the cytoplasm was occupied by granule-containing gelatinous masses composed of a deformed portion (arrowheads on Fig. 4G).

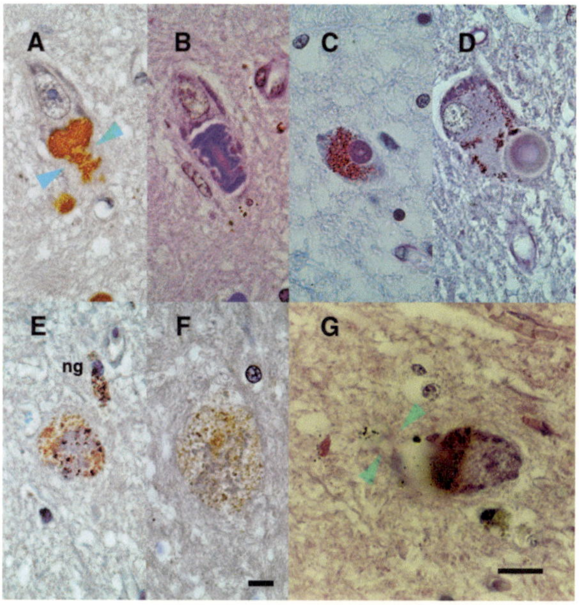

Fig. 4. Light micrographs of the VM and VL pars compacta neurons in PD patient 2. Immunostained (A) and PAS-stained next (B) sections of the VM pars compacta. PAS-stained sections (C) of the VM pars compacta and that (D) of the VL pars compacta. Immunostained sections (E and F) of the VL pars compacta. Magnification of panels a through f is the same (bar = 10 µm). H&E-stained section (G) of the VL pars compacta. Bar = 10 µm. ng; neuroglia.

3.5 Immunoreactive and PAS-positive corpora in the VM pars compacta of the substantia nigra of PD patients

The blue spots, probably identical to astroglia, were predominantly present in the VM pars compacta of PD patient 1 (Fig. 5A). In the same location, many PAS-positive spots were present among the blue spots (Fig. 5B). In higher magnification of the nigral region shown by an arrowhead on Fig. 5A or Fig. 5B, faintly immunoreactive (Fig. 5C) and PAS-positive (Fig. 5D) corpora were seen among the blue spots of which size was similar to that of corpora. An examination of other tissue section reveals that several immunoreactive (Fig. 5E) and many PAS-positive (Fig. 5F) spots were present. In higher magnification of the nigral region shown by an arrowhead on Fig. 5E or Fig. 5F, immunoreactive granule-containing (Fig. 5G) and PAS-positive corpora (Fig. 5H) were seen. Many immunoreactive (Fig. 6A & 6E) and PAS-variable (Fig. 6B) spots were seen in PD patient 2. In higher magnification of the nigral region shown by an arrowhead on Fig. 6A, 6E, 6B or 6F, immunoreactive (Fig. 6C & 6G) or PAS-positive (Fig. 6D) granule-containing corpora were observed. Faintly PAS-positive corpora were present (Fig. 6H). Several corpora were likely

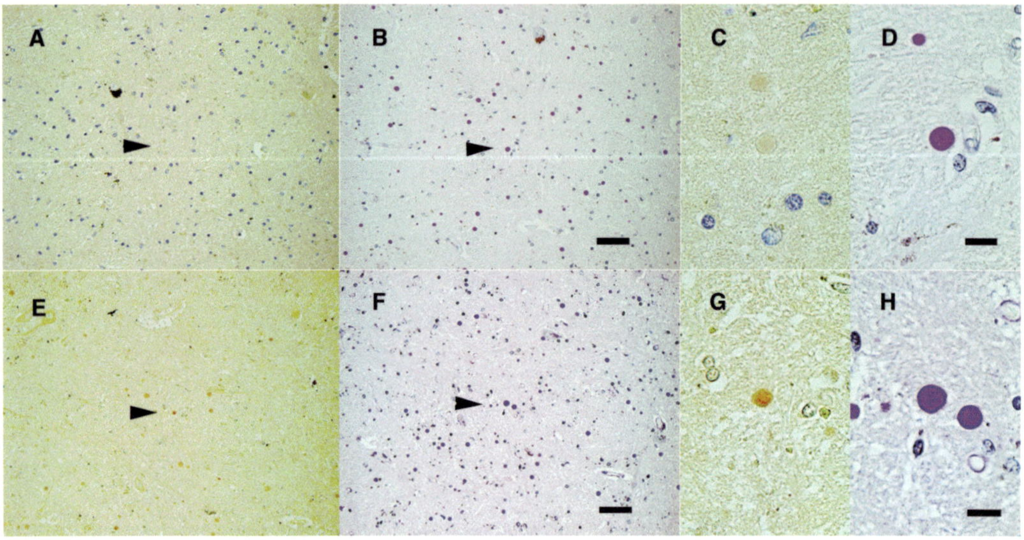

Fig. 5. Light micrographs of the VM pars compacta of the substantia nigra in PD patient 1. Immunostained sections (A, C, E, & G). PAS-stained sections (B, D, F, & H). Panels A, B, E, and F are the same magnification (bar = 50 µm). Panels C, D, G, and H are the same magnification (bar = 10 µm). The section composed of panels A through D is 120 µm-distant from other section of panels E through H in paraffin sections.

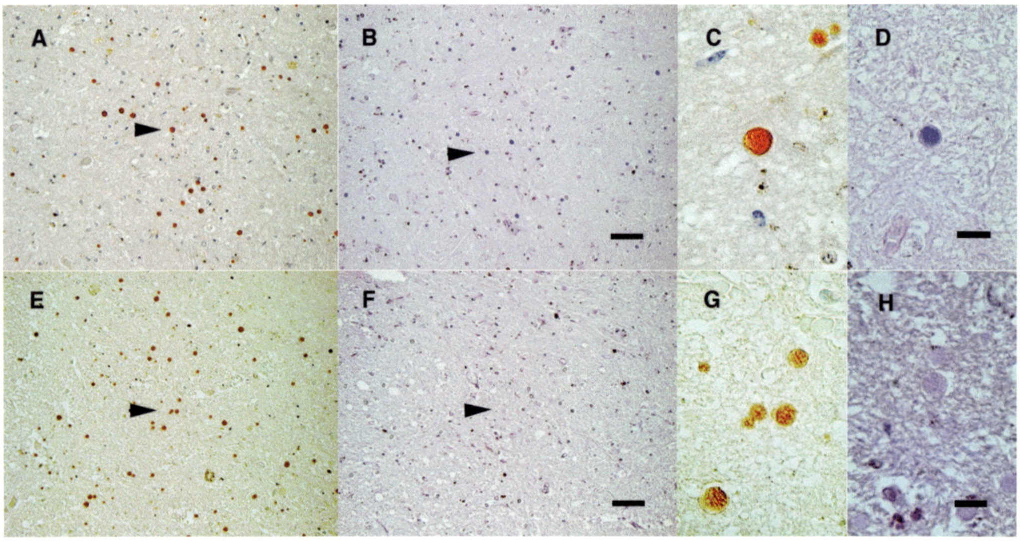

Fig. 6. Light micrographs of the VM pars compacta of the substantia nigra in PD patient 2. Immunostained sections (A, C, E & G). PAS-stained sections (B, D, F, & H). Panel A, B, E, and F are the same magnification (Bar = 50 µm). Panel C, D, G, and H are the same magnification (bar = 10 µm). The section composed of panels A through D is 285 m-distant from other section of panels E through H in paraffin sections.

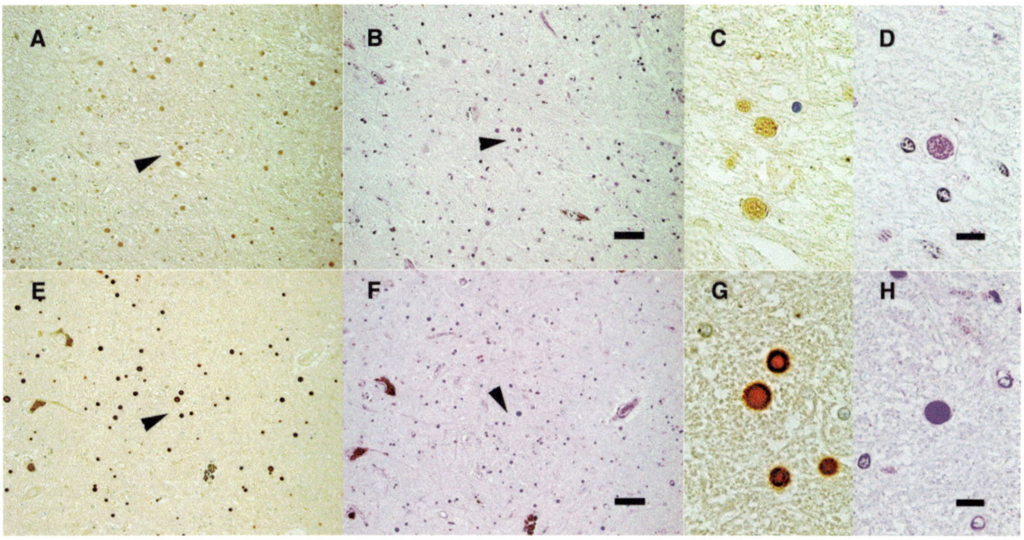

Fig. 7. Light micrographs of the VM pars compacta of the substantia nigra in PD patients 4 and 5. Immunostained sections of PD patients 4 (A & C) and 5 (E & G). PAS-stained sections of PD4 (B & D) and PD 5 (F & H). Panels A, B, E, and F are the same magnification (Bar = 50 μm). Panels C, D, G, and H are the same magnification (bar = 10 μm).

composed of immunoreactive granules. Many immunoreactive (Fig. 7A) and PAS-positive (Fig. 7B) spots were seen in PD patient 4. In higher magnification of the nigral region shown by an arrowhead on Figs. 7A or 7B, immunoreactive and PAS-positive granule-containing corpora were observed (Figs. 7 C & 7D). The same corpora were present in the VM compacta of PD patient 3. Many immunoreactive (Fig. 7E) and PAS-positive (Fig. 7F) spots were seen. In higher magnification of the nigral region shown by arrowhead on Fig, 7E or Fig. 7F, immunoreactive and PAS-positive corpora were observed (Figs. 7G & 7H). The same corpora were present in PD patient 6. A few immunoreactive spots were seen (Fig. 8A), but PAS-positive spots were not evident (Fig. 8B). In higher magnification of the nigral region shown by an arrowhead on Fig. 8A or Fig. 8B, immunoreactive (Fig. 8C) or pink-colored (Fig. 8D) corpora were present in control patient 1. In control patient 2, several immunoreactive (Fig. 8E) and PAS-positive (Fig. 8F) spots were seen. In higher magnification of the nigral region shown by an arrowhead on Fig. 8E or Fig. 8F, immunoreactive granule-containing (Fig. 8G) and pink-colored (Fig. 8H) corpora were observed. The same corpora were seen sparsely present in the substantia nigra of control patients 3 and 4.

3.6 PAS-positive corpora and gelatinous mass harboring acid-fast or AO-positive granules in the midbrain of PD patient 1

Many PAS-positive granule-bearing neuroglia (arrows on Fig. 9A), clusters of PAS-positive granules (Fig. 9B), PAS-positive large corpora (Fig. 9C), and acid-fast granule-containing gelatinous masses (Fig. 9D) were present in the VL pars compacta. When stained with AO, many fluorescent granules variable in size were seen within corpora (Fig. 9E). Near an autofluorescent granule-bearing neuron (an arrow in Fig. 9F), gelatinous masses were not autofluorescent. When stained with AO they fluoresced brilliantly nearby lipofuscin-bearing neuron (an arrow in Fig. 9G) and were found to be composed of fluorescent granules of similar size at higher magnification (Fig. 9H).

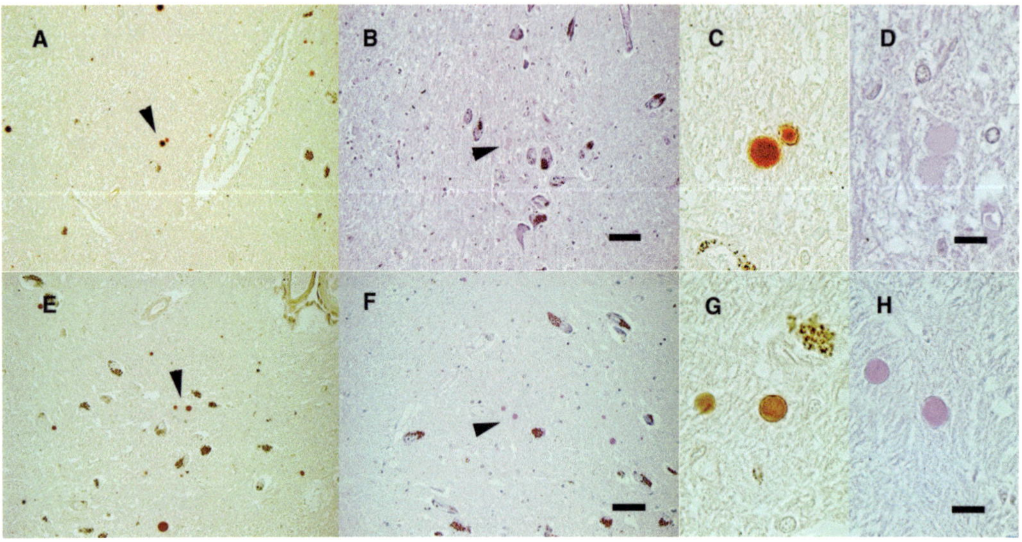

Fig. 8. Light micrographs of the VM pars compacta of the substantia nigra in control patients C1 and C2. Immunostained sections of control patients C1 (A & C) and C2 (E & G). PAS-stained sections of C1 (B & D) and C2 (F & H). Panels A, B, E, and F are the same magnification (Bar = 50 μm). Panels C, D, G, and H are the same magnification (bar = 10 μm).

3.7 Neurons connected to AO-positive gelatinous masses and degenerative neurons in the pars compacta of PD patient 1

The slide sections following that shown in Fig. 9G revealed gelatinous masses connected to the same lipofuscin-bearing neurons (arrowheads on Figs. 10A & 10B). Brilliantly yellow-fluorescent neuron-like bodies were present nearby several melanin-pigmented neurons (Fig. 10C). In H&E-stained sections, they appeared as invisible ghost cells (an arrow on Fig. 10D). Under higher magnification of the VL pars compacta shown by an arrow on Fig. 10D, they were observed as gelatinous masses containing many granules (Fig. 10E).

3.8 AO- and DAPI-positive granule-containing gelatinous masses and immunoreactive corpora connected with neurites in PD patients 2, 3, and 5

AO- and DAPI-positive granules were localized within gelatinous masses in the same section of PD patient 2 (Figs. 11A and 11B). In PD patient 5, gelatinous masses containing AO- and DAPI-positive granules were also observed. Immunoreactive corpora (Fig. 11C) were observed to be connected with neurites containing PAS-positive granules on the next section (an arrowhead on Fig. 11D). Immunoreactive corpora were composed of a deformed portion (an arrowhead on Fig. 11E) where PAS-positive granule-bearing neurites connected on the next section (an arrowhead on Fig. 11F).

4. Discussion

4.1 Isolation study of the nigral tissue samples

Gram-negative, immunoreactive, and PAS-positive granular cells were observed in broth cultures of PD patient 1 filtrates. Gram-negative and immunoreactive granular cells were

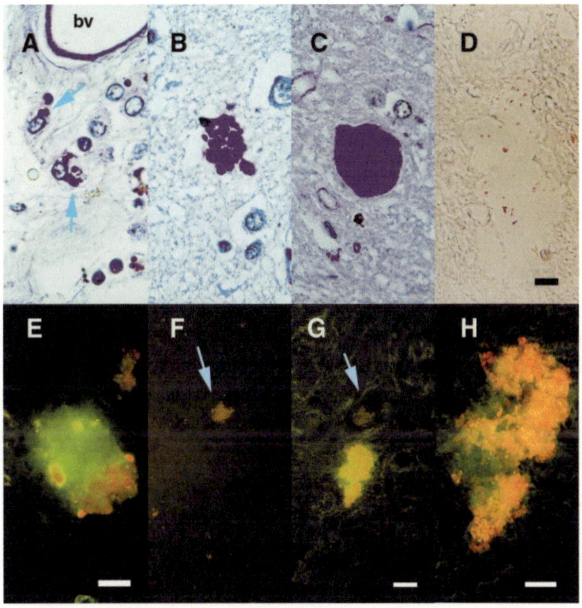

Fig. 9. Light micrographs of the VL and VM pars compacta and the central gray area of PD patient 1. PAS-stained sections (A, B, and C) and acid fast-stained section (D) of the VL pars compacta. Panels A through D are the same magnification (Bar = 10 µm). Acridine orange-stained sections from the central gray area under ultraviolet light (E). Bar = 10 µm. Unstained (F) and acridine orange-stained (G) sections from the VM pars compacta under ultraviolet light. Panels F and G are the same magnification (bar = 25 µm). Acridine orange-stained section from the VM pars compacta under ultraviolet light (H). Bar = 10 µm. bv; blood vessel.

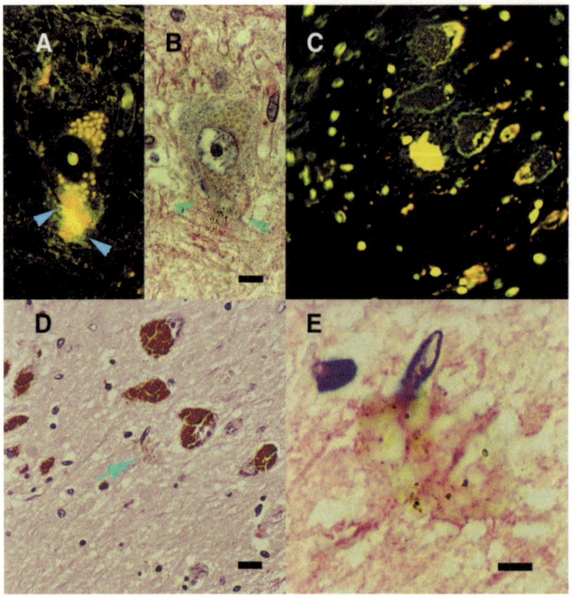

Fig. 10. Light micrographs of the different VM and VL pars compacta of PD patient 1. Acridine orange-stained (A) under ultraviolet light and H&E-stained (B) sections from the VM pars compacta. Panels A & B are the same magnification (Bar = 10 µm). Acridine orange-stained section under ultraviolet light (C) and H&E-stained (D) section from the pars compacta. Panels C and D are the same magnification (bar = 25 µm). H&E-stained section (E) from the pars compacta. Bar = 10 µm.

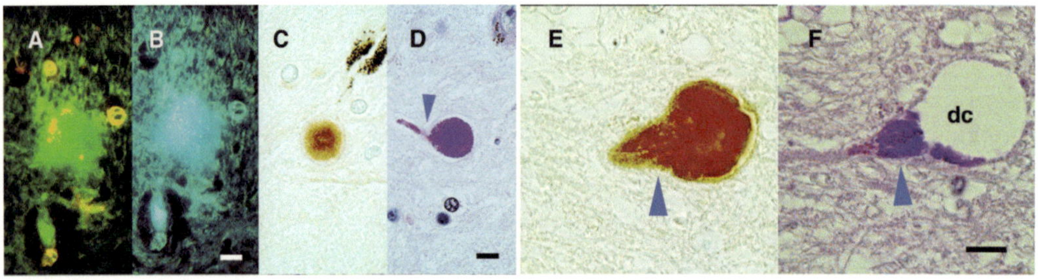

Fig. 11. Micrographs of the VM and VL pars compacta of PD patients2, 3, and 5. Acridine orange-stained (A) and DAPI-stained (B) sections of the VM pars compacta of PD2 under ultraviolet light. Panels A and B are the same magnification (bar = 10 µm). Immunostained (C) and PAS-stained (D) sections of the VM pars compacta in PD3. Panels C and D are the same magnification (bar = 10 µm). Immunostained (E) and PAS-stained (F) sections of the VL pars compacta in PD5. Panels E and F are the same magnification (bar = 10 µm). dc; detached corpora.

also observed in that of PD 4 filtrates. Both of the growth were enhanced by erythrocyte lysates supplemented. The two filterable organisms shared morphological, immunological, and physiological features with filterable nocardiae. One may postulate **first** that filterable nocardiae are likely born inside the cyst of *Nocardia* under aerated conditions and released into an environmental wind to colonize a preferable unknown site of infection (Kohbata, 1998; Kohbata et al., 2009). Filterable nocardiae may cause air-borne infection, localize within an as-yet unknown primary niche, and occupy erythrocytes as their preferred niche. Via erythrocyte, filterable nocardiae might infect other hosts horizontally or vertically. **Second**, intraerythrocytic pathogen may seed astroglia. After an invasion of astroglia, filterable nocardiae might produce cysts and preferentially multiply in the midbrain nigral tissues of PD patients, by lacking a cylindrical tubule formation. The primer, amplifying the 16S rDNA of *Nocardia,* was not effective in the detection of 16S rDNA of filterable organisms. The first trial aiming to detect of 16S rRNA, specific to gram-positive filamentous nocardiae (i.e., so-called *Nocardia*), in Lewy body-containing brain specimens did not attain satisfactory outcomes (Chapman et al., 2003; Lu et al., 2005). Filterable nocardiae might happen to be undergoing degeneration inside a new pathogenic niche.

4.2 Distribution and localization in control or PD patients

Immunoreactive and PAS-positive corpora were present in the substantia nigra of control patients. The observed corpora's morphological features are identical to those of corpora amylacea (i.e., astroglial PAS-positive inclusions). A literature reveals that corpora amylacea become microscopically detectable in the central nervous system in the first decade of life. After the age of 50, corpora amylacea increase numerous in the central nervous system (Cavanagh, 1999). Seropositivity for *Nocardia* is frequent in healthy aged as well as young subjects (Hubble et al., 1995, Kohbata & Shimokawa, 1993). Corpora amylacea are likely to be filterable nocardiae in origin. Filterable nocardiae form PAS-positive cysts at the tips of cylindrical tubules in the presence of erythrocyte lysates. Many corpora, morphologically & immunologically identical to filterable nocardiae cysts, were densely present in the substantia nigra of PD patients when compared with that of control patients. Several corpora were present in the VL pars compacta of PD patients. Gelatinous masses containing granules were connected with midbrain neurons (Figs. 10A & 10B) and present in perikarya (Fig. 4G). Immunoreactive and PAS-positive granules were present in neurites (Figs. 11C, 11D, 11E, & 11F) or perikarya (Figs. 4A & 4B). Filterable nocardiae may multiply inside astroglia, where they might invade neurons through astroglial-neuronal synapses. Immunoreactive granules were deposited in neuronal cytoplasm (Figs. 4E & 4F) as well as in various stages of Lewy body (Figs. 3E, 3F, 3G, & 3H). The gelatinous masses containing granules occupied ghost neurons (Fig. 10E). Filterable nocardiae may be involved not only in the neuronal loss but also in the Lewy body formation. Spread of Lewy bodies from the brainstem through midbrain and basal forebrain to the cerebral cortex might result from an invasion by filterable nocardiae through blood stream.

4.3 Host response to their presence

A comparison with the VL pars compacta of age-matched controls reveals that numerous melanin-pigmented neurons were absent from PD patients. The corpora in the VM pars compacta of PD patient 1 were faintly to weakly immunoreactive when compared with not only that of other PD patients but also that of control patients. In the early stage of PD, many dense clusters of acid-fast lipochrome bodies were observed. Many doughnut-like acid-fast pathogens are present on the surface or the inside of the mouse midbrain one week following the onset of movement disorder (Kohbata et al., 2009). Filterable nocardiae likely invade the midbrain substantia nigra, probably the VL pars compacta, on a massive scale from the disease onset to the early stage. Microglia, only protecting neuroglia against infection, may become activated to gather at and rapidly attack the site of infection (Verkhratsky & Butt, 2007). Faintly immunoreactive spots (Figs. 5A & 5E) may be subject to the host immune response. Filterable nocardiae's invasion and the host immune response might result in a severe loss of the VL pars compacta dopaminergic neurons, which could ensue and lead to the onset of disease. The substantia nigra of PD patients is likely to be under activated microglia in comparison to that of control patients (McGeer et al., 1998; Mirza et al., 2000). Filterable organisms, isolated from early stage PD patient 1, were PAS-positive and immunoreactive. The corpora were intensely PAS-positive and faintly immunoreactive. From the broth cultures of PAS-negative filterable organisms PD 4, sufficient amounts of genomic DNAs were obtained. Filterable organisms PD 1, under stressed conditions, were PAS-positive. The PAS-positive thick layers may inhibit yields of the genomic DNAs by using the extraction buffer.

4.4 Host intracellular digestive system

Immunoreactive and PAS-positive corpora, of which size was similar in the VM pars compacta, were different in their shape and size in the VL pars compacta. An electron microscopic study of AC-positive corpora, shown in Fig. 9E and measured as ca. 30 μm in diameter, revealed several wall-free prokaryotes measured as ca. 0.5 μm in diameter (Kohbata et al., 2005). Filterable nocardiae may penetrate perivascular astroglia, multiply to be clusters of granules with 1.0 μm in diameter and form large corpora of which diameter was 25 μm (Fig. 9C). The neuronal cytoplasm was occupied with numerous immunoreactive granules (Figs. 4E and 4F), granule-containing (Fig. 4G), and AC-positive gelatinous masses (Fig. 10E). Filterable nocardiae are not likely to be trapped into heterophagic vacuoles fused with lysosomes to be degraded, suggestive of intracellular digestive system not functional. Mutations in the glucocerebrosidase genes encoding lysosomal enzymes emerge as strong genetic determinants predisposing people to PD (Aharon-Peretz et al., 2004). Filterable organisms may be not degraded by lysosomal enzymes in astroglia as well as neurons. Corpora amylacea might be an infectious focus in the PD midbrains. Intraneuronal PAS-positive inclusions (i.e., Lafora bodies), resemble or identical with corpora amylacea, are pathologically hallmark of Lafora disease (Minassian, 2001). The digestive system of astroglia as well as neurons may be not functional by the genetic lesions including impaired autophagy and mutations in the lysosomal protein glucohydrolase (Aguado et al., 2010; Minassian el al., 2000). Lafora bodies are distributed throughout the central nervous system (Schwarz & Yanoff, 1965). Intraneuronal PAS-positive inclusions, shown in Figs. 4B & 4C, partially resemble Lafora bodies (Namba, 1968). Filterable nocardiae could potentially invade the substantia nigra, dentate nucleus, thalamus, globus pallidus, and the 3rd & 4th layers of the cerebral cortex.

4.5 Adaptation of filterable nocardiae

An intraerythrocytic pathogen may seed astroglia to form corpora amylacea through the blood-brain barrier. Ever since the first decade of life, filterable nocardiae might infect the central nervous system of normal subjects, but rapidly to be eliminated. PAS-positive granules were present within perivascular neuroglia (arrowheads on Fig. 9A). Gelatinous masses containing many acid-fast granules were present in the VL pars compacta (Fig. 9D). Acid-fast lipochrome bodies are abundantly present around blood vessels in the early stages of infection, but not in later (Kohbata et al., 1998). PAS-positive filterable nocardiae, present during all stages of PD, are likely to adapt to survive within midbrain astroglia as well as neurons. Dust-like DAPI-positive granules were present within gelatinous masses (Fig. 11B). The filterable nocardiae, as intracellular parasites, were likely to adapt and survive as PAS-, AO-, DAPI-positive, or immunoreactive small granules inside both astroglia and neurons in PD patients. DAPI staining is used for the detection of AT-rich endosymbiotic bacteria (Sun et al., 2009). *Nocardia,* closely related to *Mycobacterium,* belong to the high-G+C subdivision of gram-positive eubacteria (Woese, 1987). The leprosy-causing pathogen *Mycobacterium leprae* remains uncultivatable on artificial medium and shows a high predilection for neuroglia of the peripheral nervous system. *M. leprae* has undergone major deletions yielding a smaller genome size and lower G+C contents (Cole et al., 2001). Eight fragment sequences of filterable organisms were analyzed to be AT-rich with lower G+C contents. Most fragment contained several A/T homopolymers. The shift toward high A+T content that is common in host-restricted symbiotic bacteria leads to increased occurrence of A/T homopolymers (Moran et al., 2009). An intracellular lifestyle inside erythrocytes, astroglia, or neurons may lead to the genomic DNA degeneration by the retention of the morphological, immunological, and physiological features under host-restricted conditions. It was possible to isolate filterable organisms present in the nigral lesions for investigation of their morphological, immunological, physiological, and genomic DNA features. This will facilitate challenge and isolation studies of filterable organisms which may be a cause of PD.

5. Conclusion

An isolation study of filterable nocardiae from several frozen nigral tissue samples of PD patients was performed. A preferential site of their growth in the midbrain of six PD patients was histochemically and immunohistochemically assessed. Filterable organisms isolated from two PD patients shared the same morphological, antigenic, and physiological features with filterable nocardiae. PCR-mediated identification was not successful. The partial genomic DNAs were AT-rich with a G+C content of 41 %, containing several A/T homopolymers. Neuronal vacuoles, ghost, and shrunken nigral neurons occupied by immunoreactive, PAS-positive granules, or granule-containing gelatinous masses were present in patients with early stages of PD. Immunoreactive and PAS-positive corpora were densely distributed throughout the VM pars compacta of the substantia nigra in six PD patients. Gelatinous masses or immunoreactive corpora likely connected with midbrain neurons were observed. The results suggest that filterable organisms isolated from the nigral tissue samples likely originate from the degeneration of filterable nocardiae. Filterable nocardiae may multiply within astroglia, through which they might invade midbrain neurons, and could play a significant role in both neuronal loss and Lewy body formation.

6. Acknowledgements

We thank Dr. Ohara S (Matsumoto National Hospital, Matsumoto City, Nagano, Japan) for his help with the brain sampling. We appreciate the letter of support from European country peoples for the 0311 2011.

7. References

Aguado, C., Sarker, S., Korolchuk, VI., Criado, O., Vernia, S., Boya, P., Sanz, P., Rodriguez de Cordoba, S., Knecht, E. & Robinsztein, D.C. (2010). Laforin, the most common protein mutated in Lafora disease, regulates autophagy, *Hum Mol Genet*, Vol. 19, No. 14, pp. 2867-2876

Aharon-Peretz, J., Rosenbaum, H. & Gershoni-Baruch R. (2004). Mutations in the glucocerebrosidase gene and Parkinson's disease in Ashkenazi Jews, *New E J Med*, Vol. 351, No. 4, pp 1972-1977

Beaman, B.L. & Beaman, L. (1994). *Nocardia* species: host-parasite relationships, *Clin Microbiol Rev*, Vol. 7, No. 2, pp. 213-264

Bethlem, J. & Jager, D.H. (1960). The incidence and characteristics of Lewy bodies in idiopathic paralysis agitans (Parkinson's disease), *J Neurol Neurosurg Psychiat*, Vol. 23, pp. 74-80

Bojinov, S. (1971). Encephalitis with acute parkinsonian syndrome and bilateral inflammatory necrosis of the substantia nigra, *J Neurol Sci*, Vol. 12, No. 4, pp. 383-415

Braak, H. & Tredici, K.D. (2008). Assessing fetal nerve cell grafts in Parkinson's disease, *Nat Med*, Vol. 14, No. 5, pp. 483-485

Braak, H., Rub, U., Gai, WP. & Tredici, K.D. (2003). Idiopathic Parkinson's disease: possible routes by which vulnerable neuronal types may be subject to neuroinvasion by an unknown pathogen, *J Neural Transm*, Vol. 110, No. 5, pp. 517-536

Cavanagh, J.B. (1999). Corpora amylacea and the family of polyglucosan disease, *Brain Res Rev*, Vol 29, No. 2-3, pp. 265-95

Chapman, G., Beaman, B.L., Loeffler, D.A., Camp, D.M., Domino, E.F., Dickson, D.M., Ellis, W.G., Chen, I., Bachus, S.E. & LeWitt, P.A. (2003). In situ hybridization for detection of nocardial 16S rRNA: reactivity within intracellular inclusions in experimentally infected cynomolgus monkeys--and in Lewy body-containing human brain specimens, *Exp Neurol*, Vol. 184, No. 2, pp. 715-725

Cole, S.T., Eiglmeier, K., Parkhill, J., James, K.D., Thomson, N.R., Wheeler, P.R., Honore, N., Garnier, T., Churcher, C., Harris, D., Mungall, K., Basham, D., Brown, D., Chillingworth, T., Connor, R., Davies, R.M., Devlin, K., Duthoy, S., Feltwell, T., Fraser, A., Hamlin, N., Holroyd, S., Hornsby, T., Jagels, K., Lacroix, C., Maclean J., Moule, S., Murphy, L., Oliver, K., Quall, M.A., Rajandream, M.-A., Rutherford, K.M., Rutter, S., Seeger, K., Simon, S., Simmonds, M., Skelton, J., Squares, R., Squares, S., Stevens, K., Taylor, K., Whitehead, S., Woodward, J.R. & Barrel, B.G. (2001). Massive gene decay in the leprosy bacillus, *Nature*, Vol. 409, No. 6823, pp. 1007-1011

Fearnley, J.M. & Lees, A.J. (1991). Ageing and Parkinson's disease: substantia nigra regional selectivity, *Brain*, Vol. 114, Pt. 5, pp. 2283-2301

Greenfield, J.G. & Bosanquet, F.D. (1953). The brain-stem lesions in parkinsonism, *J Neurol Neurosurg Psychiat*, Vol. 16, No. 4, pp. 213-226

Haines, D.E. (1987). *Neuroanatomy; an atlas of structure, sections, and system* (2), Urban & Scwarzenberg, Baltimore-Munich

Hawkes, C.H. (2008). The prodromal phase of sporadic Parkinson's disease: dose it exist and is so how long is it?, *Mov Disord*, Vol. 23, No. 13, pp. 1799-1807

Hoehn, M.M. & Yahr, M.D. (1967). Parkinsonism: onset, progression, and mortality, *Neurology*, Vol. 17, No. 5, pp. 427-442

Hubble, J.P., Cao, T., Kjelstrom, J.A., Koller W.C. & Beaman, B.L. (1995). *Nocardia* species as an etiologic agent in Parkinson's disease: serological testing in a case-control study, *J Clin Microbiol*, Vol. 33, No. 10, pp. 2768-2769

Kohbata, S., Emura, S. & Kadoya, C. (2009). Filterable forms of *Nocardia*: a preferential site of infection in the mouse brain, *Microbes Infect*, Vol. 11, No. 8-9, pp. 744-752

Kohbata, S., Hayashi, R., Tamura, T., Hayashi, R. & Kadoya, C. (2005). Filterable nocardiae-like organism isolated from the midbrain nigral tissue in Parkinson's disease, *Abstracts of the 16th International Congress on Parkinson's Disease and related Disorders*, pp. 168-169, Berlin, Germany, June 5-9, 2005.

Kohbata, S., Tamura, T. & Hayashi, R. (1998). Accumulation of acid-fast lipochrome bodies in glial cells of the midbrain nigral lesion in Parkinson's disease, *Clin Diag Lab Immunol*, Vol. 5, No. 6, pp. 888-893

Kohbata, S. (1998). Tinctorial properties of spherical bodies in broth cultures of *Nocardia asteroides* GUH-2, *Microbiol Immunol*, Vol. 42, No. 3, pp. 151-157

Kohbata, S. & Shimokawa, K. (1993). Circulating antibody to *Nocardia* in the serum of patients with Parkinson's disease, *Adv Neurol*, Vol. 60, pp. 355-357

Kohbata, S. & Beaman, B.L. (1991). L-Dopa-responsive movement disorder caused by *Nocardia asteroides* localized in he brains of mice, *Infect Immunit*, Vol. 59, No. 1, pp. 181-191

Li, J-Y., Englund, E., Holton, J.L., Soulet, D., Hagell, P., Lees, A.J., Lashley, T., Quinn, N.P., Rehncrona, S., Bjorklund A., Widner, H., Revesz, T., Lindvall, O. & Brundin P. (2008). Lewy bodies in grafted neurons in subjects with Parkinson's disease suggest host to-graft disease propagation, *Nat Med*, Vol. 14, No. 5, pp. 501-503

Lu, L., Camp, D.M., Loeffler, D.A. & LeWitt, P.A. (2005). Lack of evidence for *Nocardia asteroides* in brain specimens from Lewy body-containing disorders, *Microbial Pathogenesis*, Vol. 39, No. 5-6, pp. 205-211

McGeer, P.L., Itagaki, S., Akiyama, H. & McGeer, E.G. (1988). Rate of cell death in parkinsonism indicates active neuropathological process, *Ann Neurol*, Vol. 24, No.4, pp. 574-576

Minassian, B.A. (2001). Lafora's disease: towards a clinical, pathologic, and molecular synthesis, *Pediatr Neurol*, Vol. 25, No. 1, pp. 21-29

Minassian, B.A., Ianzano L., Meloche, M., Andermann, E., Rouleau, G.A., Delgado-Escueta, A.V. & Scherer, S.W. (2000). Mutation spectrum and predicted function of laforin in Lafora's progressive myoclonus epilepsy, *Neurology*, Vol. 55, No. 3, pp. 341-346

Mirza, B., Hadberg, H., Thomsen, P. & Moos, T. (2000). The absence of reactive astrocytosis is indicative of a unique process in Parkinson's disease, *Neuroscience*, Vol. 95, No. 2, pp. 425-432

Moran, N.A., McLaughlin, H.J. & Sorek, R. (2009). The dynamics and time scale of ongoing erosion in symbiotic bacteria, *Science*, Vol. 323, No. 5912, pp. 379-382

Namba, M. (1968). Lafora disease, *Nousinkei*, Vol. 20, PP. 6-13 (in japanese).

Schwarz, G.A. & Yanoff, M. (1965). Lafora's disease, *Arch Neurol*, Vol. 12, pp. 172-188

Sun, H.Y., Noe, J., Barber, J., Coyne, R.S., Cassidy-Hanley, D., Clark, T.G., Findley, R.C. & Dickerson, H.W. (2009). Endosymbiotic bacteria in the parasitic ciliate *Ichthyophthirius*, *Appl Environ Microbiol*, Vol. 75, No. 23, pp. 7445-7452

Verkhratsky, A. & Butt, A. (2007). *Glial Neurobiology*, John Wiley & Sons, West Sussex, England

Woese, C.R. (1987). Bacterial evolution, *Microbiol Rev*, Vol. 51, No. 2, pp. 221-271

6

Parkinson's Disease and the Immune System

Roberta J. Ward[1], R.R. Crichton[1] and D.T. Dexter[2]
[1]*Universite Catholique de Louvain, Louvain-la-Neuve,*
[2]*Centre for Neuroscience, Division of Experimental Medicine,*
Hammersmith Campus, Imperial College London, London,
[1]*Belgium*
[2]*UK*

1. Introduction

The characteristic neuropathological markers of PD are the presence of Lewy bodies, containing modified α-synuclein amongst other proteins, in the surviving neurons, and the degeneration of neuromelanin-containing dopaminergic neurons in the substania nigra par compacta region of the brain. In addition, the progressive nature of PD is characterised by chronic innate inflammation with microglial activation, as well as astrogliosis and lymphocytic infiltration, which are implicated in both the initiation and progression of PD (Qin et al., 2007). Activation of microglial cells will increase the activity of NADPH-oxidase, (with the release of reactive oxygen and nitrogen species). In addition, mitochondrial dysfunction as well as cytotoxicity, (via glutamate release) will occur, which will contribute to the pro-inflammatory state. Abnormal proteasome function in PD contributes to the build up of α-synuclein aggregates within specific brain which will contribute to inflammation through the activation of microglia (reviewed in Crichton and Ward, 2006). Alterations in the innate and adaptive immune systems are reported in PD and will be reviewed in this chapter. Furthermore, considerable evidence over the past few years has indicated that there is a generalised inflammatory response in PD, that is present in both the brain and the periphery. Therapeutic intervention to retard such inflammation may reduce the progression of neurodegeneration in PD.

2. Immune system overview

The immune system is an intricate network of specialised tissues, which protects the host from infection. It can be divided into two interactive systems, innate and adaptive immunity.

2.1 Innate immune system and inflammation

Innate immunity is characterised by the immune system's ability to rapidly mobilize a response to an invading pathogen, toxin, or allergen, by distinguishing self from non-self. Toll like receptors, (TLRs), as well as nucleotide binding and oligomerization domain, (NOD-like receptors) and the cytoplasmic helicase retinoic acid inducible gene protein 1, (RIG-I-like receptors), are located on the phagocytic cell membranes, (e.g. macrophages and microglia) (**Figure 1).** These play a fundamental role in innate recognition of neuronal damage, by sensing pattern recognition receptors, (PRRs), on endogenous danger-associated molecules e.g. NOD-like receptors, (Reviewed in Ward et al., 2010). Activation of inflammatory gene transcription and post-translational processing will then occur. Innate immunity is present at birth, the effector cells being mostly myeloid cells, neutrophils, monocytes and macrophages, which on activation, release immunoactive substances such as cytokines, neurotrophic factors, chemokines, reactive oxygen and nitrogen species. In addition, a number of inhibitory pathways are induced during this pro-inflammatory stage, which ensure that the elevation in cytokine response does not overwhelm the host.

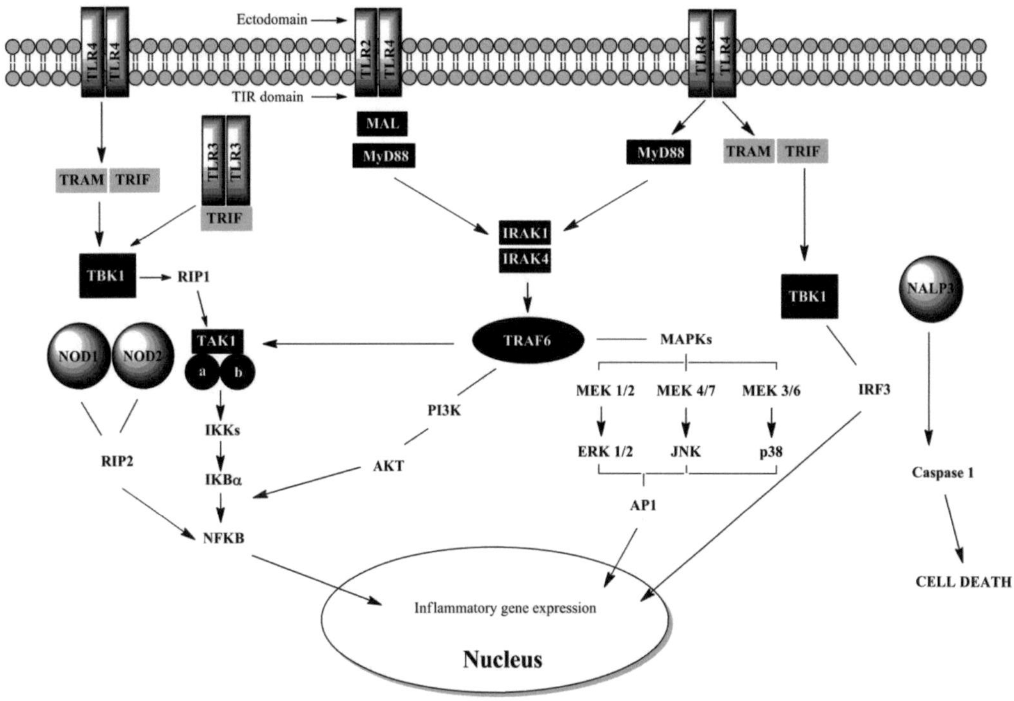

Fig. 1. Danger signals from the external environment or the cytosol are transduced through adapter protein pathways to the nucleus. TLR4 plays a major role in the activation of the immune responses.

Microglia, a subset of glial cells (the other two being oligodendrocytes and astrocytes), are regarded as the resident immuno-competent effector cells of the innate immunity in the brain. **(Figure 2).** In normal circumstances, they have two important roles; a) as surveillance cells, to regulate and supervise the removal of cell debris after neuronal death, after which the micoglia will return to their quiescent state, and b) controlling apoptosis. Microglia originate either from circulating monocytes or precursor cells that colonise the nervous system primarily during embryonic and foetal periods of development (reviewed by Chan et al., 2007). Microglia are considered to be primary mediators of neuroinflammation and, as such, have a vast repertoire of PPR as well as TLRs and phagocytic receptors. In the healthy adult brain they exist in a non-activated state, equipped with receptors for neurotransmitters, neuropeptides, hormones and immune signals. Activated microglia show a phenotypical repertoire which include the synthesis of MHC class 1 and II antigen

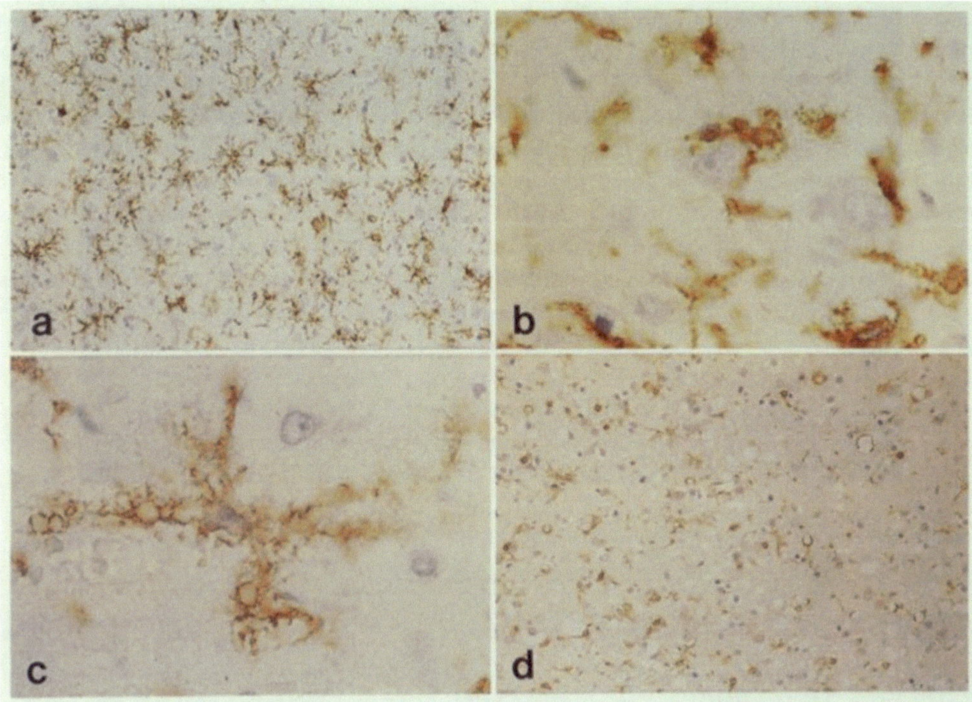

Fig. 2. Activated microglia showing highly branched processes in the ramified state.

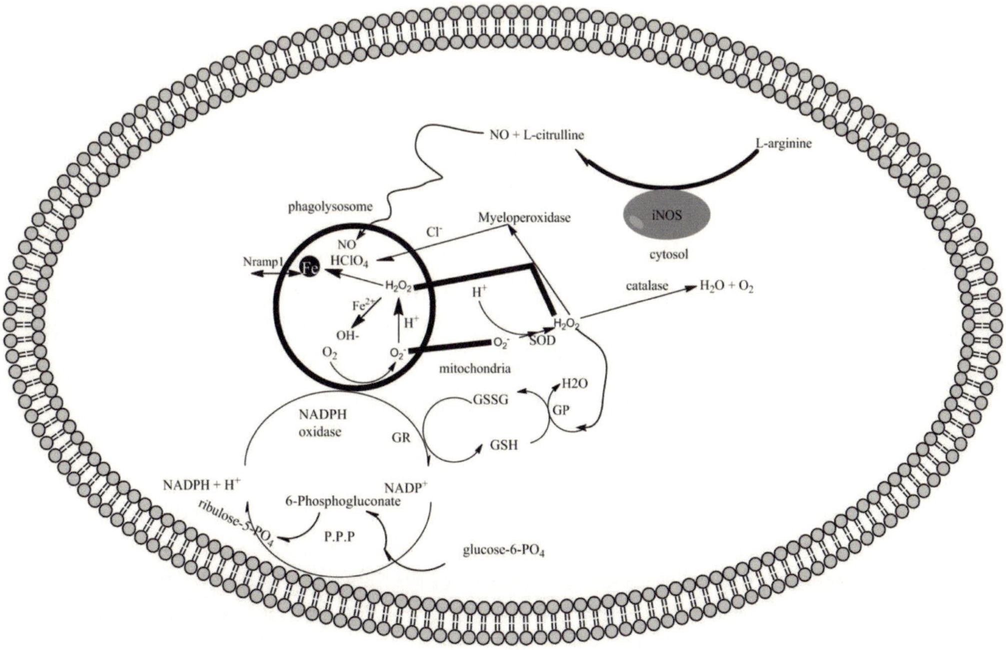

Fig. 3. Activated microglia showing NADPH oxidase activation and the subsequent generation of superoxide and nitric oxide.

presenting proteins, release cytokines such as IL-1, IL-2, IL-6. TGF-α1, CREB, the synthesis of complement components and their receptors, together with the mitogens M-CSF, GM-CSF and IL-3, **Table 1**. Cytokines are low molecular weight proteins, which modulate microglial activation by binding to their receptors, which are expressed on microglia. Pro-inflammatory cytokines e.g. IL-6, have the ability to elicit a sustained immune response while anti-inflammatory cytokines e.g. IL-10, down-regulate the immune response by binding to appropriate receptors on microglia and initiating an autocrine signalling process. Cytokine effects on the CNS function include growth promotion, inhibition and proliferation of astrocytes and oligodendrocytes, modulation of neurotransmitter release, long term potentiation which is linked to memory formation, and anxiety. Microglia also show a strong respiratory burst capacity, via NADPH oxidase, as well as the ability to release cytotoxic cytokines such as TNFα, and can produce both reactive nitrogen and oxygen species, **(Figure 3).** In normal circumstances, the inflammatory response would be rapid, decisive and then decline. In PD it is hypothesised that microglia priming may alter brain homeostasis. Furthermore, Perry (2004) proposed that chronic exposure to pro-inflammatory signals from systemic infection during an individual's lifetime, might promote an exaggerated microglial response that could contribute to neuronal deterioration, instead of facilitating a protective homeostatic response.

Cytokines	**Chemokines**	**Receptors**	**Additional factors**
IL-1	IP-10	CCR2, 3, 5	MHCI, II
IL-6	MIP1a	IL10R	CD80,86
IL-10	MIP1b	IL12R	CD95, 178
IL-12	MCP1	IL18R	Complements
IL-18	IL-8	IFN R	COX-2
TNF	RANTES	F	
TGF		TGF R	Superoxide
		FCyRI-III	Hydroxyl radical
		CR1 3,4	PGE2
		Prostaglandin receptors	PGD2
			NGF, BDNF

Table 1. Changes in mRNA expression of iron genes involved in iron homeostasis in the substantia nigra and cortex of PD patients compared with controls in post mortem tissue

3. Inflammation in PD brain-innate immune response

In early studies, McGeer et al., (1998) presented evidence for neuro-inflammation in the substantia nigra, (SNc) of PD patients with high numbers of activated microglia particularly in the vicinity of the degenerating neurons. This has been substantiated in many other studies (Dauer and Przedborski 2003; Bartels and Leenders 2007; Gao and Hong 2008). Furthermore increased levels of pro-inflammatory cytokines, e.g. TNFα, IL1β, IL-2 and IL-6, as well as β2 microglobulin, epidermal growth factor, transforming growth factor, cyclooxygenase 2 and reactive oxygen and nitrogen species are evident, post mortem, in PD brains (reviewed by Qian et al., 2010), as well as the cerebrospinal fluid (Hald and Lotharius, 2005). More recently, single positron emission tomography (PET) has shown that levels of

[11C] (*R*)-PK11195, an isoquinoline carboxamide which binds selectively to the peripheral benzodiazepine receptor (PBR), (also known as the mitochondrial 18 kDa translocator protein or TSPO) a selective marker for activated microglia is significantly higher in PD patients than control subjects and correlated with dopaminergic terminal loss, as assayed by [11C] CFT BP (Ouchi et al., 2009). Whether the activation of microglia is an initial event in the development of PD or as a consequence of the degeneration of dopaminiergic neurons remains unclear. However it would seem that there is a self perpetuating cycle whereby microglia remain continuously activated and hence represent a suitable drug target. A variety of factors will contribute to this inflammatory process:

Release of ATP from damaged neurons and/or astrocytes will initiate a rapid microglial response towards the site of injury (Davalos et al., 2005), **Figure 4**. In culture it has been shown that extracellular ATP will induce rapid microglia ruffling and whole cell migration, which is mediated via G-protein-coupled P2Y receptors (Honda et al., 2001). Extracellular ATP is also released from $CD4^+$ helper T cells, upon stimulation of the T cell receptor. This also plays a crucial role in protracting the TCR-initiated activity of MAPK and secretion of IL-2, thus determining productive T cell activation. Recent published research indicated that ATP also inhibits the generation and function of regulatory T cells via the activation of purinergic P2X receptors (Shenk et al., 2011). Release of ATP from damaged neurons and/or astrocytes will initiate a rapid changes in astrocyte function. Activated astrocytes are present in the regions of the degenerating SNc, which will contribute to the elevated cytokine

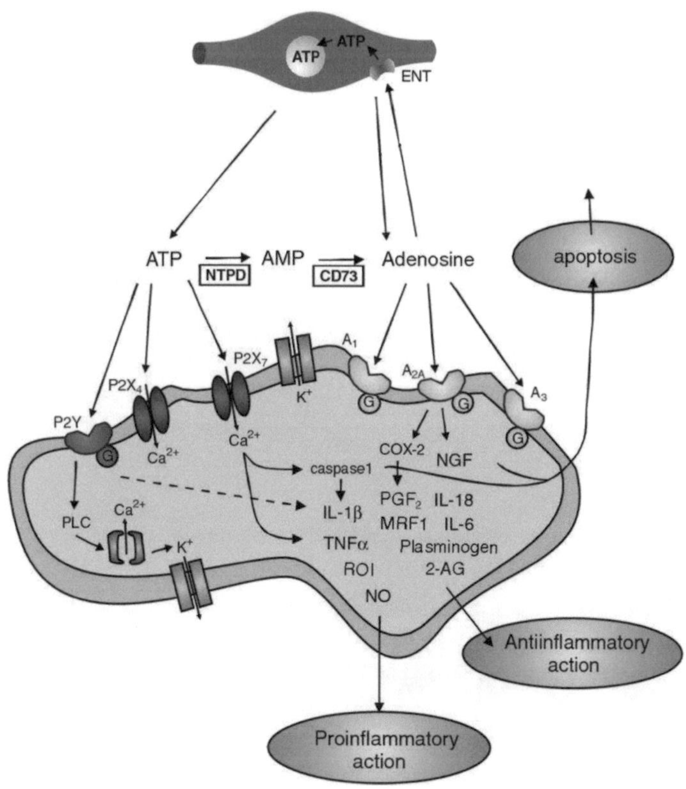

Fig. 4. Release of ATP from damaged neurons (adapted from Davalos et al., 2005).

content in this region (Forno et al., 1992). Some studies have identified a loss of astrocytes in the substatia nigra pars compacta of PD brains by comparison to controls (Damier et al., 1993). Such losses of astrocytes may imply a loss of neurotrophic support for neurons. However this has not been confirmed in other studies of PD brains (Mirza et al., 2000).

Abnormal accumulation and aggregation of α-synuclein occurs in PD. The amyloid fibril of α -synuclein will aggregate to form Lewy bodies, **Figure 5.** Such Lewy bodies will attract activated microglia (McGeer et al., 1988). Iron, which is increased in PD, will enhance intracellular aggregation of α-synuclein which leads to the formation of advanced glycation end products. In addition, there maybe an interaction between α -synuclein and Fe^{2+} to liberate hydroxy radicals, thereby contributing to the oxidative stress (Crichton & Ward, 2006).

Matrix metalloproteins, (MMPs) are proteolytic enzymes which activate microglia. Neuronal cells, in particular in dopaminergic neurons, release MMP-3 which is increased in response to various forms of cellular stress (Kim and Hwang, 2011). Thus will activate microglial cells with the production of TNFα and IL-1β as well as superoxide. The molecular mechanisms involved are unknown but may involve cleavage of surface proteins on microglial cells such as receptors, cell-cell interaction proteins, cytokines and chemokines (reviewed by Kim and Hwang 2011).

Neuromelanin, a granular dark brown pigment, is produced in catecholaminergic neurons of the SNc and locus coeruleus and is possibly the product of reactions between oxidised catechols with a variety of nucleophiles, including thiols from glutathione and proteins (Götz et al., 2004). The function of neuromelanin in the pigmented neurons is unknown but it could play a protective role via attenuation of free radical damage by binding transition metals, particularly iron. In normal individuals, the neuromelanin-iron complex is found in

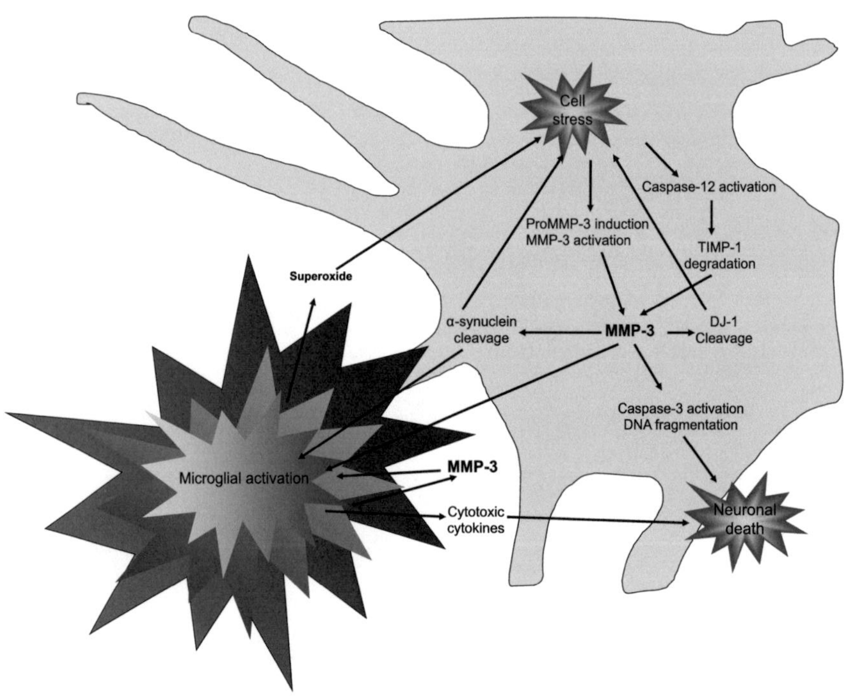

Fig. 5. Possible action of MMP-3 in neurodegeneration (adapted from Kim and Hwang, 2011)

both the SNc and locus coeruleus and increases linearly with age in the SNc. Whether the ability of the neurones to synthesis neuromelanin is impaired in PD patients is unknown, since it has been reported in some studies that the absolute concentration of nigral neuromelanin in individual neurons is less than 50% in PD with respect to age matched controls. However it is considered that when neuromelanin is released from the damaged neurons this will trigger microgliosis, microglial chemotaxis and microglial activation in PD with the subsequent release of neurotoxic mediators (reviewed in Crichton and Ward, 2006).

3.1 Stress

Stress will also have a major effect on microglial cells. Glucocorticoids are the major effector hormones of the stress system and act by binding to intracellular receptors within the cell, which are then translocated to the nucleus and act as regulators of gene expression. Generally female mammals show more robust behavioural and somatic responses to stress as well as more potent and inflammatory reactions than males (Chrousos, 2010). Stress hormones target glial cells, as well as neurons. (Jauregui-Huerta et al., 2010). Evidence that stress may contribute to the development of PD is unclear. However chronic stress will directly activate microglia as well as facilitating neuronal degeneration, which would activate microglia. Although psychological stress and glucocorticoids are reported to suppress immune function, (e.g. produce anti-inflammatory cytokines and reduce toxic radicals), possibly via glucocorticoid receptors on dopaminergic neurons, (Barcia et al., 2009), recent studies have indicated that glucocorticoids can enhance immune function in the brain (Reviewed by Jauregui-Huerta et al.,2010). This may be dependent upon the levels of glucocorticoids; i.e. high levels are pro-inflammatory while basal or low stress levels have traditional anti-inflammatory action. Such results may be important in that such stress-induced microglial activation may be involved in the progression of neurodegenerative diseases. Of the 13 epidemiological studies where the effect of stress has been studied as a possible contributory cause of PD, twelve of these studies were positive.
Serum factors, thrombin and immunoglobulins can initiate activation through protease-activated receptor 1 and Fc receptors, possibly after their passage across the BBB.

4. Polymorphisms of pro-and anti-inflammatory genes

Other contributory factors to the inflammation in PD could be functional DNA polymorphisms in some of the pro-inflammatory and anti-inflammatory cytokines which include TNF-α and IL-1β genes (Wahner et al., 2007), IL-18 607C/A polymorphism and allele 1 (C) of IL-1β (-511) (Arman et al., 2010), all of which are associated with an increased risk of PD in different populations. In contrast, the 2/2 (T/T) genotype of IL-1β (-511) may protect individuals from PD (Arman et al., 2010). Genetic variations may also be present in the HLA (human leukocyte antigen) region, where there are numerous immune related genes, which would increase the risk of PD (Hamza et al., 2010: Wahner et al., 2007). The importance of TLR4 polymorphisms in modulating the inflammatory responses has been identified.

5. Apoptosis

Neurons and glia express cellular death signalling pathways which include CD95 (Fas) /CD95L, (FasL), TNF-TNFR-1, tumor necrosis factor- tumor necrosis factor receptor 1, and TNF-related apoptosis-inducing ligand (TRAIL), with which they are able to trigger apoptosis in T cells and other infiltrating cells (Griffiths et al., 2009). Glia also express pentraxins and complement proteins. C1q, C3b and iC3b. . Hence, the rapid destruction of infiltrating T cells as well as injured neurons can be achieved by apoptosis in normal circumstances. Since apoptotic cells contain potentially neurotoxic proteins and cytokines their presence must be rapidly detected and cleared to prevent tissue damage. Such cells will express cell surface apoptotic cell-associated molecule patterns (ACAMPs) (that are comparable to PRPs), thereby identifying these cells for rapid removal from CNS to protect further damage. Failure to clear these apoptotic cells, which occurs in PD, will result in their accumulation within specific CNS tissues. Secondary necrosis of these cells will result in the release of their toxic contents thus enhancing tissue damage. Both CD47 and CD200 are expressed on microglia and are up-regulated during apoptosis, thereby inhibiting pro-inflammatory microglial cytokine expression. Apoptosis is a highly orchestrated form of cell death when a number of caspases are activated in a sequential manner. Inappropriate activation in the brain will have deleterious consequences. Apoptotic death is involved in the pathogenesis of PD.

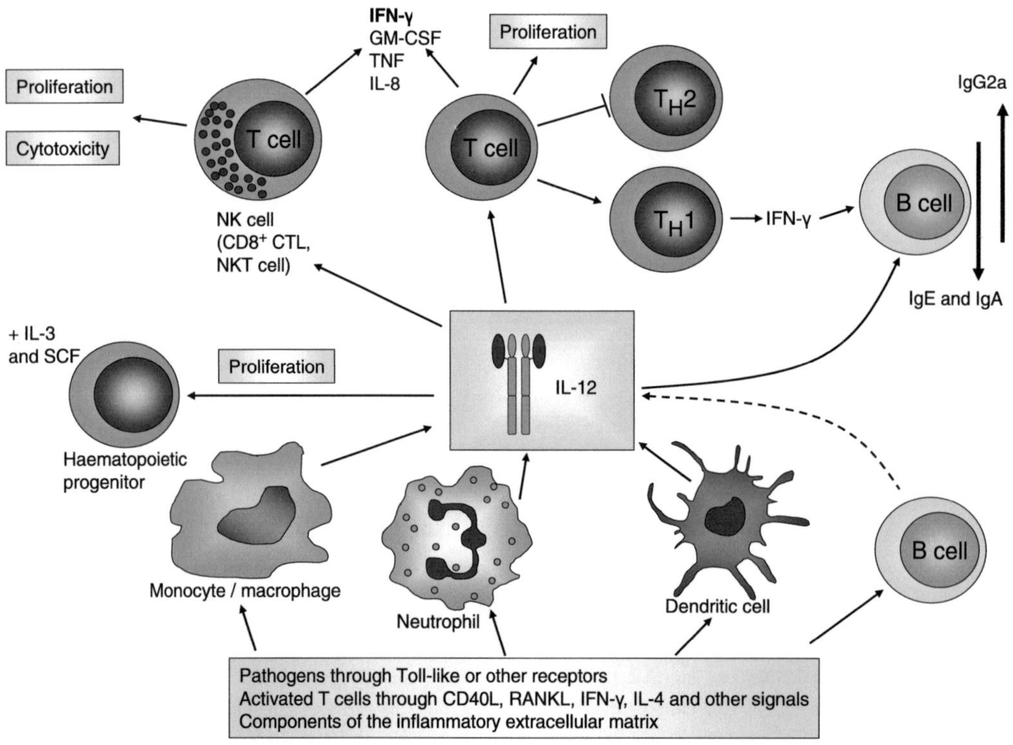

Fig. 6. Summary of the biology of Il-12 (adapted from Trinchieri, 2003)

6. Adaptive immunity and inflammation

Adaptive immunity is involved in the elimination of pathogens during the later phase of infection, (i.e. after activation of the innate immune system) and is elicited by B and T lymphocytes, which utilize immunoglobulins and T cell receptors, respectively, as antigen receptors to recognize "non self" molecules **(Figure 6).** These receptors are generated through DNA rearrangement and respond to a wide range of potential antigens. Adaptive immunity is acquired after a longer period in later life.

Lymphocytes, B-cells and T-cells are capable of responding rapidly to these specific insults/pathogens when the insult is again encountered. This mechanism allows a small number of genes to generate a large number of different antigen receptors which are expressed on each individual lymphocyte. This information will be inherited in all of the progeny, which includes memory B cells and memory T cells to give long-lived specific immunity. B cells play an important role in the humoral immune response while T-cells are intimately involved in cell -mediated immune responses. B cells are involved in the creation of antibodies that circulate in the blood and lymph which is known as humoral immunity. There are five types of antibodies, IgA, IgD, IgE, IgG and IgM. Upon activation, B cells produce antigen specific antibodies which in conjunction with the expression of unique B cell receptor (BCR), allow the identification of specific antigens.

6.1 CD8+ T lymphocytes and cytotoxicity

Naive cytotoxic T cells are activated when their T-cell receptor (TCR) strongly interacts with a peptide-bound MHC class I molecule. This affinity will depend on the type and orientation of the antigen/MHC complex. Once activated, the cytotoxic T cell undergoes a process known as clonal expansion in which it gains functionality, and divides rapidly, to produce a donor army of "armed"-effector cells which can travel throughout the body in search of cells bearing that unique MHC Class I + peptide. CD8 refers to a transmembrane glycoprotein which is a co-receptor for the T cell receptor. CD8 will bind to class I MHC protein.

6.2 $CD4^+$ lymphocytes

CD4+ lymphocytes, (helper T cells), are immune response mediators which play an important role in establishing and maximizing the capabilities of the adaptive immune response. These cells have no cytotoxic or phagocytic activity but orchestrate the immune response by directing other cells to perform these tasks. $CD4^+$ T helper cells can be induced to differentiate to specific lineages according to the local cytokine milieu, towards T helper type 1 Th1, Th2, Th17 and regulatory T cell (T_{reg}) phenotypes.

Microglial activation is propagated by T-cell releasing interferon-γ. This will sensitise the microglia by upregulating the expression of various immunoregulatory molecules including CD40 on their cell surfaces. Activation of the Janus kinase/signal transducer and activator of transcription (JAK/STAT) signalling pathway plays a central role in this IFN-γ induced CD40 expression. Modulation of the JAK/STAT signalling pathway may suppress the microglial-mediated inflammation.

7. Adaptive immunity in PD

Extraneuronal nitrated α-synuclein is able to cross the BBB to the CSF where it will activate antigen presenting cells, (reviewed by Kosloski et al., 2010), i.e. naïve T cells. With appropriate co-stimulatory signals these cells will diferentiate into Teffs that will expand into different effector cell subtypes, e.g. Th1 and Th17 cells (Reviewed by Kosloski et al., 2010). Such cells will drive the disease processes towards a pro-inflammatory situation. Th1 cells express IL-2, IFN-γ and TNFα that are pro-inflammatory and will activate microglia. Th17 also elicits a pro-inflammatory effect (Kosloski et al., 2010) and will also secrete granzyme B, a cytolytic enzyme (Kebir et al., 2007). Th2 effectors release IL-4, IL-5 and IL-13 and support anti-inflammatory responses. In addition Th1, Th2 and Th17 help in the production of antibodies which specifically target modified proteins for their removal by microglia. Th1 and Th17 Teffs are synthesied in the periphery and traverse the BBB to the inflammatory foci of the nigrostriatum and identify the N-α-synuclein/major histocompatibility complex II which are presented by the antigen presenting microglia. The induction of Teffs will drive the microglia and the innate immune responses.

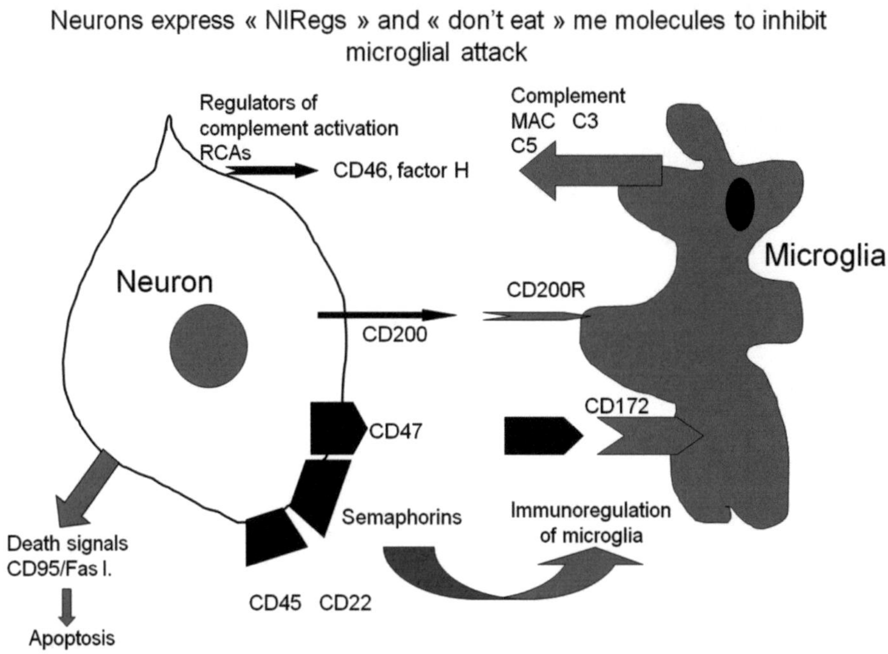

Fig. 7. Neurons express many 'self defence' proteins and receptors to prevent attack from microglia (adapted from Griffiths et al., 2010)

T cell infiltration is present in the CNS tissue of PD. Nitrated α-synuclein may activate peripheral leucocytes and mediate the adaptive immune system to potentiate mictoglial activation. Several changes in cellular and humoral immune reponses are reported to occur in the peripheral immune system of PD patients, although no clear demonstration of leucocyte involvement at the site of the neuronal damage has been reported (Brochard et al., 2009). However McGeer et al., (1998) identified cytotoxic T cells in the SNc of one PD patient while Hunot et al (1999) showed a dramatic increase of IFN-γ positive cells in brains of PD patients indicating that T cells mobilisation could be involved in the nigrostriastal injury in PD. In one further study by Brochard et al., (2009), higher densities of $CD8^+$ and $CD4^+$ T cell were present post mortem in PD brains. This may indicate that there are changes in the function of the blood brain barrier and that peripheral cells are entering the brain parenchyma. In a recent study, (Castellani et al., 2011) identified a subunit of CD3, part of the T receptor complex (TRC) on mature T cells, in Lewy bodies in PD. This subunit of CD3 has also been shown to be involved in dendritic outgrowth and synaptic formation thus raising the possibility that CD3 dysregulation as a pathogenic factor in PD.

8. Anti-inflammatory systems to regulate microglia activation

There are several anti-inflammatory systems that play a role in regulating microglia activation which include CD200/CD200 receptor, vitamin D receptor, peroxisome proliferator-activated receptors and soluble receptor for advanced glycation end products (Lue et al., 2020)

8.1 CD200/CD200 receptor

CD200 is a highly glycosylated protein. Its expression is primarily located to neurons and oligodentrocytes in human brain although both astrocytes and brain endothelial cells also express CD200 (Koning et al., 2007: Walker et al., 2009) With increasing age a loss of mRNA CD200 expression is reported in cells of rodents (Frank et al., 2006) which may also occur in humans. CD200R expression is found on many inflammatory cells which include macrophages, neutrophils, microglia, granulocytes, T lymphocytes, astrocytes and oligodentrocytes (Rijkers et al., 2008). The only known function for CD200 is to bind to CD200R. This ensures that the microglia remain in the resting state, **Figure 8.** The binding at the N-teminal of each of these molecules activates specific anti-inflammatory signalling pathways in CD200R expressing cells, thereby down regulating the pro-inflammatory response (Hatherley and Barclay, 2004). Loss of CD200, which is evident in PD brain regions where there is a loss of neurons, will induce an accelerated microglia response (Hoek et al., 2000) In addition, the activation of the extracellular signal-regulated kinase (ERK), c-Jun N-terminal kinase (JNK) and p38 mitogen activated protein kinase (MAPK) pathways will be inhibited by such binding (Zhang et al., 2004). Treatment of microglia and macrophages with IL-4 and IL-13 significantly increased expression of CD200R, in vitro. However expression of these cytokines was not generally detectable in brain (Walker et al., 2009). These anti-inflammatory cytokines bind to the same receptor complex and can activate the STST-6 transcription factor. Activation of STST-6 occurs in IL-4 stimulated human brain microglia which correlates with increased expression of CD200R. IL-4 exerts a powerful control over CD200 expression and hence modifies microglial activation. Therefore enhancing levels of IL-4 in the brain would be advantageous. Both statins and Vitamin D(3) will enhance IL-4 levels and thereby enhance an anti-inflammatory effect.

8.2 Vitamin D receptor (VDR)

Vitamin D3 plays a central role in immunity by a) modulating the production of several neurotrophins, (b) upregulating IL-4, and c) inhibiting the differentiation and survival of dendritic cells (Fernandes de Abreu, et al., 2009). Deficiency of vitamin D3 maybe associated with increased CNS diseases including PD (reviewed by Annweiler et al., 2009). The cellular receptor for vitamin D3, the vitamin D3 receptor (VDR), (nuclear receptor subfamily, group 1, member 1 (NR111) and calcitriol receptor is a member of the nuclear receptor family of transcription factors. Upon activation by vitamin D, the VDR forms a heterodimer with the retinoid-X-receptors which binds to hormone responsive elements on DNA, which causes an increased expression or repression of specific genes. Indirect evidence has suggested that PD have lower serum vitamin D than age matched controls (Sato et al., 2005). In a longitudinal study of 3000 participants in Finland, higher vitamin D levels were associated with a reduced risk of PD (Knekt et al., 2010).

8.3 Peroxisome proliferators activated receptors

The peroxisome proliferator-activated receptors, PPARs, belong to a superfamily of nuclear hormone receptors **(Figure 8).** Their main function is to regulate glucose and lipid metabolism and their subsequent storage. However, they also play a key role in the regulation of immune and inflammatory responses. PPARs can stimulate gene expression through binding to peroxisome-proliferator response elements, which are present in the promoter regions of target genes. The PPAR subfamily is comprised of three isoforms, PPAR-α, PARβ/δ and PPAR-γ. PPAR are activated by small lipophilic compounds and form heterodimers with the retinoid receptor-α (RXR) in the cytoplasm for full activation. Specific binding of PPAR onto DNA sequences leads to the activation of gene cascades involved in several biological processes (Reviewed by Chaturvedi and Beal, 2008). In the absence of ligands, PPAR and RXR heterodimers bind to co-repressor complexes and suppress gene transcription (Reviewed by Chaturvedi and Beal, 2008). PPARS also downgrade the production of MMPs, known activators of microglia and PPAR-γ agonists have been shown to be neuroprotective in a number of PD models.

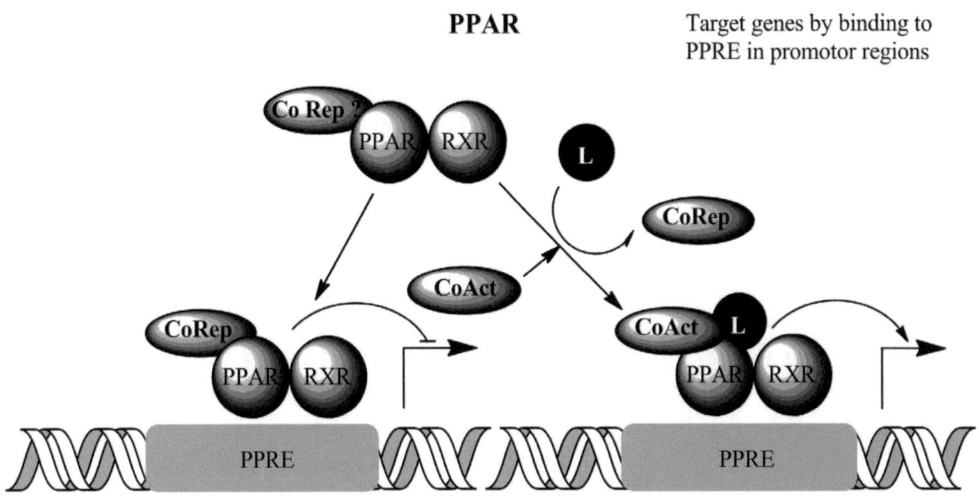

Fig. 8. Schematic representation of the PPAR signalling pathway (Adapted from Michalik et al., 2004)

9. Role of iron in inflammation in PD

There is an increased burden of iron, approximately 2 fold, compared to controls, in specific brain regions, the SNc and lateral globus pallidus of PD brains which will enhance oxidative stress (Gotz et al., 2004). H-ferritin rather than L-ferritin is present in the iron loaded SNc and lateral pallidus of PD brain (Dexter, et al., 1990) with large amounts of iron being sequestered into neuromelanin in dopaminergic neurons. Furthermore, since the SNc has a relatively high metabolic rate, with a high content of dopamine, neuromelanin, polyunsaturated fatty acids and iron, but low antioxidant protection, e.g. reduced glutathione (Sian et al., 1994) oxidative stress will be enhanced. Both reactive oxygen and nitrogen intermediates will contribute to the demise of the dopaminergic neurons, leading to the formation of lipid peroxidation products, as well as protein carbonyls and DNA damage (Alam et al., 1997). In addition, ROS, generated as a result of mitochondrial malfunction, will contribute to this toxicity. The etiology of this enhanced brain iron content may be attributable to a variety of factors which include changes in iron release mechanisms across the blood brain barrier, BBB, or perhaps more likely, a mis-regulation of iron homeostatic control in the SNc.

The control of iron homeostasis within microglia remains undefined. It is of interest that both microglia and iron deposits co-accumulate at the site of damage in PD. Whether these accumulations are a cause or effect of the disease is currently unknown. In our recent study (Ward et al., 2007) mRNA was isolated from two regions of Parkinson's brain, the SNc and the cortex, and the expression of a number of iron genes quantitated and compared with those from control post mortem material. A significant number of genes were specifically up-regulated in the substantia nigra in comparison to the cortex in the PD brains as well as controls, **Table 2.** Such up-regulation of both transferrin and transferrin receptor2 in other cell types is associated with iron deficiency, and inflammation, respectively. The high iron content of the SNc might have been expected to diminish IRP1 and IRP2 activity. However IRP-1 expression did not alter significantly whilst IRP2, which dominates post-transcriptional regulation of brain iron metabolism was up-regulated. A previous study, (Faucheux et al., 2002) reported no alteration of IRP-1 in SNc of Parkinsonian brain. The increased mRNA expression of ferroportin in SN might indicate an elevated flux of iron from certain cell types within the SNc.

Descriptor	Gene	SnM p-value	Sni	Cortex
UPREGULATED				
IRP-binding protein 1	IRP1	ns	ns	ns
IRP-binding protein 2	IRP2	0.025	ns	ns
Transferrin	Tf	0.0001	0.0030	ns
Transferrin receptor 2	TfR2	ns	0.0017	ns
Transferrin receptor 2	TfR2	ns	0.0184	ns
Ferritin H	FTH1	0.0019	ns	ns
Ferritin H pseudogene 1	FTHP1	0.0010	0.0348	ns
Ferritin L	FTL	0.0291	ns	ns
FerritinL	FTL	0.0335	ns	ns
Ferritin L	FTL	ns	0.006	ns
Caeruloplasmin	Cp	0.0276	0.0276	ns
Caeruloplasmin	Cp	ns	0.0343	ns
Caeruloplasmin	Cp	ns	0.0336	ns
Hephastin	HEPH	ns	0.009	ns
Haemochromatosis	HFE	0.0416	0.0005	ns
Haemochromatosis	HFE	ns	0.0111	ns
Haemochromatosis	HFE	ns	0.0295	ns
Haemochromatosis	HFE	ns	0.0039	ns
Ferroportin	FPN1	0.0192	ns	ns
Ferroportin	FPN1	0.0353	ns	ns
Solutecarrier family11	SLC11A2	ns	ns	0.0291
DOWNREGULATED				
Ferrochetalase		0.006	0.0223	ns
Sideroflexin 1		0.006	0.0314	ns
Friedreich ataxia		0.031	ns	ns

Table 2. Activated microglia secrete a number of factors which include cytokines, chemokines and receptors

10. Role of blood brain barrier in inflammation

The exact role played by the blood brain barrier (BBB) in excluding and permitting various molecules to cross the membrane remains an enigma. In early studies, molecular size was considered to be an important factor. However later studies have identified that passive diffusion across the blood brain barrier is very slow and that various transporters, solute carriers, as well as transcytosis, play important roles in determining whether molecules traverse the BBB. Furthermore endothelial astrocytes and neurons which are in contact with the cells of the BBB will influence intra and intercellular signalling (Neuwelt et al., 2011). The function of the BBB may be altered by inflammation in the periphery with inflammatory mediators inducing a significant paracellular leak. Immune cells are able to penetrate BBB, either at the endothelial BBB or the epithelial blood-CSF barrier. Interaction of endothelial cells with extracellular matrix will induce cross talk with adjacent cells which are pre-requisite for barrier function. For example α4β-1integrin/VCAM-1 is involved in leucocyte interaction with BBB. Inflammation and generation of ROS and RNS can acutely disrupt BBB at tight junction. Stress related pathways target nuclear transcription factors to increase P-glycoprotein expression in blood capillaries. There is altered expression of p-glycoprotein at BBB in PD. Therefore BBB function may contribute to neuro-inflammation via deregulated entry of antigen-specific T cells, via compromised removal of toxic products of neuronal damage and death and lead to disease progression via signalling of systemic inflammation. It remains unclear whether there is BBB leakage in PD patients. Polymorphism in the P-glycoprotein drug transporter MDR1 gene association and ABCB1 gene encoding the P-glycoprotein may alter the properties of the BBB in PD patients (Reveiwed by Neuwelt et al., 2011).

11. Inflammation in the periphery

Possible biofluids which can be used in the search for pertinent PD biomarkers are the cerebrospinal fluid, plasma and urine. It would be advantageous clearly to identify markers which precede the degeneration of nigrostriatal dopaminergic neurons. For example it is known that an impaired sense of smell is prevalent prior to and during the clinical motor stages of PD. Odour discrimination performance strongly correlates with risk of future PD (Berendse and Ponsen, 2009). In addition reduced striatal dopamine transporter SPECT imaging was also identified in subjects, who later developed PD. Biomarkers which correlated with these early physical symptoms would be of paramount important for early therapeutic intervention. In a small study of 84 subjects, (Chen et al., 2008), plasma inflammatory biomarkers were assessed approximately 4 years before PD diagnosis, IL-6 was associated with a greater risk of PD. Other inflammatory markers such as C-reactive protein, fibrinogen, and TNF-α were not related with risk. In contrast, analysis of serum and cerebrospinal fluid from PD patients which have active and progressive PD, it was not surprising that increased levels of the inflammatory cytokines TNFα, IL-1β, IL-2, IL-4, IL-6 and interferon γ were observed (Bacia et al., 2009). Similarly, increased oxidative damage is involved in the progression of PD and plasma levels of F(2)-Isoprostanes, hydroxyeicosatetraenoic acid products, 7 beta and 27-hydroxycholesterol, 7 ketocholesterol, F(4)-neuroprostanes and urinary 8-hydroxy-2′-deoxyguanosine were elevated in PD patients while plasma levels of phospholipase A(2) and platelet activating factor acetylhydrolase activities were lower (Seef et al., 2010).

CSF may be the most promising biological fluid since it is in closer contact with degenerating neurons. The assay of both alpha-synuclein and DJ-1 have been shown to be good biomarkers for PD but larger clinical trials as to their potential use are needed. Although some studies have advocated the assay of a pattern of inflammatory cytokines, further investigations are required to ascertain their specificity for PD.

Plasma homocysteine was increased in PD patients (Obeid et al., 2009) while platelet levels of amyloid precursor proteins and alpha synuclein may be pertinent markers of methylation. In addition various polymorphisms have been identified in the genes of TNFα and its receptor, as well as IL-1α and IL-1β (Wahner et al., 2007). All of these studies have been on small numbers of PD patients. However other studies have not confirmed the associations of such polymorphisms with PD disease (Reviewed by Hirsch and Hunot, 2009) which may indicate that such polymorphisms are involved in susceptibility to the causative agent of PD. More importantly such polymorphisms may reflect the basal levels of the inflammatory status of an individual or reflect the ability of phagocytic cells to respond to an inflammatory stimulus.

Various changes in antibodies have been identified in the serum of PD patients although these have not been confirmed in all studies (reviewed by Hirsch and Hunot, 2009). Increased numbers of circulating CD4+ bright and CD8+ dull lymphocytes are detectable in the serum of PD patients (Hisanaga et al., 2001). Since the counts of these lymphocytes increase after viral infection, this could indicate that viral infections contribute to the pathogenesis of PD.

12. Therapeutic aspects

There have been some discussions as to whether improvements in the ability of the immune system to respond to the inflammatory turmoil maybe of importance in preventing the progression of PD. Probiotics, are dietary supplements which contain beneficial bateria, (lactobacillus and bifidobacterium), or yeast. They are administered in different quantities to allow for colon colonization. They help by stimulating health promoting flora as well as suppressing pathogenic colonisation and disease. It is claimed that probiotics will strengthen the immune system to combat allergies, stress and possibly neurodegenerative diseases (Saraf et al., 2010).

12.1 Anti-inflammatory agents

Some epidemiological studies have indicated that people who regularly use anti-inflammatory drugs have less risk of developing clinical PD (Chen et al 2003., Chen., 2005), although this has not been confirmed in other studies (Ton et al., 2006; Bornebroek et al., 2007; Hancock et al., 2007). Anti-inflammatory drugs may retard the progression of the degeneration although it remains to be elucidated whether their use would be an additional therapy in diagnosed PD patients. Inhibition of inflammation is associated with reduced neuronal impairment in various PD models (Gao et al., 2003; Wu et al., 2003) as discussed below.

Non-steroidal anti-inflammatory (NSAI) drugs act by inhibiting the enzyme cyclooxygenase COX-1 and COX-2. While aspirin will inhibit both COX-1 and COX-2, ibuprufen will inhibit COX-2 only. COX-2 is specifically involved in dopaminergic degeneration. COX-2 inhibitors have been demonstrated to specifically inhibit microglia activation. NSAI may be effective in decreasing the incidence of PD which has been associated with the COX-inhibiting effect of these compounds (Chen et al., 2005). Minocycline may be effective in delaying PD progression by suppressing the formation of IL-1β and the activation of NADPH-oxidase and iNOS which are potent activators of microglia (NINDS 2006; Couzin 2007). The presence of polymorphisms of pro-inflammatory genes such as COX-2 genes may provide a genetic predisposition to initiate microglial activation.

12.2 Antioxidants

Antioxidants may reduce the progression of the neurodegenerative process. Lipoic acid is a universal antioxidants. Lipoic acid in its reduced form dihrolipoic acid is active against ROS and will reduce oxidative stress. (De Araujo et al., 2011). However peripherally administered antioxidant will need to be targeted to specific regions of the brain where oxidative stress occurs.

12.3 Vitamins and mineral

Micronutrients such as the Vitamins A, B_6, B_{12}, C, D and E, folic acid as well as iron, zinc, copper and selenium, are involved in the synergy to support the protective properties of the immune system and most are also essential for antibody production (Maggini et al., 2007). Supplementation with these micronutrients may enhance immunity.

12.4 Steroid hormones

Steroid hormones, such as 17 beta oestradiol or progesterone protect against dopaminergic degeneration which may explain why woman are less affected by PD. In addition oestrogens may reduce inflammatory processes in the brain (Reviewed by Barcia et al., 2009) diminishing glial cell activation around dopaminergic neurons possibly mediated by differential expression of oestrogen receptors on glial cells and neurons (Reviewed by Barcia et al., 2009).

12.5 Flavonoids

Flavonoids, a group of phenolic phytochemicals are abundant in various spices, vegetables and fruit. Several medicinal properties have been ascribed to flavonoids which include anti-oxidants, anti-inflammatory and anti carcinogenic. Apigenin and its phase I metabolite, luteolin reduce CD40 and CD40L expression on dentritic cells and basophils. In our recent investigation of apigenin and luteolin in cultured microglia it was demonstrated that both of these compounds significantly reduced CD40 expression induced by IFN-γ. This was paralleled by significant decreases in the release of pro-inflammatory cytokines IL-6 and TNFα by microglia. Such changes were due to inactivation of STAT1 (Datla et al., 2001, 2007; Zbarsky et al., 2005).

12.6 Taurine and taurine prodrugs

In our recent studies we have shown that taurine has an anti-inflammatory action by stabilistaion of IkappaBα in macrophages and microglia (Ward et al., 2011). This in turn will reduce NFkappaB translocation to the nucleus and will prevent the release of pro-inflammatory cytokines. In earlier animal studies the protective effect of taurine in the 6-hydroxy dopamine model was reported (Ward et al., 2006). In the later studies, prodrugs of taurine have been developed, notably ethane-β-sultam, which reduce microglial activation in the brain of an animal model of neurodegeneration (Ward, Della Corte, Dexter unpublished data).

12.7 Iron chelators

The iron content of the SNc increases in the brains of PD patients and is associated with the progression of the inflammatory process. Hence, it's chelation may prevent the progression of the disease. Two clinically used iron chelators, namely the hexadendate, deferrioxamine and the tridendate chelator deferasirox have been investigated for their efficacy to induce neuroprotection in the 6-hydroxy dopamine (6-OHDA) animal model of PD. Acute administration of desferrioxamine, 0.4 mM or desferasirox, 1 mM, via a microdialysis probe into the striatum immediately prior to a dose of 6-OHDA, prevented the generation of hydroxyl radicals, as well as reducing bio-available iron. Intraperitoneal injection of the iron chelators, desferasirox, 20 mg/kg or desferrioxamine, 30 mg/kg or deferriprone 10mg/kg, to the 6-OHDA rat model, significantly attenuated the loss of tyrosine hydroxylase positive cells as well as elevating dopamine content in the lesioned striatum (Dexter et al., 2010). Such results would confirm that the administration of these chelators show therapeutic efficacy and should be considered to be an additional therapy for the treatment of PD. Clinical trials of deferiprone are now underway in a group of drug-naïve PD patients.

12.8 MMP-3 inhibitors

The development of selective MMP-3 inhibitors has proved difficult. It is unlikely that relatively large peptide based inhibitors of MMP-3 would cross BBB. Doxycycline, a tetracycline derivative that crosses the BBB can down regulate cell stress induced MMP-3 expression and release and can therefore attenuate apoptosis in dopaminergic neurons (Cho et al., 2009). Minocycline protection of neurones from a variety of insults may in part be due to down regulation of MMP-3. However early clinical trials in PD patients were stopped because of unwanted side effects (NINDS NET-PD Investigators 2008). Preliminary studies of ghrelin, glycitein and exendin-4 have also shown down regulation of MMP-3 expression (reviewed by Kim and Hwang, 2011).

12.9 PPAR modifications

Several non-steroidal anti-inflammatory drugs bind to PPAR-α and PPAR-γ. thereby activating their receptors. PPAR regulate the transcriptional activity of several transcription factors which include NFkappaB, the signal transducer factor-1 (STAT) and the activating transcription factor-1, ATF-1 and ATF-4. PPAR function by competing with NFkappaB for binding to the overlapping series of co-activators, i.e. cAMP-response element-binding protein (CREB), and inhibiting the NFkB mediated inflammatory response. PPAR also directly interacts with p65/p50/IkBα suppressing the DNA binding activity of NFkB. PPAR also inhibit NFkB and AP-1 signal-dependent transcriptional activation of inflammatory genes by transrepression (Reviewed by Chaturvedi and Beal, 2008). Modulation of iNOS and cyclooxygenase may also occur. PPAR may play a role in improving mitochondrial function. The neuro-protective role of PPAR agonists have been evaluated in PD patients. Agonists such as pioglitazone and rosiglitazone, may be able to protect against oxidative stress, apoptosis and inflammation in CNS (Reviewd by Chaturvedi and Beal, 2008).

13. Inflammation in animal models of PD

Activation of microglia has been identified in the SNc and /or striatum in various animal models of PD, which include the MPTP and lipopolysaccharides models (reviewed by Marinova-Mutafchieva et al., 2009). In addition, in the medial forebrain bundle axotomised model, brain activation of microglia precedes neuronal loss (Gao et al., 2003). In the 6-hydroxy dopamine models significant microglia activation was evident 48h after it's administration as well as NADPH- derived free radicals prior to dopamine cell death in the SNc. In our recent studies unilateral injection of 6-OHDA into the medial forebrain bundle, activation of microglia occurred rapidly, which selectively adhered to degenerating axons dentrites and apoptotic dopamine neurons in the SNc after 7 days.(Dexter et al 2011). After this time, there was a progressive loss of tyrosine hydroxlase positive neurons. These results indicated that microglia activation precedes dopamine neuronal cell loss. Furthermore neurons undergoing degeneration may be removed prematurely by microglia phagocytosis. (Marinova-Mutafchieva et al., 2009). In vitro it has also been shown that the toxicity of LPS to immortalised dopaminergic neurons was evident only when microglia were present in the cell culture (Gao et al., 2003). These results clearly indicate that activated microglia play an important role in the early stage of the disease pathogenesis.

This review has confirmed that in PD there is a persistent and progressive inflammation both in the periphery and brain which is caused by changes in both the innate and adaptive immune systems which fuel the degeneration. The factors involved in the initiation of this cycle remains unknown. Although therapeutic intervention may diminish such inflammatory pathways, the goal for future researchers will be to identify the cause of such perturbations. Only then will there be the opportunity to develop new drugs which will cure PD.

14. References

Alam ZI., Jenner A., Daniel SE., Lees AJ., Cairns N., Marsden CD., Jenner P., Halliwell B. J Neurochem. (1997) Oxidative DNA damage in the parkinsonian brain: an apparent selective increase in 8-hydroxyguanine levels in substantia nigra J Neurochem 69:1196-203

Annweiler C., Allali G., Allain P., Bridenbaugh S., Schott AM., Kressig RW., Beauchet O. (2009) Vitamin D and cognitive performance in adults: a systematic review. Eur J Neurol 16: 1083-1089.

Arman A., Isik N., Candan F., Becit KS., List EO. (2010) Association between sporadic Parkinson disease and interleukin-1 beta-511 gene polymorphisms in the Turkish population. Eur Cytokine Netw 21: 116-121.

Barcia C., Ros F., Carrillo MA., Aguado-Llera D., Ros CM., Gomez A., Nombela C., de Pablos V., Fernandez-Villalba E., Herrero M-T. (2009) Inflammatory responses in Parkinsonism in Birth, Life and death of dopaminergic neurons in the substatia nigra G di Giovanni et al Eds J Neural Transm 73: 245-252.

Bartels AL., Leenders KL. (2007) Neuroinflammation in the pathophysiology of Parkinson's Disease: evidence from animal models to human in vivo studies with [11C]-PK11195 PET. Mov Disord 22: 1852-1856.

Berendse HW., Ponsen MM. (2009) Diagnosing premotor Parkinson's Disease using a two-step approach combing olfactory testing and DAT SPECT imaging. Parkinsonism Relat Disord 15 Suppl 3: S26-S30.

Bornebroek M., de Lau LM., Haag MD., Koudstaal PJ., Hofman A., Stricker BH., Breteler MM. (2007) Non-steroidal anti-inflammatory drugs and the risk of Parkinson's disease. Neuroepidemiology 28: 193-196.

Brochard V., Combadiere B., Prigent A. et al., (2009) Infiltration of CD4+ lymphocytes into the brain contributes to neurodegeneration in a mouse model of Parkinson Disease J Clin Invest 119: 182-192.

Castellani RJ., Nugent SL., Morrison AL., Zhu X., Lee HG., Bajic V. et al (2011) CD3 in Lexy pathology: does the abnormal recall of neurodevelopmental processes underlie Parkinson's Disease J Neural Transm 118: 23-26
Chan WY., Kohsaka S., Rezaie P.(2007) The origin and cell lineage of microglia: new concepts. Brain Res Rev. 53:344-54
Chaturedi RK,, Beal MF. (2008) PPAR: a therapeutic target in Parknison's Disease. J Neurochem 106: 506-518.
Chen H., Zhang BY., Hernan MA., Schwarzschild MA., Willett WC., Colditz GA., Speizer FE., Ascherio A. (2003) Non-steroidal anti-inflammatory drugs and the risk of Parkinson's disease. Arch Neurol 60: 1059-1064.
Chen H., Jacobs E., Schwarzschild MA., McCullough ML., Calle EE., Thun MJ., Ascherio A. (2005) Non-steroidal anti-inflammatory drug use and the risk for Parkinson's disease Ann Neurol 58: 963-967.
Chen H., O'Reilly EJ., Schwarzschild MA., Ascherio A. (2008) Periphereal inflammatory markers and risk of Parkinson's disease. Am J Epidemiol 167: 90-95.
Chrousos GP., (2010) Stress and sex versus immunity and inflammation Sci Signal 3 pe36.
Cho Y., Son HJ., Kim EM., Choi JH., Kim ST., Ji IJ., Choi DJ., Joh TH., Kim YS., Hwang O (2009) Doxycycline is neuroprotective against nigral dopaminergic degeneration by a dual mechanism involving MMP-3 Neurotox Res 16: 361-371.
Couzin J. (2007) Clinical research. Testing a novel strategy against Parkin's disease Science 315: 1778.
Crichton RR., Ward RJ. (2006) Metal based neurodegeneration. Publ Wiley and Sons. Pp 1-269.
Crichton RR., Dexter DT., Ward RJ. (2008) Molecular-based neurodegenerative diseases: from molecular mechanisms to therapeutic strategies Coordination Chemistry Reviews 252:1189-1199.
Crichton RR., Dexter DT., Ward RJ. (2008) Molecular-based neurodegenerative diseases: from molecular mechanisms to therapeutic strategies. Coordination Chem Reviews 252:1189-1199
Damier P., Hirsch EC., Zhang P., Agid Y., Javoy-Agid F. (1993) Glutathione peroxidase, glial cells and Parkisnon's Disease Neuroscience 52: 1-6.
Datla KP., Christidou M., Widmer WW., Rooprai HK., Dexter DT. (2001) Tissue distribution and neuroprotective effects of citrus flavonoid tangeretin in a rat model of Parkinson's disease. Neuroreport.2:3871-5
Datla KP., Zbarsky V., Rai D., Parkar S., Osakabe N., Aruoma OI., Dexter DT.(2007) Short-term supplementation with plant extracts rich in flavonoids protect nigrostriatal dopaminergic neurons in a rat model of Parkinson's disease. J Am Coll Nutr.;26:341-9
Dauer W., Przedborski S. (2003) Parkinson's disease: mechanisms and models Neuron: 889-909.
Davelos D., Grutzendler J., Yang G., Kim JV., Zuo Y., Jung S. et al. (2005) ATP mediates rapid microglial response to local brain injury in vivo. Nat Neuroscience 8: 752-758.
De Araujo DP., Lobato Rde F., Cavalcanti JR., Sampaio LR., Araujo PV., Silva MC., Neves KR., Fonteles MM., Sousa FC., Vasconcelos SM (2011) The contributions of antioxidant activity of lipoic acid in reducing neurogenerative progression of Parkinson's disease: a review.Int J Neurosci 121: 51-57.
Dexter DT., Carayon A., Vidailhet M., Ruberg M., Agid F., Agid Y., Lees AJ., Wells FR., Jenner P., Marsden CD. (1990) Decreased ferritin levels in brain in Parkinson's diseaseJ Neurochem. 55:16-20.
Dexter DT., Statton SA., Whitmore C., Freinbichler W., Weinberger P., Tipton KT., Della Corte L., Ward RJ., Crichton RR. (2011) Clinically available iron chelators induce

neuroprotection in gthe 6-OHDA model of Parkinson's disease after periphereal administration. J Neural Transm 118:223-231.

Forno LS., DeLanney LE., Irwin I., Di Monte D., Langston JW. (1992) Astrocytes and Parkinson's disease. Prog Brain Res 94: 429-436.

Frank MG., Barrientos RM., Biedenkapp JC., Rudy JW., Warkins LR., Maier SF. (2006) mRNA up-regulation of MHC II and pivotal pro-inflammatory genes in normal brain aging. Neurobiol Aging 27; 717-722.

Faucheux BA., Martin ME., Beaumont C., Hunot S., Hauw JJ., Agid Y., Hirsch EC. (2002) Lack of up-regulation of ferritin is associated with sustained iron regulatory protein-1 binding activity in the substantia nigra of patients with Parkinson's disease. J Neurochem. 83:320-30.

Fernandes de Abreu DA., Eyles D., Féron F. (2009) Vitamin D, a neuro-immunomodulator: implications for neurodegenerative and autoimmune diseases. Psychoneuroendocrinology. Suppl 1:S265-77.

Gao HM., Liu B., Zhang W., Hong JS. (2003) Novel; anti-inflammatory therapy for Parkinson's disease. Trends Pharmacol Sci 24: 395-401.

Gao HM., Hong JS. (2008) Why neurodegenerative diseases are progressive: uncontrolled inflammation drives disease progression Trends Immunol 29: 357-365.

Götz ME., Double K., Gerlach M., Youdim MB., Riederer P. (2004) The relevance of iron in the pathogenesis of Parkinson's disease Ann N Y Acad Sci. 1012:193-208.

Griffiths MR., Gasque P., Neal JW. (2009) The multiple roles of the innate immune system in the regulation of apoptosis and inflammation in the brain. J Neuropathol Exp neurol 68: 217-226.

Hald A., Lotharius J. (2005) Oxidative stress and inflammation in Parkinson's disease: Is there a causal link? Exp Neurol 193: 279-290.

Hamza TH., Zabetian CP., Tenesa A., Laederach A., Montimurro J., Yearout D. et al. (2010) Common genetic variation in the HLA region is associated with late-onset sporadic Parkinson's disease Nat Gener 42: 781-785.et al., 2010

Hancock DB., Martin ER., Stajich JM., Jewett R., Stacy MA., Scott BL., Vance JM., Scott WK. (2007) Smoking, caffeine and non-steroidal anti-inflammatory drugs in families with Parkinson's disease Arch Neurol 64: 576-580.

Hirsch E., Hunot S. (2009) Neuroinflammation in Parkinson's disease: a target for neuroprotection. Lancet Meurology 8: 382-397.

Hatherley D., Barclay AN. (2004) The CD200 and CD200 receptor surface cell surface proteins interact through their N-terminal immunoglobulin-like domains. Eur J immunol 34: 1688-1694.

Hisanaga K., Asagi M., Itoyama Y., Iwasaki Y. (2001) Increase in peripheral CD4 bright+ CD adult T cells in Parkinson's disease Arch Neurol 58: 1580-1583.

Hoek RM., Ruuls SR., Murphy CA., Wright GJ., Goddard R., Zurawski SM., Blom B., Homola ME., Streit WJ., Brown MH., Barclay AN., Sedgwick JD. (2000) Downregulation of the macrophage lineage through interaction with OX2 (CD200) Science 290: 1768-1771.

Honda S., Sasaki ., Ohsawa K., Imai Y., Nakamura Y. et al. (2001) Extracellular ATP or ADP induce chemotaxis of cultured microglia through Gi/o-coupled P2Y receptors. J Neurosci 21: 1975-1982.

Hunot S., Dugas N., Faucheux B., Hartmann A., Tardieu M., Debré P., Agid Y., Dugas B., Hirsch EC. (1999) FcepsilonRII/CD23 is expressed in Parkinson's disease and induces, in vitro, production of nitric oxide and tumor necrosis factor-alpha in glial cells. J Neurosci 19: 3440-3447

Jauregui-Huerta F., Ruvalcaba-Delgadillo Y., Gonzalez-Castaneda R., Garcis-Estrada J., Gonzalez-Perez O., Luguin S. (2010) Responses of glial cells to stress and glucocorticoids. Curr Immunol Rev 6: 195-204.

Kebir H., Kreymborg K., Ifergan I., Dodelet-Devilliers A., Cayrol R. et al (2007) Human Th17 lymphocytes promote blood brain barrier disruption and central nervous system inflammation Nat Med 13: 1173-1175.

Kim E-M., Hwang O. (2011) Role of matrix metalloproteinase-3 in neurodegeneration. J Neurochem 116: 22-32.

Knekt P., Kikkinen A., Rissanen H., Marniemi J., Saaksjarvi K., Heliovaara M. (2010) Serum vitamin D and the risk of Parkinson disease. Arch Neurol 67: 808-811

Koning N., Swaab DF., Hoek RM., Huitinga I. (2009) Distribution of the immune inhibitory molecules CD200 and CD200R in the normal central nervous system and multiple sclerosis lesions suggest neuron-glia and glia-glia interactions J Neuropathol Exp Neurol 68: 159-167

Koning N., Bo L., Hoek RM., Huitinga I. (2007) Downregulation of macrophage inhibitory molecules in multiple sclerosis lesions. Ann Neurol 62: 504-514

Kosloski LM., Ha DM., Huttler JA., Stone DK., Reynolds AD., Gendelman HE., Mosley RL (2010)Adaptive immune regulation of glial homeostasis as an immunization strategy for neurodegenerative diseases J Neurochem 114: 261-276.

Lue LF., Kuo YM., Beach T., Walker DG. (2010) Microglia activation and anti-inflammatory regulation in Alzheimer's disease Mol Neurobiol 41:115-128.

McGeer PL., Itagaki S., Boyes BE.,McGeer EG. (1998) Reactive microglia are positive for HLA-DR in the substantia nigra of Parkinson's and Alzheimer's disease brains. Neurology 38: 1285-1291.

Maggini S., Wintergerst ES., Beveridge S., Hornig DH. (2007) Selected vitamins and trace elements support immune function by strengthening epithelial barriers and cellular and humoral immune responses B J Nutrition 98: Suppl 1, S29-S35.

Marinova-Mutafchieva L., Sadeghian M., Broom L., Davis JB., Medhurst AD., Dexter DT. (2009) Relationship between microglial activation and dopaminergic neuronal loss in the substantia nigra: a time course study in a 6-hydroxydopamine model of Parkinson's disease. J Neurochem 110: 966-975.

Michalik L., Desvergne B., Wahli W. (2004) Peroxisome-proliferator-activated receptors and cancers: complex stories Nature Rev Cancer 4: 61-70.

Mirza B., Hadberg H., Thomsen P., Moos T. (2000) The absence of reactive astrocytosis is indicative of a unique inflammatory process in Parkinson's Disease Neuroscience 95:425-432.

Neuwelt EA., Bauer B., Fahlke C., Fricker G., Iadecola C., Janigro D., Leybaert L. et al (2011) engaging neuroscience to advance translational research in brain barrier biology Nature Reviews neuroscience 12: 169-182.

NINDS, NET-PD (2008) Investigators A randomised double-blind futility clinical trial of creatine and minocycline in early Parkinson disease Neurology: 66: 664-671.

Obeid R., Schadt A., Dillmann U., Kostopoulos P., Fassbender K., Herrmann W. (2009) Methylation status and neurodegenerative markers in Parkinson disease. Clin Chem 55: 1852-1860

Ouchi Y., Yagi S., Yokokura M., Sakamoto M. (2009) neuroinflammation in the living brain of Parkinson's disease. Parkinsonism Related Disord 15S3 S200-S204.

Perry VH. (2004) The influence of systemic inflammation in the braim: implications for chronic neurodegenerative disease, Brain Behav Immun 18: 407-413

Praczko T., Kostka T. (2006). Infections in the elderly. Part II Prevention and treatment. Wiad Lek 59: 692-696.

Qin L., Wu X., Block ML., Liu Y., Bresse GR., Hong JS., Knapp DJ., Crews FT. (2007) Systemic LPS causes chronic neuroinflammation and progressive neurodegeneration. Glia 55: 453-462.

Rijkers ES., de Ruiter T., Baridi A., Veninga H., Hoek RM., Meyaard L. (2008) The inhibitory CD200R is differentially expressed on human and mouse T and B lymphocytes.Mol Immunol. 2008 Feb;45(4):1126-35.

Sato Y., Honda Y., Iwamoto J., Kanoko T., Satoh K. (2005) Abnormal bone and calcium metabolism in immobilized Parkinson's disease patients Mov Disord. 20:1598-603

Seef RC., Lee CY., Tan JJ., Quek AM., Chong WL., Looi WF., Huang SH., Wang H., Chan YH., Halliwell B. Oxidative damage in Parkinson disease: Measurement using accurate biomnarkers. Free Radic Biol Med 48: 560-566.

Saraf K., Shashikanth MC., Priy T., Sultana N., Chaitanya NC. (2010) Probiotics--do they have a role in medicine and dentistry J assoc Physicians India 58: 488-490

Shenk U., Frascoli M., Proietti M., Geffers R., Traggiai E., Buer J., Ricordi C., Westendorf AM., Graasi F., (2011) ATP Inhibits the Generation and Function of Regulatory T Cells Through the Activation of Purinergic P2X Receptors. Sci Signal 4: ra12.

Sian J., Dexter DT., Lees AJ., Daniel S., Agid Y., Javoy-Agid F., Jenner P., Marsden CD. (1994) Alterations in glutathione levels in Parkinson's disease and other neurodegenerative disorders affecting basal ganglia. Ann Neurol. 36:348-55

Ton TG., Heckbert SR., Longstreth WT Jr, Rossing MA., Kukull WA., Franklin GM., Swanson PD., Smith-Weller T., Checkoway H. (2006) Non-steroidal anti-inflammatory drugs and risk of Parkinson's disease Mov Disord 21: 964-969.

Trinchiere G. (2004) Interleukin-12 and the regulation of innate resistance and adaptive immunity Nature Rev Immunology 3: 133-146.

Wahner AD., Sinsheimer JS., Bronstein JM., Ritz B. (2007) Inflammatory cytokine gene polymorphisms and increased risk of Parkinson disease. Arch Neurol 64: 836-840.

Walker DG., Sing-Hernandez JE., Campell NA., Lue LF. (2009) Decreased expression of CD200 and CD200 receptor in Alzheimer's Disease: a potential mechanism leading to chronic inflammation. Exp Neurol 215:5-19.

Ward R., Cirkovic-Vellichovia T., Ledeque F., Tirizitis G., Dubars G., Datla K., Dexter D., Heushling P., Crichton R. (2006) Neuroprotection by taurine and taurine analogues. Adv Exp Med Biol. 583:299-306.

Ward RJ., Crichton RR., Taylor DL., Della Corte L., Srai SK., Dexter DT. (2010). Iron and the immune system. J Neural Trans 118: 15-28.

Ward RJ, Lallemand F., De Witte P., Crichton RR., Piette J., Della Corte L., Hemmings K., Page M., Taylor D., Dexter DT. (2011)Anti-inflammatory actions of taurine analogues in phagocytic cells Biochem Pharmacol 81: 743-751

Wu DC., Teismann P., Tieu K., Vila M., Jackson-Lewis V., Ischiropoulos H. etal (2003) NADPH oxidase mediates oxidative stress in the 1-methyl-4-phenyl-1,2,3,6-tetrahydrapyridine model of Parkinson's disease Proc Natl Acad Sci USA 100: 6145-6150.

Zbarsky V., Datla KP., Parkar S., Rai DK., Aruoma OI., Dexter DT.(2005) Neuroprotective properties of the natural phenolic antioxidants curcumin and naringenin but not quercetin and fisetin in a 6-OHDA model of Parkinson's disease. Free Radic Res.;39:1119-25

Zhang S., Cherwinski H., Sedgwick JD., Phillips JH. (2004) Molecular mechanisms of CD200 inhibition of mast cell activation. J Immuno 173(11):6786-93

7

Cyclin-Dependent Kinase 5 – An Emerging Player in Parkinson's Disease Pathophysiology

Zelda H. Cheung and Nancy Y. Ip
Division of Life Science, State Key Laboratory of Molecular Neuroscience and Molecular Neuroscience Center, Hong Kong University of Science and Technology, Clear Water Bay, Kowloon, Hong Kong, China

1. Introduction

Parkinson's disease (PD) is the most common neurodegenerative movement disorder that affects 1% of the general population at age 65, with the prevalence rising to 4-5% by age 85 (de Rijk *et al.* 1997). Symptoms of PD include muscle rigidity, resting tremor, bradykinesia, postural instability, speech impediment and cognitive decline. At the cellular level, PD is characterized by selective degeneration of dopaminergic neurons in the substantia nigra, and the presence of cytoplasmic inclusions known as Lewy bodies in the brains of PD patients (Levy *et al.* 2009). Despite the prevalence of PD, therapeutic agents that slow or halt disease progression are lacking. Current treatments for PD are highly limited and focus predominantly on symptomatic relief. For example, the most effective treatment for ameliorating PD symptoms is administration of levodopa, a precursor that is converted to dopamine in the brain, to restore dopamine levels in PD patients. Nonetheless, the efficacy of levodopa wears off with prolonged treatment, in addition to triggering dyskinesia as a side effect (Obeso *et al.* 2010, Poewe *et al.* 2010). There is thus an urgent need to elucidate the cellular mechanism underlying PD pathology for the development of more effective treatments.

The etiopathology of PD has remained largely enigmatic. Majority of the PD cases are idiopathic, although familial cases of PD with identifiable mutations also account for about 5% of all PD cases (Dauer and Przedborski 2003). Prior to the identification of these missense mutations, nonetheless, scientists have predominantly focused on the two known cellular hallmarks of PD, namely the degeneration of dopaminergic neurons and the presence of Lewy bodies. Since majority of the motor deficits exhibited by PD patients is reversed by elevating dopamine levels in the brain, it is believed that the motor symptoms of PD are due mostly to the loss of dopaminergic neurons in the substantia nigra (Obeso et al. 2010). This has sparked extensive research aimed at elucidating the mechanisms implicated in the degeneration of these neurons. Abnormality in various cellular processes have been linked to neuronal loss in PD, such as oxidative stress, mitochondrial dysfunction, aberrant proteasomal degradation and deregulation of the autophagy pathway (Levy et al. 2009). On the other hand, the precise role of Lewy bodies has become a little controversial. While protein aggregates and the presence of cytoplasmic inclusions have long been considered as toxic, recent evidence suggests that the aggregates may also exhibit neuroprotective roles by serving as traps for the toxic oligomeric forms (Rubinsztein 2006).

With the dawn of the molecular era, knowledge on the pathogenic mechanisms also shifted from detection of aberrant cellular processes to the identification of molecules implicated in the pathological pathways. Importantly, unraveling of mutations associated with familial cases of PD enabled the mapping of genes and signaling pathways to the dysfunction of various cellular processes. A number of genes were found to be mutated in familial PD, including α-synuclein, Parkin, PINK1, DJ-1, leucine rich repeated kinase 2 (LRRK2), ubiquitin-C-terminal hydrolase-L1 (UCH-L1), synphilin-1 and HtrA2/Omi (Schulz 2008). These studies also led to the identification of α-synuclein as the main constituent of Lewy bodies (Levy et al. 2009). This new wave of information prompted scientists to address the signaling events that are upstream of the elimination of the diseased neurons. Among the long list of molecules that were found to contribute to PD pathology, cyclin-dependent kinase 5 (Cdk5) has emerged as an important player through its implication in multiple cellular events that are altered in PD.

Cdk5 is a serine/threonine kinase that is essential for the migration, survival and differentiation of developing neurons (Cheung and Ip 2007, Dhavan and Tsai 2001). Activated through binding to its activator p35 or p39, Cdk5/p35 activity is important for the regulation of neuronal survival during physiological and pathological states (Cheung and Ip 2004). Cdk5 was first implicated in dopaminergic neuron loss in PD when injection of MPTP, a neurotoxin that selectively eliminates neurons in the substantia nigra, was demonstrated to increase Cdk5 activity (Smith et al. 2003). Inhibition of Cdk5 activity markedly attenuates MPTP-induced degeneration of dopaminergic neurons, thus revealing the involvement of Cdk5 in PD pathogenesis (Smith et al. 2003). Interestingly, Cdk5 expression is also associated with Lewy bodies (Takahashi et al. 2000). Since then, accumulating studies have identified additional Cdk5 substrates that may contribute to PD pathology. These findings revealed that Cdk5 regulates neuronal death through modulating multiple signaling pathways and cellular events in PD, and suggests that Cdk5 may emerge as a suitable target for development of PD therapeutics.

2. Cdk5 – a multi-faceted kinase

Cdk5 was identified based on sequence homology to cell cycle regulator cdc2 as a cdc2-related kinase (Lew *et al.* 1992, Meyerson *et al.* 1992) and also as a tau kinase (Kobayashi *et al.* 1993). Cdk5 is not activated by cyclins despite its structural similarity with other cyclin-dependent kinases. Rather, it is activated upon binding to activators p35 or p39. Cdk5 is ubiquitously expressed, but its activity is mostly limited to the nervous system due to the predominantly neural-specific expression of p35 and p39. Nonetheless, accumulating evidence demonstrates that Cdk5 activity can also be detected outside the nervous system, such as at the neuromuscular junction, pancreatic cells, adipose tissue and myeloid cells (Fu *et al.* 2001, Lilja *et al.* 2001, Choi *et al.* 2010, Arif *et al.* 2011). The importance of p35 and p39 as Cdk5 activators is further demonstrated by the comparable phenotype exhibited by Cdk5-deficient mice and p35/p39 double knock-out mice. Both exhibit perinatal death and severe cortical lamination defects (Ohshima *et al.* 1996, Ko *et al.* 2001). This is in contrast to single knock-out animals lacking p35 or p39, which survive through adulthood. In addition, aberrant cortical lamination was observed only in p35 knock-out mice (Ohshima *et al.* 1996, Ko *et al.* 2001, Chae *et al.* 1997). These observations indicate that while there is some redundancy, p35 and p39 are critical for the function of Cdk5.

2.1 Regulation of Cdk5 activity

Given the pivotal role of p35 and p39 in Cdk5 activation, changes in the expression level of p35 and p39 constitute one of the major mechanisms by which Cdk5 activity is regulated. Interestingly, Cdk5 activity is also regulated by calpain-mediated cleavage of p35 and p39 into p25 and p29, respectively. These fragments retain Cdk5-activating capability but exhibit significantly longer half-lives than p35 and p39, which are rather short-lived proteins (Patrick *et al.* 1999, Patzke and Tsai 2002). Cdk5 itself was found to contribute to the short half-life of p35 through phosphorylation of p35, which promotes its degradation by the proteasome pathway (Patrick *et al.* 1998). In addition, cleavage by calpain removes the myristoylation signal from p35 and p39, thus resulting in a redistribution of Cdk5 activity within the cell. Since p25 generation has been associated with excessive Cdk5 activation and neuronal loss in neurodegenerative disease (Patrick *et al.* 1999, Cruz and Tsai 2004), it has been speculated that Cdk5-p25 may be catalytically more active than Cdk5-p35. Nonetheless, a recent study demonstrated that the activity of Cdk5 is comparable regardless of whether it is associated with p35 or p25 (Peterson *et al.* 2010). These findings collectively suggest that the aberrant Cdk5 activity associated with p25 generation is likely due to prolonged activation of Cdk5, and not an elevated Cdk5 catalytic activity.

Aside from the regulation of p35 or p39 expression, and their degradation or cleavage, direct phosphorylation of Cdk5 also modulates its activity. Phosphorylation of Cdk5 at Tyr15 has been demonstrated to enhance Cdk5 activity (Sasaki *et al.* 2002, Fu *et al.* 2007, Cheung *et al.* 2007). This mechanism is particularly important for trophic factor-mediated regulation of Cdk5 activity, as a number of trophic factor receptors are receptor tyrosine kinases. Ligand binding triggers tyrosine kinase activation, which directly phosphorylates Cdk5 at Tyr15 to enhance Cdk5 activity. This phosphorylation was found to be crucial for the effect of Cdk5 on the signaling of trophic factors such as Ephrin A1 and BDNF (Cheung *et al.* 2007, Fu *et al.* 2007). Interestingly, S-nitrosylation of Cdk5 was also recently demonstrated to reduce Cdk5 activity (Zhang et al. 2010b). These findings indicate that post-translational modification of Cdk5 also constitutes an important mechanism for controlling Cdk5 activity.

2.2 Cdk5 as a regulator of neuronal survival

Despite being a member of the cyclin-dependent kinase family, Cdk5 is unique in several aspects. Not only is its mechanism of activation different, but its action in cell cycle regulation is also distinct from other cyclin-dependent kinases. Cyclin-dependent kinases are important enzymes that ensure the proper progression of cell cycle (Nguyen *et al.* 2002). The lack of Cdk5 expression in proliferating cells led to the conclusion that Cdk5 is not involved in the regulation of cell cycle progression (Tsai *et al.* 1993). Nonetheless, recent evidence indicates that Cdk5 also takes part in cell cycle control, acting as a suppressor of cell cycle re-entry in post-mitotic neurons (Zhang and Herrup 2008). Through the identification of a myriad of Cdk5 substrates, Cdk5 has been implicated in multiple aspects of neuronal development and neuronal functions. Aside from an obvious role of Cdk5 in neuronal migration as revealed by the severe cortical lamination defects in Cdk5-deficient mice (Ohshima *et al.* 1996), Cdk5 is also involved in neuronal differentiation and synapse formation during development (Cheung and Ip 2007). Furthermore, emerging evidence indicates that Cdk5 plays a critical role in synaptic function, synaptic plasticity and learning (Lai and Ip 2009, Hawasli and Bibb 2007).

The role of Cdk5 in neuronal survival is slightly more complex, and accumulating evidence suggests that Cdk5 functions as a double-edged sword. Following the identification of Cdk5 as a tau kinase (Kobayashi et al. 1993), deregulation of Cdk5 activity was found to contribute to neuronal loss in Alzheimer's disease (Patrick et al. 1999). Elevation of Cdk5 activity that is accompanied by p25 generation leads to neuronal death (Patrick et al. 1999). Although conflicting data have been obtained regarding the increase in p25 levels in post-mortem samples of Alzheimer's disease patients (Patrick *et al.* 1999, Li *et al.* 2003b, Tandon *et al.* 2003), subsequent studies have demonstrated augmented p25 expression and Cdk5 activity in response to a large number of pro-apoptotic agents or cell death stimuli, including MPTP (reviewed in Cheung and Ip 2004). These observations collectively establish a death-inducing role of Cdk5-p25. Interestingly, a pro-survival role of Cdk5 is also gaining recognition. Indeed, nuclear margination and cell swelling were observed in brainstem and spinal cord neurons in Cdk5-deficient brains (Ohshima et al. 1996). In addition, knock-down of Cdk5 expression alone results in apoptosis in developing retinal neurons (Cheung et al. 2008). Several mechanisms likely mediate the survival-maintaining property of Cdk5. For example, Cdk5 has been reported to be required for neuregulin-induced elevation of survival signaling pathway PI3K/Akt (Li et al. 2003a). In addition, phosphorylation of Bcl-2 at Ser70 by Cdk5 is essential for its anti-apoptotic property, which is pivotal for the maintenance of neuronal survival during development (Cheung et al. 2008). Cdk5 has also been demonstrated to exhibit a neuroprotective role through suppression of cell cycle re-entry, which is associated with cell death in post-mitotic neurons (Zhang et al. 2010a).

How Cdk5 manages to mediate both cell death and survival signals is incompletely understood. It is generally believed that while basal level of Cdk5 activity is required for neuronal survival, excessive activation, particularly in the presence of p25, leads to neuronal death. In addition, recent studies suggest that the subcellular localization of Cdk5 activity may also determine whether it serves a protective or detrimental role. Cdk5 activity has been demonstrated in the cytoplasm and nucleus. Myristoylation of p35 and p39 has been shown to regulate the distribution of Cdk5, with non-myristoylated p35 and p39 preferentially accumulated in the nucleus (Asada et al. 2008). Previously it has been suggested that nuclear Cdk5 may be selectively associated with neuronal loss, while cytoplasmic Cdk5 activity is linked to neuroprotection (O'Hare et al. 2005). Nonetheless, recent studies indicate that both cytoplasmic and nuclear Cdk5 activity can contribute to neuronal loss (Rashidian et al. 2009) or neuronal survival (Zhang et al. 2010a). It appears that the differential distribution of Cdk5 in the cytoplasm and nucleus, and their respective functions, depend on the types of insults that are being inflicted. Additional studies will be required to further delineate the precise involvement of nuclear and cytoplasmic Cdk5 in the regulation of neuronal survival.

3. Cdk5 in PD pathology

In agreement with the essential role of Cdk5 as a regulator of neuronal survival, Cdk5 is also implicated in neuronal loss in PD, with elevation of Cdk5 consistently associated with cell death in different PD models. Cdk5 was first linked to PD when inhibition of Cdk5 activity reduces neuronal loss in MPTP-injected mice (Smith et al. 2003). MPTP injection increases Cdk5 activity and p25 levels in the substantia nigra of the injected mice, and attenuating this increase with Cdk5 inhibitor or adenovirus-mediated overexpression of dominant-negative Cdk5 attenuates dopaminergic neuronal loss (Smith et al. 2003). Although treatment with

MPP^+, the metabolized form of MPTP in the brain, has also been demonstrated to reduce Cdk5 activity through proteasome-dependent degradation of p35 (Endo et al. 2009), majority of the studies reported increase in Cdk5 activity following MPTP injection or MPP^+ treatment (Smith *et al.* 2003, Wong *et al.* 2011, Smith *et al.* 2006, Qu *et al.* 2007, Huang *et al.* 2010), possibly due to the use of different toxin dosages. Interestingly, additional studies aimed at elucidating the mechanisms by which Cdk5 regulates neuronal loss implicate Cdk5 in multiple cellular processes that were found to be altered in PD. Here we summarize the role of Cdk5 in several pathogenic mechanisms postulated to contribute to PD pathology.

3.1 Autophagy deregulation

Autophagy, a homeostatic process for the turnover of cytoplasmic content and organelles, is increasingly implicated in neurodegenerative diseases. Currently three types of autophagy are identified based on the mechanisms by which cargo is delivered, namely macroautophagy, microautophagy and chaperone-mediate autophagy (CMA). Macroautophagy is initiated with the formation of autophagosome, a double-membraned vesicle that is formed through the extension of isolation membrane (also known as phagophore), to encircle part of the cytoplasm for degradation. Subsequent fusion of autophagosome with lysosome leads to the formation of autolysosome, where the cargo of the autophagosome is degraded by lysosomal enzymes (Mizushima 2007). Microautophagy also entails bulk sequestration of cytoplasmic content, but instead of acting through the formation of autophagosomes, it is directly sequestered into lysosomes. CMA, on the other hand, involves selective translocation of soluble target proteins, which usually contain the KFERQ motif, to the lysosomes. Heat-shock cognate 70 (hsc70) and lysosomes-associated membrane protein 2A (LAMP2A) are important chaperones for selective transport of cargo into the CMA pathway (Cheung and Ip 2009, Mizushima *et al.* 2008, Rubinsztein 2006).

While autophagy has long been regarded as a homeostatic cellular event, recent studies revealed that deregulation of the autophagic pathway also contributes to neurodegeneration. Transgenic animals lacking Atg5 or Atg7, genes that are critical for macroautophagy, develop neurodegeneration (Hara *et al.* 2006, Komatsu *et al.* 2006). In addition, activation of macroautophagy in a drosophila model of Huntington's disease significantly reduces huntingtin toxicity (Ravikumar et al. 2004), consistent with a role of macroautophagy in the clearance of protein aggregates. Deregulation of the autophagic pathway is also demonstrated in PD (Cheung and Ip 2009). For example, accumulation of autophagosomes is evident in post-mortem brains of PD patients (Mizushima et al. 2008). In addition, both CMA and macroautophagy were implicated in the regulation of α-synuclein level, the major constituent of Lewy body. In particular, CMA is required for the degradation of wildtype soluble α-synuclein (Cuervo *et al.* 2004, Vogiatzi *et al.* 2008, Webb *et al.* 2003). Interestingly, A53T and A30P mutants of α-synuclein, which are associated with familial PD, inhibit CMA-mediated degradation of wildtype α-synuclein. These mutants are in turn degraded by macroautophagy (Cuervo et al. 2004). Furthermore, inhibition of CMA by A53T α-synuclein mutant also impairs degradation of pro-survival transcription factor MEF2D (Yang et al. 2009). Reduced degradation of MEF2D results in accumulation of MEF2D in the cytoplasm and inhibition of MEF2D activity, leading to cell death (Yang et al. 2009). Interestingly, Cdk5 has been demonstrated to phosphorylate MEF2D at S444 to inhibit its activity and facilitate its cleavage by caspases (Tang *et al.* 2005, Gong *et al.* 2003), and is required for neuronal loss triggered by MPTP injection (Smith et al. 2006). It will be interesting to examine whether phosphorylation of MEF2D by Cdk5 plays a role in its degradation by CMA. Moreover, we have recently demonstrated that overexpression of A53T α-synuclein increases Cdk5 activity (Wong et al. 2011). It is tempting to speculate that in addition to the inhibition of CMA-mediated degradation of MEF2D by α-synuclein expression, elevated phosphorylation of MEF2D by Cdk5 may also contribute to cell loss triggered by α-synuclein expression. Studies aimed at addressing this possibility will provide important insights regarding the pathogenic mechanisms of PD.

It should be noted that overexpression of A53T and A30P mutants of α-synuclein also induces activation of macroautophagy (Wong *et al.* 2011, Cuervo *et al.* 2004, Vogiatzi *et al.* 2008). While induction of macroautophagy may facilitate clearance of these mutant α-synucleins, several studies suggest that elevation of macroautophagy in response to A53T α-synuclein expression or MPP^+ treatment may be associated with neuronal loss (Wong *et al.* 2011, Yang *et al.* 2009, Xilouri *et al.* 2009, Stefanis *et al.* 2001, Kirik *et al.* 2002, Choubey *et al.* 2011). Whether this induction serves a protective or detrimental role in PD thus remains unresolved. We have recently discovered a role of Cdk5 in the regulation of macroautophagy through its phosphorylation of lipid-binding protein endophilin B1 (Wong et al. 2011). Endophilin B1, also known as Bax-interacting factor 1 (Bif-1), was previously implicated in autophagy induction in fibroblasts through its association with autophagy machinery UVRAG and Beclin 1 (Takahashi et al. 2007). We demonstrated that Cdk5-mediated phosphorylation of endophilin B1 at T145 is required for starvation-induced macroautophagy in neurons. More importantly, our findings revealed that this phosphorylation event is critical for the activation of macroautophagy in response to MPP^+ stimulation or overexpression of A53T α-synuclein (Wong et al. 2011). Attenuation of macroautophagy induction significantly reduces neuronal loss in these PD models, suggesting that activation of macroautophagy in PD may contribute to neuronal loss. Remarkably, inhibition of Cdk5 activity or endophilin B1 T145 phosphorylation concomitantly reduces macroautophagy activation or neuronal loss (Wong et al. 2011). Collectively, our findings reveal that macroautophagy activation in PD may serve a detrimental role, with Cdk5 and endophilin B1 being the essential mediators of this induction.

Deregulation of autophagy in PD also occurs in the form of impaired mitophagy, the removal of mitochondria through macroautophagy (Youle and Narendra 2011). Recent evidence reveals that two genes that are mutated in cases of familial PD, PINK1 and Parkin, are critical for mitophagy (Narendra *et al.* 2008, Geisler *et al.* 2010, Lee *et al.* 2010, Jin *et al.* 2010, Ziviani *et al.* 2010). PINK1, a serine/threonine kinase that is expressed on the outer membrane of the mitochondria, is constitutively degraded in healthy mitochondria in a voltage-dependent manner. The high level of PINK1 on damaged mitochondria will then result in the recruitment of Parkin, a ubiquitin E3 ligase, to the mitochondria. Subsequent ubiquitination of the damage mitochondria, Parkin itself and VDAC is required for the removal of damaged mitochondria via mitophagy (Narendra *et al.* 2010, Geisler *et al.* 2010, Lee *et al.* 2010, Jin *et al.* 2010). Importantly, various PD-associated missense mutations have been demonstrated to trigger different extent of mitophagy impairment (Lee et al. 2010), suggesting that aberrant mitophagy may represent one of the mechanisms by which these mutations lead to PD. Interestingly, Cdk5 has been demonstrated to phosphorylate Parkin at S131 to reduce its E3 ubiquitin ligase activity, with the S131A mutant of Parkin more prone to accumulate into inclusions (Avraham et al. 2007). In addition, phosphorylation of Parkin by Cdk5 and casein kinase I also augments its aggregation and inactivation (Rubio de la Torre et al. 2009). It will be interesting to examine whether Cdk5-mediated inhibition of Parkin activity affects the mitophagy of damaged mitochondria in PD models.

3.2 Oxidative stress

Oxidative stress has long been demonstrated to play an essential role in PD pathogenesis. Lipid peroxidation, DNA damage and protein oxidation are all evident in PD brains (Levy et al. 2009). In support of the involvement of oxidative stress in PD, familial PD-associated missense mutations were identified in DJ-1, an atypical peroxiredoxin-like peroxidase with antioxidant activity (Andres-Mateos et al. 2007). In addition, mitochondrial dysfunction, which could directly lead to generation of reactive oxygen species, is also detected in PD. These findings collectively suggest that preserving the anti-oxidative machinery in PD will be critical for limiting PD pathology.

Interestingly, an anti-oxidative peroxidase peroxiredoxin 2 (Prx2) was found to be phosphorylated by Cdk5 in response to MPTP toxicity (Qu et al. 2007). Phosphorylation of Prx2 at T89 by Cdk5 reduces its peroxidase activity. In addition, treatment with MPP^+ increases Cdk5 activity and phospho-T89 Prx2 level, while concomitantly decreasing Prx2 peroxidase activity. Importantly, the protective effect of Prx2 against MPP^+-induced cell death is attenuated when a T89 phospho-mimetic mutant of Prx2 is expressed, suggesting that phosphorylation of Prx2 at T89 abrogates its protective effect (Qu et al. 2007). These observations collectively revealed that Cdk5 may contribute to neuronal loss in PD through inhibiting the peroxidase activity of Prx2, thus rendering the cells more susceptible to oxidative stress.

DNA damage is a frequent consequence of oxidative stress and is a known factor for triggering cell death. A recent study revealed that Cdk5 also mediates neuronal loss in PD through phosphorylation of apurinic/apyrimidinic endonuclease 1 (Apel), an enzyme implicated in DNA repair (Huang et al. 2010). Cdk5-mediated phosphorylation of Apel at T232 reduces its endonuclease activity and abolishes its neuroprotective effect against MPP^+-triggered neuronal death (Huang et al. 2010). Interestingly, another enzyme implicated in DNA damage response, ataxia telangiectasia mutated (ATM), is also identified as a Cdk5 substrate (Tian et al. 2009). ATM is a phosphoinositide-3-kinase related kinase that plays critical role in the mediation of DNA damage signals, and has been implicated in neuronal loss triggered by DNA damage (Herzog *et al.* 1998, Kruman *et al.* 2004, Lee *et al.* 2001). Elevation of Cdk5 activity in response to DNA damage results in phosphorylation of ATM at S1981, an event that is critical for the activation of ATM. Interestingly, inhibition of Cdk5 activity attenuates neuronal loss induced by DNA damaging agent camptothecin (Tian et al. 2009). Although whether ATM phosphorylation is triggered in PD models remains unexplored, given the implication of DNA damage and the potential induction of Cdk5 activity in PD, it will be interesting to further dissect the precise role of Cdk5 in regulating the anti-oxidative machinery of the cells.

3.3 Mitochondrial dysfunction

Mitochondrial dysfunction has emerged as an important pathogenic mechanism in PD. Reduced mitochondrial complex I activity was detected in PD patients (Levy et al. 2009). In addition, MPTP was demonstrated to inhibit complex I of the mitochondrial respiratory chain (Levy et al. 2009). More importantly, gene products of a number of the familial PD-associated missense mutations are found to be localized to the mitochondria, including PINK1, Parkin, LRRK2, DJ-1 and HtrA2/Omi (Knott et al. 2008). In particular, recent studies revealed PINK1 and Parkin as important regulators of mitochondrial morphology through facilitating mitochondrial fission (Cho et al. 2010). Given the association of neuronal apoptosis with elevated mitochondrial fission, regulation of mitochondrial fusion/fission event by PINK1 and Parkin may also contribute to neuronal loss in PD. In addition, as mentioned above, PINK1 and Parkin are also required for the selective mitophagy of mitochondria with low membrane potential (Youle and Narendra 2011). With Parkin identified as a Cdk5 substrate (Avraham et al. 2007) and the observed expression of Cdk5 and p35 in the mitochondrial fraction of cortical neurons (Cheung et al. 2008), it is tempting to speculate that Cdk5 may also regulate mitochondrial homeostasis during PD through controlling mitochondrial fission/fusion or mitophagy. In support of this possibility, Cdk5 has also been implicated in mitochondrial fission during apoptosis (Meuer et al. 2007). In addition, another Cdk5 substrate endophilin B1 is also demonstrated to regulate mitochondrial morphology (Wong *et al.* 2011, Karbowski *et al.* 2004). It is therefore important to further delineate the role of Cdk5 in mitochondrial morphogenesis and mitophagy in PD models.

Aside from being the powerhouse of the cell and a potential source of reactive oxygen species, the mitochondria also plays a central role in the intrinsic apoptotic pathway. Release of cytochrome c from the intermembrane space of mitochondria triggers caspase activation and apoptosis (Bredesen et al. 2006). Indeed, neuronal loss in PD has been attributed at least in part to the apoptotic pathway (Levy et al. 2009). Identification of Bcl-2, a key anti-apoptotic regulator of cytochrome c release from the mitochondria, as a Cdk5 substrate suggests that Cdk5 may also regulate neuronal loss in PD through phosphorylation of Bcl-2 (Cheung et al. 2008). Furthermore, Cdk5 substrate endophilin B1, being an interacting protein of pro-apoptotic Bcl-2 family member Bax (Wong *et al.* 2011, Cuddeback *et al.* 2001), has also been demonstrated to play a role in apoptosis. Inhibition of endophilin B1 expression attenuates cytochrome c release and caspase-3 activation in HeLa cells (Takahashi et al. 2005). Although whether endophilin B1 similarly regulates apoptosis in neurons remains to be explored, these observations suggest that Cdk5-mediated phosphorylation of endophilin B1 and Bcl-2 may regulate the mitochondrial apoptotic pathway in PD. Additional studies will be required to address this hypothesis.

3.4 Proteasomal pathway anomaly

The proteasome pathway has also been demonstrated to contribute to degradation of α-synuclein (Webb *et al.* 2003, Rubinsztein 2006), suggesting that reduction in proteasomal activity may contribute to α-synuclein aggregation. Strikingly, a 40% decrease in proteasome activity has been demonstrated in the substantia nigra of PD patients post-mortem brains (McNaught and Jenner 2001). Indeed, mutation in E3 ubiquitin ligase Parkin and ubiquitin-C-terminal hydrolase-L1 (UCH-L1), a protein implicated in the degradation of poly-ubiquitin chains, are evident in familial PD cases (Kitada *et al.* 1998, Leroy *et al.* 1998). Familial PD-associated missense mutation of Parkin reduces its enzyme activity (Shimura et al. 2000). With Cdk5-mediated phosphorylation of Parkin also demonstrated to reduce its E3 ubiquitin ligase activity, it will be important to investigate if Cdk5 is involved in the deregulation of the proteasomal pathway in PD.

4. Future perspectives

It has become increasingly clear that Cdk5 plays a pivotal role in neuronal loss in PD. Using both *in vivo* and *in vitro* cell-based systems, inhibition of Cdk5 consistently attenuates neuronal loss in various PD models. The identification of multiple Cdk5 substrates that directly participates in known pathogenic mechanisms of PD has provided the much needed mechanistic insights regarding the alteration of these processes in PD, and the precise involvement of Cdk5 (Figure 1). Nonetheless, our understanding is far from complete. In particular, in light of the convergence of several pathogenic mechanisms onto the mitochondria and the identification of a number of mitochondria-associated proteins as Cdk5 substrates, it is important to further delineate how Cdk5 regulates the signaling cascades at the mitochondria during PD. In addition, Cdk5 has also been demonstrated to

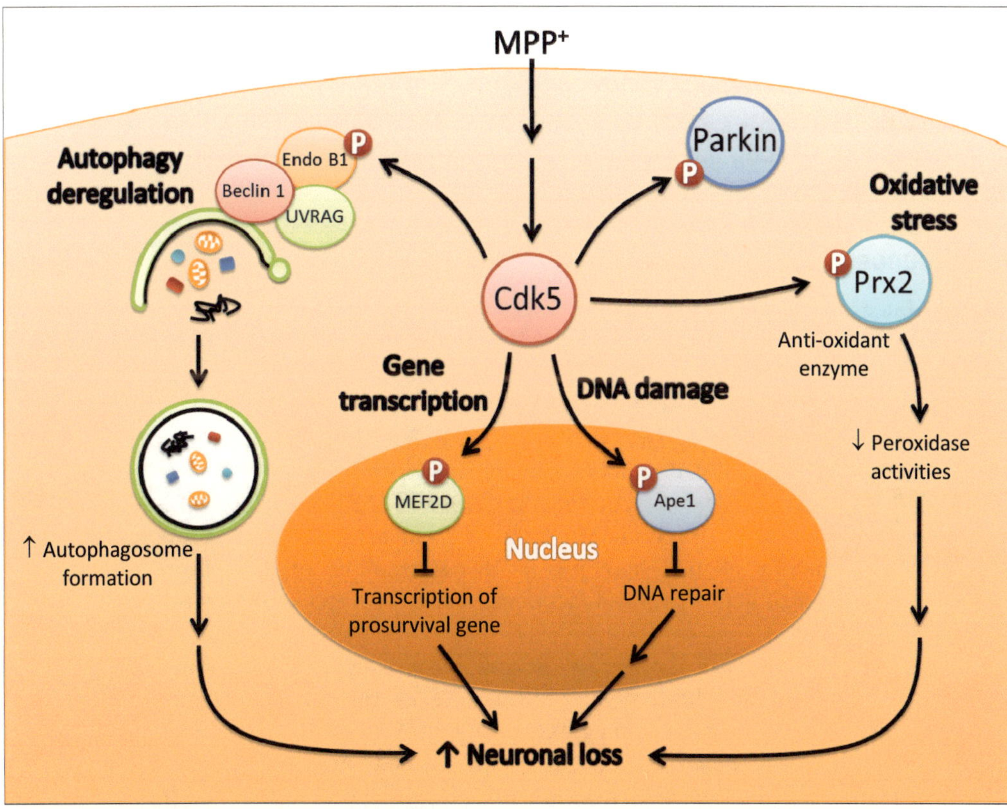

Fig. 1. Implication of Cdk5 in neuronal loss in PD through phosphorylation of multiple substrates. MPTP injection or MPP^+ treatment elevates Cdk5 activity, which in turn phosphorylates a number of cellular proteins. Phosphorylation of endophilin B1 by Cdk5 is required for macroautophagy induction in PD models, which contributes to neuronal loss. Cdk5 also phosphorylates pro-survival transcription factor MEF2D and DNA repair enzyme Ape1 to inhibit their activities, thereby leading to cell death. Phosphorylation of anti-oxidant enzyme Prx2 by Cdk5 attenuates its peroxidase activity, leaving the cell more prone to oxidative stress. Cdk5-mediated phosphorylation of Parkin also reduces its E3 ubiquitin ligase activity, but how this directly contributes to neuronal loss remains to be explored.

regulate dopaminergic transmission and dopamine downstream signaling through phosphorylation of DARPP-32 (Chergui *et al.* 2004, Bibb *et al.* 1999). Furthermore, both dopamine and tyrosine hydroxylase have been identified as Cdk5 substrates (Zhen *et al.* 2004, Kansy *et al.* 2004). It will thus be important to further examine the effect of Cdk5 on dopaminergic transmission in PD models, and investigate the possibility that Cdk5 modulators may regulate dopamine levels to alleviate PD symptoms. Together with the apparent neuroprotective effect of Cdk5 against neuronal loss in PD through acting on multiple cellular events that are aberrant in PD, Cdk5 may emerge as an important target for future development of therapeutics against PD.

5. Acknowledgement

We apologize to the many researchers whose works were not cited due to space limitation. We would like to thank Ka-Chun Lok for his excellent help on preparing the figure. The studies by Z.H. Cheung and N.Y. Ip were supported in part by the Research Grants Council of Hong Kong (HKUST 661007, 660309, 661109, 660810 and 660210), the Area of Excellence Scheme of the University Grants Committee (AoE/B-15/01) and Hong Kong Jockey Club. N.Y. Ip and Z.H. Cheung are Croucher Foundation Senior Research Fellow and Croucher Foundation Fellow, respectively.

6. References

Andres-Mateos, E., Perier, C., Zhang, L., Blanchard-Fillion, B., Greco, T. M., Thomas, B., Ko, H. S., Sasaki, M., Ischiropoulos, H., Przedborski, S., Dawson, T. M. and Dawson, V. L. (2007) DJ-1 gene deletion reveals that DJ-1 is an atypical peroxiredoxin-like peroxidase. *Proc Natl Acad Sci U S A* 104, 14807-14812.

Arif, A., Jia, J., Moodt, R. A., DiCorleto, P. E. and Fox, P. L. (2011) Phosphorylation of glutamyl-prolyl tRNA synthetase by cyclin-dependent kinase 5 dictates transcript-selective translational control. *Proc Natl Acad Sci U S A* 108, 1415-1420.

Asada, A., Yamamoto, N., Gohda, M., Saito, T., Hayashi, N. and Hisanaga, S. (2008) Myristoylation of p39 and p35 is a determinant of cytoplasmic or nuclear localization of active cyclin-dependent kinase 5 complexes. *J Neurochem* 106, 1325-1336.

Avraham, E., Rott, R., Liani, E., Szargel, R. and Engelender, S. (2007) Phosphorylation of Parkin by the cyclin-dependent kinase 5 at the linker region modulates its ubiquitin-ligase activity and aggregation. *J Biol Chem* 282, 12842-12850.

Bibb, J. A., Snyder, G. L., Nishi, A., Yan, Z., Meijer, L., Fienberg, A. A., Tsai, L. H., Kwon, Y. T., Girault, J. A., Czernik, A. J., Huganir, R. L., Hemmings, H. C., Jr., Nairn, A. C. and Greengard, P. (1999) Phosphorylation of DARPP-32 by Cdk5 modulates dopamine signalling in neurons. *Nature* 402, 669-671.

Bredesen, D. E., Rao, R. V. and Mehlen, P. (2006) Cell death in the nervous system. *Nature* 443, 796-802.

Chae, T., Kwon, Y. T., Bronson, R., Dikkes, P., Li, E. and Tsai, L. H. (1997) Mice lacking p35, a neuronal specific activator of Cdk5, display cortical lamination defects, seizures, and adult lethality. *Neuron* 18, 29-42.

Chergui, K., Svenningsson, P. and Greengard, P. (2004) Cyclin-dependent kinase 5 regulates dopaminergic and glutamatergic transmission in the striatum. *Proc Natl Acad Sci U S A* 101, 2191-2196.

Cheung, Z. H., Chin, W. H., Chen, Y., Ng, Y. P. and Ip, N. Y. (2007) Cdk5 is involved in BDNF-stimulated dendritic growth in hippocampal neurons. *PLoS Biol* 5, e63.

Cheung, Z. H., Gong, K. and Ip, N. Y. (2008) Cyclin-dependent kinase 5 supports neuronal survival through phosphorylation of Bcl-2. *J Neurosci* 28, 4872-4877.

Cheung, Z. H. and Ip, N. Y. (2004) Cdk5: mediator of neuronal death and survival. *Neurosci Lett* 361, 47-51.

Cheung, Z. H. and Ip, N. Y. (2007) The roles of cyclin-dependent kinase 5 in dendrite and synapse development. *Biotechnol J.*

Cheung, Z. H. and Ip, N. Y. (2009) The emerging role of autophagy in Parkinson's disease. *Mol Brain* 2, 29.

Cho, D. H., Nakamura, T. and Lipton, S. A. (2010) Mitochondrial dynamics in cell death and neurodegeneration. *Cell Mol Life Sci* 67, 3435-3447.

Choi, J. H., Banks, A. S., Estall, J. L., Kajimura, S., Bostrom, P., Laznik, D., Ruas, J. L., Chalmers, M. J., Kamenecka, T. M., Bluher, M., Griffin, P. R. and Spiegelman, B. M. (2010) Anti-diabetic drugs inhibit obesity-linked phosphorylation of PPARgamma by Cdk5. *Nature* 466, 451-456.

Choubey, V., Safiulina, D., Vaarmann, A., Cagalinec, M., Wareski, P., Kuum, M., Zharkovsky, A. and Kaasik, A. (2011) Mutant A53T {alpha}-synuclein induces neuronal death by increasing mitochondrial autophagy. *J Biol Chem.*

Cruz, J. C. and Tsai, L. H. (2004) A Jekyll and Hyde kinase: roles for Cdk5 in brain development and disease. *Curr Opin Neurobiol* 14, 390-394.

Cuddeback, S. M., Yamaguchi, H., Komatsu, K., Miyashita, T., Yamada, M., Wu, C., Singh, S. and Wang, H. G. (2001) Molecular cloning and characterization of Bif-1. A novel Src homology 3 domain-containing protein that associates with Bax. *J Biol Chem* 276, 20559-20565.

Cuervo, A. M., Stefanis, L., Fredenburg, R., Lansbury, P. T. and Sulzer, D. (2004) Impaired degradation of mutant alpha-synuclein by chaperone-mediated autophagy. *Science* 305, 1292-1295.

Dauer, W. and Przedborski, S. (2003) Parkinson's disease: mechanisms and models. *Neuron* 39, 889-909.

de Rijk, M. C., Tzourio, C., Breteler, M. M., Dartigues, J. F., Amaducci, L., Lopez-Pousa, S., Manubens-Bertran, J. M., Alperovitch, A. and Rocca, W. A. (1997) Prevalence of parkinsonism and Parkinson's disease in Europe: the EUROPARKINSON Collaborative Study. European Community Concerted Action on the Epidemiology of Parkinson's disease. *J Neurol Neurosurg Psychiatry* 62, 10-15.

Dhavan, R. and Tsai, L. H. (2001) A decade of CDK5. *Nat Rev Mol Cell Biol* 2, 749-759.

Endo, R., Saito, T., Asada, A., Kawahara, H., Ohshima, T. and Hisanaga, S. (2009) Commitment of 1-methyl-4-phenylpyrinidinium ion-induced neuronal cell death by proteasome-mediated degradation of p35 cyclin-dependent kinase 5 activator. *J Biol Chem* 284, 26029-26039.

Fu, A. K., Cheung, J., Smith, F. D., Ip, F. C. and Ip, N. Y. (2001) Overexpression of muscle specific kinase increases the transcription and aggregation of acetylcholine receptors in Xenopus embryos. *Brain Res Mol Brain Res* 96, 21-29.

Fu, W. Y., Chen, Y., Sahin, M., Zhao, X. S., Shi, L., Bikoff, J. B., Lai, K. O., Yung, W. H., Fu, A. K., Greenberg, M. E. and Ip, N. Y. (2007) Cdk5 regulates EphA4-mediated dendritic spine retraction through an ephexin1-dependent mechanism. *Nat Neurosci* 10, 67-76.

Geisler, S., Holmstrom, K. M., Skujat, D., Fiesel, F. C., Rothfuss, O. C., Kahle, P. J. and Springer, W. (2010) PINK1/Parkin-mediated mitophagy is dependent on VDAC1 and p62/SQSTM1. *Nat Cell Biol* 12, 119-131.

Gong, X., Tang, X., Wiedmann, M., Wang, X., Peng, J., Zheng, D., Blair, L. A., Marshall, J. and Mao, Z. (2003) Cdk5-mediated inhibition of the protective effects of transcription factor MEF2 in neurotoxicity-induced apoptosis. *Neuron* 38, 33-46.

Hara, T., Nakamura, K., Matsui, M., Yamamoto, A., Nakahara, Y., Suzuki-Migishima, R., Yokoyama, M., Mishima, K., Saito, I., Okano, H. and Mizushima, N. (2006) Suppression of basal autophagy in neural cells causes neurodegenerative disease in mice. *Nature* 441, 885-889.

Hawasli, A. H. and Bibb, J. A. (2007) Alternative roles for Cdk5 in learning and synaptic plasticity. *Biotechnol J* 2, 941-948.

Herzog, K. H., Chong, M. J., Kapsetaki, M., Morgan, J. I. and McKinnon, P. J. (1998) Requirement for Atm in ionizing radiation-induced cell death in the developing central nervous system. *Science* 280, 1089-1091.

Huang, E., Qu, D., Zhang, Y., Venderova, K., Haque, M. E., Rousseaux, M. W., Slack, R. S., Woulfe, J. M. and Park, D. S. (2010) The role of Cdk5-mediated apurinic/apyrimidinic endonuclease 1 phosphorylation in neuronal death. *Nat Cell Biol* 12, 563-571.

Jin, S. M., Lazarou, M., Wang, C., Kane, L. A., Narendra, D. P. and Youle, R. J. (2010) Mitochondrial membrane potential regulates PINK1 import and proteolytic destabilization by PARL. *J Cell Biol* 191, 933-942.

Kansy, J. W., Daubner, S. C., Nishi, A., Sotogaku, N., Lloyd, M. D., Nguyen, C., Lu, L., Haycock, J. W., Hope, B. T., Fitzpatrick, P. F. and Bibb, J. A. (2004) Identification of tyrosine hydroxylase as a physiological substrate for Cdk5. *J Neurochem* 91, 374-384.

Karbowski, M., Jeong, S. Y. and Youle, R. J. (2004) Endophilin B1 is required for the maintenance of mitochondrial morphology. *J Cell Biol* 166, 1027-1039.

Kirik, D., Rosenblad, C., Burger, C., Lundberg, C., Johansen, T. E., Muzyczka, N., Mandel, R. J. and Bjorklund, A. (2002) Parkinson-like neurodegeneration induced by targeted overexpression of alpha-synuclein in the nigrostriatal system. *J Neurosci* 22, 2780-2791.

Kitada, T., Asakawa, S., Hattori, N., Matsumine, H., Yamamura, Y., Minoshima, S., Yokochi, M., Mizuno, Y. and Shimizu, N. (1998) Mutations in the parkin gene cause autosomal recessive juvenile parkinsonism. *Nature* 392, 605-608.

Knott, A. B., Perkins, G., Schwarzenbacher, R. and Bossy-Wetzel, E. (2008) Mitochondrial fragmentation in neurodegeneration. *Nat Rev Neurosci* 9, 505-518.

Ko, J., Humbert, S., Bronson, R. T., Takahashi, S., Kulkarni, A. B., Li, E. and Tsai, L. H. (2001) p35 and p39 are essential for cyclin-dependent kinase 5 function during neurodevelopment. *J Neurosci* 21, 6758-6771.

Kobayashi, S., Ishiguro, K., Omori, A., Takamatsu, M., Arioka, M., Imahori, K. and Uchida, T. (1993) A cdc2-related kinase PSSALRE/cdk5 is homologous with the 30 kDa subunit of tau protein kinase II, a proline-directed protein kinase associated with microtubule. *FEBS Lett* 335, 171-175.

Komatsu, M., Waguri, S., Chiba, T., Murata, S., Iwata, J., Tanida, I., Ueno, T., Koike, M., Uchiyama, Y., Kominami, E. and Tanaka, K. (2006) Loss of autophagy in the central nervous system causes neurodegeneration in mice. *Nature* 441, 880-884.

Kruman, II, Wersto, R. P., Cardozo-Pelaez, F., Smilenov, L., Chan, S. L., Chrest, F. J., Emokpae, R., Jr., Gorospe, M. and Mattson, M. P. (2004) Cell cycle activation linked to neuronal cell death initiated by DNA damage. *Neuron* 41, 549-561.

Lai, K. O. and Ip, N. Y. (2009) Recent advances in understanding the roles of Cdk5 in synaptic plasticity. *Biochim Biophys Acta* 1792, 741-745.

Lee, J. Y., Nagano, Y., Taylor, J. P., Lim, K. L. and Yao, T. P. (2010) Disease-causing mutations in parkin impair mitochondrial ubiquitination, aggregation, and HDAC6-dependent mitophagy. *J Cell Biol* 189, 671-679.

Lee, Y., Chong, M. J. and McKinnon, P. J. (2001) Ataxia telangiectasia mutated-dependent apoptosis after genotoxic stress in the developing nervous system is determined by cellular differentiation status. *J Neurosci* 21, 6687-6693.

Leroy, E., Boyer, R., Auburger, G., Leube, B., Ulm, G., Mezey, E., Harta, G., Brownstein, M. J., Jonnalagada, S., Chernova, T., Dehejia, A., Lavedan, C., Gasser, T., Steinbach, P. J., Wilkinson, K. D. and Polymeropoulos, M. H. (1998) The ubiquitin pathway in Parkinson's disease. *Nature* 395, 451-452.

Levy, O. A., Malagelada, C. and Greene, L. A. (2009) Cell death pathways in Parkinson's disease: proximal triggers, distal effectors, and final steps. *Apoptosis* 14, 478-500.

Lew, J., Beaudette, K., Litwin, C. M. and Wang, J. H. (1992) Purification and characterization of a novel proline-directed protein kinase from bovine brain. *J Biol Chem* 267, 13383-13390.

Li, B. S., Ma, W., Jaffe, H., Zheng, Y., Takahashi, S., Zhang, L., Kulkarni, A. B. and Pant, H. C. (2003a) Cyclin-dependent kinase-5 is involved in neuregulin-dependent activation of phosphatidylinositol 3-kinase and Akt activity mediating neuronal survival. *J Biol Chem* 278, 35702-35709.

Li, G., Faibushevich, A., Turunen, B. J., Yoon, S. O., Georg, G., Michaelis, M. L. and Dobrowsky, R. T. (2003b) Stabilization of the cyclin-dependent kinase 5 activator, p35, by paclitaxel decreases beta-amyloid toxicity in cortical neurons. *J Neurochem* 84, 347-362.

Lilja, L., Yang, S. N., Webb, D. L., Juntti-Berggren, L., Berggren, P. O. and Bark, C. (2001) Cyclin-dependent kinase 5 promotes insulin exocytosis. *J Biol Chem* 276, 34199-34205.

McNaught, K. S. and Jenner, P. (2001) Proteasomal function is impaired in substantia nigra in Parkinson's disease. *Neurosci Lett* 297, 191-194.

Meuer, K., Suppanz, I. E., Lingor, P., Planchamp, V., Goricke, B., Fichtner, L., Braus, G. H., Dietz, G. P., Jakobs, S., Bahr, M. and Weishaupt, J. H. (2007) Cyclin-dependent kinase 5 is an upstream regulator of mitochondrial fission during neuronal apoptosis. *Cell Death Differ* 14, 651-661.

Meyerson, M., Enders, G. H., Wu, C. L., Su, L. K., Gorka, C., Nelson, C., Harlow, E. and Tsai, L. H. (1992) A family of human cdc2-related protein kinases. *Embo J* 11, 2909-2917.

Mizushima, N. (2007) Autophagy: process and function. *Genes Dev* 21, 2861-2873.

Mizushima, N., Levine, B., Cuervo, A. M. and Klionsky, D. J. (2008) Autophagy fights disease through cellular self-digestion. *Nature* 451, 1069-1075.

Narendra, D., Tanaka, A., Suen, D. F. and Youle, R. J. (2008) Parkin is recruited selectively to impaired mitochondria and promotes their autophagy. *J Cell Biol* 183, 795-803.

Narendra, D. P., Jin, S. M., Tanaka, A., Suen, D. F., Gautier, C. A., Shen, J., Cookson, M. R. and Youle, R. J. (2010) PINK1 is selectively stabilized on impaired mitochondria to activate Parkin. *PLoS Biol* 8, e1000298.

Nguyen, M. D., Mushynski, W. E. and Julien, J. P. (2002) Cycling at the interface between neurodevelopment and neurodegeneration. *Cell Death Differ* 9, 1294-1306.

O'Hare, M. J., Kushwaha, N., Zhang, Y., Aleyasin, H., Callaghan, S. M., Slack, R. S., Albert, P. R., Vincent, I. and Park, D. S. (2005) Differential roles of nuclear and cytoplasmic cyclin-dependent kinase 5 in apoptotic and excitotoxic neuronal death. *J Neurosci* 25, 8954-8966.

Obeso, J. A., Rodriguez-Oroz, M. C., Goetz, C. G., Marin, C., Kordower, J. H., Rodriguez, M., Hirsch, E. C., Farrer, M., Schapira, A. H. and Halliday, G. (2010) Missing pieces in the Parkinson's disease puzzle. *Nat Med* 16, 653-661.

Ohshima, T., Ward, J. M., Huh, C. G., Longenecker, G., Veeranna, Pant, H. C., Brady, R. O., Martin, L. J. and Kulkarni, A. B. (1996) Targeted disruption of the cyclin-dependent kinase 5 gene results in abnormal corticogenesis, neuronal pathology and perinatal death. *Proc Natl Acad Sci U S A* 93, 11173-11178.

Patrick, G. N., Zhou, P., Kwon, Y. T., Howley, P. M. and Tsai, L. H. (1998) p35, the neuronal-specific activator of cyclin-dependent kinase 5 (Cdk5) is degraded by the ubiquitin-proteasome pathway. *J Biol Chem* 273, 24057-24064.

Patrick, G. N., Zukerberg, L., Nikolic, M., de la Monte, S., Dikkes, P. and Tsai, L. H. (1999) Conversion of p35 to p25 deregulates Cdk5 activity and promotes neurodegeneration. *Nature* 402, 615-622.

Patzke, H. and Tsai, L. H. (2002) Calpain-mediated cleavage of the cyclin-dependent kinase-5 activator p39 to p29. *J Biol Chem* 277, 8054-8060.

Peterson, D. W., Ando, D. M., Taketa, D. A., Zhou, H., Dahlquist, F. W. and Lew, J. (2010) No difference in kinetics of tau or histone phosphorylation by CDK5/p25 versus CDK5/p35 in vitro. *Proc Natl Acad Sci U S A* 107, 2884-2889.

Poewe, W., Antonini, A., Zijlmans, J. C., Burkhard, P. R. and Vingerhoets, F. (2010) Levodopa in the treatment of Parkinson's disease: an old drug still going strong. *Clin Interv Aging* 5, 229-238.

Qu, D., Rashidian, J., Mount, M. P., Aleyasin, H., Parsanejad, M., Lira, A., Haque, E., Zhang, Y., Callaghan, S., Daigle, M., Rousseaux, M. W., Slack, R. S., Albert, P. R., Vincent, I., Woulfe, J. M. and Park, D. S. (2007) Role of Cdk5-mediated phosphorylation of Prx2 in MPTP toxicity and Parkinson's disease. *Neuron* 55, 37-52.

Rashidian, J., Rousseaux, M. W., Venderova, K., Qu, D., Callaghan, S. M., Phillips, M., Bland, R. J., During, M. J., Mao, Z., Slack, R. S. and Park, D. S. (2009) Essential role of cytoplasmic cdk5 and Prx2 in multiple ischemic injury models, in vivo. *J Neurosci* 29, 12497-12505.

Ravikumar, B., Vacher, C., Berger, Z., Davies, J. E., Luo, S., Oroz, L. G., Scaravilli, F., Easton, D. F., Duden, R., O'Kane, C. J. and Rubinsztein, D. C. (2004) Inhibition of mTOR induces autophagy and reduces toxicity of polyglutamine expansions in fly and mouse models of Huntington disease. *Nat Genet* 36, 585-595.

Rubinsztein, D. C. (2006) The roles of intracellular protein-degradation pathways in neurodegeneration. *Nature* 443, 780-786.

Rubio de la Torre, E., Luzon-Toro, B., Forte-Lago, I., Minguez-Castellanos, A., Ferrer, I. and Hilfiker, S. (2009) Combined kinase inhibition modulates parkin inactivation. *Hum Mol Genet* 18, 809-823.

Sasaki, Y., Cheng, C., Uchida, Y., Nakajima, O., Ohshima, T., Yagi, T., Taniguchi, M., Nakayama, T., Kishida, R., Kudo, Y., Ohno, S., Nakamura, F. and Goshima, Y. (2002) Fyn and Cdk5 mediate semaphorin-3A signaling, which is involved in regulation of dendrite orientation in cerebral cortex. *Neuron* 35, 907-920.

Schulz, J. B. (2008) Update on the pathogenesis of Parkinson's disease. *J Neurol* 255 Suppl 5, 3-7.

Shimura, H., Hattori, N., Kubo, S., Mizuno, Y., Asakawa, S., Minoshima, S., Shimizu, N., Iwai, K., Chiba, T., Tanaka, K. and Suzuki, T. (2000) Familial Parkinson disease gene product, parkin, is a ubiquitin-protein ligase. *Nat Genet* 25, 302-305.

Smith, P. D., Crocker, S. J., Jackson-Lewis, V., Jordan-Sciutto, K. L., Hayley, S., Mount, M. P., O'Hare, M. J., Callaghan, S., Slack, R. S., Przedborski, S., Anisman, H. and Park, D. S. (2003) Cyclin-dependent kinase 5 is a mediator of dopaminergic neuron loss in a mouse model of Parkinson's disease. *Proc Natl Acad Sci U S A* 100, 13650-13655.

Smith, P. D., Mount, M. P., Shree, R., Callaghan, S., Slack, R. S., Anisman, H., Vincent, I., Wang, X., Mao, Z. and Park, D. S. (2006) Calpain-regulated p35/cdk5 plays a central role in dopaminergic neuron death through modulation of the transcription factor myocyte enhancer factor 2. *J Neurosci* 26, 440-447.

Stefanis, L., Larsen, K. E., Rideout, H. J., Sulzer, D. and Greene, L. A. (2001) Expression of A53T mutant but not wild-type alpha-synuclein in PC12 cells induces alterations of the ubiquitin-dependent degradation system, loss of dopamine release, and autophagic cell death. *J Neurosci* 21, 9549-9560.

Takahashi, M., Iseki, E. and Kosaka, K. (2000) Cyclin-dependent kinase 5 (Cdk5) associated with Lewy bodies in diffuse Lewy body disease. *Brain Res* 862, 253-256.

Takahashi, Y., Coppola, D., Matsushita, N., Cualing, H. D., Sun, M., Sato, Y., Liang, C., Jung, J. U., Cheng, J. Q., Mul, J. J., Pledger, W. J. and Wang, H. G. (2007) Bif-1 interacts with Beclin 1 through UVRAG and regulates autophagy and tumorigenesis. *Nat Cell Biol* 9, 1142-1151.

Takahashi, Y., Karbowski, M., Yamaguchi, H., Kazi, A., Wu, J., Sebti, S. M., Youle, R. J. and Wang, H. G. (2005) Loss of Bif-1 suppresses Bax/Bak conformational change and mitochondrial apoptosis. *Mol Cell Biol* 25, 9369-9382.

Tandon, A., Yu, H., Wang, L., Rogaeva, E., Sato, C., Chishti, M. A., Kawarai, T., Hasegawa, H., Chen, F., Davies, P., Fraser, P. E., Westaway, D. and St George-Hyslop, P. H. (2003) Brain levels of CDK5 activator p25 are not increased in Alzheimer's or other neurodegenerative diseases with neurofibrillary tangles. *J Neurochem* 86, 572-581.

Tang, X., Wang, X., Gong, X., Tong, M., Park, D., Xia, Z. and Mao, Z. (2005) Cyclin-dependent kinase 5 mediates neurotoxin-induced degradation of the transcription factor myocyte enhancer factor 2. *J Neurosci* 25, 4823-4834.

Tian, B., Yang, Q. and Mao, Z. (2009) Phosphorylation of ATM by Cdk5 mediates DNA damage signalling and regulates neuronal death. *Nat Cell Biol* 11, 211-218.

Tsai, L. H., Takahashi, T., Caviness, V. S., Jr. and Harlow, E. (1993) Activity and expression pattern of cyclin-dependent kinase 5 in the embryonic mouse nervous system. *Development* 119, 1029-1040.

Vogiatzi, T., Xilouri, M., Vekrellis, K. and Stefanis, L. (2008) Wild type alpha-synuclein is degraded by chaperone-mediated autophagy and macroautophagy in neuronal cells. *J Biol Chem* 283, 23542-23556.

Webb, J. L., Ravikumar, B., Atkins, J., Skepper, J. N. and Rubinsztein, D. C. (2003) Alpha-Synuclein is degraded by both autophagy and the proteasome. *J Biol Chem* 278, 25009-25013.

Wong, A. S., Lee, R. H., Cheung, A. Y., Yeung, P. K., Chung, S. K., Cheung, Z. H. and Ip, N. Y. (2011) Cdk5-mediated phosphorylation of endophilin B1 is required for induced autophagy in models of Parkinson's disease. *Nat Cell Biol.*

Xilouri, M., Vogiatzi, T., Vekrellis, K., Park, D. and Stefanis, L. (2009) Abberant alpha-synuclein confers toxicity to neurons in part through inhibition of chaperone-mediated autophagy. *PLoS One* 4, e5515.

Yang, Q., She, H., Gearing, M., Colla, E., Lee, M., Shacka, J. J. and Mao, Z. (2009) Regulation of neuronal survival factor MEF2D by chaperone-mediated autophagy. *Science* 323, 124-127.

Youle, R. J. and Narendra, D. P. (2011) Mechanisms of mitophagy. *Nat Rev Mol Cell Biol* 12, 9-14.

Zhang, J. and Herrup, K. (2008) Cdk5 and the non-catalytic arrest of the neuronal cell cycle. *Cell Cycle* 7, 3487-3490.

Zhang, J., Li, H. and Herrup, K. (2010a) Cdk5 nuclear localization is p27-dependent in nerve cells: implications for cell cycle suppression and caspase-3 activation. *J Biol Chem* 285, 14052-14061.

Zhang, P., Yu, P. C., Tsang, A. H., Chen, Y., Fu, A. K., Fu, W. Y., Chung, K. K. and Ip, N. Y. (2010b) S-nitrosylation of cyclin-dependent kinase 5 (cdk5) regulates its kinase activity and dendrite growth during neuronal development. *J Neurosci* 30, 14366-14370.

Zhen, X., Goswami, S., Abdali, S. A., Gil, M., Bakshi, K. and Friedman, E. (2004) Regulation of cyclin-dependent kinase 5 and calcium/calmodulin-dependent protein kinase II by phosphatidylinositol-linked dopamine receptor in rat brain. *Mol Pharmacol* 66, 1500-1507.

Ziviani, E., Tao, R. N. and Whitworth, A. J. (2010) Drosophila parkin requires PINK1 for mitochondrial translocation and ubiquitinates mitofusin. *Proc Natl Acad Sci U S A* 107, 5018-5023.

8

Regulation of α-Synuclein Membrane Binding and Its Implications

Robert H.C. Chen[1], Sabine Wislet-Gendebien[1,2], Howard T.J. Mount[1] and Anurag Tandon[1]
[1]*Tanz Centre for Research in Neurodegenerative Diseases, University of Toronto,*
[2]*GIGA Neurosciences, University of Liège,*
[1]*Canada*
[2]*Belgium*

1. Introduction

1.1 Parkinson's disease and Lewy bodies

Parkinson's disease (PD) is the most prevalent neurodegenerative disease that affects motor control, although dementia, depression, and other psychiatric symptoms are occasionally present (reviewed in Jankovic, 2008). The motor symptoms include resting tremors, bradykinesia/akinesia, rigidity, and postural instability, and are associated with the death of dopaminergic neurons in the substantia nigra pars compacta (SNpc) (Lloyd and Hornykiewicz, 1970; reviewed in Saper, 1999) and noradrenergic neurons in the locus coeruleus (Mann and Yates, 1983; Gaspar et al., 1991). Degeneration of these neurons disrupts basal ganglia circuitry of the brain and interferes with the initiation of voluntary movement (Levy et al., 1997).

Another pathological characteristic of the disease is the presence of the intracellular protein aggregates known as Lewy bodies and Lewy neurites (Hughes et al., 1992), described initially by Frederick Lewy in 1912, that were associated with dying dopaminergic neurons in the SNpc by Tretiakoff (reviewed in Holdorff, 2006). Lewy bodies are also present in other brain regions outside the SNpc, and may appeat first in the glossopharyngeal, vagal, and olfactory centres (Braak et al., 2003). The disruption of these regions is now linked to a preclinical phase of PD that includes perturbations of smell, gastrointestinal motility, and sleep patterns prior to the development of motor impairments coincident with neurodegeneration and inclusions in the midbrain. These intraneuronal aggregates are composed of lipids and various proteins including α-synuclein, ubiquitin, and neurofilaments (Spillantini et al., 1998; reviewed in Cookson, 2005). Whether Lewy bodies directly cause cytotoxicity or are formed as compensatory activation of survival pathways remains under debate. Nevertheless, the presence of Lewy bodies is an essential component of post-mortem diagnoses of PD (Christine and Aminoff, 2004; reviewed in Jankovic, 2008).

1.2 α-Synuclein in Parkinson's disease

α-Synuclein is important to understanding the etiology of PD both because it is the main pathological component of Lewy bodies and because mutations and changes in its expression are linked to familial PD. Three missense mutations causing single amino acid substitutions in α-synuclein are linked to autosomal dominant forms of familial PD: A53T, A30P, and E46K (Polymeropoulos et al., 1997; Kruger et al., 1998; Zarranz et al., 2004). Interestingly, in many mammalian species, including mice and new world primates, threonine is the normal residue at position 53, which suggest some kind of corrective mechanism elsewhere in the coding sequence to reduce the toxicity of the A53T mutation (Hamilton, 2004). Elevated expression of normal α-synuclein is also pathogenic as gene triplication or duplication is linked to early- or late-onset PD, respectively (Singleton et al., 2003; Chartier-Harlin et al., 2004).

Despite the efforts of many research laboratories since its initial discovery as an abundant presynaptic protein in cholinergic nerve terminals innervating the *Torpedo* electric organic (Maroteax et al, 1988), α-synuclein's function still remains somewhat of a mystery. Mice deficient in α-synuclein are unremarkable, but exhibit increased release of dopamine under paired-pulse stimuli and reduced striatal tissue content of dopamine (Abeliovich et al., 2000). Over-expression of α-synuclein in yeast leads to aggregation of vesicles, disruption in vesicular transport, and death (Gitler et al., 2008; Soper et al., 2008). Similarly, moderate α-synuclein over-expression in mammalian neurons reduces transmitter release and the number of synaptic vesicles arrayed at presynaptic active zones (Nemani et al., 2010). These reports clearly implicate α-synuclein in synaptic vesicle mobilization or fusion, but offer little information about its pathogenic role.

In vitro studies revealed that A30P and A53T mutant α-synuclein form oligomers at a faster rate than wild-type α-synuclein (Conway et al., 2000). Post-translational modifications may also affect α-synuclein aggregation, as phosphorylation of serine at position 129 is highly upregulated in Lewy bodies (Fujiwara et al., 2002). Phosphomimic residue changes, such as serine 129 to aspartate, which simulates the charge distribution of phosphorylation, cause neuronal loss in fruit flies and substitution of serine 129 with alanine, which prevents phosphorylation, rescues this cell loss (Chen and Feany, 2005). However, experimental evidence for the toxicity of serine 129 phosphorylation is somewhat equivocal in rodents, because expression of α-synuclein with alanine 129 is as toxic as aspartate 129 (Gorbatyuk et al, 2008; McFarland et al., 2009).

Although α-synuclein is decreased in the cerebrospinal fluid of PD patients (Mollenhauer et al, 2011), there is an increase in α-synuclein oligomers suggesting that α-synuclein aggregation and its leakage from neurons is accelerated in PD (Tokuda et al., 2010). However, the mechanistic contribution of α-synuclein to neuronal death in PD still remains unclear. Low nanomolar concentrations of α-synuclein are neuroprotective against the oxidative insults of hydrogen peroxide and 6-hydroxydopamine, whereas higher micromolar concentrations are toxic (Batelli et al., 2008). This suggests that α-synuclein may be neuroprotective and toxic at low and high levels, respectively, and is in accord with the pathogenic effects of SNCA duplication or triplication. α-Synuclein has also been shown to cause oxidative stress through direct damage to mitochondria. For example, mitochondrial import of α-synuclein mediated by a cryptic targeting signal can disrupt complex 1 activity (Devi et al., 2008), and α-synuclein over-expression in nematodes and mammalian cells induced fragmentation of mitochondria (Kamp et al., 2010; Nakamura et al., 2011). Co-expression of PINK1, parkin, and DJ-1 protect against mitochondrial fragmentation, consistent with the notion that these three proteins function in a common mitochondrial pathway leading to PD pathology. The convergence of α-synuclein to a mitochondrial role when expressed at sufficient levels could therefore be viewed as a pathogenic pathway that diverges from its normal physiological role in vesicle trafficking.

1.3 α-Synuclein outside of disease

A role in synaptic function is implicated from the observation that α-synuclein is highly concentrated in pre-synaptic terminals (Jakes et al., 1994; George et al., 1995) and that α-synuclein disperses reversibly from these presynaptic terminals in response to brief neural activity (Fortin et al., 2005). The dispersion is attenuated by tetanus toxin, which inactivates vesicle fusion but not the preceding ion fluxes, suggesting that α-synuclein solubility is directly linked to exocytosis. While these results do not suggest a presynaptic function for α-synuclein, other studies with α-synuclein knockout mice reveal increased nigrostriatal dopamine release induced by paired-pulse stimuli (Abeliovich et al., 2000), implicating α-synuclein as a negative regulator of a readily-releasable vesicle pool of dopamine. In contrast, another line of α-synuclein null mice showed normal response to single or paired stimuli, but deficits in response to trains of stimuli which rely on reserve vesicle recruitment and a reduction in the number distal vesicles (Cabin et al., 2002). To explore whether β-synuclein compensates for loss of α-synuclein, removal of both α- and β-synuclein decreased total brain dopamine by 20% as well as complexins and 14-3-3 proteins (Chandra et al., 2004). Complexins are a regulatory component of the SNARE (soluble N-ethylmaleimide-sensitive attachment protein receptor) complexes involved in synaptic vesicle fusion (Hu et al., 2002). However, the other previously described aberrations such as synaptic vesicle reduction, electrophysiological changes, and dopamine re-uptake were not observed in these α-synuclein knockout mice. Despite the differences, α-synuclein knockout mice display subtle alterations in vesicle storage and dynamics.

The converse experimental paradigm using over-expression of α-synuclein also suggests that it inhibits synaptic transmission in primary neurons and intact *ex vivo* brain (Nemani et al., 2010). Morphological and electrophysiological analyses indicate that the reduction was due to decreased readily-releasable synaptic vesicles, but not the overall number of synaptic vesicles, consistent with the notion that α-synuclein is a negative regulator of the synaptic vesicle mobilization.

Recent studies using biochemical approaches have reported that α-synuclein disrupts arachidonic acid-mediated stabilization of soluble N-ethylmaleimide sensitive fusion protein receptor (SNARE) complex (comprised of syntaxin-1, SNAP25, and synaptobrevin-2) that is essential for synaptic vesicle fusion (Darios et al., 2010). Although this study did not co-immunoprecipitate α-synuclein with members of the SNARE complex, thus suggesting an indirect interaction, others have reported α-synuclein binding with synaptobrevin-2 and proposed that this binding stabilizes the SNARE complex (Burre et al., 2010). Interestingly, loss of assembled SNARE complexes in mice deficient for cysteine-string protein alpha (CSPα) can be rescued by α-synuclein over-expression and worsened by its knockdown. The loss of all three synucleins (α-, β-, and γ-) causes premature death due to neurological symptoms, suggesting that β- and/or γ-synuclein perform redundant functions and compensate for α-synuclein deficiency in the single knockout animals. Thus, α-synuclein exerts a regulatory effect on SNARE complex formation, but its mechanism remains poorly defined.

Some studies have suggested that α-synuclein may regulate vesicle trafficking more broadly that just in synaptic transmission. Expression of α-synuclein in yeast and mammalian cells causes delays in ER-to-Golgi vesicle trafficking, an effect that was more striking with the A53T mutant (Cooper et al., 2006; Thayanidhi et al., 2010). These changes in ER-to-Golgi trafficking by α-synuclein may be caused by immobilizing vesicles in the cytoplasm (Soper et al., 2008). The mechanism appears to involve rab proteins, small GTPases that regulate vesicle trafficking, as the impairment is rescued by overexpressing certain rab proteins (Gitler et al., 2008). Furthermore, as yeast do not express α-synuclein endogenously, these studies suggest that α-synuclein can interact with both constitutive and Ca^{2+}-dependent vesicle trafficking machineries that is conserved between yeast and higher organisms.

2. α-Synuclein and membrane-binding

2.1 The structure of α-synuclein and how it contributes to membrane-binding

The structure of α-synuclein can be divided into three domains: an amino-terminal domain with seven imperfect KTKEGV repeats, a central domain essential for aggregation called the non-amyloidβ component (NAC), and a hydrophilic carboxyl-terminal tail (Clayton and George, 1998) (**Fig. 1.1A**). The amino-terminal repeats, which are similar to sequences found in apolipoproteins, form amphipathic helices with polar and non-polar residues aligned in opposing direction and allow α-synuclein to immerse partially into lipid membranes (**Fig. 1.1B**). The capacity of α-synuclein to bind freely to membranes has been demonstrated (Jo et al., 2000; Conway et al., 2000). The helical structure of α-synuclein upon binding to sodium dodecyl sulfate (SDS)-soluble micelles has been established using nuclear magnetic

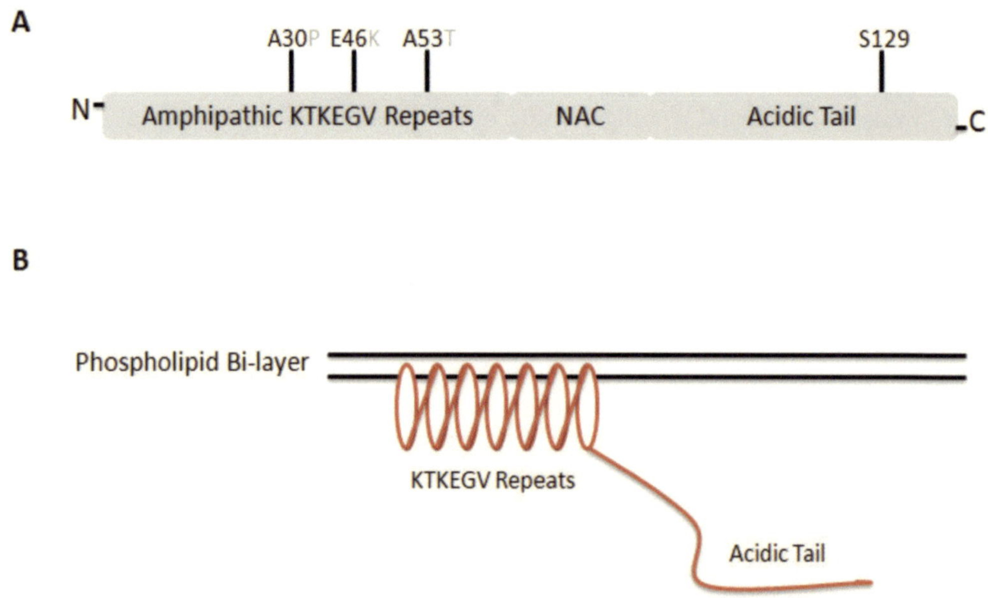

Fig. 1. The primary structure of human α-synuclein. (A) The structure itself can be divided into three unequal regions: the imperfect KTKEGV repeats believed to form a helical structure on phospholipid membranes, the non-Aβ component (NAC) seen in Alzheimer disease-associated plaques, and a non-membrane-associated acidic c-terminal tail. (B) Upon binding to membranes, α-synuclein assumes a helical conformation due to the amphipathic nature of the KTKEGV repeats. All three amino acid substitution sites associated with familial forms of PD (A30P, E46K, and A53T) can be found in the amphipathic repeat region. The serine 129 site commonly found to be phosphorylated in Lewy bodies can be found in the acidic tail. Note that the residue in position 53 is naturally a threonine instead of an alanine in many mammalian species, including rodents.

resonance and electron spin resonance studies (Jao et al., 2004; Ulmer et al., 2005; Borbat et al., 2006). The helical conformation is energetically favourable when compared to the unstructured conformation of cytosolic α-synuclein.

2.2 Implications of α-synuclein membrane-binding

Binding to and dissociation from the synaptic membrane may be linked to regulating the still-undefined function of α-synuclein. Using fluorescent imaging to visualize GFP-tagged α-synuclein, depolarization reversibly induced the redistribution of α-synuclein from synaptic boutons to the perisynaptic region (Fortin et al., 2005), consistent with the dissociation of α-synuclein from synaptic vesicles prior to exocytosis. This link between α-synuclein, its membrane binding, and exocytosis is consistent with other reports that α-synuclein regulates SNARE complex assembly (Darios et al., 2010; Burre et al, 2010).

The membrane-binding properties of α-synuclein may also have implications in PD pathogenesis. The addition of lipid vesicles causes a greater proportion of α-synuclein to assume an α-helical conformation and decreases the fibrillization of α-synuclein (Zhu et al., 2003); Jo et al., 2004), suggesting that increased membrane binding may be protective against Lewy body pathology. However, other studies adding phospholipids to α-synuclein induced fibril formation (Narayanan and Scarlata, 2001; Cole et al., 2002). Mutant A30P α-synuclein exhibits a lower propensity to bind to phospholipid membranes as determined in vitro (Jo et al., 2002), but forms oligomers faster than wild-type or A53T α-synuclein (Conway et al., 2000). Nevertheless, the A53T mutant α-synuclein forms fibrils (the likely precursor to Lewy bodies) at a higher rate. Furthermore, a rotenone model of PD revealed that lipids co-stained with α-synuclein aggregates (Lee et al., 2002), suggesting that lipids may enable Lewy body formation. Taken together, the evidence is conflicting on whether the membrane-bound or cytosolic α-synuclein is the precursor for aggregated α-synuclein and Lewy body pathology, although it remains possible that oligomerization and fibrillization could occur in distinct cellular compartments (Auluck et al., 2010).

2.3 Regulation of α-synuclein membrane-binding

While there remains some uncertainty as to whether the membrane-bound or cytosolic α-synuclein is more pathologically relevant, it is also important to understand the mechanisms regulating the exchange between these two pools. We have previously suggested that brain cytosolic factors are critical in facilitating α-synuclein dissociation and association from synaptic membranes (Wislet-Gendebien et al., 2006; 2008). The remainder of this chapter will be devoted to describing some of these cytosolic factors that were characterized using our cell-free assays.

3. Key techniques for examining the regulation of membrane-binding

3.1 Fractionation into membrane-bound and cytosolic proteins

Much of our current understanding of α-synuclein conformation and membrane interactions are based on studies with recombinant α-synuclein purified from bacteria and bound to artificial membranes. This approach has yielded a wealth of information on the biophysical characteristics of normal and mutant α-synuclein and their affinity for specific lipids. However, recombinant α-synuclein and artificial membranes provide no basis for the understanding α-synuclein behaviour *in vivo*, in particular its ability to exchange between membrane and cytosol within neurons, where the compartmentalization of α-synuclein is modulated by intracellular components and neuronal activity.

To understand endogenous intracellular regulation of α-synuclein dynamics, reconstitution of its membrane binding and dissociation can be studied using semi-intact or cell-free assays. For example, the use of hypotonic lysis to disrupt neuronal plasma membrane releases freely-diffusible cytoplasmic components and permits measurement of subtle shifts in α-synuclein membrane-binding (Fig. 2). Experiments of this type are best done with endogenously expressed α-synuclein, although where exogenous expression is required, consideration should be given to the extent of α-synuclein overexpression so as not to saturate the membrane compartment and cause artifactually low membrane-bound to cytosolic ratio of α-synuclein, as excess α-synuclein will accumulate in cytosol. Measurement of α-synuclein dynamics in intact cells may be limited by an inability to assess whether changes in membrane-bound and cytosolic α-synuclein are caused by perturbations in α-synuclein dissociation or binding kinetics. This can be overcome by using cell-free assays (such as those described below) that monitor the unidirectional movement of α-synuclein from a "donor" fraction expressing α-synuclein to an "acceptor" fraction derived from an α-synuclein-deficient mouse or cells.

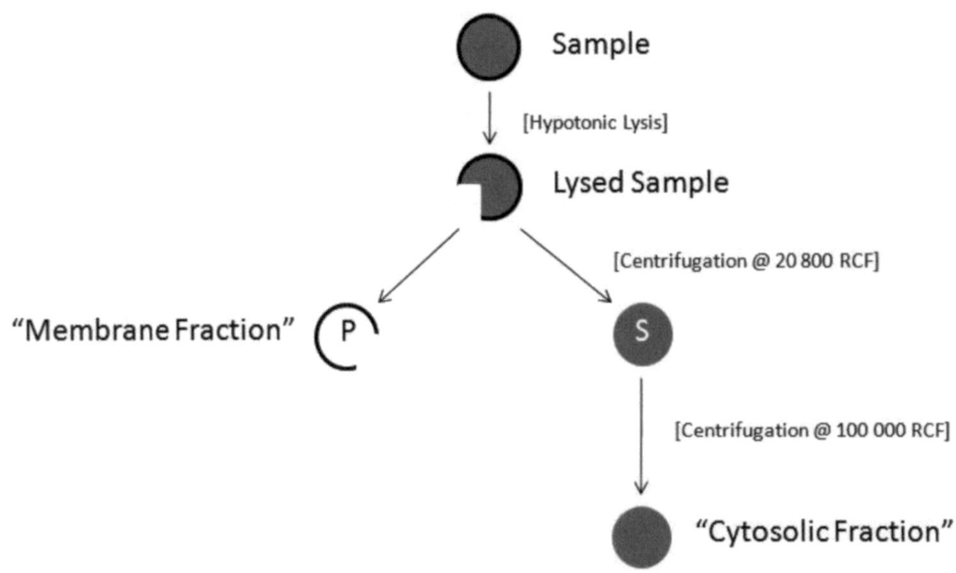

Fig. 2. A schematic overview of fractionation. Synaptosomes or cells were hypotonically lysed in either distilled water or a hypotonic buffer. The lysates were centrifuged and the supernatant (S) and pellet (P) fractions were processed separately. S fractions were centrifuged again to remove residual synaptic vesicles and supernatants were kept as cytosolic fractions. The P fractions were resuspended in buffer containing 1% CHAPS or 1% Triton X-100. Lysates were centrifuged and the supernatants were kept as membrane fraction.

3.2 α-Synuclein dissociation and binding assays

While analyzing the ratio of membrane-bound to cytosolic α-synuclein can yield useful data in an *in-vivo* or *ex-vivo* setting, it does not provide information on whether effects are taking place in the membrane-dissociation or membrane-binding step of α-synuclein dynamics. This question can be answered by employing cell-free assays we have previously published

(Wislet-Gendebien et al., 2006). To measure α-synuclein dissociation, synaptosomal membranes from either non-transgenic or α-synuclein transgenic mice are incubated with brain cytosol isolated from α-synuclein deficient mice. By measuring the amount of α-synuclein dissociated from the membrane and into the cytosol under different conditions, it is possible to determine whether specific cellular factors affect α-synuclein membrane-dissociation.

A converse protocol was developed to assess α-synuclein binding to synaptic membrane (Wislet-Gendebien et al., 2008). In this assay, α-synuclein can be prepared from 2 different origins: either 1) purified *E.coli*-expressed α-synuclein mixed with cytosol from α-synuclein deficient mouse brains, or 2) cytosol prepared from transgenic mice overexpressing the human form of wild-type or mutant α-synuclein. Either of the two sources of α-synuclein is then combined with synaptic membrane prepared from α-synuclein deficient mouse synaptosomes. Membrane-bound α-synuclein can then be analyzed as a measure of α-synuclein membrane-binding in response to various controlled factors such as pharmacological agents or lipids. This assay can provide information on whether a certain condition or factor is affecting α-synuclein membrane-binding.

The key benefit of these dissociation and binding assays is the ability to probe the intracellular milieu with specific reagents, such as antibodies, recombinant mutants, or peptide domains, which are membrane impermeant. However, because these assays depends on mixing separately-derived membrane and cytosolic fractions, one of which must be α-synuclein-deficient, there is an inherent limitation to assess the dissociation or binding of other synaptic proteins due to their presence in both the membrane and the cytosol of both assays. However, these assays can be adapted to analyze the dissociation and binding of other synaptic proteins provided that transgenic animals deficient in the protein of interest are available.

4. Factors involved in regulating α-synuclein membrane-binding

4.1 Brain cytosol

The α-synuclein dissociation assay revealed that stably membrane-bound α-synuclein can be recruited into the cytosol in the presence of brain cytosolic proteins (Wislet-Gendebien et al., 2006). Pre-digestion with trypsin or preheating at 95 °C of the cytosol eliminated its ability to induce α-synuclein dissociation, directly implicating a role for specific cytosolic proteins in controlling α-synuclein solubility. Moreover, the permissive factors required to mediate α-synuclein dissociation from the membrane appeared to be enriched in brain cytosol, as a 6-fold greater concentration of liver cytosol was required to achieve equivalent α-synuclein dissociation using brain cytosol. The proteins triggering α-synuclein dissociation were in limited quantity in cytosol and were not regenerated under our assay conditions. A single exposure to synaptosomal membranes was sufficient to deplete the capacity of the cytosol to extract membrane α-synuclein so that subsequent incubations with fresh membranes yielded no additional dissociated α-synuclein. In contrast, presynaptic membranes retained ample extractable α-synuclein, which could be dissociated with subsequent applications of fresh cytosol. We also showed that the cytosolic activity that mediated α-synuclein dissociation clearly distinguished between wild-type α-synuclein and PD-associated mutants. The cytosol-dependent off-rate for both A30P and A53T α-synuclein mutant was double that of the wild-type, but had no effect on cytosol-independent dissociation.

4.2 Cytosolic lipids

Using our α-synuclein binding assay, we observed that cytosol-mediated α-synuclein membrane-binding was heat stable and protease insensitive. Further characterization revealed that ATP and lipids are two of the main cytosolic components that modulate α-synuclein binding to synaptic membranes (Wislet-Gendebien et al., 2008). We proposed that endogenous cytosolic lipids transferred to membranes prior to α-synuclein recruitment or bound directly to cytosolic α-synuclein may aid α-synuclein folding at the lipid-cytoplasm interface so that it is more amenable to binding directly to synaptic membranes. To provide further insight into this novel protein-lipid-protein interaction, we profiled glycerophosphocholines bound to proteins in α-synuclein-deficient cytosol by nanoflow LC-ESI-MS and precursor ion scan. Our analysis identified 24 species that can potentially affect α-synuclein membrane interactions, including platelet activating factor, which was able to reconstitute the activity of delipidated cytosol.

4.3 Rab3a

Interestingly, our binding experiments also revealed that the association of α-synuclein to synaptic membranes could be stabilized by brief formaldehyde-induced cross-linking, which generates very short intermolecular covalent bonds. This suggested that α-synuclein binding is partly dependent on one or more synaptic vesicle proteins for recruitment. There are several candidate vesicular proteins that have been proposed to interact with α-synuclein, including cysteine string protein, rab3a, and synaptobrevin-2 (Chandra et al., 2005; Gitler et al., 2008; Burre et al., 2010). As a potential test to identify the α-synuclein receptive component on synaptic vesicles, when we screened the ability of antibodies against synaptic vesicle proteins to inhibit α-synuclein membrane binding, rab3a antibodies effectively reduced α-synuclein membrane binding. Moreover, exposure of membranes to rab3a antibody prior to incubation with α-synuclein was sufficient, whereas treatment of α-synuclein-containing cytosol with the antibody has no effect, suggesting that α-synuclein binding is facilitated by vesicle bound rab3a (Chen and Tandon, unpublished).

Similarities in localization and membrane-binding have previously suggested an interaction between rab3a and α-synuclein, at least under pathological conditions. Immunoprecipitation studies revealed α-synuclein interaction with rabphilin in brains from individuals with diffuse Lewy body disease and multiple system atrophy (Dalfo et al., 2004a; 2005). In addition, A30P α-synuclein in transgenic mouse brain was found to co-elute with rab3a, rab5, and rab8, suggesting that α-synuclein may interact with a broad range of rab proteins (Dalfo et al., 2004b). From a functional perspective, α-synuclein appears to antagonize rab3a function. For example, over-expression of α-synuclein in yeast interfered with ER-to-Golgi vesicle trafficking that was corrected by the simultaneous over-expression of the yeast homologue of rab1 (Cooper et al., 2006; Soper et al., 2008). Similarly, elevated toxicity in nematodes and rat primary neurons engineered to express wild-type or A53T α-synuclein was rescued by the addition of rab8 or rab3a (Gitler et al., 2008). In all these studies, α-synuclein toxicity was corrected by over-expressing rab proteins, suggesting that the over-expression of α-synuclein disrupted rab-mediated vesicle targeting and docking.

Rab3a is a small GTPase that regulates synaptic vesicle targeting, docking, and fusion, and like other members of the rab family, it's cycling between vesicles and cytosol is regulated by the phosphorylation state of its guanine nucleotide (GTP/GDP). Dissociation of rab3a from synaptic vesicles is coupled to the calcium-influx that initiates exocytosis (Fischer von

Mollard et al., 1991). The molecular machinery that mediates rab3a cycling has been extensively characterized. After GTP cleavage, rab3a is retrieved off vesicles by guanine-nucleotide dissociation inhibitor (GDI) complex that includes Hsp90, such that the Hsp90 inhibitors radicicol and geldanamycin prevent rab3a dissociation from synaptic membranes (Sakisaka et al., 2002). Using our α-synuclein dissociation assay, we found that the Hsp90 inhibitors also caused an accumulation of α-synuclein on synaptic membranes, providing support for argument that α-synuclein membrane association is closely linked to that of rab3a and is regulated by the GDI/Hsp90 chaperone complex (Chen and Tandon, unpublished). In accordance with this, expression of a constitutively GTP-bound, dominant-negative rab3a mutant also induced an increase in membrane-bound α-synuclein suggesting that GTP/GDP conversion by rab3a is a precondition for the liberation of vesicular α-synuclein. Together, our results suggest that rab3a and its recycling machinery regulate α-synuclein membrane-binding and dissociation (Fig. 3).

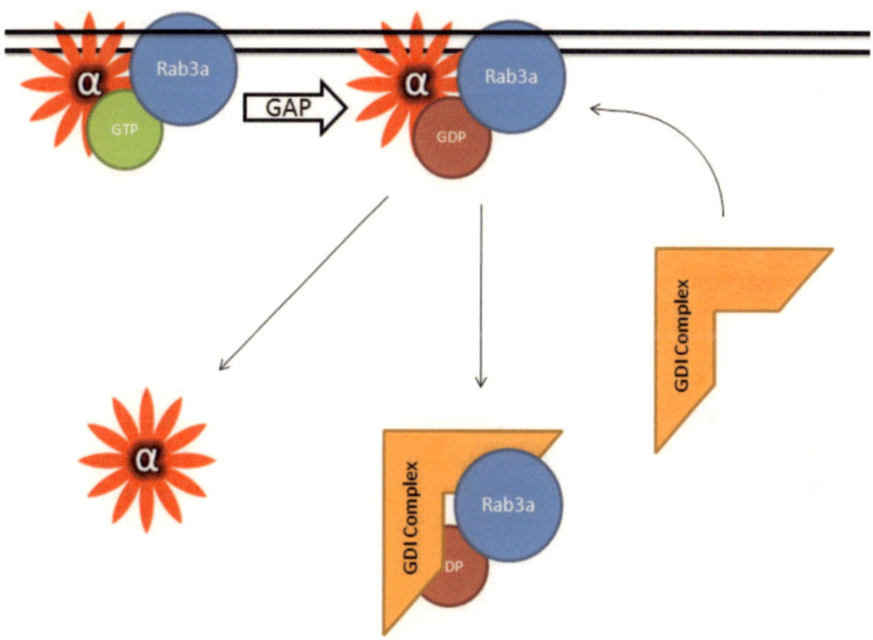

Fig. 3. A model whereby rab3a regulates dissociation of α-synuclein from synaptic membranes. GTP-bound rab3a binds to α-synuclein on the membrane. After GTP-hydrolysis mediated by a GTPase activating protein (GAP), rab3a is chaperoned off of the membrane by the GDP-dissociation inhibitor complex (GDI complex) and α-synuclein also dissociates from the membrane. Whether α-synuclein dissociation is transiently mediated by the GDI complex or is because of the loss of membrane-bound rab3a is yet to be determined.

Whether these results have any implications on the etiology of synucleinopathies is unclear and there are no rab3a mutations linked to PD. However, the interaction with rab3a reinforces α-synuclein's close relationship with the machinery controlling synaptic vesicle trafficking. Further research is needed on how α-synuclein fits into the broader picture of the exocytic pathway and how subtle changes to α-synuclein disposition may disturb vesicle dynamics and lead to pathology.

5. Conclusion

There is now ample evidence that α-synuclein is involved in the regulation of synaptic vesicle trafficking and, more recently, in mitochondrial fission/fusion machinery. Whether its role in maintaining these different organelles occurs concurrently in healthy neurons is not known, though it may be instructive to consider the levels of expression required for apparent modulation of vesicle mobilization or mitochondrial dynamics. The effects of α-synuclein on mitochondrial morphology have been noted in only two studies thus far, both requiring transient overexpression and not in models of normal or stable α-synuclein expression (Kamp et al., 2010; Nakamura et al., 2011). If this observation holds in future analyses, it may represent a segregation of α-synuclein activity based on its expression level, whereby lower levels of α-synuclein impart direct effects on synaptic vesicle behaviour and high α-synuclein concentration disrupts normal mitochondrial division and turnover. This dual activity may also explain the biphasic nature of α-synuclein toxicity, being beneficial at lower expression levels and increasing in toxicity at higher concentration, particularly in combination with oxidative stress. Moreover, a gain-of-function pathogenic link between α-synuclein and mitochondria fits well into a biological cascade that is opposed by expression of PINK1, parkin, or DJ-1, which are now recognized as controlling mitochondrial fission/fusion and mitophagy.

It is clear that direct interaction of α-synuclein with lipid membranes is necessary to propagate its biological function. Regardless of the organelle interaction, it is reasonable to assume that the binding α-synuclein to various organelle membranes is likely to involve a common mechanism whereby the amino-terminal half of α-synuclein folds into an amphipathic α-helix for partial immersion into the lipid bilayer. However, additional selective molecular requirements for stable α-synuclein binding and retrieval may vary between different organelles, such as vesicles or mitochondria, each regulated by organelle-specific factors present on the membrane or in the cytosol. One potential means to characterize α-synuclein compartmentalization on discrete organelles is by further refining the cell-free binding and dissociation assays, as described above using hypotonically permeabilized mouse brain synaptosomes, to specific organelles that are first isolated by differential density and centrifugation protocols. Alternatively, detection of organelle-specific interactors could be done by using inhibitory antibodies to screen for candidates known to exist only on defined organelles, as we have done to identify rab3a as an α-synuclein binding partner on synaptic vesicles. Finally, these cell-free assays also offer an approach to validate the functional effects of α-synuclein interactions identified by various genetic or biochemical methodologies by characterizing their consequences on α-synuclein membrane distribution.

6. Acknowledgements

This work was supported by operating grants to AT from the Canadian Institutes for Health Research and from the Parkinson Society of Canada.

7. References

Abeliovich, A., Schmitz, Y., Farinas, I., Choi-Lundberg, D., Ho, W. H., Castillo, P. E., Shinsky, N., Verdugo, J. M., Armanini, M., Ryan, A., Hynes, M., Phillips, H., Sulzer,

D., and Rosenthal, A. (2000). Mice lacking alpha-synuclein display functional deficits in the nigrostriatal dopamine system. *Neuron* 25(1), 239-52.

Auluck, P. K., Caraveo, G., and Lindquist, S. (2010). alpha-Synuclein: membrane interactions and toxicity in Parkinson's disease. *Annu Rev Cell Dev Biol* 26, 211-33.

Batelli, S., Albani, D., Rametta, R., Polito, L., Prato, F., Pesaresi, M., Negro, A., and Forloni, G. (2008). DJ-1 modulates alpha-synuclein aggregation state in a cellular model of oxidative stress: relevance for Parkinson's disease and involvement of HSP70. *PLoS ONE* 3(4), e1884.

Borbat, P., Ramlall, T. F., Freed, J. H., and Eliezer, D. (2006). Inter-helix distances in lysophospholipid micelle-bound alpha-synuclein from pulsed ESR measurements. *J Am Chem Soc* 128(31), 10004-5.

Braak, H., Del Tredici, K., Rub, U., de Vos, R. A., Jansen Steur, E. N., and Braak, E. (2003). Staging of brain pathology related to sporadic Parkinson's disease. *Neurobiol Aging* 24(2), 197-211.

Burre, J., Sharma, M., Tsetsenis, T., Buchman, V., Etherton, M., and Sudhof, T. C. (2010). {alpha}-Synuclein Promotes SNARE-Complex Assembly in Vivo and in Vitro. *Science*.

Cabin, D. E., Shimazu, K., Murphy, D., Cole, N. B., Gottschalk, W., McIlwain, K. L., Orrison, B., Chen, A., Ellis, C. E., Paylor, R., Lu, B., and Nussbaum, R. L. (2002). Synaptic vesicle depletion correlates with attenuated synaptic responses to prolonged repetitive stimulation in mice lacking alpha-synuclein. *J Neurosci* 22(20), 8797-807.

Chandra, S., Chen, X., Rizo, J., Jahn, R., and Sudhof, T. C. (2003). A broken alpha -helix in folded alpha -Synuclein. *J Biol Chem* 278(17), 15313-8.

Chandra, S., Fornai, F., Kwon, H. B., Yazdani, U., Atasoy, D., Liu, X., Hammer, R. E., Battaglia, G., German, D. C., Castillo, P. E., and Sudhof, T. C. (2004). Double-knockout mice for alpha- and beta-synucleins: effect on synaptic functions. *Proc Natl Acad Sci U S A* 101(41), 14966-71.

Chandra S, Gallardo G, Fernandez-Chacon R, Schluter OM, Sudhof TC (2005) Alpha-synuclein cooperates with CSP alpha in preventing neurodegeneration. Cell, 123:383-396.

Chartier-Harlin, M. C., Kachergus, J., Roumier, C., Mouroux, V., Douay, X., Lincoln, S., Levecque, C., Larvor, L., Andrieux, J., Hulihan, M., Waucquier, N., Defebvre, L., Amouyel, P., Farrer, M., and Destee, A. (2004). Alpha-synuclein locus duplication as a cause of familial Parkinson's disease. *Lancet* 364(9440), 1167-9.

Chen, C. Y., and Balch, W. E. (2006). The Hsp90 chaperone complex regulates GDI-dependent Rab recycling. *Mol Biol Cell* 17(8), 3494-507.

Chen, C. Y., Sakisaka, T., and Balch, W. E. (2005). Use of Hsp90 inhibitors to disrupt GDI-dependent Rab recycling. *Methods Enzymol* 403, 339-47.

Chen, L., and Feany, M. B. (2005). Alpha-synuclein phosphorylation controls neurotoxicity and inclusion formation in a Drosophila model of Parkinson disease. *Nat Neurosci* 8(5), 657-63.

Christine, C. W., and Aminoff, M. J. (2004). Clinical differentiation of parkinsonian syndromes: prognostic and therapeutic relevance. *Am J Med* 117(6), 412-9.

Clayton, D. F., and George, J. M. (1998). The synucleins: a family of proteins involved in synaptic function, plasticity, neurodegeneration and disease. *Trends Neurosci* 21(6), 249-54.

Cole, N. B., Murphy, D. D., Grider, T., Rueter, S., Brasaemle, D., and Nussbaum, R. L. (2002). Lipid droplet binding and oligomerization properties of the Parkinson's disease protein alpha-synuclein. *J Biol Chem* 277(8), 6344-52.

Conway, K. A., Lee, S. J., Rochet, J. C., Ding, T. T., Williamson, R. E., and Lansbury, P. T., Jr. (2000). Acceleration of oligomerization, not fibrillization, is a shared property of both alpha-synuclein mutations linked to early-onset Parkinson's disease: implications for pathogenesis and therapy. *Proc Natl Acad Sci U S A* 97(2), 571-6.

Cookson, M. R. (2005). The biochemistry of Parkinson's disease. *Annu Rev Biochem* 74, 29-52.

Cooper, A. A., Gitler, A. D., Cashikar, A., Haynes, C. M., Hill, K. J., Bhullar, B., Liu, K., Xu, K., Strathearn, K. E., Liu, F., Cao, S., Caldwell, K. A., Caldwell, G. A., Marsischky, G., Kolodner, R. D., Labaer, J., Rochet, J. C., Bonini, N. M., and Lindquist, S. (2006). Alpha-synuclein blocks ER-Golgi traffic and Rab1 rescues neuron loss in Parkinson's models. *Science* 313(5785), 324-8.

Dalfo, E., Barrachina, M., Rosa, J. L., Ambrosio, S., and Ferrer, I. (2004a). Abnormal alpha-synuclein interactions with rab3a and rabphilin in diffuse Lewy body disease. *Neurobiol Dis* 16(1), 92-7.

Dalfo, E., and Ferrer, I. (2005). Alpha-synuclein binding to rab3a in multiple system atrophy. *Neurosci Lett* 380(1-2), 170-5.

Dalfo, E., Gomez-Isla, T., Rosa, J. L., Nieto Bodelon, M., Cuadrado Tejedor, M., Barrachina, M., Ambrosio, S., and Ferrer, I. (2004b). Abnormal alpha-synuclein interactions with Rab proteins in alpha-synuclein A30P transgenic mice. *J Neuropathol Exp Neurol* 63(4), 302-13.

Darios, F., Ruiperez, V., Lopez, I., Villanueva, J., Gutierrez, L. M., and Davletov, B. (2010). Alpha-synuclein sequesters arachidonic acid to modulate SNARE-mediated exocytosis. *EMBO Rep* 11(7), 528-33.

Davidson, W. S., Jonas, A., Clayton, D. F., and George, J. M. (1998). Stabilization of alpha-synuclein secondary structure upon binding to synthetic membranes. *J Biol Chem* 273(16), 9443-9.

Devi, L., Raghavendran, V., Prabhu, B. M., Avadhani, N. G., and Anandatheerthavarada, H. K. (2008). Mitochondrial import and accumulation of alpha-synuclein impair complex I in human dopaminergic neuronal cultures and Parkinson disease brain. *J Biol Chem* 283(14), 9089-100.

Fischer von Mollard, G., Sudhof, T. C., and Jahn, R. (1991). A small GTP-binding protein dissociates from synaptic vesicles during exocytosis. *Nature* 349(6304), 79-81.

Fortin, D. L., Nemani, V. M., Voglmaier, S. M., Anthony, M. D., Ryan, T. A., and Edwards, R. H. (2005). Neural activity controls the synaptic accumulation of alpha-synuclein. *J Neurosci* 25(47), 10913-21.

Fujiwara, H., Hasegawa, M., Dohmae, N., Kawashima, A., Masliah, E., Goldberg, M. S., Shen, J., Takio, K., and Iwatsubo, T. (2002). alpha-Synuclein is phosphorylated in synucleinopathy lesions. *Nat Cell Biol* 4(2), 160-4.

George, J. M., Jin, H., Woods, W. S., and Clayton, D. F. (1995). Characterization of a novel protein regulated during the critical period for song learning in the zebra finch. *Neuron* 15(2), 361-72.

Georgieva, E. R., Ramlall, T. F., Borbat, P. P., Freed, J. H., and Eliezer, D. (2010). The lipid-binding domain of wild type and mutant alpha-synuclein: compactness and interconversion between the broken and extended helix forms. *J Biol Chem* 285(36), 28261-74.

Geppert, M., Bolshakov, V. Y., Siegelbaum, S. A., Takei, K., De Camilli, P., Hammer, R. E., and Sudhof, T. C. (1994). The role of Rab3A in neurotransmitter release. *Nature* 369(6480), 493-7.

Geppert, M., Goda, Y., Stevens, C. F., and Sudhof, T. C. (1997). The small GTP-binding protein Rab3A regulates a late step in synaptic vesicle fusion. *Nature* 387(6635), 810-4.

Gitler, A. D., Bevis, B. J., Shorter, J., Strathearn, K. E., Hamamichi, S., Su, L. J., Caldwell, K. A., Caldwell, G. A., Rochet, J. C., McCaffery, J. M., Barlowe, C., and Lindquist, S. (2008). The Parkinson's disease protein alpha-synuclein disrupts cellular Rab homeostasis. *Proc Natl Acad Sci U S A* 105(1), 145-50.

Gorbatyuk, O. S., Li, S., Sullivan, L. F., Chen, W., Kondrikova, G., Manfredsson, F. P., Mandel, R. J., and Muzyczka, N. (2008). The phosphorylation state of Ser-129 in human alpha-synuclein determines neurodegeneration in a rat model of Parkinson disease. *Proc Natl Acad Sci U S A* 105(2), 763-8.

Hamilton, B. A. (2004). alpha-Synuclein A53T substitution associated with Parkinson disease also marks the divergence of Old World and New World primates. *Genomics* 83(4), 739-42.

Hashimoto, M., Hsu, L. J., Rockenstein, E., Takenouchi, T., Mallory, M., and Masliah, E. (2002). alpha-Synuclein protects against oxidative stress via inactivation of the c-Jun N-terminal kinase stress-signaling pathway in neuronal cells. *J Biol Chem* 277(13), 11465-72.

Holdorff, B. (2006). Fritz Heinrich Lewy (1885-1950). *J Neurol* 253(5), 677-8.

Hu, K., Carroll, J., Rickman, C., and Davletov, B. (2002). Action of complexin on SNARE complex. *J Biol Chem* 277(44), 41652-6.

Jakes, R., Spillantini, M. G., and Goedert, M. (1994). Identification of two distinct synucleins from human brain. *FEBS Lett* 345(1), 27-32.

Jao, C. C., Der-Sarkissian, A., Chen, J., and Langen, R. (2004). Structure of membrane-bound alpha-synuclein studied by site-directed spin labeling. *Proc Natl Acad Sci U S A* 101(22), 8331-6.

Jankovic, J. (2008). Parkinson's disease: clinical features and diagnosis. *J Neurol Neurosurg Psychiatry* 79(4), 368-76.

Jo, E., McLaurin, J., Yip, C. M., St George-Hyslop, P., and Fraser, P. E. (2000). alpha-Synuclein membrane interactions and lipid specificity. *J Biol Chem* 275(44), 34328-34.

Jo, E., Fuller, N., Rand, R. P., St George-Hyslop, P., and Fraser, P. E. (2002). Defective membrane interactions of familial Parkinson's disease mutant A30P alpha-synuclein. *J Mol Biol* 315(4), 799-807.

Jo, E., Darabie, A. A., Han, K., Tandon, A., Fraser, P. E., and McLaurin, J. (2004). alpha-Synuclein-synaptosomal membrane interactions: implications for fibrillogenesis. *Eur J Biochem* 271(15), 3180-9.

Johannes, L., Doussau, F., Clabecq, A., Henry, J. P., Darchen, F., and Poulain, B. (1996). Evidence for a functional link between Rab3 and the SNARE complex. *J Cell Sci* 109 (Pt 12), 2875-84.

Johannes, L., Lledo, P. M., Roa, M., Vincent, J. D., Henry, J. P., and Darchen, F. (1994). The GTPase Rab3a negatively controls calcium-dependent exocytosis in neuroendocrine cells. *Embo J* 13(9), 2029-37.

Kamp, F., Exner, N., Lutz, A. K., Wender, N., Hegermann, J., Brunner, B., Nuscher, B., Bartels, T., Giese, A., Beyer, K., Eimer, S., Winklhofer, K. F., and Haass, C. (2010). Inhibition of mitochondrial fusion by alpha-synuclein is rescued by PINK1, Parkin and DJ-1. *Embo J* 29(20), 3571-89.

Kanda, S., Bishop, J. F., Eglitis, M. A., Yang, Y., and Mouradian, M. M. (2000). Enhanced vulnerability to oxidative stress by alpha-synuclein mutations and C-terminal truncation. *Neuroscience* 97(2), 279-84.

Kruger, R., Kuhn, W., Muller, T., Woitalla, D., Graeber, M., Kosel, S., Przuntek, H., Epplen, J. T., Schols, L., and Riess, O. (1998). Ala30Pro mutation in the gene encoding alpha-synuclein in Parkinson's disease. *Nat Genet* 18(2), 106-8.

Lee, H. J., Choi, C., and Lee, S. J. (2002). Membrane-bound alpha-synuclein has a high aggregation propensity and the ability to seed the aggregation of the cytosolic form. *J Biol Chem* 277(1), 671-8.

Leenders, A. G., Lopes da Silva, F. H., Ghijsen, W. E., and Verhage, M. (2001). Rab3a is involved in transport of synaptic vesicles to the active zone in mouse brain nerve terminals. *Mol Biol Cell* 12(10), 3095-102.

Maroteaux L, Campanelli JT, Scheller RH (1988). Synuclein: a neuron-specific protein localized to the nucleus and presynaptic nerve terminal. *J Neurosci* 8, 2804-2815.

McFarland, N. R., Fan, Z., Xu, K., Schwarzschild, M. A., Feany, M. B., Hyman, B. T., and McLean, P. J. (2009). Alpha-synuclein S129 phosphorylation mutants do not alter nigrostriatal toxicity in a rat model of Parkinson disease. *J Neuropathol Exp Neurol* 68(5), 515-24.

Mollenhauer, B., Locascio, J. J., Schulz-Schaeffer, W., Sixel-Doring, F., Trenkwalder, C., and Schlossmacher, M. G. (2011). alpha-Synuclein and tau concentrations in cerebrospinal fluid of patients presenting with parkinsonism: a cohort study. *Lancet Neurol* 10(3), 230-40.

Nakamura, K., Nemani, V. M., Azarbal, F., Skibinski, G., Levy, J. M., Egami, K., Munishkina, L., Zhang, J., Gardner, B., Wakabayashi, J., Sesaki, H., Cheng, Y., Finkbeiner, S., Nussbaum, R. L., Masliah, E., and Edwards, R. H. (2011). Direct membrane association drives mitochondrial fission by the Parkinson Disease-associated protein {alpha}-synuclein. *J Biol Chem* (Epub ahead of print).

Narayanan, V., and Scarlata, S. (2001). Membrane binding and self-association of alpha-synucleins. *Biochemistry* 40(33), 9927-34.

Nemani, V. M., Lu, W., Berge, V., Nakamura, K., Onoa, B., Lee, M. K., Chaudhry, F. A., Nicoll, R. A., and Edwards, R. H. (2010). Increased expression of alpha-synuclein reduces neurotransmitter release by inhibiting synaptic vesicle reclustering after endocytosis. *Neuron* 65(1), 66-79.

Polymeropoulos, M. H., Lavedan, C., Leroy, E., Ide, S. E., Dehejia, A., Dutra, A., Pike, B., Root, H., Rubenstein, J., Boyer, R., Stenroos, E. S., Chandrasekharappa, S., Athanassiadou, A., Papapetropoulos, T., Johnson, W. G., Lazzarini, A. M., Duvoisin, R. C., Di Iorio, G., Golbe, L. I., and Nussbaum, R. L. (1997). Mutation in the alpha-synuclein gene identified in families with Parkinson's disease. *Science* 276(5321), 2045-7.

Sakisaka, T., Meerlo, T., Matteson, J., Plutner, H., and Balch, W. E. (2002). Rab-alphaGDI activity is regulated by a Hsp90 chaperone complex. *Embo J* 21(22), 6125-35.

Saper, C. B. (1999). 'Like a thief in the night': the selectivity of degeneration in Parkinson's disease. *Brain* 122 (Pt 8), 1401-2.

Singleton, A. B., Farrer, M., Johnson, J., Singleton, A., Hague, S., Kachergus, J., Hulihan, M., Peuralinna, T., Dutra, A., Nussbaum, R., Lincoln, S., Crawley, A., Hanson, M., Maraganore, D., Adler, C., Cookson, M. R., Muenter, M., Baptista, M., Miller, D., Blancato, J., Hardy, J., and Gwinn-Hardy, K. (2003). alpha-Synuclein locus triplication causes Parkinson's disease. *Science* 302(5646), 841.

Soper, J. H., Roy, S., Stieber, A., Lee, E., Wilson, R. B., Trojanowski, J. Q., Burd, C. G., and Lee, V. M. (2008). Alpha-synuclein-induced aggregation of cytoplasmic vesicles in Saccharomyces cerevisiae. *Mol Biol Cell* 19(3), 1093-103.

Spillantini, M. G., Crowther, R. A., Jakes, R., Hasegawa, M., and Goedert, M. (1998). alpha-Synuclein in filamentous inclusions of Lewy bodies from Parkinson's disease and dementia with lewy bodies. *Proc Natl Acad Sci U S A* 95(11), 6469-73.

Thayanidhi, N., Helm, J. R., Nycz, D. C., Bentley, M., Liang, Y., and Hay, J. C. (2010). Alpha-synuclein delays endoplasmic reticulum (ER)-to-Golgi transport in mammalian cells by antagonizing ER/Golgi SNAREs. *Mol Biol Cell* 21(11), 1850-63.

Ulmer, T. S., Bax, A., Cole, N. B., and Nussbaum, R. L. (2005). Structure and dynamics of micelle-bound human alpha-synuclein. *J Biol Chem* 280(10), 9595-603.

Wislet-Gendebien, S., D'Souza, C., Kawarai, T., St George-Hyslop, P., Westaway, D., Fraser, P., and Tandon, A. (2006). Cytosolic proteins regulate alpha-synuclein dissociation from presynaptic membranes. *J Biol Chem* 281(43), 32148-55.

Wislet-Gendebien, S., Visanji, N. P., Whitehead, S. N., Marsilio, D., Hou, W., Figeys, D., Fraser, P. E., Bennett, S. A., and Tandon, A. (2008). Differential regulation of wild-type and mutant alpha-synuclein binding to synaptic membranes by cytosolic factors. *BMC Neurosci* 9, 92.

Zarranz, J. J., Alegre, J., Gomez-Esteban, J. C., Lezcano, E., Ros, R., Ampuero, I., Vidal, L., Hoenicka, J., Rodriguez, O., Atares, B., Llorens, V., Gomez Tortosa, E., del Ser, T., Munoz, D. G., and de Yebenes, J. G. (2004). The new mutation, E46K, of alpha-synuclein causes Parkinson and Lewy body dementia. *Ann Neurol* 55(2), 164-73.

Zhu, M., and Fink, A. L. (2003). Lipid binding inhibits alpha-synuclein fibril formation. *J Biol Chem* 278(19), 16873-7.

9

Role of FKBPs in Parkinson's Disease

Souvik Chattopadhaya, Amaravadhi Harikishore and Ho Sup Yoon
School of Biological Sciences, Nanyang Technological University
Singapore

1. Introduction

Parkinson's disease (PD) is the second most common neurodegenerative disease among the elderly. While sporadic PD constitutes 99% of the cases, the remaining 1% is of genetic origin. The neuropathological hallmarks of PD are progressive degeneration of dopaminergic (DA) neurons and presence of Lewy neurites and Lewy bodies (LBs) - intracytoplasmic proteinaceous inclusions that contain α-synuclein (SYN), synphilin-1, components of the ubiquitin proteasomal pathway and parkin (Dawson, 2006). The loss of DA neurons in substantia nigra pars compacta (SNpc) results in decreased signalling in the striatum thereby giving rise to motor defects like resting tremor, bradykinesia, rigidity and posture instability. Besides DA neuronal loss, microglial activation and increased astroglial and lymphocyte infiltration also occur in PD. A role for inflammation in PD has been inferred from the identification of human leukocyte antigen (HLA)-DR positive reactive microglia in the brains of PD patients (McGeer *et al.*, 1988). Additionally, levels of pro-inflammatory cytokines like IL-6, IL-1β, TNFα have been found to be elevated in the blood and cerebrospinal fluid (CSF) of PD patients (Nagatsu & Sawada, 2005; Dawson, 2006) Although these inflammatory components might serve as useful biomarkers, the aetiology of striatal DA degeneration still remains enigmatic.

In the last decade, identification of mutations in several distinct genes (*LRRK2, parkin, PINK1, DJ-1, α-synuclein, MAPT, UCHL1* etc) linked to different forms of familial Parkinsonism has imparted a new direction to understanding PD pathogenesis (Tong & Shen, 2009). The question as to how seemingly divergent genes cause PD still remains unanswered, as there is no common molecular pathway involving these gene products. While parkin, α-synuclein (SYN) and ubiquitin C-terminal hydrolase L1 (UCHL1) are functionally associated with the cellular ubiquitin proteasomal system (UPS), DJ-1 and PINK1 protect against oxidative stress and mitochondrial dysfunction. More recently, microarray analysis of SNpc from parkinsonian brain (Mandel *et al.*, 2005) has shown that 68 genes related to protein degradation, signal transduction, dopaminergic transmission, iron transport and glycolysis are downregulated. Prominent among these are the protein chaperone HSC-70, subunits of the UPS and SKP1A, a member of the E3 ubiquitin ligase complex. Therefore, it is most likely that impairment in energy metabolism and/or alterations in UPS are the underlying mechanisms for PD pathogenesis (Eriksen *et al.*, 2005; Mandel *et al.*, 2005).

Current PD treatment regimes can be divided into three categories: symptomatic, protective and restorative. Only symptomatic treatment via the administration of L-dopa and other drugs affecting neurological transmission have shown efficacy. However, side effects like dyskinesia, motor fluctuations and neurological complications limit their long-term use (Gold & Nutt, 2002). The neuroimmunophilins ligands (NILs) are a promising new class of drugs for treatment of PD as well as other neurodegenerative diseases. NILs are derived from the immunosuppressant, FK506 (tacrolimus) and exert their activity not via any cellular mechanism involving the immune system but by binding to a group of proteins termed FK506 binding proteins (FKBPs). When compared to the immune system, FKBP expression levels are highly enriched (10-50 fold greater) in both the central and peripheral nervous system. In this chapter, we review our current understanding of the role of FKBPs in the nervous system with an emphasis on the protein partners that interface with FKBPs inside cells. For brevity, we limit our discussions to FKBPs that are enriched in the nervous systems and may have important role in Parkinson's disease pathogenesis. We also highlight the mode of action of the NILs with the hope that knowledge of such interaction will enable rationale design of new drugs with improved efficacy for treatment of Parkinson's disease as well as other neurodegenerative disorders.

2. Role of FKBPs in the nervous system

FKBPs together with cyclophilins (CyPs) comprise a family of phylogenetically conserved immunophilins that have peptidyl prolyl isomerase activity (PPIase; EC 5.2.1.8), producing the *cis-trans* isomerization of X-Pro peptide bond, an essential but rate-limiting step in the protein folding process (Barik, 2006). Initial isolation and purification of immunophilins were based on their differential affinity towards the principal immunosuppressant drugs - rapamycin, FK506 and cyclosporin A (CsA). While CyPs bind to only CsA, FKBPs have affinities for both FK506 and rapamycin. Immunosuppressive activity mediated by these drugs is brought about by their binding to the cognate immunophilins. The FK506/FKBP or CsA/CyP binary complexes bind to the Ca^{2+}/calmodulin dependent protein serine/threonine phosphatase, calcineurin (CaN) and inhibit its phosphatase activity. The resulting FKBP-FK506-CaN ternary complex cannot dephosphorylate the key transcription factor, nuclear factor of activated T-cells (NF-AT). Inactive NF-AT remains in the cytoplasm thereby preventing interleukin-2 (IL-2) secretion (**Figure 1**). Consequently, both T-cell activation and proliferation is inhibited. On the other hand, FKBP-rapamycin complex exerts immunosuppression by inhibiting the serine/threonine kinase activity of mammalian target of rapamycin (mTOR) (Sharma *et al.*, 1994).

The role of FKBPs in the nervous system was initiated by observations that the brain is abundantly enriched in CyPs and FKBPs (Maki *et al.*, 1990; Steiner *et al.*, 1992; Dawson *et al.*, 1994). The importance of immunophilins in the nervous system was firmly established from studies showing that FK506 potently (as low as 0.1 nM) increases neurite outgrowth in both PC-12 (Lyons *et al.*, 1994) and SH-SY5Y cell culture models as well as in primary cultures of chick dorsal root ganglion and hippocampal neurons (Hamilton and Steiner, 1998). Efforts to explain this neurotrophic effect focussed on the calcineurin-dependent pathway involving the CaN substrate, GAP-43 (growth-associated protein-43). GAP-43 selectively localizes to developing neurons and its phosphorylation is known to enhance its neurite extension activity (Meiri *et al.*, 1991). Though initially tenable, the hypothesis was challenged when it was shown that both CsA (Gold, 1997) and non-immunosuppressive (hence non-calcineurin binding) derivatives of FK506 exhibit neurotrophic effect with similar potencies as that of FK506. Therefore, it is most likely that nerve growth proceeds via a calcineurin-independent pathway.

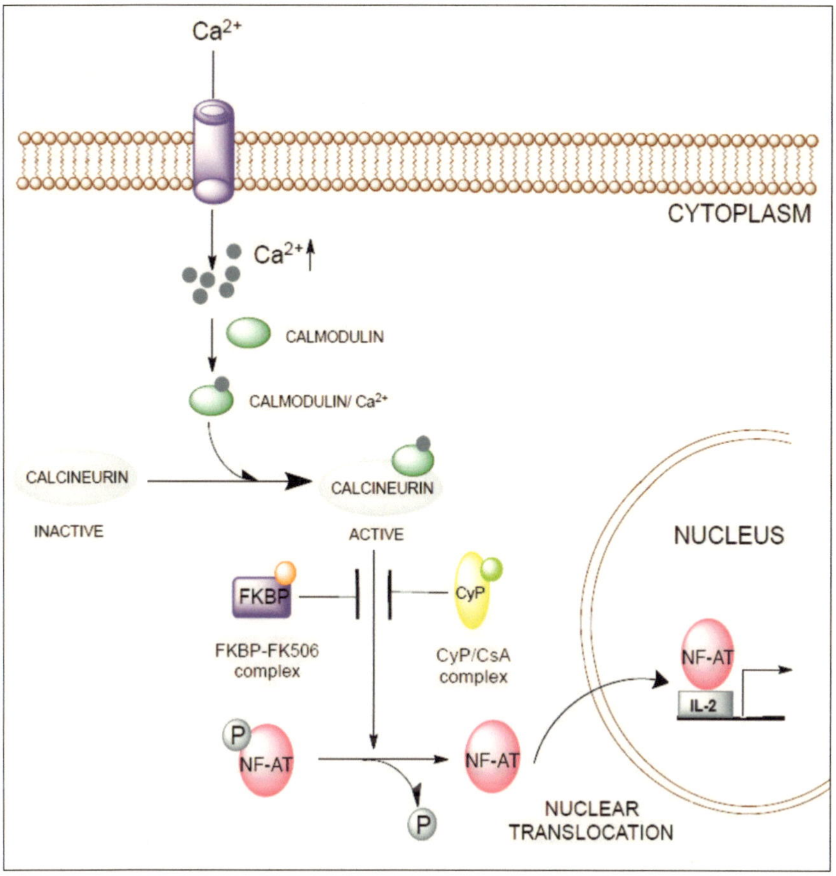

Fig. 1. Immunosuppressive effect of neuroimmunophilin ligands: T-cell receptor activation leads to a rapid increase in intracellular calcium levels with concomitant activation of the Ca^{2+}/calmodulin-dependent phosphatase, calcineurin (CaN). Active CaN dephosphorylates the transcription factor NF-AT, allowing its nuclear translocation and thereby upregulating IL-2 expression. Addition of FK506 or CsA results in formation of FKBP-FK506-CaN/CyP-CsA-CaN ternary complexes that inhibits CaN-dependent NF-AT dephosphorylation, as a result T-cell activation and IL-2 secretion does not occur.

When FK506-treated brain lysates were probed for proteins with increased phosphorylation levels, one of the identified targets was neuronal nitric oxide synthase (nNOS). In the brain, nNOS catalyzes the formation of nitric oxide (NO) from arginine and its catalytic activity is inhibited by phosphorylation. Following cerebral vascular occlusion, there is a massive increase in the excitatory neurotransmitter glutamate. Elevated glutamate levels, acting through the N-methyl-D-aspartate (NMDA) receptor, activates nNOS resulting in increased NO formation and neurotoxicity **(Figure 2)**. Toxicity may involve NO itself or its combination with superoxide free radical (O_2^-) to form peroxy-nitrite that decomposes to hydroxide (OH^-) and NO_2 (NO_2^-) free radicals with subsequent cellular damage by oxidation of nucleic acids, proteins and membrane lipids (Snyder, 1992). By enhancing phospho nNOS levels, FKBPs inhibit NO formation and thereby attenuate glutamate toxicity following vascular stroke (Snyder *et al.*, 1998). Contrary to nerve regeneration, FKBP-mediated neuroprotection proceeds via calcineurin inhibition as anti-stroke effects were also seen with CsA.

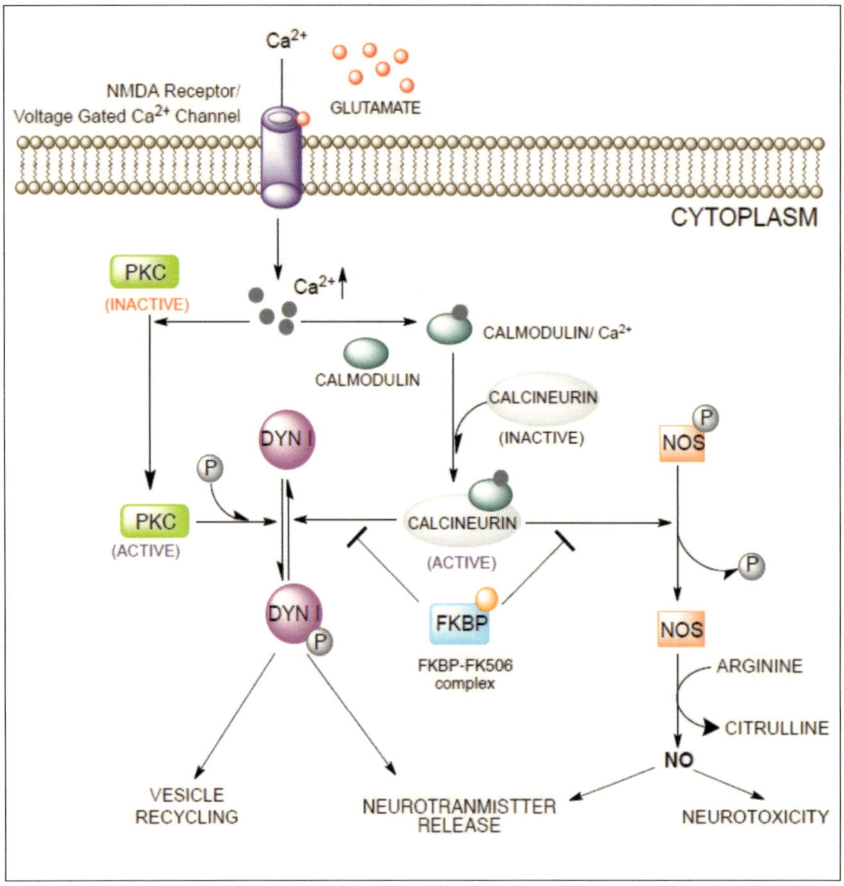

Fig. 2. NILs regulate neurotoxicity and neurotransmitter release: Glutamate-mediated influx of calcium through the NMDA receptor activates calcineurin (CaN) that in turn dephosphorylates nNOS and increases its catalytic activity. nNOS activation leads to increased NO formation and subsequent neurotoxicity and neurotransmitter release. FK506/CsA can counteract this neuronal toxicity by inhibiting CaN-dependent nNOS activation. Influx of Ca2+ also activates PKC and CaN that have opposing effect on phosphorylation state of the GTPase, dynamin I. While PKC-mediated phosphorylation of dynamin I increases its GTPase activity and leads to increased neurotransmitter release, CaN dephosphorylates and inactivates dynamin I. By inhibiting CaN, FK506 and CsA enhances phospho-dynamin I levels and subsequent depolarization-evoked neurotransmitter release.

FK506 has contradictory roles in neurotransmitter release - it inhibits NMDA induced neurotransmitter release while augmenting depolarization-induced release. Since neurotransmitter release proceeds via calcineurin-dependent pathway, this discrepancy in FK506 response can be attributed to the involvement of distinct calcineurin substrates, nNOS and dynamin I **(Figure 2)**. FK506 reduces glutamate release from NMDA-stimulated striatal synaptosomes as well as acetylcholine and dopamine release from PC12 cells that have been differentiated by NGF (Steiner *et al.*, 1996). Similar reductions seen with the nNOS inhibitor, nitro-L-arginine, indicates that NO regulates neurotransmitter release in PC12 and synaptosomes. In presence of FK506 and CsA, inhibition of calcineurin and subsequent reduction of nNOS activity results in decreased NO levels and therefore reduced neurotransmitter release.

In contrast, FK506 fails to inhibit potassium depolarization-evoked neurotransmitter release. Both CsA and L-683590 (FK506 analog that inhibits calcineurin), augment glutamate release from synaptosomes that have been treated with the K^+-channel blocker, 4-aminopyridine. In this case, the *bona fide* calcineurin substrate, dynamin I and not nNOS is involved (Nichols *et al.*, 1994). Dynamin I, a GTPase that regulates vesicular recycling, is active in its phosphorylated form; enhanced GTPase activity results in greater synaptic vesicular trafficking and increased rate of neurotransmitter release. CsA and FK506 mediated inhibition of calcineurin enhances dynamin I phosphorylation and hence its activity.

FK506 and its derivatives have also shown neuroprotective activity in neuropathy models mimicking stroke and dementia. For example, FK506-mediated calcineurin inhibition protects against ischemic brain injury (Sharkey & Butcher, 1994), desensitizes NMDA receptors (Tong *et al.*, 1995), prevents long-term depression (LTD) in rat hippocampus (Hodgkiss & Kelly, 1995) and modulates long-term potentiation (LTP) in rat visual cortex (Funauchi *et al.*, 1994). Stabilization of mitochondrial function was suggested to account for the anti-ischemic activities of FK506. FK506 does not target the mitochondrial potential transition pore (MTP) but prevents deterioration in mitochondrial respiration while maintaining cellular ATP levels and Ca^{2+} homeostasis. Furthermore, the role of FKBPs in the central nervous system has been extensively probed using 1-methyl-4-phenyl-1,2,3,6-tetrahydropyridine (MPTP) or 6-hydroxydopamine (6-OHDA) induced lesions of dopaminergic neurons. Both agents cause massive degeneration of nigrostriatal DA neurons thereby making MPTP and 6-OHDA treatment experimental paradigms for Parkinson's disease (Gerlach *et al.*, 1991). Treatment with GPI-1046, a FK506 analog was able to substantially recover the MPTP-damaged DA neurons as evidenced by increased tyrosine hydroxylase staining while rats lesioned with 6-OHDA showed morphological and functional recovery with increased striatal catecholamine levels and reduced amphetamine-induced rotations (Steiner *et al.*, 1997).

How might immunophilin ligands exert their neurotrophic and neuroprotective actions? The data suggests that PPIase activity of FKBPs maybe involved but no conclusive evidence has been provided so far. Several studies have tried to identify the FKBP(s) involved and elucidate the mechanism-of-action. This has proved particularly difficult as (1) most of the FKBP family members bind FK506 or its derivatives, albeit with varying degrees of affinity; (2) activities of both FKBPs and the protein phosphatase, calcineurin are inhibited by FK506 and its analogues and (3) FKBPs perform multifarious roles in protein folding, translocation and regulation as well as have a wide range of tissue/organellar distribution. Initial studies implicated a role for FKBP12 as elevated mRNA and proteins levels were observed in 6-OHDA model of PD (Nilsson *et al.*, 2007). Moreover, higher levels of FKBP12 have also been reported in brains of PD patients (Avramut & Achim, 2002). Therefore, a possible link between FKBPs and PD might stem from the increase in expression or redistribution of chaperone proteins in stress conditions. In addition to FKBP12, the human brain is enriched in FKBP38, FKBP51, FKBP52 and FKBP65 (Charters *et al.*, 1994; Coss *et al.*, 1998; Chambraud *et al.*, 2010; Jinwal *et al.*, 2010). Collectively, these immunophilins enriched in the nervous system are termed neuroimmunophilins. In the following sections, we will discuss the role of only those neuroimmunophilins that may be important for PD pathogenesis.

3. Molecular interacting partners of neuroimmunophilins

The neuroprotective and neurotrophic functions observed with NILs together with studies showing that chaperone proteins like HSP70 can suppresses α-synuclein (α-SYN) mediated loss of dopaminergic neurons in Drosophila model of PD (Auluck *et al.*, 2002; Muchowski, 2002), posits that FKBPs may have important role(s) in preventing PD-associated neurodegeneration. FKBPs, together with other chaperones may convert the toxic conformations of misfolded proteins to non-toxic form that is tolerated by cells. Alternatively, they may prevent the formation of toxic pre-fibrillar intermediates, or accelerate their conversion to nontoxic, amorphous aggregates that can be degraded by the cellular proteolytic machinery.

3.1 FKBPs interact with α-synuclein both *in vitro* and *in vivo*

α-SYN is a small (140 amino acid) intrinsically disordered protein predominantly localized to the presynaptic terminals. α-SYN regulates the functions of several other proteins - synphilin-1, parkin, tyrosine hydroxylase, dopamine transporter and phospholipase D, via stoichiometric protein-protein and protein-lipid interactions (Goedert, 2001; Ischiropoulos, 2003). In PD, α-SYN aggregates into characteristic fibrillar β-pleated structures in Lewy bodies. Besides LBs, α-SYN also forms intermediate-state oligomers that when released from the neurons activate microglia leading to an increased production of ROS and proinflammatory cytokines (Glass *et al.*, 2010). Activated microglia further amplifies this inflammatory response in a positive feedback loop. In α-SYN, the ability of the central hydrophobic NAC (non Aβ-component of amyloid plaques in Alzheimer's disease) domain to aggregate is normally counteracted by the highly charged hydrophilic C-terminal domain. Interestingly, all 5 proline residues (Pro^{108}, Pro^{117}, Pro^{120}, Pro^{128}, Pro^{138}) of α-SYN are located at the C-terminal of the protein. Changes to the C-terminal domain through deletion, point mutations or via posttranslational modifications such as phosphorylation (Kragh *et al.*, 2009) expose the NAC domain leading to hydrophobic interaction driven aggregation. For example, the E3-ubiquitin ligase, parkin can protect against α-SYN-induced toxicity by altering the phosphorylation levels of α-SYN (**Figure 3**). By simultaneously reducing PLK2 levels and activating PP2A, parkin decreases Ser^{87} and Ser^{129} phosphorylation thereby decreasing aggregation of phosphorylated α-SYN in LBs (Khandelwal *et al.*, 2010). The role of FKBPs in synucleinopathy has been probed both *in vitro* (Gerard *et al.*, 2006) and *in vivo* (Gerard *et al.*, 2010). *In vitro*, fluorescence correlation spectroscopy (FCS) measurements showed that addition of FKBP12 accelerates α-SYN aggregation into fibrillar structures that mimic aggregates formed in LBs. FKBP12 significantly alters the rate for both the nucleation and fibril formation stages (Gerard *et al.*, 2008). Since FKBPs catalyze the cis-trans isomerization of X-Pro peptide bond, the importance of C-terminal proline residues of α-SYN was also investigated. Changing one or more proline residues to alanine increased the aggregation kinetics of mutant α-SYN (Meuvis *et al.*, 2010). Additionally, FKBP12 did not interact with a proline deficient α-SYN mutant and this mutant was also found to be more structured.

Using a neuronal model of synucleinopathy in which α-SYN aggregation and cell death was induced by oxidative stress, Gerard and coworkers have shown that both FK506 and knockdown of FKBP12/FKBP52 can counter the effects of oxidative stress. Likewise, it was shown that overexpression of FKBP12 and -52 enhances α-SYN aggregation. FKBP52 was less potent than FKBP12 in inducing fibrillar aggregation. *In vivo*, FKBP12 was shown to colocalize with α-SYN in the brain of A30P-α-SYN transgenic mice model. Furthermore, FK506 administration reduced both the α-SYN aggregation in cells as well as increased survival of α-SYN overexpressing neurons in the striatum. Collectively, these studies validate FKBPs as a novel target for PD.

Besides α-SYN, other interacting partners of FKBP12 identified from 6-OHDA treated rat model of PD include 1-*cys* peroxyredoxin, HSP70, 14-3-3 zeta, M2-type pyruvate kinase (PKM2), annexin A2 and α-enolase (ENO1) (Nilsson *et al.*, 2007). It has been known that levels of PKM2, 14-3-3 zeta and ENO1 are altered during neurodegenerative diseases like PD and Alzheimer's (Poon *et al.*, 2006).

Given that FKBPs are chaperone proteins having important roles in protein folding, it is counterintuitive to note that the interaction between FKBP(s) and α-SYN results in α-SYN aggregation. Its is likely that α-SYN inclusions may not result simply from precipitated misfolded protein but rather from an active process meant to sequester soluble misfolded proteins from the cellular milieu (Kopito, 2000). Accordingly, inclusion body formation might serve as a cellular defense mechanism aimed at removing toxic insoluble proteins.

3.2 FKBP52 interacts with RET51 in a phosphorylation-dependent manner

RET51, a tyrosine kinase (TK) receptor, has important roles in the development and maintenance of the nervous system. Recently, FKBP52 was found to be novel interacting partner for RET51 in a split ubiquitin two-hybrid screen (Fusco *et al.*, 2010). Neurotrophins like NGF and glial-cell line derived neurotrophic factor (GDNF) promote the phosphorylation driven formation of RET51/FKBP52 complex; phosphorylation occurs on Tyr^{905} within the TK domain of RET51 and is a pre-requisite for complex formation. Association of RET51 with FKBP52 does not depend on HSP90 or other chaperones. The involvement of RET51 in PD comes from the genetic analysis of an early onset-PD patient heterozygous for mutations on both *RET51* and *FKBP52* genes (Fusco *et al.*, 2010). Mutations on both proteins disrupt formation of RET51/FKBP52 complex and its downstream signaling pathway. The detail of this signaling mechanism remains to be elucidated.

3.3 FKBP38 promotes trafficking of membrane channels

FKBP38 is distributed to both the mitochondria (Shirane & Nakayama, 2003) and endoplasmic reticulum (Wang *et al.*, 2005). Only the C-terminal tail is membrane anchored while the bulk of the protein is exposed to the cytosol. The unique topology of FKBP38 allows it to juxtapose between cytosolic and ER chaperone proteins. FKBP38 functions as a co-chaperone to HSC70/HSP90 complex to mediate proper folding and trafficking of membrane proteins like the multidomain cAMP-regulated chloride channel, CFTR (Wang *et al.*, 2006) and the voltage-dependent K^+ channel, HERG (Walker *et al.*, 2007). The immature form of HERG localizes to the endoplasmic reticulum whereas the fully glycosylated mature protein is present in the Golgi or the cell surface. While siRNA mediated knockdown of FKBP38 reduced HERG maturation, overexpression of FKBP38 was able to rescue the HERG F805C trafficking mutant. FKBP38 is involved in the late stages of HERG folding and ER export, as majority of FKBP38 has been found to associate with immature HERG. It is likely that natively folded HERG is released from its final chaperone complex while still attached with FKBP38. The bound FKBP38 could further mediate the attachment of HERG with the motor protein kinesin for transport to the plasma membrane. HERG mutations have been associated with the Long QT syndrome, a cardiac disorder characterized by long QT intervals. PD patients have an increased susceptibility to cardiac arrest as is evident from a prolongation of the QT interval (Hurst *et al.*, 2003). Therefore, it is likely that FKBP38-mediated HERG trafficking plays an important role in PD pathogenesis.

3.4 FKBP mediated regulation of Tau function and its effect on microtubule dynamics

Tau, a member of the microtubule-associated protein family (MAP), binds and stabilizes microtubules (MTs) and is therefore intrinsically linked with MT dynamics. Six isoforms of tau are present in humans, the longest one having four MT-binding repeat motifs. Normal biological functions of tau are dependent on its phosphorylation state. Involvement of tau in PD pathogenesis comes from the observations that (1) it accumulates in LBs together with α-SYN (Ishizawa *et al.*, 2003); (2) analysis of synapse-enriched fractions from PD brains show an increased phosphorylation for both tau and α-SYN (Muntane *et al.*, 2008) and (3) tau and synuclein synergistically promote *in vitro* fibrillization of each other (Giasson *et al.*, 2003). α-SYN mediates tau phosphorylation at $Ser^{262/356}$ by activating protein kinase A (PKA)(Jensen *et al.*, 1999) while in MPTP models of PD, α-SYN recruits GSKβ3 kinase to phosphorylate tau at $Ser^{396/404}$ (Duka *et al.*, 2009). Hyperphosphorylation of tau results in MT destabilization by interfering with its binding.

Recent studies have shown that both FKBP51 (Jinwal *et al.*, 2010) and FKBP52 *(Chambraud et al.*, 2007; Chambraud *et al.*, 2010) can interact with tau. FKBP52 preferentially binds to hyperphosphorylated tau and colocalizes with tau at the growth cones in both cortical neurons and PC12 cells. Interestingly, FKBP52 could inhibit tau-mediated tubulin polymerization *in vitro*. This is consistent with the observation that overexpression of FKBP52 impairs neurite outgrowth in cultured neurons (Chambraud *et al.*, 2010). Interaction of FKBP52 with tau was mapped to the C-terminal TPR domain of FKBP52 (Chambraud *et al.*, 2007). Currently it is not known if the neuroprotection mediated by "anti-tau" activity of FKBP52 is linked to proteasomal degradation of hyperphosphorylated tau via enhanced trafficking or by increased aggregation of toxic tau into fibrillary tangles.

FKBP51, a member of the HSP90 chaperone complex, directly associates with tau and its overexpression significantly increases the levels of phospho- and total tau in cells. Contrary to FKBP52, FKBP51 enhances the tau-mediated MT polymerization and the PPIase activity of FKBP51 is crucial for its function in tau processing. The data by Dickey and coworkers suggest a model whereby binding of FKBP51-HSP90 complex to phosphorylated tau triggers its dephosphorylation and recycling to the microtubules thereby facilitating MT polymerization and stabilization (Jinwal *et al.*, 2010). HSP90-FKBP51 binding also shields tau from CHIP (carboxy terminus of the HSC70-interacting protein) mediated ubiquitination and subsequent proteasomal degradation (**Figure 3).**

3.5 FKBP38 anchors Bcl-2 to the mitochondria and regulates apoptosis

The C-terminal tail of the noncanonical FKBP, FKBP38, localizes the protein to the ER and mitochondrial membrane where it interacts with the anti-apoptotic proteins, Bcl-2 and Bcl-x_L and regulates their functions. FKB38 is critical for the mitochondrial localization of Bcl-2 and Bcl-$x_{L;}$ expression of mitochondrial targeting defective FKBP38 mutants and RNAi mediated

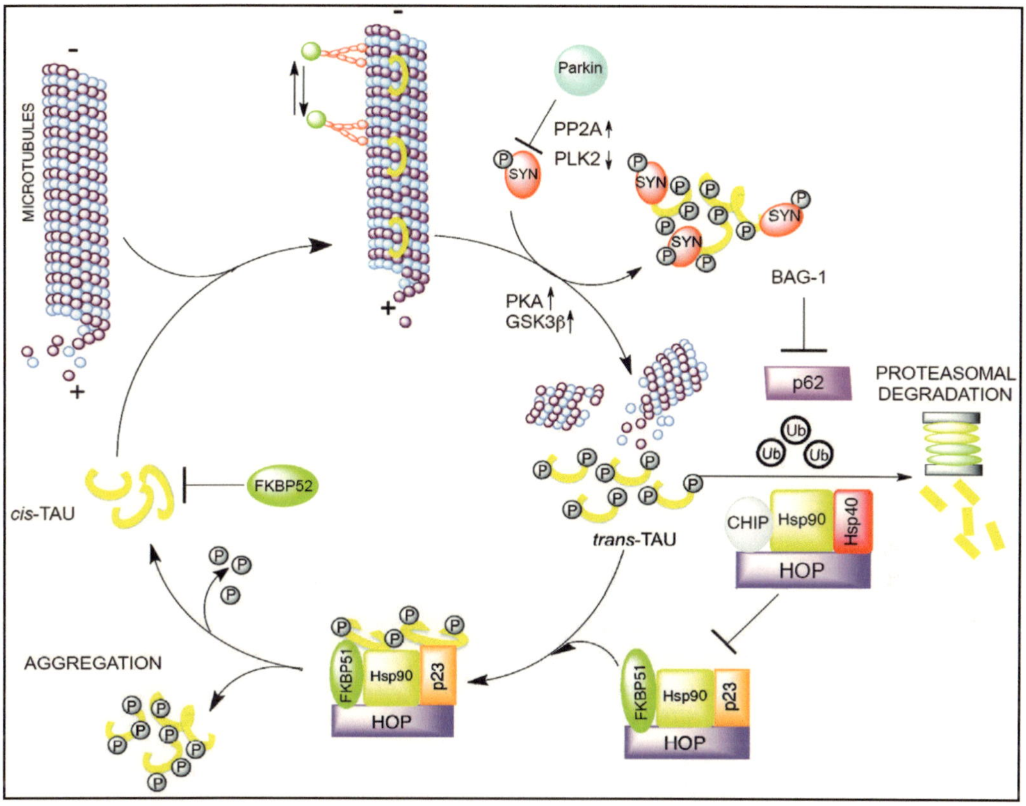

Fig. 3. FKBPs regulate microtubule stability by interacting with the microtubule-associated protein, tau. FKBP51 and FKBP52 have opposing effects on microtubule (MT) stability. FKBP52 exhibits "anti-tau" activity; by sequestering tau, it prevents its association with MT thereby destabilizing MTs. Together with the HSP90 complex, FKBP51 binds phosphorylated tau in its *trans*-conformation, isomerizes it to the *cis*-form and recycles it back to the MTs. Alternatively FKBP51 can accelerate aggregation of phospho-tau species. Phospho-tau can also be degraded by the cellular proteasomal system following CHIP-mediated polyubiquitination. Binding of FKBP51 and CHIP to phosphorylated tau is mutually exclusive. By recruiting PKA/GSK3β, α-SYN promotes tau-phosphorylation within the MT-binding domain and its subsequent removal from MTs. Activity of α-SYN is in turn regulated by the E3 ubiquitin ligase, Parkin. By inhibiting PLK2 kinase and enhancing PP2A phosphatase activity, Parkin decreases α-SYN phosphorylation and interferes with its activity.

knockdown of FKBP38 causes the cellular redistribution of these proteins. Furthermore FKBP38-mediated mitochondrial targeting is responsible for the anti-apoptotic activity of FKBP38 (Shirane & Nakayama, 2003; Kang *et al.*, 2005). Nishimura and colleagues have shown FKBP38 is a *bona fide* substrate for the aspartyl protease, presenilin 1 and 2 (PS1/2) (Wang *et al.*, 2005). Under physiological conditions PS1/2 forms macromolecular heteromeric complexes with FKBP38 and Bcl-2 and sequesters them in the ER/Golgi via a γ-secretase independent mechanism. Thus by inhibiting the FKBP38 mediated mitochondrial targeting of Bcl-2, PS1/2 antagonizes the anti-apoptotic effect of FKBP38.

In neuroblastoma cells, FKBP38 exhibits Ca2+/CaM stimulated PPIase activity and the FKBP38/Ca2+/CaM ternary complex binds Bcl-2. This binding is interrupted by GPI-1046, indicating that the active site of FKBP38 is involved in Bcl-2 interaction. HSP90 in the HSP90/Bcl-2/Ca^{2+}/CaM ternary complex has also been shown to inhibit the Bcl-2-FKBP38 interaction by blocking access to the enzyme active site (Edlich *et al.*, 2007). GPI-1046 and RNAi-mediated depletion of FKBP38 activity was able to promote neuronal cell survival thus indicating that, in neuronal cells, FKBP38 has proapoptotic function. This observation contradicts earlier reports wherein it was shown that FKBP38 has anti-apoptotic effect (Shirane & Nakayama, 2003; Kang *et al.*, 2005). One plausible explanation for this discrepancy could be explained on the basis of the different cell lines, neuronal versus non-neuronal, used in these studies. The potent neuroprotective and neuroregenerative effects of low molecular weight FKBP38 inhibitors in neuroblastoma cells concur well with the proapoptotic role of FKBP38. Furthermore, the ability of the FKBP38 inhibitor - *N*-(*N'*,*N'*-dimethylcarboxamidomethyl)-cycloheximide to elicit neural stem proliferation and neuronal differentiation in a rat model of transient cerebral ischemia underscores the importance of FKBP38 in neuronal apoptosis (Edlich *et al.*, 2006).

4. Neuroimmunophilin ligands as therapeutics for PD

Currently available drugs aimed at PD treatment do not have the capacity to inhibit PD progression but can only alleviate symptoms and/or delay neuronal atrophy by altering neurotransmitter metabolism. Neuroimmunophilin ligands are non-immunosuppressive and mediate the beneficial effects by multiple mechanisms that include inhibition of apoptosis, increased neurotrophic signaling and/or reducing oxidative stress by interfering with mitochondrial dysfunction (Tanaka & Ogawa, 2004). Several groups have reported that NILs like FK506, GPI-1046 and V-10367 (**Figure 4A**) promote striatal dopaminergic innervations in MPTP- or 6-OHDA models of PD (Kitamura *et al.*, 1994; Steiner *et al.*, 1997; Costantini *et al.*, 1998; Guo *et al.*, 2001). Studies have also shown that GPI-1046 protects against the *p*-chloroamphetamine-induced destruction of central serotoninergic neurons and

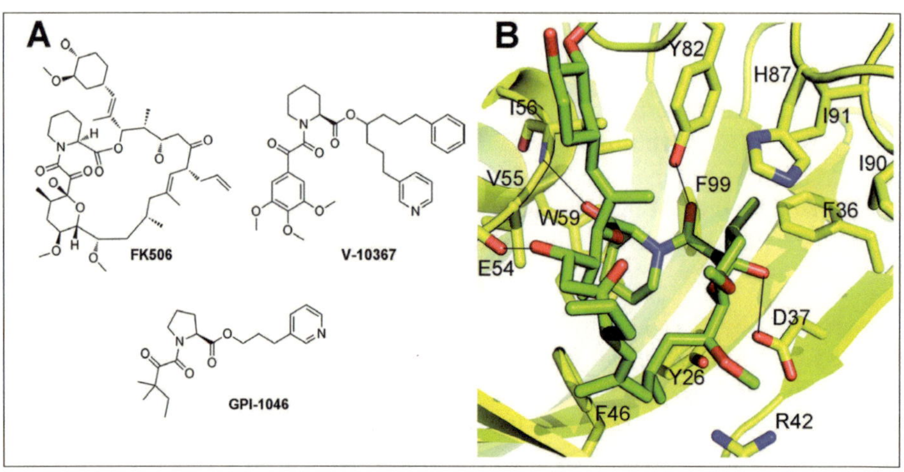

Fig. 4. (A) Structure of the neuroimmunophilin ligand FK506 and its non-immunosuppressive derivatives, GPI-1046 and V-10367. (B) Binding of FK506 (green) into the active site pocket of FKBP12 "(represented by cartoon model).

senescence-related atrophy of medial septal cholinergic neurons (Sauer *et al.*, 1999). Furthermore, rotational behavior and loss of corticostriatal long-term potentiation (LTP) in 6-OHDA treated rats was alleviated by GPI-1046. However, as similar efficacy was obtained with an analog that does not bind FKBP12 (V-13670), the importance of FKBP12 in mediating neurotrophic effects is debatable. Besides FK506 derivatives, CsA has been shown to protect against dopaminergic degeneration, promote regeneration of DA neurons and even suppress microglial cytotoxicity, as activated microglia has been known to generate free radicals (Banati *et al.*, 1993).

The binding mode of FK506 and its non-immunosuppressive counterpart, GPI-1046 has been elucidated (Van Duyne *et al.*, 1993; Sich *et al.*, 2000). Minimal binding motif comprises of the central pipecolic acid ring, the α-dicarbonyl amide linkage and pyranose ring. In the FK506-FKBP12 crystal structure (Van Duyne *et al.*, 1993), the pipecoline ring sits in the cavity defined by Trp^{59} and Tyr^{26}, Phe^{46}, Val^{55}, Ile^{56}, Phe^{99} side chains, whereas the α-dicarbonyl amide is hydrogen-bonded to -COOH and -OH group of Asp^{37} and Tyr^{82}, respectively (**Figure 4B**). The hydrophobic pocket formed by Phe^{36}, Asp^{37}, Tyr^{82}, His^{87}, Ile^{90} and Ile^{91} buries the pyranose ring while the cyclohexyl ester chain is engaged in hydrophobic interactions within a shallow surface groove. SAR studies have shown that the α-dicarbonyl amide functionality is indispensible for enzyme inhibition as replacement of either one or both carbonyl groups reduces potency. Similarly, pipecolic ring opening drastically increases the inhibition constant of the derivatives. GPI-1046 binds in a manner analogous to that of FK506 with the amide bond in *trans* configuration; the only exception being the replacement of pipecolyl moiety of FK506 by the prolyl ring of GPI-1046. Even though GPI-1046 has fewer favorable protein-ligand interactions, its effect on protein dynamics is essentially same as FK506, that is, stabilize the conformation of solvent exposed residues that are important in protein-protein and protein-ligand interactions.

The therapeutic utility of NILs has been questioned by work from other groups (Harper *et al.*, 1999; Parker *et al.*, 2000; Bocquet *et al.*, 2001) as many of the initial observations could not be replicated in identical systems. For instance, Harper and colleagues observed that GPI-1046 causes only a marginal increase in neurite outgrowth of chick dorsal root ganglia in culture under conditions where a very robust effect of nerve growth factor was seen. GPI-1046 did not restore tyrosine hydroxylase-positive fibers after 6-OHDA administration neither did it protect cultured dopaminergic neurons against MPTP induced toxicity. One possibility for the observed differences could be the levels of dopaminergic dysfunction. GPI-1046 provided neuroprotection in cases when the degradation was mild to moderate; it has no effect in severe cases when DA neuron levels deplete to 20% of that in normal controls. Other parameters like variability in culture conditions, differences in days *in vitro* prior to experimentation, can potentially account for the contrasting observations (Pong and Zaleska, 2003). Furthermore, neuroprotective effects of GPI-1046 could not be replicated in monkey model of MPTP toxicity (Emborg *et al.*, 2001) suggesting species-specific differences with respect to GPI-1046 activity.

5. Conclusion

FKBPs have emerged as novel cellular target for treatment of Parkinson's disease and other neurological disorders. The extraordinary unmet need for therapeutic intervention in PD continues to drive the search for potential drug candidates. Non-immunosuppressive NILs with their small size, target specificity, bioavailability and stability provide excellent scaffolds for the development of new drugs. Although our present knowledge of the mode of action of NILs is still fragmentary, there is increasing evidence that the neurotrophic, neuroprotective and restorative potential of these compounds is mediated by signaling pathways that can have antagonistic or additive effect. For example, multiple pathways may crosstalk via common integral components such as c-Jun (Gold *et al.*, 1999; Winter *et al.*, 2000). So far, the nervous system has been found to be enriched in only five FKBPs - FKBP-12, -38, -51, -52 and -65. Much work needs to be done so as to identify unique neuroimmunophilins and their interacting partners, assess their cellular function as well as their response to injury. Furthermore, issues such as reproducibility of pre-clinical data, structure-activity relationship studies, drug evaluation in appropriate animal models, and implementation of proper clinical designs and endpoints needs immediate attention as such information will aid in the development of novel NILs with improved efficacies, target selectivity and potency. FKBPs and NILs seem to be a promising area for therapeutic intervention of PD and other neurodegenerative disorders.

6. Acknowledgment

The authors would like to acknowledge the support from Ministry of Health-National Medical Research Council, Singapore for funding (NMRC/1177/2008).

7. References

Auluck, P.K., Chan, H.Y., Trojanowski, J.Q., Lee, V.M. & Bonini, N.M. (2002). Chaperone suppression of alpha-synuclein toxicity in a Drosophila model for Parkinson's disease. *Science,* Vol 295, pp 865-868.

Avramut, M. & Achim, C.L. (2002). Immunophilins and their ligands: insights into survival and growth of human neurons. *Physiol Behav,* Vol 77, pp 463-468.

Banati, R.B., Gehrmann, J., Schubert, P. & Kreutzberg, G.W. (1993). Cytotoxicity of microglia. *Glia,* Vol 7, pp 111-118.

Barik, S. (2006). Immunophilins: for the love of proteins. *Cell Mol. Life Sci.,* Vol 63, pp 2889-2900.

Bocquet, A., Lorent, G., Fuks, B., Grimee, R., Talaga, P., Daliers, J. & Klitgaard, H. (2001). Failure of GPI compounds to display neurotrophic activity in vitro and in vivo. *Eur. J Pharmacol.,* Vol 415, pp 173-180.

Chambraud, B., Belabes, H., Fontaine-Lenoir, V., Fellous, A. & Baulieu, E.E. (2007). The immunophilin FKBP52 specifically binds to tubulin and prevents microtubule formation. *FASEB J.,* Vol 21, pp 2787-2797.

Chambraud, B., Sardin, E., Giustiniani, J., Dounane, O., Schumacher, M., Goedert, M. & Baulieu, E.E. (2010). A role for FKBP52 in Tau protein function. *Proc. Natl. Acad. Sci. USA,* Vol 107, pp 2658-2663.

Charters, A.R., Kobayashi, M. & Butcher, S.P. (1994). Immunochemical analysis of FK506 binding proteins in neuronal cell lines and rat brain. *Biochem. Soc. Trans.,* Vol 22, pp 411S.

Coss, M.C., Stephens, R.M., Morrison, D.K., Winterstein, D., Smith, L.M. & Simek, S.L. (1998). The immunophilin FKBP65 forms an association with the serine/threonine kinase c-Raf-1. *Cell Growth Differ.,* Vol 9, pp 41-48.

Costantini, L.C., Chaturvedi, P., Armistead, D.M., McCaffrey, P.G., Deacon, T.W. & Isacson, O. (1998). A novel immunophilin ligand: distinct branching effects on dopaminergic neurons in culture and neurotrophic actions after oral administration in an animal model of Parkinson's disease. *Neurobiol. Dis* Vol 5, pp 97-106.

Dawson, T.M., Steiner, J.P., Lyons, W.E., Fotuhi, M., Blue, M. & Snyder, S.H. (1994). The immunophilins, FK506 binding protein and cyclophilin, are discretely localized in the brain: relationship to calcineurin. *Neuroscience,* Vol 62, pp 569-580.

Dawson, T.M. (2006). Parkin and defective ubiquitination in Parkinson's disease. *J. Neural Transm. Suppl*, Vol 209-213.

Duka, T., Duka, V., Joyce, J.N. & Sidhu, A. (2009). Alpha-Synuclein contributes to GSK-3beta-catalyzed Tau phosphorylation in Parkinson's disease models. *FASEB J*, Vol 23, pp 2820-2830.

Edlich, F., Weiwad, M., Erdmann, F., Fanghanel, J., Jarczowski, F., Rahfeld, J.U. & Fischer, G. (2005). Bcl-2 regulator FKBP38 is activated by Ca2+/calmodulin. *EMBO J*, Vol 24, pp 2688-2699.

Edlich, F., Weiwad, M., Wildemann, D., Jarczowski, F., Kilka, S., Moutty, M.C., Jahreis, G., Lucke, C., Schmidt, W., Striggow, F. & Fischer, G. (2006). The specific FKBP38 inhibitor N-(N',N'-dimethylcarboxamidomethyl)cycloheximide has potent neuroprotective and neurotrophic properties in brain ischemia. *J Biol. Chem.* Vol 281, pp 14961-14970.

Edlich, F., Erdmann, F., Jarczowski, F., Moutty, M.C., Weiwad, M. & Fischer, G. (2007). The Bcl-2 regulator FKBP38-calmodulin-Ca2+ is inhibited by Hsp90. *J Biol. Chem.*, Vol 282, pp 15341-15348.

Emborg, M.E., Shin, P., Roitberg, B., Sramek, J.G., Chu, Y., Stebbins, G.T., Hamilton, J.S., Suzdak, P.D., Steiner, J.P. & Kordower, J.H. (2001). Systemic administration of the immunophilin ligand GPI 1046 in MPTP-treated monkeys. *Exp. Neurol.*, Vol 168, pp 171-182.

Eriksen, J.L., Wszolek, Z. & Petrucelli, L. (2005). Molecular pathogenesis of Parkinson disease. *Arch. Neurol.* Vol 62, pp 353-357.

Funauchi, M., Haruta, H. & Tsumoto, T. (1994). Effects of an inhibitor for calcium/calmodulin-dependent protein phosphatase, calcineurin, on induction of long-term potentiation in rat visual cortex. *Neurosci. Res.*, Vol 19, pp 269-278.

Fusco, D., Vargiolu, M., Vidone, M., Mariani, E., Pennisi, L.F., Bonora, E., Capellari, S., Dirnberger, D., Baumeister, R., Martinelli, P. & Romeo, G. (2010). The RET51/FKBP52 complex and its involvement in Parkinson disease. *Hum. Mol. Genet.*, Vol 19, pp 2804-2816.

Gerard, M., Debyser, Z., Desender, L., Kahle, P.J., Baert, J., Baekelandt, V. & Engelborghs, Y. (2006). The aggregation of alpha-synuclein is stimulated by FK506 binding proteins as shown by fluorescence correlation spectroscopy. *FASEB J.*, Vol 20, pp 524-526.

Gerard, M., Debyser, Z., Desender, L., Baert, J., Brandt, I., Baekelandt, V. & Engelborghs, Y. (2008). FK506 binding protein 12 differentially accelerates fibril formation of wild type alpha-synuclein and its clinical mutants A30P or A53T. *J Neurochem.*, Vol 106, pp 121-133.

Gerard, M., Deleersnijder, A., Daniels, V., Schreurs, S., Munck, S., Reumers, V., Pottel, H., Engelborghs, Y., Van den Haute, C., Taymans, J.M., Debyser, Z. & Baekelandt, V. (2010). Inhibition of FK506 binding proteins reduces alpha-synuclein aggregation and Parkinson's disease-like pathology. *J Neurosci.*, Vol 30, pp 2454-2463.

Gerlach, M., Riederer, P., Przuntek, H. & Youdim, M.B. (1991). MPTP mechanisms of neurotoxicity and their implications for Parkinson's disease. *Eur. J Pharmacol.*, Vol 208, pp 273-286.

Giasson, B.I., Forman, M.S., Higuchi, M., Golbe, L.I., Graves, C.L., Kotzbauer, P.T., Trojanowski, J.Q. & Lee, V.M. (2003). Initiation and synergistic fibrillization of tau and alpha-synuclein. *Science*, Vol 300, pp 636-640.

Glass, C.K., Saijo, K., Winner, B., Marchetto, M.C. & Gage, F.H. (2010). Mechanisms underlying inflammation in neurodegeneration. *Cell*, Vol 140, pp 918-934.

Goedert, M. (2001). Alpha-synuclein and neurodegenerative diseases. *Nat. Rev. Neurosci.*, Vol 2, pp 492-501.

Gold, B.G. (1997). FK506 and the role of immunophilins in nerve regeneration. *Mol. Neurobiol.*, Vol 15, pp 285-306.

Gold, B.G. & Nutt, J.G. (2002). Neuroimmunophilin ligands in the treatment of Parkinson's disease. *Curr. Opin. Pharmacol.*, Vol 2, pp 82-86.

Gold, B.G., Densmore, V., Shou, W., Matzuk, M.M. & Gordon, H.S. (1999). Immunophilin FK506-binding protein 52 (not FK506-binding protein 12) mediates the neurotrophic action of FK506. *J Pharmacol. Exp. Ther.*, Vol 289, pp 1202-1210.

Guo, X., Dawson, V.L. & Dawson, T.M. (2001). Neuroimmunophilin ligands exert neuroregeneration and neuroprotection in midbrain dopaminergic neurons. *Eur. J Neurosci.*, Vol 13, pp 1683-1693.

Hamilton, G.S. & Steiner, J.P. (1998). Immunophilins: beyond immunosuppression. *J Med. Chem.*, Vol 41, pp 5119-5143.

Harper, S., Bilsland, J., Young, L., Bristow, L., Boyce, S., Mason, G., Rigby, M., Hewson, L., Smith, D., O'Donnell, R., O'Connor, D., Hill, R.G., Evans, D., Swain, C., Williams, B. & Hefti, F. (1999). Analysis of the neurotrophic effects of GPI-1046 on neuron survival and regeneration in culture and in vivo. *Neuroscience*, Vol 88, pp 257-267.

Hodgkiss, J.P. & Kelly, J.S. (1995). Only 'de novo' long-term depression (LTD) in the rat hippocampus in vitro is blocked by the same low concentration of FK506 that blocks LTD in the visual cortex. *Brain Res.*, Vol 705, pp 241-246.

Hurst, R.S., Higdon, N.R., Lawson, J.A., Clark, M.A., Rutherford-Root, K.L., McDonald, W.G., Haas, J.V., McGrath, J.P. & Meglasson, M.D. (2003). Dopamine receptor agonists differ in their actions on cardiac ion channels. *Eur. J Pharmacol.*, Vol 482, pp 31-37.

Ischiropoulos, H. (2003). Oxidative modifications of alpha-synuclein. *Ann. N. Y. Acad. Sci.*, Vol 991, pp 93-100.

Ishizawa, T., Mattila, P., Davies, P., Wang, D. & Dickson, D.W. (2003). Colocalization of tau and alpha-synuclein epitopes in Lewy bodies. *J Neuropathol. Exp. Neurol.*, Vol 62, pp 389-397.

Jensen, P.H., Hager, H., Nielsen, M.S., Hojrup, P., Gliemann, J. & Jakes, R. (1999). Alpha-synuclein binds to Tau and stimulates the protein kinase A-catalyzed tau phosphorylation of serine residues 262 and 356. *J Biol. Chem.*, Vol 274, pp 25481-25489.

Jinwal, U.K., Koren, J., Borysov, S.I., Schmid, A.B., Abisambra, J.F., Blair, L.J., Johnson, A.G., Jones, J.R., Shults, C.L., O'Leary, J.C., Jin, Y., Buchner, J., Cox, M.B. & Dickey, C.A. (2010). The Hsp90 cochaperone, FKBP51, increases Tau stability and polymerizes microtubules. *J Neurosci.*, Vol 30, pp 591-599.

Kang, C.B., Feng, L., Chia, J. & Yoon, H.S. (2005). Molecular characterization of FK-506 binding protein 38 and its potential regulatory role on the anti-apoptotic protein Bcl-2. *Biochem. Biophys. Res. Commun.*, Vol 337, pp 30-38.

Khandelwal, P.J., Dumanis, S.B., Feng, L.R., Maguire-Zeiss, K., Rebeck, G., Lashuel, H.A. & Moussa, C.E. (2010). Parkinson-related parkin reduces alpha-Synuclein phosphorylation in a gene transfer model. *Mol. Neurodegener.* Vol 5, pp 47.

Kitamura, Y., Itano, Y., Kubo, T. & Nomura, Y. (1994). Suppressive effect of FK-506, a novel immunosuppressant, against MPTP-induced dopamine depletion in the striatum of young C57BL/6 mice. *J Neuroimmunol.*, Vol 50, pp 221-224.

Kopito, R.R. (2000). Aggresomes, inclusion bodies and protein aggregation. *Trends Cell Biol.*, Vol 10, pp 524-530.

Kragh, C.L., Lund, L.B., Febbraro, F., Hansen, H.D., Gai, W.P., El-Agnaf, O., Richter-Landsberg, C. & Jensen, P.H. (2009). {alpha}-Synuclein Aggregation and Ser-129 Phosphorylation-dependent Cell Death in Oligodendroglial Cells. *J Biol. Chem.*, Vol 284, pp 10211-10222.

Lyons, W.E., George, E.B., Dawson, T.M., Steiner, J.P. & Snyder, S.H. (1994). Immunosuppressant FK506 promotes neurite outgrowth in cultures of PC12 cells and sensory ganglia. *Proc. Natl. Acad. Sci. USA,* Vol 91, pp 3191-3195.

Maki, N., Sekiguchi, F., Nishimaki, J., Miwa, K., Hayano, T., Takahashi, N. & Suzuki, M. (1990). Complementary DNA encoding the human T-cell FK506-binding protein, a peptidylprolyl cis-trans isomerase distinct from cyclophilin. *Proc. Natl. Acad. Sci. USA,* Vol 87, pp 5440-5443.

Mandel, S., Grunblatt, E., Riederer, P., Amariglio, N., Jacob-Hirsch, J., Rechavi, G. & Youdim, M.B. (2005). Gene expression profiling of sporadic Parkinson's disease substantia nigra pars compacta reveals impairment of ubiquitin-proteasome subunits, SKP1A, aldehyde dehydrogenase, and chaperone HSC-70. *Ann. N. Y. Acad. Sci.,* Vol 1053, pp 356-375.

McGeer, P.L., Itagaki, S., Boyes, B.E. & McGeer, E.G. (1988). Reactive microglia are positive for HLA-DR in the substantia nigra of Parkinson's and Alzheimer's disease brains. *Neurology,* Vol 38, pp 1285-1291.

Meiri, K.F., Bickerstaff, L.E. & Schwob, J.E. (1991). Monoclonal antibodies show that kinase C phosphorylation of GAP-43 during axonogenesis is both spatially and temporally restricted in vivo. *J Cell Biol.,* Vol 112, pp 991-1005.

Meuvis, J., Gerard, M., Desender, L., Baekelandt, V. & Engelborghs, Y. (2010). The conformation and the aggregation kinetics of alpha-synuclein depend on the proline residues in its C-terminal region. *Biochemistry,* Vol 49, pp 9345-9352.

Muchowski, P.J. (2002). Protein misfolding, amyloid formation, and neurodegeneration: a critical role for molecular chaperones? *Neuron,* Vol 35, pp 9-12.

Muntane, G., Dalfo, E., Martinez, A. & Ferrer, I. (2008). Phosphorylation of tau and alpha-synuclein in synaptic-enriched fractions of the frontal cortex in Alzheimer's disease and in Parkinson's disease and related alpha-synucleinopathies. *Neuroscience,* Vol 152, pp 913-923.

Nagatsu, T. & Sawada, M. (2005) Inflammatory process in Parkinson's disease: role for cytokines. *Curr. Pharm. Des.,* Vol 11, pp 999-1016.

Nichols, R.A., Suplick, G.R. & Brown, J.M. (1994). Calcineurin-mediated protein dephosphorylation in brain nerve terminals regulates the release of glutamate. *J Biol. Chem.,* Vol 269, pp 23817-23823.

Nilsson, A., Skold, K., Sjogren, B., Svensson, M., Pierson, J., Zhang, X., Caprioli, R.M., Buijs, J., Persson, B., Svenningsson, P & Andren, P.E. (2007). Increased striatal mRNA and protein levels of the immunophilin FKBP-12 in experimental Parkinson's disease and identification of FKBP-12-binding proteins. *J Proteome Res.,* Vol 6, pp 3952-3961.

Parker, E.M., Monopoli, A., Ongini, E., Lozza, G. & Babij. C.M. (2000). Rapamycin, but not FK506 and GPI-1046, increases neurite outgrowth in PC12 cells by inhibiting cell cycle progression. *Neuropharmacology,* Vol 39, pp 1913-1919.

Pong, K. & Zaleska, M.M. (2003). Therapeutic implications for immunophilin ligands in the treatment of neurodegenerative diseases. *Curr. Drug Targets CNS Neurol. Disord .,* Vol 2, pp 349-356.

Poon, H.F., Shepherd, H.M., Reed, T.T., Calabrese, V., Stella, A.M., Pennisi, G., Cai, J., Pierce, W.M., Klein, J.B. & Butterfield, D.A. (2006). Proteomics analysis provides insight into caloric restriction mediated oxidation and expression of brain proteins associated with age-related impaired cellular processes: Mitochondrial dysfunction, glutamate dysregulation and impaired protein synthesis. *Neurobiol. Aging.,*Vol 27, pp 1020-1034.

Sauer, H., Francis, J.M., Jiang, H., Hamilton, G.S. & Steiner, J.P. (1999). Systemic treatment with GPI 1046 improves spatial memory and reverses cholinergic neuron atrophy in the medial septal nucleus of aged mice. *Brain Res.*, Vol 842, pp 109-118.

Sharkey, J. & Butcher, S.P. (1994). Immunophilins mediate the neuroprotective effects of FK506 in focal cerebral ischaemia. *Nature*, Vol 371, pp 336-339.

Sharma, V.K., Li, B., Khanna, A., Sehajpal, P.K. & Suthanthiran, M. (1994). Which way for drug-mediated immunosuppression? *Curr. Opin. Immunol.*, Vol 6, pp 784-790.

Shirane, M. & Nakayama, K.I. (2003). Inherent calcineurin inhibitor FKBP38 targets Bcl-2 to mitochondria and inhibits apoptosis. *Nat. Cell Biol.*, Vol 5, pp 28-37.

Sich, C., Improta, S., Cowley, D.J., Guenet, C., Merly, J.P., Teufel, M & Saudek, V. (2000). Solution structure of a neurotrophic ligand bound to FKBP12 and its effects on protein dynamics. *Eur. J Biochem.*, Vol 267, pp 5342-5355.

Snyder, S.H. (1992). Nitric Oxide: first in a new class of neurotransmitters. *Science*, Vol 257, pp 494-496.

Snyder, S.H., Lai, M.M. & Burnett, P.E. (1998). Immunophilins in the nervous system. *Neuron*, Vol 21, pp 283-294.

Steiner, J.P., Dawson, T.M., Fotuhi, M., Glatt, C.E., Snowman, A.M., Cohen, N & Snyder, S.H. (1992). High brain densities of the immunophilin FKBP colocalized with calcineurin. *Nature*, Vol 358, pp 584-587.

Steiner, J.P., Dawson, T.M., Fotuhi, M & Snyder, S.H. (1996). Immunophilin regulation of neurotransmitter release. *Mol. Med.*, Vol 2, pp 325-333.

Steiner, J.P., Hamilton, G.S., Ross, D.T., Valentine, H.L., Guo, H., Connolly, M.A., Liang, S., Ramsey, C., Li, J.H., Huang, W., Howorth, P., Soni, R., Fuller, M., Sauer, H., Nowotnik, A.C. & Suzdak, P.D. (1997). Neurotrophic immunophilin ligands stimulate structural and functional recovery in neurodegenerative animal models. *Proc. Natl. Acad. Sci. USA*, Vol 94, pp 2019-2024.

Tanaka, K. & Ogawa, N. (2004). Possibility of non-immunosuppressive immunophilin ligands as potential therapeutic agents for Parkinson's disease. *Curr. Pharm. Des.*, Vol 10, pp 669-677.

Tong, G., Shepherd, D. & Jahr, C.E. (1995). Synaptic desensitization of NMDA receptors by calcineurin. *Science*, Vol 267, pp 1510-1512.

Tong, Y. & Shen, J. (2009). Alpha-synuclein and LRRK2: partners in crime. *Neuron*, Vol 64, pp 771-773.

Van Duyne, G.D., Standaert, R.F., Karplus, P.A., Schreiber, S.L. & Clardy, J. (1993). Atomic structures of the human immunophilin FKBP-12 complexes with FK506 and rapamycin. *J Mol. Biol.*, Vol 229, pp 105-124.

Walker, V.E., Atanasiu, R., Lam, H. & Shrier, A. (2007). Co-chaperone FKBP38 promotes HERG trafficking. *J Biol. Chem.*, Vol 282, pp 23509-23516.

Wang, H.Q., Nakaya, Y., Du, Z., Yamane, T., Shirane, M., Kudo, T., Takeda, M., Takebayashi, K., Noda, Y., Nakayama, K.I. & Nishimura, M. (2005). Interaction of presenilins with FKBP38 promotes apoptosis by reducing mitochondrial Bcl-2. *Hum. Mol. Genet.*, Vol 14, pp 1889-1902.

Wang, X., Venable, J., LaPointe, P., Hutt, D.M., Koulov, A.V., Coppinger, J., Gurkan, C., Kellner, W., Matteson, J., Plutner, H., Riordan, J.R., Kelly, J.W., Yates, JR. & Balch, W.E. (2006). Hsp90 cochaperone Aha1 downregulation rescues misfolding of CFTR in cystic fibrosis. *Cell*, Vol 127, pp 803-815.

Winter, C., Schenkel, J., Burger, E., Eickmeier, C., Zimmermann, M & Herdegen, T. (2000). The immunophilin ligand FK506, but not GPI-1046, protects against neuronal death and inhibits c-Jun expression in the substantia nigra pars compacta following transection of the rat medial forebrain bundle. *Neuroscience*, Vol 95, pp 753-762.

10

Targeting Tyrosine Hydroxylase to Improve Bradykinesia

Michael F. Salvatore
Louisiana State University Health Sciences Center-Shreveport
USA

1. Introduction

The product of the tyrosine hydroxylase (TH) catalyzed conversion of L-tyrosine, L-DOPA, has been the gold standard for treating Parkinson's disease (PD) for half a century (Birkmayer and Hornykiewicz, 1961; Calne and Sandler, 1970). While L-DOPA therapy can improve locomotor disability in PD, it does not arrest the course of PD progression. Furthermore, dyskinesia is a debilitating side-effect of L-DOPA use over time. There have been promising results from preclinical and clinical studies for PD treatment. In fact, preclinical work indicates that enhanced TH protein expression accompanies locomotor improvements. Furthermore, the fact that L-DOPA treatment alone can improve locomotor dysfunction in PD is, by itself, a testimony to the critical importance of TH function in the nigrostriatal pathway for maintaining the capacity for initiating and maintaining normal locomotor activity. Clearly the major loss of TH, the rate-limiting enzyme of DA biosynthesis, in PD diminishes the capacity for locomotor activity. Surprisingly, efforts to treat PD symptoms have not deliberately focused on restoration of TH protein or its activity. Nonetheless, the rationale to focus on improving TH function to reduce the motor deficits associated with PD has been developed serendipitously over the past decade. Notably, research studying the neurobiological basis of how growth factors can improve locomotor activity in both Parkinson's disease and aging-related bradykinesia has revealed that increasing TH protein and its activity, through enhanced phosphorylation, should be a central feature of therapies intended to restore locomotor function in PD and aging-related Parkinsonism. Furthermore, these studies have led to the prospect that increasing DA tissue content in the substantia nigra alone could improve locomotor activity. Taken together, the possibility that increasing TH protein and activity in the substantia nigra could, by itself, restore locomotor deficits must be explored and no longer ignored.

2. The importance of tyrosine hydroxylase in Parkinson's disease

Undoubtedly, research in Parkinson's disease (PD) is flourishing on multiple fronts and substantial progress has been made in understanding PD and determining rationale for its treatment. Numerous studies have produced intriguing results on PD etiology from environmental, genetic, and aging-related associations. There has also been considerable focus upon PD treatment, from restoration of nigrostriatal neuropil function by increasing the expression of dopamine (DA)-regulating proteins with growth factors to understanding the impact of extrinsic forces (such as the physical activity and diet) on PD prevention or improvement of symptoms. There is also a rich literature on defining the role of not only DA regulation in PD, but also the involvement of other neurotransmitters, particularly glutamate, in PD progression. The awesome breadth and depth of this work precludes discussion for the purposes of this chapter. The goal of the chapter is to provide evidence that one way to understand PD and determine an accurate treatment is to examine post-translational events in the nigrostriatal pathway and its allied tissue during PD progression. Defining these cellular and biochemical processes could unravel a therapeutic avenue that would facilitate these post-translational events, which may already be at work to correct PD-related deficiencies in the nigrostriatal pathway. The brain is indeed a robust organ capable of plasticity to accommodate insults in order to maintain as normal of function that is possible. During PD progression, there is evidence of dopaminergic compensation which may maintain sufficient levels of DA necessary for normal locomotor activity until major loss of TH (>70%) occurs. Thus, a major theme of this article is to focus on how the dopamine-regulating proteins of the nigrostriatal pathway, in particular tyrosine hydroxylase (TH), are functioning during PD progression and to propose that targeting TH should be a major priority in treating the PD patient. It will be proposed that the insights gained, and still to be gained, from understanding TH regulation during PD progression or in aging-related Parkinsonism will yield molecular targets for accurate treatment of the locomotor dysfunction accompanying these conditions.

The theme of this chapter does not infer that PD can be simply resolved by targeting TH. Certainly there are a number of molecular events and deficiencies that occur in PD, including the devastating non-motor symptoms of PD, as highlighted in several recent and comprehensive reviews (Obeso et al., 2010; Lim and Lang, 2010). However, with regard to the goal of improving compromised locomotor activity and execution, it cannot be ignored that, at the very least, a partial restoration of the expression or enhancement of function of the dopamine-regulating proteins (TH, dopamine transporter, and vesicular monoamine transporter) is important to reclaim a normal locomotor phenotype in the PD patient. This should be obvious since DA has an established role in the modulation of locomotor activity (Rech et al., 1966; Calne and Sandler, 1970; Brown and Robbins, 1991).

The dopaminergic neuropil of the nigrostriatal pathway modulates the basal ganglia circuitry to affect locomotor activity. The modulation of DA signaling in the striatum, the terminal field region of the nigrostriatal pathway, has engaged most research efforts to define the role of DA in locomotor activity. Thus the current model of how DA modulates basal ganglia output to impact locomotor activity is based upon DA release and modulation of post-synaptic DA receptor-regulation of the activity of the striatal medium spiny neurons. Conversely, the attention paid to DA in the somatodendritic region has been spent on measures of viability of the nigrostriatal neuropil in post-mortem tissue from PD patients, models of PD, and in aging related Parkinsonism by quantification of TH protein levels in the substantia nigra (SN). In subsequent sections, it should become evident to the reader that measures of nigral TH should not be considered to be static index of nigrostriatal viability, but rather a possible measure of the remaining functional capacity of DA biosynthesis that could affect locomotor capacity. Indeed, a distinct minority of studies have shown that interference with dopamine signaling in the somatodendritic region of the nigrostriatal pathway in the SN does impact locomotion.

This chapter is also intended to present and discuss research of TH, an extraordinary enzyme with regard its multiple phosphorylation sites, and what phosphorylation of TH does to modulate its activity. Tyrosine hydroxylase is a vastly studied enzyme and its function in the CNS has been of great interest in the neurosciences. It is well known that TH protein levels precipitously decrease in PD progression. However, this decline is considerable prior to the presentation of PD symptoms (Bernheimer et al., 1973). While this curious observation led to examination of TH function in PD models, it has been a rather neglected area of study since. It is a major intent of this chapter to re-energize interest in studying the importance of TH function, through its post-translational modifications in PD progression and in aging-related Parkinsonism or bradykinesia, and how agents such as growth factors mechanistically improve its activity. There is a caveat in these studies of TH protein and function in the CNS, largely because we simply do not know at the present time (2011) the extent that site-specific phosphorylation of TH affects its activity *in vivo*. However, strides have been made to identify the post-translational changes in TH function, through phosphorylation assessment, that are associated with behavioral outcomes. However, the role TH phosphorylation may play in compensating for TH loss occurring during PD progression is poorly understood. This is ultimately a vital question for accurate therapies for PD and aging-related Parkinsonism because it may define what phosphorylation site could be targeted to enhance synthesis capabilities. Certainly, increasing TH protein expression is also a vital goal, at least in PD. Again, the fact that L-DOPA, the product of TH catalysis of tyrosine, is an effective treatment for PD symptoms belies the critical importance of TH in maintaining dopamine in quantities sufficient for normal locomotor activity.

3. Site-specific tyrosine hydroxylase phosphorylation *in vivo:* current status

The phosphorylation of TH is a well-established mechanism of regulating its activity. It is unique in that there are three physiologically-regulated sites in brain, ser19, ser31, and ser40 (Haycock and Haycock, 1991). As to be discussed, there is plenty of evidence from cellular work that increased phosphorylation at ser40 can regulate L-DOPA biosynthesis. However, there is also evidence that ser31 also plays a role and furthermore, there is recent evidence that ser31 phosphorylation status has a significant role in regulating basal levels of DA in terminal field and somatodendritic regions of DA pathways (including the nigrostriatal pathway) in brain (Salvatore et al., 2009b). Yet, the question remains today as to how phosphorylation at each site can regulate its activity *in vivo*. The answer to this question will provide insight in how to most efficiently activate TH in the face of its progressive loss as seen in PD. Significant momentum and insight to answer this question has been gained from growth factor studies, as to be discussed in later sections. If TH activity can be enhanced from a treatment, then perhaps only partial restoration of TH protein in PD may be sufficient to maintain the levels of DA that are necessary for locomotion. However, again, the questions are 1) at which phosphorylation site can or should this be achieved and, 2) as recent work is telling us, where, neuroanatomically, should this restoration of DA biosynthesis capabilities be targeted: the terminal fields in striatum or somatodendritic region on the substantia nigra?

The discovery of cAMP-dependent protein kinase (PKA) in brain (Miyamoto et al., 1969) and that PKA could activate TH in brain homogenates (Morgenroth et al. 1975) set forth an explosion of research to identify TH-phosphorylating protein kinases and TH phosphorylation sites that were later characterized to be ser8, ser19, ser31, and ser40; with ser40 being a PKA-phosphorylation site (Haycock, 1990). However, the focus of TH activation has predominated around PKA-mediated ser40 phosphorylation, with the long-standing assumption that any increase in ser40 phosphorylation increases TH activity. One could argue that because of the dominating attention the PKA-targeted phosphorylation site received, it has became virtual dogma that this phosphorylation site is the most critical site for regulation of TH activity. Yet it was also apparent, as studies went forward, that TH activation could occur on one of these phosphorylation sites not associated with PKA-mediated phosphorylation. Shortly after the discovery of ser31 as a TH phosphorylation site (Haycock, 1990), evidence suggested its phosphorylation could affect TH activity (Haycock et al., 1992). This supported an earlier observation, before ser31 was identified, that the peptide fragment associated with TH activation had ser31 in the sequence (Tachikawa et al., 1987). Indeed, increased ser31 phosphorylation, alone from NGF treatment or in conjunction with depolarization-stimulated ser19 phosphorylation, enhances L-DOPA accumulation and is independent of any affect on ser40 phosphorylation (Mitchell et al., 1990; Harada et al., 1996; Salvatore et al., 2001).

There certainly is substantial evidence that ser40 phosphorylation can modulate TH activity from *in vitro* and *in situ* work. Phosphorylation at ser40 reduces catecholamine-influenced end-product inhibition of TH (Fitzpatrick et al., 1999). It was also shown that the temporal dynamics of VIP-stimulation of PKA-activation and the associated increase in TH phosphorylation and activation were matched in chromaffin cells (Waymire et al., 1991), one of several studies to show that PKA activity could enhance TH activity. The identification of ser40 phosphorylation as the PKA-targeted site (Haycock, 1990) then firmly established the notion that ser40 phosphorylation was the key regulatory site of TH. The notion that ser40 is the sole regulator of TH activity has expanded into *in vivo* and *in situ* studies, as there are numerous reports detailing phosphorylation assessment only at ser40, to the exclusion of ser31 and ser19. While evidence supports that ser40 phosphorylation can regulate TH activity, including *in vivo* (Leviel et al., 1991), a critical threshold of phosphorylation may be necessary for an impact on biosynthesis. In PC12 cells, a two-fold increase in ser40 phosphorylation has no affect on L-DOPA biosynthesis, whereas a three-fold increase is associated with an increase (Salvatore et al, 2001). However, in the case of ser31, a two-fold increase may be sufficient to increase L-DOPA biosynthesis (Salvatore et al., 2001). These observations are highly relevant when applied to interpreting the impact of changes in ser31 and ser40 phosphorylation observed *in vivo*. Indeed, the results obtained in PC12 cells may have direct relevance to the *in vivo* situation because the basal phosphorylation of TH at ser31 and ser40 in the PC12 cell line versus that in the CNS are very similar, ranging from a phosphorylation stoichiometry of 0.02-0.05 for ser40 compared to 0.05 to 0.35 for ser31 (Salvatore et al., 2001; 2004; 2005; 2009a; 2009b) (Table 1). Therefore, in order to definitively answer whether any change in ser40 phosphorylation observed *in vivo* is of any consequence to L-DOPA biosynthesis capabilities, we must first define how much phosphorylation is necessary at ser40 and ser31 to affect L-DOPA biosynthesis capabilities *in vivo*.

Phosphorylation site	PC12 cells	striatum	Substantia nigra
Ser19	0.049	0.02 – 0.10	0.08 - 0.25
Ser31	0.088	0.15 – 0.35	0.05 - 0.10
Ser40	0.033	0.01 – 0.03	0.02 - 0.04

Table 1. **Tyrosine hydroxylase phosphorylation stoichiometry *in situ* and *in vivo*.** A comparison of TH phosphorylation in PC12 cells (Salvatore et al., 2001) versus the ranges reported in the nigrostriatal pathway *in vivo* (Salvatore et al., 2000; 2004; 2005; 2009a; 2009b). The *in vivo* TH phosphorylation ranges in striatum and substantia nigra represents results from mice (C57B1/6) and rats (Sprague-Dawley, Fischer 344, and Brown-Norway/Fischer 344 F_1 hybrid).

The first indication that increased ser40 phosphorylation might not necessary for activation of TH came from a study wherein depolarizing stimulation produced increased L-DOPA biosynthesis, even though the cells expressed TH with leucine substitution at ser40 (Harada et al., 1996). This study was the first to challenge the notion that only ser40 phosphorylation was important for regulation of TH activity. Yet, this conclusion was supported by earlier evidence to show that enhanced ser31 phosphorylation (or the peptide later found to correspond to ser31 in tryptic digest) alone was associated with enhanced TH activity (Tachikawa et al., 1987; Haycock et al., 1992). After the study by Harada and colleagues, it was shown in a cell line wherein PKA could not be activated (the A126 PC12 cell line) that a depolarization stimulated increase in ser31 phosphorylation could increase L-DOPA biosynthesis. Specifically, in both the wild-type PC12 and A126 cell line, the inhibition of mitogen-activated protein kinase produced a selective decrease in depolarization-stimulated ser31 phosphorylation accompanied by a reduction in depolarization-stimulated L-DOPA biosynthesis (Salvatore et al., 2001). This effect was later observed in striatal slices (Lindgren et al., 2002).

The finding that an increase in ser31 phosphorylation alone could enhance L-DOPA biosynthesis has significant impact for understanding how growth factors may improve locomotor activity (as to be discussed in the next section). Nearly two decades earlier, Greene and colleagues reported that the PC12 cell line was responsive to nerve growth factor (NGF) (Greene and Tischler, 1976). Furthermore, treatment with NGF increased TH activity for out to 1 hour (Greene et al., 1984). Subsequent studies indicated that the effect of NGF on TH phosphorylation is solely due to enhanced ser31 phosphorylation (Haycock 1990; Salvatore et al., 2001). There is also evidence that NGF-signaling can increase TH promoter activity (Suzuki et al., 2004). These findings are tremendously relevant for the evidence that growth factors can improve deficient locomotor activity in both PD and aging models. The synthesis of these three findings that 1) ser31 phosphorylation alone can increase L-DOPA biosynthesis in response to depolarizing stimulation, 2) a growth factor could accomplish the same end result, and 3) a growth factor like NGF can induce TH gene expression all make it plausible that the mechanism by which growth factors increase locomotor activity could be related to enhanced ser31 TH phosphorylation and regulation of TH protein expression, both of which would serve to regulate DA levels in a quantity sufficient to enhance locomotor capabilities.

While there is evidence for ser31 and ser40 phosphorylation in regulating TH activity, the role for ser19 phosphorylation *in vivo* is yet unknown. However, insights from cellular work indicate ser19 phosphorylation may be a sentinel for increased depolarizing activity, thus signaling that increased TH activity would be required to replenish DA lost from release.

Indeed, phosphorylation of ser19 requires Ca^{2+} (Waymire et al., 1988; Salvatore et al., 2001). Although ser19 does not directly influence TH activity (Sutherland et al.,1993; Haycock et al., 1998), it has been shown to facilitate ser40 phosphorylation *in situ* (Bevilaqua et al., 2001). To date, there are no reports on how ser19 phosphorylation may influence ser31 phosphorylation.

To date, there is evidence that ser31 may regulate basal DA biosynthesis capabilities *in vivo* (Salvatore et al., 2009b). We have recently shown that the differences in ser31 phosphorylation, but not ser40 phosphorylation, co-vary with differences in DA tissue content (Figure 1).

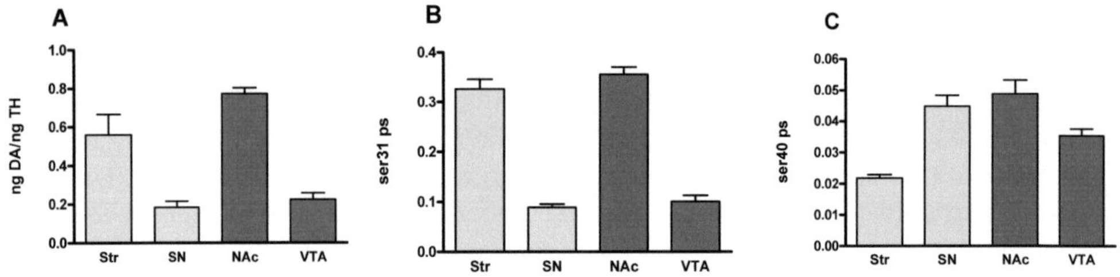

Fig. 1. **Relationship of DA tissue content with tyrosine hydroxylase ser31 and ser40 phosphorylation stoichiometry *in vivo*.** Four dopaminergic regions, striatum (Str), substantia nigra (SN), nucleus accumbens (NAc), and ventral tegmental area (VTA) were dissected from Brown-Norway/Fischer F344 F_1 hybrid rats and DA tissue content and TH protein inherent for each sample were analyzed from the same samples. **A)** The total recovered DA was normalized to total recovered TH protein to reveal differences in DA tissue content that could not be accounted for due to differences in TH protein recovery. To determine if phosphorylation at ser31 or ser40 could account for the differences in DA tissue content, we determined phosphorylation stoichiometry in each region. The differences in ser31 phosphorylation stoichiometry **(B)**, but not ser40 **(C)**, were similar to the differences in DA tissue content seen in **A.** *From Salvatore et al., 2009b*

In summary, there is no question that either increased ser31 or ser40 phosphorylation of TH can increase the biosynthesis of L-DOPA, leading to increased DA. There are still issues to be resolved. The first challenge lies in the acceptance of and practice of assessing ser31 phosphorylation in addition to ser40 phosphorylation in CNS studies of TH function or its role in behavioral paradigms. The second challenge is to ascertain how much phosphorylation at each site is necessary to produce an increase in L-DOPA biosynthesis.

4. Growth factors: dopamine & tyrosine hydroxylase

The objective in treating Parkinson's disease and aging-related Parkinsonism is to increase locomotor execution by increasing overall locomotor activity levels and the speed of execution. The discovery that glial cell line-derived neurotrophic factor (GDNF) delivery in CNS tissue can produce significant improvement in locomotor activity measures that are compromised in both aging and in PD models has revealed the critical importance of GDNF-signaling in maintenance of the nigrostriatal pathway (Hoffer et al., 1994; Gash et al., 1996; Gerhardt et al. 1999; Grondin et al 2003). There have also been successful outcomes to improve locomotor deficiencies from GDNF delivery via the use of viral-vectors. Delivery of GDNF using lentiviral vectors augments DA function in aged monkeys and reverses functional deficits caused by MPTP (Kordower et al., 2000). In fact, the precise delivery of specific quantities of the protein in the sub-nanogram quantities has shown promise for optimal outcomes in locomotor function and TH expression (Eslamboli et al., 2005). In the clinic, the outcomes from GDNF delivery on PD patients have been mixed (Gill et al., 2003; Slevin et al., 2005; Lang et al., 2006). There is evidence that the manner in which GDNF is infused into the brain may have significant impact on the clinical outcome due to the volume of distribution obtained following infusion (Hamilton et al., 2001; Ai et al., 2003; Gash et al., 2005; Salvatore et al., 2006). Notwithstanding the critical technical issues involved with GDNF delivery into the brain, there is substantial evidence that the neurobiological events triggered by GDNF delivery can have a positive influence on compromised locomotor function in PD and aging models, and possibly PD patients.

Recent work clearly indicates that maintaining GNDF signaling in the nigrostriatal pathway is critical for maintaining the DA phenotype into and beyond adulthood, as well as normal locomotor activity (Pascual et al., 2008; Nevalainen et al., 2010). Furthermore, there is definite evidence that GDNF-signaling regulates the DA phenotype through its impact on TH regulation. The mechanism by which GDNF signaling maintains or, in the case of treating PD, restores the DA phenotype involves its impact on TH expression and even TH phosphorylation. The partial depletion of the GDNF gene (GDNF +/- genotype) leads to a locomotor deficit at an earlier age during the course of aging (Boger et al., 2006). Not only is this deficit produced in the GDNF heterozygotes, but it is also observed in GDNF receptor (GFR α-1) heterozygote mice (Zaman et al., 2008). In both cases, there is significantly greater loss of TH protein with advancing age. These data suggest that there is a definite relationship between GDNF-signaling and locomotor activity, in which TH protein expression plays a vital mechanistic link. Other trophic factors can also enhance locomotor activity and DA signaling. Neurturin, an analog of GDNF, also enhances DA signaling and can protect against PD-like lesion (Gasmi et al., 2007; Cass and Peters, 2010). Most recently, there is evidence that another trophic factor, brain-derived neurotrophic factor (BDNF), also influences dopaminergic function and locomotor functions, as BDNF heterozygote mice exhibit declines in striatal DA release but, notably, without impact on TH protein expression (Boger et al., 2011). The possibility remains that diminished BDNF-signaling could affect TH phosphorylation, however, as GDNF has such effects, particularly on ser31 phosphorylation (Salvatore et al., 2004; 2009a).

Clearly the GDNF-related increase in DA tissue content or release capabilities seen in the nigrostriatal pathway has implications for involvement of enhanced tyrosine hydroxylase phosphorylation or TH protein biosynthesis. Indeed, in neuroblastoma and primary mesencephalic neurons it was shown that GDNF could increase TH phosphorylation (Kobori et al., 2003). The first *in vivo* study of the impact of GDNF on TH phosphorylation showed significant increases in TH phosphorylation in both striatum and substantia nigra, but the impact on specific phosphorylation sites showed a dichotomous result (Salvatore et al., 2004). In the substantia nigra, there was a profound increase in ser31, and only ser31 phosphorylation, the magnitude of which exceeded all other changes in TH phosphorylation examined (Salvatore et all, 2004). In striatum, all phosphorylation sites exhibited an increase in phosphorylation (Salvatore et al., 2004). Notably, this treatment also reduced TH protein levels in the nigrostriatal pathway, an effect which has also been reported in other studies in *intact,* but not lesioned, tissue (Georgievska et al., 2004). There is also evidence that the impact of GDNF on TH protein and phosphorylation is dose-dependent (Aoi et al., 2000; Salvatore et al., 2009a).

It is particularly notable that increased locomotor activity produced by GDNF is accompanied by increased DA tissue content in the SN, but not in striatum, regardless of the model of locomotor dysfunction, be it aging or a PD model (Hoffer et al., 1994; Gash et al., 1996; Hebert and Gerhardt, 1997; Gerhardt et al. 1999; Grondin et al 2003). However, the synaptic levels of striatal DA are affected following perburbations in GDNF-, BDNF-, or neurturin-related gene expression or delivery of these agents *in vivo* (Salvatore et al., 2004; Cass and Peters, 2010; Boger et al., 2011). These observations naturally raise the question of whether enhancement of locomotor activity by growth factors requires elevated DA-signaling in the striatum or SN. Furthermore, there is the question of how TH function in either region would ultimately affect DA signalling to affect locomotor activity. Bilateral improvement of locomotor activity after unilateral delivery of GDNF in striatum has been reported in clinical trials (Slevin et al., 2005) and bilateral effects on DA-regulating proteins like TH by unilateral GDNF have been shown to be limited to the SN (Salvatore et al., 2009a). Thus the increase in ser31 phosphorylation of TH, specifically in the SN, could be a critical molecular source to provide DA necessary for generating locomotor activity. This possibility leads to the necessity of asking how DA in striatum and the SN impact locomotor activity.

5. Tyrosine hydroxylase regulation in Parkinson's disease: role in dopaminergic compensation

It has been long noted that the pathological sequelae of PD include a major loss of TH protein in both the striatum and SN. There is evidence that TH activity may increase during PD progression, as increased DA release and TH activity occur in PD models (Snyder et al., 1990). TH activity may also be negatively affected by alpha-synuclein (to be discussed). Post-mortem analysis of PD brain tissue revealed the profound and yet unresolved finding that symptoms of PD were not apparent until the patient had at least 70% loss of the dopaminergic neuropil (Bernheimer et al., 1973). This observation led to formulating the concept of dopaminergic compensation, whereby locomotor functions continue normally in spite of loss of TH and other dopamine-regulating proteins until the 70-80% threshold is reached. One of the earliest observations to support dopaminergic compensation led to two hypotheses: one, that this mechanism was driving normal locomotion until the majority of the dopamine-regulating proteins were lost, but, two, at the same time could contribute to PD pathological progression (Agid et al., 1973). Other reports also suggest this compensatory mechanism may exacerbate toxicity to the nigrostriatal pathway (Zigmond et al, 2002). The human condition has been verified in MPTP-lesioned rhesus monkey in that the locomotor symptoms of PD are not present until there is nearly 80% loss of striatal DA (Bezard et al., 2001; Pifl et al., 2006). It is currently being debated as to whether or not increased striatal DA turnover can be observed during the asymptomatic stages of the disease or if, in fact, increased DA turnover is even a relevant index of dopaminergic compensation. There is support for dopaminergic compensation to maintain normal locomotion by evidence of enhanced striatal DA release (Perez et al., 2008). How TH activity is actually regulated by phosphorylation in a PD model is the subject of current investigation in this laboratory. Increased TH activity may be critical for ultimately maintaining normal locomotor activity during its progressive loss in PD. Infusion of the TH inhibitor AMPT hinders locomotor activity following nigrostriatal lesion (Leng et al, 2005), which argues that *de novo* DA biosynthesis is critical for dopaminergic compensation. As such, insights into which signaling pathway is more or less active could be made by determining how TH phosphorylation changes at each phosphorylation site in a PD model. This information, such as a decrease in ser31 phosphorylation for example, could be a guide to determining where deficiencies in signaling exist and reveal a therapeutic target.

The regulation of TH during PD progression may also be affected by alpha-synuclein. Not only has this ubiquitous protein been well-studied in *in vitro, in situ,* and in animal models for potential involvement in PD pathogenesis, but there is evidence that it may control TH activity and expression. Indeed, perhaps the strongest evidence to date that implicates alpha-synuclein in PD vulnerability is a report that in both aged monkeys and humans, there is a strong correlation to nigral TH protein loss with aging-related accumulation of non-aggregated alpha-synuclein (Chu and Kordower, 2007). Under specific conditions, there is evidence that alpha-synuclein can act as a molecular chaperone to regulate TH activity through phosphorylation (Perez et al., 2002; Peng et al., 2005; Drolet et al., 2006). Therefore, the adverse impact of this protein on TH activity or its ability to be activated by phosphorylation may be considered when determining therapeutic options involving the targeting of TH.

These considerations must also include consideration of where TH could be best targeted, either in the terminal fields or somatodendritic region. As already mentioned in the discussion on growth factors, targeting TH may be best in the SN. There is evidence that the compensatory response is greater in the SN than in striatum, because extracellular DA levels in the SN are maintained despite 90% cell loss (Sarre et al., 2004). Furthermore, prevention of rotational behavior induced by L-DOPA can be blocked by intranigral infusion of a DA D_1 antagonist, and is more effective on blocking rotational behavior than striatal infusion (Robertson and Robertson, 1989). Thus, it may be possible that elevated TH activity in the SN could produce DA in quantities sufficient enough to sustain locomotion until a critical amount of TH protein is lost during PD progression.

6. Tyrosine hydroxylase regulation in aging-related Parkinsonism

Aging is a significant risk factor for developing Parkinson's disease. However, aging-related Parkinsonism is a much greater risk factor associated with aging, with up to 50% of the elderly developing bradykinesia after reaching age 80 (Bennet et al., 1996; Prettyman, 1998; Murray et al., 2004; Fleischman et al., 2007). However, unlike the loss of TH seen in PD, over the course of the lifespan the loss of striatal TH in humans is very minor and nowhere near the >70% loss seen in symptomatic PD (Haycock et al., 2003). It might be argued that there is a decrease in striatal TH phosphorylation during aging, which would support the evidence of striatal DA loss in human (Kish et al., 1992; Haycock et al., 2003), but the rodent models do not consistently support this possibility (Cruz-Muros et al., 2007; Salvatore et al., 2009b). Thus, the dominating hypothesis that >70% loss of striatal DA must be present for the emergence of locomotor symptoms associated with PD are challenged when viewed from the standpoint of striatal TH regulation during aging. In animal model studies of aging effects on DA regulation, no study has shown loss of DA or TH to reach that of the symptomatic threshold of striatal DA or TH loss. In fact, while some studies do show loss of DA or TH approaching that seen in PD, ~60% (Collier et al., 2007)), many studies report much less, if any, loss of striatal DA or TH (Ponzio et al., 1982; Marshall and Rosenstein, 1990; Emerich et al., 1993; Irwin et al, 1994; Hebert and Gerhardt, 1998; Yurek et al., 1998; Gerhardt et al., 2002; Haycock et al., 2003; Cruz-Muros et al., 2007; Salvatore et al., 2009). In fact, 60% striatal DA loss still does not produce bradykinesia in a PD model (Bezard et al., 2001).

Two fundamental observations should prompt us to pause and consider the prospect that nigral DA affects locomotor activity. First, GDNF enhances nigral DA tissue content in both aging and PD models in conjunction with increases locomotor activity. Second, aging work reveals that little or no striatal TH loss occurs with advanced age and there is a highly variable but consistently less than 60% DA loss in aging. A deficiency in nigral DA in either PD or in aging may contribute to decreased locomotor activity. Two aging studies have reported loss of both DA and ser31 TH phosphorylation of a 30-50%magnitude in the midbrain or SN (Cruz-Muros et al., 2007; Salvatore et al., 2009b). Loss of TH in the SN of aged non-human primates has been reported to be ~50% (Emborg et al., 1998). In a PD model, bradykinesia is present when nigral TH loss is at 50% (Bezard et al., 2001). Human data also indicate loss of DA neuropil of this magnitude in the SN in aging (Fearnley and Lees, 1991; Ross et al., 2004) or with PD (Marsden, 1990). Clinical studies of TH function in movement disorders is quite limited, but recent work in post-mortem tissue of Restless Leg Syndrome patients indicates that there is increased TH activity not only in putamen, but also in the SN (Connor et al., 2009). The possible importance of targeting the SN for treating PD has also been suggested for future work, as suggested in a recent report of a clinical trial involving the bilateral AAV-mediated gene delivery of neurturin in the putamen (Marks et al., 2010).

The abundance of GDNF-impact data has pointed to the possibility that DA regulation in the SN affects locomotor activity. In fact, a recent report has shown there is an aging-related decrease in the expression of the soluble isoform of the GDNF receptor, GFRα-1 only in the substantia nigra (Pruett and Salvatore, 2010). Taken together, these results all point to the possibility that TH regulation in the SN may be an important target for improving aging- or PD-related locomotor deficits, particularly bradykinesia. Thus, if deficits in nigral TH expression or phosphorylation in PD and aging are involved with locomotor dysfunction, an important question to ask is whether interference with DA signaling, specifically in the SN, could affect locomotor activity in otherwise normal rats.

7. Proposed role for nigral tyrosine hydroxylase function in locomotor activity

When it comes to defining how exactly DA modulates basal ganglia function, and hence locomotor activity, there is a wide consensus that DA function in the striatum is most critical. Yet, ever since somatodendritic DA release was reported (Cheramy et al., 1981), there have been reports from a variety of paradigms to suggest nigral DA alone can influence locomotor behavior. This possibility is a critical perspective to recognize if we are to understand how to successfully treat PD or aging-related bradykinesia. Specifically, from the perspective of striatal DA loss in PD and in aging, if striatal DA is most critical for bradykinesia arising from aging or PD, then there is a critical discrepancy at hand. That is, even though both conditions share a common symptom of bradykinesia, there is a starkly different magnitude of striatal DA loss in some cases and furthermore, no aging study has reported striatal DA to reach this critical threshold. Thus, if we are to accept that PD symptoms like bradykinesia are not present until there is 70% loss of TH or DA, which is supported by human PD pathology and PD models (Berheimer et al., 1973; Bezard et al., 2001), then how does bradykinesia come about in aging? Furthermore, do we dare ask if

70% striatal loss of TH or DA is really the threshold for symptom manifestation in PD, or is loss in another region like the SN more critical?

Observations in intact rats suggest that this question should be asked. Nigral application of DA modulates the output of the pars reticulata output (Waszczak and Walters, 1983; Kleim et al., 2007). Nigral infusion of a D_1 receptor antagonist suppresses operant behavior and open-field locomotion (Trevitt et al., 2001), and execution of motor performance (Bergquist et al., 2003). Depletion of nigral DA stores with tetrabenazine also hinders the ability to negotiate simple motor tasks (Andersson et al., 2006). We have most recently shown in longitudinally-characterized locomotor activity in rats that nigral DA correlates to lifetime locomotor activity initiation and maintenance, but not speed (Salvatore et al., 2009b).

These observations suggest that nigral TH function, as governed by TH protein expression and phosphorylation, may play a critical role in regulating the capacity for locomotor activity. The combination of phosphorylation at ser31 and the protein levels of TH may be a significant molecular source of producing DA that impacts the capacity for locomotor activity with regard to its initiation and frequency. Thus, the amount of local release of DA is proposed to be regulated by TH protein and phosphorylation. The released DA is proposed to act upon post-synaptic DA D_1 receptors. This local action in the SN increases GABA release from the striatonigral terminals, and disinhibits the inhibitory output neurons of the pars reticulata, thus facilitating locomotor activity. It is proposed that aging or PD-related deficits in locomotor activity may stem from deficiencies in either TH protein or TH phosphorylation at ser31 in the SN (Figure 2).

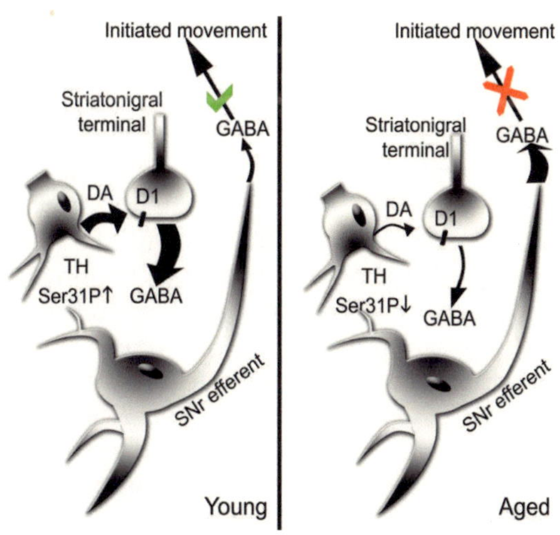

Fig. 2. **Proposed role of nigral DA leading to bradykinesia in aging.** It is proposed that inhibition of locomotion (bradykinesia) may occur by diminished local release of DA in the SN. Normally (as depicted in the young rat scenario on the left), released DA, acting upon post-synaptic D_1 receptors of the striatonigral terminals, promotes GABA release, which in turn reduces tonic release of GABA from the SNr efferent. This facilitates locomotor activity. When DA release capacity is deficient (as depicted in the aged rat scenario on the right), as proposed to be due to decreased TH protein or ser31 phosphorylation levels, the ability to promote GABA release from the striatonigral terminals is diminished, thereby removing an inhibition of GABA release from the SNr efferent, which promotes excess GABA release and inhibits locomotor activity.

8. Non-invasive approaches to target tyrosine hydroxylase function

The impact of exogenous sources of growth factors upon locomotor activity, DA tissue content and release, TH protein and phosphorylation is well-established. These observations allow us to question whether any non-invasive means exist to influence DA regulation *in vivo*. Increased production of growth factors from forced exercise, caloric restriction, and even components of the diet *in vivo* have been observed. Their impact on locomotor activity is an emerging and exciting topic as to the non-invasive measures we can take to improve locomotor deficits in PD or stave-off deficits produced by aging. Indeed, the enhancement of TH protein or its activity by phosphorylation may be a central mediator of the benefits to locomotor function realized by these non-invasive practices.

8.1 Exercise

Exercise is an activity that can be done at will with varying degrees of intensity, frequency, and longevity. Human and preclinical studies of exercise are revealing that these three variables associated with exercise have a significant impact upon our cognition and ability to move with advancing age and in the PD patient. For example in human studies, the volume of the hippocampus can increase and resist aging-related loss in volume as a result of aerobic exercise. Such changes are associated with improved memory function (Erickson et al., 2011). Exercise can prevent or reduce the risk of PD, as some longitudinal human studies support that regular exercise may lower the risk of PD (Chen et al., 2005). Other such studies do not support this hypothesis, with the caveat that study size was limited (Logroscino et al., 2006). The incidence of aging-related Parkinsonism and the disabilities arising from it may also be reduced from the quantity of physical activity that begins in midlife of healthy individuals (Savela et al., 2010). In the PD patient, there are definite benefits of exercise, and the frequency and intensity of it may be critical for its benefit. Exercise can improve motor performance and the physical activities of daily living in PD patients (Crizzle and Newhouse, 2006) and improve the efficacy of L-DOPA to improve motor performance (Muhlack et al., 2007). Most recently, the results of a forced exercise paradigm in human PD patients has shown that patients choosing to exercise on a bike with a trainer at a rate 30% greater than their preferred voluntary rate had a 35% improvement in their Unified Parkinson's Disease Rating Scale motor scores (Ridgel et al., 2009). Indeed, there is evidence from human studies that the intensity, frequency, and longevity of exercise may influence our innate capacity to move normally. The exciting aspect of this work is that exercise can be beneficial over short or long-term, even in a motorically-compromised state as seen in PD and may diminish the incidence of aging-related Parkinsonism.

The molecular events triggered in the CNS from exercise have been the subject of much study and appear to be related to growth factor production. An increase in mild cellular stress and angiogenesis are also thought to initiate signaling cascades that can be protective of DA neurons (rev. Zigmond et al., 2009). It is certainly believed that a relationship between innate DA function and physical activity exists (Knab and Lightfoot, 2010), and a number of studies examining this relationship supports this idea. Perhaps the single most compelling observation is that exercise does show a positive correlation to locomotor capabilities, which have a well-established relationship with DA regulation in the nigrostriatal pathway. Thus, the impact of exercise on TH regulation in aging and in PD models has been studied in several exercise paradigms. In animal studies, exercise paradigms are divided into voluntary or forced paradigms. In voluntary exercise, test subjects are given free access (within defined periods of time allowed for access) to an apparatus that permits and engages physical activity, most commonly a running wheel (Gerecke et al., 2010). In forced exercise, the test subjects are placed onto a treadmill on a near-daily basis and are coerced to run at a given rate of speed (12 - 20 meters/min) within a specific period of time that is typically much shorter that that used in voluntary (Tajari et al., 2010).

Regardless of the exercise paradigm used in animal studies, there is strong evidence of enhanced growth factor production, notably brain-derived neurotrophic factor (BDNF) and glial cell line-derived neurotrophic factor (GDNF) (Tajiri et al., 2010). In humans, there is a two- to three-fold increase in BDNF release from the human brain during exercise (Rasmussen et al., 2009) and endurance training also enhances the quantity of normal BDNF release compared to that seen at rest (Seifert et al., 2010). Given the well-established relationship of growth factors with TH and DA modulation, it would therefore be expected that exercise could affect TH and DA. Treadmill exercise in both PD and aging models does modulate DA tissue content and TH protein. In PD models, the impact of chemical lesions to the nigrostriatal pathway is lessened by treadmill exercise as evidenced by increased TH protein in the striatum and SN (Yoon et al., 2007). However, other reports show that despite locomotor activity improvements from exercise, no change in striatal DA or TH is observed (O'Dell et al., 2007; Petzinger et al., 2007), leaving open the possibility that enhancement of nigral TH function may be involved with locomotor activity effect. In fact, others have shown that extended periods of exercise (4-12 weeks), either treadmill (forced) or voluntary, increase nigral TH mRNA expression (Foley and Fleshner, 2008) or TH expression (Tumer et al., 2001; Gerecke et al., 2010; Tajiri et al., 2010). Thus, frequent exercise may enhance DA tone in the nigrostriatal pathway through enhancement of TH expression.

8.2 Diet: caloric restriction

The relationship of caloric intake with regulation of nigrostriatal DA function is becoming established. Seminal work showed aged rats that underwent calorie restriction (CR) had locomotor performances equal to that of younger adult rats. Furthermore, these CR aged rats had a 5-fold improvement in locomotor performance compared to age-matched controls, fed *ad libitum*. This work indicates that an innate molecular process associated with aging is hindered or diminished by CR. Calorie restriction increases striatal expression of GDNF in non-human primates (Maswood et al., 2004). Thus, if GDNF signaling is sufficiently active from CR, the impact of CR on locomotor activity could again, as in the case proposed in exercise, increase TH expression or activity enough to maintain DA signaling necessary for normal locomotor activity. Caloric restriction (CR) improves locomotor capabilities in PD models (Maswood et al., 2004) and preserves locomotor capabilities in aging models (Ingram et al., 1987; Weed et al., 1997; Kastman et al., 2010). Striatal DA loss from lesion is less severe in MPTP-treated monkeys on a 30% CR for about 6 months (Maswood et al., 2004) and amphetamine produces a marked enhancement locomotor activity in CR rats compared to rats fed *ab libitum* (Mamczarz et al., 2005; Marinkovic et al., 2007). An increase in DA release capacity from CR, as suggested by the Mamczarz study, strongly suggests an increase in DA biosynthesis capacity via increased TH protein or phosphorylation. The impact of CR on TH function has been studied sparingly. In fact, literature search yielded just one paper on the effect of 30 days CR on TH protein and ser40 phosphorylation (ser31 not studied). There was a trend toward increased TH protein in the SN. There was also an increase in striatal TH protein. There was no significant effect on ser40 phosphorylation of TH (Pan et al., 2006). However, through enhancement of GDNF expression, CR could increase TH activity via ser31 phosphorylation, which is increased by exogenous GDNF delivery *in vivo* (Salvatore et al., 2004). This would improve locomotor activity by enhancement of DA signaling, as already demonstrated in the Mamczarz and Marinkovic studies.

8.3 Diet: nutritive substances

There is an emerging literature on the relationship of fatty acid and cholesterol intake and the risk of PD (Liu et al., 2010; Miyake et al., 2010). Inhibition of cholesterol synthesis can reduce the severity of L-DOPA-induced dyskinesia in 6-OHDA lesioned rats (Schuster et al., 2008). A high-fat diet has been recently shown to promote greater DA depletion in both the striatum and SN following 6-OHDA (Morris et al., 2010). Cholesterol metabolites (oxysterols) do cross the blood-brain barrier and thus could interact with nigrostriatal neurons, possibly through liver X receptors (Sacchetti et al., 2009). Indeed, there is evidence that these oxysterols can modulate TH expression in neuroblastoma cells (Rantham Prabhakara et al., 2008). However, there is also evidence that a high dietary intake of omega-3 polyunsaturated fatty acids (PUFA), as found in fish oil extracts, is reported to be effective to sparing MPTP-induced loss of dopaminergic neuropil in the somatodendritic region of the nigrostriatal pathway (Bousquet et al., 2008). Furthermore, while the high PUFA was without effect on preventing MPTP-induced loss of TH protein in the striatum, there was a significant effect of the high PUFA diet on protecting against striatal DA loss (Bousquet et al., 2008). This exciting result may signify that high PUFA diet can activate signaling pathways to increase TH phosphorylation when loss of TH protein is occurring. The high-PUFA diet can increase BDNF expression in the striatum (Bouquet et al., 2009). Given that BDNF can increase ERK activity (Jovanovic et al., 2004), an increase in ERK activity would increase TH phosphorylation at ser31. Thus, a common denominator in enhancement or protection against nigrostriatal DA loss in a PD model, once again, appears to be an enhancement of ERK-signaling, via increased growth factor production, which could ultimately increase TH activity.

9. Future directions

Certainly there is evidence that the non-invasive lifestyle habits of exercise, caloric restriction, and diet could achieve a desirable end result of activating nigrostriatal TH to amounts sufficient to produce levels of DA necessary for normal locomotor activity. However, it is clear that the impact of these strategies upon striatal DA and TH have yielded ambiguous results and their relative impact on nigral DA and TH has yet to be fully revealed. Nonetheless, these lifestyle strategies can enhance growth factor expression. Growth factors also can enhance DA signaling and TH expression or phosphorylation *in vivo,* in conjunction with their locomotor benefits. Thus, it is an exciting prospect that TH function could be regulated from a non-invasive approach. Still, it is likely that some motorically-compromised individuals would be incapable of performing the rigorous demands of exercise required to yield an improvement in locomotor capabilities; certainly this would be the case for one afflicted with moderate-severe stage PD or one who has a physical impairment that prevents exercise. Thus the therapeutic options for such individuals, when removing the prospect of surgical approaches, are currently non-existent. Therefore, the ultimate challenge to maintain locomotor activity to conduct normal daily activities may be to take a pharmacological approach that targets TH and augments its expression and activity.

Clearly there is a critical battery of studies to support that augmenting nigral DA tissue content through enhancement of TH protein and phosphorylation could be the approach to improving the locomotor deficits seen in PD and aging. We have also known of the existence of somatodendritic DA release since the late 70s. There are handful of studies spanning nearly 30 years to support that nigral DA can influence aspects of locomotor activity. Clearly, there are still challenges in understanding the role of TH phosphorylation *in vivo,* notably, defining how much phosphorylation at TH is necessary at ser31 and ser40 to affect TH activity. Nonetheless, research efforts from a variety of angles that have been intended to improve locomotor impairment in PD and aging-related bradykinesia have shown, perhaps serendipitously, that targeting TH protein and its phosphorylation may be a promising molecular target to combat the locomotor deficits of PD and in aging.

10. References

Agid, Y, Javoy, F, & Glowinski, J. (1973). Hyperactivity of remaining dopaminergic neurones after partial destruction of the nigrostriatal dopaminergic system in the rat. *Nature New Biology* 245, 150-151. ISSN 0028-0836

Ai, Y, Markesbery, W, Zhang, Z, Grondin, R, Elseberry, D, Gerhardt, GA, & Gash, DM. (2003) Intraputamental infusion of GDNF in aged Rhesus monkeys: Distribution and dopaminergic effects. *J Comp Neurol* 461, 250-261. ISSN 0021-9967

Andersson, DR, Nissbrandt, H, & Bergquist, F. (2006). Partial depletion of dopamine in substantia nigra impairs motor performance without altering striatal dopamine neurotransmission. *Eur J Neurosci* 24, 617-624. ISSN 0953816X

Aoi, M, Date, I, Tomita, S, & Ohmoto, T. (2000). The effect of intrastriatal single injection of GDNF on the nigrostriatal dopaminergic system in hemiparkinsonian rats: behavioral and histological studies using two different dosages. *Neurosci Res* 36, 319-325. ISSN 1097-4547

Bennet, DA, Beckett, LA, Murray, AM, Shannon, KM, & Goetz, CG, Pilgrim, DM, & Evans, DA. (1996). Prevalence of Parkinsonian signs and associated mortality in a community population of older people. *New England J Med* 334, 71-76. ISSN 0028-4793

Bergquist, F, Shahabi, HN, & Nissbrandt, H. (2003). Somatodendritic dopamine release in rat substantia nigra influences motor performance on the accelerating rod. *Brain Res* 973, 81-91. ISSN 0006-8993

Bernheimer, H, Birkmayer, W, Hornykiewicz, O, Jellinger, K, & Seitelberger F, (1973). Brain dopamine and the syndromes of Parkinson and Huntington. Clinical, morphological and neurochemical correlations. *J. Neurological Sci.* 20, 415-455. ISSN 1302-1664

Bevilaqua, LRM, Graham, ME, Dunkley, PR, von Nagy-Felsobuki, EI, & Dickson, PW. (2001). Phosphorylation of Ser19 alters the conformation of tyrosine hydroxylase to increase the rate of phosphorylation of ser40. *J Biol Chem* 276, 40111-40116. ISSN 0021-9258

Bezard, E, Dovero, S, Prunier, C, Ravenscroft, P, Chalon, S, Guilloteau, D, Crossman, AR, Bioulac, B, Brotchie, JM, & Gross, CE. (2001). Relationship between the appearance of symptoms and the level of nigrostriatal degeneration in a progressive 1-methyl-

4-phenyl-1,2,3,6-tetrahydropyridine-lesioned Macaque model of Parkinson's disease. *J Neurosci* 21, 6853-6861. ISSN 0270-6474

Birkmayer, W, & Hornykiewicz, O. (1961). The L-3,4-dioxyphenylalanine (DOPA)-effect in Parkinson-akinesia. *Wien Klin Wochenschr* 73, 787-788. ISSN 0043-5325

Boger, HA, Middaugh, LD, Huang, P, Zaman, V, Smith, AC, Hoffer, BJ, Tomac, AC, & Granholm, AC. (2006). A partial GDNF depletion leads to earlier age-related deterioration of motor function and tyrosine hydroxylase expression in the substantia nigra. *Exp Neurol* 202, 336-347. ISSN 0014-4886

Boger, HA, Mannangatti, P, Samuvel, DJ, Saylor, AJ, Bender, TS, McGinty, JF, Fortress, AM, Zaman, V, Huang, P, Middaugh, LD, Randall, PK, Jayanthi, LD, Rohrer, B, Helke, KL, Granholm, AC, & Ramamoorthy, S. (2011). Effects of brain-derived neurotrophic factor on dopaminergic function and motor behavior during aging. *Genes, Brain, and Behavior* 10, 186-198. ISSN 1601-183X

Bousquet, M, Saint-Pierre, M, Julien, C, Salem, N, Cicchetti, F, & Calon, F. (2008). Beneficial effects of dietary omega-3 polyunsaturated fatty acid on toxin-induced neuronal degeneration in an animal model of Parkinson's disease. *FASEB J.* 22, 1213-1225. ISSN 1530-6860

Bousquet, M, Gibrat, C, Saint-Pierre, M, Julien, C, Calon, F, & Cicchetti, F. (2009). Modulation of brain-derived neurotrophic factor as a potential neuroprotective mechanism of action of omega-3 fatty acids in a parkinsonian animal model. *Prog Neuro-Psychopharm & Biol Psych* 33, 1401-1408. ISSN 0278-5846

Brown, VJ, & Robbins, TW. (1991). Simple and choice reaction time performance following unilateral striatal dopamine depletion in the rat. Impaired motor readiness but preserved response preparation. *Brain* 114, 513-525. ISSN 0006-8950

Calne, DB, & Sandler, M. (1970). L-DOPA and Parkinsonism. *Nature* 226, 21-24. ISSN 0028-0836

Cass, WA, & Peters, LE. (2010). Neurturin protects against 6-hydroxydopamine-induced reductions in evoked dopamine overflow in rat striatum. *Neurochem Int* 57, 540-546. ISSN 1872-9754

Chen, H, Zhang, SM, Schwarschild, MA, Hernan, MA, & Ascherio, A. (2005). Physical activity and the risk of Parkinson's disease. *Neurology* 64, 664-669. ISSN 0028-3878

Cheramy, A, Leviel, V, & Glowinski, J. (1981). Dendritic release of dopamine in the substantia nigra. *Nature* 289, 537-542. ISSN 0028-0836

Chu, Y, & Kordower, JH. (2007). Age-associated increases of a-synuclein in monkeys and humans are associated with nigrostriatal dopamine depletion: Is this the target for Parkinson's disease? *Neurobiol Aging* 25, 134-149. ISSN 0197-4580

Collier, TJ, Lipton, J, Daley, BF, Palfi, S, Chu, Y, Sortwell, C, Bakay, RA, Sladek, JR, & Kordower, JH. (2007). Aging-related changes in the nigrostriatal dopamine system and the response to MPTP in nonhuman primates: Diminished compensatory mechanisms as a prelude to parkinsonism. *Neurobiol Dis* 26, 56-65. ISSN 0969-9961

Connor, JR, Wang, X-S, Allen, RP, Beard, JL, Wiesinger, JA, Felt, BT, & Earley, CJ. (2009). Altered dopaminergic profile in the putamen and substantia nigra in restless leg syndrome. *Brain* 132, 2403-2412. ISSN 0006-8950

Crizzle, AM, & Newhouse, IJ. (2006). Is physical exercise beneficial for persons with Parkinson's disease? *Clin J Sport Med* 16, 422-425. ISSN 1050-642X

Cruz-Muros, I, Afonso-Oramas, D, Abreu, P, Barroso-Chinea, P, Rodríguez, M, Gonzalez, MC, & Hernandez, TG. (2007). Aging of the rat mesostriatal system: Differences between the nigrostriatal and the mesolimbic compartments. *Exp. Neurol.* 204, 147-161. ISSN 0014-4886

Drolet, RE, Behrouz, B, Lookingland, KJ, & Goudreau, JL. (2006). Substrate-mediated enhancement of phosphorylated tyrosine hydroxylase in nigrostriatal dopamine neurons: evidence for a role of alpha-synuclein. *J Neurochem* 96, 950-959. ISSN 0022-3042

Emborg, ME, Ma, SY, Mufson, EJ, Levey, AI, & Taylor, MD, Brown, WD, Holden, JE, & Kordower, JH. (1998). Age-related declines in nigral neuronal function correlate with motor impairments in rhesus monkeys. *J Comp Neurol* 401, 253-265. ISSN 0021-9967

Emerich, DF, McDermott, P, Krueger, P, Banks, M, Zhao, J, Marszalkowski, J, Frydel, B, Winn, SR, & Sanberg, PR. (1993). Locomotion of aged rats: Relationship to neurochemical but not morphological changes in nigrostriatal dopaminergic neurons. *Brain Res Bull* 32, 477-486. ISSN 0361-9230

Erickson, KI, Voss, MW, Prakash, RS, Basak, C, Szabo, A, Chaddock, L, Kim, JS, Heo, S, Alves, H, White, SM, Wojcicki, TR, Mailey, EL, Vieira, VJ, Martin, SA, Pence, BD, Woods, JA, McAuley, E, & Kramer, AF. (2011). Exercise training increases size of hippocampus and improves memory. *Proc Nat Acad Sci* 108, 3017-3022. ISSN 0027-8424

Eslamboli, A, Georgievska, B, Ridley, RM, Baker, HF, Muzyczka, N, Burger, C, Mandel, RJ, Annett, L, & Kirik, D. (2005). Continuous low-level glial cell line-derived neurotrophic factor delivery using recombinant adeno-associated viral vectors provides neuroprotection and induces behavioral recovery in a primate model of Parkinson's disease. *J Neurosci* 25, 769-777. ISSN 0270-6474

Fearnley, JM, & Lees, AJ. (1991). Ageing and Parkinson's disease: Substantia nigra regional selectivity. *Brain* 114, 2283-2301. ISSN 0006-8950

Fitzpatrick, PF. (1999). Tetrahydropterin-dependent amino acid hydroxylases. *Ann RevBiochem* 68, 355-381. ISSN 0066-4154

Fleischman, DA, Wilson, RS, Schneider, JA, Beinias, JL, & Bennet, DA. (2007). Parkinsonian signs and functional disability in old age. *Exp Aging Res*, 33, 59-76. ISSN 0361-073X

Foley, TE & Fleshner MR. (2008). Neuroplasticity of dopamine circuits after exercise: implications for central fatigue. *Neuromolec Med* 10: 67-80, 2008. ISSN 1535-1084

Gash, DM, Zhang, Z, Ai, Y, Grondin, R, Coffey, R, & Gerhardt, GA. (2005). Trophic factor distribution predicts functional recovery in Parkinsonian monkeys. *Ann Neurol* 58, 224-233. ISSN 0364-5134

Gash, DM, Zhang, Z, Ovadia, A, Cass, WA, Ai, Y Simmerman, L, Russell D, Martin, D, Lapchak, PA, Collins, F, Hoffer, BJ, & Gerhardt, GA. (1996). Functional recovery in parkinsonian monkeys treated with GDNF. Nature 380: 252-255. ISSN 0028-0836

Gasmi, M, Brandon, EP, Herzog, CD, Wilson, A, Bishop, KM, Hofer, EK, Cunningham, JJ, Printz, MA, Kordower, JH, & Bartus, RT. (2007). AAV2-mediated delivery of human neurturin to the rat nigrostriatal system: long-term efficacy and tolerability of CERE-120 for Parkinson's disease. *Neurobiol Dis* 27, 67-76. ISSN 0969-9961

Georgievska, B, Kirik, D, & Bjorklund, A. (2004). Overexpression of glial cell line-derived neurotrophic factor using a lentiviral vector induces time- and dose-dependent downregulation of tyrosine hydroxylase in the intact nigrostriatal dopamine system. *J Neurosci* 24, 6437-6445. ISSN 0270-6474

Gerecke, KM, Jiao, Y, Pani, A, Pagala, V, & Smeyne, RJ. (2010). Exercise protects against MPTP-induced neurotoxicity in mice. *Brain Res* 1341, 72-83. ISSN 0006-8993

Gerhardt, GA, Cass WA, Huettl P, Brock S, Zhang Z, & Gash,D.M. (1999).GDNF improves dopamine function in the substantia nigra but not the putamen of unilateral MPTP-lesioned rhesus monkeys. *Brain Res* 817, 163-171. ISSN 0006-8993

Gerhardt, GA, Cass, WA, Yi, A, Zhang, Z, & Gash, DM. (2002). Changes in somatodendritic but not terminal dopamine regulation in aged rhesus monkeys. *J Neurochem* 80, 168-177. ISSN 0022-3042

Gill, SS, Patel, NK, Hotton, GR, O'Sullivan, K, McCarter, R, Bunnage, M, Brooks, DJ, Svendsen, CN, & Heywood, P. (2003). Direct brain infusion of glial cell line-derived neurotrophic factor in Parkinson disease. *Nature Med* 9, 589-595. ISSN 1078-8956

Greene LA, & Tischler AS. (1976). Establishment of a noradrenergic clonal line of rat adrenal pheochromocytoma cells which respond to nerve growth factor. *Proc Nat Acad Sci* 73, 2424-2428. ISSN 0027-8424

Greene, LA, Seeley, PJ, Rukenstein, A, DiPiazza, M, & Howard, A. (1984). Rapid activation of tyrosine hydroxylase in response to nerve growth factor. *J Neurochem* 42, 1728-1734. ISSN 0022-3042

Grondin, R, Cass, WA, Zhang, Z, Stanford, JA, Gash, DM, & Gerhardt, GA. (2003). Glial Cell Line-Derived Neurotrophic Factor Increases Stimulus-Evoked Dopamine Release and Motor Speed in Aged Rhesus Monkeys. *J Neurosci* 23, 1974-1980. ISSN 0270-6474

Hamilton, JF, Morrison, PF, Chen, MY, Harvey-White, J, Pernaute, RS, Phillips, H, Oldfield, E, & Bankiewicz, KS. (2001). Heparin coinfusion during convection-enhanced delivery (CED) increases the distribution of the glial-derived neurotrophic factor (GDNF) ligand family in rat striatum and enhances the pharmacological activity of neurturin. *Exp Neurol* 168, 155-161. ISSN 0014-4886

Harada, K, Wu, J, Haycock, JW, & Goldstein, M. (1996). Regulation of L-DOPA biosynthesis by site-specific phosphorylation of tyrosine hydroxylase in AtT-20 cells expressing wild-type and serine 40-substituted enzyme. *J Neurochem* 67, 629-635. ISSN 0022-3042

Haycock, JW. (1990). Phosphorylation of tyrosine hydroxylase *in situ* at serine 8, 19, 31, and 40. *J Biol Chem* 265, 11682-11691. ISSN 0021-9258

Haycock, JW, & Haycock, DA. (1991). Tyrosine hydroxylase in rat brain dopaminergic nerve terminals: Multiple-site phosphorylation *in vivo* and in synaptosomes. *J Biol Chem* 266, 5650-5657. ISSN 0021-9258

Haycock, JW, Ahn, NG, Cobb, MH, & Krebs, EG. (1992) ERK1 and ERK2, two microtubule-associated protein 2 kinases, mediate the phosphorylation of tyrosine hydroxylase at serine-31 in situ. *Proc Natl Acad Sci* 89, 2365-2369. ISSN 0027-8424

Haycock, JW, Lew, JY, Garcia-Espana, A, Lee, KY, Harada, K, Meller, E, & Goldstein, M. (1998). Role of Serine-19 phosphorylation in regulating tyrosine hydroxylase studied with site- and phosphospecific antibodies and site-directed mutagenesis. *J Neurochem* 71, 1670-1675. ISSN 0022-3042

Haycock, JW, Becker, L, Ang, L, Furukawa, Y, Hornykiewicz, O, & Kish, SJ. (2003). Marked disparity between age-related changes in dopamine and other presynaptic dopaminergic markers in human striatum. *J Neurochem* 87, 574-585. ISSN 0022-3042

Hebert, MA, & Gerhardt, GA. (1998). Normal and drug-induced locomotor behavior in aging: comparison to evoked DA release and tissue content in Fischer 344 rats. *Brain Res* 797, 42-54. ISSN 0006-8993

Hoffer, BJ, Hoffman, AF, Bowenkamp, KE, Huettl, P, Hudson, J, Martin, D, Lin, LF, & Gerhardt, GA (1994). Glial cell line-derived neurotrophic factor reverses toxin-induced injury to midbrain dopaminergic neurons in vivo. *Neurosci Lett* 182:107-111. ISSN 0304-3940

Ingram, DK, Weindruch, RH, Spangler, EL, Freeman, JR, & Walford, RL. (1987). Dietary restriction benefits learning and motor performance of aged mice. *J Gerontol* 42, 78-81. ISSN 0022-1422

Irwin, I, DeLanney, LE, McNeill, T, Chan, P, Forno, LS, Murphy, GM, DiMonte, DA, Sandy, MS, Langston, JW. (1994). Aging and the nigrostriatal dopamine system: a non-human primate study. *Neurodegeneration* 3, 251-265. ISSN 1522-9661

Jovanovic, JN, Czernik, AJ, Fienberg, AA, Greengard, P, & Sihra, TS. (2004). Synapsins as mediators of BDNF-enhanced neurotransmitter release. *Nat Neurosci* 3, 323-329. ISSN 1097-6256

Kastman, EK, Willette, AA, Coe, CL, Bendlin, BB, Kosmatka, KJ, McLaren, DG, Xu, G, Canu, E, Field, AS, Alexander, AL, Voytko, ML, Beasley, TM, Colman, RJ, Weindruch, RH, & Johnson, SC. (2010). A calorie-restricted diet decreases brain iron accumulation and preserves motor performance in old rhesus monkeys. *J Neurosci* 30, 7940-7947. ISSN 0270-6474

Kish, SJ, Shannak, K, Rajput, A, Deck, JH, & Hornykiewicz, O. (1992). Aging produces a specific pattern of striatal dopamine loss: Implications for the etiology of idiopathic Parkinson's disease. J *Neurochem* 58, 642-648. ISSN 0022-3042

Kliem, MA, Maidment, NT, Ackerson, LC, Chen, S, Smith, Y, & Wichmann, T. (2007). Activation of nigral and pallidal dopamine D1-like receptors modulates basal ganglia outflow in monkeys. *J Neurophysiol* 98, 1489-1500. ISSN 0022-3077

Kobori, N, Waymire, JC, Haycock, JW, Clifton, GL, & Dash, PK. (2003). Modulation of tyrosine hydroxylase phosphorylation and activity by glial cell line-derived neurotrophic factor. *J Biol Chem* 279, 2182-2191. ISSN 0021-9258

Kordower, JH, Emborg, ME, Bloch, J, Ma, SY, Chu, Y, Leventhal, L, McBride, J, Chen, E-Y, Palfi, S, Roitberg, BZ, Brown, WD, Holden, JE, Pyzalski, R, Taylor, MD, Carvey, P, Ling, Z, Trono, D, Hantraye, P, Deglon, N, & Aebischer, P. (2000). Neurodegeneration prevented by lentiviral vector delivery of GDNF in primate models of Parkinson's disease. *Science* 290, 767-773. ISSN 0036-8075

Knab, AM, & Lightfoot, JT. (2010). Does the difference between physically active and couch potato lie in the dopamine system? *Int J Biol Sci* 6, 133-150. ISSN 1449-2288

Lang, AE, Gill, SS, Patel, NK, Lozano, A, Nutt, JG, Penn, R, Brooks, DJ, Hotton, G, Moro, E, Heywood P, Brodsky MA, Burchiel K, Kelly P, Dalvi A, Scott B, Stacy M, Turner D, Wooten, GF, Elias, WJ, Laws, ER, Dhawan, V, Stoessl, AJ, Matcham, J, Coffey, RJ, & Traub, M. (2006). Randomized controlled trial of intraputamenal glial cell line-derived neurotrophic factor infusion in Parkinson's disease. *Ann Neurol* 59, 459-466. ISSN 0364-5134

Leng, A, Mura, A, Hengerer, B, Feldon, J, & Ferger, B. (2005). Effects of blocking the dopamine biosynthesis and of neurotoxic dopamine depletion with 1-methyl-4-phenyl-1,2,3,6-tetrahydropyridine (MPTP) on voluntary wheel running in mice. *Behav Brain Res* 154, 375-383.

Leviel, V, Guibert, B, Mallet, J, & Faucon-Biguet, N. (1991). Induction of Tyrosine Hydroxylase in the Rat Substantia Nigra by Local Injection of Forskolin. *J Neurosci Res* 30, 427-432. ISSN 0360-4012

Lim, S-Y, & Lang, AE. (2010). The nonmotor symptoms of Parkinson's disease-an overview. *Movt Disord* 25, S123-S130. ISSN 1531-8257

Lindgren, N, Goiny, M, Herrera-Marschitz, M, Haycock ,JW, Hokfelt, T, Fisone, G (2002) Activation of extracellular signal-regulated kinases 1 and 2 by depolarization stimulates tyrosine hydroxylase phosphorylation and dopamine synthesis in rat brain. *Eur J Neurosci* 15, 769-773. ISSN 0953-816X

Liu, JP, Tang, Y, Zhou, S, Toh, BH, McLean, C, &Li, H. (2010). Cholesterol involvement in the pathogenesis of neurodegenerative diseases. *Mol Cell Neurosci* 43, 33-42. ISSN 1095-9327

Logroscino, G, Sesso, HD, Paffenbarger, RS, & Lee, I-M. (2006). Physical activity and risk of Parkinson's disease: a prospective cohort study. *J Neural Neurosurg Psychiatry* 77, 1318-1322.

Mamczarz, J, Bowker, JL, Duffy, K, Zhu, M, Hagepanos, A, & Ingram, DK. (2005). Enhancement of amphetamine-induced locomotor response in rats on different regimens of diet restriction and 2-deoxy-D-glucose treatment. *Neuroscience* 131, 451-464. ISSN 1873-7544

Marinkovic, P, Pesic, V, Loncarevic, N, Smiljanic, K, Kanazir, S, & Ruzdijic, S. (2007). Behavioral and biochemical effects of various food-restriction regimens in the rats. *Physiol Behav* 92, 492-499. ISSN 0031-9384

Marks, WJ, Bartus, RT, Siffert, J, Savis, CS, Lozano, A, Boulis, N, Vitek, J, Stacy, M, Turner, D, Verhagen, L, Bakay, R, Watts, R, Guthrie, B, Jankovic, J, Simpson, R, Tagliati, M, Alterman, R, Stern, M, Baltuch, G, Starr, PA, Larson, PS, Ostrem, JL, Nutt, J, Kieburtz, K, Kordower, JH, & Olanow, CW. (2010). Gene delivery of AAV2-neurturin for Parkinson's disease: a double-blind, randomised, controlled trial. *Lancet Neurology* 9, 1164-1172. ISSN 1474-4422

Marsden, CD. (1990). Parkinson's disease. *The Lancet* 335, 948-952. ISSN 0099-5355

Marshall, JF, & Rosenstein, AJ. (1990). Age-related decline in rat striatal dopamine metabolism is regionally homogeneous. *Neurobiol Aging* 11, 131-137. ISSN 0197-4580

Maswood, N, Young, J, Tilmont, E, Zhang, Z, Gash, DM, Gerhardt, GA, Grondin, R, Roth, GS, Mattison, JA, Lane, MA, Carson, RE, Cohen, RM, Mouton, PR, Quigley, C, Mattson, MP, & Ingram, DK. (2004). Caloric restriction increases neurotrophic factor levels and attenuates neurochemical and behavioral deficits in a primate model of Parkinson's disease. *Proc Natl Acd Sci* 100, 18171-18176. ISSN 0027-8424

Mitchell JP, Hardie DG, Vulliet PR (1990) Site-specific phosphorylation of tyrosine hydroxylase after KCl depolarization and nerve growth factor treatment of PC12 cells. *J Biol Chem* 265, 22358-22364. ISSN 0021-9258

Miyake, Y, Sasaki, S, Tanaka, K, Fukushima, W, Kiyohara, C, Tsuboi, Y, Yamada, T, Oeda, T, Miki, T, Kawamura, N, Sakae, N, Fukuyama, H, Hirota, Y, &Nagai, M. (2010).

Dietary fat intake and risk of Parkinson's disease: a case-control study in Japan. *J Neurol Sci* 288(1-2), 117-122. ISSN 1302-1664

Miyamoto, E, Kuo, JF, & Greengard, P. (1969). Adenosine 3′,5′-monophosphate-dependent proteín kinase from brain. *Science* 165, 63-65. ISSN 0036-8075

Morgenroth, VH, Hegstrand, LR, Roth, RH, & Greengard, P. (1975). Evidence for involvement of protein kinase in the activation by adenosine 3':5'-monophosphate of brain tyrosine 3-monooxygenase. *J Biol Chem.* 250, 1946-1948. ISSN 0021-9258

Morris, JK, Bomhoff, GL, Stanford, JA, & Gieger, PC. (2010). Neurodegeneration in an animal model of Parkinson's disease is exacerbated by a high-fat diet. *Am J Physiol Integr Comp Physiol* 299, R1082-1090. ISSN 0363-6119

Muhlack, S, Welnic, J, Woitalla, D, & Muller, T. (2007). Exercise improves the efficacy of levodopa in patients with Parkinson's disease. *Movement Disord* 22,427-430. ISSN 1531-8257

Murray, AM, Bennet, DA, Mendes, de Leon CF, Beckett, LA, & Evans, DA. (2004). A longitudinal study of Parkinsonism and disability in a community population of older people. *J Gerontol Medical Sciences* 59A, 864-870. ISSN 1079-5006

Nevalainen, N, Chermenina, M, Rehnmark, A, Berglof, E, Marschinke, F, & Stromberg, I. (2010). Glial cell line-derived neurotrophic factor is crucial for long-term maintenance of the nigrostriatal system. *Neuroscience* 171, 1357-1366. ISSN 1873-7544

Obeso, JA, Rodriguez-Oroz, MC, Goetz, CG, Marin, C, Kordower, JH, Rodriguez, M, Hirsch, EC, Farrer, M, Schapira, AHV, & Halliday, G. (2010). Missing pieces in the Parkinson's disease puzzle. *Nat Medicine* 16, 653-661. ISSN 1078-8956

O'Dell, SJ, Gross, NB, Fricks, AN, Casiano, BD, Nguyen, TB, & Marshall JF. (2007). Running wheel exercise enhances recovery from nigrostriatal dopamine injury without inducing neuroprotection. *Neuroscience* 144, 1141-1151. 1873-7544

Pan, Y, Berman, Y, Haberny, S, Meller, E, & Carr, KD. (2006). Synthesis, protein levels, activity, and phosphorylation state of tyrosine hydroxylase in mesoaccumbens and nigrostriatal dopamine pathways of chronically food-restricted rats. *Brain Res* 1122, 135-142. ISSN 0006-8993

Pascual, A, Hidalgo-Figueroa, M, Piruat, JI, Pintaldo, CO, Gomez-Diaz, R, & Lopez-Barneo, J. (2008). Absolute requirement of GDNF for adult catecholaminergic neuron survival. *Nat Neurosci* 11, 755-761. ISSN 1097-6256

Peng, XM, Tehranian, R, Dietrich, P, Stefanis, L, & Perez, RG. (2005). alpha-synuclein activation of protein phosphatase 2A reduces tyrosine hydroxylase phosphorylation in dopaminergic cells. *J Cell Sci* 118, 3523-3530. ISSN 0021-9533

Perez, RG, Waymire, JC, Lin, E, Liu, JJ, Guo, F, & Zigmond, MJ. (2002). A Role for alpha - Synuclein in the Regulation of Dopamine Biosynthesis. *J Neurosci* 22,3090-3099. ISSN 0270-6474

Perez, XA, Parameswaran, N, Huang, L, O'Leary, KT, & Quik, M. (2008). Pre-synaptic dopaminergic compensation after moderate nigrostriatal damage in non-human primates. *J Neurochem* 105, 1861-1872. ISSN 0022-3042

Petzinger, GM, Walsh, JP, Akopian, G, Hogg, E, Abernathy, A, Arevalo, P, Turnquist, P, Vuckovic, M, Fisher, BE, Togasaki, DM, Jakowec, MW. (2007). Effects of treadmill exercise on dopaminergic transmission in the 1-methyl-4-phenyl-1,2,3,6-tetrahydropyridine-lesioned mouse model of basal ganglia injury. *J Neurosci* 27, 5291-5300. ISSN 0270-6474

Pifl, C, & Hornykiewicz, O. (2006). Dopamine turnover is upregulated in the caudate putamen of asymptomatic MPTP-lesioned rhesus monkeys. *Neurochem Int* 49, 519-524. ISSN 0197-0186

Ponzio, F, Calderini, G, Lomuscio, G, Vantini, G, Toffano, G, & Algeri, S. (1982). Changes in monoamines and their metabolite levels in some brain regions of aged rats. *Neurobiol Aging* 3, 23-29. ISSN 0197-4580

Prasanthi, JR, Huls, A, Thomasson, S, Thompson, A, Schommer, E, & Ghribi, O. (2008). Differential effects of 24-hydroxycholesterol and 27-hydroxycholesterol on beta-amyloid precursor protein levels and processing in human neuroblastoma SH-SY5Y cells. *J Neurochem* 107, 1722-1729. ISSN 0022-3042

Prettyman, R. (1998). Extrapyramidal signs in cognitively intact elderly people. *Age and Ageing* 27, 557-560. ISSN 0002-0729

Pruett, BS, & Salvatore, MF. (2010). GFRα-1 receptor expression in the aging nigrostriatal and mesoaccumbens pathways. *J Neurochem*, 115, 707-715. ISSN 0022-3042

Rantham Prabhakara, JP, Feist, G, Thomasson, S, Thompson, A, Schommer, E, & Ghribi, O. (2008). Differential effects of 24-hydroxycholesterol and 27-hydroxycholesterol on tyrosine hydroxylase and alpha-synuclein in human neuroblastoma SH-SY5Y cells. *J Neurochem* 107, 1722-1729. ISSN 0022-3042

Rasmussen, P, Brassard, P, Adser, H, Pedersen, MV, Leick, L, Hart, E, Secher, NH, Pedersen, BK, & Pilegaard, H. (2009). Evidence for a release of brain-derived neurotrophic factor from the brain during exercise. *Exp Physiol* 94, 1062-1069. ISSN 0958-0670

Rech, RH, Borys, HK, & Moore, KE. (1966). Alterations in behavior and brain catecholamine levels in rats treated with alpha-methyltyrosine. *J Pharmacol Exp Ther*, 153, 412-419. ISSN 0022-3565

Ridgel, AL, Vitek, JL, & Alberts, JL. (2009). Forced, not voluntary, exercise improves motor function in Parkinson's disease patients. *Neurorehabil Neural Repair* 23, 600-608. ISSN 1545-9683

Robertson, GS, & Robertson, HA. (1989). Evidence that L-DOPA-induced rotational behavior is dependent on both striatal and nigral mechanisms. *J Neurosci* 9, 3326-3331. ISSN 0270-6474

Ross, GW, Petrovich, H, Abbott, RD, Nelson, J, Markesbery, W, Davis, D, Hardman, J, Launer, L, Masaki, K, Tanner, CM, & White, LR. (2004). Parkinsonian signs and substantia nigra neuron density in decendents elders without PD. *Ann Neurol* 56, 532-539. ISSN 0364-5134

Sacchetti, P, Sousa, KM, Hall, AC, Liste, I, Steffensen, KR, Theofilopoulos, S, Parish, CL, Hazenberg, C, Richter, LA, Hovatta, O, Gustafsson, J-A, & Arenas, E. (2009). Liver X receptors and oxysterols promote ventral midbrain neurogenesis in vivo and in human embryonic stem cells. *Cell Stem Cell* 5, 409-419. ISSN 1934-5909

Salvatore, MF, Garcia-Espana, A, Goldstein, M, Deutch, AY, & Haycock, JW. (2000). Stoichiometry of tyrosine hydroxylase phosphorylation in the nigrostriatal and mesolimbic systems *in vivo*: Effects of acute haloperidol and related compounds. *J Neurochem* 75, 225-232. ISSN 0022-3042

Salvatore, MF, Waymire, JC, & Haycock, JW. (2001). Depolarization-stimulated catecholamine biosynthesis: involvement of protein kinases and tyrosine hydroxylase phosphorylation sites *in situ*. *J Neurochem* 79, 349-360. ISSN 0022-3042

Salvatore, MF, Zhang, JL, Large, DM, Wilson, PE, Gash, CR, Thomas, TC, Haycock, JW, Bing, G, Stanford, JA, Gash, D, & Gerhardt, GA. (2004). Striatal GDNF administration increases tyrosine hydroxylase phosphorylation in the rat striatum and substantia nigra. *J Neurochem* 90, 245-254. ISSN 0022-3042

Salvatore, MF, Fisher, B, Surgener, SP, Gerhardt, GA, & Rouault, TA. (2005). Neurochemical investigations of dopamine neuronal systems in iron-regulatory protein 2 (IRP-2) knockout mice. *Mol Brain Res* 139, 341-347. ISSN 0169-328X

Salvatore, MF, Ai, Y, Fischer, B, Zhang, A, Grondin, RC, Zhang, Z, Gerhardt, GA, & Gash, DM. (2006). Point source concentration of GDNF may explain failure of phase II clinical trial. *Exp Neurol* 202, 497-505. ISSN 0014-4886

Salvatore, MF, Gerhardt, GA, Dayton, RD, Klein, RL, & Stanford, JA. (2009a). Unilateral striatal GDNF bilaterally affects nigrostriatal dopamine-regulating proteins in substantia nigra and GABA-regulating proteins in striatum. *Exp Neurol*, 219, 197-207. ISSN 0014-4886

Salvatore, MF, Pruett, BS, Spann, SL, & Dempsey, C. (2009b). Aging reveals a role for nigral tyrosine hydroxylase ser31 phosphorylation in locomotor activity generation. *PLoS ONE*, 4 (12), e8466. ISSN 1932-6203

Sarre, S, Yuan, H, Jonkers, N, Van Hemelrijck, A, Ebinger, G, & Michotte, Y. (2004). *In vivo* characterization of somatodendritic dopamine release in the substantia nigra of 6-hydroxydopamine-lesioned rats. *J Neurochem* 90, 29-39. ISSN 0022-3042

Savela, SL, Koistinen, P, Tilvis, RS, Strandberg, AY, Pitkala, KH, Salomaa, VV, Miettinen, TA, & Strandberg, TE. (2010). Physical activity at midlife and health-related quality of life in older men. *Arch Intern Med* 170, 1171-1172. ISSN 0003-9926

Schuster, S, Nadjar, A, Guo, JT, Li, Q, Ittrich, C, Hengerer, B, &Bezard, E. (2008). The 3-hydroxy-3-methylglutaryl-CoA reductase inhibitor lovastatin reduces severity of L-DOPA-induced abnormal involuntary movements in experimental Parkinson's disease. *J Neurosci* 28, 4311-4316. ISSN 0270-6474

Seifert, T, Brassard, P, Wissenberg, M, Rasmussen, P, Nordby, P, Stallknecht, B, Adser, H, Jakobsen, AH, Pilegaard, H, Nielsen, HB, & Secher, NH. (2010). Endurance training enhances BDNF release from the human brain. *Am J Physiol Regul Integr Comp* Physiol 298, R372-R377. ISSN 0363-6119

Slevin, JT, Gerhardt, GA, Smith, CD, Gash, DM, Kryscio, R, & Young,B. (2005). Improvement of bilateral motor functions in patients with Parkinson disease through the unilateral intraputamenal infusion of glial cell line-derived neurotrophic factor. *J Neurosurg* 102, 216-222. ISSN 0022-3085

Snyder, GL, Keller, RW, & Zigmond, MJ. (1990). Dopamine efflux from striatal slices after intracerebral 6-hydroxydopamine: evidence for compensatory hyperactivity of residual terminals. *J Pharm Exp Ther* 253, 867-876. ISSN 0022-3565

Sutherland, C, Alterio, J, Campbell, DG, LeBourdelles, B, Mallet, J, Haavik, J, & Cohen, P. (1993). Phosphorylation and activation of human tyrosine hydroxylase in vitro by mitogen-activated protein (MAP) kinase and MAP-kinase-activated kinases 1 and 2. *Eur J Biochem* 217, 715-722. ISSN 0014-2956

Suzuki, T, Kurahashi, H, & Ichinose, H. (2004). Ras/MEK pathway is required for NGF-induced expression of tyrosine hydroxylase gene. *Biochem Biophys Res Comm*. 315, 389-396. ISSN 0006-291X

Tachikawa, E, Tank, AW, Weiner, DH, Mosimann, WF, Yanagihara, N, & Weiner, N. (1987). Tyrosine hydroxylase is activated and phosphorylated on different sites in rat pheochromocytoma PC12 cells treated with phorbol ester and forskolin. *J Neurochem* 48, 1366-1376. ISSN 0022-3042

Tajari, N, Yasuhara, T Shingo, T, Kondo, A, Yuan, W, Kadota, T, Wang, F, Baba, T, Tayra, JT, Morimoto, T, Jing, M, Kikuchi, Y, Kuramoto, S, Agari, T, Miyoshi, Y, Fujino, H, Obata, F, Takeda, I, Furuta, T, & Date, I. (2010). Exercise exerts neuroprotective effects on Parkinson's disease model of rats. *Brain Res* 1310, 200-207. ISSN 0006-8993

Trevitt, JT, Carlson, BB, Nowend, K, & Salamone, JD. (2001). Substantia nigra pars reticulate is a highly potent site of action for the behavioral effects of the D1 antagonist SCH23390 in rat. *Psychopharmacol* 156, 32-41. ISSN 1432-2072

Tümer, N, Demirel, HA, Serova, L, Sabban, EL, Broxson, CS, & Powers, SK. (2001) Gene expression of catecholamine biosynthetic enzymes following exercise: modulation by age. *Neuroscience* 103: 703-711, 2001. ISSN 0306-4522

Waszczak, BL & Walters,J.R. (1983). Dopamine modulation of the effects of gamma-aminobutyric acid on substantia nigra pars reticulata neurons. *Science* 220, 218-221. ISSN 0036-8075

Waymire, JC, Johnston, JP, Hummer-Lickteig, K, Lloyd, A, Vigny, A, & Craviso, GL. (1988). Phosphorylation of bovine adrenal chromaffin cell tyrosine hydroxylase. Temporal correlation of acetylcholine's effect on site phosphorylation, enzyme activation, and catecholamine synthesis. *J Biol Chem* 263, 12439-12447. ISSN 0021-9258

Waymire, JC, Craviso, GL, Lichteig, K, Johnston, JP, Baldwin, C, Zigmond, RE. (1991). Vasoactive intestinal peptide stimulates catecholamine biosynthesis in isolated adrenal chromaffin cells: Evidence for a cyclic AMP-dependent phosphorylation and activation of tyrosine hydroxylase. J Neurochem 57, 1313-1324. ISSN 0022-3042

Weed, JL, Lane, MA, Roth, GS, Speer, DL, & Ingram, DK. (1997). Activity Measures in Rhesus Monkeys on Long-Term Calorie Restriction. *Physiology and Behavior* 62, 97-103. ISSN 0031-9384

Yoon, MC, Shin, MS, Kim, TS, Kim, BK, Ko, IG, Sung, YH, Kim, SE, Lee, HH, Kim, YP, & Kim, CJ. (2007). Treadmill exercise suppresses nigrostriatal dopaminergic neuronal loss in 6-hydroxydopamine-induced Parkinson's rats. *Neurosci Lett* 423, 12-17. ISSN 0304-3940

Yurek, M, Hipkens, SB, Hebert, MA, Gash, DM, & Gerhardt, GA. (1998). Age-related decline in striatal dopamine release and motoric function in Brown Norway/Fischer 344 hybrid rats. *Brain Res* 791, 246-256. ISSN 0006-8993

Zaman, V, Boger, HA, Granholm, AC, Rohrer, B, Moore, A, Buhusi, M, Gerhardt, GA, Hoffer, BJ, & Middaugh, LD. (2008). The nigrostriatal dopamine system of aging GFRalpha-1 heterozygous mice: neurochemistry, morphology and behavior. *Eur J Neurosci* 28, 1557-1568. ISSN 0953-816X

Zigmond, MJ, Hastings, TG, & Perez, RG. (2002). Increased dopamine turnover after partial loss of dopaminergic neurons: compensation or toxicity? *Parkinsonism & Related Dis* 8, 389-393. ISSN 1353-8020

Zigmond, MJ, Cameron, JL, Leak, RK, Mirnics, K, Russell, VA, Smeyne, RJ, & Smith, AD. (2009). Triggering endogenous neuroprotective processes through exercise in models of dopamine deficiency. *Parkinsonism & Related Dis* 15S3, S42-S45. ISSN 1353-8020

11

Wading into a Theoretical Model for Parkinson's Disease

Diana W. Verzi
San Diego State University-Imperial Valley Campus
USA

1. Introduction

While a lot of work has been done on theoretical models for learning and memory, with implications for Alzheimer's disease, little mathematical modeling has been offered for Parkinson's disease, a neurodegenerative disorder of the basal ganglia. The disease is characterized by progressive loss of dopaminergic neurons in the substantia nigra pars compacta, and movement disorders are associated with abnormalities in electrical activity within the substantia nigra pars reticulata. (Brown et al., 1982; Guatteo et al., 2005)

An early study implicated a thermoregulatory role for dopamine receptors in the substantia nigra, but the functional significance of this location in temperature regulation remained to be elucidated (Brown et al., 1982). More recently, changes in temperature of up to several degrees have been reported in different brain regions during various behaviors or in response to environmental stimuli. This lead to the conclusion that temperature-gated TRPV3 and TRPV4 cationic channels are expressed in nigral dopaminergic neurons, and they are active in brain slices at near physiological temperatures, affecting neuronal excitability and calcium homeostasis (Guatteo et al., 2005).

A reduction in the frequency of neuron firing within the striata nigra has been linked to a loss of dopaminergic neurons. A study of spontaneous neuron firing, cell membrane potential and currents, and intracellular calcium levels in dopaminergic neurons of the rat substantia nigra was conducted under varying temperature controls (Guatteo et al., 2005). Cooling evoked slowing of firing, cell membrane hyperpolarization, increase in cell input resistance, and outward current under voltage clamp, along with a decrease in intracellular Ca2+. Warming induced an increase in firing frequency, a decrease in input resistance, an inward current and a rise in Ca2+. Neurons within the globus pallidus and substantia nigra form a functional network that ideally resonates around *70Hz* for normal voluntary movement. However, this network has been observed to oscillate at frequencies below *30Hz* in Parkinson patients, and these oscillations are believed to disrupt normal motor function (Basu et al., 2010).

Post-morten cortices from Parkinson patients exhibit biochemical and physical alterations within dendritic arbors (Patt et al., 1991; Stephens et al., 2005), and it has been suggested that activity-dependent intraspine calcium may regulate dendritic morphology, affecting the synaptic connection between neurons (Stephens et al., 2005). One theory holds that sporadic Parkinson's involves a breakdown of the mitochondria (Surmeier et al., 2010), and recent experimental work implicates mitochondrial Ca2+ dysregulation (Celsi et al., 2009). In particular, the Cav1.3 calcium channel on striatopallidal neurons expressing the D2 dopamine receptor has been linked to the degeneration of dendritic spines on striatal projection neurons. Particular to this chapter, the density of spines within the striata nigra have been found to be greatly reduced for Parkinson's patients, along with a reduction in their dendritic arbors (Gerfen, 2006).

Earlier theoretical models have studied how activity-dependent calcium release from mitochondria may alter dendritic spine morphology (Verzi et al., 2004; Verzi & Baer, 2005), and how activity may directly affect the density and distribution of spines along the dendrite (Verzi et al., 2004). Models have demonstrated that in dendrites with excitable spines, generation and propagation of action potentials depend on the morphology and spatial distribution of spines (Verzi et al., 2004; Verzi & Baer, 2005). A wave can propagate if localized excitatory synaptic input into spine heads causes a few excitable spines to fire, initiating a chain reaction of spine firings along the dendrite. Baer and Rinzel (1991) found that a sustained wavelike response is possible for a certain range of spine densities and electrical parameters. They found that propagation is precluded when spine stem resistance is either too small or too large and that success or failure of local excitation to spread as a chain reaction depends on the spatial distribution of spines (Baer and Rinzel, 1991).

It is painfully obvious that Parkinson's is a complex disorder, involving alterations in brain chemistry, morphology and activity, and an enhanced understanding of the interdependence of these processes will increase our understanding of this devastating disease. This chapter will offer several models to consider these relationships within the striata nigra.

2. Methods

This section develops variations on models for activity-dependent and calcium-regulated spine density and morphology, with age-, temperature- and disease-related changes in the dendritic arbor of the Parkinsonian striata nigra. Dopamine has been implicated as a thermoregulator for dopaminergic neurons (Brown et al., 1982), along with the observation of localized variations in neuronal temperature (Guatteo et al, 2005). Since ionic activity is the driving force in the following models, a study of how temperature may affect the magnitude and frequency of activity is an implicit model for dopamine-dependent levels of neuronal activity.

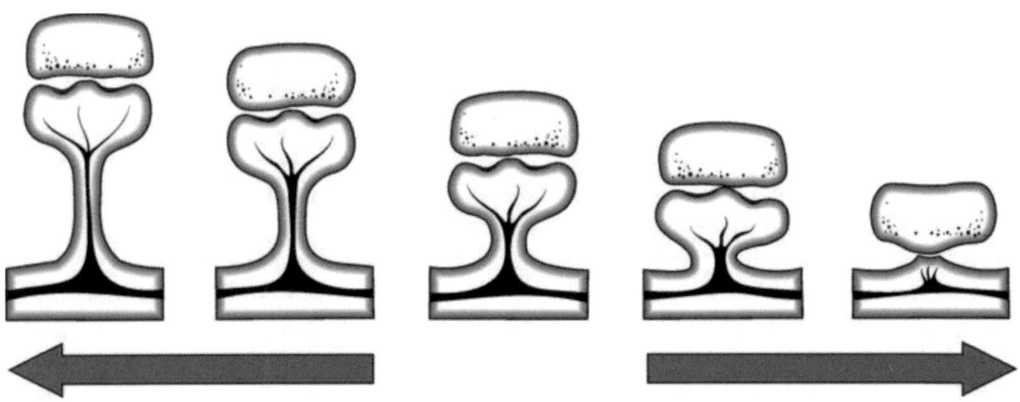

Fig. 1. **Spine loss as a contributor in neuronal death.** Spines may be reabsorbed into the dendrite, or stretch to a point where resistance from the spine stem hinders signal transduction, contributing to neuronal isolation.

2.1 Activity-dependent spine densities

Spines are mushroom shaped protrusions from the soma or dendritic arbor of a neuron, and the loci of 90% of excitatory synaptic connections. Spine loss is observed in normal aging, with an accelerated loss for patients with Parkinson's disease. A dendrite may be populated with thousands of spines of different sizes, shapes and configurations. The basic model for a dynamic distribution of spines is based on Baer and Rinzel's cable theory (1991), where the membrane potentials vary continuously in space and time. Spines interact indirectly by voltage spread along the dendritic cable.

Consider a dendrite with passive membrane properties of a prescribed (dimensionless) electrotonic length (*el*), studded with a population of spines. The spine density $\bar{n}(X,t)$ represents the average number of spines per unit *el*. At each location X, the spines deliver current $\bar{n}I_{ss}$, where I_{ss} represents the current flowing through an individual spine stem. The spine stem is modeled as a lumped Ohmic resistor, (Segev & Rall, 1988), so that the stem current is expressed as a voltage drop across the resistor, $R_{ss}(M\Omega)$:

$$I_{ss}(X,t) = \frac{V_{sh}(X,t) - V_d(X,t)}{R_{ss}}. \tag{1}$$

The variables V_{sh} (mV) and V_d (mV) are, respectively, the membrane potential in the head and dendritic base. If potential in the spine head is larger than in the dendrite, I_{ss} >0.0, then the current is flowing from spine head to base. Conversely, if the potential in the base is larger than in the spine head, I_{ss} <0.0, then current flow is from base to head. The spine stem resistance (R_{ss}) represents the ratio of specific cytoplasmic resistance to cross-sectional area, integrated over the length of the stem. A constriction at any location along the stem would decrease the cross sectional area, significantly increasing R_{ss}. Likewise, a stem occlusion could significantly increase internal cytoplasmic resistance, and increase R_{ss}.

The electrical potential in a passive dendrite, studded with $\bar{n}$ spines per unit length, satisfies the cable equation

$$\tau_m \frac{\partial V_d}{\partial t}(X,t) = \frac{\partial^2 V_d}{\partial X^2} - V_d + R_\infty \bar{n} I_{ss}, \tag{2}$$

where τ_m is the membrane time constant, R_∞ is the cable input resistance, and $\bar{n}$ is the average density of spines at each location $X = x/\lambda$, with $\lambda(\mu m)$ the physical length. The model assumes that the dendrite has sealed-end boundary conditions and that both the dendrite and spines have zero resting potentials.

An equation for the membrane potential in each spine head is obtained from a current-balance relation for the capacitive, ionic, synaptic and spine stem currents:

$$C_{sh} \frac{\partial V_{sh}}{\partial t}(X,t) = -I_{syn} - I_{ion} - I_{ss}. \tag{3}$$

The term I_{ion} represents ionic currents passing through the spine head membrane and I_{syn} the synaptically applied current. In a simulation involving spines with passive membrane properties, the ionic current is modeled simply as the ratio of head potential to resistance:

$$I_{ion}(X,t) = \frac{V_{sh}(X,t)}{R_{sh}}. \tag{4}$$

If the spines are considered to have excitable membrane properties, Hodgkin-Huxley kinetics model temperature- and voltage-dependent ion channel currents (Hodgkin & Huxley, 1952), and

$$I_{ion}(X,t) = \gamma A_{sh}\left[g_{NA}m^3h(V_{sh}-V_{NA}) + g_K n^4(V_{sh}-V_K) + g_L(V_{sh}-V_L)\right]. \tag{5}$$

The parameters γ and A_{sh} represent channel density and spine head area, and the gate activation/inactivation variables *m, n* and *h* satisfy first-order rate equations with voltage-dependent time constants and steady-state functions (Hodgkin & Huxley, 1952). The parameters V_{Na}, V_K and V_L are synaptic reversal potentials for sodium, potassium and leakage currents, with maximal conductances of g_{Na}, g_K and g_L, respectively .

Synapses over a small interval are activated by applying a brief synaptic conductance to the spines in that interval

$$I_{syn} = g_p \frac{t}{t_p}\exp\left(1-\frac{t}{t_p}\right)\left(V_{sh}-V_{syn}\right), \tag{6}$$

where V_{syn} is the synaptic reversal potential. The synaptic current is applied periodically, maximizing to g_p, when $t = t_p$ in each period.

Let I_{ss} , the spine stem current from Eq. (1), be a measure for local activity. Then, the density of spines at any location X along the dendrite is assumed to be a dynamic variable that changes slowly over time and depends on electrical interactions between the spine head and dendritic shaft, as measured by the spine stem current. Let $\bar{n}(X,t)$ the average density of spines per unit *el* be a dynamic variable that changes slowly over time and space, and depends on electrical interactions between the spine head and the dendritic base. In general, the change in $\bar{n}$ is assumed to be bounded and proportional to I_{ss}. Then,

$$\frac{\partial \bar{n}}{\partial t}(X,t) = \varepsilon_n \mathrm{K}_n I_{ss}\left(1-\frac{\bar{n}}{n_{\max}}\right)\left(\bar{n}-n_{\min}\right), \tag{7}$$

describes this change, where $\varepsilon_n << 1$ is dimensionless, and K_n is a positive parameter scaled to cable input resistance. Density increases in response to local synaptic activity, decreases in response to centripedal flow, and remains unchanged in regions experiencing no measurable level of activity. Changes in spine density depend on changes in I_{ss}, which in turn depend on the integrative properties of the surrounding membrane and synaptic activity. A more detailed derivation of this model may be found in Verzi et al. (2004).

2.2 A model of dendritic spine loss with age and Parkinsonism

An early model for idiopathic Parkinsonism considered the temporal profile for neurodegeneration in dopaminergic neurons, assuming a linear loss for normal aging, and a quadratic or exponential loss consistent with the duration of symptoms (Schulzer et al., 1994). Since ten percent of these neurons seem to survive, a lower bound was placed on the temporal function. A reduction in dendritic spines may be considered as a reduction in axo-dendritic synapses, and a total loss of synaptic contact may be considered as neuronal isolation or cell death.

To consider the implications of activity-dependent spine densities in the substantia nigra, consistent with age-related linear and Parkinson-related quadratic loss of dopaminergic neurons, one could remove the upper bound for spine density, and append linear and quadratic terms to Eq. (7), replacing it with

$$\frac{\partial \bar{n}}{\partial t}(X,t) = \varepsilon_n \mathrm{K}_n I_{ss}\left(\bar{n} - n_{\min}\right) - \delta\left(\bar{n} - n_{\min}\right) - \theta\left(\bar{n} - n_{\min}\right)^2 . \quad (8)$$

2.3 A model for the interdependence of activity, calcium and dendritic spine morphology

While activity affects, and is affected by the distribution and density of spines along the dendrite, so also are the structures of individual spines. Earlier theoretical models (Verzi et al., 2004; Verzi & Baer, 2005) have considered how activity-dependent calcium-regulated dendritic morphology could alter neuronal firing patterns to enhance or impede the efficacy of a neuronal network. This was based on experimental observations that a moderate amount of neuronal activity may release Ca2+ from mitochondria, reshaping dendritic spines to increase synaptic efficacy, but that too much activity may raise Ca2+ within the cytosol to a caustic level and cause the spines to pull away from the synaptic connection, thereby contributing to isolation of the neuron (Harris, 1999).

This section considers how activity-dependent free intraspine calcium may function as a second messenger in regulating continuous changes in dendritic spine morphology. For a fixed distribution of spines along the dendrite, let the spine stem resistance R_{ss} (reciprocal of conductance) be a measure for dynamic spine stem morphology. Spines with longer and thinner stems, or those deformed by organelle occlusions, such as mitochondria or endoplasmic reticula, generally have higher measures of stem resistance and are more isolated from the dendrite, while those with shorter and wider stems generally have lower input resistance, and may be more electrically connected to the dendrite. A continuum model consistent with the above assumptions utilizes Eqs. (1-6), replacing Eq. (7) in the model for activity-dependent dendritic spine densities with the following slow subsystem for calcium-regulated dendritic spine morphology:

$$\frac{\partial C_a}{\partial t}(X,t) = -\varepsilon_C\left(C_a - C_{\min}\right) + \left|I_{ss}\right| / \mathrm{K}_C \quad (9)$$

$$\frac{\partial R_{ss}}{\partial t}(X,t) = -\varepsilon_R\left(\frac{C_a}{C_{crit}} - 1\right)\left(\frac{C_a}{C_{\min}} - 1\right)\left(1 - \frac{R_{ss}}{R_{\max}}\right)\left(R_{ss} - R_{\min}\right) \quad (10)$$

In this model, local activity is measured by the magnitude, or absolute value, of the spine stem current, regardless of direction. Local calcium levels increase, so long as $\left|I_{ss}\right|$ is large enough, with respect to the current saturation of calcium, relative to a minimum amount. The parameter K_C scales this relationship. The model prescribes a critical intraspine calcium level (C_{crit}), consistent with Harris (1999), as threshold for whether or not local spines become long and thin or short and stubby. The stem resistance increases for $C_a < C_{crit}$

(subcritical), modeling spine stem elongation, and decreases for $C_a > C_{crit}$ (supercritical), modeling spine stem shortening.
Now the spine density ($\bar{n}$) is no longer dynamic, but the spine stem resistance ($R_{ss}(X,t)$) is a bounded, dynamic function of activity and free intraspine calcium, relative to some minimal level. When synaptic activity is present, stem resistance approaches steady-state if R_{ss} approaches the bounds of R_{max} or R_{min}, or if I_{ss} drives C_a to C_{crit}.
For ε_C and $\varepsilon_R << 1$, the slow subsystem described in Eqs. (9-10) connects to the fast equations for activity (Eq. 1-6) by I_{ss} in Eqs. 2, 3 and 9, and by R_{ss} in Eqs. 1 and 10. In the absence of activity, the system approaches equilibrium, since C_a approaches C_{min} when $I_{ss} = 0$, and $\partial R_{ss} / \partial t = 0$ when $C_a = C_{min}$. In the model, the cable input resistance (R_∞) is fixed, while R_{ss} varies over time and space. The difference between spine head and base potentials in Eq. (1) becomes negligible since $V_{sh} \to V_d$ in Eq. (1) as $R_{ss} \to R_{min}$, imposing a kinetic upper bound on calcium (i.e. $|I_{ss}| = |V_{sh} - V_d| / R_{ss}$ becomes small enough that Eq. (9) is negative).

2.4 A discussion of temperature-dependent neuronal firing patterns

Hodgkin & Huxley (1952) hypothesized in their famous study of the squid giant axon that sodium movement depends on the distribution of charged particles that allow sodium to pass through the membrane, so that changes in membrane permeability are a function of membrane potential, rather than current. They supposed that the rate of movement of the activating particles determined the rate at which the sodium conductance approached its maximum, concluding that temperature had a large effect on this rate, and the frequency for repetitive firing and recovery. While of opposite charge, similar statements were made about changes in sodium permeability.
Many theoretical models utilize Hodgkin-Huxley kinetics for excitable (or active) membrane response, with an implicit adjustment for temperature. The gating variables *m, n* and *h* in Eq. (5) consider the voltage-dependent probability that the sodium and potassium channels are open as

$$
\begin{aligned}
\frac{dm}{dt} &= \alpha_m(V_{sh})(1-m) - \beta_m m \\
\frac{dh}{dt} &= \alpha_h(V_{sh})(1-h) - \beta_h h \\
\frac{dn}{dt} &= \alpha_n(V_{sh})(1-n) - \beta_n n
\end{aligned}
\tag{11}
$$

where the voltage-dependent, gating functions $\alpha_i(V_{sh})$ and $\beta_i(V_{sh})$ *for i=m, n* and *h*

$$
\begin{aligned}
\alpha_m(T,V_{sh}) &= \Phi(T)\frac{0.1(25-V_{sh})}{\exp(0.1(25-V_{sh})-1)} \\
\beta_m(T,V_{sh}) &= \Phi(T)\exp(-V_{sh}/18) \\
\alpha_h(T,V_{sh}) &= \Phi(T)0.07\exp(-V_{sh}/20) \\
\beta_h(T,V_{sh}) &= \Phi(T)\frac{1}{\exp(0.1(30-V_{sh})+1)} \\
\alpha_n(T,V_{sh}) &= \Phi(T)\frac{0.01(10-V_{sh})}{\exp(0.1(10-V_{sh})-1)} \\
\beta_n(T,V_{sh}) &= \Phi(T)0.125\exp(-V_{sh}/80)
\end{aligned}
\tag{12}
$$

are adjusted for variation from Hodgkin & Huxley (1952) results obtained at $T = 6.3$ Celsius (C), by the factor:

$$\Phi(T) = 3^{\left(\frac{T-6.3}{10}\right)}. \tag{13}$$

Modeling an increase in temperature in Eq. (13) decreases the time-duration for an action potential, with a decrease in maximal amplitude (see Fig. 2 below). Conversely, a decrease in temperature stretches out the action potential over time and increases the maximum membrane potential. Increasing temperature also raises the voltage threshold for action potential generation, and decreasing temperature lowers this threshold (Fitzhugh, 1966).

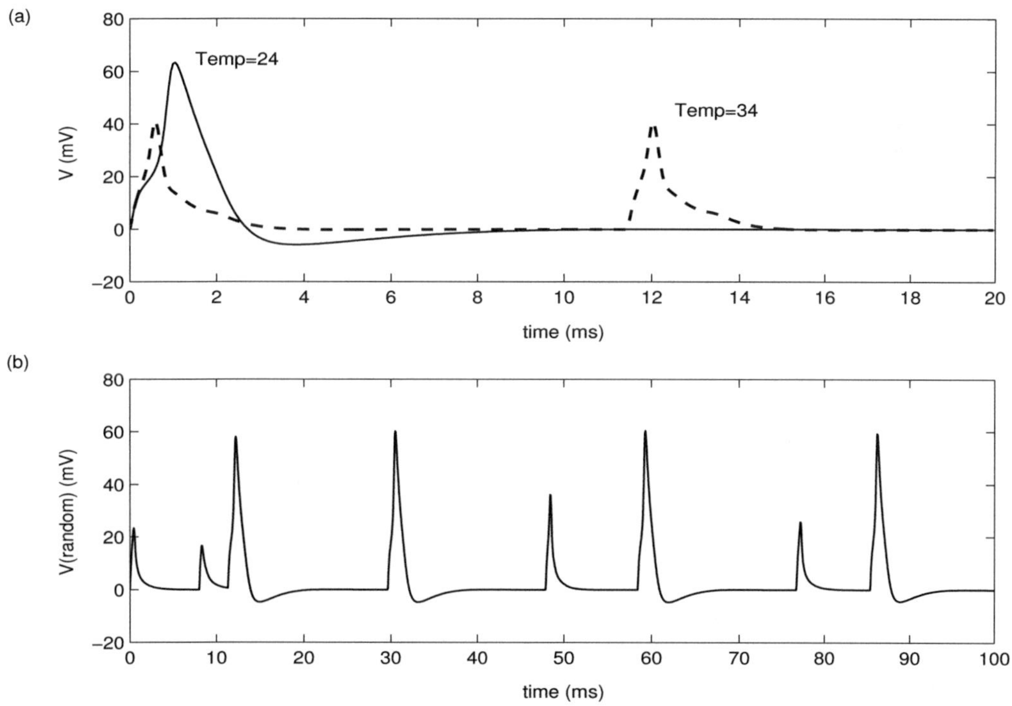

Fig. 2. **Temperature-dependent variations in neuronal activity.** The magnitude and shape of neuronal response depends on localized membrane temperature. Periodic synaptic activation is temperature-dependent.

Earlier theoretical studies demonstrated the interdependence of dendritic activity, morphology and chemistry for fixed temperature and activation periods (Verzi et al., 2004; Verzi & Baer, 2005). This chapter considers how slow changes in morphology and chemistry affect and are affected by temperature-dependent changes in ionic activity. In most of the simulations, temperature is defined iteratively for each activation cycle, remaining constant for the duration of a cycle k as

$$T(1) = \omega, \text{ and } T(k+1) = T(k) + \sigma. \tag{14}$$

For $|\sigma| << 1$, continuous changes in temperature describe a simulation for warming if $\sigma > 0$ and cooling for $\sigma < 0$. Since studies have observed a decrease in temperature and firing frequency in Parkinsonism (Guatteo et al., 2005), simulations will, likewise, consider the effect of temperature-dependent continuous changes in activation frequency, describing the period between synaptic firings from Eq. (6) as

$$P = \upsilon - \rho T \ . \tag{15}$$

For $\rho > 0$, the length of an activation cycle is inversely proportional to temperature for an increasing period during gradual cooling, and decreasing period for warming. Figure 2a displays two temperature-dependent magnitudes for excitable membrane response (Eq. 5). Note the slower rise in sodium to a greater maximum for cooler temperatures (Fitzhugh, 1966). In Fig. 2b, temperature is random on T in [24,39] to display the range of magnitudes and frequencies from Eq. (15).

3. Results

In the simulations that follow, the models are numerically integrated using a semi-implicit Crank-Nicholson/Adams-Bashforth finite differencing method. The spatial step is set to $\Delta X = 0.4$, with a corresponding time step of $\Delta t = .005$ for simulations with R_{ss} of higher values, and $\Delta X = 0.1$, with $\Delta t = .0005$ to maintain stability for R_{ss} of lower values. Computations are performed in Fortran double-precision on a *Sun-Solaris 9* computer. Since, in reality, a significant increase in spine density takes place on a time scale of hours to days and individual action-potentials are on a time scale of milliseconds, the computation time for a simulation could be on the order of hours. For most simulations, the synaptic input is repeated at greater than or equal to 8 *ms*, long enough to allow potentials in the head and dendrite to return to resting values. For each of the time scaling values that define slowly changing variables, one must identify a value that preserves the basic dynamics of the system as $\varepsilon_i \to 0$. Using a computer animation program with uniform activation periods, an initial value is chosen to animate the time course at three spatial locations over 60 synaptic events for a typical run involving the development of a propagating wave. Then each ε_i is halved, and simulations are repeated for 120 activation cycles. The results are superimposed, using every-other cycle of the 120-cycle simulation. The process is repeated several times, successively halving ε_i and doubling superimposed cycles, until the animations converge at ε_i^*. Then ε_i is set to ε_i^* for each *i*, sufficiently small and computationally efficient, without compromising the integrity of the dynamics for smaller values that define chemical and morphological changes over hours to days.

3.1 Dendritic spine loss with age and Parkinsonism

Equations (1-3) and (8) are used in four separate simulations, with initially 23 spines/unit *el*, uniformly distributed over a dendrite of length 3. Spines over X in [0, 0.2] are activated every 10 *ms* with Eq. (6). In two of the simulations, the spines are considered to have passive membrane properties, merely passing the signal along the dendrite, so that the ionic membrane current is modeled with Eq. (4). In the other two simulations, the spines are considered to have excitable, or active membrane properties to modulate a signal on its way

Cable and Spine Model	τ_m	Membrane time constant	$2.5ms$
	R_∞	Cable input resistance	$1233M\Omega$
	λ	Physical length	$180\mu m$
	C_{sh}	Spine head capacitance	$C_m A_{sh}$
	C_m	Membrane capacitance	$1mF / cm^2$
	A_{sh}	Spine head surface area	$1.31 / \mu m^2$
	R_{sh}	Spine head membrane resistance	$10.02 \cdot 10^{11}\Omega$
	R_{ss}	Spine stem resistance	See simulations
Spine Density Models	ε_n	Density time constant	$8.02 \cdot 10^{-6}$
	K_n	Scaling parameter	10^9
	$n_{\max}$	Upper bound	$50 / e.l.$
	$n_{\min}$	Lower bound	$0 / e.l.$
	δ	Linear rate of loss	10^{-3}
	θ	Quadratic rate of loss	10^{-4} or 0
Calcium-Morphology	ε_C	Calcium time constant	$3 \cdot 10^{-3}$
	ε_R	Resistance time constant	$7.5 \cdot 10^{-5}$
	K_C	Scaling parameter	$3.3 \cdot 10^{-10}$
	$C_{\min}$	Calcium lower bound	$5nM$
	C_{crit}	Calcium critical level	$300nM$
	$R_{\min}$	Stem resistance lower bound	$90M\Omega$
	$R_{\max}$	Stem resistance upper bound	$2000M\Omega$
Kinetics	γ	Channel density scale factor	2.5
	g_{NA}	Maximal sodium conductance	$120mS / cm^2$
	g_K	Maximal potassium conductance	$36mS / cm^2$
	g_L	Maximal leakage conductance	$0.3mS / cm^2$
	V_{NA}	Sodium reversal potential	$115mV$
	V_K	Potassium reversal potential	$-12mV$
	V_L	Leakage reversal potential	$10.5989mV$
Synaptic activation	g_p	Peak synaptic conductance	$0.074nS$
	t_p	Time to peak synaptic conductance	$0.2ms$
	V_{syn}	Synaptic reversal potential	$100mV$
Temperature and Period	ω	Initial temperature	See simulations
	σ	Rate of change in temperature	See simulations
	υ	Period scaling constant	40
	ρ	Rate of change in period	0.8

Table 1. Table of model parameters

to the soma, modeled here with kinetics from Eq. (5). Figure 3 graphs results for two passive simulations (left) and two active simulations (right), reporting results for spines "downstream" of the synaptic activation at *X=0.5,* to observe local response without input current from the axon.

In Eq. (8), spine density may increase for sufficiently high levels of activity to offset linear and/or quadratic loss due to age or the onset of Parkinson's disease, respectively. The spine density over time is graphed in Fig. 3a for two passive (left) and two active (right) simulations, superimposing results for linear assumptions for aging only (*NL*) over linear and quadratic assumptions for both aging and Parkinsonism (*NQ*).

Simulations with passive or active membrane in dendritic spines shows a linear decrease when $\theta = 0$, to model only age-related loss of spines in Eq. (8), and a quadratic decrease in spine density when θ is positive, modeling the effect of both aging and Parkinson's disease on the loss of synaptic connections. Parameter values chosen here are set to emphasize qualitative differences for age- and Parkinson-related spine loss, and results are observed over a relatively short period of time. Since the action potential is rapidly shut down by spine loss, the rate of spine loss is similar from passive to active simulation.

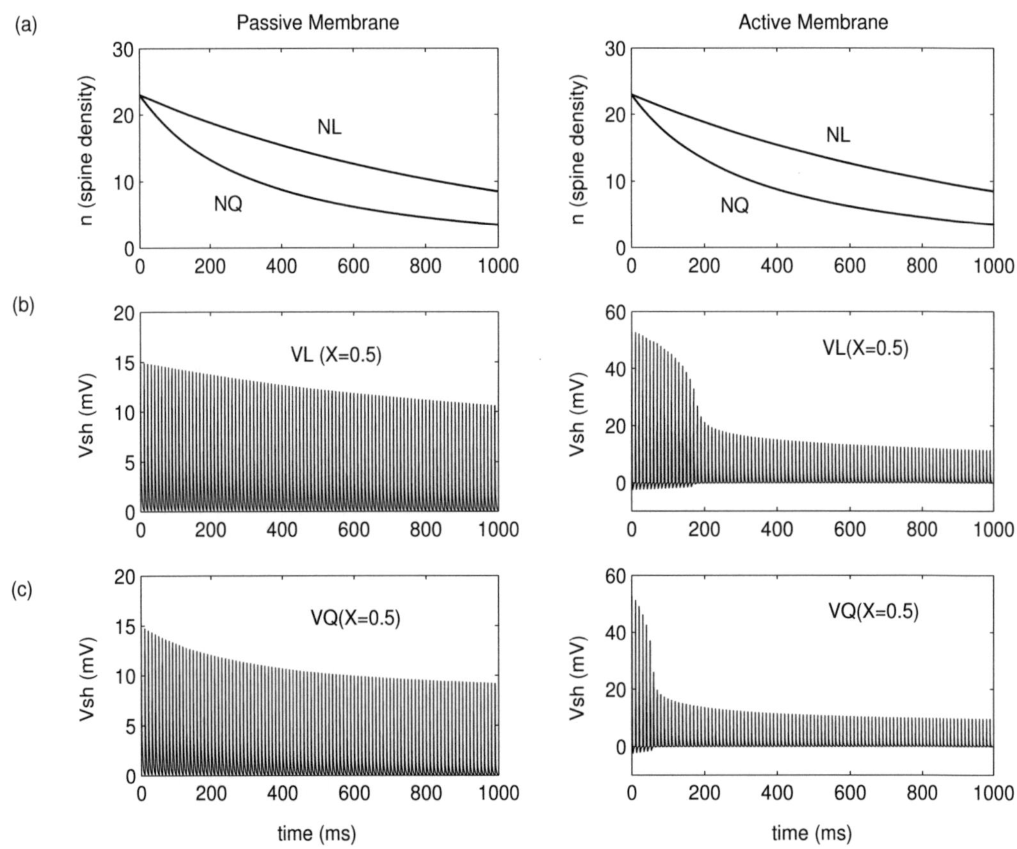

Fig. 3. **Age- and Parkinson- related dendritic spine loss**. Spine density is modeled to decrease linearly with age, and quadratically after the onset of Parkinson's disease.

Figure 3b graphs the time course for spine head potential in the linear simulation (*VL*). In the passive simulation (left) peak potential in each 10-*ms* activation cycle decreases linearly with *NL* (above). Spine density is initially large enough to cause an action potential in the active spine simulation (right), but quickly decreases below threshold *NL*=20, so that maximum potentials decrease linearly for the duration of the simulation. In Fig. 3c, potential in the spine heads is graphed over time for the quadratic simulation (*VQ*). Peak potentials decrease quadratically with *NQ* in Fig. 3a for the passive simulation (left). In the active simulation (right), *VQ* loses its nonlinear response much earlier, when *NQ* falls below threshold to generate an action potential for spines with stem resistance uniformly set to $R_{ss} = 1240M\Omega$. Spine density decreases at each time step linearly or quadratically, with a decrease in the rate of change as $\bar{n} \to n_{\min} = 0$. The strength of the signal passed to the dendrite decreases proportional to the density of spines.

3.2 Temperature-regulated dendritic spine density

To model how cooling temperatures due to dopamine depletion affect the density of spines and resultant efficacy of signal transduction in the dendrite, Equations (1-3) and Eq. (7) are used in a single simulation for spines with excitable membrane properties. The initial spine density is set to 23 spines/unit *el*, uniformly distributed over a dendrite of length 3. Since the spines are assumed active, I_{ion} from Eq. (5) models voltage-dependent membrane kinetics. Spines are stimulated over *X* in [0, 0.2] with I_{syn} from Eq. (6) that peaks at $t_p = 0.2ms$ in each activation cycle. Different in this simulation, the period between activations is temperature-dependent from Eq. (15) with υ and ρ chosen to vary the period from 8 to 20 *ms* over a temperature range of 39 to 24° C. The temperature decreases from $\omega = 39$ in Eq. (14) at a rate of $\alpha = -0.05$.

In Fig. 4a (left) temperature changes with each cycle, with the rate of change decreasing as cycles grow longer for cooler temperatures. On the right side of Fig. 4a, spine density is graphed in a spatial profile over the entire dendrite at three frozen moments in time: The initial condition is indicated by the top dashed line at $\bar{n} = 23$, with a slight rise in density over the activation site at *t*=1000 *ms*, with a decrease in densities downstream. After 5000 *ms*, density has significantly decreased over the entire length of the dendrite.

In Fig. 4b, spine head potential is graphed over time within the activation site (left) and downstream (right). Downstream, $I_{ss} \leq 0$ until the spines initiate their own action potential to propagate the signal. At *t*=1000 *ms*, action potential generation begins at X=1.0, but spine densities continue to decrease across the dendrite (4a right) , even in the presence of a propagating wave, due to the increasingly longer periods with little or no activity. Shorter cycles for higher temperatures may be observed in the dark shading (*t*<800*ms*), compared to the shading for longer periods (*t*>3000).

Spine density is an important parameter for action potential generation and propagation, since more spines increase membrane potential per location X. While the initial density of 23 would be sufficient for an action potential under normal temperatures, the higher voltgage-threshold for *T=39* degrees prevents generation at the beginning of the simulation. The voltage-dependent gating functions α_i and β_i from Eq. (12) contain a temperature-dependent factor from Eq. (13) that increases the magnitude and decreases the voltage-threshold for action potential response under cooler temperatures (Fitzhugh, 1966). Figure

4c graphs the change in density over time within the activation site (left) and downstream (right). Note the rate of decrease is constant in the activation site (left), but greater downstream (right) in the absence of local action potential generation.

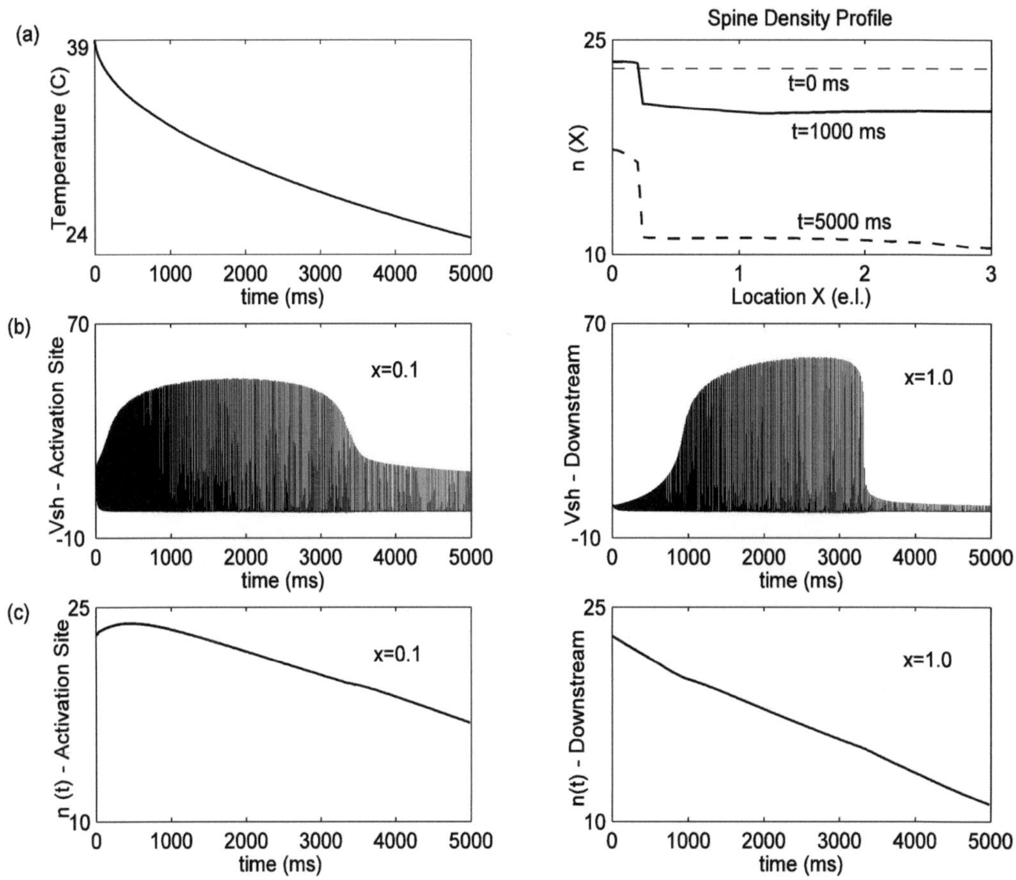

Fig. 4. **Temperature regulated excitable dendritic spine densities.** Spine densities decrease for cooler temperatures and longer activation cycles, even in the presence of action potential generation and propagation.

3.3 Steady-state calcium regulated spine morphology

The model for calcium-regulated spine morphology demonstrates how variations in the frequency of synaptic activation may affect the shape and efficacy of dendritic spines (Verzi et al., 2004; Verzi & Baer, 2005). Eqs. (1-3) and (9-10) model the interdependence of activity, chemistry and morphology for a fixed population of spines along the dendrite. Using the stem resistance as a measure for morphology, the model identifies a variation in steady-states for calcium and spine shape, based on the frequency of activation.

Figure 5 illustrates two such steady-states. A uniform density of 23 spines/unit *el* are distributed along a dendrite of length 3. They are assumed passive, so that Eq. (4) describes the ionic current. Now the spine density is fixed, but the morphology of each spine is a dynamic variable, measured by the spine stem resistance, $R_{ss}(X,t)$. The morphology depends on the local level of calcium $C_a(X,t)$ (Eq. 10), which, in turn, is regulated by the magnitude of local activity, as measured by $|I_{ss}|$ (Eq. 9). Initially, stem resistance and calcium are uniformly set to $R_{ss} = 750M\Omega$, and $C_a = 15nM$. Spines are activated over X in [0, 0.2] with Eq. (6) every 20 *ms* or 50 *Hz* (left), and every 8 *ms* or 125 *Hz* (right), and results are shown for spines under synaptic activation. The parameter $C_{crit} = 300nM$ for Eq. (10), so that R_{ss} increases when C_a is below the dashed line in Fig. 5a, and decreases when C_a is above the dashed line.

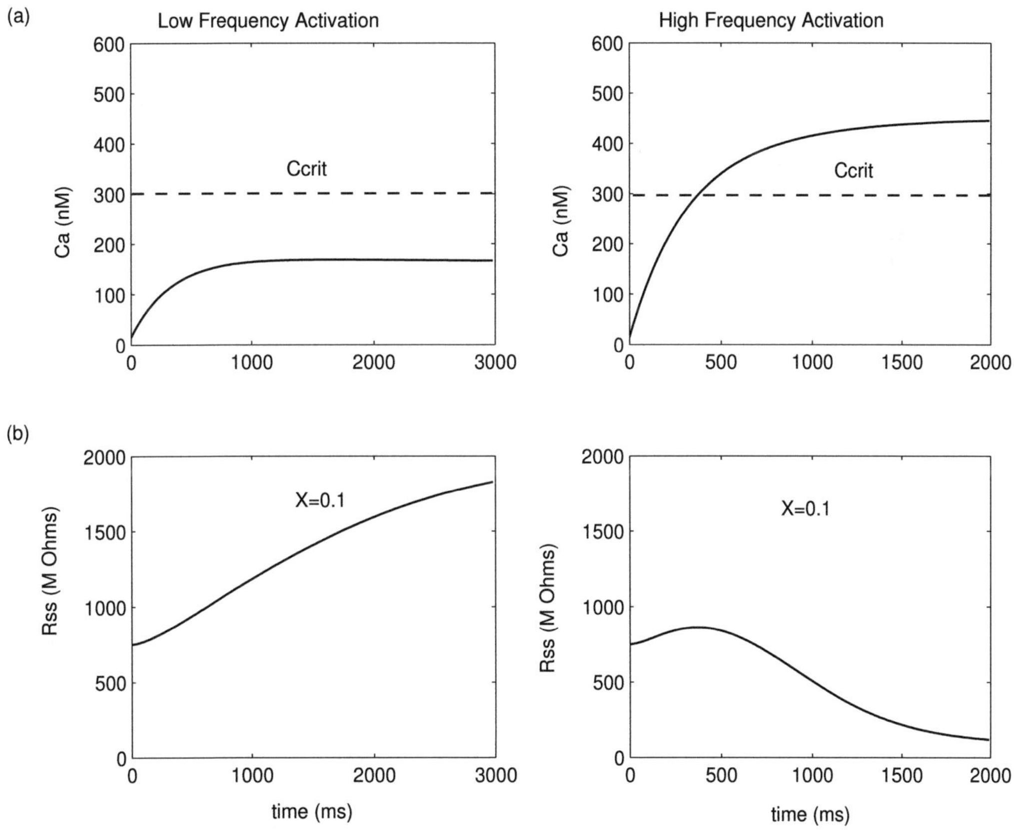

Fig. 5. **Calcium-regulated dendritic spine morphology.** Steady-state solutions depend on the frequency of synaptic activation. If calcium is supercritical/subcritical, the spines display higher/lower input resistance.

The upper bound for free intraspine calcium settles to a sub-critical steady-state for low-frequency activation (Fig. 5a left) and a super-critical steady-state for high-frequency activation (Fig. 5a right). In Fig. 5b (left), stem resistance rises rapidly as calcium increases, but reaches an inflection point to slow its ascent toward $R_{\max}$ as calcium approaches steady-state, for low-frequency synaptic activation. In Fig. 5b (right), stem resistance increases while calcium is below C_{crit}, and begins to decrease toward $R_{\min}$ when calcium becomes super-critical for high-frequency stimulation.

3.4 Frequency-dependent calcium regulation for spines with passive membrane properties

It has been observed in Parkinson's disease that a decrease in temperature causes a reduction in the frequency of neuronal firing in the striata nigra, along with a decrease in the amount of free interstitial calcium. Likewise, an increase in temperature has been shown to cause an increase in the frequency of firing, with an increase in free calcium, citing temperatures ranging from -10 to +5 degrees from 34 *C* (Guatteo et al., 2005). While temperature is not explicit in the model for spines with passive membrane properties, it may be inferred from the positive correlation between temperature and firing frequency.

Figure 6 illustrates two simulations to study the effect of a continuous change in temperature-dependent frequency variations from Eq. (15) for the calcium-regulated spine morphology model, using Eqs. (1-3) to model rapid changes in activity and Eqs. (9-10) for the slow subsystem of calcium and spine stem resistance, as in the steady-state simulations from Fig. 5 above. Once again, a dendrite of length 3 is assumed to have a fixed density of 23 uniformly distributed passive spines/unit *el*, with initial uniform morphology $R_{ss} = 750M\Omega$. This time, initial free calcium is uniformly set to $C_a = 150nM$. Since the spines are assumed to have passive membrane properties, the ionic current is modeled with Eq. (4).

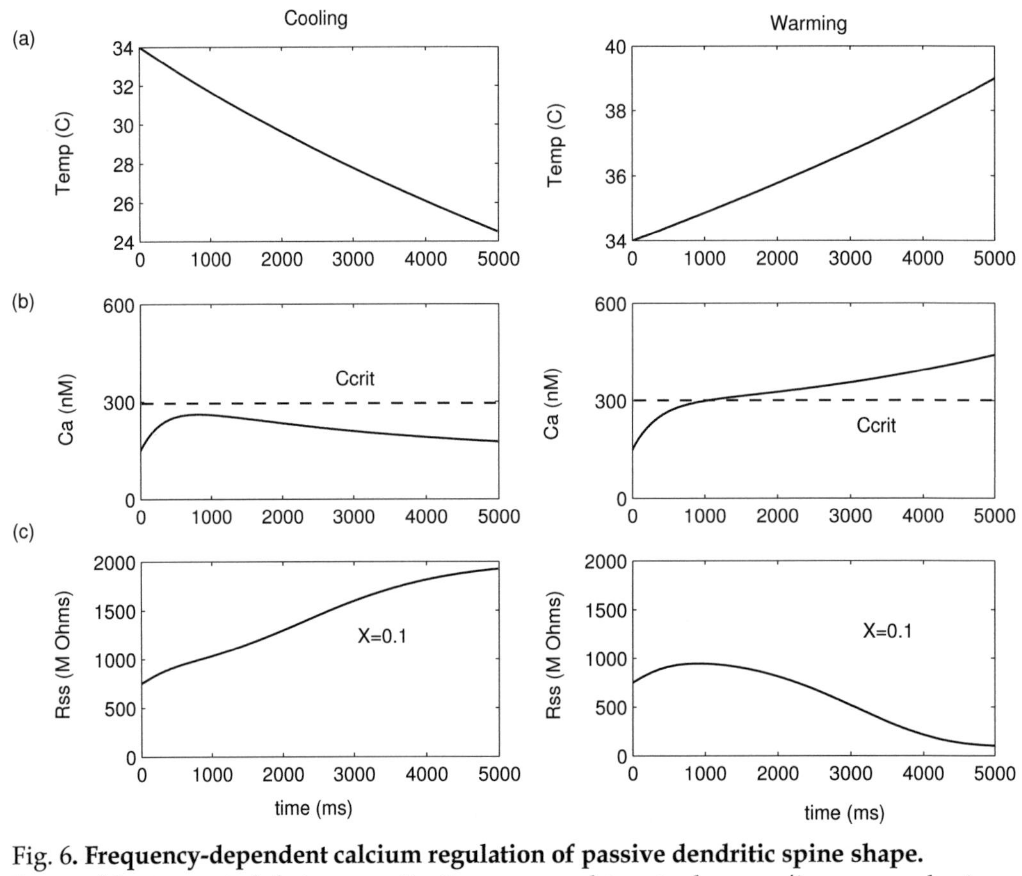

Fig. 6. **Frequency-dependent calcium regulation of passive dendritic spine shape.** Longer/shorter periods between activations cause calcium to decrease/increase and spine length to increase/decrease.

The period between activations is modeled to be temperature-dependent from Eq. (15), with υ and ρ chosen to, again, vary the period from 8 to 20 *ms* over a temperature range of 39 to 24 degrees. Figure 6a graphs temperature over 5000 *ms* for cooling (left) and warming (right). The initial temperature is set to change from $\omega = 34$ in Eq. (14) at a rate of $\alpha = -0.03$ in each activation period for the simulation over 10 degrees of cooling in Fig. 6 (left), and $\alpha = 0.01$ for the simulation over 5 degrees of warming in Fig. 6 (right), since activation cycles are much shorter over time for warmer temperatures.
In Fig. 6b, calcium does not approach equilibrium, but remains subcritical during cooling (left), and climbs steadily beyond C_{crit} as both the temperature and frequency of activation increase during warming (right). In response, Fig. 6c displays an increase in stem resistance toward maximum as the temperature cools (longer activation period) and decreases toward its minimum under warming conditions (shorter activation period), consistent with experimental observations (Guatteo et al., 2005). It is interesting to note that the balance between local activity and free intraspine calcium from Eq. (9) changes sign so that calcium begins to decrease (6b left) when the length of each activation period equals 13.6 *ms* (*T*=*32 C*). It is also interesting to observe that calcium increases almost linearly with warming (6b right) after stem resistance begins to decrease.

3.5 Temperature-dependent calcium regulation for spines with active membrane properties

Different from the previous simulation for calcium regulated passive spine morphology, a simulation of the same model for spines with active membrane properties has a direct link to temperature. Recall that the gating functions in the Hodgkin-Huxley kinetics are adjusted for temperature by Eq. (13). Once again, Eqs. (1-3) and (9-10) model activity-dependent calcium, and calcium-regulated spine morphology, under the assumption that the period between synaptic activations is a function of temperature from Eq. (15). Twenty-five spines/unit *el* with excitable membrane properties are uniformly distributed across a dendrite of length 3. Spines over X in [0, 0.2] are activated with I_{syn} from Eq. (6), and the active ionic membrane currents are modeled by Eq. (5).
Figure 7 illustrates results from a simulation for temperatures cooling (Eq. 14) from $\omega = 34$ to 24 degrees at a rate of $\sigma = -0.03$ degrees/activation cycle. Initial values for calcium and spine stem resistance are uniformly 15 *nM* and 900 $M\Omega$, respectively. While the rate of cooling is constant between cycles, Fig. 7a (left) again shows a reduction in the rate of cooling over time, since the length of activation cycles lengthens as the temperature cools. In Fig. 7a (right) calcium rises quickly to supercritical, since voltage is above threshold to generate an action potential for the current values of stem resistance and temperature. Voltage in the spine heads under synaptic activation rises in the presence of an action potential briefly in Fig. 7b (left) until the temperature drops below. It is interesting that the magnitude of an action potential may be higher for cooler temperatures, but the voltage threshold for generation decreases as temperatures cool (Fitzhugh, 1966).
Stem resistance rises when calcium is below the dashed line for C_{crit} and falls when calcium is above it in Fig. 7 (right). When action potential generation ceases, $|I_{ss}| / K_c < \varepsilon_c (C_a - C_{\min})$ in Eq. (9), so that the change in calcium is negative and calcium falls below subcritical to a steady-state balance between these two terms. However, since the steady-state is subcritical, as in Fig. 5 for low frequency activation, R_{ss} continues to rise for the duration of the simulation. After

6500 *ms*, stem resistance has returned to its initial value of 900 $M\Omega$ (7b right), but the maximum spine head potential has fallen from 28 mV to 13 mV for the same number of spines with the same morphology. The temperature has fallen from 34 to 24, affecting voltage threshold to generate an action potential. Note also the hyperpolarization of head potential in the presence an action potential at the beginning of the simulation, and after 2500 *ms*, when the temperature has fallen below 30. Compare this result with Figs. 3 and 4 for dynamic spine density where there is no hyperpolarization for passive membrane simulations, and only in the presence of an action potential for active simulations.

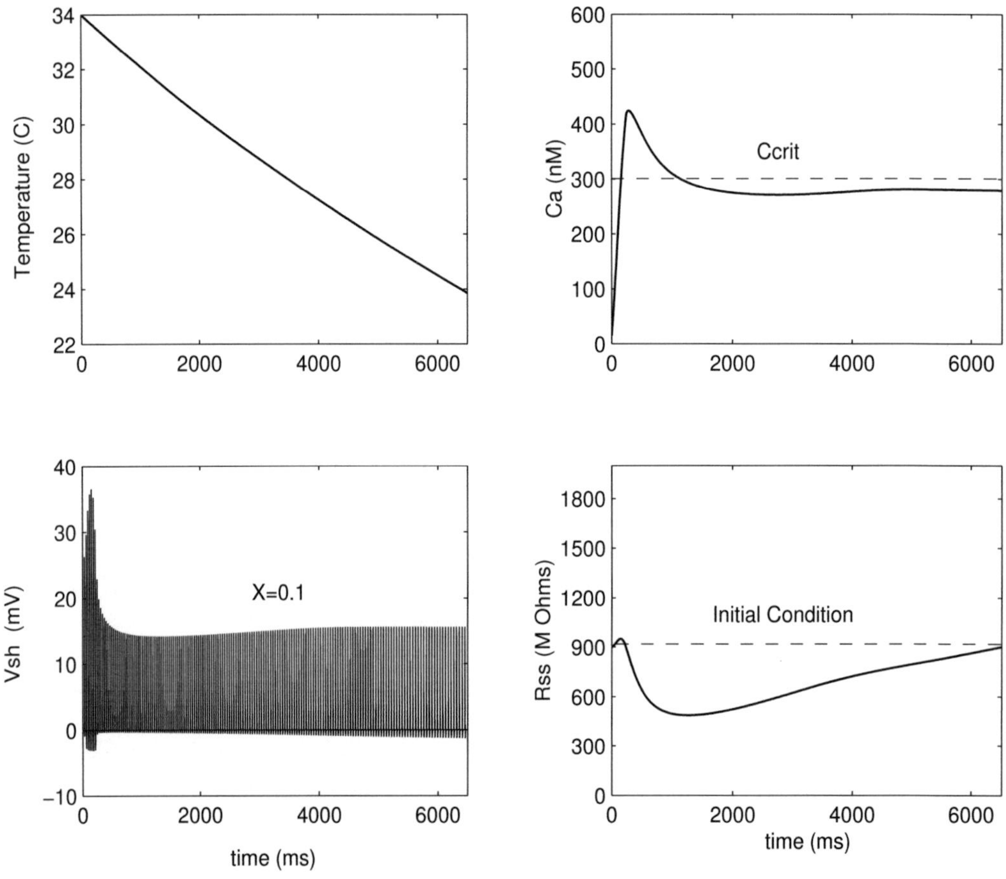

Fig. 7. **Temperature-dependent calcium regulation of active dendritic spine morphology.** Cooler temperatures lengthen the period between synaptic activations, decreasing the amount of local activity and free intraspine calcium levels, which increases spine stem length and input resistance.

4. Conclusions

It is challenging to consider the long-term effect over months to years of activity that scales on the order of milliseconds. The length of time for density and structural transition in the models presented depends on the magnitude of ε_i, for $i=n$, C, R, selected here for computational efficiency. To achieve the results shown in this paper over several months, one would need to set the rate of change in spine structure on the order of 10^{-25}. An alternative to speed up computation time in systems with periodic activation would be to exploit the fact that the slow variables are piecewise continuous over time and relatively constant within each activation cycle. One might then use the average measure of local activity (such as I_{ss}) in each cycle to compute changes in the slow system at the end of each cycle of length P, rather than integrating the entire system at each time step. While simulations in this paper consider repetitive input to a fixed site along the dendrite, an interesting question for future work is to observe long term effects for simulations where the activation site is randomly selected in each cycle.

The results in this chapter agree with earlier generalized neuronal studies for spine density (Annis et al., 1994) and morphology (Harris, 1999), and specifically to recent studies within the striata nigra for Parkinsonism (Guatteo et al., 2005; Patt et al., 1991; Schulzer et al., 1994). Earlier studies (Verzi et al., 2004; Verzi & Baer, 2005) identified both analytic and numeric equilibria, centers and limit cycles for calcium and stem resistance that coincide with healthy or ailing spine morphologies illustrated in this chapter, and suggested in the literature (Guatteo et al., 2005; Harris, 1999). There are numerous observations about spine loss in the literature (Gerfen, 2006, Patt et al., 1991, and Schulzer et al., 1994), and studies that involve the thermoregulatory role of dopamine within the striata nigra suggest cooling, a reduction in firing frequency, and a decrease in cell input resistance (Brown et al., 1982, Guatteo et al., 2005). The model for calcium and spine morphology uses stem resistance as a measure for cell shape, suggesting long, thin spines under warming conditions and short stubby spines under cooling conditions. One cannot help but wonder what is the morphological precursor to the loss of a dendritic spine? Do spines die as a result of stretching out their stems and increasing input resistance (under cooling and low frequency activation) to the point that the synaptic connection is isolated from the dendrite? Or do they die as a result of being driven down into the dendrite, decreasing input resistance (under warming and high frequency activation) to the point that they can no longer boost or modulate a signal? These are interesting questions that beg more study.

With evidence that ion channel proteins within the dendritic arbor play an important role in thermoregulation (Geffen et al., 1976; Simon, 2006), experimentalists will need to work closely with theoretical biologists to include components within ionic membrane modeling to include dopamine uptake and release, as well as TRPV3 and TRPV4 channel function. Likewise, mathematical modelers need to include components to more accurately capture important dynamics within the striata nigra. A recent Ranvier node model (Smit et al., 2009), based on a modification of the Hodgkin-Huxley model accurately captures excitable membrane properties within the range for human temperatures for large-diameter nerve fibres. Likewise, a model by Moore (1958, as cited in Fitzhugh, 1966) suggests that sodium and potassium conductances (g_{NA} and g_K) in Eq. (5) increase linearly with temperature, where the Hodgkin-Huxley model (1952) assumes they are independent of temperature. Since temperature has been shown to be a significant variable in the study of Parkinson's disease, it may be prudent to multiply these conductances by

$$\eta = A\left[1 + B(T - 6.3)\right], \tag{16}$$

where A is the ratio between ionic conductions of the axon at *6.3 C* and the values used by Hodgkin & Huxley (1952), and B is the rate of change in conductance with temperature, (Fitzhugh, 1966). Measurement data within the striata nigra will be required to accurately fit the parameters A and B. Moreover, with the recent identification of variations in intracellular calcium levels as a contributor to mitochondrial damage (Celci et al, 2009), it is important to include calcium as a component of activity, as well as a consequence. Calcium currents should be included in further theoretical studies to consider the effect of calcium influx to localized cell deterioration.

Patients not adequately controlled with medication may be treated with deep brain stimulation, a current that is thought to block abnormal nerve signals (Benabid, 2003). Other work has demonstrated that high frequency electro-acupucture stimulation could enhance survival of dopamineric neurons and interfere with abnormal signaling (Jia et al., 2010). These studies suggest that high-frequency stimulation may result in changes in neuronal activity within the basal ganglia, by correcting signal rather than chemical abnormalities. Deep brain stimulation or high frequency electro-acupuncture may induce an inhibitory current, blocking abnormal synaptic activation and excitation (Benabid, 2003, Ascoli et al., 2010). Synaptic inhibition may be thought of as increased membrane permeability to negatively charged ions such as potassium and chloride, which tend to extinguish excitation. Inhibitory conductance in the spine head creates a current path to ground, shunting local currents. For an inhibitory reversal potential, it produces a hyperpolarizing inhibitory postsynaptic potential in the spines. In the presence of synaptic excitation, it reduces the net depolarizing current produced by both the excitatory input and the active channels (Segev & Rall, 1988). Theoretical biologists need to address the connection between deep brain stimulation and Parkinson's disease.

Because a neuron may have as many as ten or twenty thousand spines, small changes in one or more spine parameters could affect the relative weighting of several different synaptic inputs. Nonlinear dynamics in thousands of these compartments along a dynamic geometry within the dendritic arbor may change a single neuron's response to varying input patterns, as well as the dynamic behavior of the entire neuronal subsystem (Segev & Rall, 1988). Severe pathological changes, such as decrease of dendritic length, loss of dendritic spines, and several types of dendritic varicosities have been found in the melanin-containing neurons of substantia nigra pars compacta for Parkinson's patients (Patt et al., 1991). Continuing theoretical studies of action potential generation and propagation under geometric and chemical fluctuations will give insight to the pathology of this complex and devastating disease.

5. Acknowledgments

The author gratefully acknowledges Frank Perez of Frank's Graffik Graffiti in Brawley, California, for illustrations; SM Baer of Arizona State University for inspiration; and Oliver Velarde of San Diego State University-Imperial Valley Campus for technical assistance. This work was supported by National Institutes of Mental Health Grant MH1065515 to Terry Cronan of SDSU.

6. References

Annis, C. M.; O'Dowd, D. K. & Robertson, R. T. (1994). Activity-dependent regulation of dendritic spine density on cortical pyramidal neurons in organotypic slice cultures. *Journal of Neurobiology,* 25(12), (December, 1994), pp. 1483-1493.

Ascoli, G. A.; Gasparini, S., Medinilla, V.; & Migliore, M. (2010). Local control of postinhibitory rebound spiking in CA1 pyramidal neuron dendrites. *Journal of Neuroscience,* 30(18), (May, 2010), pp. 6434-6442.

Basu I., Graupe, D; Tuninetti, D. & Slavin, K. V. (2010). Stochastic modeling of the neuronal activity in the subthalamic nucleus and model parameter identification from Parkinson patient data. *Biological Cybernetics,* 103(6), (June, 2010) pp. 273-283.

Benabid, A. L. (2003). Deep brain stimulation for Parkinson's disease. *Current Opinion in Neurobiology,* 13(6), (December, 2003), pp. 696-706.

Brown, S. J.; Gisolfi, C. V. & Mora, F. (1982). Temperature regulation and dopaminergic systems in the brain: does the substatia nigra play a role? *Brain Research,* 234(2), (February, 1982), pp. 275-286.

Celsi, F.; Pizzo, P.; Brini, M.; Leo, S.; Fotino, C.; Pinton, P. & Rizzuto, R. (2009). Mitochondria, calcium and cell death: a deadly triad in neurodegeneration. *Biochimica, Biophysica Acta.* 1787(5), (May, 2009), pp. 335-344.

Fitzhugh, R. (1966). Theoretical effect of temperature on threshold in the Hodgkin-Huxley nerve model. *General Physio*logy, 49(5), (May, 1966), pp. 989-1005.

Geffen, L. B.; Jessell, T. M.; Cuello, A. C.; & Iversen, L. L. (1976). Release of dopamine from dendrites in rat substantia nigra. *Nature,* (March, 1976), 260(3), pp. 258-260.

Gerfen, C. R. (2006). Indirect-pathway neurons lose their spines in Parkinson disease. *Nature Neuroscience,* 9(2), (February, 2006), pp. 157-158.

Guatteo, E.; Chung, K. K.; Bowala, T. K.; Bernardi, G.; Mercuri, N.B. & Lipski, J. J. (2005). Temperature sensitivity of dopaminergic neurons of the substantia nigra pars compacta: involvement of transient receptor potential channels. *Journal of Neurophysio*logy, 94(5), (May, 2005), pp. 3069-80.

Harris, K. M. (1999). Calcium from internal stores modifies dendritic spine shape. *Proceedings of the National Academy of Sciences, USA,* 96(22), (October, 1999), pp. 12213-12215.

Hodgkin, A. L. & Huxley, A. F. (1952). A quantitative description of membrane current and its application to conduction and excitation in nerves. *Journal of Physio*logy, 117, (March, 1952), pp. 500-544

Jia, J.; Li, B.; Sun, Z. L.; Yu, F.; Wang, X.; & Wang, X. M. (2010). Electro-acupuncture stimulation acts on the basal ganglia output pathway to ameliorate motor impairment in Parkinsonian model rats. *Behavioral Neuroscience,* 124(2), (February, 2010), pp. 305-310.

Patt, S.; Gertz, H. J.; Gerhard, L. & Cervos-Navarro, J. (1991). Pathological changes in dendrities of substantia nigra neurons in Parkinson's diseases: a Golgi study. *Journal of Histology and Histopathology,* 6(3), (July, 1991), pp. 373-380.

Schulzer, M.; Lee, C. S.; Mak, E. K.; Vingerhoets, F. J. G.; & Calne, D. B. (1994). A mathematical model of pathogenesis in idopathic parkinsonism. *Brain,* 117(3), (March, 1994), pp. 509-516.

Segev, I & Rall, W. J. (1988). Computational study of an excitable dendritic spine. *Journal of Neurophysio*logy, 60(2), (February, 1988), pp. 499-523.

Simon, E . (2006). Ion channel proteins in neuronal temperature transduction: from inferences to testable theories of deep body thermosensitivity. *American Journal of Physiology: Regulatory, Integraative and Comparative Physiology* , 291(4), (April, 2006), pp. 273-283.

Smit , J. E.; Hanekom, T.; & Hanekom, J. J. (2009). Modelled temperature-dependent excitability behavior of a generalised human peripheral sensory nerve fibre. *Biological Cybernetics,* 101(7), (July, 2009), pp. 115-`30.

Stephens, B; Mueller, A. J.; Shering, A. F.; Hood, S. H.; Taggart, P.; Arbuthnott, G. W.; Bell, J. E.; Kilford, L; Kingsbury, A. E.; Daniel, S. E.; & Ingham, C. A. (2005). Evidence of a breakdown of corticostriatal connections in Parkinson's disease. *Neuroscience,* 132(3), (March, 2005), pp. 741–754.

Surmeier, D. J.; Guzman, J. N.; Sanchez-Padilla, J. & Goldberg, J. A. (2010). What causes the death of dopaminergic neurons in Parkinson's disease? *Progress in Brain Research,* 183(1), (January, 2010), pp. 59-77.

Verzi, D. W.; Rheuben, M. B. & Baer, S. M. (2004). Impact of time-dependent changes in spine density and spine shape on the input-output properties of a dendritic branch: A computational study. *Journal of Neurophysiology,* 93(12), (December, 2004), pp. 2073-2089.

Verzi, D. W. & Baer, S. M. (2005). Calcium-mediated spine stem restructuring. *Journal of Mathematical and Computer Modelling,* 42(1), (February, 2004), pp. 151-165.

12

Successes of Modelling Parkinson Disease in Drosophila

Brian E. Staveley
Memorial University of Newfoundland
Canada

1. Introduction

Over one hundred years of innovative experimentation with the "common fruit fly" or *Drosophila melanogaster* has placed this remarkable organism at the forefront of contemporary biological research. Whether we consider the implications of modern genetic technologies and comprehensive genomic research, or we are interested in leading-edge aspects of molecular and cellular biology or complex developmental biology systems, or our studies range from the pin-point accuracy of proteomics to the large-scale questions of population biology, research with fruit flies has made very significant contributions to our understanding of the basic and complex functions of life. Although research into a wide range of biological questions has benefited greatly from experimentation with Drosophila, it never fails to surprise how often an approach that uses this model organism is undervalued or ignored. Any experimental system can be and should be criticized; however the opportunity to explore the biological basis of disease should never be missed. One shining example of this point is our understanding of Parkinson disease which has expanded through and continues to benefit from basic research into the biology of Drosophila, a model organism whose genome has been so thoroughly understood as to make it indispensable for medical research. These recent advances provide significant support for the use of *Drosophila melanogaster* models in the study of the biological basis of many human diseases and disorders.

Parkinson disease is the most common movement disorder and the second most common neurodegenerative disorder. Most apparent to even the most casual of observers is the fact that patients with Parkinson disease present with symptoms that are related to locomotion and motor control. These symptoms include resting tremor, slowness of movement, rigidity and postural instability. As the common underlying source that gives rise to these movement difficulties, Parkinson disease is most often associated with and distinguished by the degeneration of neurons, especially the dopamine-producing, or dopaminergic, neurons in the *substantia nigra* of the midbrain and the subsequent loss of dopamine (Dauer & Przedborski, 2003). Associated with these degenerating neurons is the appearance in many cases of the disease of large aggregates of proteins that are often referred to as the Lewy bodies. Often ignored are the additional non-motor symptoms, where non-dopaminergic neurons including olfactory and brain stem neurons, can frequently deteriorate before the dopaminergic neurons show signs of loss (Braak et al., 2003). Additional Parkinson disease symptoms are common and comprise a number of behavioural symptoms that include dementia, depression, anxiety and difficulties with sleep, plus non-behavioural symptoms such as the development of muscular and skeletal anomalies and skin lesions (Simuni & Sethi, 2008). Given the importance and the complexity of this disease, the application of a multifaceted, interdisciplinary approach to understanding the biological basis of Parkinson disease, including the modelling of the disease in well-known genetically versatile organisms, cannot be stressed enough.

The inherited or familial forms of Parkinson disease are, for the most part, indistinguishable in nature and severity from the sporadic forms of the disease (Hardy et al., 2009). As of only a few years ago, Parkinson disease was believed to be completely sporadic in nature, yet the identification of the inherited forms of the disease along with subsequent characterization of the causative genetic defects has revolutionized this area of research. It is now known that the familial cases comprise approximately 10 to 15% of the cases and arise from mutations in several identified genes with new loci associated with Parkinson disease being routinely discovered. Of the loci identified early in this process, mutations in the *alpha-synuclein* gene (designated as both *PARK1/PARK4*) (Polymeropoulos et al., 1997; Singleton et al., 2003) and *Leucine-rich repeat kinase 2* or *LRRK2* (identified as *PARK8*) (Paisan-Ruiz et al., 2004; Zimprich et al., 2004) cause autosomal dominant or "gain-of-function" forms of the disease. Mutations in the *parkin* gene (designated as *PARK2*)(Kitada et al., 1998), *PTEN-induced kinase 1* or *Pink1* (*PARK6*)(Valente et al., 2004), and *Dj-1* (*PARK7*) (Bonifati et al., 2003) are associated with autosomal recessive or "loss-of-function" forms of Parkinson disease. With the identification of the underlying genetic contributions to, at the very least, a sizable proportion of the incidents of Parkinson disease, it has become possible to apply the principles of disease modelling in genetically tractable animal systems to the study of this disease.

To demonstrate the great utility of the application of research into *Drosophila melanogaster* in the modelling of Parkinson disease, I will describe some of the most exciting recent advances in this field. To begin, a brief description of the wealth of genetic and transgenic approaches that are most commonly used to model aspects of human disease in Drosophila will be provided as an introduction to the organism. The first model of Parkinson disease, one based upon the toxic expression of the human *alpha-synuclein* gene, the first gene identified as a genetic cause of Parkinson disease, will be discussed. This model offered the opportunities to study a wide range of biological contributions to Parkinson disease including aspects of protein structural stability, oxidative stresses and other disease genes. Investigation of *Lrrk/LRRK2* in flies has revealed roles in dopamine distribution, protein synthesis and cell death in another model of a dominant form of Parkinson disease. Then, the processes of modelling Parkinson disease through examination of the loss-of-function of the Drosophila homologues of the *parkin* and *Pink1* genes, both responsible for recessive forms of Parkinson disease will be detailed. Of a very significant nature, this area of research has lead to the fundamental understanding the activity of these gene products at the mitochondria. Furthermore, recent studies have lead to the proposal of a mechanism that outlines the normal role of *parkin* and *Pink1* in mitochondrial dynamics. It is very likely that the loss of this mechanism leads to failure of the cell's ability to clear damaged mitochondria and ultimately results in the degeneration of these cells and, subsequently, the disease state. Finally, continued study of Drosophila models of Parkinson disease is clearly well positioned to contribute a great deal to the future of research into the basis of this disease.

2. The Drosophila approach to model human disease

Drosophila melanogaster has been extensively studied and a wealth of genetic, genomic, cellular and developmental knowledge and reagents are readily available. Drosophila are inexpensive to propagate and can produce a large number of genetically homogenous progeny. Flies display surprisingly intricate behaviours and have complicated brain and nervous systems. For many purposes, the fly provides a well-characterized system that is relatively easy to manipulate but complex enough to be relevant to the development of human disease models.

Often, once a gene has been implicated in a given disease, a bioinformatic search of genomic sequences can readily identify a potential homologue or orthologue from among the genes that comprise the well-characterized genome of *Drosophila melanogaster* as well as the genomes of a number of other Drosophila species for comparison. Application of reverse genetics can lead the production of both loss-of-function and gain-of-function phenotypes that may recapitulate symptoms of a given disease. Loss-of-function can be achieved either through the creation of mutations that lower or abolish gene activity or through the directed expression of an interfering RNAi transgene. A gain of function phenotype can be generated by the directed expression of a gene to where there is normally low or no expression or by inducing elevated levels of expression far above the norm. As a very well studied system, the Drosophila's pre-existing loss-of-function mutations, as well as transposon-bearing lines that can be employed to direct the expression, are available through stock centres and individual research laboratories from around the world. Due to the genomics projects, it is easy to access cDNA and genomic clones along with various vectors for generation of a variety of transgenic animals.

2.1 Drosophila genetics: genes, mutants and transgenics

In most cases, genes that have been identified as playing a role in human disease have counterparts in the genome of *Drosophila melanogaster*. Through the analysis of pre-existing mutants, the application of genetic screens to generate novel loss-of-function mutants and the implementation of "interfering RNA" or RNAi technology to reduce or eliminate gene activity can mimic the effect of recessively inherited diseases. For dominantly inherited disease, some pre-existing dominantly inherited alleles may exist in the stock centre collections. However, hypermorphic gain-of-function phenotypes can be generated by the directed overexpression of a transgene introduced into the fly genome through germ-line transformation. In addition, neomorphic and antimorphic gain-of-function phenotypes may be produced by *in vitro* construction and transformation of Drosophila transgenes that replicate molecular defects that have been determined to cause disease in people. Alternatively, a transgene that can express a variant form of a human gene can be fashioned and transformed. This approach has been applied to study the function and the potential contribution of genes to a number of diseases, including Parkinson disease. This approach can be instrumental in providing insight into the function of an identified gene involved in a human disease when the function is difficult to determine.

To produce the gain-of-function or the RNAi loss-of-function phenotypes described above, the Gal4/UAS system has been widely employed for the ectopic expression of specific genes in Drosophila (Brand & Perrimon 1993). For the most part, a gene of interest is cloned within a P element transposon-bearing plasmid containing several copies of the DNA-binding target of the yeast transcription factor GAL4 designated as the 'Upstream Activating

Sequence' (UAS) along with a selectable marker to readily track the presence of the transgene. As there is no Drosophila transcription factor that acts though binding of this sequence, in the absence of GAL4 these fusion transgenes are mostly inactive. Once established, individuals bearing a responsive transgene can be mated to specific lines that express Gal4 in any one or combination of expression patterns. Many choices of expression are available including ubiquitous, pan-neural, dopaminergic neuron-specific, early or late in eye development, inducible by heat shock, and many more. When the Gal4 transgene and the UAS target gene are combined in the offspring of the controlled breeding experiments, the gene of interest is subject to control of expression with regard to level, timing and tissue specificity. Analyses of these progeny provide the opportunity to approach a wide range of fundamental biological investigations including the detailed modelling of human disease.

When dealing with living systems, and in particular when carrying out complex manipulation of a model organism, careful evaluation and consideration of the techniques employed are necessary. With this in mind, it is important to note that a very limited number of Gal4 transgenes had been demonstrated to lead to cell death: first in the neuron-rich compound eye (Kramer & Staveley, 2003) and later in the nervous system (Rezaval et al., 2007). This suggests that the use of the Gal4/UAS system requires some caution because there may be a compounding Gal4-effect in some experiments when interpreting experimental observations. As always, control experiments must be subjected to proper evaluation and scrutiny. Nevertheless, the Gal4/UAS ectopic gene expression system in Drosophila is an extremely powerful tool and is one of the reasons that modelling human disease in flies is such an attractive pursuit.

2.2 Drosophila dopaminergic neurons

For a model system to functionally approach a condition as complex as Parkinson disease, changes to specific tissues that result in recapitulation of phenotypes that resemble symptoms of the disease are key. The Drosophila adult brain has been characterized to contain clusters of dopaminergic neurons (Nassel & Elekes, 1992). The feeding of rotenone, the complex I inhibitor that initiates degeneration of dopaminergic neurons in mammals, can cause the loss of these clusters of dopaminergic neurons in flies (Coulom & Birman, 2004). This demonstrates that there is a susceptibility of dopamine-producing neurons to toxins that is conserved between mammals and flies. As described below, altering the expression of selected genes in these dopaminergic neurons has resulted in loss of the neurons coupled with an age-dependent loss of locomotor abilities. The basic similarities between the genetically manipulated Drosophila models and Parkinson disease patients, given that the loss of the dopamine-producing neurons and the subsequent change in behaviour occurs over time, suggests that significant aspects of the disease may be well modelled in flies.

3. The alpha-synuclein-dependent Drosophila model of Parkinson disease

Once the genetic basis of a familial form of Parkinson disease was identified (the *alpha-synuclein* gene or *PARK1* and, later, *PARK4* as well) and the molecular basis of the defect determined (as specific changes to the protein), exploring the function or dysfunction of this gene was greatly aided by study in the Drosophila system.

3.1 The alpha-synuclein gene (PARK1) models Parkinson disease in Drosophila

Although instances are rare, mutations that result in substitution of amino acid residues within the human alpha-synuclein protein, specifically A30P, A53T and E46K, produce a dominant autosomally inherited version of Parkinson disease (PARK1; Polymeropoulos et al. 1997; Kruger et al. 1998; Zarranz et al. 2004). An early onset familial version of Parkinson disease results when a duplication of the region bearing this gene produces an increase in gene copy number (PARK4; Singleton et al. 2003). Although abundant in Lewy bodies, the precise physiological function of alpha-synuclein is uncertain. Because two of the original designated PARK loci (PARK1 and PARK4) have mapped to the *alpha-synuclein* gene, the native role and consequences of dysfunction appear complex and deserve to undergo extensive evaluation.

It is of extreme importance to the modelling of Parkinson disease in Drosophila that the first and most exploited Drosophila model of Parkinson disease depends upon the Gal4/UAS system for the ectopic expression of various forms of the human alpha-synuclein gene (Feany & Bender, 2000). Expression of human wild-type and Parkinson disease-causing mutant forms of *alpha-synuclein* in Drosophila results in the loss of the dopamine-producing neurons. The loss of neurons is coupled with the loss of the ability to climb over time in adult flies. As well, the development of Lewy body-like cytoplasmic inclusions and degeneration of the retina occurs with the expression of A30P, A53T and wild-type versions of *alpha-synuclein* using different Gal4 drivers. The observed phenotypic end-points produced by the disease-associated forms of the alpha-synuclein protein appear to display some differences and may mirror aspects of the toxicity that lead to various sub-types of Parkinson disease. To be clear, bioinformatic analysis of the genome of *Drosophila melanogaster* has not identified genes that encode any member of the synuclein family of proteins, including alpha synuclein. However, the recapitulation of phenotypes in Drosophila caused by the toxicity of *alpha-synuclein* gene product that somewhat mimic the consequences of Parkinson disease certainly seems to validate such study in this model organism. As with Parkinson disease patients, Drosophila models of Parkinson disease involve multiple defects, the cellular basis that provides insight into the pathogenesis of Parkinson disease.

3.2 Controversial detection of neurodegeneration in the model

Briefly, visualization of the dopaminergic neurons in Drosophila brains or brain sections has been accomplished through two main methods: detection of the tyrosine hydroxylase enzyme via immunohistochemistry, or detection of a *green fluorescent protein* or *GFP* reporter gene placed under the control of the *tyrosine hydroxylase-Gal4* transcription factor. For the most part, the determination of the specific death of dopaminergic neurons over time in response to the expression of *alpha-synuclein* has been demonstrated reproducibly since development of the alpha-synuclein-induced Drosophila model of Parkinson disease (Feany & Bender, 2000; Auluck et al., 2002; Cooper et al., 2006; Wassef et al., 2007; Botella et al., 2008; Trinh et al., 2008). Not all studies could detect dopaminergic neurodegeneration using anti-tyrosine hydroxylase immunostaining (Pesah et al., 2005) or detection of transgenic GFP (Whitworth et al. 2006). Clearly differences in the approach or methodology used to measure loss of dopaminergic neurons can influence the sensitivity of the assay (Auluck et al., 2005). In addition, as a definite decrease in the strength of the nuclear GFP signal has been observed the dopaminergic neurons of ageing flies that express *alpha-synuclein*, (Botella et al. 2008) a significant proportion of the differences could have easily been overlooked. In primary cultures of neurons cultivated from Drosophila that express *alpha-synuclein*, an *in vitro* model for Parkinson disease that shows great potential, the observed decrease in detection of GFP in these cultured neurons has been strongly associated with the early stages of apoptosis and signs of neurodegeneration (Park et al., 2007). Although this has been a contentious issue, the loss of immunological staining of the tyrosine hydroxylase enzyme, or detection of the tyrosine hydroxylase-responsive GFP reporter, seems to be very well correlated to neuronal dysfunction and degeneration.

This controversy highlights one great advantage of the study of Parkinson disease in an organism that presents complex phenotypes that reflect the consequences of the disease in humans. Of great importance, experiments where the loss of neurons is correlated to the loss of locomotor ability over time have provided sufficient comparison. For example, when oxidative stress is prevented, the loss of locomotor activity and the loss of dopaminergic neurons are diminished together in flies expressing alpha-synuclein (Pendleton et al., 2002, Yang et al., 2003, Wassef et al., 2007, Botella et al., 2008). As such, the loss of climbing ability seems to be a meaningful and modifiable phenotype that allows for the detection and validation of subtle influences.

3.3 Mechanisms to prevent alpha-synuclein-dependent toxicity

To address the possibility that chaperone activity may actively counteract protein toxicity, elevated expression of Heat Shock Protein 70 (HSP70) was demonstrated to toxicity of a-synuclein expression although aggregates were found (Auluck et al., 2002). Reduced chaperone activity contributed to increased loss of neurons resulting from expression of alpha-synuclein. Providing transgenic flies with geldanamycin, an inducer of chaperone activity, added to the food source contributed to survival of *alpha-synuclein*-expressing neurons (Auluck et al., 2005). The phosphorylation of alpha-synuclein at residue Serine residue-129, a modification often found in brains from Parkinson disease patients, apparently leads to toxicity (Fujiwara et al., 2002). In *Drosophila melanogaster*, study of the consequences of *in vivo* alteration of this site of phosphorylation suggests that this amino-acid residue is responsible for keeping the alpha-synuclein protein in a soluble form instead of in a state of aggregation (Chen & Feany, 2005). Prevention of phosphorylation at this site results in aggregation and reduced toxicity. This observation supports the hypothesis that the soluble form of the protein has a much greater potential for toxicity than does the non-phosphorylated form. Taken all together, this suggests that the process of aggregation acts as a protective cellular mechanism that works to neutralize the toxic forms of the alpha-synuclein protein.

While oxidative stress seems to contribute to Parkinson disease, a relationship to the mechanism behind alpha-synuclein toxicity is unclear. The degeneration of neuronal phenotypes induced by expression of mutant forms of *alpha-synuclein* is enhanced growth under conditions of hyperoxia while the elevated expression of the oxygen free radial scavenger superoxide dismutase suppresses the neuronal degeneration and the loss of locomotor activity over the lifespan of alpha-synuclein-expressing flies (Botella et al., 2008). To support the role of oxidative insult in the disease process, the alpha-synuclein-induced phenotypes are suppressed by other known antioxidants. These include the overexpression of methionine sulfoxide reductase and the supplementation of the Drosophila growth medium with S-methyl-L-cysteine (Wassef et al., 2007), and the induction of glutathione synthesis or glutathione conjugation activity (Trinh et al., 2008). As the toxicity of alpha-synuclein is sensitive to oxidative stress, manipulation of antioxidants may make a significant contribution to modify these effects.

One of the great advantages of employing the Drosophila model is the ability to combine and evaluate various components identified to contribute to Parkinson disease in an animal model organism. The first example of combining gene products that are known to cause inherited forms of Parkinson disease was the demonstration that the overexpression of *parkin* can act to counteract the toxic effects of both wild type and mutant forms of alpha-synuclein to restore climbing ability and to prevent degeneration of the retina when co-expressed in the eye (Haywood & Staveley, 2004; 2006). Similarly, the directed expression of *Pink1*, an upstream activator of *parkin*, acts to restore locomotor abilities and prevent subtle developmental defects in the eye (Todd & Staveley, 2008). This approach demonstrates that the directed expression of some of the recessive Parkinson genes can act to balance defects caused by a dominantly inherited Parkinson disease gene.

4. The LRRK2/Lrrk (PARK8) models of Parkinson disease in Drosophila

Leucine-rich repeat kinase 2 or *LRRK2* (first identified as *PARK8*) causes an autosomal dominant or "gain-of-function" form of Parkinson disease (Paisan-Ruiz et al., 2004; Zimprich et al., 2004). Dysfunction of LRRK2 has been mapped to several amino-acid substitutions in the protein and is very prominent among sporadic and inherited forms of Parkinson disease. The *LRRK2* gene encodes a very large protein with a leucine-rich repeat (LRR) domain, a kinase domain, a RAS-like GTPase domain and WD-40 domain and is very similar to an orthologous gene *LRRK1*.

There is a single homologue, *Lrrk*, in *Drosophila melanogaster*. Perhaps due to difficulties in the detection of neurodegeneration, as discussed above, there has been some confusion with studies of *Lrrk/LRRK2* in flies. In one case, Lrrk mutant flies display impaired locomotive activity and a reduction in the immunostaining of tyrosine hydroxylase in dopaminergic neurons (Lee et al., 2007). While the dopaminergic neurons display abnormal morphologies, the absolute number of the neurons appears to be unchanged although they may be degenerating slowly. Under other circumstances, *Lrrk* mutants seemed relatively normal which lead to the claim that *Lrrk* is not required for the survival of dopaminergic neurons (Wang et al., 2008). Directed expression of wild type of *Lrrk* did not lead to detectable degeneration of dopaminergic neurons (Lee et al., 2007). However, expression of mutant forms of both human (G2019S) and Drosophila (I2020T) did lead to documented loss of dopaminergic neurons (Imai et al., 2008; Liu et al., 2008). Nevertheless, the few studies of Lrrk/LRRK2 in flies have revealed a great deal that may influence our understanding of Parkinson disease.

The *Lrrk* mutants undergo lipid peroxidation and mutant flies containing the carboxy-terminal kinase domain truncated Lrrk transgene are sensitive to hydrogen peroxide (Wang et al., 2008). However, *Lrrk* mutants seem to be reasonably resistant to the oxidative stresses presented by paraquat and hydrogen peroxide (Imai et al., 2008). The relationship between Lrrk/LRRK2 and oxidative stress is unclear for now.

Lrrk/LRRK2 has been demonstrated to be involved in the negative regulation of normal levels of dopamine. The over expression of select mutants of Lrrk, but not wild-type Lrrk, causes a severe reduction in the dopamine levels of the brain (Imai et al., 2008). Treatment with I -DOPA causes improvement in movement not survival of dopaminergic neurons (Liu et al., 2008). Conversely, dopamine content is highly elevated in *Lrrk* mutants, as changes in dopamine levels must not be due to survival neurons but due to either defects in metabolism or processing and handling.

The eukaryotic initiation factor 4E (eIF4E)-binding protein, a major controller of protein synthesis and as such a key regulator of responses to cellular stress is phosphorylated by the Lrrk/LRRK2 kinase (Imai et al., 2008). This strongly suggests that the survival of dopaminergic neurons is compromised by pathogenic forms of Lrrk/LRRK2 through the deregulation or mis-regulation of protein translation. The Lrrk and LRRK2 proteins have been shown to phosphorylate and activate the transcription factor foxo (Kanao et al., 2010). This suggests that downstream targets of foxo, such as *hid* in flies (and *Bim* in humans), act to activate the apoptotic machinery to cause the neurodegeneration in Lrrk/LRRK2 models of PD. These research findings demonstrate a very meaningful connection between the control of protein synthesis, activation of cell death programs and the development of Parkinson disease.

5. The parkin/Pink1-dependent Drosophila models of Parkinson disease

5.1 The consequences of parkin and Pink1 loss in Drosophila

The loss-of-function in the *parkin* gene (PARK2), which encodes a highly conserved ubiquitin E3 ligase, is responsible for a rare autosomal recessive subtype of Parkinson disease. The Drosophila *parkin* gene is highly expressed in the Drosophila central nervous system (Horowitz et al. 2001; Bae et al. 2003). In *parkin* mutants, the dopaminergic neurons degenerate (Greene et al., 2003; Cha et al., 2005; Whitworth et al., 2005; Wang et al., 2007). In flies that that overexpress some mutant forms of *parkin*, dopaminergic neurons degeneration occurs (Sang et al., 2007). Although viable, *parkin* mutants present with a reduction in life-span, locomotor defects and extensive degeneration of muscle fibres, the latter is clearly associated with mitochondrial deterioration (Greene et al., 2005). The male *parkin* mutants are sterile due to failure of mitochondrial activities during spermatogenesis (Riparbelli and Callaini, 2007). Reduction of neuronal-specific staining (either GFP or TH) and/or cell death has been reported in these *parkin* mutants (Greene et al., 2003; Cha et al., 2005; Whitworth et al., 2005; Wang et al. 2007). The localization of this protein to the mitochondria (Darios et al., 2003) coupled with the consequences of *parkin* loss is a strong indication that it protects this organelle.

Mutations in the *PTEN-induced kinase 1* (*Pink1* or PARK6) gene are a common cause of autosomal recessive Parkinson disease (Valente et al., 2004). In flies, the *Pink1* gene, like *parkin*, is highly expressed in adult heads and testes (Park et al. 2006). The Pink1 serine–threonine kinase, along with a kinase domain, contains a mitochondrial-targeting signal (Clark et al., 2006). A decrease in the levels of dopamine with age plus a somewhat limited loss of dopaminergic neurons was found in the *Pink1* mutants along with the presence of abnormal mitochondria in the surviving dopaminergic neurons. When the function of *Pink1* was inhibited through the directed expression of an RNAi transgene, loss of dopaminergic neurons as well as the age-dependent degeneration of ommatidia was observed (Wang et al. 2006; Yang et al. 2006). The potential for a functional association with the mitochondria and the similarity in the consequences of dysfunction clearly suggest a shared role for these two proteins.

5.2 The parkin and Pink1 proteins act in one pathway

Although not identical, the flies that have lost *Pink1* function share a number of defects found in the *parkin* mutants including shortened lifespan, apoptotic muscle degeneration, male sterility, defects in mitochondrial morphology and disruption of locomotor abilities. These mitochondria are lost with age from the dopaminergic neurons of Pink1 mutants. While, for the most part, double *Pink1-parkin* mutants show the same phenotypes as either of the single mutants, the overexpression of *parkin* is able to rescue the mitochondrial defects found in *Pink1,* whereas *Pink1* overexpression does not rescue the *parkin* phenotypes. The parkin and Pink1 proteins have been reported to interact physically in at least some contexts (Kim et al., 2008; Xiong et al., 2009). This, at least in part, indicates that the Pink1 and parkin proteins function in the same pathway with Pink1 functioning upstream of parkin activity. This Pink1/parkin pathway is necessary for the integrity of dopaminergic neurons, because the loss of neurons due to loss of *Pink1* function could be rescued by additional expression of parkin (Clark et al., 2006; Park et al., 2006). The contribution of the study of the relationship between *parkin* and *Pink1* to our understanding of mitochondrial pathology in Parkinson disease highlights the utility of Drosophila to model Parkinson disease.

Similar to *parkin* and *Pink1,* mutations in the *Dj-1* gene cause autosomal recessive forms of Parkinson disease (Bonifati et al., 2003) and it has been suggested that they will become another potential component of this pathway. *Drosophila melanogaster* has two homologues of Dj-1 and is viable when both are deleted or silenced by RNAi transgenes (Menzies et al., 2005; Meulener et al., 2005; 2006). The loss of *Dj-1* activities leads to increased sensitivity to oxidative stress when exposed to paraquat or rotenone. However, the overexpression of *Dj-1* does not rescue the *Pink1* mutant phenotypes (Yang et al., 2006). The possibility exists that *Dj-1* may act much further upstream or through a parallel mechanism. However, at this time the relationship in unclear and *Dj-1* may or may not influence the Pink1/parkin pathway.

5.3 The parkin and Pink1 proteins co-operate at the mitochondria

Mitochondria undergo fission and fusion to change shape and share components (Chen & Chan, 2009). The fusion of mitochondria requires fusion of both the inner and outer mitochondrial membranes. The control of outer membrane fusion requires the activity of the protein mitofusin, and the inner membrane fusion requires the product of the *Optic atrophy-1* gene. Mitochondrial fission is promoted by the recruitment of dynamin-related protein 1 (Drp1) to the mitochondria, and this recruitment requires the activity of Fis1, a mitochondrial outer membrane protein. The regulation of this process is essential to the maintenance of a healthy cell.

To focus upon the mitochondria, in the dopaminergic neurons and the adult flight muscles of *parkin* mutants, the mitochondria are swollen with fragmented cristae (Greene et al., 2003; Pesah et al., 2004). A similar phenomenon is observed in flies that have lost the function of *Pink1* (Clark et al., 2006; Park et al., 2006; Yang et al., 2006). During Drosophila spermatogenesis, the spermatid's mitochondria aggregate and fuse to produce the nebenkern, a structure composed of two entangled strings of fused mitochondria. During subsequent elongation, the nebenkern disentangles to yield two fused structures that are maintained throughout the process of spermatogenesis. Whether due to reduced mitochondrial fission or excess fusion, in *parkin* and *Pink1* mutants only one mitochondrial fusion product has been detected (Deng et al., 2008). These mitochondrial defects, along with locomotion defects, flight muscle degeneration, cell death and diminishment of dopamine levels in heads, are suppressed both by the directed expression of the pro-fission genes *drp1* or *fis1* and by decreasing levels of the pro-fusion genes *mitofusin* or *opa1* (Deng et al., 2008; Park et al., 2009; Poole et al., 2008; Yang et al., 2008). In a *Pink1* mutant background, a reduction in the gene copy number of *drp1*, as seen with mutant heterozygotes, causes lethality (Deng et al., 2008; Poole et al., 2008). This clearly suggests that *parkin* and *Pink1* must act to promote mitochondrial fission. It is extremely important to point out that the phenotypes that arise from the loss of *parkin* or *Pink1* are very different from the loss of *drp1* (Deng et al., 2008). This is a strong indication that the Pink1-parkin pathway acts to regulate mitochondrial fission machinery.

5.4 The regulation of Mitophagy by parkin and Pink1 proteins

The process of mitophagy is a recently described specialized mitochondrial-specific version of autophagy (Goldman et al., 2010). In this procedure, the mitochondria undergo engulfment by autophagosomes and are degraded. This essential mechanism is absolutely dependent upon the dynamics of the continual fission and fusion of the mitochondria that alter the size and shape of the organelle and allow the exchange of components. With the failure of mitophagy, the quality of cellular respiration is severely diminished as is illustrated through the accumulation of oxidized proteins. Through the regulation of the fission/fusion dynamics of the cellular mitochondria, the Pink1 and parkin collaborate to contribute to this process.

First of all, although the parkin E3 ubiquitin ligase can target toxic proteins for proteasomal degradation, as the loss of *parkin* results in the accumulation of toxic proteins and overexpression can suppress toxicity of potential targets, other cellular processes can be regulated by ubiquitination by parkin (Geisler et al., 2009). With this in mind, a mechanism has been proposed that outlines the potential roles of the parkin and Pink1 proteins in the regulation of mitochondrial dynamics, changes in which can lead to alterations in the process of mitophagy (Geisler et al., 2009; Narendra et al., 2009; Vives-Bauza et al., 2010; Ziviani et al., 2010). The recruitment of parkin from the cytoplasm to the mitochondria depends on the activity of the Pink1 kinase. Pink1 is localized to the outer mitochondrial membrane through a well-conserved mitochondrial targeting signal peptide located near the amino-terminus of the protein (Zhou et al., 2008). This arrangement leaves the carboxy-terminal kinase-containing remainder of the protein exposed to the cytoplasm. It is proposed that under normal conditions, the tethered Pink1 protein is cleaved in a constitutive way to release the portion of Pink1 that contains the kinase activity into the cytoplasm (Narendra et al., 2009; Vives-Bauza et al., 2010; Ziviani et al., 2010). As a result, under standard conditions, Pink1 activity at the mitochondrial membrane is maintained at a steady but low level.

However, when stressed mitochondria undergo a critical amount of damage, the routine degradation of the Pink1 kinase is discontinued (Narendra et al., 2009; Vives-Bauza et al., 2010; Ziviani et al., 2010). This leaves intact and active versions of Pink1 to accumulate at the mitochondrial membrane in response to the termination of Pink1 inactivation. The initiation and maintenance of the accumulation of Pink1 may depend upon a signal generated when the mitochondria are not able to maintain membrane potential. Although the Rhomboid-7 protease is a candidate enzyme that can cleave Pink1 (Whitworth et al., 2008), this protease may not be the one responsible for this activity in response to mitochondria signalling for destruction. In the first major step of this process, the result is the differential identification of damaged mitochondria through the build up of active Pink1 activity bound and secured to the outer mitochondrial membrane. According to this mechanism, the next step in the regulation of mitophagy depends upon the recruitment of the parkin E3 ubiquitin ligase though Pink1 activity to the outer mitochondrial membrane (Narendra et al., 2009; Vives-Bauza et al., 2010; Ziviani et al., 2010). Recruitment of parkin to the mitochondrial membrane depends upon the localization of the Pink1 kinase to the mitochondria. An alternative method of mitochondrial targeting of Pink1 also recruits parkin (Narendra et al., 2009). Finally, the presence of the parkin ligase at the mitochondria results in the ubiquitination and subsequent degradation of the fusion-promoting outer mitochondrial membrane protein mitofusin (Ziviani et al., 2010). The mitofusin protein has been shown to accumulate with the loss of *Pink1* and *parkin* gene functions. If this proposal holds true, the initiation of mitophagy may very well depend upon signaling through the ubiquitination of mitofusin. In turn, whether mitofusin is targeted for degradation or modified to a form that no longer contributes to the process, this situation leads to the prevention of the fusion of the outer mitochondrial membrane. Although there is no evidence that fission is directly influenced, the subsequent failure of damaged mitochondria to be isolated would likely result from their loss of the ability to undergo proper segregation.

In summary, when mitochondria accumulate sufficient damage, the Pink1 protein becomes stabilized at the mitochondria. This acts to recruit parkin to the damaged mitochondria that in turn causes degradation or modification of mitofusin to promote mitochondrial fission and mitophagy to remove these damaged mitochondria. In Pink1/parkin mediated Parkinson disease, the damaged mitochondria are not cleared as efficiently to result in cellular damage.

6. The future of drosophila models of Parkinson disease

Drosophila is proving to have great advantages in the genetic and cell biological study of Parkinson disease. As more genes are found to be associated with Parkinson disease, further applications of reverse genetics should lead to greater understanding of the disease. The Drosophila phenotypes offer many diverse clues that may benefit from greater scrutiny. As well as future screens that modify the more obvious phenotypes such as male sterility, muscle degeneration, abnormal wing positioning, locomotion defects as well as mitochondrial defects in multiple tissues in young adults, these can be examined/scored for suppression or enhancement without having to carry out aging studies that can span months. Studies of candidate genes that may modify the activities of genes that mediate familial Parkinson disease are rigorous, but allow for rapid and straightforward means to deduce mechanisms. Given that mitochondria defects accumulate during normal aging, identification of multiple means to activate mitophagy may have applications to many aspects of aging. Drosophila provides an indispensable and unique opportunity to contribute to the Parkinson disease field.

7. Conclusion

To summarize, the recent expansion of research interest in the well understood laboratory organism *Drosophila melanogaster* to provide highly informative models of Parkinson disease demonstrates some of the great advantages that this system has to offer. The first model of Parkinson disease, one based on the toxic expression of the human *alpha-synuclein* gene, has allowed a great deal of investigation into various biological factors, such as protein folding, oxidative stress and protein detoxification, that may contribute to the disease. Studies of

Lrrk/LRRK2 have revealed roles for the management of dopamine handling, the control of protein synthesis and the initiation of programmed cell death in models of Parkinson disease. Further modelling of Parkinson disease through careful evaluation of *parkin* and *Pink1* loss-of-function in Drosophila has revealed that these two genes contribute to a pathway where the parkin E3 ubiquitin ligase is under the regulatory control of the Pink1 protein kinase. In flies, the relationship between *parkin* and *Pink1* has been extended from the neurons to other tissues including the mitochondrial-rich flight muscle and the male gametes. This has led to investigation of the products of these highly conserved genes in the processes that promote mitochondrial survival. The routine participation of *parkin* and *Pink1* in mitochondrial activities reveals that the loss of the fusion/fission dynamic can result in the failure of the cells to adequately deal with mitochondria that present a burden to the health of the cell. Future study of Parkinson disease in Drosophila models will continue to reveal much about the basis of this disease. As the past century has made clear, over and over again, investigations that apply our collective knowledge of the genetics and biology of *Drosophila melanogaster* to explore the fundamentals of disease, such as Parkinson disease, are very difficult to ignore.

8. Acknowledgments

I wish to thank the Natural Sciences and Engineering Research Council of Canada (NSERC) Discovery Grants, NSERC Research Tool Instruments Grants, and Parkinson Society Canada Friedman Pilot Project Grants for funding my research programs. In a special acknowledgement, I wish to thank the family of Jerry Friedman for supporting Parkinson disease research in Canada. I wish to thank the School of Graduate Studies at Memorial University of Newfoundland and the NSERC post-graduate scholarship and NSERC undergraduate scholarship programs for funding the students that have studied aspects of Parkinson disease in Drosophila in my laboratory. I thank the talented technical and the patient administrative support staff within the Department of Biology, the Faculty of Science and the Office of Research at Memorial University of Newfoundland. I thank Annika F.M. Haywood, Amy M. Todd, Githure (Peter) M'Angale, Lisa Baker (Saunders), Gillian Sheppard, Sharleen Hoffe, Michael Nightingale, Jo-Anna Clark, Kevin Mitchell, Greg Dale, Meghan O'Leary, Kate Bassett, Heather Stone, Kimberley Chafe, David Lipsett and Jamie M. Kramer for participation in modelling Parkinson disease in *Drosophila melanogaster* in my laboratory.

Finally, as the recent progress in this field has been extensive, I must offer my sincere apologies to those colleagues whom I have failed to include in this discussion. There are many research groups that have made and continue to make extremely significant contributions to the study of Parkinson disease through the study of the Drosophila model system.

9. References

Auluck, P.K.; Chan, H.Y., Trojanowski, J.Q., Lee, V.M. & Bonini, N.M. (2002). Chaperone suppression of alpha-synuclein toxicity in a Drosophila model for Parkinson's disease. *Science*, 295, pp. 865-8.

Auluck, P.K.; Meulener, M.C. & Bonini, N.M. (2005). Mechanisms of suppression of {alpha}-synuclein neurotoxicity by geldanamycin in Drosophila. *J Biol Chem*, 280, pp. 2873-8.

Bae, Y.J.; Park, K.S. & Kang, S.J. (2003). Genomic organization and expression of parkin in Drosophila melanogaster. *Exp Mol Med*, 35, pp. 393-402.

Bonifati, V.; Rizzu, P., van Baren, M.J., Schaap, O., Breedveld, G.J., Krieger, E., Dekker, M.C., Squitieri, F., Ibanez, P., Joosse, M., van Dongen, J.W., Vanacore, N., van Swieten, J.C., Brice, A., Meco, G., van Duijn, C.M., Oostra, B.A. & Heutink, P. (2003). Mutations in the DJ-1 gene associated with autosomal recessive early-onset parkinsonism. *Science*, 299, pp. 256-9.

Botella, J.A.; Bayersdorfer, F. & Schneuwly, S. (2008). Superoxide dismutase overexpression protects dopaminergic neurons in a Drosophila model of Parkinson's disease. *Neurobiol Dis*, 30, pp. 65-73.

Braak, H.; Del Tredici, K., Rüb, U., de Vos, R.A., Jansen Steur, E.N. & Braak, E. (2003). Staging of brain pathology related to sporadic Parkinson's disease. *Neurobiol Aging*, 24, pp. 197-211.

Brand, A.H.; & Perrimon, N. (1993). Targeted gene expression as a means of altering cell fates and generating dominant phenotypes. *Development*, 118, pp. 401-15.

Cha G.H.; Kim, S., Park, J., Lee, E., Kim, M., Lee, S.B., Kim, J.M., Chung, J. & Cho K. S. (2005), Parkin negatively regulates JNK pathway in the dopaminergic neurons of Drosophila. *Proc Natl Acad Sci U S A*, 102, pp. 10345-50.

Chen, H.; & Chan, D.C. (2009), Mitochondrial dynamics--fusion, fission, movement, and mitophagy-in neurodegenerative diseases. *Hum Mol Genet*, 18, pp. R169-76.

Chen, L.; & Feany, M.B. (2005). Alpha-synuclein phosphorylation controls neurotoxicity and inclusion formation in a Drosophila model of Parkinson disease. *Nat Neurosci*, 8, pp. 657-63.

Clark, I.E.; Dodson, M.W., Jiang, C., Cao, J.H., Huh, J.R., Seol, J.H., Yoo, S.J., Hay, B.A. & Guo, M. (2006). Drosophila pink1 is required for mitochondrial function and interacts genetically with parkin. *Nature*, 441, pp. 1162-6.

Cooper, A.A.; Gitler, A.D., Cashikar, A., Haynes, C.M., Hill, K.J., Bhullar, B., Liu, K., Xu, K., Strathearn, K.E., Liu, F., Cao, S., Caldwell, K.A., Caldwell, G.A., Marsischky, G., Kolodner, R.D., Labaer, J., Rochet, J.C., Bonini, N.M. & Lindquist, S. (2006). Alpha-synuclein blocks ER-Golgi traffic and Rab1 rescues neuron loss in Parkinson's models. *Science*, 313, pp. 324-8.

Coulom H.; & Birman S. (2004). Chronic exposure to rotenone models sporadic Parkinson's disease in Drosophila melanogaster. *J Neurosci*, 24, pp. 10993-8.

Darios, F.; Corti, O., Lücking, C.B., Hampe, C., Muriel, M.P., Abbas, N., Gu, W.J., Hirsch, E.C., Rooney, T., Ruberg, M., & Brice, A. (2003). Parkin prevents mitochondrial swelling and cytochrome c release in mitochondria-dependent cell death. *Hum Mol Genet*, 12, pp. 517-26.

Dauer, W.; & Przedborski, S. (2003). Parkinson's disease: mechanisms and models. Neuron, 39, pp. 889-909.

Deng, H.; Dodson, M.W., Huang, H. & Guo, M. (2008). The Parkinson's disease genes pink1 and parkin promote mitochondrial fission and/or inhibit fusion in Drosophila. *Proc Natl Acad Sci U S A*, 105, pp. 14503-8.

Feany, M.B.; & Bender, W.W. (2000). A Drosophila model of Parkinson's disease. Nature, 404, pp. 394-8.

Fujiwara, H.; Hasegawa, M., Dohmae, N., Kawashima, A., Masliah, E., Goldberg, M.S., Shen, J., Takio, K. & Iwatsubo, T. (2002). alpha-Synuclein is phosphorylated in synucleinopathy lesions. *Nat Cell Biol*, 4, pp. 160-4.

Geisler, S.; Holmström, K.M., Skujat, D., Fiesel, F.C., Rothfuss, O.C., Kahle, P.J. & Springer W. (2010). PINK1/Parkin-mediated mitophagy is dependent on VDAC1 and p62/SQSTM1. *Nat Cell Biol*, 12, pp. 119-31.

Goldman, S.J.; Taylor, R., Zhang, Y. & Jin, S. (2010). Autophagy and the degradation of mitochondria. *Mitochondrion*, 10, pp. 309-15.

Greene, J.C.; Whitworth, A.J., Kuo, I., Andrews, L.A., Feany, M.B. & Pallanck, L.J. (2003). Mitochondrial pathology and apoptotic muscle degeneration in Drosophila parkin mutants. *Proc Natl Acad Sci U S A*, 100, pp. 4078-83.

Greene, J.C.; Whitworth, A.J., Andrews, L.A., Parker, T.J. & Pallanck, L.J. (2005). Genetic and genomic studies of Drosophila parkin mutants implicate oxidative stress and innate immune responses in pathogenesis. *Hum Mol Genet*, 14, pp. 799-811.

Hardy, J.; Lewis, P., Revesz, T., Lees, A. & Paisan-Ruiz, C. (2009). The genetics of Parkinson's syndromes: a critical review. *Curr Opin Genet Dev*, 19, pp. 254-65.

Haywood, A.F.; & Staveley, B.E. (2004). Parkin counteracts symptoms in a Drosophila model of Parkinson's disease. *BMC Neurosci*, 5:14.

Haywood, A.F.; & Staveley, B.E. (2006). Mutant alpha-synuclein-induced degeneration is reduced by parkin in a fly model of Parkinson's disease. *Genome*, 49, pp. 505-10.

Horowitz, J.M.; Vernace, V.A., Myers, J., Stachowiak, M.K., Hanlon, D.W., Fraley, G.S. & Torres, G. (2001). Immunodetection of Parkin protein in vertebrate and invertebrate brains: a comparative study using specific antibodies. *J Chem Neuroanat*, 21, pp. 75-93.

Imai, Y.; Gehrke, S., Wang, H.Q., Takahashi, R., Hasegawa, K., Oota, E. & Lu B. (2008). Phosphorylation of 4E-BP by LRRK2 affects the maintenance of dopaminergic neurons in Drosophila. *EMBO J*, 27, pp. 2432-43.

Kanao, T.; Venderova, K., Park, D.S., Unterman, T., Lu, B. & Imai Y. (2010). Activation of FoxO by LRRK2 induces expression of proapoptotic proteins and alters survival of postmitotic dopaminergic neuron in Drosophila. *Hum Mol Genet*, 19, pp. 3747-58.

Kim, Y.; Park, J., Kim, S., Song, S., Kwon, S.K., Lee, S.H., Kitada, T., Kim, J.M. & Chung, J. (2008). PINK1 controls mitochondrial localization of Parkin through direct phosphorylation. *Biochem Biophys Res Commun*, 377, pp. 975-80.

Kitada, T.; Asakawa, S., Hattori, N., Matsumine, H., Yamamura, Y., Minoshima, S., Yokochi, M., Mizuno, Y. & Shimizu N. (1998). Mutations in the parkin gene cause autosomal recessive juvenile parkinsonism. *Nature*, 392, pp. 605-8.

Kramer, J.M.; & Staveley, B.E. (2003). GAL4 causes developmental defects and apoptosis when expressed in the developing eye of Drosophila melanogaster. *Genet Mol Res*, 2, pp. 43-7.

Krüger R.; Kuhn, W., Müller, T., Woitalla, D., Graeber, M., Kösel, S., Przuntek, H., Epplen, J.T., Schöls, L. & Riess, O. (1998). Ala30Pro mutation in the gene encoding alpha-synuclein in Parkinson's disease. *Nat Genet*, 18, pp. 106-8.

Lee, S.B.; Kim, W., Lee, S. & Chung J. (2007). Loss of LRRK2/PARK8 induces degeneration of dopaminergic neurons in Drosophila. *Biochem Biophys Res Commun*, 358, pp. 534-9.

Liu, Z.; Wang, X., Yu, Y., Li, X., Wang, T., Jiang, H., Ren, Q., Jiao, Y., Sawa, A., Moran, T., Ross, C.A., Montell, C. & Smith, W.W. (2008). A Drosophila model for LRRK2-linked parkinsonism. *Proc Natl Acad Sci U S A*, 105, pp. 2693-8.

Menzies, F.M.; Yenisetti, S.C. & Min, K.T. (2005). Roles of Drosophila DJ-1 in survival of dopaminergic neurons and oxidative stress. *Curr Biol*, 15, 1578-82.

Meulener, M.; Whitworth, A.J., Armstrong-Gold, C.E., Rizzu, P., Heutink, P., Wes, P.D., Pallanck, L.J. & Bonini, N.M. (2005). Drosophila DJ-1 mutants are selectively sensitive to environmental toxins associated with Parkinson's disease. *Curr Biol*, 15, pp. 1572-7.

Meulener, M.C.; Xu, K., Thomson. L., Ischiropoulos, H. & Bonini, N.M. (2006). Mutational analysis of DJ-1 in Drosophila implicates functional inactivation by oxidative damage and aging. *Proc Natl Acad Sci U S A*, 103, pp. 12517-22.

Narendra, D.P.; Jin, S.M., Tanaka, A., Suen, D.F., Gautier, C.A., Shen, J., Cookson, M.R. & Youle, R.J. (2010). PINK1 is selectively stabilized on impaired mitochondria to activate Parkin. *PLoS Biol*, 8, pp. e1000298.

Nässel, D.R.; & Elekes, K. (1992). Aminergic neurons in the brain of blowflies and Drosophila: dopamine- and tyrosine hydroxylase-immunoreactive neurons and their relationship with putative histaminergic neurons. *Cell Tissue Res*, 267, pp. 147-67.

Paisán-Ruíz, C.; Jain, S., Evans, E.W., Gilks, W.P., Simón, J., van der Brug, M., López de Munain, A., Aparicio, S., Gil, A.M., Khan, N., Johnson, J., Martinez, J.R., Nicholl, D., Carrera, I.M., Pena, A.S., de Silva, R., Lees, A., Martí-Massó, J.F., Pérez-Tur, J. & Wood, N.W. & Singleton, A.B. (2004). Cloning of the gene containing mutations that cause PARK8-linked Parkinson's disease. *Neuron*, 44, pp. 595-600.

Park, J.; Lee, S.B., Lee, S., Kim, Y., Song, S., Kim, S., Bae, E., Kim, J., Shong, M., Kim, J.M. & Chung, J. (2006). Mitochondrial dysfunction in Drosophila PINK1 mutants is complemented by parkin. *Nature*, 441, pp. 1157-61.

Park, J.; Lee, G. & Chung, J. (2009). The PINK1-Parkin pathway is involved in the regulation of mitochondrial remodeling process. *Biochem Biophys Res Commun*, 378, pp. 518-23.

Park, S.S.; Schulz, E.M. & Lee, D. (2007). Disruption of dopamine homeostasis underlies selective neurodegeneration mediated by alpha-synuclein. *Eur J Neurosci*, 26, pp. 3104-12.

Pendleton, R.G.; Parvez, F., Sayed, M. & Hillman R. (2002). Effects of pharmacological agents upon a transgenic model of Parkinson's disease in Drosophila melanogaster. *J Pharmacol Exp Ther*, 300, pp. 91-6.

Pesah, Y.; Pham, T., Burgess, H., Middlebrooks, B., Verstreken, P., Zhou, Y., Harding, M., Bellen, H. & Mardon G. (2004). Drosophila parkin mutants have decreased mass and cell size and increased sensitivity to oxygen radical stress. *Development*, 131, pp. 2183-94.

Polymeropoulos, M.H.; Lavedan, C., Leroy, E., Ide, S.E., Dehejia, A., Dutra, A., Pike, B., Root, H., Rubenstein, J., Boyer, R., Stenroos, E.S., Chandrasekharappa, S., Athanassiadou, A., Papapetropoulos, T., Johnson, W.G., Lazzarini, A.M., Duvoisin, R.C., Di Iorio, G., Golbe, L.I. & Nussbaum, R.L. (1997). Mutation in the alpha-synuclein gene identified in families with Parkinson's disease. *Science*, 276, pp. 2045-7.

Poole, A.C.; Thomas, R.E., Andrews, L.A., McBride, H.M., Whitworth, A.J. & Pallanck, L.J. (2008). The PINK1/Parkin pathway regulates mitochondrial morphology. *Proc Natl Acad Sci U S A*, 105, pp. 1638-43.

Rezával, C.; Werbajh, S. & Ceriani, M.F. (2007). Neuronal death in Drosophila triggered by GAL4 accumulation. *Eur J Neurosci*, 25, pp. 683-94.

Riparbelli, M.G.; & Callaini, G. (2007). The Drosophila parkin homologue is required for normal mitochondrial dynamics during spermiogenesis. *Dev Biol*, 303, pp. 108-20.

Sang, T.K.; Chang, H.Y., Lawless, G.M., Ratnaparkhi, A., Mee, L., Ackerson, L.C., Maidment, N.T., Krantz, D.E. & Jackson, G.R. (2007). A Drosophila model of mutant human parkin-induced toxicity demonstrates selective loss of dopaminergic neurons and dependence on cellular dopamine. *J Neurosci*, 27, pp. 981-92.

Simuni, T.; & Sethi, K. (2008). Nonmotor manifestations of Parkinson's disease. *Ann Neurol*, 64, pp. S65-80.

Singleton, A.B.; Farrer, M., Johnson, J., Singleton, A., Hague, S., Kachergus, J., Hulihan, M., Peuralinna, T., Dutra, A., Nussbaum, R., Lincoln, S., Crawley, A., Hanson, M., Maraganore, D., Adler, C., Cookson, M.R., Muenter, M., Baptista, M., Miller, D., Blancato, J., Hardy, J., & Gwinn-Hardy, K. (2003). alpha-Synuclein locus triplication causes Parkinson's disease. *Science*, 302, pp. 841.

Todd, A.M.; & Staveley, B.E. (2008). Pink1 suppresses alpha-synuclein-induced phenotypes in a Drosophila model of Parkinson's disease. *Genome*, 51, pp. 1040-6.

Trinh, K.; Moore, K., Wes, P.D., Muchowski, P.J., Dey, J., Andrews, L. & Pallanck LJ. (2008). Induction of the phase II detoxification pathway suppresses neuron loss in Drosophila models of Parkinson's disease. *J Neurosci*, 28, pp. 465-72.

Valente, E.M.; Abou-Sleiman, P.M., Caputo, V., Muqit, M.M., Harvey, K., Gispert, S., Ali, Z., Del Turco, D., Bentivoglio, A.R., Healy, D.G., Albanese, A., Nussbaum, R., González-Maldonado, R., Deller, T., Salvi, S., Cortelli, P., Gilks, W.P., Latchman, D.S., Harvey, R.J., Dallapiccola, B., Auburger, G. & Wood N.W. (2004). Hereditary early-onset Parkinson's disease caused by mutations in PINK1. *Science*, 304, pp. 1158-60.

Vives-Bauza, C.; Zhou, C., Huang, Y., Cui, M., de Vries, R.L., Kim, J., May, J., Tocilescu, M.A., Liu, W., Ko, H.S., Magrané, J., Moore, D.J., Dawson, V.L., Grailhe, R., Dawson, T.M., Li, C., Tieu, K. & Przedborski, S. (2010). PINK1-dependent recruitment of Parkin to mitochondria in mitophagy. *Proc Natl Acad Sci U S A*, 107, pp. 378-83.

Wang, D.; Qian, L., Xiong, H., Liu, J., Neckameyer, W.S., Oldham, S., Xia, K., Wang, J., Bodmer, R.& Zhang, Z. (2006). Antioxidants protect PINK1-dependent dopaminergic neurons in Drosophila. *Proc Natl Acad Sci U S A*, 103, pp. 13520-5.

Wang, C.; Lu, R., Ouyang, X., Ho, M.W., Chia, W., Yu, F. & Lim, K.L. (2007). Drosophila overexpressing parkin R275W mutant exhibits dopaminergic neuron degeneration and mitochondrial abnormalities. *J Neurosci*, 27,pp. 8563-70.

Wassef, R.; Haenold, R., Hansel, A., Brot, N., Heinemann, S.H. & Hoshi, T. (2007). Methionine sulfoxide reductase A and a dietary supplement S-methyl-L-cysteine prevent Parkinson's-like symptoms. *J Neurosci*, 27, pp. 12808-16.

Whitworth, A.J.; Theodore, D.A., Greene, J.C., Benes, H., Wes, P.D. & Pallanck, L.J. (2005). Increased glutathione S-transferase activity rescues dopaminergic neuron loss in a Drosophila model of Parkinson's disease. *Proc Natl Acad Sci U S A*, 102, pp. 8024-9.

Whitworth, A.J.; Wes, P.D. & Pallanck, L.J. (2006). Drosophila models pioneer a new approach to drug discovery for Parkinson's disease. *Drug Discov Today*, 11, pp. 119-26.

Whitworth, A.J.; Lee, J.R., Ho, V.M., Flick, R., Chowdhury, R. & McQuibban, G.A. (2008). Rhomboid-7 and HtrA2/Omi act in a common pathway with the Parkinson's disease factors Pink1 and Parkin. *Dis Model Mech*, 1, pp. 168-74.

Xiong, H.; Wang, D., Chen, L., Choo, Y.S., Ma, H., Tang, C., Xia, K., Jiang, W., Ronai, Z., Zhuang, X. & Zhang, Z. (2009). Parkin, PINK1, and DJ-1 form a ubiquitin E3 ligase complex promoting unfolded protein degradation. *J Clin Invest*, 119, pp. 650-60.

Yang, Y.; Nishimura, I., Imai, Y., Takahashi, R. & Lu, B. (2003). Parkin suppresses dopaminergic neuron-selective neurotoxicity induced by Pael-R in Drosophila. *Neuron*, 37, pp. 911-24.

Yang, Y.; Gehrke, S., Imai, Y., Huang, Z., Ouyang, Y., Wang, J.W., Yang, L., Beal, M.F., Vogel, H. & Lu, B. (2006). Mitochondrial pathology and muscle and dopaminergic neuron degeneration caused by inactivation of Drosophila Pink1 is rescued by Parkin. *Proc Natl Acad Sci U S A*, 103, pp. 10793-8.

Yang, Y.; Ouyang, Y., Yang, L., Beal, M.F., McQuibban, A., Vogel, H. & Lu, B. (2008). Pink1 regulates mitochondrial dynamics through interaction with the fission/fusion machinery. *Proc Natl Acad Sci U S A*, 105, pp. 7070-5.

Zarranz, J.J.; Alegre, J., Gómez-Esteban, J.C., Lezcano, E., Ros, R., Ampuero, I., Vidal, L., Hoenicka, J., Rodriguez, O., Atarés, B., Llorens, V., Gomez Tortosa, E., del Ser, T., Muñoz, D.G. & de Yebenes, J.G. (2004). The new mutation, E46K, of alpha-synuclein causes Parkinson and Lewy body dementia. *Ann Neurol*, 55, pp. 164-73.

Zhou, C.; Huang, Y., Shao, Y., May, J., Prou, D., Perier, C., Dauer, W., Schon, E.A. & Przedborski, S. (2008). The kinase domain of mitochondrial PINK1 faces the cytoplasm. *Proc Natl Acad Sci U S A*, 105, pp. 12022-7.

Zimprich, A.; Biskup, S., Leitner, P., Lichtner, P., Farrer, M., Lincoln, S., Kachergus, J., Hulihan, M., Uitti, R.J., Calne, D.B., Stoessl, A.J., Pfeiffer, R.F., Patenge, N., Carbajal, I.C., Vieregge, P., Asmus, F., Müller-Myhsok, B., Dickson, D.W., Meitinger, T., Strom, T.M., Wszolek, Z.K. & Gasser, T. (2004). Mutations in LRRK2 cause autosomal-dominant parkinsonism with pleomorphic pathology. *Neuron*, 44, pp. 601-7.

Ziviani, E; Tao, R.N. & Whitworth, A.J. (2010). Drosophila parkin requires PINK1 for mitochondrial translocation and ubiquitinates mitofusin. *Proc Natl Acad Sci U S A*, 107, pp. 5018-23.

13

Parkinson's Disease and Parkin: Insights from *Park2* Knockout Mice

Sarah E.M. Stephenson[1,2], Juliet M. Taylor[2] and Paul J. Lockhart[1,2]
[1]*Murdoch Childrens Research Institute*
[2]*University of Melbourne*
Australia

1 Introduction

Parkinson's disease (PD) is a neurodegenerative movement disorder distinguished by resting tremor, bradykinesia, rigidity, postural instability and gait disturbances. Non-motor symptoms including dysfunction of the autonomic nervous system, neuropsychiatric changes, sensory and sleep disturbances are also common. PD may be diagnosed at any age but is most common in aged populations - affecting approximately 1% of individuals over 60 years of age and rising to approximately 4% in age groups above 85 years of age (de Lau and Breteler, 2006; Van Den Eeden et al., 2003). It has become apparent that differential subgroups may be categorised by age of onset, dominant symptoms and progression. Two key subsets include late- and early-onset PD. Late-onset PD is typically identified in individuals over the age of 70 and is characterised by postural imbalance and gait impairment with accompanying rigidity and akinesia. Early-onset PD is typified by a dominant tremor and slow progression in motor decline, and is primarily identified in individuals less than 50 years of age (Lewis et al., 2005; Selikhova et al., 2009).

The lead pathological identifier of PD is moderate to severe dopaminergic neuronal loss within the substantia nigra pars compacta with accompanying Lewy pathology in surviving neurons (Daniel and Lees, 1993; Dickson et al., 2009; Gelb et al., 1999). It is thought that the combination of Lewy pathology and dopaminergic cell loss in PD leads to striatal dopamine depletion, and this accounts for the motor symptoms (Obeso et al., 2008). Earlier diagnosis of PD is important as motor symptoms do not become apparent until approximately 60% of dopaminergic neurons are lost (Fearnley and Lees, 1991; Pakkenberg et al., 1991).

Current treatments are available to manage the symptoms of PD. Medications such as the dopamine precursor L-3,4-dihydroxyphenylalanine (L-DOPA) and inhibitors of dopamine metabolism are used to supplement the reduced dopamine level. Deep brain stimulation is an alternative treatment. The patient undergoes surgery to implant an electrical stimulation device into the affected region of the basal ganglia. The electrical impulses generated by the device interfere with the abnormal signals that are causing the tremor, thereby alleviating some of the symptoms of the disease (reviewed in (Hurelbrink and Lewis, 2010)). To identify treatments that address or arrest the progressive nature of PD, an understanding of the molecular mechanisms responsible for the loss of nigrostriatal dopaminergic neurons and associated Lewy pathology must be delineated.

The aetiology of the majority of PD cases remain unknown, however, gene mutations in familial forms of PD account for up to 10% of cases. Over 15 PD loci have been reported and greater than 10 genes have been identified (reviewed in (Shulman et al., 2010)). Mutations in *alpha synuclein* and *LRRK2* are the predominant cause of autosomal dominant PD, while mutations in *parkin* and *PINK1* cause autosomal recessive PD. Several genome wide association studies using large idiopathic PD cohorts have demonstrated an unequivocal role for common genetic variation in familial PD genes in the aetiology of idiopathic PD, and identified new genetic players including *microtubule associated protein tau* in sporadic disease aetiology (Satake et al., 2009; Simon-Sanchez et al., 2009).

Mutations in *PARK2* (*parkin)* account for 50% of all familial early-onset PD cases, at least 20% of young-onset sporadic PD and also contribute to late onset sporadic disease (Foroud et al., 2003; Lucking et al., 2000; Mata et al., 2004). *Parkin* encodes a 465 amino acid multi-domain protein with homology to a class of enzymes termed E3 ubiquitin-protein ligases that function in the ubiquitin proteasome system (UPS) (Shimura et al., 2000). The UPS is the predominant cellular pathway for the turnover of misfolded and short-lived intracellular proteins (Ciechanover et al., 2000). Parkin mediates the formation of a lysine-48 polyubiquitin chain linked to the target protein, which functions as a signal for degradation by the proteasome. Parkin is also capable of alternative modes of ubiquitination including monoubiquitination and lysine-63 polyubiquitination, which appear to function in signalling and autophagy, respectively (Chew et al., 2011; Olzmann and Chin, 2008).

The pathological hallmark of many neurodegenerative diseases is the accumulation of proteins in aggregates/inclusions. There is very little information about the neuropathology observed in the brains of individuals with *parkin*-proven PD as only a seven cases have gone to autopsy. These cases displayed variable degree of cell loss in the substantia nigra pars compacta, and in some cases the locus coeruleus. Several cases displayed evidence of gliosis and astrocytosis. With the exception of two cases, Lewy pathology was not identified. Evidence of other types of protein aggregation including neurofibrillary tangles, alpha-synuclein-positive dendritic inclusions and tau accumulation were evident to varying degrees (reviewed in (Cookson et al., 2008)). As Lewy pathology is often cited as a significant pathological difference between idiopathic and *parkin*-proven PD some have hypothesised that parkin may play an integral role in Lewy formation (von Coelln et al., 2006). However, due to the small number of autopsies and the limitations of studying end stage disease tissues, animal and cell models provide a more detailed mechanistic understanding of *parkin*-mediated PD and the contribution of parkin to idiopathic PD.

A number of animal and cellular models of parkin dysfunction have been described. Parkin knockout flies demonstrated a reduced lifespan, muscle degeneration mitochondrial abnormalities, sensitivity to oxidative stress and male infertility (Greene et al., 2003; Pesah et al., 2004). While the first reports suggested *parkin* deficient drosophila did not have significant loss of dopaminergic neurons, a subsequent study utilising more sensitive analytical techniques indicated a reduction in the number of a subtype of dopaminergic neurons (Whitworth et al., 2005). *Park2* knockout mice did not appear to display extensive behavioural or dopaminergic abnormalities. As such the utility of such models to evaluate new pharmaceutical agents is unclear. A number of independent *parkin* deficient mouse models have now been generated. This review will outline the insights provided and look ahead to how *Park2* knockout mice may help to better understand *parkin*-mediated PD and by extension idiopathic PD.

2. *Parkin* mouse models

To date, eleven models of parkin dysfunction have been reported, seven of which are independently generated *Park2* knockout models. Studies on these mice will provide the basis of the discussion within. Models noted that are outside the scope of this paper include the quaking viable mouse which is a knockout of *parkin* and *PArkin Co-Regulated Gene* with dysregulation of *quaking* gene (Lockhart et al., 2004; Lorenzetti et al., 2004;), a recently identified spontaneous CH3-*Park2*^{E398Q} mutant (Ramsey and Giasson, 2010), a model of transgenic overexpression of a parkin truncated mutant (Lu et al., 2009) and a model of overexpression of wildtype parkin (Yoshida et al., 2010).
The majority of *parkin*-proven PD cases are the result of large genomic alterations (deletion, duplication or inversion) that affect one or more exons. *PARK2* spans an exaggerated genomic interval of approximately 1.4 Mb due to super-expanded introns and is located in a region of genomic instability (Denison et al., 2003; Palumbo et al., 2010). Several mouse models were generated to replicate known deletions that affect a single exon. Exons targeted in the *Park2* knockout models were exon 2, exon 3 or exon 7, which are predicted to result in a peptide/protein of 4aa, 57aa or 243aa truncated, respectively (Table 1). This suggests that parkin function would be abrogated in all of these models in the event translation occurs. Consistent with loss of function, immunoreactivity corresponding to full length parkin could not be detected in any of the knockout mice lines (Table 1 for references).

2.1 Behavioural characteristics

PD is a progressive adult onset neurodegenerative disorder, therefore, it would be anticipated that disease associated mutations within animal models would replicate this feature. For this reason it is important to consider mouse to human age equivalents. It is generally considered that between the ages of 3-6 months mice have finished development, the rapid maturational growth of most biological processes and structures, but are not affected by senescence. These mice are considered to represent 'mature adults' equivalent to a 20-30 year old human. Changes in senescence can be detected in some but not all mice between the ages of 10-15 months, which is considered 'middle age' and corresponds to 38-47 years in humans. Senescence markers can be detected in almost all 'old' mice between 18-24 months of age and these represent approximately 56-69 years in humans. Although for each inbred strain it varies, the average life span (50% survivorship) of a laboratory mouse is 28 months and the upper limit near 36 months, considered the equivalent of approximately 78 and 94 human years, respectively (Harrison, 2011).
Park2 knockout mice appear to develop normally, have normal general motor function and do not show any obvious clinical phenotype or behavioural abnormality. In one study, Kaplan-Meier survival analysis using the *Park2*^{tm1Roo} knockout model suggested an increase in mortality, which is consistent with data from PD patients' pre-L-DOPA therapy (Rodriguez-Navarro et al., 2007). However, in another study using the *Park2*^{tm1Roo} knockout model on a different background a difference in survival was not found (Guerrero et al., 2008). A reduction in body weight was identified in three lines but was not replicated in three other lines (Table 2) (Itier et al., 2003; Oyama et al., 2010; Palacino et al., 2004; Perez and Palmiter, 2005; Von Coelln et al., 2004; Zhu et al., 2007). In addition, a reduced body temperature was detected in *Park2*^{tm1Roo} knockout mice but was not replicated in the *Park2*^{tm1Rpa} knockout line. The findings for adhesive-removal tests and acoustic-startle were also conflicting (Goldberg et al., 2003; Itier et al., 2003; Perez and Palmiter, 2005; Von Coelln et al., 2004).

B6;129S2-*Park2*^{tm1Roo} (Itier et al., 2003)[1] Partial replacement of exon 3 with PGK-Neo^R cassette resulting in a truncated protein. If exon 3 is skipped, the predicted result is a frame shift after parkin amino acid 57 with the addition of 49 novel amino acids.
B6;129S4-*Park2*^{tm1Shn} (Goldberg et al., 2003) Partial replacement of exon 3 with in frame insertion of EGFP followed by PGK-Neo^R cassette resulting in a truncated protein consisting of the first 95 amino acids of parkin followed by EGFP (expression of EGFP protein was not detected). If exon 3 skipping occurs, the predicted result is a frameshift after parkin amino acid 57 with the addition of 49 novel amino acids.
B6;129S7/S4-*Park2*^{tm1Tmd} (Von Coelln et al., 2004)[2] Cre-mediated deletion of exon 7 resulting in a frameshift after parkin amino acid 243 with the addition of 8 novel amino acids.
B6;129S4-*Park2*^{tm1Rpa} (Perez and Palmiter, 2005)[1] Complete replacement of exon 2 with Polr2a-Neo^R cassette. If exon 2 is skipped, the predicted result would be a change in the reading frame producing a 4-aa peptide.
B6;CBA-*Park2*^{tm1Hn} (Sato et al., 2006)[3] Partial replacement of exon 2 with in frame insertion of tauGFP fusion protein followed by MC1-Neo^R cassette to produce tauGFP driven by the parkin promoter (expression of tauGFP protein was not detected). If exon 2 skipping occurs, the predicted result would be a change in the reading frame producing a 4-aa peptide.
B6;129P2-*Park2*^{tm1Oga}(Kitao et al., 2007) Complete replacement of exon 3 with PGK-Neo^R cassette. If exon 3 is skipped, the predicted result is a frame shift after parkin amino acid 57 with the addition of 49 novel amino acids.
B6;129S1/X1-*Park2*^{tm1Ccs} (Stichel et al., 2007) Complete replacement of exon 3 with a Neo^R cassette. If exon 3 is skipped, the predicted result is a frame shift after parkin amino acid 57 with the addition of 49 novel amino acids.

Table 1. *Park2* knockout mouse models
Nomenclature guidelines for naming genetically modified mouse strains were followed. Information regarding the genetic background of the mouse strain was extracted from the embryonic stem cell line strain and strain used in initial chimeric breeding. Only the first reported mouse strain is indicated, mutant alleles may have subsequently been bred to other strains or isogenicity for subsequent publications. [1]Also reported the allele on 129 isogenic background but unless indicated experiments were performed on a mixed background. [2]Strain information was obtained from Perez and Palmiter (2005) Supplementary Table 3. [3]A laboratory code for Nobutaka Hattori, the corresponding author of the publication by Sato et al., (2006) could not be identified with the Institute for Laboratory Animal Research (ILAR) therefore his initials (Hn) were used. This is only for the purposes of differentiating these strains in this chapter and does not represent the true allele designation.

It was anticipated that *parkin*-deficient mouse models would display motor defects, which would validate their suitability for PD research. Initial experiments indicated that only *Park2*^{tm1Roo} knockout line showed a basal reduction in locomotion (Table 3) (Itier et al., 2003). However, when investigated in the same line at 24 months, only a non-significant tendency for reduced locomotion was reported (Rodriguez-Navarro et al., 2007). The *Park2* knockout lines did not show significant deficits on the rotarod, which is used to measure balance,

	Body weight		*Body temperature*		*Adhesive-removal*		*Acoustic-startle*	
$Park2^{tm1Roo}$	↓	1-16	↓	4				
$Park2^{tm1Shn}$	↓	1-12			↓[3]	2-7		
$Park2^{tm1Tmd}$	–	NA					↓	9
$Park2^{tm1Rpa}$	–[1]	3-24	–	3, 22	–	19	–[2]	12-15
$Park2^{tm1Hn}$								
$Park2^{tm1Oga}$	↓	NA						
$Park2^{tm1Ccs}$	–	6, 18						

Table 2. General behavioural attributes of *Park2* knockout mice
Attributes investigated in two or more *Park2* knockout models. *Park2* knockout showed no difference (-) or a significant difference compared to wildtype (decreased = ↓, increased = ↑). The age(s) of mice (in months) is indicated, if unreported it is shown as not available (NA). Gray cells indicate that attribute has not been reported. [1]Decrease in weight was identified at 6 months of age in the B6:129S4 background but was not reproduced in the 129S4 background. [2]An increased sensitivity was detected in the B6:129S4 background but was not reproduced in the 129S4 background. [3]A significant decrease was not identified at 18 months. The table should be used as a guide only as methodology and analysis varies for each model.

	Locomotion		*Amphetamine response*		*Rotarod*		*Balance-beam*		*Pole Test*	
$Park2^{tm1Roo}$	↓	6	↓	6						
$Park2^{tm1Shn}$	–	6-18			–	6-18	↓	2-18		
$Park2^{tm1Tmd}$	–	18			–	3-24				
$Park2^{tm1Rpa}$	–[1]	3-22	–	3	–[3]	3-18	–	19	↓	6, 18
$Park2^{tm1Hn}$	–	12	–	12	–	12				
$Park2^{tm1Oga}$					–	3-12			–	3-12
$Park2^{tm1Ccs}$	–	6-21	↓[2]	3	–	6-24				

Table 3. Motor function of *Park2* knockout mice.
Attributes investigated in two or more *Park2* knockout models. *Park2* knockout showed no difference (-) or a significant difference compared to wildtype (decreased = ↓, increased = ↑). The age(s) of mice (in months) is indicated. Gray cells indicate that attribute has not been reported. [1]$Park2^{tm1Rpa}$ knockout mice exhibited greater locomotor activity specifically during the second dark cycle at 12 months only. [2]Reported as a lack of amphetamine to induce thigmotaxic behaviour. [3]$Park2^{tm1Rpa}$ knockout mice were more likely to grip the rotarod at 6 months. The table should be used as a guide only as methodology and analysis varies for each model.

coordination, physical condition, and motor-planning (Goldberg et al., 2003; Oyama et al., 2010; Perez and Palmiter, 2005; Sato et al., 2006; Von Coelln et al., 2004; Zhu et al., 2007). Two of the *Park2* knockout models appeared to have a reduced response to amphetamine, which increases the amount of dopamine in the synaptic cleft and enhances the response of post-synaptic neurons, whereas another two did not (Itier et al., 2003; Perez and Palmiter, 2005; Sato et al., 2006; Zhu et al., 2007). Furthermore, alternative results were reported for motor co-ordination determined by the balance beam test and the pole test (Goldberg et al., 2003; Oyama et al., 2010; Perez and Palmiter, 2005).

Cognitive function has been investigated in three of the *Park2* knockout lines (Table 4). Two of the models displayed a reduction in exploratory behaviour which was suggestive of an increased anxiety (Itier et al., 2003; Zhu et al., 2007). However, in other tests of cognition, including light/dark exploration and T-maze alteration the finding varied depending on the *Park2* knockout model analysed (Itier et al., 2003; Perez and Palmiter, 2005; Zhu et al., 2007).

For the most part, based on the aforementioned investigations of the behavioural attributes of the *Park2* knockout mouse lines it would appear that *parkin* deficiency does not cause a PD-like phenotype in mice. The discrepancies reported for the *Park2* knockout lines may be attributable to the genetic background of the mouse strain harbouring the mutant allele (discussed in (Perez and Palmiter, 2005)). The relative inability to identify a significant difference from wildtype for a number of the attributes investigated may be because the effect of parkin deficiency is very subtle and the experimental approach lacks the required sensitivity. As PD is a progressive disorder, an alternative explanation may be the age of *Park2* knockout model when the attribute was investigated. For example, 18 month old *Park2^tm1Roo^* knockout mice showed a significant decrease in the length of their hind limb stride, and at 24 months a number of motor and non-motor irregularities were apparent in the *Park2^tm1Roo^* knockout line that were suggested to parallel symptoms observed in PD sufferers (Rodriguez-Navarro et al., 2007). Further investigation when *parkin* deficiency is combined with old age in the *Park2* knockout models is required to address this issue.

	Refuse to perform tests		*T-maze alternation*		*Exploratory behaviour*		*Light/dark exploration*		*Morris water maze*	
Park2^{tm1Roo}	↓	15	↓	4	↓	6				
Park2^{tm1Shn}										
Park2^{tm1Tmd}										
Park2^{tm1Rpa}	–	3-22	–	12-20			–	12,18	–	18
Park2^{tm1Hn}										
Park2^{tm1Oga}										
Park2^{tm1Ccs}					↓	3	↓	3	↑	NA

Table 4. Cognitive-related behaviour in *Park2* knockout mice.
Attributes investigated in two or more *Park2* knockout models. *Park2* knockout showed no difference (-) or a significant difference compared to wildtype (decreased = ↓, increased = ↑). The age(s) of mice (in months) is indicated, if age was unreported it is shown as not available (NA). Gray cells indicate that attribute has not been reported. The table should be used as a guide only as methodology and analysis varies for each model.

2.2 Pathology

The pathological hallmark of PD is the loss of dopaminergic neurons within the substantia nigra and Lewy pathology. Other regions may also display loss of neurons and/or Lewy pathology, including the locus ceruleus, the hypothalamus and some regions of the cortex (Halliday and McCann, 2010). The cell body of dopaminergic neurons are predominantly localised to three regions of the brain: the substantia nigra pars compacta, the ventral tegmental area and the hypothalamus. These neurons project into the putamen to form the nigrostriatal dopaminergic system, the ventral striatum or the cortex to form the mesolimbic or the mesocortical dopaminergic pathways, and the pituitary gland to form the tuberoinfundibular pathway, respectively. In contrast, the largest population of noradrenergic neurons is found in the locus ceruleus, and these project to most central nervous system areas (Grimm et al., 2004).

The number and morphology of tyrosine hydroxylase staining neurons in the substantia nigra of *Park2* knockout mice was not found to be remarkably different from wildtype mice (Table 5). However, in the $Park2^{tm1Roo}$ knockout line age was an important factor influencing loss of dopaminergic neurons. When examined at 2 or 15 months there was no difference in the

	Morphology of tyrosine hydroxylase staining neurons			*Number of tyrosine hydroxylase staining neurons*		
	Result	Age	Region	Result	Age	Region
$Park2^{tm1Roo}$	–	2, 15	C, BS, H, SN, ST	– ; ↓[1]	2, 15 ; 18, 24	SN
$Park2^{tm1Shn}$	–	NA	LC, SN, ST	–	12-24	SN
$Park2^{tm1Tmd}$	–	18	SN, ST	– ; ↓[2]	12-18 ; 2,12-18	SN ; LC
$Park2^{tm1Rpa}$	–	NA	SN	–	NA	SN
$Park2^{tm1Hn}$	–	3	SN	–	3	LC, SN
$Park2^{tm1Oga}$				–	26	SN
$Park2^{tm1Ccs}$	–	6-18	LC, SN, ST	–	6-18	LC, SN

Table 5. Catecholaminergic neuron pathology in *Park2* knockout mice.

The morphology and number of catecholaminergic neurons in *Park2* knockout mice were identified by staining with anti-tyrosine hydroxylase antibody. *Park2* knockout showed no difference (-) or a significant difference compared to wildtype (decreased = ↓, increased = ↑) The age(s) of mice (in months) is indicated, if unreported it is shown as not available (NA). Gray cells indicate that attribute has not been reported. Brain stem (BS), cerebellum (C), locus ceruleus *(LC),* hippocampus (H), substantia nigra (SN), striatum (ST). [1]Significant reduction in the number of tyrosine hydroxylase staining neurons at 18 month was only identified in female $Park2^{tm1Roo}$ knockout mice. [2]Phenotype shows reduced penetrance, ~30% of $Park2^{tm1Tmd}$ knockout do not show a significant reduction in the number of tyrosine hydroxylase staining neurons in the LC. The table should be used as a guide only as methodology and analysis varies for each model.

number of dopaminergic neurons in the substantia nigra, but when investigated at 24 months a loss of ~35% of neurons was detected (Itier et al., 2003; Rodriguez-Navarro et al., 2007). In addition, a significant loss of tyrosine hydroxylase reactivity was demonstrable at 18 months in females but not males mice (Rodriguez-Navarro et al., 2008). Notably, in two other models examined at or above 24 months no significant loss of dopamineric neurons in the substantia nigra was reported (Goldberg et al., 2003; Kitao et al., 2007). Alternatively, in ~70% of *Park2*^{tm1Tmd} knockout mice there was significant reduction in the number of catecholaminergic neurons in the locus coeruleus. Such pathology was present at 2 months of age, suggesting dysfunctional development of catecholaminergic neurons in the locus ceruleus (Von Coelln et al., 2004). As ~30% *Park2*^{tm1Tmd} knockout mice showed no significant decrease, it is indicative of reduced penetrance and suggests other factors must also influence the trait.

It is generally considered that *parkin* deletion alone in humans is sufficient to cause PD with the onset of symptoms typically earlier than observed for idiopathic PD. The analyses summarised in Tables 2 to 5 suggests mouse models of *parkin* deficiency do not replicate this phenotype. However, some of the *Park2* knockout models display subtle behavioural and pathological phenotypes that parallel PD. Therefore, *parkin* deficiency in the mouse may alter pathways common to human pathogenesis but for as yet unknown reasons do not cause a pronounced PD-like phenotype. Observations reported suggest that the mechanistic pathways in which parkin functions are conserved between the human and mouse, and *Park2* knockout mice may be a useful model to further refine the function of parkin and its role in disease pathogenesis.

2.3 Neurochemistry

It is hypothesised that dysfunction in dopamine metabolism may precede loss of dopaminergic neurons and represent a presymptomatic disease state. This is supported by studies of dopamine metabolism using positron emission tomography in both *parkin*-proven and idiopathic Parkinson's disease, and unaffected individuals with heterozygous mutations in *Parkin* and *PINK1* (Guo et al., 2010; Sioka et al., 2010; Tang et al., 2010). The biosynthetic pathway for dopamine production in catecholaminergic neurons is the sequential conversion of phenylalanine to tyrosine, dihydroxyphenylalanine (L-DOPA) and dopamine. In dopaminergic neurons the synthesis of dopamine is the final product of the process whereas in noradrenergic neurons dopamine may be further modified to norepinephrine (Daubner et al., 2011). Within dopaminergic neurons, newly synthesised cytoplasmic dopamine is translocated by vesicular monoamine transporter 2 (VMAT2) into vesicles for storage until synaptic release. Synaptic dopamine interacts with D1 and D2 receptors on postsynaptic neurons in the striatum, which mediate the direct and indirect dopaminergic pathways, respectively. Within the substantia nigra and the basal ganglia synaptic dopamine is inactivated primarily via reuptake by the dopamine transporter (DAT) on presynaptic neurons. Intracellular dopamine is then sequestered in vesicles via VMAT for re-use or converted by monoamine oxidase (MAO) to 3,4-dihydroxyphenylacetic acid (DOPAC) for degradation. DOPAC then diffuses out of the nerve terminal and into the extracellular space, where it can be transformed into the more stable metabolite homovanillic acid (HVA) via catechol-*O*-methyltransferase (COMT). To a lesser extent, extracellular dopamine can be metabolised without reuptake into presynaptic neurons. In this process, extracellular dopamine is converted to 3-methoxytyramine (3-MT) by COMT then to HVA by MAO (reviewed in (Standaert and Galanter, 2007)).

Investigation of the levels of dopamine and its metabolites DOPAC and HVA in the striatum of the *Park2* knockout lines did not reveal significant alterations (Table 6) (Itier et al., 2003; Oyama et al., 2010; Palacino et al., 2004; Perez and Palmiter, 2005; Von Coelln et al., 2004). The notable exception was the increase in HVA in the $Park2^{tm1Ccs}$ model (Zhu et al., 2007). In addition, in a later study, a significant increase in DOPAC and HVA in the striatum at 3 months old $Park2^{tm1Roo}$ knockout mice was reported (omitted from table) (Menendez et al., 2006). This may be reflective of an increase dopamine metabolism. Likewise, an increase in the ratio of DOPAC to dopamine or 3-MT was identified in the striatum of the $Park2^{tm1Roo}$ knockout line, perhaps indicative of increased intracellular dopamine metabolism via MAO as opposed to extracellular metabolism via COMT (Itier et al., 2003). Although no significant difference of total dopamine levels were identified in the striatum of the $Park2^{tm1Shn}$ knockout model, the amount of extracellular dopamine in this region was significantly increased. In addition, dopamine reuptake was unaltered, which suggests that the increased extracellular dopamine was due to increased release of dopamine from presynaptic dopaminergic neurons (Goldberg et al., 2003). In contrast, in the striatum of the $Park2^{tm1Hn}$ knockout model a reduction in dopamine synthesis and an increase in D1 and D2 receptor

	Dopamine	DOPAC	HVA	Noradrenaline
$Park2^{tm1Roo}$	– 11 BS, D, ST; ↑ 11 L	– 11 BS, D, ST; ↑ 11 L	– 11 BS, D, L, ST	– 11 BS, D, L, ST
$Park2^{tm1Shn}$	– 6-24 ST	– 6-24 ST		
$Park2^{tm1Tmd}$	– 18 ST	– 18 ST	– 18 ST	– 18 BS, C, CC, D, H, PC; ↓ 18 OB, SC
$Park2^{tm1Rpa}$	– 22 ST	– 22 MB, ST	– 22 ST	– 18-22 OB, SC, ST
$Park2^{tm1Hn}$	↑ 12 MB; – 12 ST	– 12 MB, ST	– 12 MB, ST	
$Park2^{tm1Oga}$	– 3-12 ST	– 3-12 ST	– 3-12 ST	
$Park2^{tm1Ccs}$	– NA ST	– NA ST	↑ NA ST	

Table 6. Neurochemical analysis of *Park2* Knockout mice
The level of dopamine, its metabolites 3,4-Dihydroxyphenylacetic acid (DOPAC) and homovanillic acid (HVA) and its derivate noradrenaline were analysed. *Park2* knockout showed no difference (-) or a significant difference compared to wildtype (decreased = ↓, increased = ↑). The age(s) of mice (in months) is indicated, if unreported it is shown as not available (NA). Gray cells indicate that attribute has not been reported. Brain stem (BS), cerebral cortex (CC), cerebellum (C), diencephalon (D), hippocampus (H), limbic region (L), olfactory bulb (OB), midbrain (MB), prefrontal cortex (PC), spinal cord (SC), substantia nigra (SN), striatum (ST). The table should be used as a guide only as methodology and analysis varies for each model.

binding was detected using receptor specific antagonists. This suggests decline in striatal dopamine release may result in decreased synaptic dopamine (Sato et al., 2006). Similar analysis in the *Park2*^{tm1Shn} knockout line however, did not indicate an alteration in the amount of D1 or D2 receptor binding in the striatum (Goldberg et al., 2003; Kitada et al., 2009a). In the *Park2*^{tm1Hn} line the binding index of DAT and VMAT was unchanged and suggests that the levels of these proteins are not altered (Sato et al., 2006). Likewise, the level of DAT in the *Park2*^{tm1Shn} knockout mice, measured using radiolabeled dopamine uptake, suggested that DAT levels were not altered (Kitada et al., 2009a). However, a reduction of the DAT and VMAT protein levels were identified in the *Park2*^{tm1Roo} line (Itier et al., 2003).
Alterations in dopamine metabolism were also found in other brain regions. An increase in the level of dopamine and DOPAC was identified in the limbic region from *Park2*^{tm1Roo} knockout mice, and an increase in dopamine but not DOPAC was identified in the midbrain, which includes the limbic region, from the *Park2*^{tm1Hn} knockout line (Itier et al., 2003; Sato et al., 2006). In addition, in the *Park2*^{tm1Tmd} knockout model, which showed loss of noradrenergic neurons within the locus coeruleus, a significant reduction in the dopamine derivative norepinephrine was identified in two regions that are innervated by the locus ceruleus, the olfactory bulb and the spinal cord (Von Coelln et al., 2004). Although a number of discrepancies related to dopamine metabolism are evident between the different *Park2* knockout models, collectively these analyses have suggested parkin may play a role in the presynaptic release of dopamine. The loss of parkin function may alter dopamine release, potentially by affecting vesicular packaging. Furthermore, they suggest that alterations in presynaptic dopamine function are evident prior to the development of PD-associated pathology.

2.4 Synaptic transmission

Deficits in dopamine-related synaptic transmission have been identified in *parkin*-mediated PD (Guo et al., 2010). Studies in a number of the *Park2* knockout lines suggest the presynaptic dopamine transmission is perturbed. In the *Park2*^{tm1Shn} knockout line, the evoked dopamine signal of medium spiny-neurons, the major class of striatal neurons whose excitability is influenced by dopamine levels, was reduced and could not be restored with DAT inhibition, suggesting dopamine re-uptake was not affected (Goldberg et al., 2003). Long term depression (LTD), which is activity-dependent reduction in the efficacy of neuronal synapses that lasts for an extended period, was also found to also be dysfunctional in these neurons. LTD could be restored by increasing synaptic dopamine with amphetamine but not by inhibition of dopamine re-uptake by antagonism of DAT. In addition, simultaneous antagonism of both D1 and D2 receptors, but not individual receptor antagonism, was required to restore LTD, and L-DOPA treatment was also effective. Furthermore, using primary dissociated adrenal chromaffin cells, which enable real time analysis of catecholamine release from single vesicles, exocytosis was found to be reduced (Kitada et al., 2009a). These observations suggest neurons from *Park2*^{tm1Shn} knockout have an intrinsic impairment in synaptic transmission that may result from defective presynaptic dopamine release.
The amplitude and half-life of evoked dopamine overflow was reduced in nigrostriatal fibers of the medial forebrain bundle of *Park2*^{tm1Oga} knockout mice. These are reflective of competing mechanisms of synaptic release and re-uptake, indicating that these mice also have alterations in dopamine synaptic transmission. Furthermore, a progressive age related

reduction in facilitation of these neurons was identified, which may be reflective of presymptomatic age-related changes (Oyama et al., 2010). The synaptic strength of hippocampal neurons from *Park2*^{tm1Rpa} line was significantly weaker in mice carrying one *Park2*^{tm1Rpa} mutant allele but not two mutant alleles. Hemizygous mice consistently showed reduced pair-pulse ratio whereas *Park2*^{tm1Rpa} knockout mice were only affected under small inter-stimulus ranges. Changes in pulse-pair ratio are consistent with presynaptic abnormalities, suggesting that in *Park2*^{tm1Rpa} mouse line parkin deficiency also affects presynaptic process.

Long term potentiation (LTP) is a long-lasting enhancement in signal transmission between two neurons that results from stimulating them synchronously, and is considered one of the major cellular mechanisms that underlies learning and memory. In the *Park2*^{tm1Rpa} knockout line, the LTP of 24 month old, but not 2 month old, appeared to be more robust, which may suggest that there is an absence of normal age related decline in the hippocampus of these mice (Hanson et al., 2010). In contrast, LTP was unchanged in the hippocampus of *Park2*^{tm1Roo} knockout line of a similar age (Itier et al., 2003). Furthermore, LTP was also unaltered in the hippocampus of *Park2*^{tm1Shn} knockout mice but could not be induced in striatal medium spiny neurons (Kitada et al., 2009a). Studies carried out to date on *Park2* knockout mice suggest that these mice have presynaptic abnormalities affecting dopamine function, which may be differentially modulated by the homozygous or heterozygous state of the mutant allele, cellular and regional specificity and/or age.

2.5 Neuroinflammation

Neuroinflammation is the chronic presence of activated microglia and reactive astrocytes, and associated mediators of the immune response in the central nervous system (reviewed in (Lee et al., 2009)). Postmortem analyses have demonstrated activated glia in both the striatum and in the substantia nigra of patients with idiopathic PD and in *parkin*-proven PD (reviewed in (Cookson et al., 2008; Lee et al., 2009)).

In vivo, *Park2*^{tm1Ccs} and *Park2*^{tm1Roo} knockout mice did not appear to have increased astrocytic or microglial markers in the substantia nigra, striatum or midbrain (Rodriguez-Navarro et al., 2007; Schmidt et al., 2011). However, a significant increase in the number of astrocytes in the striatum and the number of microglia in the midbrain occurs with age in the *Park2*^{tm1Roo} mice, independent of parkin deficiency, indicating an age-associated increase in the inflammatory environment may contribute to neuronal degeneration (Rodriguez-Navarro et al., 2007). *In vitro* however, alterations of glial populations are evident. Neuronal enriched cultures derived from *Park2*^{tm1Roo} knockout embryos appear to be enriched for microglial and glial progenitor cells (Casarejos et al., 2005), and glial cultures appear to have a reduced proportion of astrocytes compared to wildtype derived cultures (Solano et al., 2008). Furthermore, glial conditioned medium from *Park2*^{tm1Roo} and *Park2*^{tm1Ccs} knockout mice were found to have reduced neuroprotective capabilities that suggest a reduction in a trophic factor production or excretion by astrocytes (Schmidt et al., 2011; Solano et al., 2008).

Park2^{tm1Shn} knockout mice have been used to investigate if parkin deficiency can affect vulnerability to inflammation-mediated dopaminergic degeneration, using sustained low dose intraperitoneal injection of lipopolysaccaride (LPS). LPS is a bacterial endotoxin that is used as a glial activator for the induction of inflammatory dopaminergic neurodegeneration (Dutta et al., 2008). *Park2*^{tm1Shn} knockout mice showed increased vulnerability to LPS treatment and developed fine motor deficits and a loss of dopaminergic neurons (Frank-

Cannon et al., 2008). This suggests that *parkin* deficiency selectively increases the vulnerability of dopaminergic neurons to the effects of LPS induced inflammatory dopaminergic neurodegeneration. Collectively, these studies suggest that there may be inherent dysregulation of glial cells in *parkin* deficiency. Alterations in the function of these mediators of neuroinflammation within *parkin*-proven PD, together with endogenous age related changes in the neuroimmune system may play a role in the pathogenesis of PD.

2.6 Oxidative stress

Oxidative stress occurs when there is an imbalance between the production of reactive oxygen species (ROS) and the ability to rapidly detoxify the reactive intermediates or repair the resulting damage to cellular constituents. Markers of oxidative stress are increased in PD patients (reviewed in (Tobon-Velasco et al., 2010)), and dopamine metabolism facilitates production of ROS (Lotharius and Brundin, 2002). Glutathione (GSH) is a free radical scavenger that acts on redox reactive molecules. Both astrocytes and neurons have the capacity to synthesis GSH, but astrocytes are known to play an important role in supply of GSH and other substrates to neurons. One of the earliest biochemical changes observed in PD patients is a decrease in GSH levels. It is thought the decrease in GSH levels may be due to increased oxidative stress and recent research suggests that GSH depletion itself may have a role in the pathogenesis of PD (reviewed in (Martin and Teismann, 2009)).

Park2^{tm1Roo} knockout mice aged 2 months were found to have significantly increased GSH in the midbrain, striatum and limbic system (Itier et al., 2003; Rodriguez-Navarro et al., 2007). However, when GSH levels were investigated in *Park2*^{tm1Roo} knockout mice aged 24 months, the level of GSH in the midbrain was not significantly different from either the 24 month old wildtype or 2 month old knockout mice. While GSH levels in the striatum of 24 month *Park2*^{tm1Roo} knockout mice were significantly reduced compared to 2 month old knockout mice they were not significantly different to 24 month old wildtype mice. In the limbic system of 24 month old *Park2*^{tm1Roo} knockout mice the level of GSH was significantly increased compared to 24 month old wildtype mice. Therefore, regional and age-related alterations of GSH are present in the *Park2*^{tm1Roo} knockout mouse line. Consistent with these observations, *in vitro* age-related studies of alterations in GSH levels have been identified in glial cells derived from *Park2*^{tm1Roo} knockout mice. When knockout glia are cultured for an extended period (6-9 months) the intracellular levels of GSH were significantly reduced compared to wildtype control glia, whereas knockout glia cultured for a shorter time (1-3 months) were shown to have a significant increase in the level of intracellular GSH compared to wildtype (Solano et al., 2008). However, conditioned media generated from glial cultures derived from *Park2*^{tm1Roo} knockout mice that had been cultured for a shorter period had lower levels of GSH and higher levels of hydrogen peroxide, and appeared to be less neuroprotective to wildtype neurons than conditioned media from wildtype glial cultures (Solano et al., 2008). These observations suggest that although intracellular GSH levels are increased in 2 month old *Park2*^{tm1Roo} knockout, there may be defective exocytosis of GSH out of the glia and into the extracellular space.

Mitochondria are a major source of ROS within cells and mitochondrial dysfunction has been robustly implicated with PD. The capacity for electron transport in mitochondria was found to be impaired in the *Park2*^{tm1Shn} and *Park2*^{tm1Ccs} knockout mice (Palacino et al., 2004; Stichel et al., 2007). Dopaminergic neurons in the *Park2*^{tm1Rpa} and *Park2*^{tm1Tmd} knockout lines do not appear to be more sensitive to the mitochondrial toxin MPTP (Perez et al., 2005;

Thomas et al., 2007). However, glial cultures derived from *Park2^{tm1Roo}* knockout mice appeared more sensitive to MPTP (Solano et al., 2008). Furthermore, neuronal cultures derived from *Park2^{tm1Roo}* knockout mice were more sensitive to the mitochondrial toxin rotenone. Co-culture of glia from *Park2^{tm1Roo}* knockout mice with neurons derived from wildtype mice increased the sensitivity of wildtype neurons to rotenone (Casarejos et al., 2006). Furthermore, wildtype neurons exhibited significantly shorter processes and smaller neuronal areas when they were co-cultured with *Park2^{tm1Ccs}* knockout derived astrocytes as opposed to wildtype astrocytes (Schmidt et al., 2011). Collectively, this suggests that lack of parkin leads to a functional disturbance of neuron-glia interactions, and that environmentally induced mitochondrial dysfunction when combined with parkin deficiency may be detrimental to dopaminergic neurons and stimulatory of neuroinflammatory processes.

The ultrastructure of mitochondria from *Park2^{tm1Ccs}* knockout mouse has been investigated in both neuronal and glial populations *in vivo*. Compared to 3 month old mice, neurons in the substantia nigra of 12 month old *Park2^{tm1Ccs}* knockout mice displayed an increased proportion of abnormal mitochondria. This age related change was not identified in wildtype mice (Stichel et al., 2007). Mitochondria within glial populations of *Park2^{tm1Ccs}* knockout mice were found to exhibit an elevated number of structural deficits that included abnormal disintegration, a reduction of mitochondrial cristae and mitochondrial enlargement. The proportion of abnormal mitochondria identified in *Park2^{tm1Ccs}* knockout glia depended on both age and glial cell type. Nonetheless, the amount of mitochondrial damage was significant at just 16 days of age in all glial cell types, and the mitochondrial burden was much greater in glial than neuronal cells (Schmidt et al., 2011). Oxidative stress is thought to be a major contributor to the development of PD. Several pathways associated with oxidative stress, notably GSH and the mitochondria, may be dysfunctional within *Park2* knockout mice. Furthermore, it appears that a number of factors including age and cell type may mediate the extent of dysfunction associated with lack of parkin.

2.7 Ubiquitin Proteasome System (UPS)

Parkin was originally identified as an E3 ubiquitin ligase that functions in the UPS, and a number of putative interacting proteins and substrates have subsequently been identified (reviewed in (Dawson and Dawson, 2010)). Knockout mice allow the *in vivo* analysis of interacting proteins, substrates and pathway deficits that have been identified *in vitro*. A simple working hypothesis is that if a protein is a substrate of parkin mediated ubiquitination and subsequent degradation via the UPS, that protein would be expected to accumulate in a *Park2* knockout mouse model. A number of groups have investigated some of the putative parkin substrates in *Park2* knockout mice, but in general very few studies have replicated the *in vitro* results and shown increased levels of putative substrates *in vivo*.

Two comprehensive analyses of parkin substrates have been reported using the *Park2^{tm1Tmd}* knockout mice. The steady state level of aminoacyl-tRNA synthetase cofactor (AIMP2) was increased in the ventral midbrain/hindbrain of *Park2^{tm1Tmd}* knockout mice but no alteration in the amount of seven other putative parkin substrates, including β-tubulin and α-synuclein, was identified. An accumulation of AIMP2 in brain tissue from individuals with *parkin*-proven PD was also shown, and AIMP2 was shown to interact with parkin *in vitro*, suggesting that AIMP2 is an authentic substrate of parkin (Ko et al., 2005). AIMP2 is a known interacting protein of far upstream element (FUSE)-binding protein 1 (FBP1), promoting its ubiquitination and degradation. Subsequent studies demonstrated that the level of FBP1 was increased in the brain stem and cortex of *Park2^tm1Tmd^* knockout mice and also patients with *parkin*-proven PD (Ko et al., 2006). In contrast to the results in the ventral midbrain/hindbrain of *Park2^tm1Tmd^* knockout mice, the level of AIMP2 in the cortex, cerebellum, brain stem, and striatum, and the level of FBP1 in the ventral midbrain, cerebellum or striatum was not altered (Ko et al., 2006; Ko et al., 2005). This may imply functional redundancy for turnover of these proteins in some regions of the brain. However, an alternative explanation may be that the rate of new protein synthesis is greater than the rate of protein degradation in these regions and so the effect of parkin absence is masked. A similar phenomenon was observed with estrogen related receptor (ERR) isoforms and α-tubulin. The consequence of loss of parkin on accumulation of ERRs and α-tubulin was only demonstrated after new protein synthesis was inhibited by treatment with puromycin (Ren et al., 2010).

In general, *in vitro* studies suggesting a role for parkin in the turnover of putative substrates have not been replicated in the different *in vivo* models. However the extent to which investigation has been reported is limited. Such apparent discrepancy between *in vitro* and *in vivo* models may due in part to experimental methodology. For example, the *in vitro* data suggesting a role for parkin in ubiquitin-proteasome mediated degradation may be an artefact of exogenous expression of parkin and putative substrates, or due to specificity of the cell type utilised. In addition, there is compelling evidence to suggest that parkin is able to function as a multifaceted ubiquitin ligase, capable of modulating alternative forms of ubiquitination not associated with ubiquitin-proteasome mediated degradation of proteins.

2.8 Autophagy

For a substrate to be recognised by the proteasome it needs to labelled with at least four ubiquitin molecules attached via lysine-48 linkage. Most recently, parkin-mediated lysine-63 polyubiquitylation was shown to be an important mediator of the aggregation and turnover of damaged mitochondria via autophagy (Geisler et al., 2010; Narendra et al., 2008; Narendra et al., 2010; Suen et al., 2010). Autophagy is the major pathway involved in the degradation of long-lived proteins and organelles and has been shown to play an integral role in protection against neurodegeneration (Hara et al., 2006; Komatsu et al., 2006). It is comprised of three distinct pathways, macroautophagy, microautophagy and chaperone-mediated autophagy. Macroautophagy (hereafter referred to as autophagy) involves the sequestration of organelles and proteins in a double-membrane vesicle, called an autophagosome or autophagic vacuole, which subsequently fuses with a lysosome and the contents are degraded by lysosomal hydrolases (reviewed in (Klionsky and Emr, 2000)). Emerging data suggests that the UPS and autophagy are functionally coupled and inhibition of the UPS can result in aggresome formation and elevated autophagy (Pandey et al., 2007). Several markers of the autophagic pathway have been shown to be elevated in the substantia nigra of PD cases and it has been proposed that Lewy bodies may be the *in vivo* representation of aggresome. It is not yet clear if the elevated numbers of autophagosomes identified in PD brains represent increased autophagy induction or impaired completion of autophagic degradation (reviewed in (Chu, 2011)). However, the ability of the autophagic vacuole to engulf organelles and large protein aggregates suggests upregulation of autophagy may represent a therapeutic target for PD (reviewed in ((Arduino et al., 2010; Banerjee et al., 2010)). Recent studies have defined a pathway linking parkin and PINK1 to mitophagy, a form of autophagy selective for mitochondria. Depolarisation of mitochondria results in the accumulation of parkin at the mitochondrion in a PINK1-dependent manner with subsequent degradation via mitophagy (Kawajiri et al., 2010; Narendra et al., 2008; Narendra et al., 2010; Vives-Bauza et al., 2010).

The effect of parkin deficiency on autophagy in *Park2* knockout mice has not been extensively reported. However, one study has investigated autophagy in neuronal cultures derived from *Park2*^{tm1Roo} knockout mice. Midbrain neuronal cultures derived from *Park2*^{tm1Roo} knockout mice were treated with epoxomicin to partially inhibit the proteasome. *Park2*^{tm1Roo} knockout cultures appeared to be less susceptible to the toxic effects of proteasomal inhibition. The autophagic substrate p62 was increased in wildtype neuronal cultures but not in *Park2*^{tm1Roo} knockout neuronal cultures, suggestive of increased autophagic activity. A second indicator of autophagic activity is the relative ratio of LC3I and LC3II. LC3 II is generated by site specific proteolysis and lipidation of LC3I and serves as a specific marker of autophagic activation. In basal conditions, the LC3II/I ratio was unchanged in neuronal cultures derived from wildtype mice, but it was significantly increased in cultures from derived *Park2*^{tm1Roo} knockout mice, and this was further potentiated by epoxomicin treatment. These observations suggest that neuronal cultures derived from *Park2*^{tm1Roo} knockout mice have increased autophagy and that partial proteasomal inhibition further potentiates autophagy in this model (Casarejos et al., 2009). The majority of cell culture models have suggested that Parkin regulates mitochondrial degradation through autophagy, and an early step in this process is the requirement for PINK1 to recruit Parkin to the mitochondria (Vives-Bauza et al., 2010). Therefore, it seems counter intuitive that neuronal cultures derived from *Park2*^{tm1Roo} knockout mice would display increased autophagy following proteasomal inhibition. However, a study of neurons taken from rat substantia nigra suggested that mitophagy was parkin independent in these cells. It was suggested that the difference in neurons may be due to the high dependence of neurons on mitochondrial respiration (Van Laar et al., 2011). Much of what is currently understood about the potential role of parkin in autophagy is derived from studies in cell culture models. However, this is an expanding field in PD research and future studies utilising *Park2* knockout mice will provide considerable insight into the significance of this role *in vivo*.

2.9 Trafficking/signalling

Parkin-mediated ubiquitination has also been suggested to play a role in signal transduction and trafficking. Monoubiquitination is associated with the regulation of endocytosis of membrane proteins and signalling (Mukhopadhyay and Riezman, 2007). The interaction between parkin and PICK1 is an example of this function. PICK1 regulates the trafficking and stability of a number of synaptic proteins, including neurotransmitter receptors, transporters and ion channels (Madsen et al., 2005). *In vitro* analysis suggested that parkin monoubiquitinated rather than polyubiquitinated PICK1. In neurons derived from *Park2*^{tm1Roo} knockout mice steady-state PICK1 levels were not altered, suggesting turnover of the protein is independent of parkin. PICK1 has been shown to interact with the proton-gated ion channel ASIC2a, and potentiation of ASIC2a currents is suggested to be PICK1 dependent. Hippocampal neurons from *Park2*^{tm1Roo} knockout mice show deficits of ASIC2a current potentiation, which suggest that monoubiquitination of PICK1 by parkin is required for ASIC2a channel function (Joch et al., 2007).

The interaction of parkin and the endocytic protein Endophilin A1 provides additional evidence that the ubiquitination activity of parkin is not limited to proteasome turnover. Endophilin A1 is a protein that is abundant in neural synapses and is involved in formation of presynaptic endocytic vesicles. Limited ubiquitination of Endophilin A1 by parkin was shown *in vitro* and Endophilin A1 did not appear to accumulate in synapses from *Park2*^{tm1Roo} knockout mice. *In vivo* the interaction of the two proteins appears to promote co-localisation from the cytosol to the plasma membrane and synaptic vesicle enriched fractions. In synaptosome preparations from wildtype mice relocalisation leads to increased ubiquitination of synaptic proteins, however, this effect is abrogated in *Park2tm1Roo* knockout mice (Trempe et al., 2009). Further understanding of the functional deficits associated with this loss of relocalisation and ubiquitination activity in *Park2* knockout mice may shed light on the defects in synaptic transmission observed in both *Park2* knockout mice and *parkin*-mediated PD.

2.10 Genetic modification of *Park2* knockout mice

Mutations in the genes *parkin, PINK1* and *DJ-1* have been associated with familial recessive early-onset PD. A number of lines of evidence suggest that these genes may function in a common pathway(s) important for mitochondrial function (Geisler et al., 2010; Narendra et al., 2010; Thomas et al., 2011). The effect of knockout of all three genes in a single mouse model revealed that *Park2*^{tm1Shn}*/Pink1/Dj-1* knockout mice at 24 months of age do not show significant dopaminergic degeneration (Kitada et al., 2009b). This may suggest a functional redundancy between these genes. An alternative interpretation may be that these genes are not essential for neuronal survival, but rather may play a protective role against cellular insults.

A major component of Lewy bodies in PD is alpha-synuclein, which is also genetically linked with autosomal dominant PD and sporadic PD (reviewed in (Obeso et al., 2010). The effect of parkin deficiency combined with dysregulation of α-synuclein has been reported for three *Park2* knockout mouse lines. The *Park2*^{tm1Tmd} knockout mouse was crossed with a transgenic mouse overexpressing familial mutant A53T α-synuclein under the control of the mouse prion promoter [Tg(PRP-SNCA^{A53T})]. In this model, parkin deficiency did not appear to exacerbate attributes previously recognised in Tg(PRP-SNCA^{A53T}) mice. Likewise, Tg(PRP-SNCA^{A53T}) did not potentiate the locus coeruleus degeneration of the *Park2*^{tm1Tmd} knockout line (von Coelln et al., 2006). The *Park2*^{tm1Roo} knockout mouse was crossed with a transgenic mouse overexpressing familial mutant A30P α-synuclein under the control of the thymus cell antigen 1 promoter [Tg(THY1-SNCA^{A30P})]. In contrast to the previous model, parkin deficiency appeared to delay the progressive neurodegenerative motor phenotype of Tg(THY1-SNCA^{A30P}) mice, and decreased neuritic pathology that is associated with these symptoms. Furthermore, co-staining of ubiquitin with phosphorylated α-synuclein positive structures was reduced in this model (Fournier et al., 2009). The *Park2*^{tm1Ccs} knockout mouse was crossed with two different mutant α-synuclein lines. Both lines expressed human α-synuclein carrying two familial mutations, A30P and A53T, under the control of either the chicken beta-actin (BA) promoter [Tg(BA-SNCA$^{A30/PA53T}$)] or the mouse tyrosine hydroxylase (TH) promoter [Tg(TH-SNCA$^{A30/PA53T}$)]. The most prominent feature identified in neurons from these mutant mice was an age-related increase in the proportion of abnormal mitochondria and a reduction in mitochondrial complex I activity in the substantia nigra (Stichel et al., 2007). Collectively, these studies suggest that the effect of parkin deficiency on α-synuclein mediated phenotypes may be independent (von Coelln et al., 2006), delayed (Fournier et al., 2009) or enhanced (Stichel et al., 2007). Whether this is related to differential attributes of the *Park2* knockout mice or the differential regional effects of α-synuclein overexpression remains to be investigated.

The normal age related increase of tau pathology is potentiated in the *Park2*^{tm1Roo} knockout mouse (Rodriguez-Navarro et al., 2007). Tauopathies are neurodegenerative diseases principally identified by dementia and Parkinsonism. Idiopathic forms are thought to be due to post-translational alteration of tau whereas familiar tauopathies are the result of mutations in the gene encoding tau, *microtubule associated protein tau* (*MAPT*) (Avila et al., 2004; Hutton et al., 1998). *MAPT* has also recently been genetically implicated in sporadic PD aetiology (Satake et al., 2009; Simon-Sanchez et al., 2009) and aggregation of tau has been shown to be a feature of some cases of *parkin*-proven PD (reviewed in (Cookson et al., 2008).

The consequence of combining the over-expression of a human 4-repeat tau isoform with known familial alterations G2727V, P301L, R406W under the control of human thymus cell antigen 1 promoter [Tg(THY1-Tau^{VLW})] with the *Park2*^{tm1Roo} knockout mouse was investigated. Like *Park2*^{tm1Roo} knockout mice, Tg(THY1-Tau^{VLW}) mice have slight behavioural and molecular changes that do not manifest in a clinical phenotype. However, when combined a number of age-progressive behavioural attributes including reduced hind limb length, uncontrolled movements, loss of balance and postural abnormalities as well as increased self-injury of the face that is a reflection of compulsive long-term grooming, were identified. This was coupled with a significant loss of motor neurons, and dopaminergic neurons in the substantia nigra. In addition, tau pathology was identified, as was abnormal expression glia in the substantia nigra and the hippocampus (Menendez et al., 2006; Rodriguez-Navarro et al., 2008a). Furthermore, phosphorylated tau plaques and tangles, as well as endogenous β-amyloid plaques were found in the hippocampus. Notably, dietary supplementation with the disaccharide trehalose, which is thought to enhance autophagy, was found to ameliorate the severity of the symptoms and pathology in this model. (Rodriguez-Navarro et al., 2010). By combining parkin deficiency with abnormal tau expression, a number of attributes that were modestly perturbed in the single monogenetic mutants were significantly dysregulated. This suggests that parkin and tau may be functionally coupled *in vivo*, and their perturbation is capable of eliciting a progressive neurodegenerative phenotype with characteristics of both PD and Alzheimer's disease.

Alzheimer disease is a degenerative dementia characterised by loss of neurons in the cerebral cortex. Pathological features include extracellular amyloid plaques, which are composed predominately of β-amyloid, and intracellular neurofibrillary tangles that mainly consist of hyperphosphorylated tau. The identification of β-amyloid plaques in the *Park2*^{tm1Roo}/Tg(THY1-Tau^{VLW}) mouse led to the investigation of the effect of parkin deficiency on β-amyloid expression. The APP_{swe} is a transgenic mouse line that overexpresses the β-amyloid precursor protein containing two mutations, K670N and M671L, under the control of the prion protein promoter. Parkin deficiency appears to reduce the severity of behavioural deficits of APP_{swe} mice including reduced weight gain, exploratory activity and working memory. Furthermore, parkin deficiency appears to reduce β-amyloid plaque pathology within the cerebral cortex and hippocampus, and in the hippocampus the amount of astrogliosis and phosphorylated tau was also reduced. This

was coupled with alterations in a number of autophagic markers consistent with induction of autophagy (Perucho et al., 2010).
Therefore, in contrast to the *Park2*^{tm1Roo}/Tg(THY1-Tau^{VLW}) mouse, where combining the two mutant alleles appeared to enhanced the disease process, parkin deficiency combined with APP_{swe} over-expression can ameliorate a number of pathological characteristics of these mice. Consequently, it appears parkin has the potential to be both neuroprotective and a neurotoxic to the neurodegenerative process, depending on context. Furthermore, the effect of active autophagy when either APP_{swe} or Tg(THY1-Tau^{VLW}) were combined with *Park2*^{tm1Roo} knockout appears to be protective. This suggests further investigation into factors that enhance autophagy may identify potential treatments for individuals with PD and other neurodegenerative disorders.

3. Discussion

PD is differentiated from other neurodegenerative disorders by defined motor disturbances resulting from the pathological loss of dopaminergic neurons. Seven *Park2* knockout models have been generated and characterised. In the current context, loss of function of parkin in these mouse models does not appear to reproduce a PD-like phenotype that is reflective of *parkin*-proven PD. However, two models showed a significant loss of catecholaminergic neurons, one in the substantia nigra and the other in the locus coeruleus. Notably, the extent of neuronal loss within the substantia nigra was not equivalent to that associated with the onset of symptomatic PD in humans. However, both neurochemical and electrophysiological studies have identified disturbances in dopamine pathways in *Park2* knockout mice that are consistent with altered presynaptic release of dopamine. Glial and redox dysfunction was also identified, indicating that the capacity to protect neurons against cellular insult may be diminished in *Park2* knockout mice. Furthermore, mitochondrial abnormalities highlight the importance of parkin function in maintaining mitochondrial integrity. Accumulation of specific proteins within *Park2* knockout mice has confirmed *in vivo* that parkin functions as an E3 ubiquitin ligase in the UPS. The additional role of parkin in autophagy and trafficking/signalling pathways are indicative of a broad role in normal cellular function. With regard to the involvement of parkin with neurodegeneration the most important findings were identified by genetic modification of *Park2* knockout mice. *Park2* knockout mice, when combined with other mutant transgenic models, appeared to have the capacity to both exacerbate and ameliorate disease associated characteristics in a context dependent manner. Therefore, dysfunction of parkin has the potential to be both neuroprotective and neurotoxic.
The inability of *Park2* knockout mice to adequately recapitulate the clinical and pathological manifestation of PD is not an isolated observation. Knockout of other PD associated genes such as *Pink1*, *α-synuclein* and *Lrrk2* also fail to produce robust PD-like phenotypes, and the results of transgenic overexpression of disease associated genes and mutants vary considerably depending on the promoter used to drive expression (reviewed in (Dawson et al., 2010)). In addition, a knockin model of a common pathogenic variant of LRRK2 does not show evidence of dopaminergic degeneration. However, like *Park2* knockout mice these *Lrrk2* knockin mice appear to have dysregulation of the dopamine system (Tong et al., 2009). In addition, a number of other features identified in *Park2* knockout mice, including

alterations of the neuroimmune system, mitochondrial dysfunction and oxidative stress are shared between the models. These observations suggest a commonality to the perturbations that occur prior to manifestation of pathogenic phenotypic features.

An explanation as to why *Park2* knockout mice fail, for the most part, to recapitulate the loss of dopaminergic neurons that is a feature of human disease may be the short lifespan of the species. Aging research carried out in mice indicate that a number of molecular markers of aging follow a similar course to that observed in humans, although over a shorter duration. (reviewed ((Yuan et al., 2011)). This suggests that at the cellular and systemic level aging follows a parallel path in mice and humans. The symptoms of *parkin*-mediated PD typically present before 45 years of age. However, there is considerable disparity in age of onset, presentation, progression and response to drug treatment, even for patients within the same sibship, with the same mutations (reviewed in (Mata et al., 2004)). Therefore, loss of function of parkin alone may not be responsible for dopaminergic neuronal loss in individuals with *parkin*-mediated PD. Three lines of evidence from studies carried out in *Park2* knockout mice support this notion. 1) A significant loss (35%), of dopaminergic neurons occurs in the substantia nigra of the $Park2^{tm1Roo}$ knockout in an age-related progressive manner over the duration of the life-span of the mouse, although not to the extent that is observed (~60%) at symptom onset in humans. This indicates that parkin deficiency can cause dopaminergic neuronal loss in a mouse model. 2) The loss of catecholaminergic neurons in the locus coeruleus in the $Park2^{tm1Tmd}$ knockout line shows reduced penetrance. This suggests that additional factors mediate this trait. 3) The increased vulnerability of $Park2^{tm1Shn}$ knockout mice to loss of dopaminergic neurons in the substantia nigra induced by repeated low-dose systemic LPS treatment. This indicates that in this model, although parkin deficiency alone was not sufficient to cause dopaminergic neuronal loss, dopaminergic integrity was compromised in a neuroinflammatory environment.

A number of the phenotypic discrepancies between the *Park2* knockout mice may be attributable to differences between the genetic background of the mouse strains used (discussed in (Perez and Palmiter, 2005)). The majority of studies used mice of variable mixed backgrounds. Isogenic strains are preferred when investigating the effect of gene knockout as genetic similarity tends to result in phenotypic uniformity, increasing the power to identify significant effects. It would be an advantage when comparing traits between different knockout mice for them to be on the same isogenic background, particularly if the genetic effect is modest, as appears to be the case of *parkin*. Therefore, until these carefully controlled studies are undertaken, it remains difficult to determine which of the identified phenotypic features are likely to be attributable to parkin.

Isogenic strains may also be a hindrance if pathogenicity has undefined multigenic influences, as potentially could be the case for parkin. During the process of generating an inbred strain, mice undergo a process called inbreeding depression. In this process the reproductive fitness reduces as homozygosity increases because repressive alleles are unmasked. Therefore, founders of an inbred strain and their offspring must be considered selective survivors of the inbreeding process, and as such have a level of fitness that does not reflect the species as a whole (McClearn and McCarter, 2011). In a multifaceted disease such as PD, other genetic factors may contribute to disease progression. Therefore, the isogenic inbred strains could limit the affect of *Park2* knockout. However, the negative effects associated with inbreeding depression can be overcome by generating F1 hybrids of two different inbred strains. In the context of the *Park2* knockout models, it may be noteworthy that the only strain that demonstrates significant loss of dopaminergic neurons in the substantia nigra, the *Park2*^{tm1Roo} knockout mouse, was reported in a mixed 129S2/C57BL6 (50/50) genetic background.

Another factor that could be significant in the development of a disease phenotype is the environmental differences between laboratory mice and humans. It is clear that environmental factors influence PD development, and in some cases may cause PD. Laboratory mice are housed in controlled environments, often pathogen free, with none or limited exposure to environmental toxins or stresses. Therefore these mice may not be exposed to the appropriate triggers that are necessary for dopaminergic protective mechanisms to fail. Loss of parkin may result in a pre-degenerative state where neurons are under stress but not sufficiently compromised as to cause significant loss. Other cues, such as pro-inflammatory factors, could provide the additional stimulus required for degeneration to occur. This model may better explain an inherited autosomal recessive trait that takes multiple decades to manifest symptoms.

The *Park2* knockout mice are useful to understand the mechanistic consequence of loss of parkin function in a mammalian species. An improved understanding of the effect of *parkin* deletion on neuron and glial populations will provide considerable insight into the pathogenesis of PD, and the contribution that dopamine dysregulation plays in the pathogenic process. Cellular models have provided a great deal of information about the role of parkin in the turnover of protein and cellular constituents, in particular mitochondria, via the UPS and autophagy. The *Park2* knockout models provide a sophisticated platform to refine and advance these studies, for example using neuronal and glial cultures derived from *Park2* knockout mice.

There are a number of avenues that can be explored to potentially develop a *Park2* knockout model with a pathological phenotype of clinical relevance. Crossing the *Park2* knockout mice with α-synuclein, tau and β-amyloid models has provided enormous insight into the role of parkin in the neurodegenerative process *in vivo*. Further research following on from these studies, including breeding to the conditional α-synuclein knockin model currently in development (NIH project No. 1R21NS057795-01A1), has the potential to develop these mice into a more clinically relevant model. Likewise, the role of neuroinflammation in the neurodegenerative process could be further explored using *Park2* knockout mice. This could be achieved by breeding to genetic models with perturbations in the inflammatory response or treatment with agents such as LPS. In addition, a second rodent model, knockout of parkin in the rat, has recently been developed (SAGE Labs). The phenotypic outcome will be of great interest to compare and contrast with the results already obtained in mouse models.

4. Conclusion

A quote by Michael FW Festing, an expert in the field of laboratory animal genetics, eloquently encapsulates the use of mouse models in disease research. "*Models are subject to improvement through further research. A lot of animal research is aimed at understanding the animal as a potential model for particular human conditions, without being too precise as to what those conditions might be. Models are not just found. They need to be developed, and this requires an understanding of the biology of the species and the effects of various interventions such as inactivating specific genes or manipulating the environment. As our understanding increases, so the chance of choosing the most appropriate models for a specific disease increases"* (Festing, 2011). To date, seven *Park2* knockout mice have been generated but *Park2* knockout models still need to be developed in order to understand the clinical manifestation of *parkin*-mediated PD and the contribution of parkin to idiopathic PD.

5. References

Chew, K.C., N. Matsuda, K. Saisho, G.G. Lim, C. Chai, H.M. Tan, K. Tanaka, and K.L. Lim. 2011. Parkin mediates apparent e2-independent monoubiquitination in vitro and contains an intrinsic activity that catalyzes polyubiquitination. *PLoS One*. 6:e19720.

Chu, C.T. 2011. Diversity in the regulation of autophagy and mitophagy: lessons from Parkinson's disease. *Parkinsons Dis*. 2011:789431.

Ciechanover, A., A. Orian, and A.L. Schwartz. 2000. Ubiquitin-mediated proteolysis: biological regulation via destruction. *Bioessays*. 22:442-51.

Cookson, M.R., J. Hardy, and P.A. Lewis. 2008. Genetic neuropathology of Parkinson's disease. *Int J Clin Exp Pathol*. 1:217-31.

Daniel, S.E., and A.J. Lees. 1993. Parkinson's Disease Society Brain Bank, London: overview and research. *J Neural Transm Suppl*. 39:165-72.

Daubner, S.C., T. Le, and S. Wang. 2011. Tyrosine hydroxylase and regulation of dopamine synthesis. *Arch Biochem Biophys*. 508:1-12.

Dawson, T.M., and V.L. Dawson. 2010. The role of parkin in familial and sporadic Parkinson's disease. *Mov Disord*. 25 Suppl 1:S32-9.

Dawson, T.M., H.S. Ko, and V.L. Dawson. 2010. Genetic animal models of Parkinson's disease. *Neuron*. 66:646-61.

de Lau, L.M., and M.M. Breteler. 2006. Epidemiology of Parkinson's disease. *Lancet Neurol*. 5:525-35.

Denison, S.R., G. Callahan, N.A. Becker, L.A. Phillips, and D.I. Smith. 2003. Characterization of FRA6E and its potential role in autosomal recessive juvenile parkinsonism and ovarian cancer. *Genes Chromosomes Cancer*. 38:40-52.

Dickson, D.W., H. Braak, J.E. Duda, C. Duyckaerts, T. Gasser, G.M. Halliday, J. Hardy, J.B. Leverenz, K. Del Tredici, Z.K. Wszolek, and I. Litvan. 2009. Neuropathological assessment of Parkinson's disease: refining the diagnostic criteria. *Lancet Neurol*. 8:1150-7.

Dutta, G., P. Zhang, and B. Liu. 2008. The lipopolysaccharide Parkinson's disease animal model: mechanistic studies and drug discovery. *Fundam Clin Pharmacol*. 22:453-64.

Fearnley, J.M., and A.J. Lees. 1991. Ageing and Parkinson's disease: substantia nigra regional selectivity. *Brain*. 114 (Pt 5):2283-301.

Festing, M.F.W. (2011) Animal models in research, In: *Isogenic.info*. May 2011, available from: http://isogenic.info/index.html

Foroud, T., S.K. Uniacke, L. Liu, N. Pankratz, A. Rudolph, C. Halter, C. Shults, K. Marder, P.M. Conneally, and W.C. Nichols. 2003. Heterozygosity for a mutation in the parkin gene leads to later onset Parkinson disease. *Neurology*. 60:796-801.

Gelb, D.J., E. Oliver, and S. Gilman. 1999. Diagnostic criteria for Parkinson disease. *Arch Neurol*. 56:33-9.

Goldberg, M.S., S.M. Fleming, J.J. Palacino, C. Cepeda, H.A. Lam, A. Bhatnagar, E.G. Meloni, N. Wu, L.C. Ackerson, G.J. Klapstein, M. Gajendiran, B.L. Roth, M.F. Chesselet, N.T. Maidment, M.S. Levine, and J. Shen. 2003. Parkin-deficient mice exhibit nigrostriatal deficits but not loss of dopaminergic neurons. *J Biol Chem*. 278:43628-35.

Greene, J.C., A.J. Whitworth, I. Kuo, L.A. Andrews, M.B. Feany, and L.J. Pallanck. 2003. Mitochondrial pathology and apoptotic muscle degeneration in Drosophila parkin mutants. *Proc Natl Acad Sci U S A*. 100:4078-83.

Grimm, J., A. Mueller, F. Hefti, and A. Rosenthal. 2004. Molecular basis for catecholaminergic neuron diversity. *Proc Natl Acad Sci U S A*. 101:13891-6.

Guerrero, R., P. Navarro, E. Gallego, J. Avila, J.G. de Yebenes, and M.P. Sanchez. 2008. Park2-null/tau transgenic mice reveal a functional relationship between parkin and tau. *J Alzheimers Dis*. 13:161-72.

Guo, J.F., L. Wang, D. He, Q.H. Yang, Z.X. Duan, X.W. Zhang, L.L. Nie, X.X. Yan, and B.S. Tang. 2010. Clinical features and [11C]-CFT PET analysis of PARK2, PARK6, PARK7-linked autosomal recessive early onset Parkinsonism. *Neurol Sci*. 32:35-40.

Halliday, G.M., and H. McCann. 2010. The progression of pathology in Parkinson's disease. *Ann N Y Acad Sci*. 1184:188-95.

Hanson, J.E., A.L. Orr, and D.V. Madison. 2010. Altered hippocampal synaptic physiology in aged parkin-deficient mice. *Neuromolecular Med*. 12:270-6.

Harrison, D.E. (2011) Maximum Lifespan As a Biomarker of Aging, In: *The Jackson Laboratory, May 2011,* available from: http://www.jax.org/

Hurelbrink, C.B., and S.J. Lewis. 2010. Pathological considerations in the treatment of Parkinson's disease: more than just a wiring diagram. *Clin Neurol Neurosurg*. 113:1-6.

Itier, J.M., P. Ibanez, M.A. Mena, N. Abbas, C. Cohen-Salmon, G.A. Bohme, M. Laville, J. Pratt, O. Corti, L. Pradier, G. Ret, C. Joubert, M. Periquet, F. Araujo, J. Negroni, M.J. Casarejos, S. Canals, R. Solano, A. Serrano, E. Gallego, M. Sanchez, P. Denefle, J. Benavides, G. Tremp, T.A. Rooney, A. Brice, and J. Garcia de Yebenes. 2003. Parkin gene inactivation alters behaviour and dopamine neurotransmission in the mouse. *Hum Mol Genet*. 12:2277-91.

Kitada, T., A. Pisani, M. Karouani, M. Haburcak, G. Martella, A. Tscherter, P. Platania, B. Wu, E.N. Pothos, and J. Shen. 2009a. Impaired dopamine release and synaptic plasticity in the striatum of parkin-/- mice. *J Neurochem*. 110:613-21.

Kitada, T., Y. Tong, C.A. Gautier, and J. Shen. 2009b. Absence of nigral degeneration in aged parkin/DJ-1/PINK1 triple knockout mice. *J Neurochem*. 111:696-702.

Kitao, Y., Y. Imai, K. Ozawa, A. Kataoka, T. Ikeda, M. Soda, K. Nakimawa, H. Kiyama, D.M. Stern, O. Hori, K. Wakamatsu, S. Ito, S. Itohara, R. Takahashi, and S. Ogawa. 2007. Pael receptor induces death of dopaminergic neurons in the substantia nigra via endoplasmic reticulum stress and dopamine toxicity, which is enhanced under condition of parkin inactivation. *Hum Mol Genet*. 16:50-60.

Klionsky, D.J., and S.D. Emr. 2000. Autophagy as a regulated pathway of cellular degradation. *Science*. 290:1717-21.

Ko, H.S., S.W. Kim, S.R. Sriram, V.L. Dawson, and T.M. Dawson. 2006. Identification of far upstream element-binding protein-1 as an authentic Parkin substrate. *J Biol Chem*. 281:16193-6.

Lee, J.K., T. Tran, and M.G. Tansey. 2009. Neuroinflammation in Parkinson's disease. *J Neuroimmune Pharmacol*. 4:419-29.

Lewis, S.J., T. Foltynie, A.D. Blackwell, T.W. Robbins, A.M. Owen, and R.A. Barker. 2005. Heterogeneity of Parkinson's disease in the early clinical stages using a data driven approach. *J Neurol Neurosurg Psychiatry*. 76:343-8.

Lotharius, J., and P. Brundin. 2002. Pathogenesis of Parkinson's disease: dopamine, vesicles and alpha-synuclein. *Nat Rev Neurosci*. 3:932-42.

Lu, X.H., S.M. Fleming, B. Meurers, L.C. Ackerson, F. Mortazavi, V. Lo, D. Hernandez, D. Sulzer, G.R. Jackson, N.T. Maidment, M.F. Chesselet, and X.W. Yang. 2009. Bacterial artificial chromosome transgenic mice expressing a truncated mutant parkin exhibit age-dependent hypokinetic motor deficits, dopaminergic neuron degeneration, and accumulation of proteinase K-resistant alpha-synuclein. *J Neurosci*. 29:1962-76.

Lucking, C.B., A. Durr, V. Bonifati, J. Vaughan, G. De Michele, T. Gasser, B.S. Harhangi, G. Meco, P. Denefle, N.W. Wood, Y. Agid, and A. Brice. 2000. Association between early-onset Parkinson's disease and mutations in the parkin gene. *N Engl J Med*. 342:1560-7.

Martin, H.L., and P. Teismann. 2009. Glutathione--a review on its role and significance in Parkinson's disease. *FASEB J*. 23:3263-72.

Mata, I.F., P.J. Lockhart, and M.J. Farrer. 2004. Parkin genetics: one model for Parkinson's disease. *Hum Mol Genet*. 13 Spec No 1:R127-33.

McClearn, G.E., and R.J. McCarter. 2011. Heterogeneous stocks and selective breeding in aging research. *ILAR J*. 52:16-23.

Menendez, J., J.A. Rodriguez-Navarro, R.M. Solano, M.J. Casarejos, I. Rodal, R. Guerrero, M.P. Sanchez, J. Avila, M.A. Mena, and J.G. de Yebenes. 2006. Suppression of Parkin enhances nigrostriatal and motor neuron lesion in mice over-expressing human-mutated tau protein. *Hum Mol Genet*. 15:2045-58.

Mukhopadhyay, D., and H. Riezman. 2007. Proteasome-independent functions of ubiquitin in endocytosis and signaling. *Science*. 315:201-5.

Obeso, J.A., M.C. Rodriguez-Oroz, B. Benitez-Temino, F.J. Blesa, J. Guridi, C. Marin, and M. Rodriguez. 2008. Functional organization of the basal ganglia: therapeutic implications for Parkinson's disease. *Mov Disord*. 23 Suppl 3:S548-59.

Obeso, J.A., M.C. Rodriguez-Oroz, C.G. Goetz, C. Marin, J.H. Kordower, M. Rodriguez, E.C. Hirsch, M. Farrer, A.H. Schapira, and G. Halliday. 2010. Missing pieces in the Parkinson's disease puzzle. *Nat Med*. 16:653-61.

Olzmann, J.A., and L.S. Chin. 2008. Parkin-mediated K63-linked polyubiquitination: a signal for targeting misfolded proteins to the aggresome-autophagy pathway. *Autophagy*. 4:85-7.

Oyama, G., K. Yoshimi, S. Natori, Y. Chikaoka, Y.R. Ren, M. Funayama, Y. Shimo, R. Takahashi, T. Nakazato, S. Kitazawa, and N. Hattori. 2010. Impaired in vivo dopamine release in parkin knockout mice. *Brain Res.* 1352:214-22.

Pakkenberg, B., A. Moller, H.J. Gundersen, A. Mouritzen Dam, and H. Pakkenberg. 1991. The absolute number of nerve cells in substantia nigra in normal subjects and in patients with Parkinson's disease estimated with an unbiased stereological method. *J Neurol Neurosurg Psychiatry.* 54:30-3.

Palacino, J.J., D. Sagi, M.S. Goldberg, S. Krauss, C. Motz, M. Wacker, J. Klose, and J. Shen. 2004. Mitochondrial dysfunction and oxidative damage in parkin-deficient mice. *J Biol Chem.* 279:18614-22.

Palumbo, E., L. Matricardi, E. Tosoni, A. Bensimon, and A. Russo. 2010. Replication dynamics at common fragile site FRA6E. *Chromosoma.* 119:575-87.

Perez, F.A., and R.D. Palmiter. 2005. Parkin-deficient mice are not a robust model of parkinsonism. *Proc Natl Acad Sci U S A.* 102:2174-9.

Perucho, J., M.J. Casarejos, I. Rubio, J.A. Rodriguez-Navarro, A. Gomez, I. Ampuero, I. Rodal, R.M. Solano, E. Carro, J. Garcia de Yebenes, and M.A. Mena. 2010. The effects of parkin suppression on the behaviour, amyloid processing, and cell survival in APP mutant transgenic mice. *Exp Neurol.* 221:54-67.

Pesah, Y., T. Pham, H. Burgess, B. Middlebrooks, P. Verstreken, Y. Zhou, M. Harding, H. Bellen, and G. Mardon. 2004. Drosophila parkin mutants have decreased mass and cell size and increased sensitivity to oxygen radical stress. *Development.* 131:2183-94.

Ren, Y., H. Jiang, D. Ma, K. Nakaso, and J. Feng. 2010. Parkin degrades estrogen-related receptors to limit the expression of monoamine oxidases. *Hum Mol Genet.* 20:1074-83.

Rodriguez-Navarro, J.A., M.J. Casarejos, J. Menendez, R.M. Solano, I. Rodal, A. Gomez, J.G. Yebenes, and M.A. Mena. 2007. Mortality, oxidative stress and tau accumulation during ageing in parkin null mice. *J Neurochem.* 103:98-114.

Rodriguez-Navarro, J.A., R.M. Solano, M.J. Casarejos, A. Gomez, J. Perucho, J.G. de Yebenes, and M.A. Mena. 2008. Gender differences and estrogen effects in parkin null mice. *J Neurochem.* 106:2143-57.

Satake, W., Y. Nakabayashi, I. Mizuta, Y. Hirota, C. Ito, M. Kubo, T. Kawaguchi, T. Tsunoda, M. Watanabe, A. Takeda, H. Tomiyama, K. Nakashima, K. Hasegawa, F. Obata, T. Yoshikawa, H. Kawakami, S. Sakoda, M. Yamamoto, N. Hattori, M. Murata, Y. Nakamura, and T. Toda. 2009. Genome-wide association study identifies common variants at four loci as genetic risk factors for Parkinson's disease. *Nat Genet.* 41:1303-7.

Sato, S., T. Chiba, S. Nishiyama, T. Kakiuchi, H. Tsukada, T. Hatano, T. Fukuda, Y. Yasoshima, N. Kai, K. Kobayashi, Y. Mizuno, K. Tanaka, and N. Hattori. 2006. Decline of striatal dopamine release in parkin-deficient mice shown by ex vivo autoradiography. *J Neurosci Res.* 84:1350-7.

Schmidt, S., B. Linnartz, S. Mendritzki, T. Sczepan, M. Lubbert, C.C. Stichel, and H. Lubbert. 2011. Genetic mouse models for Parkinson's disease display severe pathology in glial cell mitochondria. *Hum Mol Genet.* 20:1197-211.

Selikhova, M., D.R. Williams, P.A. Kempster, J.L. Holton, T. Revesz, and A.J. Lees. 2009. A clinico-pathological study of subtypes in Parkinson's disease. *Brain*. 132:2947-57.

Shimura, H., N. Hattori, S. Kubo, Y. Mizuno, S. Asakawa, S. Minoshima, N. Shimizu, K. Iwai, T. Chiba, K. Tanaka, and T. Suzuki. 2000. Familial Parkinson disease gene product, parkin, is a ubiquitin-protein ligase. *Nat Genet*. 25:302-5.

Shulman, J.M., P.L. De Jager, and M.B. Feany. 2010. Parkinson's Disease: Genetics and Pathogenesis. *Annu Rev Pathol*. 6:193-222.

Simon-Sanchez, J., C. Schulte, J.M. Bras, M. Sharma, J.R. Gibbs, D. Berg, C. Paisan-Ruiz, P. Lichtner, S.W. Scholz, D.G. Hernandez, R. Kruger, M. Federoff, C. Klein, A. Goate, J. Perlmutter, M. Bonin, M.A. Nalls, T. Illig, C. Gieger, H. Houlden, M. Steffens, M.S. Okun, B.A. Racette, M.R. Cookson, K.D. Foote, H.H. Fernandez, B.J. Traynor, S. Schreiber, S. Arepalli, R. Zonozi, K. Gwinn, M. van der Brug, G. Lopez, S.J. Chanock, A. Schatzkin, Y. Park, A. Hollenbeck, J. Gao, X. Huang, N.W. Wood, D. Lorenz, G. Deuschl, H. Chen, O. Riess, J.A. Hardy, A.B. Singleton, and T. Gasser. 2009. Genome-wide association study reveals genetic risk underlying Parkinson's disease. *Nat Genet*. 41:1308-12.

Solano, R.M., M.J. Casarejos, J. Menendez-Cuervo, J.A. Rodriguez-Navarro, J. Garcia de Yebenes, and M.A. Mena. 2008. Glial dysfunction in parkin null mice: effects of aging. *J Neurosci*. 28:598-611.

Standaert, D.G., and J.M. Galanter. (2007) Pharmacology of dopaminergic neurotransmission. In*: Principles of pharmacology: the pathophysiologic basis of drug therapy.* Golan, D.E., editor. pp. 185-200, Lippincott Williams & Wilkins, 0781783550, United Kingdom.

Stichel, C.C., X.R. Zhu, V. Bader, B. Linnartz, S. Schmidt, and H. Lubbert. 2007. Mono- and double-mutant mouse models of Parkinson's disease display severe mitochondrial damage. *Hum Mol Genet*. 16:2377-93.

Tong, Y., A. Pisani, G. Martella, M. Karouani, H. Yamaguchi, E.N. Pothos, and J. Shen. 2009. R1441C mutation in LRRK2 impairs dopaminergic neurotransmission in mice. *Proc Natl Acad Sci U S A*. 106:14622-7.

Van Den Eeden, S.K., C.M. Tanner, A.L. Bernstein, R.D. Fross, A. Leimpeter, D.A. Bloch, and L.M. Nelson. 2003. Incidence of Parkinson's disease: variation by age, gender, and race/ethnicity. *Am J Epidemiol*. 157:1015-22.

von Coelln, R., B. Thomas, S.A. Andrabi, K.L. Lim, J.M. Savitt, R. Saffary, W. Stirling, K. Bruno, E.J. Hess, M.K. Lee, V.L. Dawson, and T.M. Dawson. 2006. Inclusion body formation and neurodegeneration are parkin independent in a mouse model of alpha-synucleinopathy. *J Neurosci*. 26:3685-96.

Von Coelln, R., B. Thomas, J.M. Savitt, K.L. Lim, M. Sasaki, E.J. Hess, V.L. Dawson, and T.M. Dawson. 2004. Loss of locus coeruleus neurons and reduced startle in parkin null mice. *Proc Natl Acad Sci U S A*. 101:10744-9.

Whitworth, A.J., D.A. Theodore, J.C. Greene, H. Benes, P.D. Wes, and L.J. Pallanck. 2005. Increased glutathione S-transferase activity rescues dopaminergic neuron loss in a Drosophila model of Parkinson's disease. *Proc Natl Acad Sci U S A*. 102:8024-9.

Yoshida, T., T. Mizuta, and S. Shimizu. 2010. Neurodegeneration in mnd2 mutant mice is not prevented by parkin transgene. *Biochem Biophys Res Commun*. 402:676-9.

Yuan, R., L.L. Peters, and B. Paigen. 2011. Mice as a mammalian model for research on the genetics of aging. *ILAR J*. 52:4-15.

Zhu, X.R., L. Maskri, C. Herold, V. Bader, C.C. Stichel, O. Gunturkun, and H. Lubbert. 2007. Non-motor behavioural impairments in parkin-deficient mice. *Eur J Neurosci*. 26:1902-11.

14

Bilateral Distribution of Oxytocinase Activity in the Medial Prefrontal Cortex of Spontaneously Hypertensive Rats with Experimental Hemiparkinsonism

Manuel Ramírez[1] et al.*
[1]*Unit of Physiology, Department of Health Sciences, University of Jaén, Jaén, Spain*

1. Introduction

Oxytocin and vasopressin are important modulators of diverse social and anxiety-related behaviors (Insel, 2010). The enzyme that regulates the function of both peptides, called oxytocinase (OX) or vasopressinase, is also involved in cognitive functions (Stragier et al., 2008; Banegas et al., 2010). Normotensive male Wistar rats exhibited a marked left predominance of OX in the medial prefrontal cortex (mPFC), an area implicated in cognitive functions and reward-related mechanisms in the rat brain and characterized by its asymmetrical organization. Brain dopamine (DA) content as well as the functions in which this neurotransmitter is involved, are asymmetrically organized in physiologic conditions (reviewed by Ramírez et al., 2004). Therefore, Parkinson's disease (PD) represents a disruption of this bilateral pattern of brain DA. Indeed, the disease normally begins unilaterally in the early stages. Animals with hemi-parkinsonism, induced by unilateral nigrostratal lesions using 6-hydroxydopamine (6-OHDA), showed several behavioral abnormalities, not only linked to a disruption of the normal bilateral distribution of brain DA, but probably also by the alteration of other factors such as the disruption of the striking basal left predominance of OX observed in both the left and right sham controls. The bilateral distribution in lesioned animals was altered differently depending on the injured hemisphere. These results may reflect changes in the levels of oxytocin and vasopressin in the mPFC and consequently in the functions in which they are involved and might account, in part, for the cognitive abnormalities observed in hemi-parkinsonism (Henderson et al., 2003). The spontaneously hypertensive rat (SHR), is a recognised model for studies of hypertension. This strain of rat also display major symptoms of the attention-deficit/hyperactivity disorder (ADHD) such as deficits in attention, impulsivity and hyperactivity when compared to Wistar-Kyoto rats (Russell, 2007). Indeed, SHR have been shown to have also disturbances in the dopaminergic system (Russell, 2007). The aim of this

*Inmaculada Banegas[1], Ana Belén Segarra[1], Rosemary Wangesteen[1], Marc de Gasparo[2], Raquel Durán[3], Francisco Vives[3], Antonio Martínez[1], Francisco Alba[3] and Isabel Prieto[1]
[2]*Rue es Planches 5, 2842 Rossemaison, Switzerland.*
[3]*Instituto de Neurociencias 'Federico Oloriz', University of Granada, Granada, Spain.*

study was to analyze OX in the left and right mPFC of SHR with left or right hemi-parkinsonism, induced by intrastriatal injections of 6-OHDA, and compared with sham controls. The results dramatically differed from those obtained in Wistar normotensive rats. SHR demonstrated a slighter basal left predominance of OX, only significant in left sham controls. The bilateral distribution in lesioned animals was differently altered depending on the injured hemisphere but in a way dissimilar to the one observed in Wistar. Thus, the hemi-parkinsonism induced in animals with cognitive and behavioral abnormalities such as ADHD induces a different brain bilateral response in OX than the one observed in Wistar. These results suggest that the cognitive consequences of hemi-parkinsonism differed between both Wistar and SHR rats. It is proposed that increased OX in mPFC is related to decreased cognitive process.

1.1 Brain asymmetry and cognitive functions

The brain asymmetry, understood as an anatomical, functional or neurochemical difference between the two hemispheres, is a dynamic phenomenon, modulated by both exogenous and endogenous factors. Increasing evidences suggest that under the anatomical and functional asymmetries underlie neurochemical brain lateralizations. However, the link between these three aspects of the brain asymmetry concept as well its own physiological meaning is not yet well understood (Ramírez et al., 2004). In addition, the impairment of cognitive functions, such as occurs during aging, is linked to vascular dementia (Vallesi et al., 2010; Xu et al., 2008). This is also related to some brain disorders, such as PD or ADHD, both characterized by disruptions in the specific physiological bilateral organization of the brain (Ramírez et al., 2004; Banegas et al., 2010; Shaw et al., 2009). Analyzing how brain bilaterality changes in specific conditions may help us to understand its meaning and its importance in physiology and pathology.

1.2 Brain asymmetry and dopamine function

Numerous studies of the DA content in the striatum in relationship with the rotation (circling behaviour) that the rats exhibited spontaneously and after drug induction (Zimmerberg et al., 1974; Glick et al., 1974; Shapiro et al., 1986) were performed to attempt to relate a neurochemical asymmetry with a lateralized function in physiologic conditions. Zimmerberg et al. (1974) demonstrated that DA levels in the striatum were significantly higher in the contralateral side to which the rats choose in a T-maze test. The concentration of DA between the two hemispheres differed by 15%. However, when high doses of amphetamine were administrated to the animals, this bilateral difference was increased up to 25% (Glick et al., 1974). For these and later studies, the model of rotational behaviour in rodents was used and revised by Shapiro et al. in 1986. The animals with 6-OHDA-induced unilateral lesions of the substantia nigra exhibited a circling behavior in response to several drugs. It was postulated that animals rotated mainly contralaterally to the side containing a higher content of DA or a higher number of activate postsynaptic DA receptors. Xu et al., (2005) compared, by quantitative autoradiography, the changes in DA receptor binding in the left and right striatum in rats after unilateral DA depletion. In comparison with control levels, DA D_1-like receptor binding in the dorsal striatum was reduced 2 weeks after unilateral lesions of the substantia nigra (SN) with 6-OHDA. Remarkably, D_1-like receptor binding was decreased in the ipsilateral striatum following unilateral lesions of either the left or right SN. Also, the left and right striatum responded similarly to unilateral SN lesions, as there were no significant differences in the percent decrease in D_1-like binding in the two striata. In contrast, D_2-like receptor binding was significantly increased in the dorsal striatum following an ipsilateral SN lesion. Furthermore, the up-regulation of D_2-like receptors in the right striatum was significantly greater than that in the left striatum after an ipsilateral lesion. The authors speculated that the asymmetrical up-regulation of striatal D_2 receptors after DA depletion may contribute to the lateralization of the nigrostriatal system observed in some pathological conditions.

1.3 Parkinson's disease, brain asymmetry and cognitive functions

Parkinson's disease is the second most common neurodegenerative disorder (Dorsey et al., 2007). Despite the intensive efforts, progresses in the fight against this disease are slow and new strategies for early diagnosis and treatment to prevent its progression are required (George et al., 2009). A deep knowledge of its pathophysiology is essential to achieve this goal. Although symmetric at the later stages, the damage observed in PD begins asymmetrically (Djaldetti et al., 2006). Therefore, there exist in PD a disruption of the physiologic bilateral distribution of DA content as well as a bilateral disturbance of other neurochemical factors (Banegas et al., 2010). Animal models of PD, such as the experimental hemiparkinsonism after unilateral intrastriatal injections of 6-OHDA, could simulate the initial phase of PD. In the early stages, PD patients exhibit cognitive and behavioral impairments unrelated to the motor symptoms, and involving frontal lobe dysfunction (Brück et al., 2004; Farina et al., 1994; Zgaljardic et al., 2006). They are the result of damage of a specific hemisphere (Cubo et al., 2010). In addition, hemiparkinsonism has been associated with asymmetrical cognitive changes (Huber et al., 1992; Piacentini et al., 2010). Studies in animals with induced hemi-parkinsonism have reported several behavioral abnormalities (Henderson et al., 2003). The mPFC, a part of the mesocorticolimbic system, is involved in cognitive functions and reward-related mechanisms in the rat brain (Tzschentke, 2000). Interestingly, the mesocortical dopamine system, particularly the mPFC, is characterized by its asymmetric organization (Sullivan, 2004).

1.4 Vascular damage, cognitive impairment and brain asymmetry

Cerebral capillary damage occurs not only in neurodegenerative disorders such as in Alzheimer's disease and PD but also in hypertension. Thus, it was hypothesized that ultrastructural abnormalities of cerebral capillaries were related to decreased cerebral blood flow that favors neurodegenerative mechanisms leading to the development of dementia (Farkas et al., 2000). Clearly, hypertension is involved in the development of vascular cognitive impairment and vascular dementia (Amenta et al., 2003). Indeed, an impairment of cognitive functions was described in elderly hypertensive individuals (Vinyoles et al., 2008) as well as in childhood (Adams et al., 2010). The SHR is a recognized animal model of cognitive decline associated with hypertension (Diana, 2002). These animals present abnormal dopaminergic transmission and altered neuronal dendrite morphology of the mPFC (Sánchez et al., 2011). Therefore, there exists a connection between hypertension, vascular dementia, cognitive impairment and a modification of the basal brain asymmetry (Xu et al., 2008; Vallesi et al., 2010; Bergerbest et al., 2009).

In the ADHD, characterized by impaired sustained attention, impulsivity and hyperactivity, a disruption of the physiological cortical asymmetry has been implicated in its pathogenesis (Shaw et al., 2009). The SHR, largely used as a model for hypertension, also display major symptoms of the ADHD (Russel, 2007) when compared with normotensive rats. Indeed,

SHR have also disturbances in the dopaminergic system. Therefore, it could be hypothesized that their brain bilateral functioning for cognitive processes may differ from the brain bilateral behaviour of normotensive rats.

1.5 Oxytocin, oxytocinase, cognitive functions and brain asymmetry

It was proposed that systems other than the dopaminergic pathway may also be involved in the behavioral abnormalities observed in PD (Lang & Obeso, 2004; Banegas et al., 2010). Oxytocin and vasopressin as well as the enzyme that regulates their functions, called oxytocinase (OX) or vasopressinase are involved in cognitive functions. Normotensive male Wistar rats exhibit a marked left predominance of OX in the mPFC, an area implicated in cognitive functions and reward-related mechanisms in the rat brain and characterized by its asymmetrical organization as already mentioned (Sullivan, 2004). Changes in this basal pattern of bilateral organization may cause disorders in brain function (Ramírez et al., 2004). Normotensive animals with hemi-parkinsonism induced by unilateral nigrostratal lesions using 6-OHDA showed several behavioral abnormalities and a disruption of the striking basal left predominance of OX as observed in both the left and right sham controls. The bilateral distribution in lesioned animals was altered differently depending on the injured hemisphere. These results may reflect changes in the levels of oxytocin and vasopressin in the mPFC and consequently, in their functions. This could account, in part, for the cognitive abnormalities observed in hemi-parkinsonism (Banegas et al., 2010).

Therefore, considering that background, it was indicated to analyze OX in the left and right mPFC of SHR with left or right hemi-parkinsonism, induced by intrastriatal injections of 6-OHDA, and compare its activity in sham SHR controls. These results will be discussed with those obtained previously in normotensive rats using the same protocol (Banegas et al., 2010). This approach should give precious indications on the behavior of brain bilaterality in two strains of rat that clearly differ in their cognitive status.

2. Materials and methods

2.1 Animals

Three-month-old male SHR (systolic blood pressure: 164.1 ± 4.2 mmHg; n=40) weighing 250 g at the beginning of the study were used for both sham and lesioned groups. During the experimental period, food and water were available *ad libitum*. The animals were housed under standard conditions of light (12 h of light from 7.00 h to 19.00 h and 12 h of dark from 19.00 h to 7.00 h) and temperature (22° C).

2.2 Surgical procedure

Degeneration of the left or right nigrostriatal dopaminergic pathway was accomplished via neurochemical lesions induced with the catecholaminergic toxin 6-OHDA (Jolicoeur and Rivest, 1992). All animals were anesthetized with 2 ml/kg body weight equithensin (42.5 g/L chloralhydrate dissolved in 19.76 mL ethanol, 9.72 g/L Nembutal®, 0.396 L/L propylenglycol and 21.3 g/L magnesium sulfate in distilled water) and placed in a stereotaxic instrument (David Kopf Instruments, Palo Alto, CA, USA). A 2 mm burr hole was drilled through the skull at horizontal coordinates approximating the position of the striatum (AP 0 mm, L or R 3 mm and H -5 mm) according to the atlas by Paxinos and Watson (1998). Infusion of 4 µL of 6-OHDA (8 mg dissolved in 1 mL of cold saline with 0.02% ascorbic acid to inhibit oxidation) was administered into the left or right striatum

(Jolicoeur & Rivest, 1992). The control rats were operated the same manner but they received 4 µl of saline with 0.02% ascorbic acid.

2.3 Motor behaviour in experimental hemiparkinsonism

Normal rats exhibit a spontaneous turning behaviour, the levels of DA being higher in the contralateral striatum than the side of the turning preference (Glick, 1983). Therefore, animals with experimental hemiparkinsonism turn ipsilaterally to the side of lesion. This turning behavior was amplified after amphetamine administration that increases dopamine in the synaptic cleft. Assessment of the ipsilateral rotational behavior allowed us to verify the efficacy of the 6-OHDA-induced lesions. Four weeks post-surgery and three days before sacrifice, animals were given D-amphetamine sulfate (5 mg/kg s.c.) to enhance the turning behaviour (Robinson et al., 1994) while placed in a 30 cm diameter bowl. Number of turns was determined in 6 periods of 10 min. during 1 h. Sufficiently rotating animals were included in lesion group. Sham-lesioned rats underwent the same surgery and rotational testing but did not demonstrate sufficient rotational behaviour to qualify as parkinsonian models. Most animals exceeded the 100 % of turns from mean of control and were considered with hemiparkinson. Lesioned animals that did not presented turning behaviour but exhibited rigidity after D-amphetamine injection also were considered with hemiparkinson. Compared with sham controls, a marked ipsilateral rotational behavior was observed in left- and right-lesioned animals (Banegas et al., 2009) (figure 1).

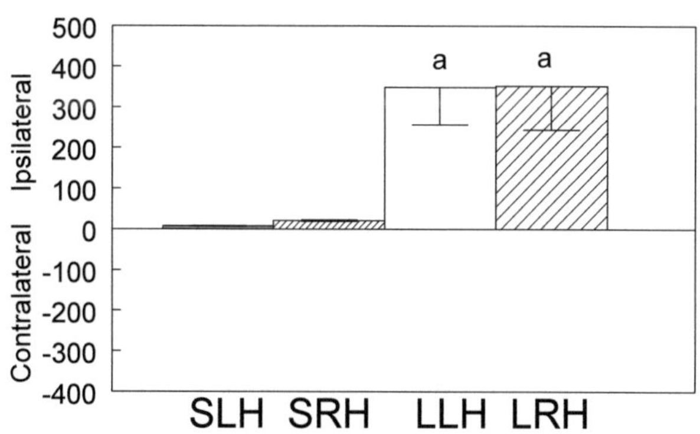

Fig. 1. Turning behaviour in the groups studied.

Turning behaviour in lesioned left (LL) or lesioned right (LR) and sham left (SL) or sham right (SR) spontaneously hypertensive rats (H). Number of turns were determined individually in 6 periods of 10 min during 1 h. Values represent mean ± SEM (n=10) of the cumulative turns recorded in the 6 periods (modified from Banegas et al., 2009 with permission). a Differences between the same side of lesioned vs sham animals. a $p<0.001$

2.4 Collection and treatment of tissue samples

The surgical procedure, sacrifice and sample collection were performed under anesthesia between 9.00 h and 11.00 h. Four weeks after receiving the injections, the animals were sacrificed and mPFC samples were obtained from each group as previously described (Banegas et al, 2005a). Briefly, the animals were perfused with saline transcardially under equithensin anaesthesia (2 ml/kg body weight). The brain was quickly removed (less than

60 s) and cooled in dry ice. Left and right brain samples were dissected according to the stereotaxic atlas of Paxinos & Watson (1998). The selected area of mPFC was between 12,70 mm and 11,70 mm anterior to the interaural line. All samples were collected the same day and frozen for assays. Tissue samples were homogenized in 400 µl of 10 mM HCl-Tris buffer (pH 7,4) and ultracentrifugated at 100,000 x g for 30 min. at 4 °C. The pellets were re-homogenized in HCl-Tris buffer (pH 7,4) plus 1% Triton-X-100 to solubilize membrane proteins. After centrifugation (100,000 x g, 30 min., 4 °C the supernatants were shaked in an orbital rotor during 2 h. at 4 °C with the polymeric adsorbent Bio-Beads SM-2 (100 mg/ml) in order to remove the detergent from the sample (Alba et al., 1995). The bio-beads were removed and the supernatants were used to measure in triplicate membrane-bound aminopeptidase activities and protein content. Left or right 6-OHDA-lesioned animals were compared with their corresponding left or right sham-operated animals in which the DA pathways were intact. Because bilateral injuries usually lead to the death of rats due to the occurrence of marked aphagia and adipsia (Ungerstedt, 1971), such control animals were not available.

2.5 Procedures for enzymatic assays

Membrane-bound oxytocinase activity was measured fluorometrically using L-Cys-β-naphthylamide as previously described (Banegas et al., 2005a). Proteins were quantified in triplicate by the method of Bradford (1976) using BSA as a standard. Specific OX was expressed as nanomoles of L-Cys-β-naphthylamide hydrolyzed per minute per milligram of protein. Fluorogenic assays were linear with respect to the time of hydrolysis and protein content.

2.6 Experimental groups

Oxytocinase activity levels were measured in mPFC of the following groups (n = 10 for all groups):

a. Simulated lesion of the left hemisphere with saline (sham left, SL)
b. Simulated lesion of the right hemisphere with saline (sham right, SR)
c. Lesion of left hemisphere with 6-OHDA (lesion left, LL)
d. Lesion of right hemisphere with 6-OHDA (lesion right, LR)

All experimental procedures involving animals, including their use and care, were in accordance with the European Communities Council Directive 86/609/EEC.

2.7 Statistical analysis

We used a one-way analysis of variance (ANOVA) to analyze differences between groups. Post-hoc comparisons were made using the paired Student's t test; p-values below 0.05 were considered significant.

3. Results

Results of the present research are represented in figures 2 and 3. There was an asymmetry of OX in the mPFC of left controls (SL) showing a significant left predominance (41% higher; $p<0.01$). The right controls (SR) showed a tendency for left predominance (15% higher) without reaching statistical significance. After left lesion (LL), there was an increased left

predominance (75% higher; $p<0.001$), whereas the OX predominance shifted slightly to the right hemisphere in right lesioned animals (LR) (19% higher; $p<0.05$) (fig. 2).
Compared with the same side of sham animals, the LL produced a significant increase in OX in the left mPFC (48% higher; $p<0.01$) and no modification in the right side. The LR decreased OX in the left mPFC (32% lower; $p<0.01$) but did not modify OX activity in the right side compared to the control.
The percentage differences ([(high/low)-1] x 100) between the left and right values of OX in mPFC for each animal in the four groups are shown in figure 3. In SL and SR, although with low level of percentage, most animals were left predominant. The differences ranged from 11% to 113% higher OX activity in the left mPFC of eight SL animals ($p<0.01$) and from 4% to 56% in seven SR animals (without significant differences between mean values). In LL animals, the level of percentage for left OX predominance increased slightly, ranging from 18% to 185% (higher) in eight animals ($p<0.001$). The SHR from the LR group shifted slightly to the right predominance ($p<0.05$) with seven animals right predominance ranging from 3% to 77%.
The present results are indicative of an influence of DA depletion on the bilateral levels of OX in the mPFC of hypertensive rats, and dramatically differ from the data observed in normotensive Wistar rats (Banegas et al, 2010). These effects are conditioned by the side in which 6-OHDA or saline was administered.

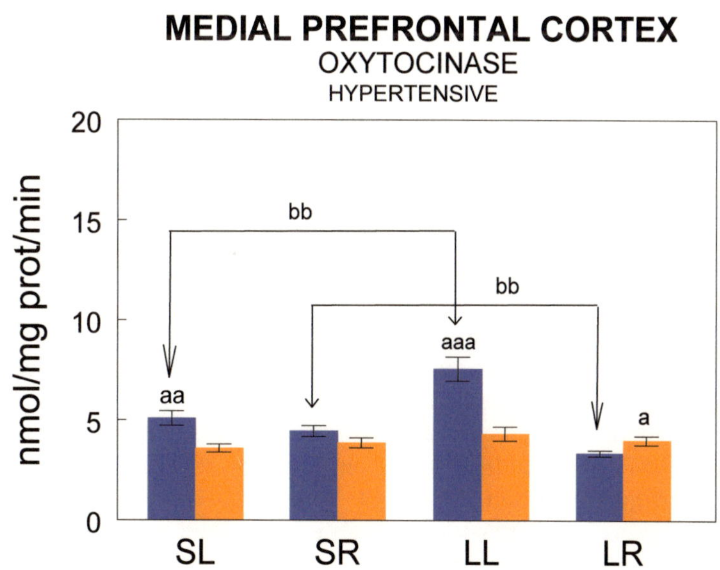

Fig. 2. Oxytocinase activity in the left and right medial prefrontal cortex of hypertensive rats.

Oxytocinase activity in the left (blue bars) and right (rose bars) medial prefrontal cortex of left (SL) or right (SR) sham-operated and left (LL) or right (LR) 6-OHDA lesioned hypertensive rats. (n=10 in each group). Values represent mean ± SEM of specific oxytocinase activity expressed as nanomoles of Cys-β-naphthylamide hydrolyzed per minute per milligram of protein. (a) Differences between left and right sides. (b) Differences in the same side between sham and lesioned animals. Single letter: $p<0.05$; double letter: $p<0.01$; triple letter: $p<0.001$.

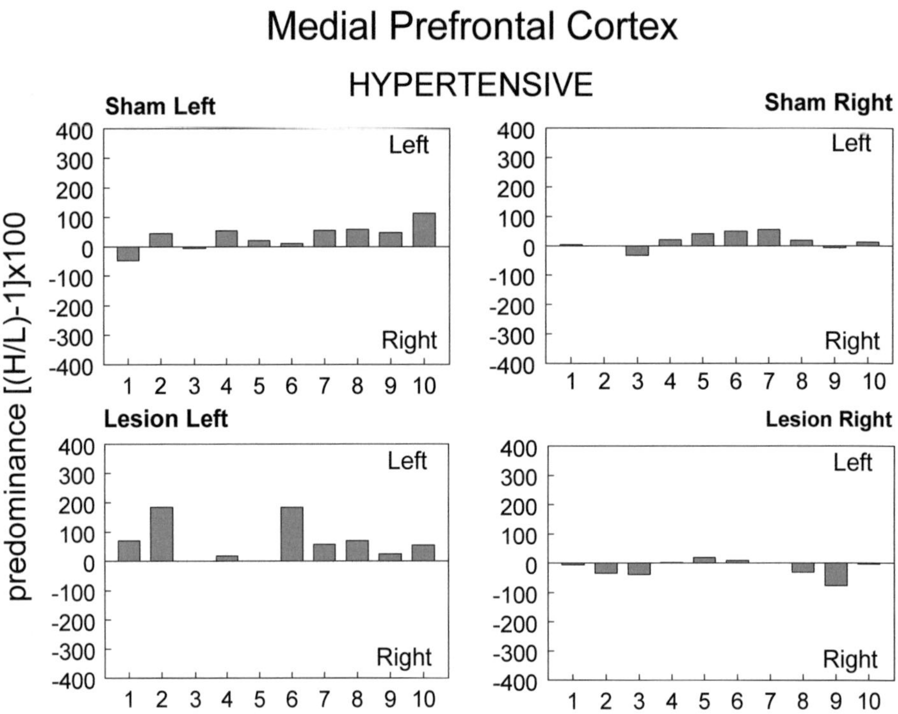

Fig. 3. Percentage differences between the left and right prefrontal cortex of hypertensive rats

Bars represent the percentage differences between the levels of oxytocinase activity of the left and right sides of the prefrontal cortex for each of the hypertensive rats studied in all four groups. H, higher value; L, lower value.

4. Discussion

It has been demonstrated that the PFC plays a critical role in the development of ADHD and that the mesocortical DA system is involved in that process. In addition, previous studies demonstrated that the laterality of the prefrontal function in the rat is also involved in ADHD, particularly the dysregulation of the right PFC having a deficit of its dopaminergic system (Sullivan & Brake, 2003). Indeed, the mPFC DA system exhibits many functional hemispheric asymmetries involving the right mesocortical DA system. Thus, 6-OHDA lesions of the right but not the left frontal cortex conducts to pronounced behavioural hyperactivity and altered subcortical catecholamine function. The right frontal systems play a key role in motor inhibition and the mesocortical DA seems to be an important part of this regulation. It is therefore expected that its impairment may led to hyperactivity behaviour. ADHD children have mainly impaired ability to keep their attention focus due to dysfunctions in the right hemisphere attention systems (Reviewed by Sullivan & Brake, 2003).

Therefore, it is interesting to compare the bilateral behavior of the mPFC after the specific lesion of the right or the left nigrostriatal dopaminergic system in normotensive rats and in an animal model of ADHD: the SHR strain. This could provide valuable information on the bilateral behaviour of the frontostriatal dopaminergic system whose operation is critical for understanding the pathogenesis of disorders such as PD or ADHD.

The present results obtained in SHR differed substantially from those previously obtained in normotensive rats (Banegas et al, 2010). Most importantly, there is a remarkable lower level of left predominance in sham hypertensive controls (figures 2 and 3), compared with the high one observed in sham normotensive controls (figures 4 and 5). This is in agreement with the reduction of the asymmetry observed in prefrontal cortex and hippocampus in ADHD (Shaw et al., 2009) and during aging and vascular dementia compared to healthy subjects (Xu et al., 2008; Vallesi et al., 2010; Bergerbest et al., 2009). Indeed, disruption of physiological asymmetry has been involved in the pathogenesis of cognitive disorders such as ADHD. An increase in the thickness of the right frontal cortex together with a left-hemispheric increase in the occipital cortical regions characterize the normal bilateral development of children. However, in ADHD, while the posterior component of this bilateral development was intact, the prefrontal one was lost (Shaw et al., 2009). The morphological asymmetry of hippocampus in healthy subjects, assessed by magnetic resonance imaging, is greater than that in Alzheimer's disease and in patients with vascular dementia (Xu et al., 2008). Studying the effects of age on the asymmetry of the motor system, Vallesi et al. (2010) reported that older adults showed a more symmetric pattern than younger subjects. Moreover, an age-associated reduction of asymmetry in prefrontal function has been related to several forms of cognitive impairment (Bergerbest et al., 2009).

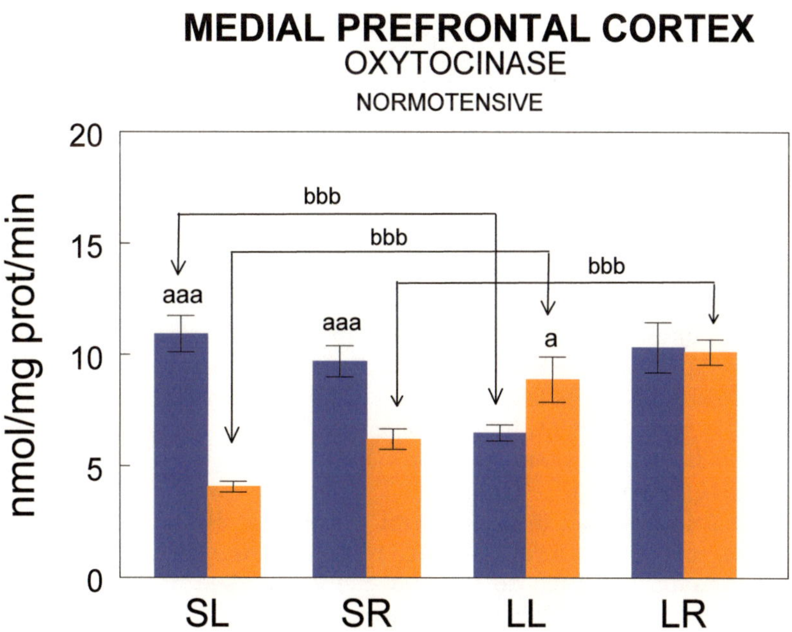

Fig. 4. Oxytocinase activity in the left and right medial prefrontal cortex of normotensive rats

Oxytocinase activity in the left (gray bars) and right (open bars) medial prefrontal cortex of left (SL) or right (SR) sham-operated and left (LL) or right (LR) 6-OHDA lesioned normotensive rats. (n=10 in each group). Values represent mean±SEM of specific oxytocinase activity expressed as nanomoles of Cys-β-naphthylamide hydrolyzed per minute per milligram of protein. (a) Differences between left and right sides. (b) Differences in the same side between sham and lesioned animals. Single letter: $p<0.05$; triple letter: $p<0.001$ (from Banegas et al, 2010 with permission).

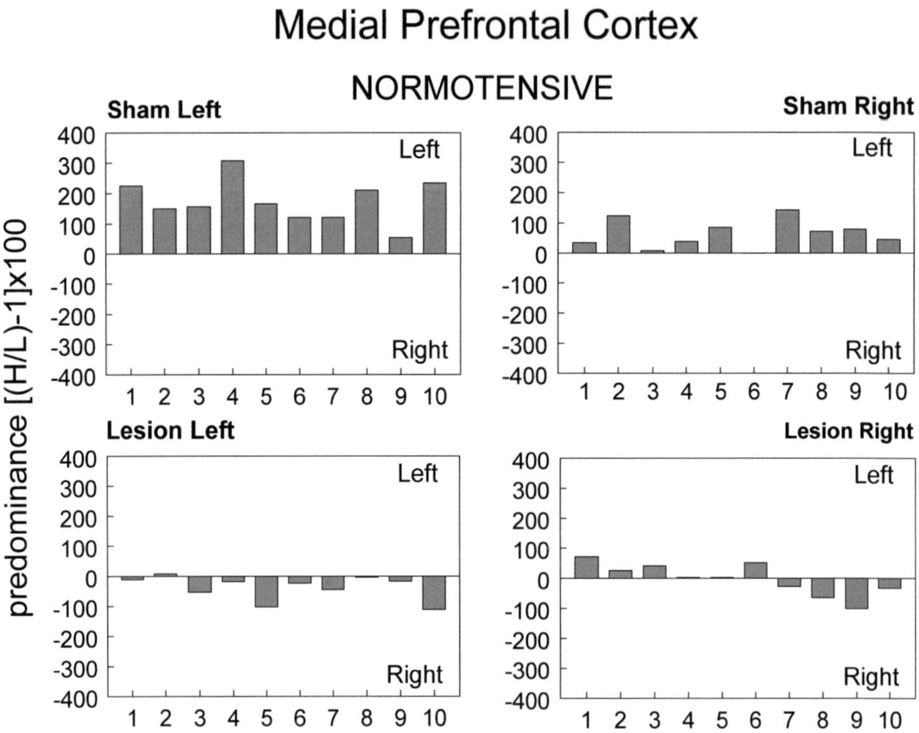

Fig. 5. Percentage differences between the left and right prefrontal cortex of normotensive rats.

Bars represent the percentage differences between the levels of oxytocinase activity of the left and right sides of the prefrontal cortex for each of the normotensive rats studied in all four groups. H, higher value; L, lower value.

Especially informative is the comparison of figures 3 and 5 in which we can notice the great difference in the bilateral response of normotensive and SHR. While in SL and SR normotensive rats virtually all the animals were left predominant with a high percentage of difference (figure 5), in SL and SR hypertensive the left predominance is substantially lower (figure 3). Whereas in LL normotensive animals, OX predominance was shifted to the right in nine animals (figure 5), in LL hypertensive rats the left predominance was increased (figure 3). The bilateral response of animals from the LR group of normotensive and hypertensive was quite similar.

The slight difference observed in the bilateral distribution of OX between SL and SR of hypertensive rats could be due to a differential response of the local inflammatory processes following the introduction of the cannula into the left or right hemisphere, as previously suggested by Banegas et al. (2009) in normotensive rats.

The direct effect of lesions in hypertensive animals on OX also differed from the previous observation in normotensive rats. OX decreased in the left side and increased in the right hemisphere of normotensive LL (figure 4). In contrast, in hypertensive LL rats, the enzyme activity increased in the left hemisphere and was not modified in the right one (figure 2).

Clearly, the response to left or right lesions in normotensive rats involved both left and right hemispheres. On the contrary, in hypertensive rats, it only implies changes in the left hemisphere. It is particularly noticeable that the right mPFC was not modified either when left or right lesions were performed, in marked contrast with the important changes that

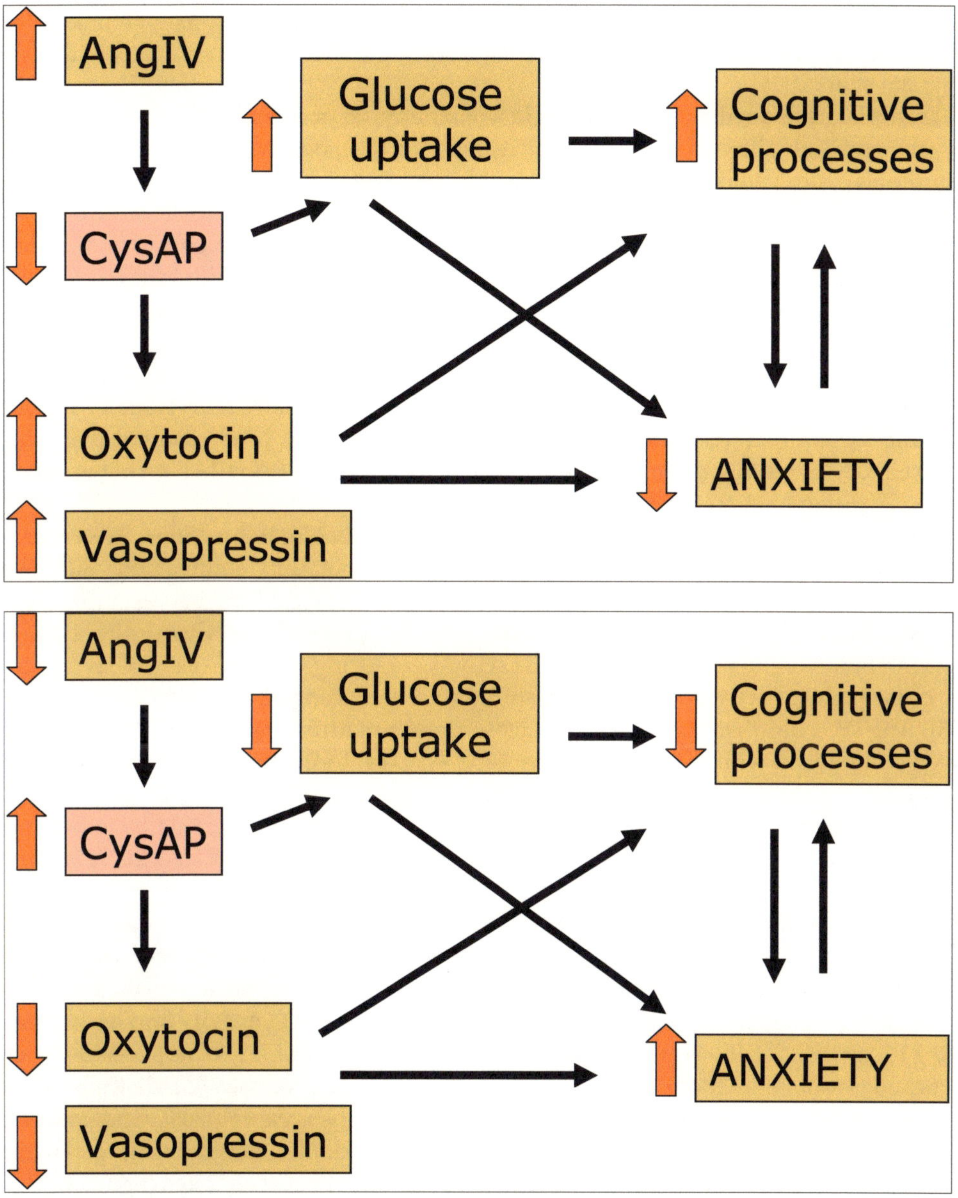

Fig. 6. Hypothetic consequences of frontal changes in CysAP/OX activity

Hypothetic consequences of a reduction (top) or increase (bottom) in the frontal levels of CysAP/OX. Decreased CysAP would imply higher availability of Ang IV as well as lower metabolism/higher availability of its substrates oxytocin and vasopressin. Higher levels of Ang IV could indicate an improvement of cognitive processes (Gard, 2008). The reduction of CysAP may also suggest increased glucose uptake which would also improve cognitive processes (Wenk, 1989). In addition, increased availability of oxytocin or vasopressin would agree with the facilitation of cognitive processes (Gulpinar and Yegen, 2004) as well as a higher anxyolitic effect (Neumann, 2009). Finally, this would support an inverse relationship between cognitive processes and anxiety level (Ouimet et al., 2009). We could suggest contrary effects for an increased frontal level of CysAP.

occurred in normotensive rats (Banegas et al., 2010). This observation may be linked to the reduced volume of right PFC and reduced metabolism in the mPFC in humans with ADHD (Viggiano et al., 2004).
While ADHD have a reduction of left/right asymmetry, as observed in SL and SR, LL return the asymmetrical difference to a degree similar to that observed in normotensive rats. Accordingly, we could hypothesize that LL but not LR balanced the asymmetrical misbalance of SHR/ADHD.
Angiotensin IV (Ang IV) binds specifically to the AT_4 receptor, which is identical to the insulin-regulated aminopeptidase (IRAP) (Albiston et al., 2001). Cystein aminopeptidase (CysAP), also called oxytocinase (OX) or vasopressinase (EC 3.4.11.3), is considered the human variant of IRAP (Stragier et al., 2008). In addition, CysAP was also reported to be identical to the placental leucine aminopeptidase (Tsujimoto et al., 1992). These enzymes can therefore be considered identical and they are located in virtually all regions of the brain, including the cortex (Fernando et al., 2005). In addition, it has been reported that Ang IV increased DA levels in striatum, this effect being mediated by OX/IRAP acting as receptor for Ang IV (Stragier et al., 2007).
Ang IV is thought to play a role in cognitive and behavioral functions. However, the mechanism by which it modulates these functions is not fully understood and several compatible hypothesis have been proposed (Stragier et al., 2008). For example, it was proposed that the binding of Ang IV to its receptor, AT_4 (oxytocinase/CysAP/IRAP), results in the inhibition of the receptor's metabolic activity, reducing the catabolism of its substrates and consequently increasing their availability and extending their action (Stragier et al., 2008). Ang IV could therefore regulate glucose uptake modulating OX activity: OX/IRAP is indeed co-localized with the glucose transporter GLUT4. In the presence of insulin, OX and GLUT4 are expressed in the plasma membrane, where GLUT4 induces glucose uptake. It was suggested that the inhibition of OX, following binding of AngIV, could increase glucose uptake in neurons leading to an improvement of cognitive processes (Gard, 2008; Stragier et al., 2008) (figure 6).
In addition to oxytocin, CysAP/OX hydrolyzes vasopressin, enkephalins and other neuropeptides also involved in cognitive processes (Gard, 2008). Indeed, oxytocin and vasopressin are important modulators of diverse social and anxiety-related behaviors (Veenema & Neumann, 2008). Therefore, a decrease in CysAP/OX activity implies high levels of Ang IV, as well as a lower metabolism and thus a higher availability of its substrates such as oxytocin or vasopressin. Both effects may facilitate cognitive processes (Gard, 2008; Gülpinar & Yegen, 2004) and reduce anxiety levels (Veenema & Neumann, 2008). The contrary is occurring in case of an increase in CysAP/OX. Indeed, the development of cognitive enhancers based on the inhibition of OX has been proposed (Chai et al., 2008) (figure 6).

5. Conclusion

The present results demonstrated that the bilateral behavior of OX in the mPFC differs between normotensive and hypertensive rats and highlights the importance of bilaterality in biology. The functional meaning of bilaterality as well as how its disruption may lead to pathological consequences are unknown. However, we can speculate that brain functions, processed with varying degrees of asymmetry for the two hemispheres, could be under an universal *modus operandi* which would consist in the reciprocal inhibition of homologous centers. The regulationof a large number of brain processes is based on a retro-inhibitor-stimulator *feed-back* system. This could explain the existence of neurochemical imbalances that arise, change their side of prevalence or increase their degree of asymmetry in specific conditions. It could be speculated that imbalances in established brain asymmetries (toward symmetry or toward increasing asymmetry) due to unilateral damage, might lead to neuropathological deviations in brain functions (Ramirez et al., 2004; Banegas-Font et al., 2005b) In any case, these results confirm that studies which are not considering the bilaterality may lead to loss of invaluable informations leading to erroneous conclusions and misinterpretations of the pathophysiological processes.

6. References

Adams, H.R., Szilagyi, P.G., Gebhardt, L. & Lande, M.B. (2010), Learning and attention problems among children with pediatric primary hypertension. *Pediatrics,* Vol. 126, No. 6, (December 2010), pp. 1425-1429. ISSN 0031-4005

Alba, F., Arenas, J.C. & López, M.A. (1995). Properties of rat brain dipeptidyl aminopeptidases in the presence of detergents. *Peptides,* Vol. 16, No. 2, pp. 325-329, ISSN 0196-9781

Albiston, A.L., Mcdowall, S.G., Matsacos, D., Sim, P., Clune, E., Mustafa, T., Lee, J., Mendelsohn, F.A., Simpson, R.J., Connolly, L.M. & Chai, S.Y. (2001), Evidence that the angiotensin IV (AT4) receptor is the enzyme insulin-regulated aminopeptidase. *Journal of Biological Chemistry,* Vol. 276, No. 52, (December 2001), pp. 48623-48626, ISSN 0021-9258

Amenta, F., Di Tullio, M.A. & Tomassoni, D. (2003) Arterial hypertension and brain damage - evidence from animal models. *Clinical and Experimental Hypertension,* Vol. 25, No. 6, (August 2003) pp. 359-380, ISSN 1064-1963

Banegas, I., Prieto, I., Alba, F., Vives, F., Araque, A., Segarra, A.B., Durán, R., de Gasparo, M. & Ramírez, M. (2005a). Angiotensinase activity is asymmetrically distributed in the amygdala, hippocampus and prefrontal cortex of the rat. *Behavioural Brain Research* Vol. 156, No. 2, (January 2005) pp. 321-326, ISSN 0166-4328

Banegas Font I, Prieto Gómez I, Araque Cuenca A, Alba Aragüez F, Vives Montero F, Segarra Robles AB, Durán Ogalla R, Ramírez Sánchez MD & Ramírez Sánchez M. (2005b). [Neurochemical asymmetries in psychiatric alterations] Spanish. *Psiquiatría Biológica,* Vol.12, No.4, (July 2005) pp. 159-165, ISSN 1134-5934

Banegas, I., Prieto, I., Vives, F., Alba, F., de Gasparo, M., Duran, R., Luna, J de D., Segarra, A.B., Hermoso, F. & Ramírez, M. (2009). Asymmetrical response of aminopeptidase A and nitric oxide in plasma of normotensive and hypertensive rats with experimental hemiparkinsonism. *Neuropharmacology,* Vol.56, No3, (Mars 2009), pp. 573-579, ISSN 0028-3908

Banegas, I., Prieto, I., Vives, F., Alba, F., de Gasparo, M., Duran, R., Segarra, A.B. & Ramírez, M. (2010). Lateralized response of oxytocinase activity in the medial prefrontal cortex of a unilateral rat model of Parkinson's disease. *Behavioural Brain Research,* Vol.213, No.2, (December 2010), pp. 328-331, ISSN 0166-4328

Bergerbest, D., Gabrieli, J.D., Whitfield-Gabrieli, S., Kim, H., Stebbins, G.T., Bennett, D.A. & Fleischman D.A. (2009). Age-associated reduction of asymmetry in prefrontal function and preservation of conceptual repetition priming. *Neuroimage.* Vol.45, No.1, (Mars 2009) pp.237-246, ISSN 1053-8119

Bradford, M.M. (1976). A rapid and sensitive method for the quantification of microgram quantities of protein utilizing the principle of protein dye binding. *Analytical Biochemistry* Vol.72, (May 1976) pp.248-254, ISSN 0003-2697

Brück, A., Kurki, T., Kaasinen, V., Vahlberg, T. & Rinne, J.O. (2004). Hippocampal and prefrontal atrophy in patients with early non-demented Parkinson's disease is related to cognitive impairment. *Journal of Neurology, Neurosurgery & Psychiatry*, Vol.75, No.10, (October 2004), pp.1467-1469. ISSN 0022-3050

Chai SY, Yeatman HR, Parker MW, Ascher DB, Thompson PE, Mulvey HT. & Albiston, A.L. (2008), Development of cognitive enhancers based on inhibition of insulin-regulated aminopeptidase. *BMC Neuroscience*, Vol. 9, Suppl. 2, (December 2008), pp. S14, ISSN 1471-2202

Cubo, E., Martin, P.M., Martin-Gonzalez, J.A., Rodriguez-Blazquez, C. & Kulisevsky, J. ELEP Group Members. (2010). Motor laterality asymmetry and nonmotor symptoms in Parkinson's disease. *Movement Disorders*, Vol.25, No.1, (January 2010), pp.70-75. ISSN 0885-3185

Diana, G. (2002). Does hypertension alone lead to cognitive decline in spontaneously hypertensive rats? *Behavioural Brain Research*, Vol.134, No.1-2, (August 2002), pp. 113-121. ISSN 0166-4328

Djaldetti, R., Ziv, I. & Melamed, E. (2006). The mystery of motor asymmetry in Parkinson's disease. *Lancet Neurology*, Vol. 5, No.9, (September 2006), pp.796-802. ISSN 1474-4422

Dorsey, E.R., Constantinescu, R., Thompson, J.P., Biglan, K.M., Holloway, R.G., Kieburtz, K., Marshall, F.J., Ravina, B.M., Schifitto, G., Siderowf, A. & Tanner, C.M. (2007). Projected number of people with Parkinson disease in the most populous nations, 2005 through 2030. *Neurology*, Vol.68, No.5, (January 2007), pp.384-386, ISSN 0028-3878

Farina, E., Cappa, S.F., Polimeni, M., Magni, E., Canesi, M., Zecchinelli, A., Scarlato, G. & Mariani, C. (1994). Frontal dysfunction in early Parkinson's disease, *Acta Neurologica Scandinavica*, Vol.90, No.1, (July 1994) pp. 34-38. ISSN 0365-5598

Farkas, E., De Jong, G.I., Apró, E., De Vos, R.A., Steur, E.N. & Luiten, P.G. (2000). Similar ultrastructural breakdown of cerebrocortical capillaries in Alzheimer's disease, Parkinson's disease, and experimental hypertension. What is the functional link? *Annals of the New York Academy of Sciences*. Vol.903, (April 2000) pp.72-82. ISSN 0077-8923

Fernando, R.N., Lara, J., Albiston, A.L. & Chai, S.Y. (2005). Distribution and cellular localization of insulin-regulated aminopeptidase in the rat central nervous system. *Journal of Comparative Neurology*, Vol.487, No.4, (July 2005), pp. 372–90. ISSN 0021-9967

Gard, P.R. (2008). Cognitive-enhancing effects of angiotensin IV. *BMC Neuroscience*, Vol.9, Suppl.2, (December 2008) pp. S15. ISSN 1471-2202

George, J.L., Mok, S., Moses, D., Wilkins, S., Bush, A.I., Cherny, R.A. & Finkelstein, D.I. (2009). Targeting the progression of Parkinson's disease. *Current Neuropharmacology*, Vol.7, No.1, (Mars 2009) pp.9-36. ISSN 1570-159X

Glick, S.D., Jerussi, T.P., Water, D.H. & Green JP. (1974), Amphetamine-induced changes in striatal dopamine and acetylcholine levels and relationship to rotation (circling behavior) in rats. *Biochemical Pharmacology*. Vol.23, No.22, (November 1974), pp. 3223-3225, ISSN 0006-2952.

Glick, S.D. (1983). Cerebral lateralization in the rat and tentative extrapolations to man. In: *Hemisyndromes: Psychobiology, Neurology, Psychiatry*. M. Myslobodsky (Ed.) pp. 7-26., ISBN 0125124600, Academic Press, London.

Gülpinar, M.A. & Yegen, B.C. (2004). The physiology of learning and memory: role of peptides and stress. *Current Protein and Peptide Science* Vol.5, No.6, (December 2004), pp. 457-473, ISSN 1098-5522

Henderson, J.M., Watson, S., Halliday, G.M., Heinemann, T. & Gerlach, M. (2003). Relationships between various behavioural abnormalities and nigrostriatal dopamine depletion in the unilateral 6-OHDA-lesioned rat. *Behavioural Brain Research*, Vol.139, No.1-2, (February 2003) pp. 105-113. ISSN 0166-4328

Huber, S.J., Miller, H., Bohaska, L., Christy, J.A. & Bornstein, R.A. (1992). Asymmetrical cognitive differences associated with hemiparkinsonism. *Archives of Clinical Neuropsychology*, Vol.7, No.6, (November 1992), pp. 471-80. ISSN 0887-6177

Insel, T.R. (2010). The challenge of translation in social neuroscience: a review of oxytocin, vasopressin, and affiliative behavior. *Neuron,* Vol.65 No.6 (Mars 2010), pp.768-779, ISSN 0896-6273.

Jolicoeur, F.B. & Rivest, R. (1992). Rodent model of Parkinson's disease, In: *Neuromethods 21, Animal Models of Neurological Disease I,* A.A. Boulto, G.B. Bakerand a R.F. Butterworth (Eds.). 135-158, Humana Press, ISBN 0-89603-198-5, Totowa, New Jersey

Lang, A.E. & Obeso, J.A. (2004), Challenges in Parkinson's disease: restoration of the nigrostriatal dopamine system is not enough. *Lancet Neurology*, Vol.3, No.5, (May 2004), pp. 309-16, ISSN 1474-4422

Neumann, I.D. (2009). The advantage of social living: brain neuropeptides mediate the beneficial consequences of sex and motherhood. *Frontiers in Neuroendocrinology,* Vol. 30, No.4, (October 2009), pp. 483-496, ISSN 0091-3022

Ouimet, A.J., Gawronski, B. & Dozois, D.J. (2009). Cognitive vulnerability to anxiety: A review and an integrative model. *Clinical Psychology Review,* Vol.29, No.6, (August 2009), pp. 459-470, ISSN 0272-7358

Paxinos, G. & Watson C. (1998). *The rat brain in stereotaxic coordinates,* Academic Press, 4th Ed. ISBN 13: 9780123742438, London, England.

Piacentini, S., Versaci, R., Romito, L., Ferré, F. & Albanese A. (2010) Behavioral and personality features in patients with lateralized Parkinson's disease. *European Journal of Neurology.* (December 2010) [Epub ahead of print], ISSN 1468-1331

Ramírez, M., Prieto, I., Vives, F., de Gasparo, M. & Alba, F. (2004). Neuropeptides, neuropeptidases and brain asymmetry. *Current Protein and Peptide Science,* Vol.5, No.6, (December 2004), pp. 497-506. ISSN 1098-5522

Robinson, T.E., Noordhoorn, M., Chan, E.M., Mocsary, Z., Camp, D.M, & Whishaw, I.Q. (1994). Relationship between asymmetries in striatal dopamine release and the direction of amphetamine-induced rotation during the first week following a unilateral 6-OHDA lesion of the substantia nigra. *Synapse,* (May 1994)Vol. 17, No.1, pp. 16-25, ISSN 0887-4476

Russell, V.A. (2007). Reprint of "Neurobiology of animal models of attention-deficit hyperactivity disorder". *Journal of Neuroscience Methods,* (November 2007), Vol.166, No.2, pp. I-XIV, ISSN 1872-678X

Sánchez, F., Gómez-Villalobos, M. de J., Juarez, I., Quevedo, L. & Flores, G. (2011). Dendritic morphology of neurons in medial prefrontal cortex, hippocampus, and nucleus accumbens in adult SH rats. *Synapse.* (Mars 2011) Vol.65, No.3, (Mars 2011), pp. 198-206. ISSN 0887-4476

Shapiro, R.M., Glick, S.D. & Hough, L.B. (1986). Striatal dopamine uptake asymmetries and rotational behavior in unlesioned rats: revising the model? *Psychopharmacology (Berl),* Vol.89, No.1, pp.25-30, *ISSN*: 0033-3158.

Shaw, P., Lalonde, F., Lepage, C., Rabin, C., Eckstrand, K., Sharp, W., Greenstein, D., Evans, A., Giedd, J.N. & Rapoport, J. (2009). Development of cortical asymmetry in typically developing children and its disruption in attention-deficit/hyperactivity disorder. *Archives of General Psychiatry,* Vol.66, No.8, (August 2009), pp.888-896, ISSN 0003-990x

Stragier, B., Demaegdt, H., De Burdel, D., Smolders, I., Sarre, S., Vauquelin, G., Ebinger, G., Micote, Y. & Vanderheyden, P. (2007), Involvement of insulin-regulated aminopeptidase and/or aminopeptidase N in the angiotensin IV-induced effect on dopamine release in the striatum of the rat. *Brain Research*, Vol. 1131 No.1 (February 2007) pp. 97-105. ISSN 00068993.

Stragier, B., De Bundel, D., Sarre, S., Smolders, I., Vauquelin, G., Dupont, A., Michotte, Y. & Vanderheyden, P. (2008). Involvement of insulin-regulated aminopeptidase in the effects of the renin-angiotensin fragment angiotensin IV: a review. *Heart Failure Reviews*, Vol.13, No.3, (September 2008), pp. 321-37. ISSN 1382-4147

Sullivan, R.M. & Brake, W.G. (2003). What the rodent prefrontal cortex can teach us about attention-deficit/hyperactivity disorder: the critical role of early developmental events on prefrontal function. *Behavioural Brain Research*, Vol.146, No.1-2, (November 2003) pp. 43-55, ISSN 0166-4328

Sullivan, R.M. (2004). Hemispheric asymmetry in stress processing in rat prefrontal cortex and the role of mesocortical dopamine. *Stress*, Vol.7, No.2, (June 2004), pp. 131-143. ISSN 1025-3890

Tsujimoto, M., Mizutani, S., Adachi, H., Kimura, M., Nakazato, H. & Tomoda, Y. (1992). Identification of human placental leucine aminopeptidase as oxytocinase. *Archives of Biochemistry and Biophysics*, Vol.292, No.2, (February 1992), pp. 388–392. ISSN 0003-9861

Tzschentke, T.M. (2000). The medial prefrontal cortex as a part of the brain reward system. *Amino Acids*, Vol.19, No.1, pp. 211-219, ISSN 0939-4451

Ungerstedt, U. (1971). Adipsia and aphagia after 6-hydroxydopamine induced degeneration of the nigro-striatal dopamine system. *Acta Physiologica Scandinavica* Vol.367, pp. 95–122, ISSN 0001-6772

Vallesi, A., McIntosh, A.R., Kovacevic, N., Chan, S.C. & Stuss, D.T. (2010). Age effects on the asymmetry of the motor system: evidence from cortical oscillatory activity. *Biological Psychology*, (October 2010) Vol.85, No.2, pp.213-218. ISSN 0301-0511

Veenema, A.H. & Neumann, I.D. (2008). Central vasopressin and oxytocin release: regulation of complex social behaviours. *Progress in Brain Research* Vol.170 pp. 261-276. ISSN 0079-6123

Viggiano, D., Ruocco, L.A., Arcieri, S. & Sadile, A.G. (2004). Involvement of norepinephrine in the control of activity and attentive processes in animal models of attention deficit hyperactivity disorder. *Neural Plasticity*. Vol.11, No.1-2, pp.133-149. ISSN 1687-5443

Vinyoles, E., De la Figuera. M. & Gonzalez-Segura, D. (2008). Cognitive function and blood pressure control in hypertensive patients over 60 years of age: COGNIPRES study. *Current Medical Research and Opinion*. Vol.24, No.12, (December 2008), pp.3331-3339, ISSN 0300-7995

Wenk, G.L. (1989) An hypothesis on the role of glucose in the mechanism of action of cognitive enhancers. *Psychopharmacology* Vol.99, No,4, pp. 431-438. ISSN 0033-3158

Xu, Z.C., Ling, G., Sahr, R.N. & Neal-Beliveau BS. (2005). Asymmetrical changes of dopamine receptors in the striatum after unilateral dopamine depletion. *Brain Research*, (Mars 2005), Vol.1038, No.2, pp.163-70, ISSN: 0006-8993

Xu, Y., Valentino, D.J., Scher, A.I., Dinov, I., White, L.R., Thompson, P.M., Launer, L.J. & Toga, A.W. (2008). Age effects on hippocampal structural changes in old men: the HAAS. *Neuroimage*, Vol.40, No.3, (April 2008) pp. 1003-1015. ISSN 1053-8119

Zgaljardic, D.J., Borod, J.C., Foldi, N.S., Mattis, P.J., Gordon, M.F., Feigin, A. & Eidelberg, D. (2006). An examination of executive dysfunction associated with frontostriatal circuitry in Parkinson's disease. *Journal of Clinical and Experimental Neuropsychology* Vol.28, No.7, (October 2006), pp. 1127-1144. ISSN 1380-3395

Zimmerberg, B., Glick, S.D. & Jerussi, T.P. (1974) Neurochemical correlate of a spatial preference in rats. *Science*. Vol.185, No.151, (August 1974), pp. 623-5, ISSN 0036-8075.

15

Dictyostelium discoideum: A Model System to Study LRRK2-Mediated Parkinson Disease

Arjan Kortholt, Bernd Gilsbach, and Peter J.M. van Haastert
Department of Molecular Cell Biology, University of Groningen
The Netherlands

1. Introduction

Parkinson disease (PD) is a neurodegenerative disease that affects more than 5 million people worldwide and one in hundred people over the age of 60. PD is both a chronic and degenerative disorder that is characterized by loss of dopaminergic neurons in the substantia nigra, associated with the formation of fibrillar aggregates composed of α-synuclein and other proteins (Lees et al., 2009). PD is clinically characterized by tremor, bradykinesia, rigidity and postural instability. Initially PD was considered to have no genetic cause, however many patients have one or more family member with the disease and genome-wide association studies identified a number of genetic factors segregating with PD (Satake et al., 2009; Simon-Sanchez et al., 2009). Therefore, it is now general believed that PD is caused by a combination of genetic and environmental factors. Recently, missense mutations in LRRK2 have been linked to autosomal-dominant, late-onset PD (Zimprich et al., 2004;Paisan-Ruiz et al., 2004). LRRK2 is a member of the novel Roco family of complex Ras-like GTPases that have an unique domain architecture (Fig. 1) (Bosgraaf and van Haastert, 2003). Roco proteins are characterized by the presence of a Ras-like Guanine nucleotide binding domain, called Roc (Ras of complex proteins), followed by a conserved stretch of 300-400 amino-acids with no significant homology to other described protein domains called the COR domain (C-terminal of Roc; Fig. 1). The Roc and COR domains always occurs as a pair, and so far no proteins have been identified containing either the Roc or COR domain alone, suggesting that these two domains function as one inseparable unit. Roco proteins were first identified in the social amoeba *Dictyostelium discoideum* and are found in prokaryotes, plants and metazoa, but not in *Plasmodium* and yeast (Bosgraaf et al., 2003). Besides a Roc and COR domain, all Roco proteins contain an N-terminal stretch of leucine-rich repeats (LRR), which are supposed to be involved in protein-protein interaction. A large group of Roco proteins, which is only present in *Dictyostelium* and metazoan, contains an additional C-terminal kinase domain of the MAPKKK subfamily of kinases. Next to this general domain composition, individual Roco proteins are found to be combined with a diversity of additional domains such as Guanine nucleotide exchange factor (GEF) and Regulator of G-protein Signalling (RGS) domains, implicating a link between traditional G-protein signalling pathways and Roco proteins (Bosgraaf et al., 2003). The identification of missense mutations in LRRK2 has redefined the role of genetic variation in PD susceptibility. LRRK2 mutations initiate a penetrant phenotype with complete clinical and neurochemical overlap with idiopathic disease (Khan et al., 2005;Hernandez et al., 2005;Aasly et al., 2005). The various mutations that have been identified in PD are concentrated in the central region of the protein: one amino acid change within the LRR domain, one amino acid change in the Roc domain, one in the COR domain that can have multiple mutations and two amino acids change in the kinase domain (Fig. 1A, (Cookson, 2010). Identified mutations outside of these domains do not segregate in a Mendelian fashion with PD. The mutations are found in 5-6 % of patients with familial PD, and importantly also have been implicated with sporadic PD with unprecedented 1-2 % prevalence (Gilks et al., 2005). Although much progress has been made during the last few years, the exact pathogenic role and associated biochemical pathways responsible for LRRK2-linked disease are slowly emerging. However, recent evidence suggests that these pathways involve other proteins that have been linked to PD, especially α-synuclein and tau (Cookson and Bandmann, 2010;Cookson, 2010). The considerable number of described disease-linked LRRK2 mutations represent an unique opportunity to biochemically explore the pathogenicity of LRRK2 and identify therapeutic targets for related neurodegenerative disorders. Importantly, all known pathogenic mutations in LRRK2 result in decreased GTPase activity and enhanced kinase activity, suggesting a possible PD-related gain of abnormal/toxic function (West et al., 2005;Greggio et al., 2006;Guo et al., 2007;Ito et al., 2007;Luzon-Toro et al., 2007;Lewis et al., 2007;Li et al., 2007;West et al., 2007). Since LRRK2 kinase activity is critically linked to clinical effects, it presents a viable target for therapeutic modulation.

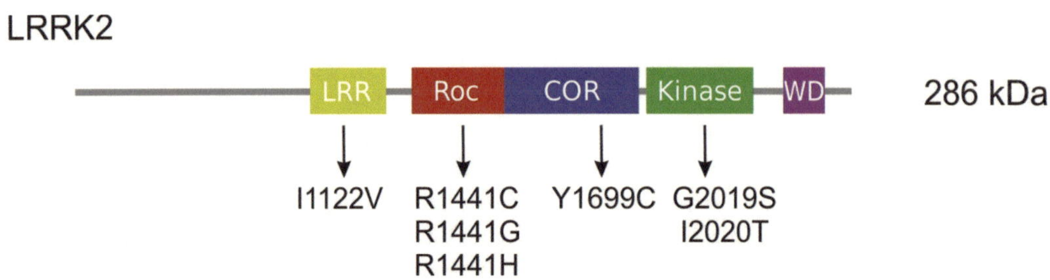

Fig. 1. Domain structure and mutations of LRRK2. The most clearly defined pathogenetic mutations are shown below the diagram.

Attempts to purify mammalian LRRK2 have failed so far in many laboratories. Therefore, the detailed biochemical and structural understanding of LRRK2 is very limited. We have used related proteins, which can serve as models to understand the complex structure and regulatory mechanism of LRRK2. Previously the structure of the Roco protein from the cyanobacterium *Chlorobium tepidum* was elucidated, which revealed that COR is a constitutive dimerization device and that Roco proteins belong to the GAD class of molecular switches (G proteins activated by nucleotide dependent dimerization) (Gotthardt et al., 2008;Gasper et al., 2009). This class also includes proteins such as signal recognition particle, dynamin and septins (Gasper et al., 2009). It is proposed that the juxtaposition of the G domains of two monomers in the complex across the GTP-binding sites activates the GTPase reaction and thereby regulate the biological function of these proteins. The *Chlorobium* Roco structure revealed that the PD-analogous mutations of the Roc and COR domain are in close proximity to each other, and are present in a region of the protein that is strongly conserved between bacteria and man. PD mutations in *Chlorobium*, like that of

LRRK2, decrease the GTPase reaction. Based on the structure and the observed effects of PD-mutations in LRRK2 it is thought that interaction with other proteins modify the dimer interactions resulting in decreased GTPases and enhanced kinase activity (Gotthardt et al., 2008;Gasper et al., 2009). This shows that mechanistic insight can even gained from very distantly related proteins

2. *Dictyostelium discoideum* as model sytem to resolve the function of Roco proteins

This chapter concentrates on *Dictyostelium discoideum* Roco proteins, which are excellent models for LRRK2 and can thus be used to answer key questions for the intramolecular regulation of LRRK2 and give insight in the function of the LRR, the mechanism by which the Roc domain regulates kinase activity, the role that COR plays in this process and how the PD-linked missense mutations alter the interactions between the different domains.

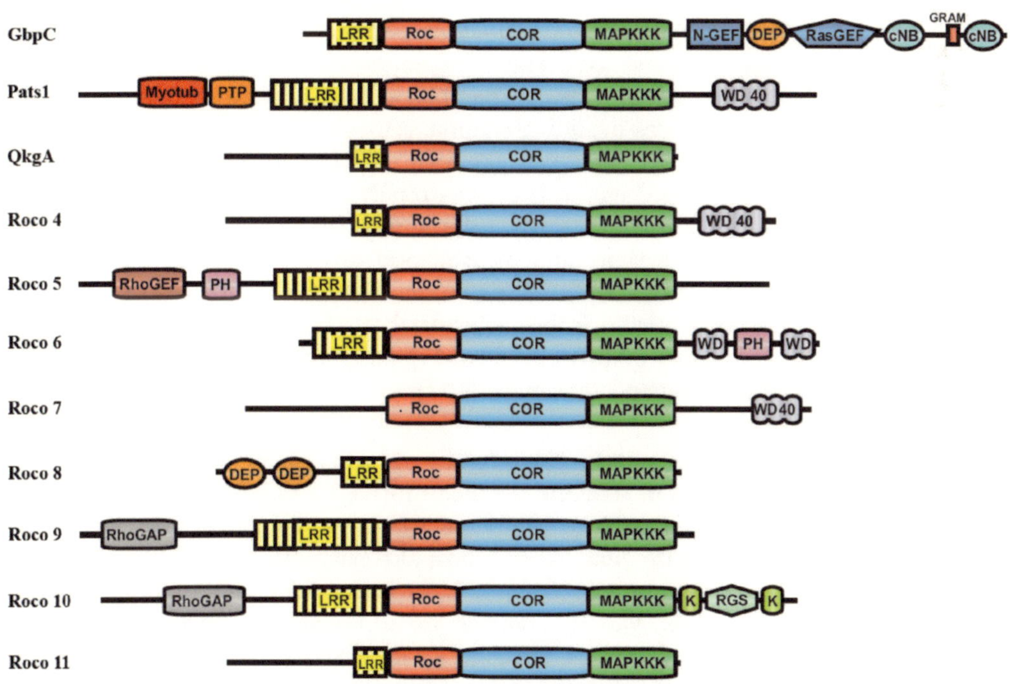

Fig. 2. Domain architecture of the *Dictyostelium* Roco proteins. All proteins contain LRR, the Roc, COR and the kinase domain. Additional a variety of domains are found in specific Roco proteins, such as RasGEFs ,RhoGEFs, RhoGAPs, Regulator of G protein signaling (RGS), and Pleckstrin homology domains (PH).

2.1 Dictyostelium discoideum

Dictyostelium discoideum is a free living soil amoeba. In nature, single *Dictyostelium* cells are feeding on bacteria. They chase bacteria by chemotaxing towards folic acid, which is secreted by the bacteria. Upon starvation cells enter the developmental stage (Kessin, 2000). During development single cells undergo a drastic change in gene expression and start to secrete cAMP. Neighbouring cells respond by migrating toward the chemoattractant cAMP and by secreting cAMP themselves. Thus a cAMP gradient is created around the initiation point. After six hours of starvation, the chemotaxing cells have formed an aggregation centre at the intiation point, which consists of up to 100.000 cells. Differentiation and morphogenesis culminate in the formation of a fruiting body, or stalks of vacuolated dead cells with a spore head on top. These spores can survive long periods without food, high temperatures and drought. Recently the assembly of the *Dictyostelium* genome was completed (Eichinger *et al.*, 2005). The thirty-four Mb genome contains many genes that are homologous to those in higher eukaryotes and are missing in other model system. Due to the availability of the genome sequence, the well established molecular cloning and imaging techniques, *Dictyostelium* provides a well-established model to study the basic aspects of directed cell movement and development (Devreotes and Zigmond, 1988;Van Haastert and Devreotes, 2004). Chemotaxis or directional movement towards a chemical compound is an essential property of many cells and is fundamentally important for processes as diverse as the sourcing of nutrients by prokaryotes, the organisation of the embryo in metazoa, the formation of multicellular structures in protazoa and the migration of lymphocytes during immune response (Baggiolini, 1998;Campbell and Butcher, 2000;Iijima *et al.*, 2002;Crone and Lee, 2002). Chemotaxis is also linked to the development and progression of many diseases including asthma, arthritis, atherosclerosis, and cancers (Trusolino and Comoglio, 2002;Charo and Taubman, 2004;Eccles, 2005). Since the key signalling pathways underlying chemotaxis are essentially similar to those of mammalian cells, *Dictyostelium* has been used to study cell-motility related pathologies, including deficiencies in the immune system and neurological disorders (Carnell and Insall, 2011;Escalante, 2011;Meyer *et al.*, 2011). *Dictyostelium* also has been used as model in pharmacogenomics and to characterize the molecular basis of human diseases associated with the endocytic and secretory pathway (Williams *et al.*, 2006;Van *et al.*, 2007;Francione *et al.*, 2011;Maniak, 2011;Alexander and Alexander, 2011).

2.2 *Dictyostelium discoideum* and the Roco family of proteins

Four Roco proteins are detected in vertebrates, called LRRK1, LRRK2, DAPK1 and MFHAS1. Remarkably, in *Dictyostelium* eleven Roco family members were identified, that all share the characteristic Roc, Cor and kinase domains and most also have LRR (Fig. 2, (Bosgraaf *et al.*, 2003)). *Dictyostelium* Roco proteins are structurally more varied than the Roco proteins found in all the other species together; various domains are additionally fused to the conserved region. Most likely all the *Dictyostelium* Roco genes have evolved quit recently by gene duplication (Marin, 2006). From a functional point of view, the *Dictyostelium* Rocos have provided the most significant data (van Egmond and van Haastert, 2010).

2.2.1 Functions for *Dictyostelium* GbpC in chemotaxis, streaming and osmotic stress

GbpC, also called Roco1, was originally identified in a bioinformatical screen for molecular targets of the second messenger cGMP and is the founding member of the Roco family of proteins (Bosgraaf *et al.*, 2002;Bosgraaf *et al.*, 2003). Besides the conserved Roco region, GbpC has a unique regulatory C-terminal region, consisting of a Ras Exchange Motif (REM), DEP, CDC25, and two cyclic nucleotide binding (cNB) domains with a GRAM domain inserted in between (Fig. 3,(Goldberg *et al.*, 2002)). In the contrary to LRRK2, the cellular function of GbpC has been characterized in detail. GbpC is the only cGMP-signal transducing protein in

Dictyostelium, it binds to cGMP with high affinity to its cNB domains (Bosgraaf *et al.*, 2002). cGMP mediated GbpC activation is essential for the proper regulation of myosin II during chemotaxis, cell streaming and osmotic-stress (Fig.3, (Kuwayama *et al.*, 1996;Bosgraaf *et al.*, 2002;Goldberg *et al.*, 2002;Veltman and van Haastert, 2008;Araki *et al.*, 2010)). Myosin II is an essential regulator of the cytoskeleton at the rear of moving cells. The establishment of a cellular gradient during chemotaxis leads to major changes in the cytoskeleton; actin polymerization occurs at the leading edge of the cell, while acto-myosin filaments are formed at the rear of the cell. The formed myosin-II filaments are preventing the formation of lateral pseudopods and providing the power to retract the uropod (Levi *et al.*, 2002). In *Dictyostelium*, myosin assembly seems to be strictly dependent on the phosphorylation state of the myosin heavy chain (MHC) (Bosgraaf and van Haastert, 2006). Phosphorylation by MHCKs inhibits filament formation (Cote and Bukiejko, 1987;Kolman *et al.*, 1996), whereas dephosphorylation by protein phosphatase 2A is essential for myosin disassembly (Murphy *et al.*, 1996). Phosphorylation of the myosin light chain (MLC) by MLCKs, promotes myosin motor activity, which is important for supplying contractile force to retract the rear of the cell (De la Roche and Cote, 2001;De la Roche *et al.*, 2002). Cells lacking cGMP formation or GbpC have an impaired recruitment of myosin II to the cytoskeleton and impaired chemotaxis. Cells with elevated levels of cGMP have increased activation of myosin-light-chain kinase A (MLCKa) and subsequently an increased myosin motor activity (Bosgraaf *et al.*, 2002). The role of GbpC, becomes even more evident in longer developed cells, which begin to secrete cAMP, neighbouring cells move towards the cAMP and relay the signal. Due to the resulting wave of cAMP through the population, cells become polarized, connect to each other in a head-to-tail fashion, and form streams of cells. Cells lacking cGMP or GbpC have a severe streaming defect; these cells show extensive stream break up due to reduced cell elongation and the inability to maintain stable head-to-tail cell contacts (Veltman *et al.*, 2008). Together these results show that cGMP and GbpC are important for the formation of stably polarized and elongated cells by regulating myosin filament formation in the posterior of the cell, which is important for both chemotaxis and cell streaming.

The cGMP pathway is not only activated in response to cAMP, but also by folic acid and osmotic stress (Hadwiger *et al.*, 1994;Kuwayama *et al.*, 1996;Kuwayama and van Haastert, 1998). *Dictyostelium* can bind folic acid, secreted by bacteria, to the so far unidentified folic acid receptor, resulting in activation of Gα4 and subsequently activation of the cGMP pathway (Hadwiger *et al.*, 1994). In the contrary, cGMP production in response to osmoshock is independent of heterotrimeric proteins (Kuwayama *et al.*, 1998). Also the kinetics of the cGMP responses are completely different, cGMP production occurs in minutes after osmoshock and in seconds after stimulation with cAMP or folic acid (Kuwayama and van Haastert, 1996). The transcription factor StatC and the protein kinase SAPKα show osmotic stressed-induced phosphorylation (Sun *et al.*, 2003;Araki *et al.*, 2003;Araki *et al.*, 2010). Phosphorylated StatC subsequently translocates to the nucleus to bind its transcriptional targets. Activation of both SAPKα and StatC occurs downstream of cGMP and GbpC; SAPKα and StatC are rapidly phosphorylated after treatment with 8-bromo-cGMP and *gbpC*-null cells are lacking the osmotic-stress-induced StatC translocation (Araki *et al.*, 2010). Although the phosphorylation state of Myosin Light Chain Kinase, the protein kinase SAPKα and transcription factor StatC are cGMP-dependent (Sun *et al.*, 2003;Bosgraaf *et al.*, 2006;Araki *et al.*, 2010), no direct binding of GbpC to these proteins could be detected. To completely understand the function of GbpC in *vivo*, it will be important to identify its direct substrates.

2.2.2 Biological role of QKGA and PATS1

Initially two proteins similar to GbpC were found in *Dictyostelium*, Qkga (now also called Roco3) and Pats1 (now also called Roco2). Qkga (Quick growth factor a) only consist of the central Roco region (Fig. 2), and was first described in a study for a new method to create gene disruptions in *Dictyostelium* (Abe et al., 2003). Cells lacking *qkgA* grow faster suggesting a role in cell proliferation. Consistently, Qkga overexpressed in *qkgA* null cells results in slower groth, indicating that higher amounts of QkgA lead to slower cell proliferation, thus confirming a role for QkgA in this process (van Egmond *et al.*, 2010).

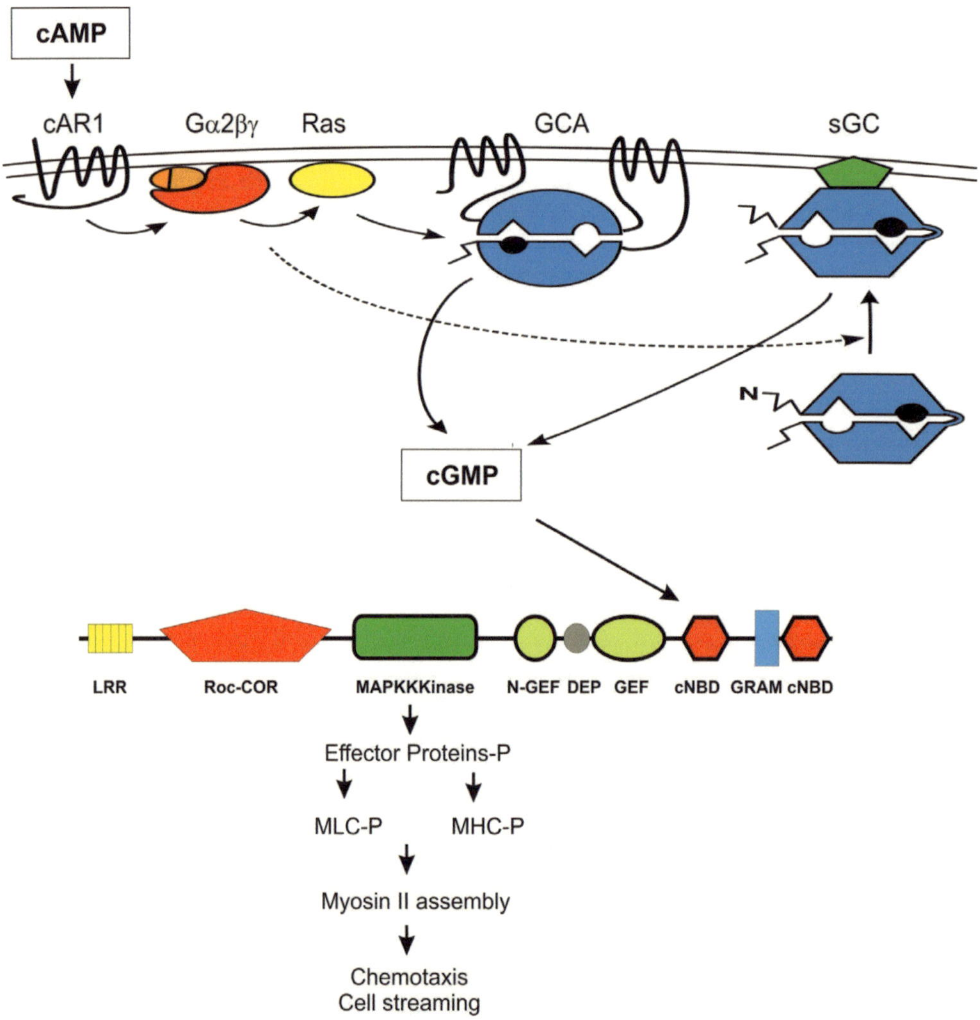

Fig. 3. The cGMP/ GbpC pathway in *Dictyostelium discoideum*. Extracellular cAMP binds to a G-protein coupled receptor cAR1 that stimulates a specific G-protein and Ras. cGMP is synthesised by two guanylyl cyclases, GCA and sGC that are unrelated to mammalian guanylyl cyclases, but are homologs of respectively mammalian membrane and soluble adenylyl cyclase. GbpC, the only target of cGMP, modulates the phosphorylation and assembly of conventional myosin into filaments.

Pats1 was identified in a screen for proteins involved in cytokinesis (Abysalh et al., 2003) and consist, like LRRK2, of LRRs, a ROC, COR, MAPKKK domain and WD40 repeats, and has additionally an N-terminal myotub-related and PTP (Protein Tyrosine Phosphatases) domain (Fig. 2). In a first study, *pats1* was disrupted in DH1 cells, resulting in large multinuclear cells in shaking culture, but these cells divide normally when grown on plate (Abysalh et al., 2003). DH1/*pats1*-null cells show improper localization of MHC to the cleavage furrow and an interaction between the WD40 repeats and the actomyosin was found, suggesting a role for Pats1 in regulating myosin II formation during cytokinesis (Abysalh et al., 2003). In a second study by van Egmond et al., where *pats1* was disrupted in an AX3 background, cells showed large multinuclear cells when grown on plate, but not in shaking culture, which is opposite to *pats1*-null cells that were created in DH1 background (van Egmond *et al.*, 2010). Furthermore, re-expression of the Pats1 kinase domain in *pats1*/DH1 cells, led to rescue of the phenotype and overexpression in DH1 resulted in large multinucleated cells again (Abysalh et al., 2003), whereas no rescue or overexpression effect was observed in the AX3 background (van Egmond *et al.*, 2010). Together these results show that Pats1 has an important role in cytokinesis, but the division-mechanism that it is involved in might vary among different wild-type strains.

2.2.3 Developmental role for Roco4

The complete Roco protein family was identified by Bosgraaf and van Haastert (2003) in a bioinformatic search with the Roc and COR domain of GbpC. Phylogenetic analysis showed that *roco4*, *qkga* and *roco11* are higly similar and are resulting from an ancestor *roco4* gene that was duplicated late in evolution (later than 300 million years ago) (van Egmond *et al.*, 2010). Interestingly, Roco4 has the same domain architecture as LRRK2 (Fig. 1 + 2). The expression of many *Dictyostelium* genes is strictly regulated during the life cycle. RT-PCR experiments showed that *roco4* expression is also developmentally regulated, with a strong elevated expression levels during the slug stage, suggesting a role for Roco4 in late development (van Egmond *et al.*, 2010). To study the function during development, the *roco4* gene was disrupted, and *roco4*-null cells were subjected to starvation on nutrient-free agar plates. During the first hours of development, no difference between *roco4*-null and wild-type could be observed. Cells start to aggregate and form characteristic streams after 6 hours starvation. After 9 hours, aggregation is complete and both cell strains have formed mounds. Developmental defects of *roco4*-null cells become visible after 12 hours of starvation, when wild-type cells are at the onset of forming slugs and form first fingers, while in *roco4*-null this process is first observed after 16 hours of starvation. After 24 hours, wild-type cells culminate in the formation of a fruiting body, while *roco4*-null slugs migrate for many hours before making multiple attempts to culminate, a process that sometimes takes up to 72 hours after the onset of starvation. Eventually, this aberrant culmination results in fruiting bodies consisting of sporeheads that are located on the agar surface, because a proper stalk is not present to lift the sporehead into the air (Fig. 4, (van Egmond *et al.*, 2010)). Re-expression of Roco4 completely rescues the phenotype of *roco4* disruption. Consistent with the developmental defects, Roco4 expression is highly enriched in the prestalk cell and *roco4*-null cells have severely reduced cellulose levels. Cellulose is known in *Dictyostelium* to be the cement of stalking cells, necessary for stability (van Egmond *et al.*, 2010). Together these results show that Roco4 is a prestalk-specific protein involved in the proper production of cellulose.

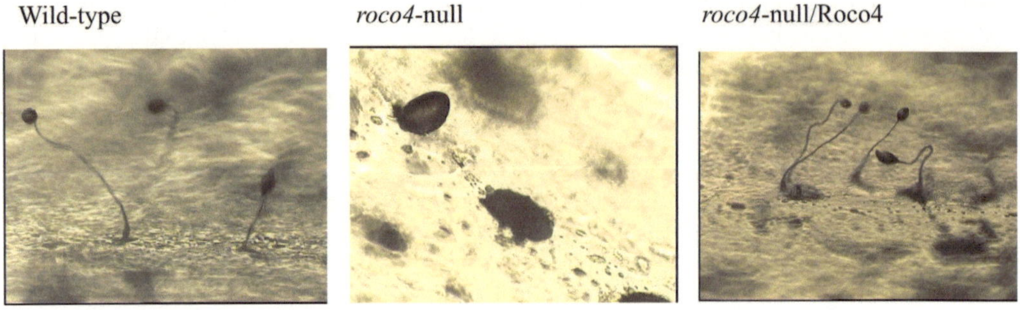

Fig. 4. Phenotype of *roco4*-null cells. Wild-type, *roco4*-null cells, and *roco4*-null cells re-expressing Roco4, were allowed to develop on nutrient-free agar. *roco4*-null cells fail to make a normal fruiting body due to defective synthesis of cellulose.

2.2.4 Function of other *Dictyostelium* Roco proteins

To further investigate the role of Roco proteins during the *Dictyostelium* life cycle, van Egmond et al., (2010) knocked out the 8 remaining *roco* genes and analysed their developmental phenotypes. *Dictyostelium* Roco proteins have distinct expression patterns during development; no major differences in expression were found for Roco5, Roco8 and Roco10 during development. In contrast, Roco6 and Roco11 show, like Pats1, QkgA and Roco4, elevated expression levels during the slug phase. Roco7 and Roco9 are expressed mostly during aggregation, similar to GbpC. Although *roco5*-null cells were previously identified in a large screen for mutants with defects in the developmental cycle (Sawai *et al.*, 2007), they did not show any recognizable developmental phenotype. In the contrary *roco11*-null cells show mild developmental defects: these cells develop significantly larger fruiting bodies; in particular, the multicellular structures have longer stalks compared to wild-type cells, re-expression of Roco11 in *roco11*-null cells rescues this defect. All other *roco*-null mutants did not show any phenotype in development and it will be interesting to see which biological function these proteins have in *Dictyostelium*.

2.3 Activation mechanism of Roco proteins

Pathogenic mutations in LRRK2 result in decreased GTPase activity (West *et al.*, 2005;Greggio *et al.*, 2006;Guo *et al.*, 2007;Ito *et al.*, 2007;Luzon-Toro *et al.*, 2007;Lewis *et al.*, 2007;Li *et al.*, 2007;West *et al.*, 2007). Furthermore, it has been shown that activity of the Roc domain is required to modulate downstream kinase activity, but kinase activity does not have a significant effect on GTP-binding of the Roc domain (Luzon-Toro *et al.*, 2007;West *et al.*, 2007). These results lead to the unifying model that the pathogenetic gain-of-function of LRRK2 relates to increased kinase activity, either directly through mutation of residues in the kinase domain, or indirectly through mutations in the GTPase domain or predicted protein binding domains. However, detailed information about the activation mechanism is missing; it is for example still unclear by which mechanism the Roc domain regulates kinase activity, the role that COR plays in this process and importantly how the PD-linked missense mutations alter the interactions between the different domains. The strong and diverse phenotypes of the *Dictyostelium* Roco disruption mutants provide a strong tool to investigate the activation mechanisms of Roco proteins.

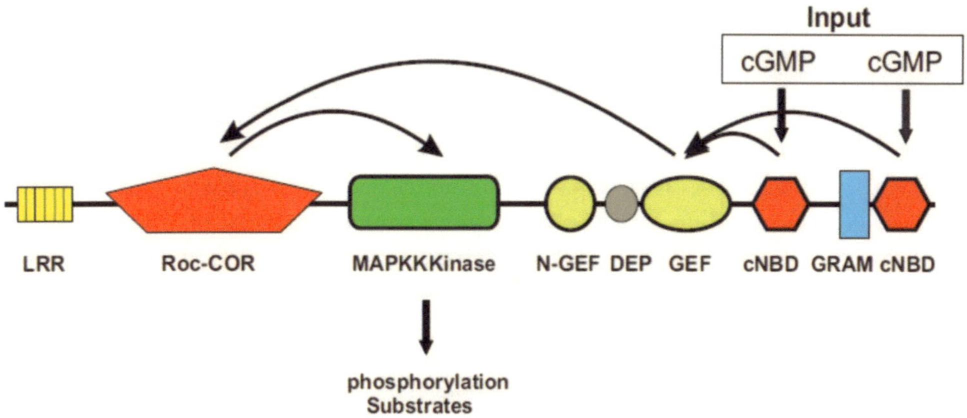

Fig. 5. GbpC: An intramolecular signalling cascade on one protein.

2.3.1 GbpC an intramolecular signaling cascade on one protein

The biochemical properties of GbpC were investigated by rescue analysis of the chemotactic defects of *gbpC*-null cells (van Egmond *et al.*, 2008). Whereas, re-expression of GbpC completely rescued the phenotype, mutants that lack a functional GEF, Roc or kinase domain are inactive. G-proteins function as molecular switches; they cycle between an active GTP- and inactive GDP-bound state. Consistently, in GbpC and LRRK2 the Roc domain is also activated upon GDP/GTP exchange, which subsequently increases kinase activity. The conventional Ras cycle is strictly regulated by guanine nucleotide exchange factors (GEFs) that catalyze the exchange of GDP for GTP, thereby activating the Ras protein. GTPase activating proteins (GAPs) stimulate an otherwise low intrinsic GTPase activity by many orders of magnitude, reverting the conformation back to the inactive GDP-bound form (Bourne *et al.*, 1991). So far it is unclear whether the GDP/GTP cycle of Roco proteins is regulated by GEFs and GAPs, and which structural consequences the GDP and GTP binding has. GbpC differs from the other Roco family members, in the sense that it already contains its own putative GEF domain (Bosgraaf *et al.*, 2003). In vitro nucleotide exchange assays showed that the RasGEF of GbpC specifically activates its own Roc domain. Furthermore, cGMP-binding to GbpC strongly stimulates binding of GbpC to GTP-agarose. Together these results suggest that GbpC contains a complete intramolecular signal transduction pathway; cGMP-binding to the cNB domains causes activation of the GEF domains, the subsequent GDP/GTP exchange of the Roc-COR domain, leading to the activation of the MAPKKK domain and phosphorylating downstream targets (Fig. 5, (van Egmond *et al.*, 2008).

2.3.2 Roc and kinase activities

Dictyostelium Roco4 has the same domain architecture as LRRK2, but in contrast to LRRK2, Roco4 is biochemically and structurally more tractable. The strong developmental phenotype of *roco4*-null cells was used to determine essential structural elements in the protein. Furthermore, high yields of Roco4 and combinations of its domains can be produced in *E. coli*. Similar to LRRK2, a functional Roco4 Roc domain is essential for kinase activity, the COR domain functions as dimerization device and disruption of Roc or the kinase domain by a single point mutation leads to the complete inactivation of the protein, which was also found for all other biochemically studied Roco proteins so far. Also, kinase inactivation does not lead to loss of GTP-binding, thus suggesting that Roc activation occurs upstream of kinase activity. These results indicate that Roco4 has properties very much resembling those described for LRRK2, indicating that Roco4 protein can serve as a valid model to understand the complex structure and regulatory mechanism of LRRK2. As to the relevance for understanding Parkinson we have demonstrated that all Roco4 PD-related mutants show a decreased GTPase and increased kinase activity, except the Roco4 L1180T mutant (LRRK2 I2020T) which shows a large decrease in kinase activity. Strikingly, also for LRRK2 I2020T a reduced kinase activity has been reported, and it has been postulated that the higher neurotoxity of this mutant might be due to a higher susceptibility of the mutant to intracellular degradation (Jaleel et al., 2007;Ohta et al., 2010).

2.3.3 Different roles for the WD40 repeats in Roco4 and LRRK2

For LRRK2 it was found that deletion of the WD40 repeats leads to lower kinase activity in vitro, which could be restored by introduction of one of the PD-mutations (Iaccarino et al., 2007). Surprisingly, we found that deletion of the Roco4 WD40 repeats does not lead to effects on Roco4 activity *in vivo* (van Egmond et al., 2010). This suggests that in the contrary to LRRK2, the WD40 repeats of Roco4 are apparently not needed for full activation of the kinase domain. A possible explanation for this discrepancy comes from phylogenetic data; Roco4, QkgA and Roco11 have a common ancestor that was duplicated only relatively recently in evolution. QkgA and Roco11 do not have the WD40 repeats that are present in all Roco4 proteins, suggesting that during or after duplication, *qkgA* and *roco11* have lost the WD40 repeats. Apparently, the WD40 repeats were not important enough for the regulation of Roco proteins, that they had to be maintained during evolution (van Egmond *et al.*, 2010).

2.3.4 The LRR are essential for biological activity

The LRR of LRRK2, and Dictyostelium GbpC and Roco4 are not involved in Roc or kinase activation in vitro, but are absolutely essential for activity of the protein in vivo (Iaccarino et al., 2007;van Egmond et al., 2008). Recent data suggest that the LRR are directly involved in determining input/output specificity of the roco proteins, most likely by binding upstream proteins that activate specifically the Roco protein and/or by selectively binding of the substrate (unpublished data).

2.3.5 Subcellular localization of Roco proteins important for activity and function

Recent data suggest that also the subcellular localization of LRRK2 is important for the activity and function. LRRK2 is present both in the cytosol and at the membrane, and the membrane-associated LRRK2 dimer most likely represents the physiologically active form of the protein (Berger *et al.*, 2010). The regulation of membrane association is not well understood, but probably includes dimerization, post-translational modifications and protein-protein interactions (Sen *et al.*, 2009;Berger *et al.*, 2010;Nichols *et al.*, 2010). To better understand the distribution of Roco proteins in the cell, we studied the localization of GbpC (ms in preparation). In resting cells, the protein is present uniformly in the cytosol, but during stream formation and osmotic stress the protein localizes to the membrane. Also

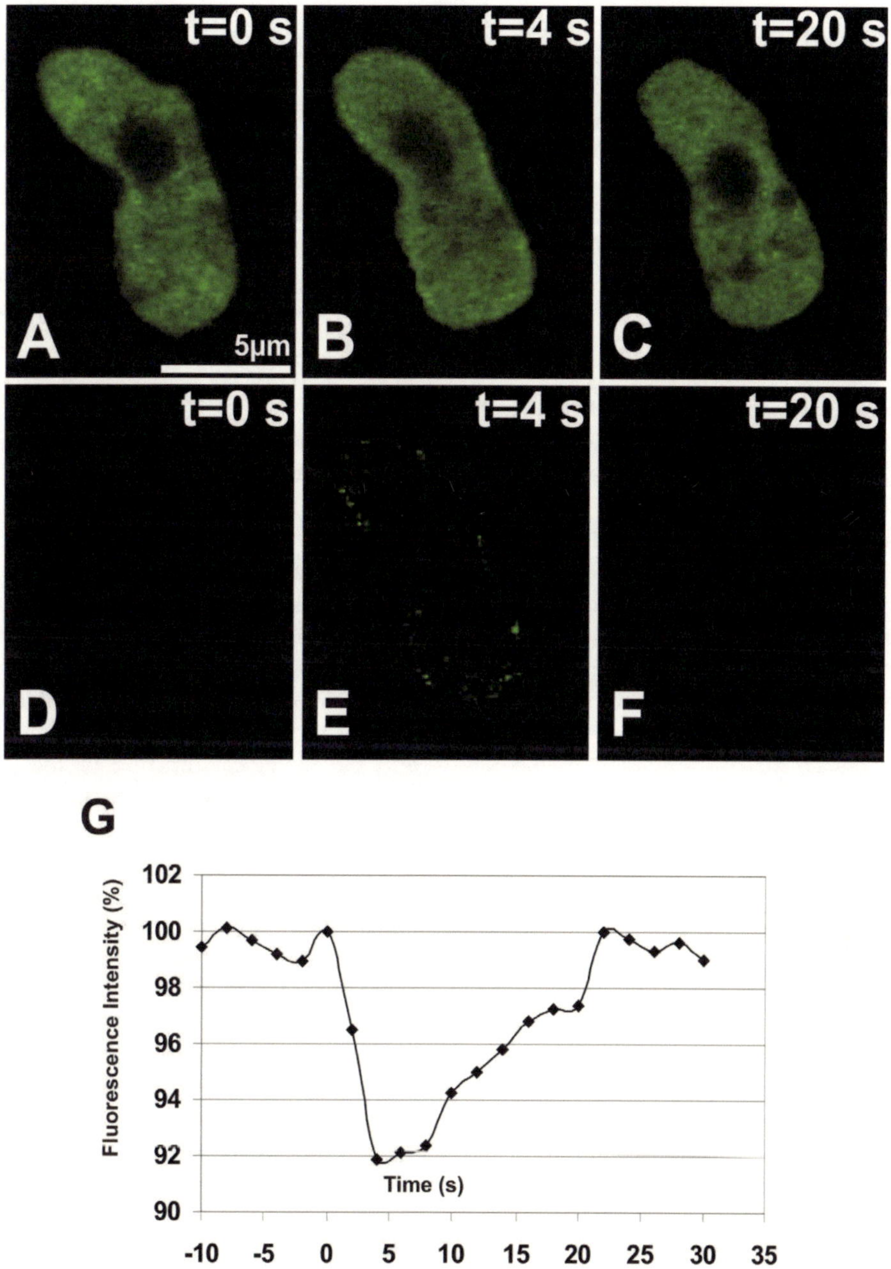

Fig. 6. GbpC translocates to the membrane upon cAMP-stimulation. Starved *gbpC*-null cells expressing GbpC-GFP were stimulated with 10^{-6} M cAMP and movies were recorded with time frames of one or two seconds. Shown are confocal images of three frames, at the point of cAMP-stimulation (A; t = 0 s), 4 seconds after stimulation (B), and 20 seconds after stimulation (C). To highlight membrane localization, D-F show equivalents of A-C after subtraction of the average cytosolic fluorescence intensity. Panel (G) shows the decrease of the fluorescence intensity of the cytosol averaged over 8 cells, which was analyzed using ImageJ

stimulation with the chemoattractant cAMP induces a rapid translocation to the cell membrane (Fig 6.). This translocation occurs independent of cGMP and the below described intramolecular signaling cascade in GbpC (van Egmond et al., 2008); GbpC still translocates in mutants that lack cGMP production or a functional GEF, Roc or kinase domain. In the contrary, mutations in the GRAM domain of GbpC lead to disturbed membrane association upon cAMP-stimulation; furthermore, the GRAM domain itself associates with cellular membranes and binds various phospholipids *in vitro*. Furthermore, mutants in the GRAM domain cause inactivation of GbpC *in vivo*. Together, the results show that GbpC receives multiple input signals: cAMP-stimulation induces a cGMP-dependent signaling cascade leading to kinase activity, and independently GRAM-dependent translocation of GbpC to the membrane is needed for proper functional activity.

2.4 Model for the activation of Roco proteins

Together these data show that although there is a high variation of additional regulatory domains among the Roco proteins, the Roco core itself functions in a similar way in all proteins. We have translated our biochemical, genetic and structural data into a model for the regulatory mechanism of LRRK2 (Fig 7). LRRK2 is a constitutive dimer by interaction of the COR domains. In the GDP-bound inactive state the G-domains are flexible, but in the active form the G-domains come in close proximity to each other. This conformational change is transmitted to the kinase domains to allow the activation loops of the two kinase protomers to be autophosphorylated and activated. The GTPase reaction is also dependent on dimerization, because efficient catalytic machinery is formed by complementation of the active site of one protomer with that of the other protomer. In this way the GTPase reaction functions as a timing device for the activation of the kinase and the biological function of the protein. Consistently, PD-related mutations have reduced GTPase activity and enhance kinase activity (unpublished data, (Cookson *et al.*, 2010)). Since the GTPase reaction is regulated by homodimerization and Roco proteins have a low nucleotide affinity (in the μM range), regulation by GEFs and GAPs is not necessary (Gotthardt *et al.*, 2008). However in some transient responses, as shown for GbpC, additional stimulation of the already high intrinsic exchange rate by GEF protein might be required. To completely understand the mechanism it will be important to know how the GDP-GTP cycle changes the RocCOR tandem and how it might influences the output of other parts of the protein. Therefore it will be important to solve structures of wild-type and/or PD-analogous mutants of Roco proteins in the different nucleotide states. The N-terminal segment, including the LRRs, is determining the input/output specificity of the proteins, but the exact mechanism is not clear. We propose two non-exclusive mechanisms: the N-terminal segment may selectively bind its substrates, brings it in close proximity of the Roco kinase domain and is subsequently phosphorylated. Alternatively, the N-terminal segment is binding upstream protein that activates specifically the Roco protein. In the context of LRRK2, 14-3-3 might be one of these upstream regulators: 14-3-3 binds in a phosphorylation dependent way to the N-terminal segment of LRRK2, thereby regulating its subcellular localization (Sen *et al.*, 2009;Nichols *et al.*, 2010).

3. Conclusion

Together, our results show that *Dictyostelium* provides an excellent model to study the function and activation mechanism of LRRK2. Roco proteins are the result of recent gene duplications, and are very homologous to mammalian LRRK2. Disruption of *Dictyostelium*

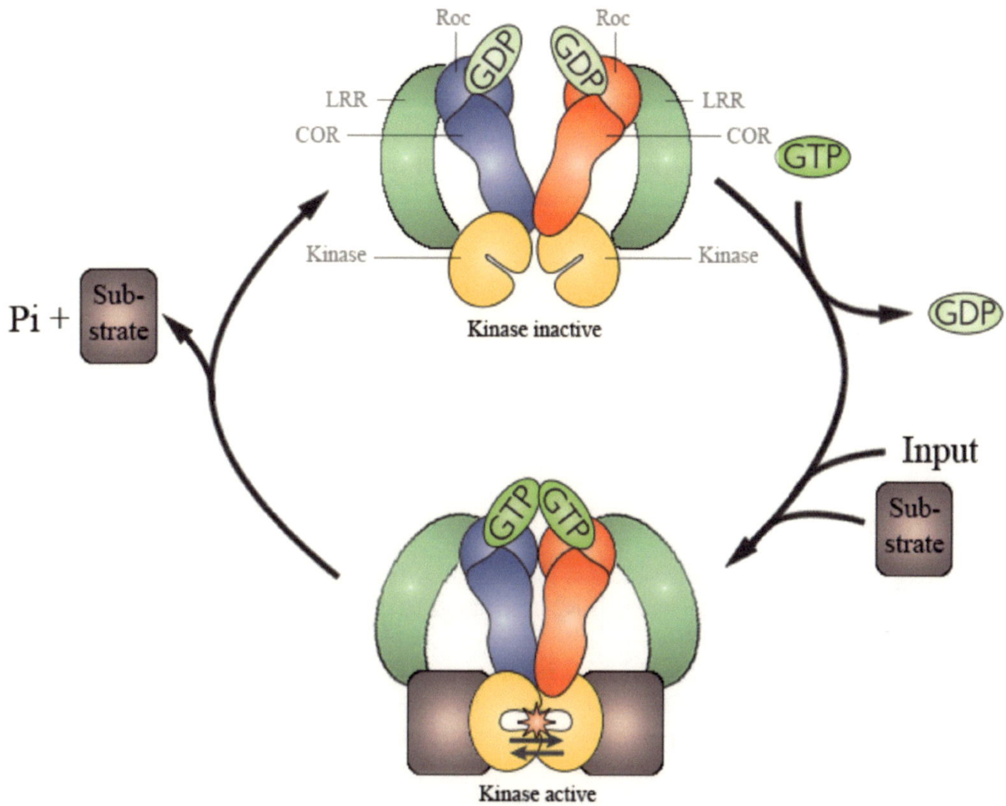

Fig. 7. Proposed model for the function and mechanism of LRRK2. GTP binding to the Roc domain results in dimerization of the Roc domain and subsequently activation of the kinase domain. The GTPase reaction is also dependent on dimerization; the efficient catalytic machinery is formed by complementation of the active site of one protomer with that of the other protomer. The LRR are directly involved in determining input/output specificity of the Roco proteins, most likely by binding upstream proteins that activate specifically the Roco protein and/or by selectively binding of the substrate.

Roco genes leads to very different phenotypes, indicating that they are involved in multiple cellular processes: they participate in cell division, osmotic-stress-response and development (van Egmond et al., 2010). The strong and diverse deletion phenotypes provide a unique opportunity to study PD-related mutations in living cells. These *roco2*- or *roco4*-null cells also provide a tool to express chimera proteins of Roco2, Roco4 and LRRK2 (full length proteins with domains derived from different sources). In contrast to LRRK2, many large parts of Roco4 can be expressed in *E.coli* to high levels in a stable and active form. Sufficient Roco4 protein and combinations of its domains could be purified for biochemical studies and crystallization. All Roco4 constructs both of wild-type and PD-related mutants show properties very much resembling those described for LRRK2. We have translated our results in a model, which can serve as a framework for the basic understanding for the complex regulatory mechanism of LRRK2, and provides a new starting point to answer major questions in the Parkinson field (Cookson, 2010): i) what are the upstream activators of Roco proteins, ii) what is the 3D structure of Roco proteins and how are they activated, iii) what are the output substrates of activated kinase, and iv) can we identify small molecule inhibitors of the activated kinase to revert the activity of the PD-associated mutations. Our studies in *Dictyostelium* might be instrumental in this enterprise and can give important insights in the molecular mechanism of LRRK2 activation, and how mutations of LRRK2 result in neuronal toxicity. In this way we hope to contribute to the understanding of the biochemical pathways responsible for LRRK2-linked PD and help to identify therapeutic targets for PD and related neurodegenerative disorders.

4. Acknowledgment

This work is done in collaboration with Dr. A Wittinghofer (MPI Dortmund) and is supported by the Alexander von Humboldt foundation and the Michael J Fox foundation for Parkinson's disease research. We want to thank Dr. Wouter van Egmond, Dr. Yiu-Fung Ho and Matthieu Bosman for their input in this the project.

5. References

[1] Aasly JO, Toft M, Fernandez-Mata I, Kachergus J, Hulihan M, White LR, and Farrer M (2005) Clinical features of LRRK2-associated Parkinson's disease in central Norway. *Ann Neurol,* 57, 762-765.

[2] Alexander S and Alexander H (2011) Lead genetic studies in Dictyostelium discoideum and translational studies in human cells demonstrate that sphingolipids are key regulators of sensitivity to cisplatin and other anticancer drugs. *Semin Cell Dev Biol,* 22, 97-104.

[3] Araki T, Tsujioka M, Abe T, Fukuzawa M, Meima M, Schaap P, Morio T, Urushihara H, Katoh M, Maeda M, Tanaka Y, Takeuchi I, and Williams JG (2003) A STAT-regulated, stress-induced signalling pathway in Dictyostelium. *J Cell Sci,* 116, 2907-2915.

[4] Araki T, van Egmond WN, van Haastert PJ, and Williams JG (2010) Dual regulation of a Dictyostelium STAT by cGMP and Ca2+ signalling. *J Cell Sci,* 123, 837-841.

[5] Baggiolini M (1998) Chemokines and leukocyte traffic. *Nature,* 392, 565-568.

[6] Berger Z, Smith KA, and Lavoie MJ (2010) Membrane localization of LRRK2 is associated with increased formation of the highly active LRRK2 dimer and changes in its phosphorylation. *Biochemistry,* 49, 5511-5523.

[7] Bosgraaf L, Russcher H, Smith JL, Wessels D, Soll DR, and van Haastert PJ (2002) A novel cGMP signalling pathway mediating myosin phosphorylation and chemotaxis in Dictyostelium. *EMBO J,* 21, 4560-4570.

[8] Bosgraaf L and van Haastert PJ (2003) Roc, a Ras/GTPase domain in complex proteins. *Biochim Biophys Acta,* 1643, 5-10.

[9] Bosgraaf L and van Haastert PJ (2006) The regulation of myosin II in Dictyostelium. *Eur J Cell Biol,* 85, 969-979.

[10] Bourne HR, Sanders DA, and Mccormick F (1991) The Gtpase Superfamily - Conserved Structure and Molecular Mechanism. *Nature,* 349, 117-127.

[11] Campbell JJ and Butcher EC (2000) Chemokines in tissue-specific and microenvironment-specific lymphocyte homing. *Current Opinion in Immunology,* 12, 336-341.

[12] Carnell MJ and Insall RH (2011) Actin on disease--studying the pathobiology of cell motility using Dictyostelium discoideum. *Semin Cell Dev Biol,* 22, 82-88.
[13] Charo IF and Taubman MB (2004) Chemokines in the pathogenesis of vascular disease. *Circ Res,* 95, 858-866.
[14] Cookson MR (2010) The role of leucine-rich repeat kinase 2 (LRRK2) in Parkinson's disease. *Nat Rev Neurosci,* 11, 791-797.
[15] Cookson MR and Bandmann O (2010) Parkinson's disease: insights from pathways. *Hum Mol Genet,* 19, R21-R27.
[16] Cote GP and Bukiejko U (1987) Purification and Characterization of A Myosin Heavy-Chain Kinase from Dictyostelium-Discoideum. *Journal of Biological Chemistry,* 262, 1065-1072.
[17] Crone SA and Lee KF (2002) The bound leading the bound: Target-derived receptors act as guidance cues. *Neuron,* 36, 333-335.
[18] De la Roche MA and Cote GP (2001) Regulation of Dictyostelium myosin I and II. *Biochim Biophys Acta,* 1525, 245-261.
[19] De la Roche MA, Smith JL, Betapudi V, Egelhoff TT, and Cote GP (2002) Signaling pathways regulating Dictyostelium myosin II. *J Muscle Res Cell Motil,* 23, 703-718.
[20] Devreotes PN and Zigmond SH (1988) Chemotaxis in Eukaryotic Cells - A Focus on Leukocytes and Dictyostelium. *Annual Review of Cell Biology,* 4, 649-686.
[21] Eccles SA (2005) Targeting key steps in metastatic tumour progression. *Curr Opin Genet Dev,* 15, 77-86.
[22] Eichinger L, Pachebat JA, Glockner G, Rajandream MA, Sucgang R, Berriman M, Song J, Olsen R, Szafranski K, Xu Q, Tunggal B, Kummerfeld S, Madera M, Konfortov BA, Rivero F, Bankier AT, Lehmann R, Hamlin N, Davies R, Gaudet P, Fey P, Pilcher K, Chen G, Saunders D, Sodergren E, Davis P, Kerhornou A, Nie X, Hall N, Anjard C, Hemphill L, Bason N, Farbrother P, Desany B, Just E, Morio T, Rost R, Churcher C, Cooper J, Haydock S, van Driessche N, Cronin A, Goodhead I, Muzny D, Mourier T, Pain A, Lu M, Harper D, Lindsay R, Hauser H, James K, Quiles M, Babu MM, Saito T, Buchrieser C, Wardroper A, Felder M, Thangavelu M, Johnson D, Knights A, Loulseged H, Mungall K, Oliver K, Price C, Quail MA, Urushihara H, Hernandez J, Rabbinowitsch E, Steffen D, Sanders M, Ma J, Kohara Y, Sharp S, Simmonds M, Spiegler S, Tivey A, Sugano S, White B, Walker D, Woodward J, Winckler T, Tanaka Y, Shaulsky G, Schleicher M, Weinstock G, Rosenthal A, Cox EC, Chisholm RL, Gibbs R, Loomis WF, Platzer M, Kay RR, Williams J, Dear PH, Noegel AA, Barrell B, and Kuspa A (2005) The genome of the social amoeba Dictyostelium discoideum. *Nature,* 435, 43-57.
[23] Escalante R (2011) Dictyostelium as a model for human disease. *Semin Cell Dev Biol,* 22, 69.
[24] Francione LM, Annesley SJ, Carilla-Latorre S, Escalante R, and Fisher PR (2011) The Dictyostelium model for mitochondrial disease. *Semin Cell Dev Biol,* 22, 120-130.
[25] Gasper R, Meyer S, Gotthardt K, Sirajuddin M, and Wittinghofer A (2009) It takes two to tango: regulation of G proteins by dimerization. *Nat Rev Mol Cell Biol,* 10, 423-429.
[26] Gilks WP, bou-Sleiman PM, Gandhi S, Jain S, Singleton A, Lees AJ, Shaw K, Bhatia KP, Bonifati V, Quinn NP, Lynch J, Healy DG, Holton JL, Revesz T, and Wood NW (2005) A common LRRK2 mutation in idiopathic Parkinson's disease. *Lancet,* 365, 415-416.

[27] Goldberg JM, Bosgraaf L, van Haastert PJ, and Smith JL (2002) Identification of four candidate cGMP targets in Dictyostelium. *Proc Natl Acad Sci U S A,* 99, 6749-6754.

[28] Gotthardt K, Weyand M, Kortholt A, van Haastert PJ, and Wittinghofer A (2008) Structure of the Roc-COR domain tandem of C. tepidum, a prokaryotic homologue of the human LRRK2 Parkinson kinase. *EMBO J,* 27, 2239-2249.

[29] Greggio E, Jain S, Kingsbury A, Bandopadhyay R, Lewis P, Kaganovich A, van der Brug MP, Beilina A, Blackinton J, Thomas KJ, Ahmad R, Miller DW, Kesavapany S, Singleton A, Lees A, Harvey RJ, Harvey K, and Cookson MR (2006) Kinase activity is required for the toxic effects of mutant LRRK2/dardarin. *Neurobiol Dis,* 23, 329-341.

[30] Guo L, Gandhi PN, Wang W, Petersen RB, Wilson-Delfosse AL, and Chen SG (2007) The Parkinson's disease-associated protein, leucine-rich repeat kinase 2 (LRRK2), is an authentic GTPase that stimulates kinase activity. *Exp Cell Res,* 313, 3658-3670.

[31] Hadwiger JA, Lee S, and Firtel RA (1994) The G alpha subunit G alpha 4 couples to pterin receptors and identifies a signaling pathway that is essential for multicellular development in Dictyostelium. *Proc Natl Acad Sci U S A,* 91, 10566-10570.

[32] Hernandez DG, Paisan-Ruiz C, Inerney-Leo A, Jain S, Meyer-Lindenberg A, Evans EW, Berman KF, Johnson J, Auburger G, Schaffer AA, Lopez GJ, Nussbaum RL, and Singleton AB (2005) Clinical and positron emission tomography of Parkinson's disease caused by LRRK2. *Ann Neurol,* 57, 453-456.

[33] Iaccarino C, Crosio C, Vitale C, Sanna G, Carri MT, and Barone P (2007) Apoptotic mechanisms in mutant LRRK2-mediated cell death. *Hum Mol Genet,* 16, 1319-1326.

[34] Iijima M, Huang YE, and Devreotes P (2002) Temporal and spatial regulation of chemotaxis. *Developmental Cell,* 3, 469-478.

[35] Ito G, Okai T, Fujino G, Takeda K, Ichijo H, Katada T, and Iwatsubo T (2007) GTP binding is essential to the protein kinase activity of LRRK2, a causative gene product for familial Parkinson's disease. *Biochemistry,* 46, 1380-1388.

[36] Jaleel M, Nichols RJ, Deak M, Campbell DG, Gillardon F, Knebel A, and Alessi DR (2007) LRRK2 phosphorylates moesin at threonine-558: characterization of how Parkinson's disease mutants affect kinase activity. *Biochem J,* 405, 307-317.

[37] Kessin RH (2000) Evolutionary biology. Cooperation can be dangerous. *Nature,* 408, 917, 919.

[38] Khan NL, Jain S, Lynch JM, Pavese N, bou-Sleiman P, Holton JL, Healy DG, Gilks WP, Sweeney MG, Ganguly M, Gibbons V, Gandhi S, Vaughan J, Eunson LH, Katzenschlager R, Gayton J, Lennox G, Revesz T, Nicholl D, Bhatia KP, Quinn N, Brooks D, Lees AJ, Davis MB, Piccini P, Singleton AB, and Wood NW (2005) Mutations in the gene LRRK2 encoding dardarin (PARK8) cause familial Parkinson's disease: clinical, pathological, olfactory and functional imaging and genetic data. *Brain,* 128, 2786-2796.

[39] Kolman MF, Futey LM, and Egelhoff TT (1996) Dictyostelium myosin heavy chain kinase A regulates myosin localization during growth and development. *Journal of Cell Biology,* 132, 101-109.

[40] Kuwayama H, Ecke M, Gerisch G, and van Haastert PJ (1996) Protection against osmotic stress by cGMP-mediated myosin phosphorylation. *Science,* 271, 207-209.

[41] Kuwayama H and van Haastert PJ (1996) Regulation of guanylyl cyclase by a cGMP-binding protein during chemotaxis in Dictyostelium discoideum. *J Biol Chem,* 271, 23718-23724.

[42] Kuwayama H and van Haastert PJ (1998) Chemotactic and osmotic signals share a cGMP transduction pathway in Dictyostelium discoideum. *FEBS Lett,* 424, 248-252.

[43] Lees AJ, Hardy J, and Revesz T (2009) Parkinson's disease. *Lancet,* 373, 2055-2066.

[44] Levi S, Polyakov MV, and Egelhoff TT (2002) Myosin II dynamics in Dictyostelium: Determinants for filament assembly and translocation to the cell cortex during chemoattractant responses. *Cell Motility and the Cytoskeleton,* 53, 177-188.

[45] Lewis PA, Greggio E, Beilina A, Jain S, Baker A, and Cookson MR (2007) The R1441C mutation of LRRK2 disrupts GTP hydrolysis. *Biochem Biophys Res Commun,* 357, 668-671.

[46] Li X, Tan YC, Poulose S, Olanow CW, Huang XY, and Yue Z (2007) Leucine-rich repeat kinase 2 (LRRK2)/PARK8 possesses GTPase activity that is altered in familial Parkinson's disease R1441C/G mutants. *J Neurochem,* 103, 238-247.

[47] Luzon-Toro B, Rubio dlT, Delgado A, Perez-Tur J, and Hilfiker S (2007) Mechanistic insight into the dominant mode of the Parkinson's disease-associated G2019S LRRK2 mutation. *Hum Mol Genet,* 16, 2031-2039.

[48] Maniak M (2011) Dictyostelium as a model for human lysosomal and trafficking diseases. *Semin Cell Dev Biol,* 22, 114-119.

[49] Marin I (2006) The Parkinson disease gene LRRK2: evolutionary and structural insights. *Mol Biol Evol,* 23, 2423-2433.

[50] Meyer I, Kuhnert O, and Graf R (2011) Functional analyses of lissencephaly-related proteins in Dictyostelium. *Semin Cell Dev Biol,* 22, 89-96.

[51] Murphy MB, Cote GP, and Egelhoff TT (1996) Purification and characterization of a myosin heavy chain phosphatase from Dictyostelium. *Molecular Biology of the Cell,* 7, 1153.

[52] Nichols RJ, Dzamko N, Morrice NA, Campbell DG, Deak M, Ordureau A, Macartney T, Tong Y, Shen J, Prescott AR, and Alessi DR (2010) 14-3-3 binding to LRRK2 is disrupted by multiple Parkinson's disease-associated mutations and regulates cytoplasmic localization. *Biochem J,* 430, 393-404.

[53] Ohta E, Kubo M, and Obata F (2010) Prevention of intracellular degradation of I2020T mutant LRRK2 restores its protectivity against apoptosis. *Biochem Biophys Res Commun,* 391, 242-247.

[54] Paisan-Ruiz C, Jain S, Evans EW, Gilks WP, Simon J, van der BM, Lopez de MA, Aparicio S, Gil AM, Khan N, Johnson J, Martinez JR, Nicholl D, Carrera IM, Pena AS, de SR, Lees A, Marti-Masso JF, Perez-Tur J, Wood NW, and Singleton AB (2004) Cloning of the gene containing mutations that cause PARK8-linked Parkinson's disease. *Neuron,* 44, 595-600.

[55] Satake W, Nakabayashi Y, Mizuta I, Hirota Y, Ito C, Kubo M, Kawaguchi T, Tsunoda T, Watanabe M, Takeda A, Tomiyama H, Nakashima K, Hasegawa K, Obata F, Yoshikawa T, Kawakami H, Sakoda S, Yamamoto M, Hattori N, Murata M, Nakamura Y, and Toda T (2009) Genome-wide association study identifies common variants at four loci as genetic risk factors for Parkinson's disease. *Nat Genet,* 41, 1303-1307.

[56] Sawai S, Guan XJ, Kuspa A, and Cox EC (2007) High-throughput analysis of spatio-temporal dynamics in Dictyostelium. *Genome Biol,* 8, R144.
[57] Sen S, Webber PJ, and West AB (2009) Dependence of leucine-rich repeat kinase 2 (LRRK2) kinase activity on dimerization. *J Biol Chem,* 284, 36346-36356.
[58] Simon-Sanchez J, Schulte C, Bras JM, Sharma M, Gibbs JR, Berg D, Paisan-Ruiz C, Lichtner P, Scholz SW, Hernandez DG, Kruger R, Federoff M, Klein C, Goate A, Perlmutter J, Bonin M, Nalls MA, Illig T, Gieger C, Houlden H, Steffens M, Okun MS, Racette BA, Cookson MR, Foote KD, Fernandez HH, Traynor BJ, Schreiber S, Arepalli S, Zonozi R, Gwinn K, van der BM, Lopez G, Chanock SJ, Schatzkin A, Park Y, Hollenbeck A, Gao J, Huang X, Wood NW, Lorenz D, Deuschl G, Chen H, Riess O, Hardy JA, Singleton AB, and Gasser T (2009) Genome-wide association study reveals genetic risk underlying Parkinson's disease. *Nat Genet,* 41, 1308-1312.
[59] Sun B, Ma H, and Firtel RA (2003) Dictyostelium stress-activated protein kinase alpha, a novel stress-activated mitogen-activated protein kinase kinase kinase-like kinase, is important for the proper regulation of the cytoskeleton. *Mol Biol Cell,* 14, 4526-4540.
[60] Trusolino L and Comoglio PM (2002) Scatter-factor and semaphorin receptors: cell signalling for invasive growth. *Nat Rev Cancer,* 2, 289-300.
[61] van Egmond WN, Kortholt A, Plak K, Bosgraaf L, Bosgraaf S, Keizer-Gunnink I, and van Haastert PJ (2008) Intramolecular activation mechanism of the Dictyostelium LRRK2 homolog Roco protein GbpC. *J Biol Chem,* 283, 30412-30420.
[62] van Egmond WN and van Haastert PJ (2010) Characterization of the Roco protein family in Dictyostelium discoideum. *Eukaryot Cell,* 9, 751-761.
[63] Van Haastert PJM and Devreotes PN (2004) Chemotaxis: Signalling the way forward. *Nature Reviews Molecular Cell Biology,* 5, 626-634.
[64] Van DN, Alexander H, Min J, Kuspa A, Alexander S, and Shaulsky G (2007) Global transcriptional responses to cisplatin in Dictyostelium discoideum identify potential drug targets. *Proc Natl Acad Sci U S A,* 104, 15406-15411.
[65] Veltman DM and van Haastert PJ (2008) The role of cGMP and the rear of the cell in Dictyostelium chemotaxis and cell streaming. *J Cell Sci,* 121, 120-127.
[66] West AB, Moore DJ, Biskup S, Bugayenko A, Smith WW, Ross CA, Dawson VL, and Dawson TM (2005) Parkinson's disease-associated mutations in leucine-rich repeat kinase 2 augment kinase activity. *Proc Natl Acad Sci U S A,* 102, 16842-16847.
[67] West AB, Moore DJ, Choi C, Andrabi SA, Li X, Dikeman D, Biskup S, Zhang Z, Lim KL, Dawson VL, and Dawson TM (2007) Parkinson's disease-associated mutations in LRRK2 link enhanced GTP-binding and kinase activities to neuronal toxicity. *Hum Mol Genet,* 16, 223-232.
[68] Williams RS, Boeckeler K, Graf R, Muller-Taubenberger A, Li Z, Isberg RR, Wessels D, Soll DR, Alexander H, and Alexander S (2006) Towards a molecular understanding of human diseases using Dictyostelium discoideum. *Trends Mol Med,* 12, 415-424.
[69] Zimprich A, Biskup S, Leitner P, Lichtner P, Farrer M, Lincoln S, Kachergus J, Hulihan M, Uitti RJ, Calne DB, Stoessl AJ, Pfeiffer RF, Patenge N, Carbajal IC, Vieregge P, Asmus F, Muller-Myhsok B, Dickson DW, Meitinger T, Strom TM, Wszolek ZK, and Gasser T (2004) Mutations in LRRK2 cause autosomal-dominant parkinsonism with pleomorphic pathology. *Neuron,* 44, 601-607.

16

Comparison of Normal and Parkinsonian Microcircuit Dynamics in the Rodent Striatum

O. Jaidar, L. Carrillo-Reid and J. Bargas
División de Neurociencias, Instituto de Fisiología Celular, Universidad Nacional Autónoma de México, Mexico City, México

1. Introduction

Experimentally, depriving the basal ganglia (BG) from their dopaminergic innervation, dramatically changes the behavior of all their circuits, neurons, and synapses in multiple ways. Dopamine afferents are received by all BG nuclei (Rommelfanger and Wichmann, 2010). In the absence of DA, BG generate enhanced pathological oscillatory patterns in the external segment of the striatum: globus pallidus (GPe), internal segment of the globus pallidus (GPi), subthalamic nucleus (STN) and substantia nigra pars reticulata (SNr) (Blandini et al., 2000). These pathological oscillatory patterns are expressed as increased cortical beta frequency coherence (Costa et al., 2006; Fuentes et al., 2009; Kozlov et al., 2009; Walters and Bergstrom, 2009) and are reflected as the inability to select, change or initiate motor actions (Magill et al., 2001; Ni et al., 2001; Wilson et al., 2006), as though all neurons were trapped in a massive oscillation that does not allow the selection of any circuit or action. Behaviorally, circuit disfunction is accompanied by bradykinesia, akinesia, tremor and muscular rigidity (Brown, 2007; Hammond et al., 2007; Galvan and Wichmann, 2008; Fuentes et al., 2009; Walters and Bergstrom, 2009; Zold et al., 2009).
One question is what are the manifestations of these changes at the level of the striatal microcircuitry (Alexander and Crutcher, 1990; Middleton and Strick, 2002), given that its neurons are the principal entrance to the BG (Alexander and Crutcher, 1990; Middleton and Strick, 2002), and DA is particularly concentrated in this nucleus (striatum); more than in any other BG nuclei (Bjorklund and Dunnett, 2007). To answer this question, here we show how the striatal microcircuit functions before and after DA depletion. The changes observed may be fundamental to understand BG activity during Parkinsonism.

2. Activity in the striatal microcircuit

The striatum integrates inputs from the cortex, the intralaminar thalamic nuclei, the dopaminergic afferents from the *substantia nigra pars compacta* (SNc) and other nuclei (Smith et al., 1994; Parr-Brownlie et al., 2009). The basic elements that configure the striatal microcircuit are the medium spiny projection neurons (MSNs) and its interneurons (Kreitzer, 2009). MSNs are the major cell population commonly being in a resting state with a polarized membrane potential (ca., -80 mV) and relatively low input resistance (ca., 100

MΩ in adult neurons) (Bargas et al., 1988; Reyes et al., 1998). Upon depolarization, these neurons fire tonically due to persistent voltage-activated K^+-currents (Galarraga et al., 1989; Nisenbaum and Wilson, 1995; Bargas et al., 1999), with a long latency to first spike due inactivating K^+-currents (Surmeier et al., 1988; Bargas et al., 1989), inward rectification (Galarraga et al., 1994; Nisenbaum and Wilson, 1995), and interspike intervals partially dependent on Ca^{2+}-activated K^+-currents (Pineda et al., 1992; Bargas et al., 1999), among other outward currents (Nisenbaum and Wilson, 1995; Shen et al., 2005).

MSNs can be classified as striatopallidal or indirect pathway neurons and striatonigral or direct pathway neurons, based on their axonal projections, receptors and peptide expression (Gerfen et al., 1990; Smith et al., 1998). Striatopallidal fibers target the GPe and striatonigral axons target the output nuclei of the BG: GPi and SNr. Interneurons are divided into genres with much intrinsic, still not-well studied variation: i) the parvalbumin-immunoreactive (PV+) or fast spiking interneurons (FS), ii) the somatostatin (SS), neuropeptide Y (NPY), tyrosine hydroxylase (TH), nitric oxide synthase (NOS)-immunoreactive populations of cells that fire with a low threshold calcium spike (LTS), iii) large cholinergic or tonic active neurons (TANs), and iv) calretinin-immunoreactive neurons (Wilson et al., 1990; Kawaguchi et al., 1995; Tepper et al., 2004; Kreitzer, 2009; Ibáñez-Sandoval et al., 2010; Tepper et al., 2010). A challenge is to find out how all these neurons process striatal inputs into coherent spatio-temporal patterned outputs: what is their role in microcircuitry processing. Thus, as a first approach we decided to observe what characteristics of the microcircuit activity are plainly evident in order to establish top-down hypothesis and experimental designs to understand the role of each neuron class during microcircuit activity (Carrillo-Reid et al., 2008).

MSNs seldom fire in physiological conditions (without a motor behavior) (Crutcher and DeLong, 1984; Kimura, 1992; Carrillo-Reid et al., 2008; Liang et al., 2008; Vautrelle, 2009; Jaidar et al., 2010), due to their intrinsic inward rectifying K^+ currents and strong depolarization-activated K^+-currents (see above and Bargas et al., 1989; Galarraga et al., 1994; Nisenbaum and Wilson, 1995; Bargas et al., 1999; Tepper et al., 2004). Since MSNs are majority, this characteristic makes the striatum to be classified as a quasi-"silent" nucleus; very different from the neurons of other BG nuclei which exhibit firing all the time (e.g., Nakanishi et al., 1987; Kita and Kitai, 1991; Ibáñez-Sandoval et al., 2007). Either activity from the cortex, thalamus, or addition of NMDA in vitro, activates the striatal microcircuits so that groups of MSNs begin to fire in a persistent or recurrent way (Vergara et al., 2003; Mahon et al., 2006; Vautrelle, 2009).

Firing in MSNs is characterized by prolonged membrane potential transitions from a hyperpolarized "down"-state to a depolarized "up"-state where bursts of action potentials are displayed (Wilson and Kawaguchi, 1996; Vergara et al., 2003; Vautrelle, 2009). In vitro, this firing pattern occurs without overt stimulation and is due to an acquired conditional bistability (Vergara et al., 2003; Carrillo-Reid et al., 2008). Because burst firing can also be recorded using calcium-imaging that allow the recording of dozens of cells simultaneously (Cossart et al., 2003), the use of this technique resulted useful to observe how burst firing can extend to neighboring neurons, and how this firing generates network dynamics, that is, to a cell assembly type of processing (Hebb, 1949).

3. The Cell Assembly hypothesis

Cell Assemblies (CAs) have been posited as the building blocks or structures capable to give support and store neuronal representations, or coding, of perceptual, cognitive, and motor processes (Grinvald et al., 2003; Harris, 2005). However, although Hebbian and non-Hebbian types of learning have been formalized and used in artificial neuronal networks under different paradigms (Bowles, 2006), the demonstration of the existence of these structures in living circuits has not been trivial and they are mostly assumed to exist using indirect evidence, such as the correlation of the firing generated by a single, or a small group of neurons, with field or multiunitary population recordings (e.g., Sakurai, 1996; Costa et al., 2006; Zold et al., 2009), or with population activity as revealed by voltage dyes (Grinvald et al., 2003; Grinvald, 2005). Numerous evidences of correlated firing in neurons, using these techniques, are available. However, an inconvenience for cell physiology is that these techniques do not achieve single cell resolution. That is, these techniques cannot identify the elements that participate in a given activity of the microcircuit. If they cannot be identified, a role for them cannot be found or assigned. On the other hand, speculations about how a circuit may function, based on cell-focused studies, are abundant and utterly speculative. Between these two extremes: system and cellular neurophysiology, respectively, there is very little work. To fill the gap we need to make a proper description of network dynamics at the cellular level while recording many cells simultaneous with single cell resolution. In the following section we will describe how this is achieved as well as some properties of the striatal microcircuit that reflect cell assembly organization and dynamics. At the same time, we will describe how these properties change in a Parkinsonian microcircuit.

4. Recurrent bursting

The first property is recurrent burst firing. Striatal neurons fire in bursts of action potentials riding on top of depolarizing plateau potentials called "up-states". This firing mode has been shown in vivo and in vitro (Wilson, 1993; Stern et al., 1997; Vergara et al., 2003). Plateau potentials underlying bursts of spikes can arise from intrinsic nonlinear properties leading to bistability (Hounsgaard and Kiehn, 1989; Hsiao et al., 1998; Kiehn, 2006), from temporal summation of excitatory and inhibitory synaptic events (Sanchez-Vives and McCormick, 2000; Yanagawa and Mogi, 2009), or both (Destexhe and Pare, 1999; Tal et al., 2008). It is possible that the same neurons can generate plateau potentials of different origin depending on network situation (Hounsgaard and Kiehn, 1989; Alaburda et al., 2005; Vautrelle, 2009).

Interestingly, recurrent bursts of action potentials on top of sustained depolarizations (up-states or plateau potentials) resemble a basic property of certain microcircuits called Central Pattern Generators (CPGs) (Grillner, 2006). The main difference between CAs and CPGs is that CPGs activity is thought to be "innate", whereas CAs are supposedly to be "acquired" through synaptic plasticity. CPGs can display their electrical behavior in the absence of afferent inputs, and in isolated tissue maintained vitro, as long as an "excitatory drive" turns them on. In the case of fictive locomotion and swimming, a physiological excitatory drive can be generated pharmacologically: by the addition of micromolar NMDA into the bath saline, a maneuver that induces conditional bistability, plateau potentials and recurrent regular bursting (Grillner et al., 1981; Guertin and Hounsgaard, 1998).

In the striatal microcircuit robust recurrent bursting is induced by the same pharmacological manipulation in vivo (Herrling et al., 1983) and in vitro (Vergara et al., 2003) obtaining an electrophysiological patterned output from spiny neurons; similar to that previously recorded in both CPGs or suspected CAs. Furthermore, unilateral NMDA administration induces contralateral turning behavior directly relating recurrent burst firing in medium spiny neurons with a rhythmic and regular motor behavior (Ossowska, 1995). Then, we can say that the striatal bursting activity under these conditions codes for movement (e.g., Hikosaka et al., 2006).

What happens when the DA is absent? A "logical" common mistake is to think that if a Parkinsonian patient or animal cannot generate movements then, the striatal microcircuit should even be more "silent" that in control conditions. However, it has been shown, *in vitro* and *in vivo*, exactly the opposite: after DA depletion the spontaneous firing and synaptic activity of striatal neurons becomes more active and noisy (Galarraga et al., 1987; Tang et al., 2001; Tseng et al., 2001; Liang et al., 2008). That is, a more robust neuronal activity and bursting can be recorded in the DA-depleted striatum.

5. Correlated firing

The next property observed during CAs physiological behavior, and which can be observed in the striatal microcircuit, is the synchronous or correlated firing of pools of neurons that here will be called "neuronal aggregates". Synchrony or correlated firing (coherence, phase locking) between these auto-associated clusters of neurons make up network states as described in many circuits (e.g., Petersen and Sakmann, 2000; Doupe et al., 2004; Carrillo-Reid et al., 2008; Li et al., 2010). In some cases, the time scale of synchronization is fast: that of synaptic and action potentials duration (Diesmann et al., 1999; Leger et al., 2005; Robbe et al., 2006). However, in most physiological conditions, a great variability in the responses of neurons at the action potential time scale is found (Calvin and Stevens, 1968; Shadlen and Newsome, 1994; Grinvald et al., 2003; Kostal et al., 2007). Thus, synchronicity in the action potential time scale is hard to record in most central nervous system circuits (Shadlen and Newsome, 1994; Arieli et al., 1996) and simulations of that activity change with minimal perturbations (Izhikevich and Edelman, 2008).

Notwithstanding, recurrent burst firing of individual neurons has been found to be synchronized and correlated among several members of a neuronal aggregate (Carrillo-Reid et al., 2008), and also in population recordings of network conditions in which a given neuron participates: its "preferred condition" (Grinvald et al., 2003). Moreover, up-states and bursting have been found to be a reflection of an attractor-like network dynamics (Cossart et al., 2003) capable to recruit connected neurons into a preferred aggregate. Connections, internal to the aggregate, can in part explain the maintenance of bursts shared by the elements of the group (Lambe and Aghajanian, 2007). That is, the up-state is a product or reflection of the correlated firing of a group of interconnected neurons.

In the striatum, correlated firing has been inferred by recording local field potentials correlated with neuronal firing (Murer et al., 2002; Berke et al., 2004; Costa et al., 2006; Mahon et al., 2006; Walters et al., 2007; Zold et al., 2009). Also, the use of calcium imaging techniques, which records bursting behavior of several cells simultaneously, reveals spontaneous peaks of burst synchronization and correlated firing after the application of NMDA (Carrillo-Reid et al., 2008) (See Figure). That is, recurrent bursting recorded in single neurons (Vergara et al., 2003) has been demonstrated to be shared by sets of neurons that spontaneously synchronize their bursts in a particular condition (Carrillo-Reid et al., 2008).

During Parkinsonism caused by DA-depletion, the recording of pathological bursting activity exhibit an increase in the number of synchrony peaks (Jaidar et al., 2010). Synchronizing events emerge spontaneously and regularly during recordings. Up-states are the manifestation of a network phenomenon linking neurons that sometimes are located far

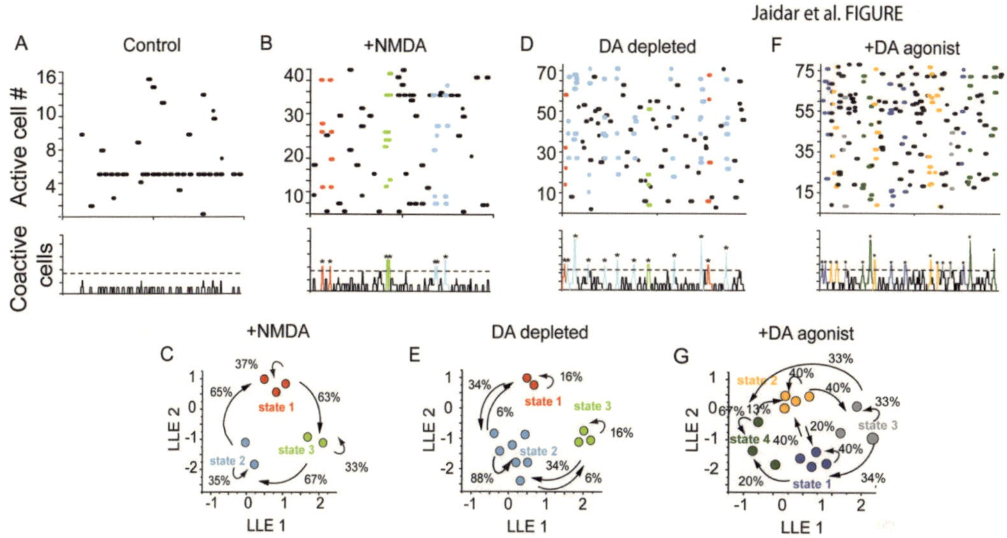

Fig. 1. Following the striatal microcircuit with calcium imaging.

A. Top: A raster plot showing the activity of a striatal slice in control conditions. It exhibits a few active neurons (y-axis = number of active neurons; files, x-axis = time = 3 min recording). No active neurons synchronized their bursting significantly with other neurons. Bottom: histogram representing activity displayed in the raster plot on top (sum of columns).

B. Top: After adding 8 μM NMDA to the bath saline more neurons become active (> 40). Colored dots shows peaks of significant spontaneous synchronization. Bottom: activity histogram shows the spontaneous peaks of synchronization (colored with asterisks) ($P<0.05$ dashed horizontal line).

C. Locally linear embedding (LLE) was used to reduce dimensions of the peaks of synchronization and to project the vectors in a two dimensional space. Column vectors representing similar neurons are represented by clusters of neighboring circles of the same color (network states). Note that neuronal aggregates follow a sequence when displaying their activity, that is, the microcircuit shows its dynamics as an activity cycle or phase sequence. This sequence of network states is robust and may repeat itself several times during about two hours of recording time (only one representative epoch = 3 min is shown).

D. Top: After dopamine depletion (DA-depletion) a striatal slice exhibits more active neurons than with NMDA (> 70). No NMDA is added to DA-depleted slices. That is, DA absence induces that more neurons in the microcircuit become active. Bottom: nevertheless, the same peak of synchrony repeats itself almost all the time during recording. That is, microcircuit dynamics is greatly lost. DA was lowered using the 6-OHDA model of Parkinsonism. The toxin was injected into the substantia nigra pars compacta and the experiments were done after observing turning behavior in lesioned animals.

E: LLE obtained from a DA-depleted slice shows that one network state becomes dominant impeding normal dynamics.

F: When a dopamine receptor agonist (1 μM SKF-81296) is administered in a slice with DA-depletion, diverse peaks of synchrony with high probability of occurrence return. However, the number of active neurons is still high.

G: LLE shows that microcircuit dynamics tends to be restored because the dominant network state is dissolved (see: Carrillo-Reid et al., 2008; Carrillo-Reid et al., 2009; Jaidar et al., 2010).

way from each other (Stern et al., 1997; Carrillo-Reid et al., 2008). Strikingly, in the striatal parkinsonian microcircuit all active neurons synchronize their bursts with one another (Jaidar et al., 2010). No matter what is the predominant component of an up-state: intrinsic, synaptic or both, the important feature is that up-states work as "windows" for synchronization and correlated activity (Yuste et al., 2005), while action potentials within the up-states need not be synchronized (Wickens and Wilson, 1998). A signature of a CAs is that its inputs do not determine all its outputs all the time, in a deterministic way. On the contrary, the spike trains are variable due to the simultaneous integration of inputs within internal circuitry states (Arieli et al., 1996; Grinvald et al., 2003; Harris, 2005).

As stated by the modified Hebbian learning theory, sets of neurons display synchronous or correlated firing because LTP has strengthened the connections among them: "neurons that fire together wire together", whereas LTD has weakened some synapses due to their uncorrelated firing leading to the separation of different neuronal aggregates. Thus, connections within a neuronal ensemble are non-random (Kozloski et al., 2001; Song et al., 2005; Planert et al., 2010). There are preferred pathways for the flow of activity (Markram et al., 1997; Ikegaya et al., 2004; Song et al., 2005) even if anatomically they seem intermingled (Grinvald et al., 2003; Harris, 2005; Song et al., 2005). In conclusion, recurrent bursting elicited in striatal neurons can be seen as the product of correlated firing among neurons belonging to groups or ensembles. The time window for synchronization is the up-state and the product of the ensemble is the same up-state shared by the neurons of the ensemble. Most probably, neurons sharing up-states do in fact maintain these plateau potentials along time due to their strong interconnections (Flores-Barrera et al., 2010).

6. Microcircuit dynamics as sequences of network states

In what follows, a peak of synchronized activity generated by the members of a neuron aggregate or cluster will be called a network state. Therefore, what is recorded using calcium imaging is sequences of network states. That is, different neuronal aggregates with correlated firing, alternate the activity among them following determined sequences (Figure). These sequences result in particular trajectories, sometimes following Hamiltonian or Eulerian rules (Carrillo-Reid et al., 2009). In the case of CPGs, it is clear that what flows through the circuit is the correlated activity of neuron pools that activate in a rhythmic, alternating and recurrent way, making up sequences of activity called "activity cycles" (Grillner, 2003). Activity cycles code for repetitive behaviors such as locomotion, deglutition, swimming, scratching and so on. Activity cycles can go on spontaneously even when the physiological stimulus is no longer active, such as in vitro "ficitive locomotion" (Guertin and Hounsgaard, 1998).

But recursive activity of this sort has also been postulated for CAs where they are called "phase sequences" by DO Hebb (1949), a term coined for chains of neuronal aggregates activated in sequence, each one displaying a network state (Harris, 2005).

In the striatum, the trajectories followed by active CAs may change as a result of the presence of particular modulatory neurotransmitters (Carrillo-Reid et al., 2008; Carrillo-Reid et al., 2009a). This quality allows the striatal circuit to generate diverse phase sequences that probably code for different behaviors while using the same neuronal aggregates.

Interestingly, in the absence of DA, phase sequences are lost. Almost all active neurons participate in the same, repetitive, network state, that apparently is not coding for a useful command or motor program (Jaidar et al., 2010). The normal dynamics of the microcircuit is

gone (Figure). Addition of DA agonists under DA depleted states is capable to modify this state of affairs and partially restore a phase sequence (Jaidar et al., 2010).
To conclude, the striatal microcircuit generates phase sequences, activity trajectories, or cycles, that are lost during DA-depletion but that can be partially restored with DA receptor agonists. Because these methods allow the visualization of these phenomena with single cell resolution, they may be used to test anti-parkinsonian drugs and to search into the details of microcircuitry processing.

7. Final remarks

Over the last century two main visions of neuronal circuits have been generated from experimental data: First, the theory of Central Pattern Generators (CPGs) and, second, the theory of Hebbian Cell Assemblies. What we would like to stress here is that the time has come for a re-synthesis of both into a new microcircuit hypothesis, while new experimental evidence arrives. For instance, their requirements are very much the same. And since they were proposed somewhat independently, we have to conclude that biological evidence that put them forward is robust. Imaging technology used in conjunction with targeted recordings will allow the discerning of their operational rules in control and in pathological situations (Cossart et al., 2003; Grinvald et al., 2003; Carrillo-Reid et al., 2008 ; 2009a; Jaidar et al., 2010). It perhaps will be possible to record, compare and describe diverse pathological microcircuits. These microcircuits could then be challenged with therapeutic manipulations of potential value.

8. References

Alaburda A, Russo R, MacAulay N, Hounsgaard J (2005) Periodic high-conductance states in spinal neurons during scratch-like network activity in adult turtles. J Neurosci 25:6316-6321.

Alexander GE, Crutcher MD (1990) Functional architecture of basal ganglia circuits: neural substrates of parallel processing. Trends Neurosci 13:266-271.

Arieli A, Sterkin A, Grinvald A, Aertsen A (1996) Dynamics of ongoing activity: explanation of the large variability in evoked cortical responses. Science 273:1868-1871.

Bargas J, Galarraga E, Aceves J (1988) Electrotonic properties of neostriatal neurons are modulated by extracellular potassium. Exp Brain Res 72:390-398.

Bargas J, Galarraga E, Aceves J (1989) An early outward conductance modulates the firing latency and frequency of neostriatal neurons of the rat brain. Exp Brain Res 75:146-156.

Bargas J, Ayala CX, Vilchis C, Pineda JC, Galarraga E (1999) Ca^{2+}-activated outward currents in neostriatal neurons. Neurosci 88:479-488.

Berke JD, Okatan M, Skurski J, Eichenbaum HB (2004) Oscillatory entrainment of striatal neurons in freely moving rats. Neuron 43:883-896.

Bjorklund A, Dunnett SB (2007) Dopamine neuron systems in the brain: an update. Trends Neurosci 30:194-202.

Blandini F, Nappi G, Tassorelli C, Martignoni E (2000) Functional changes of the basal ganglia circuitry in Parkinson's disease. Prog Neurobiol 62:63-88.

Bowles R (2006) Investigating the Storage Capacity of a Network with Cell Assemblies. In. UK: Middlesex University.
Brown P (2007) Abnormal oscillatory synchronisation in the motor system leads to impaired movement. Curr Opin Neurobiol 17:656-664.
Calvin WH, Stevens CF (1968) Synaptic noise and other sources of randomness in motoneuron interspike intervals. J Neurophysiol 31:574-587.
Carrillo-Reid L, Tecuapetla F, Ibanez-Sandoval O, Hernandez-Cruz A, Galarraga E, Bargas J (2009) Activation of the cholinergic system endows compositional properties to striatal cell assemblies. J Neurophysiol 101:737-749.
Carrillo-Reid L, Tecuapetla F, Tapia D, Hernandez-Cruz A, Galarraga E, Drucker-Colin R, Bargas J (2008) Encoding network states by striatal cell assemblies. J Neurophysiol 99:1435-1450.
Cossart R, Aronov D, Yuste R (2003) Attractor dynamics of network UP states in the neocortex. Nature 423:283-288.
Costa RM, Lin SC, Sotnikova TD, Cyr M, Gainetdinov RR, Caron MG, Nicolelis MA (2006) Rapid alterations in corticostriatal ensemble coordination during acute dopamine-dependent motor dysfunction. Neuron 52:359-369.
Crutcher MD, DeLong MR (1984) Single cell studies of the primate putamen. II. Relations to direction of movement and pattern of muscular activity. Exp Brain Res 53:244-258.
Destexhe A, Pare D (1999) Impact of network activity on the integrative properties of neocortical pyramidal neurons in vivo. J Neurophysiol 81:1531-1547.
Diesmann M, Gewaltig MO, Aertsen A (1999) Stable propagation of synchronous spiking in cortical neural networks. Nature 402:529-533.
Doupe AJ, Solis MM, Kimpo R, Boettiger CA (2004) Cellular, circuit, and synaptic mechanisms in song learning. Ann N Y Acad Sci 1016:495-523.
Flores-Barrera E, Vizcarra-Chacon BJ, Tapia D, Bargas J, Galarraga E (2010) Different corticostriatal integration in spiny projection neurons from direct and indirect pathways. Front Syst Neurosci 4:15.
Fuentes R, Petersson P, Siesser WB, Caron MG, Nicolelis MA (2009) Spinal cord stimulation restores locomotion in animal models of Parkinson's disease. Science 323:1578-1582.
Galarraga E, Bargas J, Martinez-Fong D, Aceves J (1987) Spontaneous synaptic potentials in dopamine-denervated neostriatal neurons. Neurosci Lett 81:351-355.
Galarraga E, Bargas J, Sierra A, Aceves J (1989) The role of calcium in the repetitive firing of neostriatal neurons. Exp Brain Res 75:157-168.
Galarraga E, Pacheco-Cano MT, Flores-Hernández JV, Bargas J (1994) Subthreshold rectification in neostriatal spiny projection neurons. Exp Brain Res 100:239-249.
Galvan A, Wichmann T (2008) Pathophysiology of parkinsonism. Clin Neurophysiol 119:1459-1474.
Gerfen CR, Engber TM, Mahan LC, Susel Z, Chase TN, Monsma FJ, Jr., Sibley DR (1990) D1 and D2 dopamine receptor-regulated gene expression of striatonigral and striatopallidal neurons. Science 250:1429-1432.
Grillner S (2003) The motor infrastructure: from ion channels to neuronal networks. Nat Rev Neurosci 4:573-586.
Grillner S (2006) Biological pattern generation: the cellular and computational logic of networks in motion. Neuron 52:751-766.

Grillner S, McClellan A, Sigvardt K, Wallen P, Wilen M (1981) Activation of NMDA-receptors elicits "fictive locomotion" in lamprey spinal cord in vitro. Acta Physiol Scand 113:549-551.

Grinvald A (2005) Imaging input and output dynamics of neocortical networks in vivo: exciting times ahead. Proc Natl Acad Sci U S A 102:14125-14126.

Grinvald A, Arieli A, Tsodyks M, Kenet T (2003) Neuronal assemblies: single cortical neurons are obedient members of a huge orchestra. Biopolymers 68:422-436.

Guertin PA, Hounsgaard J (1998) NMDA-Induced intrinsic voltage oscillations depend on L-type calcium channels in spinal motoneurons of adult turtles. J Neurophysiol 80:3380-3382.

Hammond C, Bergman H, Brown P (2007) Pathological synchronization in Parkinson's disease: networks, models and treatments. Trends Neurosci 30:357-364.

Harris KD (2005) Neural signatures of cell assembly organization. Nature Rev Neurosci 6:399-407.

Hebb DO (1949) The organization of behavior. New York: Wiley.

Herrling PL, Morris R, Salt TE (1983) Effects of excitatory amino acids and their antagonists on membrane and action potentials of cat caudate neurones. J Physiol 339:207-222.

Hikosaka O, Nakamura K, Nakahara H (2006) Basal ganglia orient eyes to reward. J Neurophysiol 95:567-584.

Hounsgaard J, Kiehn O (1989) Serotonin-induced bistability of turtle motoneurones caused by a nifedipine-sensitive calcium plateau potential. J Physiol 414:265-282.

Hsiao CF, Del Negro CA, Trueblood PR, Chandler SH (1998) Ionic basis for serotonin-induced bistable membrane properties in guinea pig trigeminal motoneurons. J Neurophysiol 79:2847-2856.

Ibáñez-Sandoval O, Tecuapetla F, Unal B, Shah F, Koós T, Tepper JM (2010) Electrophysiological and morphological characteristics and synaptic connectivity of tyrosine hydroxylase-expressing neurons in adult mouse striatum. J Neurosci 30:6999-7016.

Ibáñez-Sandoval O, Carrillo-Reid L, Galarraga E, Tapia D, Mendoza E, Gomora JC, Aceves J, Bargas J (2007) Bursting in substantia nigra pars reticulata neurons in vitro: possible relevance for Parkinson disease. J Neurophysiol 98:2311-2323.

Ikegaya Y, Aaron G, Cossart R, Aronov D, Lampl I, Ferster D, Yuste R (2004) Synfire chains and cortical songs: temporal modules of cortical activity. Science 304:559-564.

Izhikevich EM, Edelman GM (2008) Large-scale model of mammalian thalamocortical systems. Proc Natl Acad Sci U S A 105:3593-3598.

Jaidar O, Carrillo-Reid L, Hernandez A, Drucker-Colin R, Bargas J, Hernandez-Cruz A (2010) Dynamics of the Parkinsonian striatal microcircuit: entrainment into a dominant network state. J Neurosci 30:11326-11336.

Kawaguchi Y, Wilson CJ, Augood SJ, Emson PC (1995) Striatal interneurones: chemical, physiological and morphological characterization. Trends Neurosci 18:527-535.

Kiehn O (2006) Locomotor circuits in the mammalian spinal cord. Annu Rev Neurosci 29:279-306.

Kimura M (1992) Behavioral modulation of sensory responses of primate putamen neurons. Brain Res 578:204-214.

Kita H, Kitai ST (1991) Intracellular study of rat globus pallidus neurons: membrane properties and responses to neostriatal, subthalamic and nigral stimulation. Brain Res 564:296-305.

Kostal L, Lansky P, Rospars JP (2007) Neuronal coding and spiking randomness. Eur J Neurosci 26:2693-2701.

Kozloski J, Hamzei-Sichani F, Yuste R (2001) Stereotyped position of local synaptic targets in neocortex. Science 293:868-872.

Kozlov A, Huss M, Lansner A, Kotaleski JH, Grillner S (2009) Simple cellular and network control principles govern complex patterns of motor behavior. Proc Natl Acad Sci U S A 106:20027-20032.

Kreitzer AC (2009) Physiology and pharmacology of striatal neurons. Annu Rev Neurosci 32:127-147.

Lambe EK, Aghajanian GK (2007) Prefrontal cortical network activity: Opposite effects of psychedelic hallucinogens and D1/D5 dopamine receptor activation. Neuroscience 145:900-910.

Leger JF, Stern EA, Aertsen A, Heck D (2005) Synaptic integration in rat frontal cortex shaped by network activity. J Neurophysiol 93:281-293.

Li X, Ouyang G, Usami A, Ikegaya Y, Sik A (2010) Scale-free topology of the CA3 hippocampal network: a novel method to analyze functional neuronal assemblies. Biophys J 98:1733-1741.

Liang L, DeLong MR, Papa SM (2008) Inversion of dopamine responses in striatal medium spiny neurons and involuntary movements. J Neurosci 28:7537-7547.

Magill PJ, Bolam JP, Bevan MD (2001) Dopamine regulates the impact of the cerebral cortex on the subthalamic nucleus-globus pallidus network. Neuroscience 106:313-330.

Mahon S, Vautrelle N, Pezard L, Slaght SJ, Deniau JM, Chouvet G, Charpier S (2006) Distinct patterns of striatal medium spiny neuron activity during the natural sleep-wake cycle. J Neurosci 26:12587-12595.

Markram H, Lubke J, Frotscher M, Roth A, Sakmann B (1997) Physiology and anatomy of synaptic connections between thick tufted pyramidal neurones in the developing rat neocortex. J Physiol 500 (Pt 2):409-440.

Middleton FA, Strick PL (2002) Basal-ganglia 'projections' to the prefrontal cortex of the primate. Cereb Cortex 12:926-935.

Murer MG, Tseng KY, Kasanetz F, Belluscio M, Riquelme LA (2002) Brain oscillations, medium spiny neurons, and dopamine. Cell Mol Neurobiol 22:611-632.

Nakanishi H, Kita H, Kitai ST (1987) Electrical membrane properties of rat subthalamic neurons in an in vitro slice preparation. Brain Res 437:35-44.

Ni ZG, Bouali-Benazzouz R, Gao DM, Benabid AL, Benazzouz A (2001) Time-course of changes in firing rates and firing patterns of subthalamic nucleus neuronal activity after 6-OHDA-induced dopamine depletion in rats. Brain Res 899:142-147.

Nisenbaum ES, Wilson CJ (1995) Potassium currents responsible for inward and outward rectification in rat neostriatal spiny projection neurons. J Neurosci 15:4449-4463.

Ossowska K (1995) Interaction between striatal excitatory amino acid and gamma-aminobutyric acid (GABA) receptors in the turning behaviour of rats. Neurosci Lett 202:57-60.

Parr-Brownlie LC, Poloskey SL, Bergstrom DA, Walters JR (2009) Parafascicular thalamic nucleus activity in a rat model of Parkinson's disease. Exp Neurol 217:269-281.

Petersen CC, Sakmann B (2000) The excitatory neuronal network of rat layer 4 barrel cortex. J Neurosci 20:7579-7586.

Pineda JC, Galarraga E, Bargas J, Cristancho JM, Aceves J (1992) Charybdotoxin and apamin sensitivity of the calcium-dependent repolarization and the afterhyperpolarization in neostriatal neurons. J Neurophysiol 68:287-294.

Planert H, Szydlowski SN, Hjorth JJ, Grillner S, Silberberg G (2010) Dynamics of synaptic transmission between fast-spiking interneurons and striatal projection neurons of the direct and indirect pathways. J Neurosci 30:3499-3507.

Reyes A, Galarraga E, Flores-Hernández J, Tapia D, Bargas J (1998) Passive properties of neostriatal neurons during potassium conductance blockade. Exp Brain Res 120:70-84.

Robbe D, Montgomery SM, Thome A, Rueda-Orozco PE, McNaughton BL, Buzsaki G (2006) Cannabinoids reveal importance of spike timing coordination in hippocampal function. Nat Neurosci 9:1526-1533.

Rommelfanger KS, Wichmann T (2010) Extrastriatal dopaminergic circuits of the basal ganglia. Front Neuroanat 4:139.

Sakurai Y (1996) Hippocampal and neocortical cell assemblies encode memory processes for different types of stimuli in the rat. J Neurosci 16:2809-2819.

Sanchez-Vives MV, McCormick DA (2000) Cellular and network mechanisms of rhythmic recurrent activity in neocortex. Nat Neurosci 3:1027-1034.

Shadlen MN, Newsome WT (1994) Noise, neural codes and cortical organization. Curr Opin Neurobiol 4:569-579.

Shen W, Hamilton SE, Nathanson NM, Surmeier DJ (2005) Cholinergic suppression of KCNQ channel currents enhances excitability of striatal medium spiny neurons. J Neurosci 25:7449-7458.

Smith Y, Bevan MD, Shink E, Bolam JP (1998) Microcircuitry of the direct and indirect pathways of the basal ganglia. Neuroscience 86:353-387.

Smith Y, Bennett BD, Bolam JP, Parent A, Sadikot AF (1994) Synaptic relationships between dopaminergic afferents and cortical or thalamic input in the sensorimotor territory of the striatum in monkey. J Comp Neurol 344:1-19.

Song S, Sjostrom PJ, Reigl M, Nelson S, Chklovskii DB (2005) Highly nonrandom features of synaptic connectivity in local cortical circuits. PLoS Biol 3:e68.

Stern EA, Kincaid AE, Wilson CJ (1997) Spontaneous subthreshold membrane potential fluctuations and action potential variability of rat corticostriatal and striatal neurons in vivo. J Neurophysiol 77:1697-1715.

Surmeier DJ, Bargas J, Kitai ST (1988) Voltage-clamp analysis of a transient potassium current in rat neostriatal neurons. Brain Res 473:187-192.

Tal Z, Chorev E, Yarom Y (2008) State-dependent modification of complex spike waveforms in the cerebellar cortex. Cerebellum 7:577-582.

Tang K, Low MJ, Grandy DK, Lovinger DM (2001) Dopamine-dependent synaptic plasticity in striatum during in vivo development. Proc Natl Acad Sci U S A 98:1255-1260.

Tepper JM, Koos T, Wilson CJ (2004) GABAergic microcircuits in the neostriatum. Trends Neurosci 27:662-669.

Tepper JM, Tecuapetla F, Koos T, Ibanez-Sandoval O (2010) Heterogeneity and diversity of striatal GABAergic interneurons. Front Neuroanat 4:150.

Tseng KY, Kasanetz F, Kargieman L, Riquelme LA, Murer MG (2001) Cortical slow oscillatory activity is reflected in the membrane potential and spike trains of striatal neurons in rats with chronic nigrostriatal lesions. J Neurosci 21:6430-6439.

Vautrelle N, Carrillo-Reid, L., Bargas, J. (2009) Diversity of up-state voltage transitions during different network states. In: Cortico-Subcortical Dynamics in Parkinson Disease (Tseng KY, ed), pp 73-85. New York: Humana/Springer.

Vergara R, Rick C, Hernandez-Lopez S, Laville JA, Guzman JN, Galarraga E, Surmeier DJ, Bargas J (2003) Spontaneous voltage oscillations in striatal projection neurons in a rat corticostriatal slice. J Physiol 553:169-182.

Walters JR, Bergstrom DA (2009) Basal ganglia network synchronization in animal models of Parkinson's disease. In: Cortico-Subcortical Dynamics in Parkinson Disease (Tseng KY, ed), pp 117-142. New York: Humana/Springer.

Walters JR, Hu D, Itoga CA, Parr-Brownlie LC, Bergstrom DA (2007) Phase relationships support a role for coordinated activity in the indirect pathway in organizing slow oscillations in basal ganglia output after loss of dopamine. Neuroscience 144:762-776.

Wickens JR, Wilson CJ (1998) Regulation of action-potential firing in spiny neurons of the rat neostriatum in vivo. J Neurophysiol 79:2358-2364.

Wilson CJ (1993) The generation of natural firing patterns in neostriatal neurons. Prog Brain Res 99:277-297.

Wilson CJ, Kawaguchi Y (1996) The origins of two-state spontaneous membrane potential fluctuations of neostriatal spiny neurons. J Neurosci 16:2397-2410.

Wilson CJ, Chang HT, Kitai ST (1990) Firing patterns and synaptic potentials of identified giant aspiny interneurons in the rat neostriatum. J Neurosci 10:508-519.

Wilson CL, Cash D, Galley K, Chapman H, Lacey MG, Stanford IM (2006) Subthalamic nucleus neurones in slices from 1-methyl-4-phenyl-1,2,3,6-tetrahydropyridine-lesioned mice show irregular, dopamine-reversible firing pattern changes, but without synchronous activity. Neuroscience 143:565-572.

Yanagawa T, Mogi K (2009) Analysis of ongoing dynamics in neural networks. Neurosci Res 64:177-184.

Yuste R, MacLean JN, Smith J, Lansner A (2005) The cortex as a central pattern generator. Nat Rev Neurosci 6:477-483.

Zold CL, Belluscio M, Kasanetz F, Pomata PE, Riquelme LA, Gonon F, Murer MG (2009) Converging into a unified model of Parkinson's disease pathophysiology. In: Cortico-Subcortical Dynamics in Parkinson Disease (Tseng KY, ed), pp 143-156. New York: Humana/Springer.

17

Animal Models of Parkinson's Disease Induced by Toxins and Genetic Manipulation

Shin Hisahara and Shun Shimohama
Department of Neurology, Sapporo Medical University, Japan

1. Introduction

Parkinson's disease (PD) is one of the most common chronic neurodegenerative disorders. It is characterized by a variety of motor (bradykinesia, rigidity, tremor, and postural instability) and nonmotor (autonomic disturbances and psychosis) symptoms. Although it can be diagnosed accurately, no therapeutic strategies can cure or completely block the progression of PD. Pathologically, PD is characterized by the severe loss of dopaminergic (DAergic) neurons in the pars-compacta nigra and the presence of proteinaceous α-synuclein inclusions, called Lewy bodies (LBs), which are present in neurons of the central nervous system (specific cortical regions, brain stem, and spinal cord), peripheral autonomic nervous system, enteric nervous system (ENS), and cutaneous nerves (Braak et al., 2006; Ikemura et al., 2008; Lebouvier et al., 2009). Similar to other neurodegenerative diseases, such as Alzheimer's disease, age is the major risk factor for PD although 10% of the people with the disease are younger than 45.

Although PD is regarded as a sporadic disorder, remarkably few environmental causes or triggers have been identified (Dick et al., 2007; Tanner, 2003; Taylor et al., 2005). Pesticides and herbicides are the most likely candidates for environmental agents associated with the pathogenesis of PD. On the other hand, PD characteristics are seen in a number of familial motor disorders caused by different genetic factors. Animal models of neurodegenerative diseases, including PD, have in general been quite instructive in understanding their pathogenesis. Ideally, animal models of PD, whether induced by environmental risk factors (neurotoxins) or genetic manipulations, should faithfully reproduce the clinical manifestations (behavioral abnormalities), pathological features, and molecular dysfunctions characterizing the disease. Unfortunately, animal models rarely mimic the etiology, progression, and pathology of PD completely, and in most cases, only partial insight can be gained from these studies. Despite these difficulties, animal models are considered to be very helpful in the development of therapies to treat PD. In this paper, we discuss recently developed neurotoxin-induced and genetic model animals of PD.

Over the years, many chemical compounds and toxin have been identified causative agents of PD. 1-Methyl-4-phenyl-1,2,3,6-tetrahydropyridine (MPTP) is a representative strong neurotoxin that has been recognized from several young drug addicts developed severe parkinsonism. The addicts illegally achieved street preparations of drugs and products were contaminated with MPTP. In addition, epidemiologically, environmental neurotoxins such as agricultural chemicals (pesticides, herbicides, and fungicides) are promising candidates for causative factors of PD. Rotenone and paraquat could promote and accelerate the development of PD. Oxidative stress and mitochondrial dysfunction induced by these toxins could contribute to the progression of PD. While most cases of PD are sporadic, specific mutations in genes that cause familial forms of PD have led to provide new insights into its pathogenesis. Analysis of these gene products may provide vital clues to our understanding of the molecular pathogenesis of dopaminergic neuronal death in PD.

Over 10 causative genes for autosomal-dominant (*α-synuclein, Ubiqitin carboxy-terminal hydrolase L1 (UCHL1),* and *Leucine-rich repeat kinase 2 (LRRK2)*) or autosomal-recessive (*parkin, phosphatase and tensin homolog deleted on chromosome ten (PTEN)-induced putative kinase 1 (PINK1),* and *DJ-1* inheritance PD have been identified and classified for PARK loci. Studying animal models are important tools in experimental medical science for understanding the pathogenesis and therapeutic intervention strategies of human diseases, including neurodegenerative diseases such as PD. However, it is quite difficult to completely reproduce symptomatic and pathological features of human disorders. Since many human diseases including PD do not arise spontaneously in animals, in particular, characteristic functional changes have to be mimicked by neurotoxic agents. Nevertheless, recent studies have indicated excellent neurotoxin-induced animal models of PD. In addition, many genetic animal models of familial PD have been generated and recognized valuable tools for investigating and understanding pathophysiology of familial and even sporadic PD. Apart from the obvious preference for vertebrate (rodents and primates) models to investigate PD, an increasing number of studies have also shown a number of advantages and the utility of invertebrate (flies and nematodes) models. The central nervous system of invertebrate animal has a rather small number of neuron and glia as compared to vertebrates, however, essential functional features such as neurotransmitter system of vertebrates and invertebrates are conserved. This chapter focuses on animal models of both toxin-induced and genetically determined PD that have provided significant insight for understanding this disease. We also discuss the validity, benefits, and limitations of representative models.

2. Neurotoxin-induced animal models of PD

PD is currently viewed as a multifactorial disease. Environmental exposures, particularly to pesticides, are thought to be involved in the pathogenesis of sporadic PD. Specifically, the herbicide Paraquat (PQ) and the fungicide Maneb (manganese ethylene-bis-dithiocarbamate) have been associated with the incidence of PD (Ascherio et al., 2006; Ferraz et al., 1988). However, a causal role for pesticides in the etiology of PD has yet to be definitively established. In animal models, PD-like disorders induced by neurotoxins or other chemical compounds have led to a better understanding of the pathophysiology of PD (Table 1).

2.1 1-Methyl-4-Phenyl-1,2,3,6-Tetrahydropyridine (MPTP)

In 1979 and 1983, MPTP was initially identified as a strong neurotoxin when heroin addicts accidentally self-administered MPTP and developed an acute form of parkinsonism that was indistinguishable from idiopathic PD (Davis et al., 1979; Langston et al., 1999). A detailed neuropathological study of MPTP-induced parkinsonism in humans showed severe neuronal degeneration in the substantia nigra and the absence of LBs (Langston, et al., 1999).

Neurotoxin	Behavioral and Pathological Features	Molecular Mechanisms
MPTP	1) Parkinsonism (akinesia, rigidity, and tremor) with acute onset 2) Relatively less potent in rodents 3) Good response to L-DOPA and DA-agonists 4) Loss of TH-neurons (-fibers) and DA-content in nigrostriatal region 5) Loss of TH-neurons (-fibers) in ENS 6) α-Synuclein-positive inclusions 7) No typical LBs	1) Easily crosses the BBB 2) Converted to MPP^+ in glial cells 3) Transferred into mitochondria by transporters 4) Inhibits electron transport chain complex I 5) Upregulation of iNOS, NADPH-oxidase, and ROS 6) Microglial activation
6-OHDA	1) Intracerebral administration 2) Quantifiable locomotor abnormalities (rotation, akinsesia) 3) Good response to L-DOPA and DA-agonists 4) Loss of TH-neurons (-fibers) and DA-content in nigrostriatal region 5) No typical LBs	1) Transferred into mitochondria by transporters 2) Inhibits electron transport chain complex I 3) Microglial activation
Rotenone	1) Parkinsonism (bradykinesia, fixed posture, and rigidity) 2) Good response to L-DOPA and DA-agonists 3) Loss of TH-neurons (-fibers) and DA-content in nigrostriatal region 4) α-Synuclein-positive inclusions, resemblance to true LBs 5) Loss of myenteric neurons	1) Easily crosses the BBB 2) Inhibits electron transport chain complex I 3) Upregulation of NADPH-oxidase 4) Microglial activation
Paraquat (+ Maneb)	1) Parkinsonism similar to that of induced by MPTP 2) Loss of DA-content in nigrostriatal region 3) α-Synuclein-positive inclusions with long exposure	1) Crosses the BBB by neutral amino acid transporter 2) Inhibits electron transport chain complex I 3) Reduction of nAchR-mediated DA release 4) Inhibits complex III (Maneb)

Abbreviations: MPTP, 1-Methyl-4-phenyl-1,2,3,6-tetrahydropyridine; 6-OHDA, 6-hydroxy-dopamine; Maneb, manganese ethylene-bis-dithiocarbamate; L-DOPA, L-3,4-dihydroxy-L-phenylalanine; TH, tyrosine hydroxylase; DA, dopamine; ENS, enteric nervous system; LB, Lewy body; BBB, blood-brain barrier; MPP^+, 1-methyl-4-phenylpyridinium; iNOS, inducible nitric oxide synthase; ROS, reactive oxygen species; NADPH, nicotinamide adenine dinucleotide phosphate; nAchR, nicotinic acetylcholine receptor

Table 1. Representative neurotoxin-induced mammalian models of PD

The lack of LBs may have reflected the age of the patient and the duration of exposure to MPTP. The tragic results of MPTP poisoning in the heroin addicts led to the development of MPTP-induced rodent and nonhuman primate animal models of PD, which have proved extremely valuable (Chiueh et al., 1984; Kopin & Markey, 1988; Langston et al., 1984; Langston & Irwin, 1986; Markey et al., 1984). The MPTP-exposed primates show good response to therapy with L-3,4-dihydroxy-L-phenylalanine (L-DOPA) and dopamine (DA) receptor agonists (Kopin & Markey, 1988; Langston & Irwin, 1986). However, rats are relatively insensitive to MPTP neurotoxicity compared with primates. Rats given MPTP at doses comparable to those used in mice do not show remarkable neurodegeneration

(Giovanni et al., 1994; Giovanni et al., 1994). Only high doses of MPTP cause DAergic neurodegeneration in rats, indicating that complete blockade of the DA receptors is required for them to display signs of parkinsonism. Mice, like rats, are also less sensitive to MPTP than primates (Przedborski et al., 2001; Schmidt & Ferger, 2001). This model also shows pathological changes in the ENS, as observed in PD. In PD, gastrointestinal (GI) dysfunction was hypothesized to depend on neuronal degeneration in the ENS that is similar to that seen in the CNS. Recent studies show that the administration of MPTP results in decreased tyrosine hydroxylase- (TH-) positive enteric neurons in mice, indicating that the MPTP model mice should be suitable for understanding the extranigral pathophysiology of PD (Anderson et al., 2007; Natale et al., 2010).

2.2 6-Hydroxy-Dopamine (6-OHDA)

Like MPTP, 6-OHDA is a neurotoxin that has been successfully used in induction animal models of PD. 6-OHDA's strong neurotoxic effects were described by Ungerstedt in 1971, in a study presenting the first example of using a chemical agent to produce an animal model of PD (Ungerstedt, 1971). Since 6-OHDA cannot cross the blood-brain barrier (BBB), systemic administration fails to induce parkinsonism. This induction model requires 6-OHDA to be injected into the substantia nigra, medial forebrain bundle, and striatum (Perez & Palmiter, 2005; Przedborski et al., 1995). The effects resemble those in the acute MPTP model, causing neuronal death over a brief time course (12 hours to 2-3 days). Interestingly, the intrastriatal injection of 6-OHDA causes progressive retrograde neuronal degeneration in the substantia nigra and ventral tegmental complex (ST-VTA) (Berger et al., 1991; Przedborski, et al., 1995; Sauer & Oertel, 1994). As in PD, DAergic neurons are killed, and the non-DAergic neurons are preserved. However LBs do not form. Typically, 6-OHDA is used as a hemiparkinson model, in which its unilateral injection into the substantia nigra causes asymmetric motor behavior (turning, rotation) when apomorphine, a DAergic receptor agonist, or amphetamine, a dopamine releasing agent, is given systemically. In this model, the quantifiable motor behavior is a major advantage for screening pharmacological screening agents for their effects on the DAergic system and for testing cell replacement therapies (Beal, 2001; Deumens et al., 2002; Hirsch et al., 2003).

2.3 Rotenone

Rotenone is a naturally occurring complex ketone pesticide derived from the roots of *Lonchocarpus* species. It can rapidly cross cellular membranes without the aid of transporters, including the BBB. Rotenone is a strong inhibitor of complex I, which is located at the innermitochondrial membrane and protrudes into the matrix. In 2000, Betarbet et al. demonstrated in rats that chronic systemic exposure to rotenone causes many features of PD, including nigrostriatal DAergic degeneration (Betarbet et al., 2000). Importantly, pathological features match those seen in typical PD. For example, many of the degenerating neurons have intracellular inclusions that are morphologically similar to LBs. These inclusions also show immunoreactivity for α–synuclein and ubiquitin, like true LBs (Betarbet, et al., 2000; Sherer et al., 2003). The rotenone-administered model animals also reproduce all the behavioral and pathological features seen in the typical form of human PD. However, rotenone-injected rats without nigrostriatal DAergic neuronal loss demonstrate the same abnormal motor behaviors as those with such pathological features (Lapointe et al., 2004; Sherer, et al., 2003). This finding suggested that the abnormal behaviors of PD could depend, at least partly, on the damage to non-DAergic neurons in the nigrostriatal area. Furthermore, rotenone exposure also causes the loss of myenteric neurons in the rat (Drolet et al., 2009).

2.4 Paraquat and maneb

Because of its close structural similarity to 1-methyl-4-phenylpyridinium (MPP+, the active metabolite form of MPTP), an herbicide, 1,1′-dimethyl-4,4′-bipyridinium, named paraquat has been suggested as a risk factor for PD (Di Monte et al., 1986). The systemic administration of paraquat to adult mice results in a significant decrease in substantia nigra DAergic neurons, a decline in striatal dopamine nerve terminal density, and a neurobehavioral syndrome characterized by reduced ambulatory activity (Brooks et al., 1999). These data support the idea that paraquat crosses the BBB to cause destruction of the dopamine neurons in the substantia nigra, like MPP+ (Brooks, et al., 1999). The prolonged exposure to paraquat leads to a remarkable accumulation of α–synuclein-like aggregates in neurons of the substantia nigra pars compacta in mice (Manning-Bog et al., 2002). Chronic exposure to paraquat also reduces the expression of the nicotinic acetylcholine receptor (nAChR) subunit $\alpha 3/\alpha 6\beta 2*$ (the asterisk indicates the possible presence of additional subunits). Normally, the activation of both nAChR subtypes stimulates DA release in the striatum (Khwaja et al., 2007; McCallum et al., 2005; Wonnacott et al., 2000). The injection of paraquat selectively reduces the $\alpha 3/\alpha 6\beta 2*$-mediated DA release from the striatum in primates (O'Leary et al., 2008). Maneb is an organomanganese fungicide that is broadly used in agriculture and is a putative causative agent for PD. Surprisingly, Thiruchelvam et al. found that the neurotoxic effects of maneb or paraquat on the nigrostriatal DA system in mice are synergistically potentiated in combination (Thiruchelvam et al., 2000). Their report argued that this finding has important implications for the human risk of PD, because the marked geographical overlap in the estimated annual agricultural applications of paraquat and maneb means that people living in these areas may be exposed to the synergistic neurotoxicity of these two agents (Thiruchelvam, et al., 2000; Thiruchelvam et al., 2000).

3. Pathophysiological mechanisms of DAergic neurotoxins

All the representative neurotoxin-induced PD models described above show defective mitochondrial function, manifested by the inhibition of mitochondrial complex I or III. MPTP is a highly lipophilic agent. After its systemic administration, MPTP rapidly crosses the BBB. Once in the brain, MPTP is converted to 1-methyl-4-phenyl-2,3- dihydropyridium (MPDP+) in glial cells (astrocytes) and serotonin neurons by monoamine oxidase B (MAO-B) and then spontaneously oxidizes to MPP+ (Nicklas et al., 1985; Przedborski & Vila, 2003). Thereafter, MPP+ is released into the extracellular space. Unlike MPTP, MPP+ is a polar molecule that cannot freely enter DAergic neurons. Thus, a plasma membrane transport system is required. MPP+ has a high affinity for dopamine transporter (DAT) as well as for norepinephrine and serotonin transporters (Bezard et al., 1999; Mayer et al., 1986). Once inside DAergic neurons, MPP+ can accumulate in mitochondria and impair mitochondrial respiration by inhibiting complex I in the electron transport chain (Nicklas, et al., 1985; Ramsay & Singer, 1986), which induces the generation of reactive oxygen species (ROS). MPP+ can also bind to vesicular monoamine transporters (VMATs), which help move selected materials into synaptic vesicles containing DA (Del Zompo et al., 1993). MPP+ can also remain in the cytoplasm and interact with cytosolic enzymes (Klaidman et al., 1993).

Inducible nitric oxide synthase (iNOS) is also involved in the pathogenesis of MPP+-induced parkinsonism in animal models. Increased iNOS has also been found in the substantia nigra of autopsied PD patients, indicating that nitric oxide (NO) overproduction is a feature of the human disease (Huerta et al., 2007; Hunot et al., 1996). Excess NO could contribute to the formation of free radicals, which could damage DAergic neurons, leading to the development of PD symptoms. Mice null for iNOS show a resistance to neuronal damage by MPTP, and iNOS inhibitors protect against the degeneration of DAergic neurons in MPTP-treated mice (Dehmer et al., 2000; Liberatore et al., 1999). Furthermore, microglial cells can be activated by the formation of free radicals and iNOS-mediated damage, and thereby exacerbate the toxicity of MPTP (Barcia et al., 2004; Breidert et al., 2002; Wu et al., 2002). Finally, MPTP can also upregulate nicotinamide adenine dinucleotide phosphate (NADPH)-oxidase in the substantia nigra of mice (Wu, et al., 2002), which is significant because NADPH-oxidase appears to be ubiquitously expressed in all brain regions and metabolizes molecular oxygen, generating superoxide as a product. In fact, MPTP toxicity is diminished in mice lacking functional NADPH-oxidase, indicating a pivotal role for superoxide ions in the neurotoxicity induced by MPTP (Wu, et al., 2002).

The toxicity of 6-OHDA also involves mechanisms of oxidative stress. 6-OHDA can be taken up by DAergic neurons through DAT (Bove et al., 2005; Schober, 2004). Once transported into neurons, 6-OHDA is oxidized like DA. The oxidized molecule generates free radicals inhibits mitochondrial complex I and produces superoxide and hydroxyl radicals (Bove, et al., 2005; Schober, 2004). It is not only toxic to the DAergic neurons but can also induce microglial activation (Bove, et al., 2005).

Like MPTP, the pesticide rotenone is very lipophilic, crosses the BBB, and is distributed evenly throughout the brain (Bove, et al., 2005; Uversky, 2004). It can enter mitochondria, where it inhibits complex I of the electron transport chain with high affinity (Bove, et al., 2005). Interestingly, the inhibition of microglial activation by an antibiotic,minocycline, can attenuate the neurotoxicity of rotenone (Casarejos et al., 2006). Gao et al. also showed that the neurotoxicity of rotenone is reduced in neuron-glia cocultures from NADPH oxidase-null mice (Gao et al., 2003). The DA uptake of the neuron-enriched cultures was not affected by the addition of microglia from NADPH oxidase-null mice, the addition of microglia from wild-type (WT) mice significantly increased the sensitivity of DAergic neurons either from WT or knockout (KO) mice to rotenone neurotoxicity. These data indicate that microglial NADPH oxidase, but not neuronal NADPH oxidase, is responsible for the NADPH oxidase-mediated neurotoxicity of rotenone (Gao, et al., 2003). Paraquat mainly crosses the BBB through the neutral amino acid transporter (McCormack & Di Monte, 2003; Shimizu et al., 2003; Yang & Sun, 1998). Once in the brain, it is selectively taken up by the terminals of DA-containing neurons in the substantia nigra by the DAT, and it inhibits mitochondrial complex I (Shimizu, et al., 2003). Maneb contains a major active fungicidal component, manganese ethylene-bis-dithiocarbamate (Mn–EBDC). In a rat model in which Mn–EBDC is directly delivered to the lateral ventricles, Mn–EBDC causes selective DAergic neurodegeneration (Zhang et al., 2003). Mn–EBDC preferentially inhibits mitochondrial complex III (Zhang, et al., 2003).

4. Genetic animal models of PD

Although the etiopathogenesis (including environmental factors) of PD is not fully understood, the extensive examination of human postmortem material, the genetic analysis of patients, and the study of experimental animal models have shed significant light on the molecular mechanisms involved in its progression. However, since the number of patients with familial PD is extremely low compared to the number with sporadic PD, genetic studies in affected human families are very difficult. Therefore, the development of animal genetic models for PD is especially important, and such models provide an opportunity not only to investigate the genetic etiology of PD but also to identify new factors that could be invaluable in terms of diagnosis, drug design, and/or therapy (Gasser, 2009; Lees et al., 2009). Even invertebrate animals, for example, *Drosophila melanogaster*, are useful models for surveys of human PD. While their numbers of neurons and glia are obviously much smaller than in rodents and primates, *Drosophila* have the same types of neuron-glia systems, and a great number of genes and molecular transduction pathways are conserved between *Drosophila* and humans.

In recent years, several genetic animal models of PD have been reported, including models for autosomal-dominant (AD) inheritance patterns. The genes manipulated in these models include *α-synuclein, LRRK2, UCHL1*, and *high temperature requirement A2* (*HTRA2/Omi*) (Table 2). There are also models of autosomal-recessive (AR) inherited PD, which involve KO or knockdown genes for *parkin, DJ-1*, and *PINK1* (Table 3). In addition, we will review a PD mouse model deficient in *nuclear receptor-related 1* (*Nurr1*), also named *nuclear receptor subfamily 4, group A, member 2* (*NR4A2*), which is a susceptibility gene for familial PD (Table 3).

Gene	Animal	Manipulation	DA neuron loss	LB-like inclusions[1]	DA-responsive motor deficits[2]
α-synuclein (*PARK1*)	Nematode	Transgenic	Yes§	No	Yes
	Fly	Transgenic	Yes	Yes	Yes
	Mouse	Transgenic	No	Yes§ (PrP promoter)	Yes§ (PDGFβ promoter)
	Rat	Transgenic	Yes	No	Yes
	Monkey	Transgenic	Yes	No	ND
UCHL1 (*PARK5*)	Mouse	Transgenic	Yes	No	Yes
LRRK2 (*PARK8*)	Nematode	Transgenic	Yes	ND	ND
	Fly	Transgenic	Yes	No	Yes
	Mouse	Transgenic	No	No	Yes

Abbreviations: UCHL1, ubiqitin carboxy-terminal hydrolase L1; LRRK2, leucine-rich repeat kinase 2; DA, dopamine; LB, Lewy body; ND, not determined; PrP, prion; PDGFβ, platelet-derived growth factor β

1; LB-like inclusions by definition contain filamentous α-synuclein

2; ND could include some degree of behavioral impairment in spontaneous and locomotor activity and in response to sensory stimulation

§; Controversial. The opposite result has also been shown.

Table 2. Autosomal-dominant PD models

Gene	Animal	Manipulation	DA neuron loss	LB-like inclusion[1]	DA-responsive motor deficits[2]
parkin (*PARK2*)	Nematode	Knockout	No	No	No
	Fly	Knockout	Yes	No	Yes
		Transgenic	Yes	No	Yes
	Mouse	Knockout	No	No	ND
		Transgenic	Yes	Yes	ND
PINK1 (*PARK6*)	Fly	Knockout	Yes	No	Yes
	Mouse	Knockout	No	No	ND
DJ-1 (*PARK7*)	Fly	Knockout	Yes	No	Yes
	Mouse	Knockout	No	No	ND
HtrA2/Omi (*PARK13*)	Fly	Knockout	No	No	No
	Mouse	Knockout	No	No	ND
Nurr1 (*NR4A2*)	Mouse	Knockout	Yes	No	ND

Abbreviations: PINK1, phosphatase and tensin homolog deleted on chromosome ten (PTEN)-induced putative kinase 1; HtrA2, high temperature requirement A2; Nurr1, nuclear receptor-related 1; NR4A2, nuclear receptor subfamily 4, group A, member 2; DA, dopamine; LB, Lewy body; ND, not determined
1; LB-like inclusions by definition contain filamentous α-synuclein
2; ND could include some degree of behavioral impairment in spontaneous and locomotor activity and in response to sensory stimulation

Table 3. Autosomal-recessive PD models and other causative genes of PD

4.1 α-synuclein

α-synuclein was the first gene linked to an AD-type familial PD, called Park1. The identification of an *α-synuclein* mutation in this family revolutionized PD research, since *α*-synuclein is the main component of LBs, which are observed in the sporadic PD brain. This striking result strongly indicates that genetic and sporadic PD may share similar etiologies and that investigating *α*-synuclein-mediated pathogenesis in familial PD could uncover important information about sporadic PD. Three missense mutations of *α-synuclein*, encoding the substitutions A30P, A53T, and E46K, have been identified in familial PD (Gasser, 2009; Kruger et al., 1998; Lees, et al., 2009; Polymeropoulos et al., 1997). Furthermore, the duplication or triplication of *α-synuclein* is sufficient to cause PD, suggesting that the level of *α*-synuclein expression is a critical determinant of PD progression (Singleton, 2005; Singleton et al., 2003). Even though no direct relationship between sporadic PD and *α*-synuclein expression has yet been shown, the existence of several polymorphisms in the promoter or 3′-UTR of the *α-synuclein* gene suggests that its expression level might be a risk factor (Holzmann et al., 2003; Pals et al., 2004; Winkler et al., 2007).

Human *α*-synuclein is an abundant 140-amino acid presynaptic phosphoprotein involved in vesicle handling and neurotransmitter release. Mutations in *α*-synuclein that increase the propensity for misfolding are probably deleterious, because the misfolded forms are toxic, and they induce cell death *in vitro* (Cookson, 2005; Lee & Trojanowski, 2006). Among the variety of abnormal forms that mutant α-synuclein can adopt, protofibrils and fibrils seem to be the most toxic (Lee & Trojanowski, 2006). These demonstrations of α-synuclein toxicity *in vitro* led to the creation and extensive analysis of many *α-synuclein*-based animal models of PD.

Although flies (*Drosophila*) and nematodes (*C. elegans*) do not have complex nervous systems compared to vertebrates and do not express endogenous α-synuclein, they are useful for identifying genetic and pharmacological modifiers of *α-synuclein* and its product. In *Drosophila*, the overexpression of WT and mutated (A30P, A53T) human α-synuclein causes the age-dependent loss of dorsomedial DAergic neurons, an accumulation of LB-like filamentous inclusions with α-synuclein immunoreactivity, and compromised locomotor activity (climbing ability) (Feany & Bender, 2000). In *C. elegans*, α-synuclein overexpression leads to accelerated DAergic neuronal loss and motor impairment (Kuwahara et al., 2006; Lakso et al., 2003). However, the neurons of these nematodes do not contain notable synuclein-containing inclusions.

Many different mouse lines that overexpress α-synuclein under various promoters have been generated in the last ten years, and most have been described in recent reviews (Chesselet, 2008; Fernagut & Chesselet, 2004; Fleming & Chesselet, 2006). Mice expressing α-synuclein containing two mutations (A30P + A53T) under the TH promoter show progressive declines in locomotor activity and the loss of substantia nigra neurons and striatal DA content (Richfield et al., 2002; Thiruchelvam et al., 2004). Similarly, mice overexpressing WT human (-synuclein under the neuron-specific platelet-derived growth factor β (PDGFβ) promoter show reduced TH immunoreactivity and DA content in the striatum and impaired motor performance (Masliah et al., 2000). Mice overexpressing WT human α-synuclein under another neuron-specific promotor, Thy1, show strong widespread expression in cortical and subcortical neurons, including the substantia nigra pars compacta, but no glial, spinal, or neuromuscular pathology (Kahle et al., 2001; Rockenstein et al., 2002; Song et al., 2004). These mice have an increased sensitivity to mitochondrial damage from low doses of MPTP (Song, et al., 2004). Mice in which the mouse prion promoter (mPrP) is used to drive the expression of α-synuclein A53T show α-synuclein aggregation, fibrils and truncation, α-synuclein phosphorylation, ubiquitination, and progressive age-dependent neurodegeneration, just as in humans (Giasson et al., 2002; Lee et al., 2002).

Several viral vectors, primarily lentiviruses and adenoassociated viruses (AAVs), have been used to drive exogenous α-synuclein. Because viral vector delivery requires stereotactic injections within or near the site of the neuronal cell bodies in the substantia nigra pars compacta, rats are generally used for these studies although the model has been reproduced in other rodents (Kirik et al., 2002; Klein et al., 2002; Lauwers et al., 2003; Lo Bianco et al., 2002). The overexpression of human WT or A53T mutant α-synuclein by AAVs in the SNc neurons of rats causes the progressive age-dependent loss of DA neurons, motor impairment, and α-synuclein-positive cytoplasmic inclusions (Kirik, et al., 2002). Kirik et al. also overexpressed WT or A53T mutant α-synuclein in marmosets (Kirik et al., 2003), in which the α-synuclein protein was expressed in 90%–95% of all substantia nigra DA neurons. The transduced neurons showed evidence of severe pathology, including α-synuclein-positive cytoplasmic inclusions, granular deposits, and loss of the TH-positivity.

It is particularly notable that the phenotypic outcome of α-synuclein overexpression in mice heavily depends on the promoter used to drive transgene expression. Unfortunately, most of these models fail to accurately mimic PD in that there is no progressive loss of DA neurons. The loss of TH-positive cell bodies in the substantia nigra does not necessarily indicate cell death. Despite the lack of overt degenerative pathology in the DA-positive neurons, obvious locomoter abnormalities due to degeneration of the nigrostriatal system and a lack of DA responsiveness are observed in the various mouse α-synuclein models. Thus, most of these lines are excellent models of α-synuclein-induced neurodegenerative disorders, such as PD.

Although mutated α-synuclein causes human familial PD, α-synuclein's physiological roles in PD are not fully understood. In KO mice of α-synuclein, neuronal development and the formation of presynaptic terminals are normal (Abeliovich et al., 2000). Moreover, double KO mice that lack α- and β-synuclein exhibit normal basic brain functions and survive to adulthood (Chandra et al., 2004). Thus, the loss of α-synuclein function is unlikely to play a role in the pathogenesis of α-synuclein-induced neurodegeneration. Meanwhile, α-synuclein KO mice show reduced rearing activity in the open field, decreased DA content in the striatum, and a decrease in the reserve pool of vesicles in the hippocampus (Abeliovich, et al., 2000; Cabin et al., 2002). These results indicate that α-synuclein may play a regulatory role *in vivo*, possibly in the fine tuning of synaptic plasticity and/or vesicle maintenance. Interestingly, several lines of α-synuclein-null mice have a complete or partial resistance to the MPTP (Dauer et al., 2002; Schluter et al., 2003). Dauer et al. showed that this resistance is not due to abnormalities of the DA transporter, which appears to function normally in α-synuclein null mice (Dauer, et al., 2002). These reports indicate that α-synuclein is not obligatorily coupled to MPTP sensitivity, but can influence MPTP toxicity on some genetic background.

4.2 *UCHL1*

A rare AD-inherited form of PD, PARK5, is caused by a missense mutation in the *UCHL1* gene. UCHL1 constitutes 1%-2% of the brain proteins and functions in the ubiquitin-proteasome system. The ubiquitin hydrolase activity of UCHL1 is important for freeing reusable ubiquitin monomers. The missense mutation in PARK5 causes an Ile93Met substitution in the UCHL1 protein (UCHL1Ile93Met), and this mutant was initially shown to have decreased ubiquitin hydrolase activity (Leroy et al., 1998). Interestingly, UCHL1 is detected in LBs in sporadic PD cases (Lowe et al., 1990). These findings initiated a debate on whether the Ile93Met mutation causes a gain of function (toxicity) or loss of function (deficiency).

The gracile axonal dystrophy (*gad*) mouse is an AR-mutant that shows sensory ataxia at an early stage, followed by motor ataxia. Saigoh et al. showed that these mice exhibit spontaneous intragenic deletion of the *UCHL1* gene and do not express the UCHL1 protein (Saigoh et al., 1999). These mice do not show obvious pathological changes in the nigrostriatal DA pathway; in particular, there is no loss of DA cell bodies in the substantia nigra. Setsuie et al. generated transgenic mice that overexpressed UCHL1Ile93Met and reported a reduction in the DAergic neurons of the substantia nigra and of the DA content in the striatum (Setsuie et al., 2007). These mice show behavioral and pathological phenotypes of parkinsonism at 20 weeks of age. Moreover, recently, Yasuda et al. performed a viral vector-mediated *α-synuclein* injection into the substantia nigra of the UCHL1Ile93Met transgenic mice (Yasuda et al., 2009). These mice show a significantly enhanced loss of DA-positive cell bodies in the substantia nigra and of DA content in the striatum. The neurotoxicity is enhanced by PARK5-associated UCHL1Ile93Met mutant, but not influenced by the loss of UCH-L1 WT protein *in vivo*, indicating that the UCHL1Ile93Met toxicity results from a gain of function.

4.3 *LRRK2*

The *LRRK2* mutation is another type of ADPD, called *PARK8*. LRRK2 is a large protein containing a serine/threonine kinase and a GTPase domain that is localized to membranous structures (Biskup et al., 2006). The frequency of the common LRRK2 Gly2019Ser mutation was 1% in patients with sporadic PD and, interestingly, 4% of patients with hereditary PD (Healy et al., 2008). The risk of PD when the LRRK2 Gly2019Ser mutation was present was 28% at age 59 years, 51% at 69 years, and 74% at 79 years. The motor symptoms and non-motor symptoms of LRRK2-associated PD are more benign than those of idiopathic PD. In autopsied tissue, the LB pathology was present in a representative LRRK2 G2019S case, indicating that LRRK2 and α-synuclein share some pathogenic mechanisms (Ross et al., 2006). Yet, LRRK2 may play a role in neuronal outgrowth and guidance, and its precise physiological function remains to be clarified (MacLeod et al., 2006).

dLRRK is a *Drosophila* orthologue of LRRK2, and it shows elevated expression in DA neurons of the head (Imai et al., 2008; Lee et al., 2007). Liu et al. overexpressed constructs with mutations similar to those found in patients (G2019S), in *Drosophila* (Liu et al., 2008). The neuronal expression of LRRK2 or LRRK2-G2019S produces an adult-onset selective loss of DAergic neurons, locomotor dysfunction, and early mortality. However, the phenotype caused by the G2019S-LRRK2 mutant is more severe than that cause by the expression of equivalent levels of WT LRRK2. Treatment with L-DOPA improves the mutant LRRK2-induced locomotor impairment but does not prevent the loss of TH-positive neurons. Some fly models that overexpress other LRRK2 mutations, such as I1122V, Y1699C, and I2020T, show similar results, in terms of an age-dependent impairment of locomotor activity that improves with DA stimulation, and the loss of DA neurons (Liu, et al., 2008; Ng et al., 2009; Venderova et al., 2009). Moreover, in transgenic *C. elegans*, DA marker loss is greater in those expressing G2019S LRRK2 than WT LRRK2 (Saha et al., 2009).

Transgenic mice made using bacterial artificial chromosome (BAC) technology and expressing WT LRRK2, or the R1441G or G2091S mutation exhibit mild axonal pathology in the nigrostriatal DA projection (Li et al., 2010; Li et al., 2009). However, the conditional overexpression of neither WT LRRK2 nor its G2019S mutation causes degeneration of the DA-containing neurons (Lin et al., 2009). Interestingly, although the LRRK2 conditional transgenic mice show minimal nigrostriatal pathologies, they exhibit a progressive age-dependent motor impairment that is improved by DA stimulation. LRRK2 involvement in the pathogenesis of PD may be limited, and other genetic and/or environmental factors are probably required to trigger DA neuronal degeneration.

LRRK2 KO mice are viable, have no major abnormalities, and live to adulthood, and there is no significant difference in the susceptibility of LRRK2-deficient and WT mice to MPTP (Andres-Mateos et al., 2009). In *LRRK2*-KO *Drosophila* models, differing results on the pathology of the DA neurons have been obtained (Imai, et al., 2008; Wang et al., 2008). Lee et al. showed that *LRRK* loss-of-function mutants exhibited severely impaired locomotive activity (Lee, et al., 2007). Moreover, DAergic neurons in *LRRK* mutants showed a severe reduction in tyrosine hydroxylase immunostaining and shrunken morphology. Conversely, Wang et al. demonstrated that mutants lacking *dLRRK* kinase activity are viable with normal development and life span as well as unchanged number and pattern of DAergic neurons (Wang, et al., 2008). Nematode deletion mutants indicate that LRRK2 is dispensable for the development and maintenance of DA neurons (Sakaguchi-Nakashima et al., 2007).

4.4 *Parkin*

Parkin covers approximately 1.3 Mb of genomic DNA and is the causative gene for representative AR juvenile PD (*PARK2*). Mutations in *parkin* are not only a cause of familial PD but are also seen in 20% of young-onset sporadic PD cases (Lucking et al., 2000). Parkin is an E3 ubiquitin ligase that functions in the ubiquitin-proteasome system. The loss of parkin function is believed to result in abnormal accumulations of parkin's substrates. Springer et al. demonstrated that *pdr-1* (the nematode parkin homolog) mutants are viable and display no obvious morphological defects or alterations in motility, egg-laying behavior, brood size, or life span under standard growth conditions (Springer et al., 2005). Moreover, the authors did not detect any effect of the mutations on the survival of the DA neurons in the worms. However, overexpression of the α-synuclein A53T mutation in *pdr-1* mutants leads to developmental arrest and lethality, indicating this *C. elegans* model recapitulates parkin insolubility and aggregation similar to several AR juvenile PD-linked parkin mutations (Springer, et al., 2005).

Drosophila parkin-null mutants exhibit a reduced lifespan, locomotor defects (flight and climbing abilities), and male sterility (Greene et al., 2003; Whitworth et al., 2005). The locomotor defects derive from the apoptotic cell death of muscle subsets whereas the male sterile phenotype derives from a spermatid individualization defect at a late stage of spermatogenesis. Mitochondrial pathology is the earliest manifestation of muscle degeneration and a prominent characteristic of individualizing spermatids in parkin mutants. These mutants also display a decrement in the TH level and degeneration of a subset of DA neurons in the brain (Whitworth, et al., 2005). Several parkin-null mice have been generated and display motor and cognitive deficits including reduced locomotor activity and decreased spontaneous alteration in the T-maze; however, they show no substantial DAergic behavioral abnormalities (Goldberg et al., 2003; Itier et al., 2003; Perez & Palmiter, 2005; Von Coelln et al., 2004). Pathologically, KO mice exhibit slightly abnormal DA nigrostriatal and locus coeruleus noradrenergic regions (Goldberg, et al., 2003; Von Coelln, et al., 2004).

The overexpression of human mutant *parkin* in *Drosophila* causes an age-dependent, selective degeneration of DA neurons accompanied by progressive motor impairment (Sang et al., 2007; Wang et al., 2007). *Parkin-Q311X* mice also exhibit multiple late-onset and progressive hypokinetic motor deficits (Lu et al., 2009). Stereological analyses revealed that the mutant mice develop age-dependent DA neuron degeneration in the substantia nigra and a significant reduction of the striatal DA level, accompanied by a significant loss of DA neuron terminals in the striatum. These results indicate that *parkin* mutants may play a pivotal role in the dominant-negative etiological mechanisms of PD.

4.5 *PINK1*

PINK1 is another causative gene for the AR inherited PD called *PARK6*. PARK6 is the second most frequent early-onset AR PD. PINK1 is located in mitochondria and is a putative mitochondrial kinase, because it contains a conserved serine/threonine kinase domain with an N-terminal mitochondrial-targeting motif (Silvestri et al., 2005). Thus, the PD-causative

mutations of *PINK1* may cause loss of function. Park et al. and Clark et al. generated and characterized loss-of-function *Drosophila* PINK1 mutants (Clark et al., 2006; Park et al., 2006). These flies exhibit male sterility, apoptotic muscle degeneration, defects in mitochondrial morphology, and increased sensitivity to multiple stresses, including oxidative stress.
Park et al. showed an age-dependent decrease in DA levels and a mild loss of DA neurons in these *Drosophila* mutants (Park, et al., 2006). Notably, the PINK1mutants share marked phenotypic similarities with parkin mutants. Parkin overexpression is able to rescue the mitochondrial defects found in PINK1, although the double mutants do not show an enhanced phenotype. PINK1 overexpression does not rescue parkin phenotypes. Together, the data indicate that parkin and PINK1 function, at least partly, in a common pathway, and PINK1 acts upstream of parkin. Whereas PINK1-deficient mice show age-dependent mitochondrial dysfunction, increased sensitivity to oxidative stress, decreased evoked DA release, and DA receptor agonist-responsive impairment of striatal plasticity, the number of DA neurons, the level of striatal DA, and the level of DA receptors are the same as in WT animals (Gautier et al., 2008; Gispert et al., 2009; Kitada et al., 2007). These phenotypes are similar to those of *parkin*-KO mice.

4.6 *DJ-1*

Deletion or point mutations in *DJ-1* have been identified in early onset AR PD (*PARK7*). DJ-1 plays a role as an antioxidant and chaperone, and it is expressed ubiquitously in the cytosol, mitochondrial matrix, and intermembranous space (Zhang et al., 2005). In vitro, downregulation or KO of the endogenous DJ-1 increases cells' vulnerability to oxidative stress and proteasome inhibition, implicating it in the cellular response to oxidative stress (Martinat et al., 2004; Mitsumoto et al., 2001; Yokota et al., 2003). *Drosophila* possesses two different orthologs of the human DJ-1 gene, named *DJ-1*α and *DJ-1*β. While loss-of-function DJ-1β mutants have normal numbers of DA neurons, classical genetic analyses and RNAi experiments have yielded contradictory results regarding the function of DJ-1α in DA neuron maintenance (Lavara-Culebras & Paricio, 2007; Menzies et al., 2005; Meulener et al., 2005; Park et al., 2005; Yang et al., 2005). However, DA neuron loss cannot be detected inDJ-1α/DJ-1β double-deletion mutants, which are also viable, fertile, and have a normal life span. Some studies have reported a loss of DA neurons upon acute RNA silencing of DJ-1α (Lavara-Culebras & Paricio, 2007; Yang, et al., 2005).
Similar to α-synuclein and parkin KO mice, DJ-1 KO mice do not show major DA-agonist-responsive behavioral abnormalities or the loss of nigrostriatal DA neurons (Andres-Mateos et al., 2007; Goldberg et al., 2005; Kim et al., 2005). In particular, although the levels of striatal DA and DA receptors are unchanged, the evoked dopamine release from striatal slices is clearly reduced, most likely as a consequence of increased reuptake. DJ-1 mutant mice also show an increased sensitivity to MPTP (Kim, et al., 2005). This is rescued by restoring the DJ-1 expression in mutant mice, further indicating a role for DJ-1 in the oxidative stress response.

4.7 HtrA2/Omi

HtrA2/Omi has been identified as the causative gene for a rare inherited PD, *PARK13*. HtrA2/Omi has a PDZ (PDZ is based on three proteins that led to its discovery, postsynaptic density protein (PSD-95), *Drosophila* disc large tumor suppressor (DLG1), and zonula occludens-1 protein (ZO-1)) domain in addition to a serine protease domain and is localized to the mitochondrial intermembrane space by its mitochondria-targeting sequence. Whitworth et al. have demonstrated a genetic interaction between *HtrA2/Omi* and *PINK1*, described below, by investigating the eye phenotype of double mutant flies (Whitworth et al., 2008). Their study revealed that *HtrA2/Omi* acts downstream of *PINK1* and is independent of the *parkin* gene. Yet, Yun et al. indicated that *HtrA2/Omi* null fly mutants show neither mitochondrial morphological defects nor DAergic neuronal loss (Yun et al., 2008). They also generated a *Drosophila HtrA2/Omi* mutant analogue to the human mutation G399S, which was identified in *PARK13* patients. HtrA2/Omi G399S retains a significant, if not complete, function of HtrA2/Omi, compared with protease-compromised versions of the protein, indicating that *HtrA2/Omi* is unlikely to play a pivotal role in PD pathogenesis or as an etiological factor. The targeted deletion of *HtrA2/Omi* in mice increases their sensitivity to stress-induced cell death (Jones et al., 2003; Martins et al., 2004). Animals lacking HtrA2/Omi display a progressive movement disorder similar to progressive akinesia, a rigidity syndrome, showing lack of coordination, decreased mobility, bent posture, tremor, and a decreased number of TH-positive striatal neurons (Martins, et al., 2004).

4.8 Nurr1 (NR4A2)

Nurr1 is a member of the nuclear receptor superfamily and is involved in the differentiation and development of nigrostriatal DA neurons. Le et al. identified two mutations in *Nurr1* associated with PD (-291Tdel and -245T→G), which map to the first exon of *NR4A2* and affected one allele in 10 of 107 individuals with familial PD (Le et al., 2003). Mutations in *Nurr1* alter the transcription of *TH* and the DA transporter, suggesting that alterations in Nurr1 may cause chronic DA alterations that could increase susceptibility to PD (Sacchetti et al., 2001). Nurr1 is essential for the development of the ventral mesencephalic DA neurons, because homozygous Nurr1-KO mice do not develop DA neurons in the substantia nigra and die soon after birth (Zetterstrom et al., 1997). Heterozygous Nurr1-KO mice exhibit a significant decrease in rotarod performance and locomotor activities (Jiang et al., 2005). These phenotypes are associated with decreased DA levels in the striatum, decreased numbers of DAergic neurons, and a reduced expression of Nurr1 and DAT in the substantia nigra. Moreover, Le et al. reported that heterozygous Nurr1-KO mice show a significant decrease in the total number of TH-positive neurons in the substantia nigra and reduced DA in the striatum after MPTP administration (Le et al., 1999). Thus, these mice show a progressive DA phenotype that bears some resemblance to that found in α-synuclein-overexpressing and mutant mice. Therefore, *Nurr1*-knockdown mice may provide a good model for investigating the later stages of PD characterized by severe DA neuron loss.

5. Genetic risk factors of PD

The identification and characterization of susceptibility genes for common human disease, including PD, is a difficult challenge. The usual approach of focusing a study on just one or a few candidate genes limits our ability to identify novel genetic effects associated with disease. In addition, many susceptibility genes may exhibit effects that are partially or solely dependent on interactions with other genes and/or the environment. Recently, Genome-wide association studies (GWAS) have been proposed as a solution to these problems. GWAS analyses must embrace abundant clinical and environmental data available to complement the rich genotypic data with the ultimate goal of revealing the genetic and environmental factors important for disease risk.

In 2009, two reports of GWAS demonstrated that several genes and loci could be genetic risk factors for PD in the different population (Satake et al., 2009; Simon-Sanchez et al., 2009). These studies indicated that *α-synuclein, LRRK2,* and locus on 1q32 (designated as *PARK16*) showed strong association to PD. Interestingly, *BST1* on 4q15 is only identified a new risk locus in the Japanese study (Satake, et al., 2009) and *microtubule-associated protein tau (MAPT)* is only found association in the European study (Simon-Sanchez, et al., 2009), indicating that population-specific genetic heterogeneity involves in the pathogenesis of PD.

MAPT is primarily expressed in neurons and plays a key role in the organization and integrity of the cytoskeleton and filamentous neuronal tau inclusions define a set of neurodegenerative diseases referred to as the "tauopathies," which include Alzheimer's disease, corticobasal degeneration (CBD), progressive supranuclear palsy (PSP), and frontotemporal dementia with parkinsonism linked to chromosome 17 (FTDP-17). While tau pathology is sometimes found in PD, it is not pathognomic. Thus, the relationship between the MAPT and the pathophysiology of PD still remains to be elucidated, however, brain pathology in Alzheimer's disease cases with amyloid precursor protein mutation exhibits not only β-amyloid deposition, tangle, but also sometimes LB pathology (Hardy, 1994). This finding indicates that there are genetic pathologic connections between α-synuclein and tau.

Other GWAS demonstrated that the strongest evidence of association was obtained on chromosome 4p16 in the gene *cyclin G associated kinase (GAK)*, designated as PARK17 (Hamza et al., 2010; Pankratz et al., 2009). This gene might be a promising candidate since the expression of cell cycle regulators altered in the substantia nigra pars compacta with PD (Grunblatt et al., 2004).

More recent GWAS showed a new genetic association with PD in the *human leukocyte antigen (HLA)-DRA* region (6p21), designated as PARK18 (Hamza, et al., 2010). Interestingly, this result suggests an involvement of immune system in the pathogenesis of PD. Furthermore, genetic variability of *HLA* region potentially has impact on damage repair and cleaning up risk for disease. The adaptive or innate immune systems had previously been implicated in disease pathology in the late-onset neurodegenerative diseases such as PD and Alzheimer's disease (McGeer et al., 2005).

Gaucher disease (GD) is an autosomal recessive glycolipid storage disorder with multisystemic manifestations caused by loss of function mutations in the *glucocerebrosidase (GBA)* gene, which encodes the enzyme glucocerebrosidase. A small subset of patients with GD develops parkinsonism with brain stem or diffuses LB-related pathology (Wong et al., 2004). An increased incidence of parkinsonism has also been reported in relatives of patients with PD (Halperin et al., 2006). In 2009, multicenter analysis demonstrated that there is a strong association between GBA mutations (L444P and N370S) and PD (Sidransky et al., 2009). While both gain-of- and loss-of- function hypotheses have been proposed, he mechanism by which GBA mutations increase risk for PD is not fully known (Velayati et al., 2010).

Additional susceptibility loci will likely be uncovered in the near future, as the wealth of recent data from GWASs is further analyzed. Such efforts will include meta-analysis, consideration of gene-gene and gene -environment interaction, and analysis of copy number variation. Although important progress has been made, the mechanisms by which variation in PD-linked genes leads to neurodegeneration remains poorly understood. However, data accumulated thus far has implicated mitochondrial dysfunction, oxidative damage, aberrant protein aggregation, deficits in ubiquitin-mediated protein degradation, and malfunction of immune system as playing key roles in the etiopathogenesis of PD. Actually, animal models of these risk factor gene mutations have been described very few, but once they are available (if pathological features including LB and clinical manifestation are replicated by candidate genes manipulation), they will undoubtedly shed new light on the mechanisms of PD.

6. Concluding remarks

The symptoms of PD become apparent after more than 80% of the DA neurons have died. The rate of substantia nigral cell loss is assumed to be about 2,500 per year in normal people. The loss of DA function can be accelerated by exposure to neurotoxins and by molecular (genetic) abnormalities, leading to a fast and significant decrease in the number of DA neurons. Consequently, these pharmacological and/or genetic insults can cause early onset of PD. This scenario indicates that critical pathological changes could be initiated one or two decades prior to the onset of PD. As described above, whether the causative factor is a toxic compound or a mutated gene, we have no perfect animal models of PD. So far, the neurotoxin-induced vertebrate models of PD are suitable for investigating disease-modifying therapies, since they have already proved predictive. Several genetic animal models of PD are useful for understanding the early processes of degeneration in the nigrostriatal DA system. In particular, transgenic α-synuclein animals are valuable for researching general toxicity effects and the mechanisms of α-synuclein pathology, as well as for confirming potential therapeutic strategies.

Neurotoxic and genetic models of PD have opened new perspectives for modeling and understanding the progression of PD but the advantages and disadvantages of each approach must be carefully considered. As described above, some models of PD induced by toxins and mutations exhibit insoluble α-synuclein inclusions in the pathological feature, however, they fail to exhibit true LBs. It is important to distinguish models that reproduce the progressive degeneration of nigrostriatal DA neurons from those that model disease progression in the whole organism. Genetic modeling of nigrostriatal degeneration complements toxin-induced neuronal loss by reproducing insults that are mechanistically linked to PD in humans. These models can provide useful information on stages of neurodegeneration, in particular on the interplay between protective and detrimental mechanisms, which are likely to contribute to the late onset of the disease and the effect of aging, a main risk factor for PD.

7. References

Abeliovich, A. et al. (2000). Mice lacking alpha-synuclein display functional deficits in the nigrostriatal dopamine system, *Neuron*, Vol. 25, No. 1, pp. 239-252, ISSN 0896-6273

Anderson, G. et al. (2007). Loss of enteric dopaminergic neurons and associated changes in colon motility in an MPTP mouse model of Parkinson's disease, *Experimental Neurology*, Vol. 207, No. 1, pp. 4-12, ISSN 0014-4886

Andres-Mateos, E. et al. (2007). DJ-1 gene deletion reveals that DJ-1 is an atypical peroxiredoxin-like peroxidase, *Proceedings of the National Academy of Sciences of the United States of America*, Vol. 104, No. 37, pp. 14807-14812, ISSN 0027-8424

Andres-Mateos, E. et al. (2009). Unexpected lack of hypersensitivity in LRRK2 knock-out mice to MPTP (1-methyl-4-phenyl-1,2,3,6-tetrahydropyridine), *Journal of Neuroscience*, Vol. 29, No. 50, pp. 15846-15850, ISSN 1529-2401

Ascherio, A. et al. (2006). Pesticide exposure and risk for Parkinson's disease, *Ann Neurol*, Vol. 60, No. 2, pp. 197-203, ISSN 0364-5134

Barcia, C. et al. (2004). Evidence of active microglia in substantia nigra pars compacta of parkinsonian monkeys 1 year after MPTP exposure, *Glia*, Vol. 46, No. 4, pp. 402-409, ISSN 0894-1491

Beal, M. F. (2001). Experimental models of Parkinson's disease, *Nat Rev Neurosci*, Vol. 2, No. 5, pp. 325-334, ISSN 1471-003X

Berger, K. et al. (1991). Retrograde degeneration of nigrostriatal neurons induced by intrastriatal 6-hydroxydopamine injection in rats, *Brain Research Bulletin*, Vol. 26, No. 2, pp. 301-307, ISSN 0361-9230

Betarbet, R. et al. (2000). Chronic systemic pesticide exposure reproduces features of Parkinson's disease, *Nature Neuroscience*, Vol. 3, No. 12, pp. 1301-1306, ISSN 1097-6256

Bezard, E. et al. (1999). Absence of MPTP-induced neuronal death in mice lacking the dopamine transporter, *Experimental Neurology*, Vol. 155, No. 2, pp. 268-273, ISSN 0014-4886

Biskup, S. et al. (2006). Localization of LRRK2 to membranous and vesicular structures in mammalian brain, *Annals of Neurology*, Vol. 60, No. 5, pp. 557-569, ISSN 0364-5134

Bove, J. et al. (2005). Toxin-induced models of Parkinson's disease, *NeuroRx*, Vol. 2, No. 3, pp. 484-494, ISSN 1545-5343

Braak, H. et al. (2006). Gastric alpha-synuclein immunoreactive inclusions in Meissner's and Auerbach's plexuses in cases staged for Parkinson's disease-related brain pathology, *Neuroscience Letters*, Vol. 396, No. 1, pp. 67-72, ISSN 0304-3940

Breidert, T. et al. (2002). Protective action of the peroxisome proliferator-activated receptor-gamma agonist pioglitazone in a mouse model of Parkinson's disease, *Journal of Neurochemistry*, Vol. 82, No. 3, pp. 615-624, ISSN 0022-3042

Brooks, A. I. et al. (1999). Paraquat elicited neurobehavioral syndrome caused by dopaminergic neuron loss, *Brain Research*, Vol. 823, No. 1-2, pp. 1-10, ISSN 0006-8993

Cabin, D. E. et al. (2002). Synaptic vesicle depletion correlates with attenuated synaptic responses to prolonged repetitive stimulation in mice lacking alpha-synuclein, *Journal of Neuroscience*, Vol. 22, No. 20, pp. 8797-8807, ISSN 1529-2401

Casarejos, M. J. et al. (2006). Susceptibility to rotenone is increased in neurons from parkin null mice and is reduced by minocycline, *Journal of Neurochemistry*, Vol. 97, No. 4, pp. 934-946, ISSN 0022-3042

Chandra, S. et al. (2004). Double-knockout mice for alpha- and beta-synucleins: effect on synaptic functions, *Proceedings of the National Academy of Sciences of the United States of America*, Vol. 101, No. 41, pp. 14966-14971, ISSN 0027-8424

Chesselet, M. F. (2008). In vivo alpha-synuclein overexpression in rodents: a useful model of Parkinson's disease?, *Experimental Neurology*, Vol. 209, No. 1, pp. 22-27, ISSN 0014-4886

Chiueh, C. C. et al. (1984). Neurochemical and behavioral effects of 1-methyl-4-phenyl-1,2,3,6- tetrahydropyridine (MPTP) in rat, guinea pig, and monkey, *Psychopharmacology Bulletin*, Vol. 20, No. 3, pp. 548-553, ISSN 0048-5764

Clark, I. E. et al. (2006). Drosophila pink1 is required for mitochondrial function and interacts genetically with parkin, *Nature*, Vol. 441, No. 7097, pp. 1162-1166, ISSN 1476-4687

Cookson, M. R. (2005). The biochemistry of Parkinson's disease, *Annual Review of Biochemistry*, Vol. 74, No. pp. 29-52, ISSN 0066-4154

Dauer, W. et al. (2002). Resistance of alpha -synuclein null mice to the parkinsonian neurotoxin MPTP, *Proceedings of the National Academy of Sciences of the United States of America*, Vol. 99, No. 22, pp. 14524-14529, ISSN 0027-8424

Davis, G. C. et al. (1979). Chronic Parkinsonism secondary to intravenous injection of meperidine analogues, *Psychiatry Res*, Vol. 1, No. 3, pp. 249-254, ISSN 0165-1781

Dehmer, T. et al. (2000). Deficiency of inducible nitric oxide synthase protects against MPTP toxicity in vivo, *Journal of Neurochemistry*, Vol. 74, No. 5, pp. 2213-2216, ISSN 0022-3042

Del Zompo, M. et al. (1993). Selective MPP+ uptake into synaptic dopamine vesicles: possible involvement in MPTP neurotoxicity, *Br J Pharmacol*, Vol. 109, No. 2, pp. 411-414, ISSN 0007-1188

Deumens, R. et al. (2002). Modeling Parkinson's disease in rats: an evaluation of 6-OHDA lesions of the nigrostriatal pathway, *Experimental Neurology*, Vol. 175, No. 2, pp. 303-317, ISSN 0014-4886

Di Monte, D. et al. (1986). Comparative studies on the mechanisms of paraquat and 1-methyl-4-phenylpyridine (MPP+) cytotoxicity, *Biochem Biophys Res Commun*, Vol. 137, No. 1, pp. 303-309, ISSN 0006-291X

Dick, F. D. et al. (2007). Environmental risk factors for Parkinson's disease and parkinsonism: the Geoparkinson study, *Occupational and Environmental Medicine*, Vol. 64, No. 10, pp. 666-672, ISSN 1470-7926

Drolet, R. E. et al. (2009). Chronic rotenone exposure reproduces Parkinson's disease gastrointestinal neuropathology, *Neurobiology of Disease*, Vol. 36, No. 1, pp. 96-102, ISSN 1095-953X

Feany, M. B. & Bender, W. W. (2000). A Drosophila model of Parkinson's disease, *Nature*, Vol. 404, No. 6776, pp. 394-398, ISSN 0028-0836

Fernagut, P. O. & Chesselet, M. F. (2004). Alpha-synuclein and transgenic mouse models, *Neurobiology of Disease*, Vol. 17, No. 2, pp. 123-130, ISSN 0969-9961

Ferraz, H. B. et al. (1988). Chronic exposure to the fungicide maneb may produce symptoms and signs of CNS manganese intoxication, *Neurology*, Vol. 38, No. 4, pp. 550-553, ISSN 0028-3878

Fleming, S. M. & Chesselet, M. F. (2006). Behavioral phenotypes and pharmacology in genetic mouse models of Parkinsonism, *Behavioural Pharmacology*, Vol. 17, No. 5-6, pp. 383-391, ISSN 0955-8810

Gao, H. M. et al. (2003). Critical role for microglial NADPH oxidase in rotenone-induced degeneration of dopaminergic neurons, *Journal of Neuroscience*, Vol. 23, No. 15, pp. 6181-6187, ISSN 1529-2401

Gasser, T. (2009). Molecular pathogenesis of Parkinson disease: insights from genetic studies, *Expert Rev Mol Med*, Vol. 11, No. pp. e22, ISSN 1462-3994

Gautier, C. A. et al. (2008). Loss of PINK1 causes mitochondrial functional defects and increased sensitivity to oxidative stress, *Proceedings of the National Academy of Sciences of the United States of America*, Vol. 105, No. 32, pp. 11364-11369, ISSN 1091-6490

Giasson, B. I. et al. (2002). Neuronal alpha-synucleinopathy with severe movement disorder in mice expressing A53T human alpha-synuclein, *Neuron*, Vol. 34, No. 4, pp. 521-533, ISSN 0896-6273

Giovanni, A. et al. (1994a). Studies on species sensitivity to the dopaminergic neurotoxin 1-methyl-4-phenyl-1,2,3,6-tetrahydropyridine. Part 1: Systemic administration, *Journal of Pharmacology and Experimental Therapeutics*, Vol. 270, No. 3, pp. 1000-1007, ISSN 0022-3565

Giovanni, A. et al. (1994b). Studies on species sensitivity to the dopaminergic neurotoxin 1-methyl-4-phenyl-1,2,3,6-tetrahydropyridine. Part 2: Central administration of 1-methyl-4-phenylpyridinium, *Journal of Pharmacology and Experimental Therapeutics*, Vol. 270, No. 3, pp. 1008-1014, ISSN 0022-3565

Gispert, S. et al. (2009). Parkinson phenotype in aged PINK1-deficient mice is accompanied by progressive mitochondrial dysfunction in absence of neurodegeneration, *PLoS One*, Vol. 4, No. 6, pp. e5777, ISSN 1932-6203

Goldberg, M. S. et al. (2003). Parkin-deficient mice exhibit nigrostriatal deficits but not loss of dopaminergic neurons, *Journal of Biological Chemistry*, Vol. 278, No. 44, pp. 43628-43635, ISSN 0021-9258

Goldberg, M. S. et al. (2005). Nigrostriatal dopaminergic deficits and hypokinesia caused by inactivation of the familial Parkinsonism-linked gene DJ-1, *Neuron*, Vol. 45, No. 4, pp. 489-496, ISSN 0896-6273

Greene, J. C. et al. (2003). Mitochondrial pathology and apoptotic muscle degeneration in Drosophila parkin mutants, *Proceedings of the National Academy of Sciences of the United States of America*, Vol. 100, No. 7, pp. 4078-4083, ISSN 0027-8424

Grunblatt, E. et al. (2004). Gene expression profiling of parkinsonian substantia nigra pars compacta; alterations in ubiquitin-proteasome, heat shock protein, iron and oxidative stress regulated proteins, cell adhesion/cellular matrix and vesicle trafficking genes, *J Neural Transm*, Vol. 111, No. 12, pp. 1543-1573, ISSN 0300-9564

Halperin, A., Elstein, D. & Zimran, A. (2006). Increased incidence of Parkinson disease among relatives of patients with Gaucher disease, *Blood Cells Mol Dis*, Vol. 36, No. 3, pp. 426-428, ISSN, 1079-9796

Hamza, T. H. et al. (2010). Common genetic variation in the HLA region is associated with late-onset sporadic Parkinson's disease, *Nat Genet*, Vol. 42, No. 9, pp. 781-785, ISSN 1546-1718

Hardy, J. (1994). Lewy bodies in Alzheimer's disease in which the primary lesion is a mutation in the amyloid precursor protein, *Neurosci Lett*, Vol. 180, No. 2, pp. 290-291, ISSN 0304-3940

Healy, D. G. et al. (2008). Phenotype, genotype, and worldwide genetic penetrance of LRRK2-associated Parkinson's disease: a case-control study, *Lancet Neurol*, Vol. 7, No. 7, pp. 583-590, ISSN 1474-4422

Hirsch, E. C. et al. (2003). Animal models of Parkinson's disease in rodents induced by toxins: an update, *Journal of Neural Transmission. Supplementum*, Vol. No. 65, pp. 89-100, ISSN 0303-6995

Holzmann, C. et al. (2003). Polymorphisms of the alpha-synuclein promoter: expression analyses and association studies in Parkinson's disease, *Journal of Neural Transmission*, Vol. 110, No. 1, pp. 67-76, ISSN 0300-9564

Huerta, C. et al. (2007). No association between Parkinson's disease and three polymorphisms in the eNOS, nNOS, and iNOS genes, *Neuroscience Letters*, Vol. 413, No. 3, pp. 202-205, ISSN 0304-3940

Hunot, S. et al. (1996). Nitric oxide synthase and neuronal vulnerability in Parkinson's disease, *Neuroscience*, Vol. 72, No. 2, pp. 355-363, ISSN 0306-4522

Ikemura, M. et al. (2008). Lewy body pathology involves cutaneous nerves, *Journal of Neuropathology and Experimental Neurology*, Vol. 67, No. 10, pp. 945-953, ISSN 0022-3069

Imai, Y. et al. (2008). Phosphorylation of 4E-BP by LRRK2 affects the maintenance of dopaminergic neurons in Drosophila, *EMBO Journal*, Vol. 27, No. 18, pp. 2432-2443, ISSN 1460-2075

Itier, J. M. et al. (2003). Parkin gene inactivation alters behaviour and dopamine neurotransmission in the mouse, *Human Molecular Genetics*, Vol. 12, No. 18, pp. 2277-2291, ISSN 0964-6906

Jiang, C. et al. (2005). Age-dependent dopaminergic dysfunction in Nurr1 knockout mice, *Experimental Neurology*, Vol. 191, No. 1, pp. 154-162, ISSN 0014-4886

Jones, J. M. et al. (2003). Loss of Omi mitochondrial protease activity causes the neuromuscular disorder of mnd2 mutant mice, *Nature*, Vol. 425, No. 6959, pp. 721-727, ISSN 1476-4687

Kahle, P. J. et al. (2001). Selective insolubility of alpha-synuclein in human Lewy body diseases is recapitulated in a transgenic mouse model, *American Journal of Pathology*, Vol. 159, No. 6, pp. 2215-2225, ISSN 0002-9440

Khwaja, M. et al. (2007). Nicotine partially protects against paraquat-induced nigrostriatal damage in mice; link to alpha6beta2* nAChRs, *Journal of Neurochemistry*, Vol. 100, No. 1, pp. 180-190, ISSN 0022-3042

Kim, R. H. et al. (2005). Hypersensitivity of DJ-1-deficient mice to 1-methyl-4-phenyl-1,2,3,6-tetrahydropyrindine (MPTP) and oxidative stress, *Proceedings of the National Academy of Sciences of the United States of America*, Vol. 102, No. 14, pp. 5215-5220, ISSN 0027-8424

Kirik, D. et al. (2002). Parkinson-like neurodegeneration induced by targeted overexpression of alpha-synuclein in the nigrostriatal system, *Journal of Neuroscience*, Vol. 22, No. 7, pp. 2780-2791, ISSN 1529-2401

Kirik, D. et al. (2003). Nigrostriatal alpha-synucleinopathy induced by viral vector-mediated overexpression of human alpha-synuclein: a new primate model of Parkinson's disease, *Proceedings of the National Academy of Sciences of the United States of America*, Vol. 100, No. 5, pp. 2884-2889, ISSN 0027-8424

Kitada, T. et al. (2007). Impaired dopamine release and synaptic plasticity in the striatum of PINK1-deficient mice, *Proceedings of the National Academy of Sciences of the United States of America*, Vol. 104, No. 27, pp. 11441-11446, ISSN 0027-8424

Klaidman, L. K. et al. (1993). Redox cycling of MPP+: evidence for a new mechanism involving hydride transfer with xanthine oxidase, aldehyde dehydrogenase, and lipoamide dehydrogenase, *Free Radical Biology and Medicine*, Vol. 15, No. 2, pp. 169-179, ISSN 0891-5849

Klein, R. L. et al. (2002). Dopaminergic cell loss induced by human A30P alpha-synuclein gene transfer to the rat substantia nigra, *Human Gene Therapy*, Vol. 13, No. 5, pp. 605-612, ISSN 1043-0342

Kopin, I. J. & Markey, S. P. (1988). MPTP toxicity: implications for research in Parkinson's disease, *Annual Review of Neuroscience*, Vol. 11, No. pp. 81-96, ISSN 0147-006X

Kruger, R. et al. (1998). Ala30Pro mutation in the gene encoding alpha-synuclein in Parkinson's disease, *Nature Genetics*, Vol. 18, No. 2, pp. 106-108, ISSN 1061-4036

Kuwahara, T. et al. (2006). Familial Parkinson mutant alpha-synuclein causes dopamine neuron dysfunction in transgenic Caenorhabditis elegans, *Journal of Biological Chemistry*, Vol. 281, No. 1, pp. 334-340, ISSN 0021-9258

Lakso, M. et al. (2003). Dopaminergic neuronal loss and motor deficits in Caenorhabditis elegans overexpressing human alpha-synuclein, *Journal of Neurochemistry*, Vol. 86, No. 1, pp. 165-172, ISSN 0022-3042

Langston, J. W. et al. (1984). Selective nigral toxicity after systemic administration of 1-methyl-4-phenyl-1,2,5,6-tetrahydropyrine (MPTP) in the squirrel monkey, *Brain Research*, Vol. 292, No. 2, pp. 390-394, ISSN 0006-8993

Langston, J. W. & Irwin, I. (1986). MPTP: current concepts and controversies, *Clinical Neuropharmacology*, Vol. 9, No. 6, pp. 485-507, ISSN 0362-5664

Langston, J. W. et al. (1999). Evidence of active nerve cell degeneration in the substantia nigra of humans years after 1-methyl-4-phenyl-1,2,3,6-tetrahydropyridine exposure, *Annals of Neurology*, Vol. 46, No. 4, pp. 598-605, ISSN 0364-5134

Lapointe, N. et al. (2004). Rotenone induces non-specific central nervous system and systemic toxicity, *FASEB Journal*, Vol. 18, No. 6, pp. 717-719, ISSN 1530-6860

Lauwers, E. et al. (2003). Neuropathology and neurodegeneration in rodent brain induced by lentiviral vector-mediated overexpression of alpha-synuclein, *Brain Pathology*, Vol. 13, No. 3, pp. 364-372, ISSN 1015-6305

Lavara-Culebras, E. & Paricio, N. (2007). Drosophila DJ-1 mutants are sensitive to oxidative stress and show reduced lifespan and motor deficits, *Gene*, Vol. 400, No. 1-2, pp. 158-165, ISSN 0378-1119

Le, W. et al. (1999). Reduced Nurr1 expression increases the vulnerability of mesencephalic dopamine neurons to MPTP-induced injury, *Journal of Neurochemistry*, Vol. 73, No. 5, pp. 2218-2221, ISSN 0022-3042

Le, W. D. et al. (2003). Mutations in NR4A2 associated with familial Parkinson disease, *Nature Genetics*, Vol. 33, No. 1, pp. 85-89, ISSN 1061-4036

Lebouvier, T. et al. (2009). The second brain and Parkinson's disease, *European Journal of Neuroscience*, Vol. 30, No. 5, pp. 735-741, ISSN 1460-9568

Lee, M. K. et al. (2002). Human alpha-synuclein-harboring familial Parkinson's disease-linked Ala-53 --> Thr mutation causes neurodegenerative disease with alpha-synuclein aggregation in transgenic mice, *Proceedings of the National Academy of Sciences of the United States of America*, Vol. 99, No. 13, pp. 8968-8973, ISSN 0027-8424

Lee, S. B. et al. (2007). Loss of LRRK2/PARK8 induces degeneration of dopaminergic neurons in Drosophila, *Biochemical and Biophysical Research Communications*, Vol. 358, No. 2, pp. 534-539, ISSN 0006-291X

Lee, V. M. & Trojanowski, J. Q. (2006). Mechanisms of Parkinson's disease linked to pathological alpha-synuclein: new targets for drug discovery, *Neuron*, Vol. 52, No. 1, pp. 33-38, ISSN 0896-6273

Lees, A. J. et al. (2009). Parkinson's disease, *Lancet*, Vol. 373, No. 9680, pp. 2055-2066, ISSN 1474-547X

Leroy, E. et al. (1998). The ubiquitin pathway in Parkinson's disease, *Nature*, Vol. 395, No. 6701, pp. 451-452, ISSN 0028-0836

Li, X. et al. (2010). Enhanced striatal dopamine transmission and motor performance with LRRK2 overexpression in mice is eliminated by familial Parkinson's disease mutation G2019S, *Journal of Neuroscience*, Vol. 30, No. 5, pp. 1788-1797, ISSN 1529-2401

Li, Y. et al. (2009). Mutant LRRK2(R1441G) BAC transgenic mice recapitulate cardinal features of Parkinson's disease, *Nature Neuroscience*, Vol. 12, No. 7, pp. 826-828, ISSN 1546-1726

Liberatore, G. T. et al. (1999). Inducible nitric oxide synthase stimulates dopaminergic neurodegeneration in the MPTP model of Parkinson disease, *Nature Medicine*, Vol. 5, No. 12, pp. 1403-1409, ISSN 1078-8956

Lin, X. et al. (2009). Leucine-rich repeat kinase 2 regulates the progression of neuropathology induced by Parkinson's-disease-related mutant alpha-synuclein, *Neuron*, Vol. 64, No. 6, pp. 807-827, ISSN 1097-4199

Liu, Z. et al. (2008). A Drosophila model for LRRK2-linked parkinsonism, *Proceedings of the National Academy of Sciences of the United States of America*, Vol. 105, No. 7, pp. 2693-2698, ISSN 1091-6490

Lo Bianco, C. et al. (2002). alpha -Synucleinopathy and selective dopaminergic neuron loss in a rat lentiviral-based model of Parkinson's disease, *Proc Natl Acad Sci U S A*, Vol. 99, No. 16, pp. 10813-10818, ISSN 0027-8424

Lowe, J. et al. (1990). Ubiquitin carboxyl-terminal hydrolase (PGP 9.5) is selectively present in ubiquitinated inclusion bodies characteristic of human neurodegenerative diseases, *Journal of Pathology*, Vol. 161, No. 2, pp. 153-160, ISSN 0022-3417

Lu, X. H. et al. (2009). Bacterial artificial chromosome transgenic mice expressing a truncated mutant parkin exhibit age-dependent hypokinetic motor deficits, dopaminergic neuron degeneration, and accumulation of proteinase K-resistant alpha-synuclein, *Journal of Neuroscience*, Vol. 29, No. 7, pp. 1962-1976, ISSN 1529-2401

Lucking, C. B. et al. (2000). Association between early-onset Parkinson's disease and mutations in the parkin gene, *New England Journal of Medicine*, Vol. 342, No. 21, pp. 1560-1567, ISSN 0028-4793

MacLeod, D. et al. (2006). The familial Parkinsonism gene LRRK2 regulates neurite process morphology, *Neuron*, Vol. 52, No. 4, pp. 587-593, ISSN 0896-6273

Manning-Bog, A. B. et al. (2002). The herbicide paraquat causes up-regulation and aggregation of alpha-synuclein in mice: paraquat and alpha-synuclein, *Journal of Biological Chemistry*, Vol. 277, No. 3, pp. 1641-1644, ISSN 0021-9258

Markey, S. P. et al. (1984). Intraneuronal generation of a pyridinium metabolite may cause drug-induced parkinsonism, *Nature*, Vol. 311, No. 5985, pp. 464-467, ISSN 0028-0836

Martinat, C. et al. (2004). Sensitivity to oxidative stress in DJ-1-deficient dopamine neurons: an ES- derived cell model of primary Parkinsonism, *PLoS Biol*, Vol. 2, No. 11, pp. e327, ISSN 1545-7885

Martins, L. M. et al. (2004). Neuroprotective role of the Reaper-related serine protease HtrA2/Omi revealed by targeted deletion in mice, *Molecular and Cellular Biology*, Vol. 24, No. 22, pp. 9848-9862, ISSN 0270-7306

Masliah, E. et al. (2000). Dopaminergic loss and inclusion body formation in alpha-synuclein mice: implications for neurodegenerative disorders, *Science*, Vol. 287, No. 5456, pp. 1265-1269, ISSN 0036-8075

Mayer, R. A. et al. (1986). Prevention of the nigrostriatal toxicity of 1-methyl-4-phenyl-1,2,3,6-tetrahydropyridine by inhibitors of 3,4-dihydroxyphenylethylamine transport, *Journal of Neurochemistry*, Vol. 47, No. 4, pp. 1073-1079, ISSN 0022-3042

McCallum, S. E. et al. (2005). Decrease in alpha3*/alpha6* nicotinic receptors but not nicotine-evoked dopamine release in monkey brain after nigrostriatal damage, *Molecular Pharmacology*, Vol. 68, No. 3, pp. 737-746, ISSN 0026-895X

McCormack, A. L. & Di Monte, D. A. (2003). Effects of L-dopa and other amino acids against paraquat-induced nigrostriatal degeneration, *Journal of Neurochemistry*, Vol. 85, No. 1, pp. 82-86, ISSN 0022-3042

McGeer, E. G., Klegeris, A. & McGeer, P. L. (2005). Inflammation, the complement system and the diseases of aging, *Neurobiol Aging*, Vol. 26 Suppl 1, No. pp. 94-97, ISSN 0197-4580

Menzies, F. M. et al. (2005). Roles of Drosophila DJ-1 in survival of dopaminergic neurons and oxidative stress, *Current Biology*, Vol. 15, No. 17, pp. 1578-1582, ISSN 0960-9822

Meulener, M. et al. (2005). Drosophila DJ-1 mutants are selectively sensitive to environmental toxins associated with Parkinson's disease, *Current Biology*, Vol. 15, No. 17, pp. 1572-1577, ISSN 0960-9822

Mitsumoto, A. et al. (2001). Oxidized forms of peroxiredoxins and DJ-1 on two-dimensional gels increased in response to sublethal levels of paraquat, *Free Radical Research*, Vol. 35, No. 3, pp. 301-310, ISSN 1071-5762

Natale, G. et al. (2010). MPTP-induced parkinsonism extends to a subclass of TH positive neurons in the gut, *Brain Research*, Vol. 1355, No. pp. 195-206, ISSN 1872-6240

Ng, C. H. et al. (2009). Parkin protects against LRRK2 G2019S mutant-induced dopaminergic neurodegeneration in Drosophila, *Journal of Neuroscience*, Vol. 29, No. 36, pp. 11257-11262, ISSN 1529-2401

Nicklas, W. J. et al. (1985). Inhibition of NADH-linked oxidation in brain mitochondria by 1-methyl-4-phenyl-pyridine, a metabolite of the neurotoxin, 1-methyl-4-phenyl-

1,2,5,6-tetrahydropyridine, *Life Sciences*, Vol. 36, No. 26, pp. 2503-2508, ISSN 0024-3205

O'Leary, K. T. et al. (2008). Paraquat exposure reduces nicotinic receptor-evoked dopamine release in monkey striatum, *Journal of Pharmacology and Experimental Therapeutics*, Vol. 327, No. 1, pp. 124-129, ISSN 1521-0103

Pals, P. et al. (2004). alpha-Synuclein promoter confers susceptibility to Parkinson's disease, *Annals of Neurology*, Vol. 56, No. 4, pp. 591-595, ISSN 0364-5134

Pankratz, N. et al. (2009). Genomewide association study for susceptibility genes contributing to familial Parkinson disease, *Hum Genet*, Vol. 124, No. 6, pp. 593-605, ISSN 1432-1203

Park, J. et al. (2005). Drosophila DJ-1 mutants show oxidative stress-sensitive locomotive dysfunction, *Gene*, Vol. 361, No. pp. 133-139, ISSN 0378-1119

Park, J. et al. (2006). Mitochondrial dysfunction in Drosophila PINK1 mutants is complemented by parkin, *Nature*, Vol. 441, No. 7097, pp. 1157-1161, ISSN 1476-4687

Perez, F. A. & Palmiter, R. D. (2005). Parkin-deficient mice are not a robust model of parkinsonism, *Proceedings of the National Academy of Sciences of the United States of America*, Vol. 102, No. 6, pp. 2174-2179, ISSN 0027-8424

Polymeropoulos, M. H. et al. (1997). Mutation in the alpha-synuclein gene identified in families with Parkinson's disease, *Science*, Vol. 276, No. 5321, pp. 2045-2047, ISSN 0036-8075

Przedborski, S. et al. (1995). Dose-dependent lesions of the dopaminergic nigrostriatal pathway induced by intrastriatal injection of 6-hydroxydopamine, *Neuroscience*, Vol. 67, No. 3, pp. 631-647, ISSN 0306-4522

Przedborski, S. et al. (2001). The parkinsonian toxin 1-methyl-4-phenyl-1,2,3,6-tetrahydropyridine (MPTP): a technical review of its utility and safety, *Journal of Neurochemistry*, Vol. 76, No. 5, pp. 1265-1274, ISSN 0022-3042

Przedborski, S. & Vila, M. (2003). The 1-methyl-4-phenyl-1,2,3,6-tetrahydropyridine mouse model: a tool to explore the pathogenesis of Parkinson's disease, *Annals of the New York Academy of Sciences*, Vol. 991, No. pp. 189-198, ISSN 0077-8923

Ramsay, R. R. & Singer, T. P. (1986). Energy-dependent uptake of N-methyl-4-phenylpyridinium, the neurotoxic metabolite of 1-methyl-4-phenyl-1,2,3,6-tetrahydropyridine, by mitochondria, *Journal of Biological Chemistry*, Vol. 261, No. 17, pp. 7585-7587, ISSN 0021-9258

Richfield, E. K. et al. (2002). Behavioral and neurochemical effects of wild-type and mutated human alpha-synuclein in transgenic mice, *Experimental Neurology*, Vol. 175, No. 1, pp. 35-48, ISSN 0014-4886

Rockenstein, E. et al. (2002). Differential neuropathological alterations in transgenic mice expressing alpha-synuclein from the platelet-derived growth factor and Thy-1 promoters, *Journal of Neuroscience Research*, Vol. 68, No. 5, pp. 568-578, ISSN 0360-4012

Ross, O. A. et al. (2006). Lrrk2 and Lewy body disease, *Annals of Neurology*, Vol. 59, No. 2, pp. 388-393, ISSN 0364-5134

Sacchetti, P. et al. (2001). Nurr1 enhances transcription of the human dopamine transporter gene through a novel mechanism, *Journal of Neurochemistry*, Vol. 76, No. 5, pp. 1565-1572, ISSN 0022-3042

Saha, S. et al. (2009). LRRK2 modulates vulnerability to mitochondrial dysfunction in Caenorhabditis elegans, *Journal of Neuroscience*, Vol. 29, No. 29, pp. 9210-9218, ISSN 1529-2401

Satake, W. et al. (2009). Genome-wide association study identifies common variants at four loci as genetic risk factors for Parkinson's disease, *Nat Genet*, Vol. 41, No. 12, pp. 1303-1307, ISSN 1546-1718

Saigoh, K. et al. (1999). Intragenic deletion in the gene encoding ubiquitin carboxy-terminal hydrolase in gad mice, *Nature Genetics*, Vol. 23, No. 1, pp. 47-51, ISSN 1061-4036

Sakaguchi-Nakashima, A. et al. (2007). LRK-1, a C. elegans PARK8-related kinase, regulates axonal-dendritic polarity of SV proteins, *Current Biology*, Vol. 17, No. 7, pp. 592-598, ISSN 0960-9822

Sang, T. K. et al. (2007). A Drosophila model of mutant human parkin-induced toxicity demonstrates selective loss of dopaminergic neurons and dependence on cellular dopamine, *Journal of Neuroscience*, Vol. 27, No. 5, pp. 981-992, ISSN 1529-2401

Sauer, H. & Oertel, W. H. (1994). Progressive degeneration of nigrostriatal dopamine neurons following intrastriatal terminal lesions with 6-hydroxydopamine: a combined retrograde tracing and immunocytochemical study in the rat, *Neuroscience*, Vol. 59, No. 2, pp. 401-415, ISSN 0306-4522

Schluter, O. M. et al. (2003). Role of alpha-synuclein in 1-methyl-4-phenyl-1,2,3,6-tetrahydropyridine-induced parkinsonism in mice, *Neuroscience*, Vol. 118, No. 4, pp. 985-1002, ISSN 0306-4522

Schmidt, N. & Ferger, B. (2001). Neurochemical findings in the MPTP model of Parkinson's disease, *Journal of Neural Transmission*, Vol. 108, No. 11, pp. 1263-1282, ISSN 0300-9564

Schober, A. (2004). Classic toxin-induced animal models of Parkinson's disease: 6-OHDA and MPTP, *Cell and Tissue Research*, Vol. 318, No. 1, pp. 215-224, ISSN 0302-766X

Setsuie, R. et al. (2007). Dopaminergic neuronal loss in transgenic mice expressing the Parkinson's disease-associated UCH-L1 I93M mutant, *Neurochemistry International*, Vol. 50, No. 1, pp. 119-129, ISSN 0197-0186

Sherer, T. B. et al. (2003). Subcutaneous rotenone exposure causes highly selective dopaminergic degeneration and alpha-synuclein aggregation, *Experimental Neurology*, Vol. 179, No. 1, pp. 9-16, ISSN 0014-4886

Shimizu, K. et al. (2003). Paraquat induces long-lasting dopamine overflow through the excitotoxic pathway in the striatum of freely moving rats, *Brain Research*, Vol. 976, No. 2, pp. 243-252, ISSN 0006-8993

Sidransky, E. et al. (2009). Multicenter analysis of glucocerebrosidase mutations in Parkinson's disease, *N Engl J Med*, Vol. 361, No. 17, pp. 1651-1661, ISSN 1533-4406

Silvestri, L. et al. (2005). Mitochondrial import and enzymatic activity of PINK1 mutants associated to recessive parkinsonism, *Human Molecular Genetics*, Vol. 14, No. 22, pp. 3477-3492, ISSN 0964-6906

Simon-Sanchez, J. et al. (2009). Genome-wide association study reveals genetic risk underlying Parkinson's disease, *Nat Genet*, Vol. 41, No. 12, pp. 1308-1312, ISSN 1546-1718

Singleton, A. B. (2005). Altered alpha-synuclein homeostasis causing Parkinson's disease: the potential roles of dardarin, *Trends in Neurosciences*, Vol. 28, No. 8, pp. 416-421, ISSN 0166-2236

Singleton, A. B. et al. (2003). alpha-Synuclein locus triplication causes Parkinson's disease, *Science*, Vol. 302, No. 5646, pp. 841, ISSN 1095-9203

Song, D. D. et al. (2004). Enhanced substantia nigra mitochondrial pathology in human alpha-synuclein transgenic mice after treatment with MPTP, *Experimental Neurology*, Vol. 186, No. 2, pp. 158-172, ISSN 0014-4886

Springer, W. et al. (2005). A Caenorhabditis elegans Parkin mutant with altered solubility couples alpha-synuclein aggregation to proteotoxic stress, *Human Molecular Genetics*, Vol. 14, No. 22, pp. 3407-3423, ISSN 0964-6906

Tanner, C. M. (2003). Is the cause of Parkinson's disease environmental or hereditary? Evidence from twin studies, *Advances in Neurology*, Vol. 91, No. pp. 133-142, ISSN 0091-3952

Taylor, K. S. et al. (2005). Screening for undiagnosed parkinsonism among older people in general practice, *Age and Ageing*, Vol. 34, No. 5, pp. 501-504, ISSN 0002-0729

Thiruchelvam, M. et al. (2000a). Potentiated and preferential effects of combined paraquat and maneb on nigrostriatal dopamine systems: environmental risk factors for Parkinson's disease?, *Brain Research*, Vol. 873, No. 2, pp. 225-234, ISSN 0006-8993

Thiruchelvam, M. et al. (2000b). The nigrostriatal dopaminergic system as a preferential target of repeated exposures to combined paraquat and maneb: implications for Parkinson's disease, *Journal of Neuroscience*, Vol. 20, No. 24, pp. 9207-9214, ISSN 1529-2401

Thiruchelvam, M. J. et al. (2004). Risk factors for dopaminergic neuron loss in human alpha-synuclein transgenic mice, *European Journal of Neuroscience*, Vol. 19, No. 4, pp. 845-854, ISSN 0953-816X

Ungerstedt, U. (1971). Postsynaptic supersensitivity after 6-hydroxy-dopamine induced degeneration of the nigro-striatal dopamine system, *Acta Physiologica Scandinavica. Supplementum*, Vol. 367, No. pp. 69-93, ISSN 0302-2994

Uversky, V. N. (2004). Neurotoxicant-induced animal models of Parkinson's disease: understanding the role of rotenone, maneb and paraquat in neurodegeneration, *Cell and Tissue Research*, Vol. 318, No. 1, pp. 225-241, ISSN 0302-766X

Velayati, A., Yu, W. H. & Sidransky, E. (2010). The role of glucocerebrosidase mutations in Parkinson disease and Lewy body disorders, *Curr Neurol Neurosci Rep*, Vol. 10, No. 3, pp. 190-198, ISSN, 1534-6293

Venderova, K. et al. (2009). Leucine-Rich Repeat Kinase 2 interacts with Parkin, DJ-1 and PINK-1 in a Drosophila melanogaster model of Parkinson's disease, *Human Molecular Genetics*, Vol. 18, No. 22, pp. 4390-4404, ISSN 1460-2083

Von Coelln, R. et al. (2004). Loss of locus coeruleus neurons and reduced startle in parkin null mice, *Proc Natl Acad Sci U S A*, Vol. 101, No. 29, pp. 10744-10749, ISSN 0027-8424

Wang, C. et al. (2007). Drosophila overexpressing parkin R275W mutant exhibits dopaminergic neuron degeneration and mitochondrial abnormalities, *Journal of Neuroscience*, Vol. 27, No. 32, pp. 8563-8570, ISSN 1529-2401

Wang, D. et al. (2008). Dispensable role of Drosophila ortholog of LRRK2 kinase activity in survival of dopaminergic neurons, *Mol Neurodegener*, Vol. 3, No. pp. 3, ISSN 1750-1326

Whitworth, A. J. et al. (2005). Increased glutathione S-transferase activity rescues dopaminergic neuron loss in a Drosophila model of Parkinson's disease, *Proceedings of the National Academy of Sciences of the United States of America*, Vol. 102, No. 22, pp. 8024-8029, ISSN 0027-8424

Whitworth, A. J. et al. (2008). Rhomboid-7 and HtrA2/Omi act in a common pathway with the Parkinson's disease factors Pink1 and Parkin, *Dis Model Mech*, Vol. 1, No. 2-3, pp. 168-174; discussion 173, ISSN 1754-8411

Winkler, S. et al. (2007). alpha-Synuclein and Parkinson disease susceptibility, *Neurology*, Vol. 69, No. 18, pp. 1745-1750, ISSN 1526-632X

Wong, K. et al. (2004). Neuropathology provides clues to the pathophysiology of Gaucher disease, *Mol Genet Metab*, Vol. 82, No. 3, pp. 192-207, ISSN 1096-7192

Wonnacott, S. et al. (2000). Presynaptic nicotinic receptors modulating dopamine release in the rat striatum, *European Journal of Pharmacology*, Vol. 393, No. 1-3, pp. 51-58, ISSN 0014-2999

Wu, D. C. et al. (2002). Blockade of microglial activation is neuroprotective in the 1-methyl-4-phenyl-1,2,3,6-tetrahydropyridine mouse model of Parkinson disease, *Journal of Neuroscience*, Vol. 22, No. 5, pp. 1763-1771, ISSN 1529-2401

Yang, W. & Sun, A. Y. (1998). Paraquat-induced free radical reaction in mouse brain microsomes, *Neurochemical Research*, Vol. 23, No. 1, pp. 47-53, ISSN 0364-3190

Yang, Y. et al. (2005). Inactivation of Drosophila DJ-1 leads to impairments of oxidative stress response and phosphatidylinositol 3-kinase/Akt signaling, *Proceedings of the National Academy of Sciences of the United States of America*, Vol. 102, No. 38, pp. 13670-13675, ISSN 0027-8424

Yasuda, T. et al. (2009). Effects of UCH-L1 on alpha-synuclein over-expression mouse model of Parkinson's disease, *Journal of Neurochemistry*, Vol. 108, No. 4, pp. 932-944, ISSN 1471-4159

Yokota, T. et al. (2003). Down regulation of DJ-1 enhances cell death by oxidative stress, ER stress, and proteasome inhibition, *Biochemical and Biophysical Research Communications*, Vol. 312, No. 4, pp. 1342-1348, ISSN 0006-291X

Yun, J. et al. (2008). Loss-of-function analysis suggests that Omi/HtrA2 is not an essential component of the PINK1/PARKIN pathway in vivo, *Journal of Neuroscience*, Vol. 28, No. 53, pp. 14500-14510, ISSN 1529-2401

Zetterstrom, R. H. et al. (1997). Dopamine neuron agenesis in Nurr1-deficient mice, *Science*, Vol. 276, No. 5310, pp. 248-250, ISSN 0036-8075

Zhang, J. et al. (2003). Manganese ethylene-bis-dithiocarbamate and selective dopaminergic neurodegeneration in rat: a link through mitochondrial dysfunction, *Journal of Neurochemistry*, Vol. 84, No. 2, pp. 336-346, ISSN 0022-3042

Zhang, L. et al. (2005). Mitochondrial localization of the Parkinson's disease related protein DJ-1: implications for pathogenesis, *Human Molecular Genetics*, Vol. 14, No. 14, pp. 2063-2073, ISSN 0964-6906

18

Neuroprotective Effects of Herbal Butanol Extracts from *Gynostemma pentaphyllum* on the Exposure to Chronic Stress in a 6-Hydroxydopamine-Lesioned Rat Model of Parkinson's Disease Treated with or Without L-DOPA

Myung Koo Lee[1] et al.*
[1]*College of Pharmacy and Research Center for Bioresource and Health, Chungbuk National University, Cheongju Republic of Korea*

1. Introduction

Parkinson's disease (PD), which is characterized by the degeneration of dopaminergic neurons in the substantia nigra pars compacta, is accompanied by symptoms of muscular rigidity, bradykinesia, rest tremor, and loss of postural balance (Fearnley & Lees, 1991). Mitochondrial dysfunction by reactive oxygen species (ROS)-induced oxidative stress has also been suggested to be important in the loss of dopaminergic neurons in PD (Ozawa et al., 1990). Therefore, the degeneration of the dopaminergic nigrostriatal tracts in PD results in a corresponding decrease in the levels of dopamine and its metabolites, including 3,4-dihydroxyphenylacetic acid (DOPAC), homovanillic acid (HVA), and norepinephrine (Hornykiewicz, 1982).

3,4-Dihydroxyphenylalanine (L-DOPA), the precursor of dopamine, is the most prescribed therapy for the symptomatic relief of PD (Neil & David, 2008; Marsden, 1994). However, chronic prolonged therapy for PD with L-DOPA results in a loss of drug efficacy and irreversible adverse effects, and subsequently leads to the development of motor complications, such as fluctuation and dyskinesia (Jankovic, 2005). L-DOPA and dopamine can accelerate the degenerative process in the residual cells in patients with PD and induce oxidative stress-induced neurotoxicity by generating ROS in primary dopaminergic neurons and dopaminergic cell lines (Cheng et al., 1996). ROS generation leads to neuronal damage and apoptotic or non-apoptotic cell death (Walkinshaw & Waters, 1995). Dopaminergic neurons are in a perpetual state of oxidative stress, and this imbalance may lead to reduced levels of endogenous antioxidants (Merad-Boudia, 1998). In addition, chronic treatment with L-DOPA

*Hyun Sook Choi[1], Chen Lei[1], Kwang Hoon Suh[1], Keon Sung Shin[1], Seung Hwan Kim[2], Bang Yeon Hwang[1] and Chong Kil Lee[1]
[2]*College of Physical Education, Kyunghee University, Youngin, Republic of Korea*

leads to the production of a specific dopaminergic neurotoxin, 6-hydroxydopamine (6-OHDA), in the striatum of rodents (Borah & Mohanakumar, 2010). These results fuel the search for new agents for PD that are anti-oxidative substances or non-dopaminergic alternatives that can relieve the L-DOPA-induced cytotoxicity.

Various stressful stimuli can induce the production of many ROS and activate both the sympathetic nervous system and the hypothalamic-pituitary-adrenal-axis (Ganong, 2001), which increases the release of dopamine, norepinephrine, epinephrine, glucocorticoids, glutamate, and corticotropin releasing factor in the brain and peripheral circulation (Kandel et al., 2000). Chronic stress-induced adverse reactions are increased in neurodegenerative diseases, including anxiety disorders, depression, schizophrenia, stroke, Alzheimer's disease, and PD (Amanda et al., 2002). For example, the tremor in PD may be worsened by anxiety or anger (Schwab & Zieoer, 1965). In addition, a decrease in dopamine levels and an enhancement of dopamine turnover have been observed in 1-methyl-4-phenyl-1,2,3,6-tetrahydropyridine (MPTP)-treated mice after immersion immobilization stress, resulting in the mice being remarkably akinetic (Urakami et al., 1988). Repeated or relatively prolonged exposure to stress can also change central dopamine biosynthesis and extracellular dopamine levels in rat models (Ahmed et al., 1955), and changes in the cellular characteristics in the prefrontal cortex, such as dendritic atrophy and neuronal loss, have been found in response to stress (Rajkowska, 2000).

The stereotaxic injection of 6-OHDA into the substantia nigra, medial forebrain bundle, and striatum of the brain has been commonly used to produce experimental animal models of PD. These injections selectively injure dopaminergic neurons through the formation of various ROS (Perese et al., 1989). In addition, anti-oxidants, such as glutathione, catalase, and N-acetylcysteine, have been shown to be protective against 6-OHDA-induced cytotoxicity in PC12 and dopaminergic cells (Przedborski et al., 1995; Paxinos & Watson, 1986).

Gynostemma pentaphyllum (Cucurbitaceae; GP) is usually used as an herbal tea, and it is widely believed to result in various protective and functional improvements in diabetes, depression, anxiety, fatigue, hyperlipidemia, immunity, oxidative stress, and tumors (Razmovski-Naumovski et al., 2001). The major constituents of GP, which have been isolated, are a number of gypenoside derivatives (Razmovski-Naumovski et al., 2001). The gypenoside-rich fraction shows neuroprotective effects in the MPTP-induced mouse model of PD (Wang et al., 2010). The ethanol extract from GP has been found to have anti-stress and immunomodulatory functions in mice (Choi et al., 2008; Im et al., 2009). GP ethanol extract also exhibits protective effects against neurotoxicity by reducing tyrosine hydroxylase (TH) neuronal cell death and by normalizing dopamine levels in the 6-OHDA-lesioned rat model of PD (Choi et al., 2010). These results suggest that GP may function as a potential therapeutic and antioxidant in PD. The ethanol extract of GP was partitioned to obtain the butanol extract (GP-BX). GP-BX has been shown to have gypenoside-rich components, which were identified as gypenoside derivatives, and these include gynosaponin TN-1, gynosaponin TN-2, gypenoside XLV, and gypenoside LXXIV (Choi et al., 2010; Razmovski-Naumovski et al., 2005; Nagai et al., 1981; Takemoto et al., 1984; Yoshikawa et al., 1987).

The purpose of the present study was to investigate whether orally administered GP-BX obtained from the leaves of GP had protective effects against chronic stress in the 6-OHDA-lesioned rat model of PD with or without long-term L-DOPA treatment. Dopaminergic neuronal cell death induced by chronic stress in 6-OHDA-lesioned rats was blocked by the coadministration of GP-BX, and this was shown by histochemical (the number of surviving TH-immunopositive neuronal cells) and neurochemical (dopamine, DOPAC, HVA, and norepinephrine levels) techniques.

2. Experimental methods

2.1 Chemicals

L-DOPA, 6-OHDA, dopamine, norepinephrine, DOPAC, HVA, benserazide hydrochloride, apomorphine, and L-ascorbic acid were purchased from Sigma-Aldrich Co. (St. Louis, MO, USA). TH antibody was obtained from Millipore (Temecula, CA, USA). Anti-mouse IgG, Vectastain diaminobenzidine (DAB), and avidin/biotin complex (ABC) kits were purchased form Vector Laboratories, Inc. (Burlingame, CA, USA). All other chemicals were of analytical grade.

2.2 Preparation of GP-BX

GP was obtained from Geochang (Gyungnam, Korea), and a voucher specimen of the herbal leaves of GP was deposited at the herbarium of the College of Pharmacy, Chungbuk National University (Cheongju, Korea). The air-dried leaves of GP (10 kg) were extracted with ethanol (80%, v/v), and then the ethanol extracts were evaporated to dryness (GP ethanol extract, 1.05 kg; yield, 10.5%, w/w). The dry GP ethanol extracts (1 kg) were suspended in water and portioned subsequently with n-hexane, ethylacetate, and n-butanol. The final butanol extracts were evaporated to dryness under reduced pressure and temperature (GP-BX, 155 g; yield, 15.5%, w/w).

2.3 Animals

Rats (Sprague-Dawley, male, 200–250 g) were purchased from Samtako Co. (Animal Breeding Center, Osan, Korea). Animals were housed two per cage in a temperature-controlled environment with a 12-h light/dark cycle (lights on at 07:00) and with *ad libitum* access to standard rat food and water. All procedures were performed according to the guidelines of the Animal Ethics Committee of College of Pharmacy (Chungbuk National University).

2.4 Preparation of 6-OHDA-lesioned rats

The rats were anesthetized intraperitoneally with Zoletil 50 (100 mg/kg, Virbac, Carros, France) and placed in a stereotaxic stand (David Kopf Instruments, Tujunga, CA, USA). The coordinates for the striatum were measured accurately (antero-posterior, AP: -5.3 mm; lateral, ML: +1.9 mm; dorso-ventral, DV: -7.5 mm; relative to bregma). Next, 6-OHDA (8 µg/2 µL in saline solution containing 0.1% of L-ascorbic acid) was injected into the left substantia nigra pars compacta at 1 µL/min using a Hamilton syringe. After the injection, the needle was left in place for 5 min before being retracted in order to allow for complete diffusion of the medium. The rats were left until they had recovered from the anesthesia. Two weeks after the surgery, rats were challenged with apomorphine (0.5 mg/kg, s.c.), and the contralateral rotation was monitored. Rats showing fewer than 150 rotations per 30 min were excluded from further studies.

2.5 The exposure to chronic stress

Two weeks after the 6-OHDA lesions, the rats were placed individually in the electrified shock chamber for the exposure to chronic stress, and they received unavoidable electric footshock (EF) (intensity, 0.2 mA; duration, 10 s; interval, 10 min) at 14:00 every other day for 28 days using a shock generator (Seil Electric Co., Taejeon, Korea).

2.6 Drug treatment

Rats were divided into four groups with each group containing 7–10 rats. GP-BX (30 mg/kg), which was freshly prepared every day with water, was administered to 6-OHDA-lesioned rats orally (p.o.) once a day for 28 days. L-DOPA (10 mg/kg, i.p.) was treated with benserazide (15 mg/kg, i.p.) prepared in saline in order to prevent the peripheral decarboxylation of L-DOPA. The rats were sacrificed the day after the last exposure to stress and GP-BX administration. The experimental design was described as follows.

Experiment I:

Group I (normal rat groups): received 3 μL of saline containing 0.1% L-ascorbic acid by stereotaxic injection into the substantia nigra.
Group II (6-OHDA-lesioned rat groups): received 6-OHDA (8 μg/2 μL in saline solution containing 0.1% of L-ascorbic acid) by stereotaxic injection into the left substantia nigra.
Group III (6-OHDA-lesioned rat groups + chronic EF stress): exposed to EF stress for 28 days two weeks after receiving 6-OHDA (8 μg/2 μL).
Group IV (6-OHDA-lesioned rat groups + chronic EF stress + GP-BX): administered GP-BX (30 mg/kg) for 28 days to EF stress-exposed 6-OHDA-lesioned rat groups (Group III).

Experiment II:

Group I (L-DOPA-treated 6-OHDA-lesioned rat groups): treated with L-DOPA (10 mg/kg) for 28 days two weeks after receiving 6-OHDA (8 μg/2 μL).
Group II (L-DOPA-treated 6-OHDA-lesioned rat groups + chronic EF stress): exposed to EF stress for 28 days in L-DOPA (10 mg/kg)-treated 6-OHDA-lesioned rat groups (Group I).
Group III (L-DOPA-treated 6-OHDA-lesioned rat groups + GP-BX): administered GP-BX (30 mg/kg) for 28 days in L-DOPA-treated 6-OHDA-lesioned groups (Group I).
Group IV (L-DOPA-treated 6-OHDA-lesioned rat groups + chronic EF stress + GP-BX): administered GP-BX (30 mg/kg) for 28 days in L-DOPA-treated 6-OHDA-lesioned groups exposed to chronic EF stress (Group II).

2.7 TH-immunohistochemistry staining

For the immunohistochemical study, the rats were sacrificed 28 days after 6-OHDA lesioning and then perfused intracardially with saline, which was followed by 4% paraformaldehyde of the fixative solution. The brain was removed from the skull and placed in 30% sucrose solution. Sections of 35-μm thickness were cut with a Vibratome (Leica Microsystems GmbH, Wetzlar, Germany). The tissue sections were incubated with primary anti-TH antibody raised in rabbits and diluted in PBS containing 0.3% Triton X-100 (1:200, AB152, Millipore) overnight at 4°C. A 1:250 dilution of biotinylated anti-rabbit IgG was used as a secondary antibody, and the sections were then incubated with an ABC kit. TH immunoreactivity was visualized using a DAB kit (Vector Laboratories, Inc.). Photomicrographs of TH and digitized bright-field images were captured using a Zeiss Axiophot microscope (Carl Zeiss MicroImaging GmbH, Jena, Germany) (100X magnification). Cell counting was done using a computerized image analysis system (Axiovision software, Carl Zeiss MicroImaging GmbH). Analysis values obtained on the ipsilateral side (6-OHDA-lesioned side) were expressed as a percentage of those on the intact contralateral side (intact side).

2.8 Biochemical analysis

The brains were removed quickly, and the striatum was dissected in cold conditions. The samples were homogenized in 300 µL $HClO_4$. The homogenates were immediately centrifuged at 50,000 × *g* at 4°C for 20 min, and then, the supernatants were filtered using pore filters (0.45 µm). The levels of dopamine, DOPAC, HVA, and norepinephrine in the striatum were measured with a high-performance liquid chromatography (HPLC) system. The HPLC system consisted of a solvent delivery pump (Model 1525, Waters, Milford, MA, USA), an electrochemical detector (+0.85 V, Ag/AgCl reference electrode; Model 2465; Waters), and a Waters 120 ODS-BP column (5 µm, 50 × 4.6 mm). The mobile phase consisted of 10 mM citric acid, 0.13 mM Na_4EDTA, 0.58 mM SOS, and 10% methanol, and a flow rate of 1 mL/min. The results were expressed in terms of ng/g tissue.

2.9 Statistical analysis

All data were expressed as means ± S.E.M. Data were analyzed with an one-way analysis of variance (ANOVA) followed by a Tukey's test. P values <0.05 were considered statistically significant.

3. Results

3.1 TH-immunopositive neuronal cell survival in the substantia nigra of 6-OHDA-lesioned rats exposed to chronic EF stress and administered GP-BX

TH-immunopositive neuronal cell death by 6-OHDA lesions in the substantia nigra was ameliorated by the administration of GP-BX at 30 mg/kg (p.o.) for 28 days (Figure 1). TH-immunopositive neurons were observed consecutively in both the substantia nigra compacta and lateralis. TH-immunostained nerve fibers in the substantia nigra were tangled into a net, and the cells were either poly- or ovoid-shaped in the normal areas (Figure 1, A-I). The substantia nigra regions near the 6-OHDA-lesioned areas displayed drastic reductions in TH-immunopositive neuronal cells, and the staining intensity was decreased compared with the intact sides of the control rat groups (Figure 1, A-II). After exposure to chronic EF stress, TH-immunopositive neuronal cells were decreased in the substantia nigra of both the normal and the 6-OHDA-lesioned rats, even though the color was uneven, compared to the 6-OHDA-lesioned rat groups without chronic EF stress (Figure 1, A-II and III). However, the administration of GP-BX at 30 mg/kg (p.o.) for 28 days ameliorated the loss of TH-immunopositive neuronal cells induced by the exposure to chronic EF stress in both the intact and 6-OHDA-lesioned sides of 6-OHDA-lesioned rats (Figure 1, A-IV).

The number of TH-immunopositive neuronal cells on the ipsilateral sides (6-OHDA-lesioned sides) was analyzed as a percentage of those in the intact contralateral sides (intact sides) of 6-OHDA-lesioned rat groups. In the 6-OHDA-lesioned rat groups, 6-OHDA lesions caused a marked decrease in the number of TH-immunopositive neuronal cells in the intact and 6-OHDA-lesioned sides to 79.1% and 35.8%, respectively, compared to the normal rat groups (Figure 1, B-I and II). In addition, the exposure to chronic EF stress in the 6-OHDA-lesioned rat groups further decreased the number of TH-immunopositive neuronal cells in the intact and 6-OHDA-lesioned sides to 45.9% and 19.9%, respectively, compared to the 6-OHDA-lesioned rat groups (Figure, B-II and III). However, in the 6-OHDA-lesioned rat groups exposed to chronic EF stress, GP-BX administration (30 mg/kg) for 28 days showed a protective effect on the loss of the number of TH-immunopositive neuronal cells in the intact and 6-OHDA-lesioned sides to 63.0% and 38.1%, respectively (Figure 1, B-III and IV).

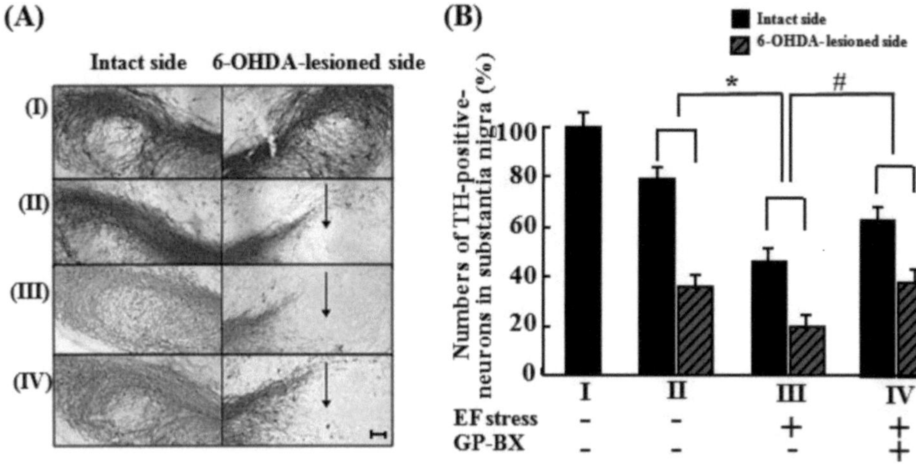

Fig. 1. Photomicrographs of tyrosine hydroxylase (TH) immunoreactivity on substantia nigra tissue sections from representative rats of each group (A), and the number of surviving TH-immunopositive neuronal cells in the ipsilateral substantia nigra [6-hydroxydopamine (6-OHDA)-lesioned side] was analyzed as a percentage of that in the intact contralateral side (intact side) (B). Normal rat groups (I), 6-OHDA-lesioned rat groups (II), 6-OHDA-lesioned rat groups + chronic electric foot (EF) stress (III), and 6-OHDA-lesioned rat groups + chronic EF stress + *Gynostemma pentaphyllum*-butanol extract (GP-BX) (IV). Rats were treated with GP-BX (30 mg/kg/day, p.o.) or vehicle (0.9% saline, p.o.) and then subjected to every-other-day sessions of EF stress (duration and interval of 10 s for 10 min, 2 mA). These data are representative of 7–10 animals per group, and the arrow indicates the 6-OHDA-lesioned side. TH-immunopositive neuronal cells were analyzed as a percentage of intact side. Scale bar is 100 µm. * $p < 0.05$ compared with 6-OHDA-lesioned rat groups; # $p < 0.05$ compared with 6-OHDA-lesioned rat groups + chronic EF stress (ANOVA followed by Tukey's test).

3.2 The levels of dopamine, DOPAC, HVA, and norepinephrine in the striatum of 6-OHDA-lesioned rats exposed to chronic EF-stress and administered GP-BX

The levels of dopamine, DOPAC, HVA, and norepinephrine in the striatum of GP-BX-administered normal rats (those without 6-OHDA lesions) were not altered compared to the GP-BX-untreated rat groups (data not shown). In addition, no differences were seen on the intact side of normal rats, 6-OHDA-lesioned rat groups, and 6-OHDA-lesioned rat groups administered GP-BX (30 mg/kg, 28 days).

A significant decrease in the levels of dopamine, DOPAC, HVA, and norepinephrine by 47.0%, 44.3%, 38.6%, and 40.5% in the 6-OHDA-lesioned sides of the 6-OHDA-lesioned rat groups, respectively, was observed (Figure 2, I and II). Chronic EF stress-exposed 6-OHDA-lesioned rat groups had a more marked decrease in the levels of dopamine, DOPAC, HVA, and norepinephrine to 71.7% and 28.2%, 66.9% and 28.3%, 61.0% and 25.3%, and 71.6% and

27.4%, respectively, in both the intact and 6-OHDA-lesioned sides, compared with 6-OHDA-lesioned rats without chronic EF stress (Figure 2, II and III). However, GP-BX administration (30 mg/kg) for 28 days resulted in an improvement in the reduced levels of dopamine, DOPAC, HVA, and norepinephrine by chronic EF stress to 84.6% and 47.8%, 79.7% and 47.9, 72.8% and 46.0%, and 88.6% and 46.8%, respectively, in the intact and 6-OHDA-lesioned sides of the 6-OHDA-lesioned rat groups (Figure 2, III and IV).

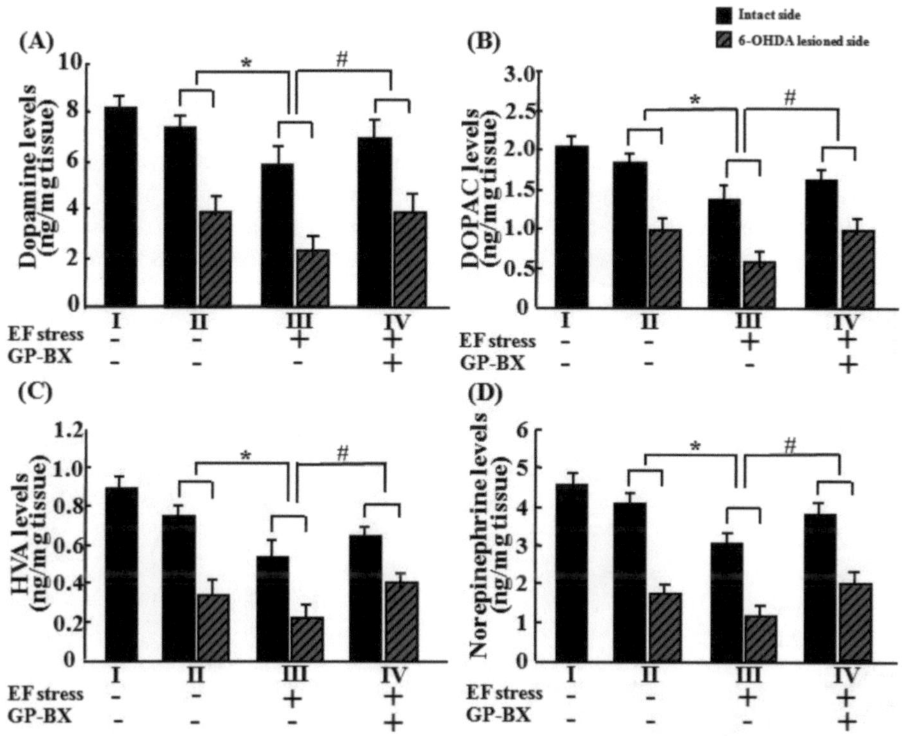

Fig. 2. Effects of GP-BX on the levels of dopamine (A), 3,4-dihydroxyphenylacetic acid (DOPAC; B), homovanillic acid (HVA; C), and norepinephrine (D) in the striatum of 6-OHDA-lesioned rats. Normal rat groups (I), 6-OHDA-lesioned rat groups (II), 6-OHDA-lesioned rat groups + chronic EF stress (III), and 6-OHDA-lesioned rat groups + chronic EF stress+ GP-BX (IV). Rats were treated with GP-BX (30 mg/kg/day, p.o.) or vehicle (0.9% saline, p.o.) and then subjected to every-other-day sessions of EF stress (duration and interval of 10 s for 10 min, 2 mA). After 4 weeks, the brains were removed, and the levels of dopamine, DOPAC, HVA, and norepinephrine were determined by a high-performance liquid chromatography (HPLC) method. Results represent means ± S.E.M. for 7–10 animals per group. * $p < 0.05$ compared with 6-OHDA-lesioned rat groups; # $p < 0.05$ compared with 6-OHDA-lesioned rat groups + chronic EF stress (ANOVA followed by Tukey's test).

3.3 TH-immunopositive neuronal cell survival in L-DOPA-treated 6-OHDA-lesioned rats exposed to chronic EF stress and administered GP-BX

Treatment with L-DOPA (10 mg/kg) for 28 days in 6-OHDA-lesioned rats slightly increased the number of TH-immunopositive neuronal cells in the 6-OHDA-lesioned sides compared to the L-DOPA-untreated 6-OHDA-lesioned rats (Figure 1-II and 3-I), indicating that a low dose of L-DOPA showed a protective and therapeutic activity. However, with exposure to chronic stress, the number of TH-immunopositive neuronal cells was significantly reduced in the substantia nigra in the L-DOPA-treated 6-OHDA-lesioned rat groups (Figure 3, A I and II). Furthermore, GP-BX administration (30 mg/kg) for 28 days protected against the loss of TH-immunopositive neuronal cells in L-DOPA-treated 6-OHDA-lesioned rat groups with or without chronic EF stress (Figure 3, A III and IV). Chronic EF stress induced the loss of a number of TH-immunopositive neuronal cells in both the intact and 6-OHDA-lesioned sides: the number of TH-immunopositive neuronal cells in the 6-OHDA-lesioned sides was decreased to 45.1% by the exposure to chronic EF stress in L-DOPA (10 mg/kg)-treated 6-OHDA-lesioned rat groups compared with those without chronic EF stress (Figure 3, A I and II). However, GP-BX administration (30 mg/kg) recovered the number of TH-immunopositive neuronal cells by 12.1% in the intact sides of L-DOPA-treated 6-OHDA-lesioned rats (Figure 3, B I and III) and also increased them by 18.6% and 36.7%, respectively, in the intact and 6-OHDA-lesioned sides of chronic EF stress-exposed 6-OHDA-lesioned rats compared with GP-BX-untreated groups (Figure 3, B II and IV).

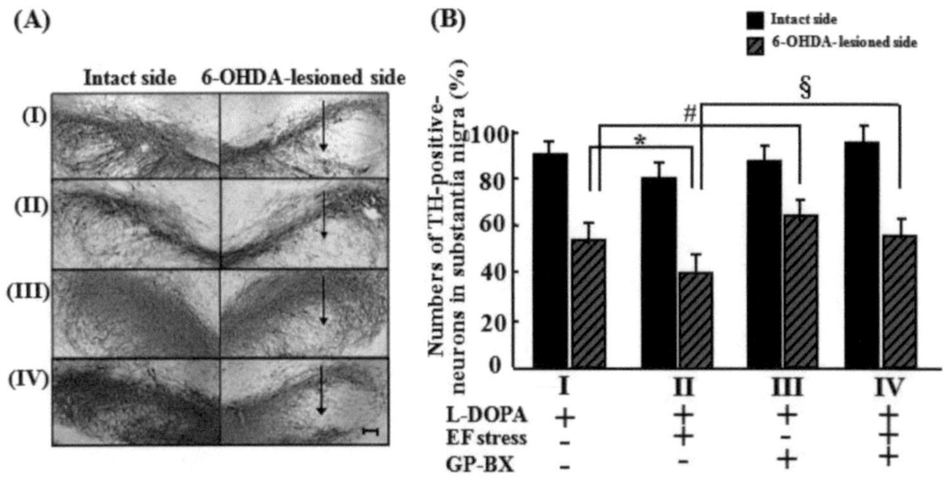

Fig. 3. Photomicrographs of TH immunoreactivity on substantia nigra tissue sections from representative rats of each group (A), and the number of surviving TH-immunopositive neuronal cells in the ipsilateral substantia nigra (6-OHDA-lesioned side) was analyzed as a percentage of that in the intact contralateral side (intact side) (B). L-DOPA-treated 6-OHDA-lesioned rat groups (I), L-DOPA-treated 6-OHDA-lesioned rat groups + chronic EF stress (II), L-DOPA-treated 6-OHDA-lesioned rat groups + GP-BX (III), and L-DOPA-treated 6-OHDA-lesioned rat groups + chronic EF stress + GP-BX (IV). Rats were treated with GP-BX (30 mg/kg/day, p.o.) or vehicle (0.9% saline, p.o.) and then subjected to every-other-day sessions of EF stress (duration and interval of 10 s for 10 min, 2 mA). L-DOPA (10 mg/kg/day, i.p.) was administered with benserazide (15 mg/kg/day, i.p.) prepared in saline. These data are representative of 7–10 animals per group, and the arrow indicates 6-OHDA-lesioned side. TH-immunopositive neuronal cells were analyzed as a percentage of intact side. Scale bar is 100 μm. * $p < 0.05$ compared with L-DOPA-treated 6-OHDA-lesioned rat groups; # $p < 0.05$ compared with L-DOPA-treated 6-OHDA-lesioned rat groups; § $p < 0.05$ compared with L-DOPA-treated 6-OHDA-lesioned rat groups + chronic EF stress (ANOVA followed by Tukey's test).

3.4 The levels of dopamine, DOPAC, HVA, and norepinephrine in the striatum of L-DOPA- treated 6-OHDA-lesioned rats exposed to chronic EF stress and administered GP-BX

The levels of dopamine, DOPAC, HVA, and norepinephrine were slightly increased in the striatal regions of the 6-OHDA-lesioned rat groups treated with L-DOPA (10 mg/kg), compared with those of the L-DOPA-untreated groups (Figures 2 and 4), but they were still decreased by 6-OHDA lesions (Figure 4, A-D I). The exposure to chronic EF stress in the L-

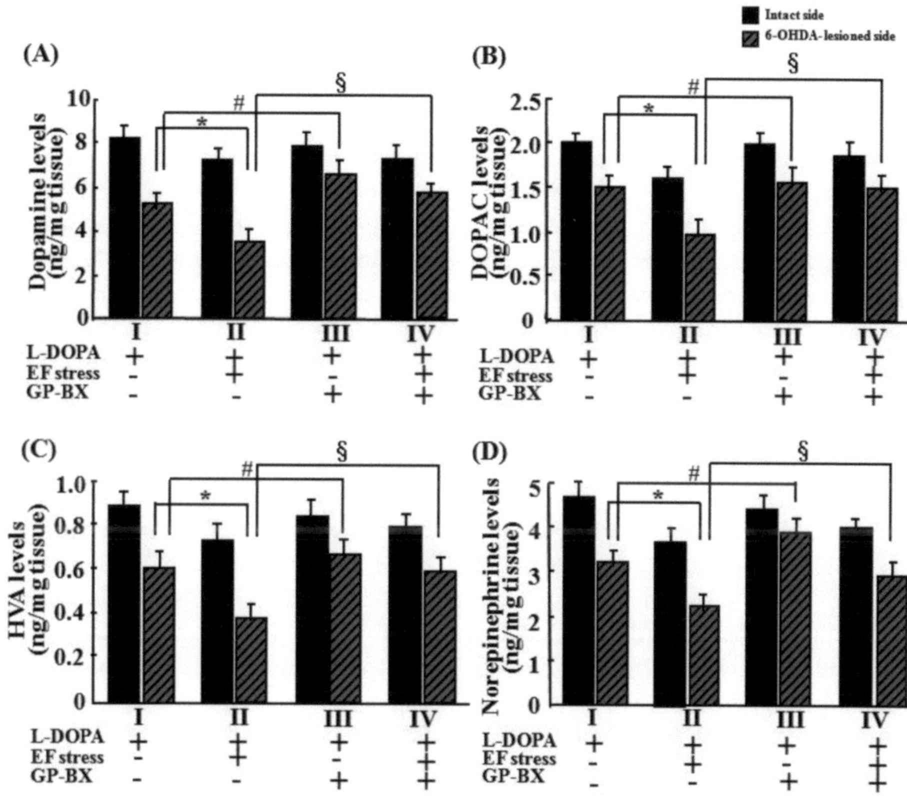

Fig. 4. Effects of GP-BX on the levels of dopamine (A), DOPAC (B), HVA (C), and norepinephrine (D) in the striatum of 6-OHDA-lesioned rats. L-DOPA-treated 6-OHDA-lesioned rat groups (I), L-DOPA-treated 6-OHDA-lesioned rat groups + chronic EF stress (II), L-DOPA-treated 6-OHDA-lesioned rat groups + GP-BX (III), and L-DOPA-treated 6-OHDA-lesioned rat groups + chronic EF stress + GP-BX (IV). Rats were treated with GP-BX (30 mg/kg/day, p.o.) or vehicle (0.9% saline, p.o.) and then subjected to every-other-day sessions of EF stress (duration and interval of 10 s for 10 min, 2 mA). L-DOPA (10 mg/kg/day, i.p.) was administered with benserazide (15 mg/kg/day, i.p.) prepared in saline. After 4 weeks, the brains were removed, and the levels of dopamine, DOPAC, HVA, and norepinephrine were determined by an HPLC method. Results represent means ± S.E.M. for 7–10 animals per group. * $p < 0.05$ compared with L-DOPA-treated 6-OHDA-lesioned rat groups; # $p < 0.05$ compared with L-DOPA-treated 6-OHDA-lesioned rat groups; § $p < 0.05$ compared with L-DOPA-treated 6-OHDA-lesioned rat groups + chronic EF stress. (ANOVA followed by Tukey's test).

DOPA (10 mg/kg)-treated 6-OHDA-lesioned rat groups showed a further significant decrease in the levels of dopamine, DOPAC, HVA, and norepinephrine in the 6-OHDA-lesioned sides of the striatal regions by 43.0%, 47.9%, 43.1%, and 47.4%, respectively, compared with those of the unstressed groups (Figure 4, A-D I and II). This was significantly recovered by 30 mg/kg GP-BX administration for 28 days (Figure 4, A-D I and III). In addition, 30 mg/kg GP-BX administration for 28 days resulted in an improvement in the levels of dopamine, DOPAC, HVA, and norepinephrine to 62.5%, 54.5%, 55.1%, and 31.7%, respectively, in the L-DOPA (10 mg/kg)-treated 6-OHDA-lesioned rat groups (Figure 4, A-D I and IV).

4. Discussion

The neurotoxin 6-OHDA is commonly used for animal models of PD, and it is believed to cause dopaminergic cell death with a unilateral destruction of the nigrostriatal system (Schober, 2004). Among the various bioactive functions of GP, it has been known to have anti-oxidant, anti-inflammatory, and immunostimulatory actions (Razmovski-Naumovski et al., 2005). In addition, GP ethanol extract has been found to have an anti-stress function against chronic EF stress in mice (Choi et al., 2008; Im et al., 2009). In this study, the neuroprotective functions of GP-BX on the exposure to chronic EF stress in the 6-OHDA-lesioned rat model of PD with or without long-term L-DOPA treatment were investigated by determining the quantities of TH-immunopositive neuronal cells surviving in the substantia nigra and the levels of dopamine, DOPAC, HVA, and norepinephrine in the striatum.

GP ethanol extracts at doses of 10–50 mg/kg/day for 28 days did not show toxic effects, such as weight loss or death in rats (Choi et al., 2008; Im et al., 2009), and the water extract (750 mg/kg) of GP also did not produce any significant toxic effects in rats during a 6-month period of treatment (Attawish et al., 2004). GP-BX (30 mg) was selected in this study, and its administration for 28 days did not exhibit adverse effects, such as weight loss, diarrhea, vomiting, or death.

The infusion of 6-OHDA into the CNS resulted in decreased rotational movements, including stereotypic behavior, by the change of monoamine contents (Deumens et al., 2002), which was recovered by GP-BX administration (data not shown). These findings suggest that GP-BX showed a preventive activity against 6-OHDA-lesioned rats.

The number of TH-immunopositive surviving cells showed a large decrease in the ventrolateral side of the substantia compacta (intact side), and their numbers were well maintained in the ventral tegmental area (VTA) of the ventral side (intact side). These findings were very similar to the pathological findings of PD. However, the number of TH-immunopositive neuronal cells in the VTA decreased slightly due to the passage of time with 6-OHDA (Figure 1, A I and II). The chronic exposure to EF stress every other day for 28 days enhanced the 6-OHDA-induced dopaminergic neuronal cell death in the 6-OHDA-lesioned rat groups used as a PD model system (Figures 1 and 2). The chronic EF stress also inhibited the therapeutic effects of L-DOPA (10 mg/kg) in the 6-OHDA-lesioned rats (Figures 3 and 4). However, GP-BX administration (30 mg/kg) for 28 days ameliorated the enhanced neurotoxic effects induced by the exposure to chronic EF stress in 6-OHDA-lesioned rats with or without L-DOPA: the number of surviving TH-immunopositive neuronal cells in the substantia nigra and the levels of dopamine, DOPAC, HVA, and norepinephrine in the striatum were recovered by GP-BX. In addition, GP-BX inhibited 6-OHDA-induced neurotoxicity in the brain regions of normal rats and 6-OHDA-lesioned rats (data not shown), which was similar to the findings with GP ethanol extract (Choi et al., 2010). These results indicate that oral administration of GP-BX exhibited a preventive and protective activity against the chronic EF stress- and/or 6-OHDA-induced dopaminergic neuronal cell death in rats.

Stressful stimuli induced the production of ROS and increased the release of catecholamines and glucocorticoids (Ganong, 2001; Kandel et al., 2000), which reduced the function of immune systems (Im et al., 2009). Immobilized stress inhibited the neuroprotective effects of free-running wheel exercise in a rat model of PD (Urakami et al,, 1988). The exposure to chronically repetitive stress also reduced dopamine levels in the rat brain, leading to decreased ambulatory activity (Ahmed et al., 1995; Rajkowska, 2000). ROS, which are generated by 6-OHDA by autoxidation, directly destroyed DNA, essential proteins, and cell lipid membranes to cause necrosis (Schober, 2004). In addition, 6-OHDA was detected in rat brain after L-DOPA treatment due to the high levels of dopamine and hydrogen peroxide (Maharaj et al., 2005), which induced dopaminergic neuronal cell death by inflammatory processes and oxidative apoptosis (Blum et al., 2004). L-DOPA treatment in MPTP-induced PD rodents increased the striatal 6-OHDA levels, which may be sensitized by monoamine oxidase inhibitor (Borah & Mohanakumar, 2010). Long-term treatment with L-DOPA caused disabling motor side effects in PD and alleviated oxidative stress-induced neurotoxicity by ROS formation against striatal dopaminergic neurons and PC12 cells (Basma et al., 1995; Walkinshaw & Waters, 1995; Migheli et al., 1999). Subchronic or chronic L-DOPA treatment resulted in increased levels of dopamine and hydroxyl-free radicals in the striatum (Pandey et al., 2009). L-DOPA also showed treatment dose-dependent dual functions, including protection and neurotoxicity, in the 6-OHDA-lesioned rat model of PD (Cenci, 2009). In addition, L-DOPA at low concentrations (3–10 μM) produced trophic or cell-protective effects on neuronal and differentiated PC12 cells (Mena et al., 1997). In this study, L-DOPA treatment of 10 mg/kg for 28 days showed a slightly protective effect by increasing TH-immunopositive surviving cells in 6-OHDA-lesioned rats. However, the TH-immunopositive surviving cells were decreased by chronic EF stress (Figures 1 and 3), suggesting that the function of L-DOPA in rat model of PD was aggravated by the exposure to chronic EF stress. Taken together, these results suggest that the formation of ROS by chronic stress can enhance dopaminergic neuronal cell death in 6-OHDA-lesioned rats with or without L-DOPA treatment. Therefore, it is proposed that antioxidants scavenging 6-OHDA- or L-DOPA-induced ROS are a key to the prevention and control of the symptoms of PD (Andrew et al., 1993).

Previously, we reported that GP ethanol extract had an anti-stress function by improving the loss of body weight and the reduction of grip strength in rodents, which was induced by chronic EF stress (Choi et al., 2008). The extract also showed an immunomodulatory activity by preventing dexamethasone-induced immunosuppression (Im et al., 2009). In addition, GP ethanol extract protected against 6-OHDA-induced neurotoxicity in 6-OHDA-lesioned rats (Choi et al., 2010). In this study, GP-BX exhibited a protective activity against chronic EF stress by reducing L-DOPA-induced neuronal cell death in 6-OHDA-lesioned rats treated with L-DOPA. These results suggest that the protective functions of GP-BX on chronic EF stress- and L-DOPA-induced neurotoxicity could be mediated by the modulation of the ROS formation and immune system in rodents.

The gypenoside-rich fraction, gypenosides, protected against oxidative neurotoxicity involving glutamate in primary cultures of rat cortical cells (Shang et al., 2006) and showed anti-inflammatory activity (Lin et al., 1993). Gypenosides also showed a protective effect on dopaminergic neuronal cell death in the MPTP-induced rat model of PD (Wang et al., 2010). It has been shown that GP-BX has several gypenoside derivatives, including gynosaponin TN-1, gynosaponin TN-2, gypenoside XLV, and gypenoside LXXIV (Choi et al., 2010; Razmovski-Naumovski et al., 2005; Nagai et al., 1981; Takemoto et al., 1984; Yoshikawa et al., 1987). These data further support that GP-BX can be applied for the prevention of the symptoms of PD by scavenging the formation of ROS.

Besides herbal GP, black tea extract exhibited neuroprotective and neurorescue effects against 6-OHDA-induced degeneration of the nigrostriatal dopaminergic system (Chaturvedi et al., 2004), and Yeoldahanso-tang, which is a Korean herbal formula containing 10 herbs, also protected against neurotoxicity in a MPTP-induced mice model of PD (Bae et al., 2011). Therefore, the comparative functions for PD among these herbal extracts, including drug interactions, adverse effects, and toxicity may need to be studied further.

5. Conclusion

GP-BX showed protective functions for dopaminergic neurons from chronic stress- and L-DOPA-induced neurotoxicity in 6-OHDA-lesioned rat model of PD. Considering our results, GP-BX may be helpful in preventing the L-DOPA-induced adverse or oxidative toxic effects for PD, especially with chronic stress, as well as slow down the progression of PD symptoms. Clinical trials for patients with PD using herbal GP extract and its bioactive components need to be studied further.

6. Acknowledgments

This work was supported by a grant of Research Center for Bioresource and Health, KIAT and MKE (2010).

7. References

Ahmed S.H.; Stinus, L., Moal, M.L. & Cador, M. (1995), Social deprivation enhances the vulnerability of male Wistar rats to stressor-and amphetamine-induced sensitization. *Psychopharmacology*, Vol.117, No.1, pp. 116-124, ISSN 0033-3158

Amanda D. S.; Sandra, L., Castro, Michael, J. & Zigmond. (2002). Stress-induced Parkinson's disease: a working hypothesis, *Physiology & Behavior*, Vol.77, No.4-5, pp. 527-531, ISSN 0031-9384

Andrew, R.; Watson, D.G., Best, S.A., Midgley, J.M, Wenlong, H. & Petty, R.K. (1993). The determination of hydroxydopamines and other trace amines in the urine of parkinsonian patients and normal controls. *Neurochemical Research,* Vol.18, No.11, pp. 1175–1177, ISSN 0364-3190

Attawish, A.; Chivapat, S., Phadungpat, S., Bansiddhi, J., Techadamrongsin, Y., Mitrijit, O., Chaorai, B. & Chavalittumrong, P. (2004). Chronic toxicity of Gynostemma pentaphyllum. *Fitoterapia,* Vol.75, No.6, pp. 539–551, ISSN 0367-326X

Bae, N.; Ahn, T., Chung, S., Oh, M.S., Ko, H., Oh, H., Park, G. & Yang, H.O. (2011). The neuroprotective effect of modified Yeoldahanso-tang via autophagy enhancement in models of Parkinson's disease. *Journal of Ethnopharmacology,* Vol.134, No.2, pp. 313-322, ISSN 0378-8741

Basma, A.N.; Morris, E.J., Nicklas, W.J. & Geller, H.M. (1995). L-DOPA cytotoxicity to PC12 cells in culture is via its autoxidation. *Journal of Neurochemistry,* Vol.64, No.2, pp. 825–832, ISSN 0022-3042

Blum, D.; Torch, S., Lambeng, N., Nissou, M., Benabid, A.L., Sadoul, R. & Verna, J.M. (2001). Molecular pathways involved in the neurotoxicity of 6-OHDA, dopamine and MPTP: contribution to the apoptotic theory in Parkinson's disease. *Progress in Neurobiology,* Vol.65, No.2, pp. 135–172, ISSN 0301-0082

Borah, A. & Mohanakumar, K.P. (2010). L-DOPA-induced 6-hydroxydopamine production in the striata of rodents is sensitive to the degree of denervation. *Neurochemistry International,* Vol.56, No.2, pp. 357-62, ISSN 0197-0186

Cenci, M.A. (2007). L-DOPA-induced dyskinesia: cellular mechanisms and approaches to treatment. *Parkinsonism & Related Disorders,* Vol.13, pp. S263–S267, ISSN 1353-8020

Cheng, N.; Maeda, T., Kume, T., Kaneko, S., Kochiyama, H., Akaike, A., Goshima, Y. & Misu. (1996). Differential neurotoxicity induced by L-DOPA and dopamine in cultured striatal neurons, *Brain Research,* Vol.16, No.743, pp. 278–283, ISSN 0006-8993

Chaturvedi RK.; Shukla, S., Seth, K., Chauhan, S., Sinha, C., Shukla, Y. & Agrawal, AK. (2006). Neuroprotective and neurorescue effect of black tea extract in 6-hydroxydopamine-lesioned rat model of Parkinson's disease. *Neurobiology of Disease,* Vol.22, No.2, pp. 421-34, ISSN 0969-9961

Choi, H.S.; Lim, S.A., Park, M.S., Hwang, B.Y., Lee, C.K., Kim, S.H., Lim, S.C. & Lee, M.K. (2008). Ameliorating effects of the ethanol extracts from Gynostemma pentaphyllum on electric footshock stress. *Korean Journal of Pharmacognosy,* Vol.39, No.4, pp. 341–346, ISSN 0253-3073

Choi H.S.; Park M.S., Kim S.H., Hwang B.Y., Lee C.K. & Lee M.K. (2010). Neuroprotective effects of herbal ethanol extracts from Gynostemma pentaphyllum in the 6-hydroxydopamine-lesioned rat model of Parkinson's disease. *Molecules,* Vol.15, No.4, pp. 2814-2824, ISSN 1420-3049

Deumens, R.; Blokland, A. & Prickaerts, J. (2002). Modeling Parkinson's disease in rats: an evaluation of 6-OHDA lesions of the nigrostriatal pathway. *Experimental Neurology,* Vol.175, No.2 pp. 303–317, ISSN 0014-4886

Fearnley, M. & Lees, A.J. (1991). Ageing and Parkinson's disease: substantia nigra regional selectivity. *Brain,* Vol.114, No.5, pp. 2283–2301, ISSN 0006-8950

Ganong, W. F. (2003). *Review of Medical Physiology*, 23th ed. pp. 359–384, McGraw-Hill, ISBN 0071287289, United States

Hornykiewicz, O. (1982). Imbalance of brain monoamines and clinical disorders. *Progress in Brain Research*, Vol.55, pp. 419–429, ISSN 0079-6123

Jankovic, J. (2005). Motor fluctuations and dyskinesias in Parkinson's disease: clinical manifestations. *Movement Disorders: Official journal of the Movement Disorder Society*, Vol.20, No.11, pp. S11–S16, ISSN 0885-3185

Im, S.A.; Choi, H.S., Hwang, B.Y., Lee, M.K. & Lee, C.K. (2009). Augmentation of immune responses by oral administration of Gynostemma pentaphyllum ethanol extract. *Korean Journal of Pharmacognosy*, Vol.40, No.1, pp. 35–40, ISSN 0253-3073

Kandel, E.R.; Schwartz, J. H. & Jessell, T.M. (2000) *Principles of Neural Science*, McGraw-Hill, ISBN 0071287289, United States

Lin, J.M.; Lin, C.C., Chiu, H.F., Yang, J.J. & Lee, S.G. (1993). Evaluation of the anti-inflammatory and liver-protective effects of Anoectochilus formosanus, Ganoderma lucidum and Gynostemma pentaphyllum in rats. *The American Journal of Chinese Medicine*, Vol.21, No.1 pp. 59–69. ISSN 0192-415X

Maharaj H.; Sukhdev Maharaj D., Scheepers M., Mokokong R. & Daya S. (2005). L-DOPA administration enhances 6-hydroxydopamine generation. *Brain Research*, Vol.1063, No.2, pp. 180-186, ISSN 0006-8993

Marsden, C.D. (1994). Parkinson's disease. *Journal of Neurology, Neurosurgery, and Psychiatry*, Vol.57, No.6, pp. 672–681, ISSN 0022-3050

Mena, M.A.; Davila, V., & Sulzer, D. (1997). Neurotrophic effects of L-DOPA in postnatal midbrain dopamine neuron/cortical historicity cocultures. *Journal of Neurochemistry*, Vol.69, pp. 1398-1408, ISSN 0022-3042

Merad-Boudia, M.; Nicole, A., Santiard-Baron, D., Saille, C. & Ceballos-Picot, I. (1998). Mitochondrial impairment as an early event in the process of apoptosis induced by glutathione depletion in neuronal cells: relevance to Parkinson's disease. *Biochemical Pharmacology*, Vol.56, No.5, pp. 645–655, ISSN 0006-2952

Migheli, R.; Godani, C., Sciola, L., Delogu, M.R., Serra, P.A., Zangani, D., De Natale, G., Miele, E. & Desole, M.S. (1999). Enhancing effect of manganese on L-DOPA-induced apoptosis in PC12 cells: role of oxidative stress. *Journal of Neurochemistry*, Vol.73, No. 3, pp. 1155-1163, ISSN 0022-3042

Nagai, M.; Izawa, K.; Nagumo, S.; Sakurai, N.; Inoue, T. (1981). Two glycosides of a novel dammarane alcohol from Gynostemma pentaphyllum. *Chemical & Pharmaceutical Bulletin*, Vol.29, pp. 779–783, ISSN 0009-2363

Neil, A. & David, B. (2008). Parkinson's disease, *Medicine*, Vol.36, No.12, pp. 630–635, ISSN 0025-7974

Ozawa, T.; Tanaka, M., Ikebe, S., Ohno, K., Kondo, T. & Mizuno, Y. (1990). Quantitative determination of deleted mitochondrial DNA relative to normal DNA in parkinsonian striatum by a kinetic PCR analysis. *Biochemical and Biophysical Research Communications*, Vol.172, No.2, pp. 483–489, ISSN 0006-291X

Paxinos, G. & Watson, C. (1986). *The Rat Brain in Stereotaxic Coordinates*, 2nd ed.; Academic Press, ISBN 0126930198, Australia

Pandey, A.; Borah, M., Varghese, P.K., Barman, K.P., Mohanakumar & R. Usha, R. (2009) Striatal dopamine level contributes to hydroxyl radical generation and subsequent neurodegeneration in the striatum in 3-nitropropionic acid-induced Huntington's disease in rats. *Neurochemistry International,* Vol.55, No.6, pp. 431–437, ISSN 0197-0186

Perese, D.A.; Ulman, J., Viola, J., Ewing, S.E. & Bankiewicz, K.S. (1989). A 6-hydroxydopamine-induced selective parkinsonian rat model. *Brain Research,* Vol.494, No.2, pp. 285–293, ISSN 0006-8993

Przedborski, S.; Levivier, M., Jiang, H., Ferreira, M., Jackson-Lewis, V., Donaldson, D. & Togasaki, D.M. (1995). Dose-dependent lesions of the dopaminergic nigrostriatal pathway induced by intrastriatal injection of 6-hydroxydopamine. *Neuroscience,* Vol.67, No.3, pp. 631–647, ISSN 0306-4522

Rajkowska G. (2000). Postmortem studies in mood disorders indicate altered numbers of neurons and glial cells. *Biological Psychiatry,* Vol.48, No.8, pp. 766-777, ISSN 0006-3223

Razmovski-Naumovski, V.; Huang, T.H-.W., Tran, V.H., Li, G.Q., Duke, C.C. & Roufogalis, B.D. (2005). Chemistry and pharmacology of Gynostemma pentaphyllum. *Phytochemistry Review,* Vol.4, pp. 197–219

Schober, A. (2004). Classic toxin-induced animal models of Parkinson's disease: 6-OHDA and MPTP. *Cell and Tissue Research,* Vol.318, No.1, pp. 215–224, ISSN 0302-766X

Schwab, R.S. & Zieoer, I. (1965) Effect of mood, motivation, stress and alertness on the performance in Parkinson's disease. *Psychiatria et Neurologia,* Vol.150, No. 6, pp. 345-357

Shang, L.; Liu, J., Zhu, Q., Zhao, L., Feng, Y., Wang, X., Cao, W. & Xin, H. (2006). Gypenosides protect primary cultures of rat cortical cells against oxidative neurotoxicity. *Brain Research,* Vol.1102, No.1, pp. 163–174, ISSN 0006-8993

Takemoto, T.; Arihara, S.; Yoshikawa, K.; Kawasaki, J.; Nakajima, T.; Okuhira, M. (1984). Studies on the constituents of Cucurbitaceae plants. XI. On the saponin constituents of Gynostemma pentaphyllum MAKINO. (7). *Yakugaku Zasshi,* Vol.104, pp. 1043–1049, ISSN 0031-6903

Urakami, K.; Masaki, N., Shimoda, K., Nishikawa, S. & Takahashi K. (1988). Increase of striatal dopamine turnover by stress in MPTP-treated mice. *Clinical Neuropharmacology,* Vol.11, No.4, pp. 360-368, ISSN 0362-5664

Walkinshaw, G. & Waters, C.M. (1995). Induction of apoptosis in catecholaminergic PC12 cells by l-DOPA. Implications for the treatment of Parkinson's disease. *The Journal of Clinical Investigation,* Vol.95, No.6, pp. 2458–2464, ISSN 0021-9738

Wang, P.; Niu, L., Gao, L., Li, WX., Jia, D., Wang, XL. & Gao, G.D. (2010). Neuroprotective effect of gypenosides against oxidative injury in the substantia nigra of a mouse model of Parkinson's disease. *The Journal of International Medical Research,* Vol.38, No.3, pp. 1084-92.

Yoshikawa, K.; Arimitsu, M. Kuki, K. Takemoto, T.; Arihara, S. (1987). Studies on the constituents of Cucurbitaceae plants. XVIII. On the saponin constituents of Gynostemma pentaphyllum MAKINO. (13). *Yakugaku Zasshi*, Vol.107, pp. 361–366, ISSN 0031-6903

19

Acetyl-L-Carnitine in Parkinson's Disease

Maria Stefania Sinicropi[1], Nicola Rovito[2],
Alessia Carocci[3] and Giuseppe Genchi[2]
[1]Department of Pharmaceutical Sciences, University of Calabria,
[2]Department of Pharmaco-Biology, University of Calabria,
[3]Department of Medicinal Chemistry, University of Bari,
Italy

1. Introduction

Parkinson's disease (PD) is the most common neurodegenerative movement disorder that is estimated to affect approximately 1% of the population older than 65 years of age (deRijk et al., 2006; Saunders, 2000). PD was first described in 1818 by the British physician J. Parkinson. Before that date, no one had ever described the symptoms of this disease; so many researchers theorize that this pathology is the product of the English Industrial Revolution (Parris, 2000; Perlmutter, 2000). Some authors speculate that new neurotoxic contaminants produced by the industries can have been the cause of this chronic and progressive disease. PD is characterized by the progressive depletion of pigmented dopamine-containing neurons in the region known as the substantia nigra pars compacta and by the presence of intraneuronal aggregates called Lewy bodies (LBs), which are enriched in filamentous α-synuclein and other proteins that are often ubiquinated (Lee & Trojanowsky, 2006). Approximately 80% of dopaminergic neurons in the substantia nigra are already irreversibly destroyed when the symptoms of PD becomes significantly visible. Depletion of dopamine causes dysregulation of the motor circuits that project throughout the basal ganglia (BG), resulting in the cardinal clinical manifestations of PD: bradykinesia (extreme slowness), tremor, rigidity, and postural instability. Consequently, patients experience increasing difficulty in daily living functions along the course of the disease. Additional neuronal fields and neurotransmitter systems are also involved in PD, including the locus coeruleus, the dorsal motor nucleus, the autonomic nervous system and the cerebral cortex. Consequently, noradrenergic, serotoninergic, and cholinergic neurons are also lost. These widespread neuronal changes led to complex and variable progressive non-motor symptoms such as cognitive decline, sleep abnormalities, and depression which dominate the later stages of PD (Braak, 2003). In any case, PD is primarily a sporadic disorder and its etiopathogenesis is still not fully understood, but the recent discovery of genes associated with rare monogenic forms of the disease, together with earlier studies and new experimental animal models, has provided important and novel insight into the molecular pathways involved in disease pathogenesis (Wood-Kaczamar, 2006). Increasing evidence indicates that deficits in mitochondrial function, oxidative and nitrosative stress, accumulation of aberrant or misfolded proteins, and ubiquitin-proteasome system dysfunction can represent the principal molecular pathways or events that commonly underlie the pathogenesis of sporadic and familial forms of PD (Schapira, 2008). However it is possible that multiple factors contribute to the cascade of events leading to cells death in patients with PD and that different factors might be more important in different individuals (Olanow, 2009) (Fig. 1).

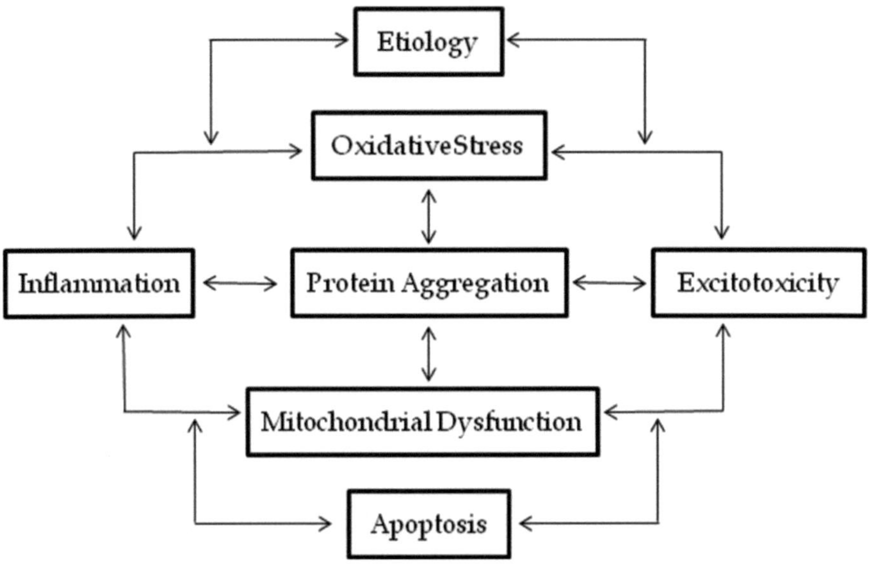

Fig. 1. Schematic illustration of factors that might be involved in the pathogenesis of cells death in PD. (Adapted from Olanow, 2007).

Several pharmacological agents are currently available for the management of PD (Table 1). These drugs can provide symptomatic relief but no agents capable to halt the progression of the neurodegenerative process or reverse the neuronal degeneration have been developed yet. Moreover, the neuroprotective effects suggested for many of the approved drugs have not been convincingly demonstrated in PD patients. Furthermore, although PD also involves degeneration of non-dopaminergic neurons, the treatment of the resulting predominantly non-motor features remains a challenge. The leading therapeutic strategy pursued in PD management is the so called dopamine replacement therapy (DRT), which employs drugs acting on dopamine (DA) circuits to restore the deficient dopaminergic tone existing in this pathology. Pharmacological agents have also been developed which can indirectly boost DA transmission, based on the functional interactions existing between DA and other neurotransmitters in the BG. L-Dopa is the key compound in the treatment of PD, acting as a precursor of DA. It has a long clinical record as the most effective antiparkinsonian drug, and it is still considered the "gold standard" in pharmacological treatment of PD (Mercuri & Bernardi, 2005). However, besides offering only symptomatic relief for patients, motor and non-motor untoward effects are often observed in the course of L-dopa therapy, which can be severe and limit its therapeutic potential (Encarnation & Hauser, 2008; Fox & Lang, 2008). Furthermore, exposure of patients to L-dopa, results in fluctuations of motor responses in approximately 30–50% of patients exposed to therapy for as little as 5 or more years. The most common fluctuation experienced is the so-called "on-

Drugs	Mechanism of action
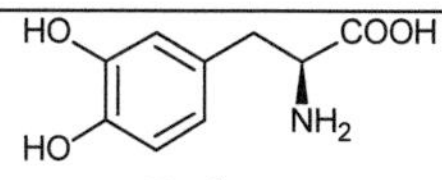 L-dopa	Precursor of DA
Ergot derivatives: 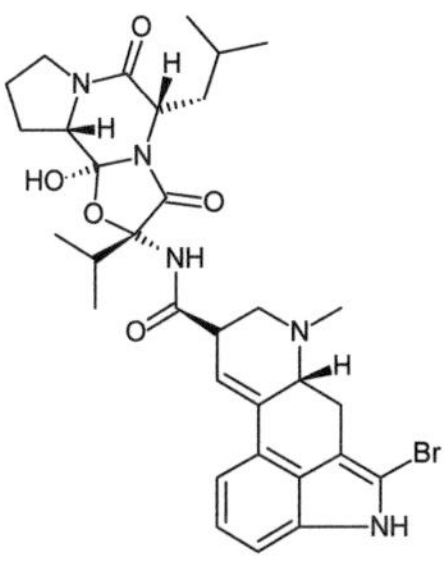 Bromocriptine; 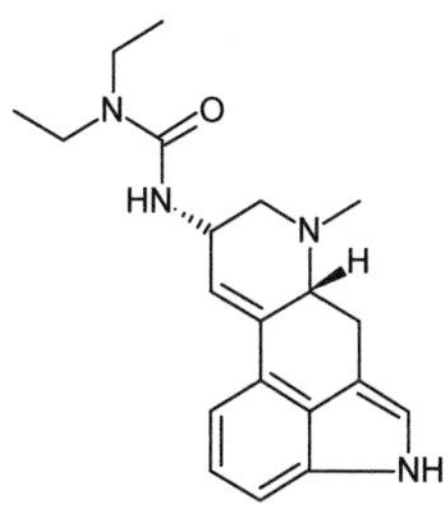 Lisuride; 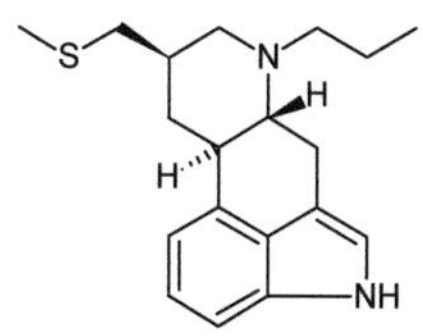 Pergolide	Agonist at D_2-like receptors
Non-Ergot derivatives: 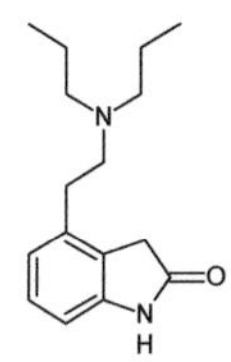 Ropinirole; 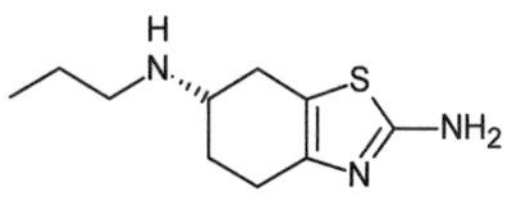 Pramipexole; 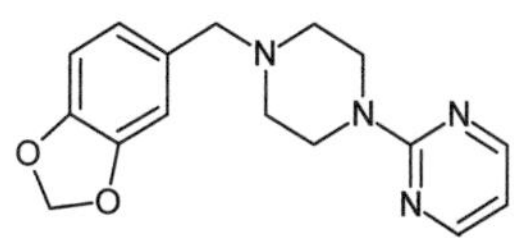 Piribedil	Agonist at D_2-like receptors
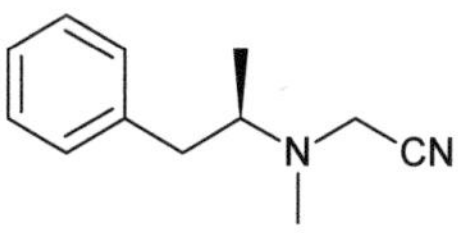 Selegiline; 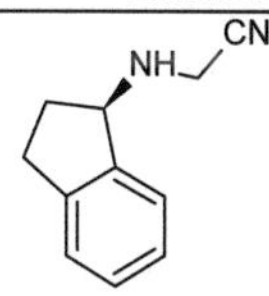 Rasagiline	MAO-B inhibitors
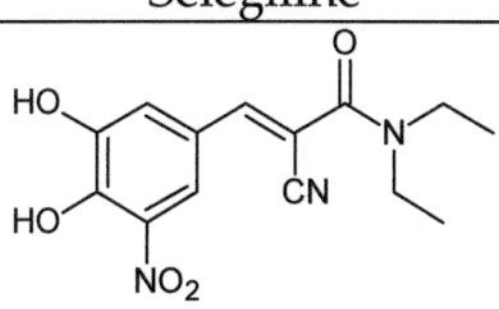 Entacapone; 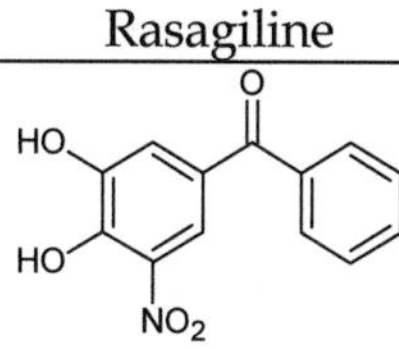 Tolcapone	COMT inhibitors
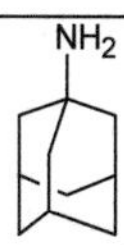 Amantadine	NMDA glutamate receptor antagonist
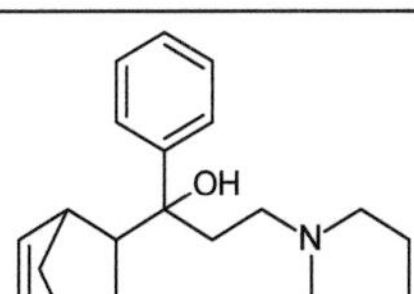 Biperiden; 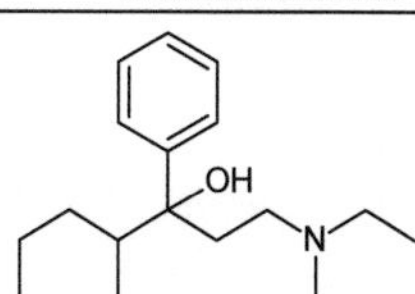 Triexyphenidyl; 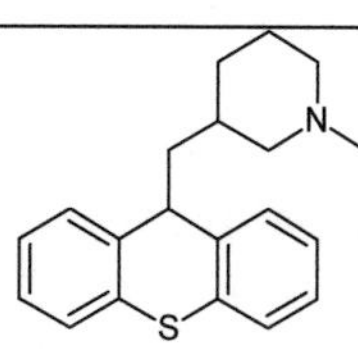 Metixene	Muscarinic receptor antagonists

Table 1. Currently available pharmacological therapies for PD treatment.

off" phenomenon that results in an unpredictable transient loss of therapeutic effect. Apart from L-dopa, drugs that are currently prescribed for the management of PD include DA receptor agonists, selective monoaminooxidase type B inhibitors (MAO-B), catecol-O-methyltransferase (COMT) inhibitors, amantadine (an antiviral agent that also bears action as an antiglutamatergic agent), and anticholinergics. DA receptor agonists counteract PD-associated motor impairment chiefly stimulating the D_2-like receptors, though some of them can also bind non–dopaminergic receptors. They may be used alone to delay the need for L-dopa or as multiple-medication therapy (MMT) with L-dopa to increase its effectiveness (Cavalli et al. 2008). Neuroprotective properties have been suggested for some dopaminergic agonists (e.g. bromocriptine and pramipexole), although the clinical evidence collected so far does not convincingly support this hypothesis (Schapira, 2003). Certain other available drugs, like MAO-B (Fernandez & Chen, 2007) and COMT inhibitors (Canesi et al., 2008; Schrag, 2005), are used mainly as MMT with L-dopa, since they alter the *in vivo* metabolism of DA by increasing its plasma half-life. Functional interactions between glutamate and DA receptors exist in BG, and evidence suggests that the loss of DA in PD may lead to glutamatergic hyperactivity, which participates in the manifestation of motor impairment accompanying the disease (Chase & Oh, 2003). On this basis, glutamatergic antagonists have been extensively investigated as potential antiparkinsonian drugs (Johnson et al. 2009). Among these, amantadine is the best characterized antiglutamatergic agent used in PD management. In addition to the blockade of ionotropic *N*-methyl-D-aspartate (NMDA) receptors, amantadine posses other mechanisms of action which contribute to its effects: anticholinergic activity, stimulation of DA release, modulation of the affinity of post-synaptic DAergic receptors for DA (Metman et al., 1998, Peeters et al., 2003). Anticholinergic compounds were the first, and for a long time the only, pharmacological agents available to treat motor deficits accompanying PD (Brocks, 1999). They were intend to correct the imbalance between DA and acetylcholine levels that take place in the BG, where a reduction of cholinergic tone may amplify DA-mediated signal (Cragg, 2006). Although these drugs produce some beneficial effects on PD symptoms, they are associated with adverse cognitive effects (Cancelli et al., 2009). All the anticholinergics used against PD bind to the central muscarinic receptors, having no affinity for the nicotinic ones, although they also block peripheral muscarinic receptors, and this triggers many of their adverse effects, which include nausea, constipation and urinary retention (Lees, 2005). Nevertheless, currently available pharmacological therapies are unable to arrest or to reverse the progression of this relentlessly progressive and severely debilitating condition. PD is currently an incurable disease, and the number of subjects afflicted with this disease is constantly increasing due to the increasing global geriatric population. Therefore, the need for newer and more effective agents is receiving a great deal of attention and, consequently, being subjected to extensive research. The vast amount of information gained regarding the pathogenesis of PD has fuelled numerous developments and vast range of investigated agents have demonstrated immense potential for preventing and eventually providing cure for this condition. Clinical and biochemical evidences suggest that PD involves multifactorial, oxidative neurodegeneration and that L-dopa therapy aggravates the oxidative burden. Strong evidence now exists to support an aberrant role for mitochondrial functions, as well as increased oxidative stress, in the pathogenesis of PD. If mitochondrial defects and oxidative damage play a role in the pathogenesis of PD, then one would suspect that agents that may improve mitochondrial function or exert antioxidative effects could be neuroprotective. There are several agents that are currently under investigation for their potential neuroprotective effects based on their capacity to modify mitochondrial dysfunction. These include creatine, coenzyme Q10, nicotinamide, lipoic acid and acetyl-L-carnitine, etc. (Table 2). These agents are therefore promising candidates for neuroprotective drugs against PD (Beal, 2003). Acetyl-L-carnitine, (3*R*)-3-(acetyloxy)-4-(trimethylammonio)butanoate (table 2), is an ester of the trimethylated amino acid, L-carnitine, and is synthesized in the brain, liver and kidney by the enzyme acetyl-L-carnitine transferase. Acetyl-L-carnitine facilitates the transport of fatty acids and other moieties across the membranes of mitochondria, thereby participating in the production of energy and mitochondrial function within the brain. Acetyl-L-carnitine has been proposed to have beneficial effects in preventing the loss of brain functions which typically occur during aging and neurodegenerative disorders. The main mechanism of action of acetyl-L-carnitine is the improvement of mitochondrial respiration which allows the neuron to produce ATP necessary to maintain the normal membrane potential. However, acetyl-L-carnitine has been shown to be neuroprotective through a variety of other effects such as the increase in protein kinase C (PKC) activity (McDaniel, et al. 2003). Moreover acetyl-L-carnitine has also been reported to attenuate the occurrence of parkinsonian symptoms associated with 1-methyl-4-phenyl-1,2,3,6-tetrahydropyridine (MPTP) *in vivo*, and protects *in vitro* against the toxicity of neurotoxic 1-methyl-4-phenylpyridinium (MPP^+), a metabolite of MPTP (Hongyu et. al., 2010). Therefore, acetyl-L-carnitine with its well known antioxidant energizing protective activities and with its trophic effects, might be an effective and safe prevention strategy for PD.

Agent	**Structure**
Coenzyme Q10	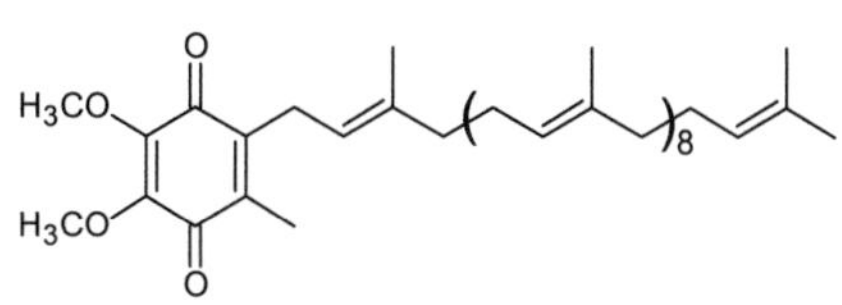
Carnitine	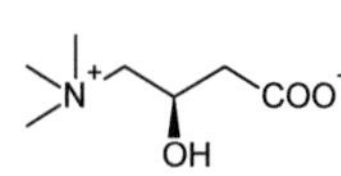
Acetyl-L-carnitine	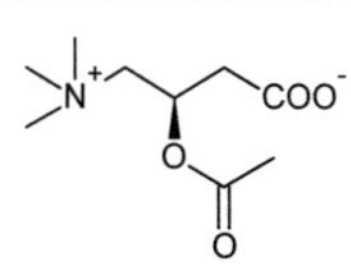
Lipoic acid	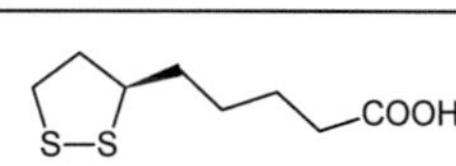

Agent	Structure
Nicotinammide	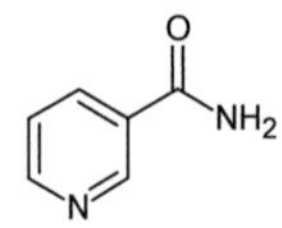
Creatine	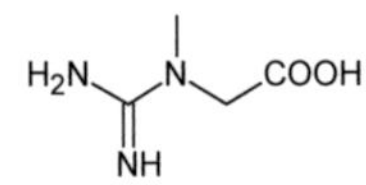
Curcumin	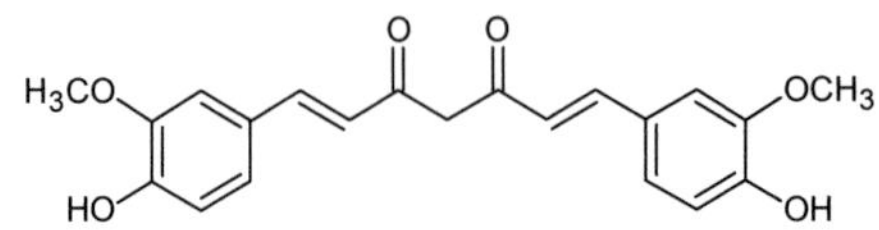
Resveratrole	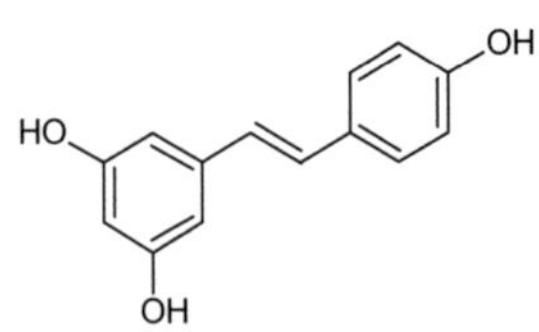
Vitamine C	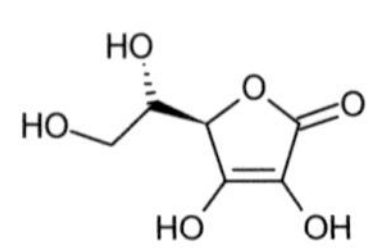
Melatonin	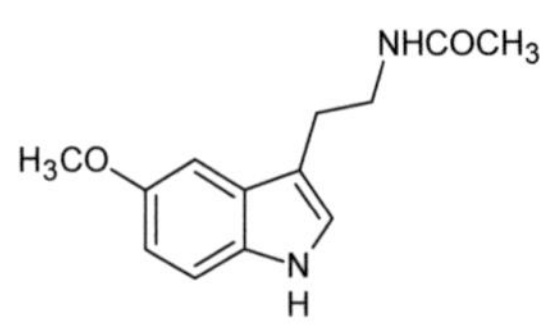
Omega-3 and Omega-6 fatty acids	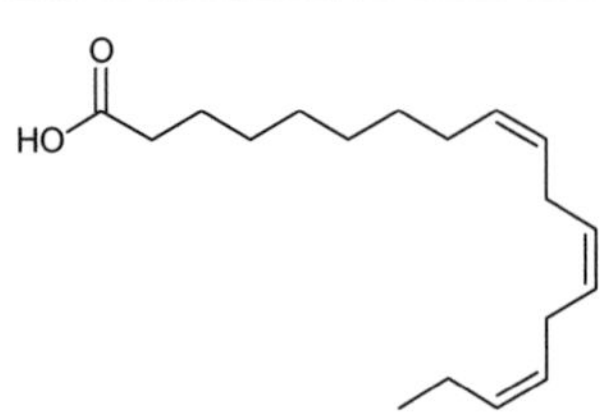 Linolenic acid 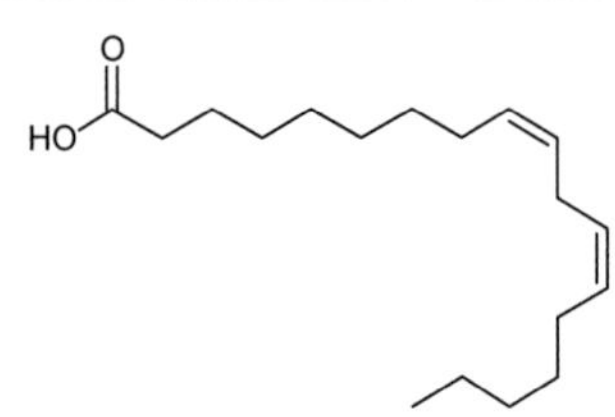 Linoleic acid
Uric acid	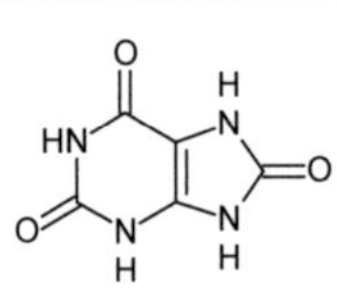

Table 2. Neuroprotective agents effective in PD models.

2. Nutritional and biochemical aspects of acetyl-L-carnitine

Carnitine has been discovered in the bovine muscle in 1905, but its structure was defined only in 1927. In 1958 the role of carnitine has been discovered by I. Frizz, who demonstrated that this substance is important in stimulating the oxidation of long chain fatty acids into the mitochondria. L-Carnitine (–)-3-hydroxy-4-(trimethylammonio)butanoate is a highly polar, water-soluble quaternary amine that exists as a zwitterion under physiological conditions. It was initially called vitamin T, because it is necessary for the growth of the *Tenebrio Molitor* warm. Although it is structurally similar to an amino acid it is not involved in the formation of proteins, and it is more similar to acetylcholine. Carnitine is synthesized *in vivo* from the amino acids lysine and methionine, especially in liver, kidney, and muscle, and it is stored mainly in skeletal and cardiac muscles (Marquis & Fritz, 1965). Exogenous carnitine, taken predominantly with the meat of the diet, is about 75% of the body carnitines, while the daily requirement is about 200—300 mg. *In vivo* synthesis of carnitine, supplemented by carnitine from diet, provides sufficient carnitine to maintain metabolic functions. However, in cases of excessive loss of carnitine (low carnitine intake with the diet, altered carnitine metabolism or disease states such as in neurodegenerative diseases and geriatric depression), supplementation with acetyl-L-carnitine may be beneficial. Tissue levels of L-carnitine in animals and humans decrease with age, due to reduced integrity of the mitochondrial membranes. Acetyl-L-carnitine, an ester of the L-carnitine, is synthesized in human brain, liver, and kidney by the enzyme acetyl-L-carnitine transferase. Carnitine, acetyl-L-carnitine and acyl-L-carnitine are responsible for many biological actions. Several authors have suggested that acetyl-L-carnitine has beneficial effects on brain functions during aging and in conditions of neurodegenerative diseases such as Parkinson's and Alzheimer's diseases. It has been demonstrated that acetyl-L-carnitine plays a role in increasing the potency of cholinergic and anti-cholinergic actions, by reacting with the electrophilic or cationic site of the cholinergic receptor (Sinicropi et al., 2010). Carnitine as acyl-L-carnitine is important in the mitochondrial process of β-oxidation of fatty acids (Bremer, 1962; Bremer et al., 1983) and the acetyl moiety can be utilized to maintain acetyl-CoA levels. Acetyl-L-carnitine promotes acetylcholine production and release, and stimulates membrane phospholipid synthesis (Pettegrew et al., 2000). In addition, the acetyl moiety of acetyl-L-carnitine can acetylate –NH_2 and/or –OH functional groups of lysine, serine, threonine, tyrosine and *N*-terminal amino acids in proteins modifying their structure, function and activity. Moreover acetyl-L-carnitine modulates glucose metabolism and stimulates glycogen synthesis, restores ammonia induced depletion of brain energy stores in sparse-fur mice with elevated ammonia and glutamine levels (Rao et al., 1997) and, with carnitine, maintains progressive spermatozoa motility (Jeulin et al., 1988). This molecule acts also on the mitochondrial redox reactions that allow neurons to produce ATP, required to maintain normal membrane potential (McDaniel et al., 2003). L-carnitine and acetyl-L-carnitine are administrated orally, intravenously and/or intramuscularly. These compounds are absorbed in the jejunum by simple diffusion. Transport into tissues and cells is via an active transport mechanism and acetyl-L-carnitine and carnitine plasma concentrations reach equilibrium via carnitine acetyl-transferase activity. Both intravenous and oral administrations result in a corresponding increase of cerebrospinal fluid (CSF) concentrations of acetyl-L-carnitine, indicating that it readily crosses the blood-brain barrier (Kido et al., 2001; Thal et al., 1996).

3. MPTP and neuroprotective effect of acetyl-L-carnitine in pathogenesis of Parkinson's disease

In the mitochondria of all cells redox reactions produce free radicals. High levels of reactive oxygen species (ROS) and reactive nitrogen species (RNS), especially in Parkinson's disease, can result in damage to phospholipids and polyunsaturated fatty acids, which are both abundant in the brain and therefore susceptible to oxidative damage. Therefore, there are many evidences for increased oxidative damage also to DNA and proteins (Dexter et al., 1994). Many evidences have accumulated implicating mitochondrial defects and oxidative stress damage in the pathogenesis of Parkinson's disease. In this contest, fundamental role is attributed to 1-methyl-4-phenyl-1,2,3,6-tetrahydropyridine (MPTP), a neurotoxin that is able to produce an experimental model of Parkinson's disease (PD) in humans and laboratory animals (such as primates and mice). It replicates most of the clinical features of PD as well as the main biochemical and pathologic hallmarks of the disease. The apparent neurotoxic specificity of MPTP is mediated through its conversion into 1-methyl-4-phenylpyridine (MPP^+) (Fig. 2) by the action of the mitochondrial enzyme MAO B (Javitch & Snyder, 1984; Javitch et al., 1985).

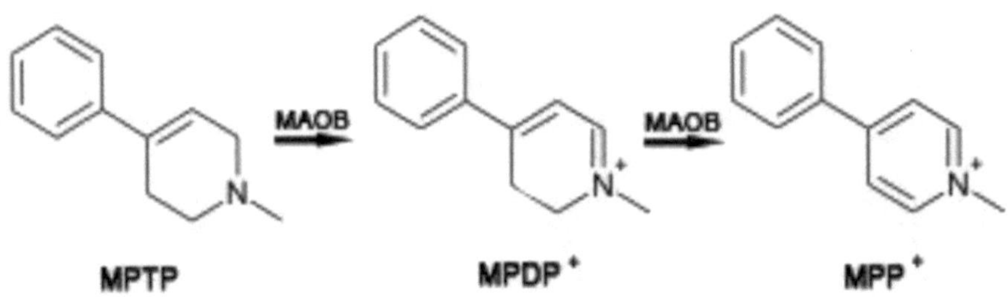

Fig. 2. Conversion of MPTP in MPP^+

The neurotoxicity of MPTP was discovered in 1976 when B. Kidstone, a 23 years old student of chemistry in Maryland, synthesized MPTP and injected it himself. He was contaminated by the MPTP and three days later he showed all the symptoms of Parkinson's disease. Studies on MPTP toxicity showed that it is mediated by inhibition of respiratory chain complex I activity (Bloem et al., 1990). There are at least three ways that MPP^+ can follow once inside dopaminergic neurons (Przedborski & Vila, 2003). It can: a) take the vesicular pathway, bind to dopamine transporters to be translocated into synaptosomal vesicles (Liu et al., 1992); b) interact with various cytosolic enzymes by remaining into the cytosol (Klaidman et al., 1993); c) be concentrated in the mitochondria (Ramsay & Singer, 1986). MPP^+ can passively enter the mitochondria through the transmembrane potential of the mitochondrial membranes and it can accumulate into the mitochondrial matrix. First of all, MPP^+, after being entered the mitochondrial matrix, inhibits the Krebs cycle enzyme α-ketoglutarate dehydrogenase (Mizuno et al., 1987), but the main cause of mitochondrial dysfunction involves the respiratory chain complex I (Ramsay et al., 1991). The MPP^+ toxicity is associated with oxidative damage. In fact MPP^+ induces superoxide production and increases lipid peroxidation. Important studies of Dexter and colleagues, showing increases in both malondialdehyde and in cholesterol hydroperoxides, led to a direct evidence of oxidative damage in Parkinson's disease (Dexter et al., 1994). Even the concentration of 8-hydroxy-2'-deoxyguanosine has been found three to four times higher in the caudate and substantia nigra of Parkinson's disease subjects (Sancher-Ramos et al., 1994). Shergill and co-authors have found a significant increase of nitrosyl complexes in Parkinson's disease substantia nigra (Shergill, 1996). However, recent studies suggest that MPP^+ toxicity, at least in the initial stages, is primarily due to a decrease in mitochondrial ATP synthesis rather than the formation of free radicals (Fonck & Baudry, 2003). Subsequently, the protective effect of acetyl-L-carnitine in Parkinson's disease, induced by MPTP, has been studied in a group of primates by the research group of Bodis-Wolner (Bodis-Wolner et al., 1991). For their studies Bodis-Wolner and colleagues used three groups of primates, the first of which was treated just with MPTP. To the second group was administered acetyl-L-carnitine before the MPTP, while the third group had a control role. Their results have shown that primates treated only with MPTP developed the classic symptoms of parkinsonism. In the second group, only in a primate a weak form of Parkinson's disease has evolved to signify the protective effect of acetyl-L-carnitine on the disease development. It is conceivable that the effect of MPP^+ results in altering the mitochondrial respiration processes linked to NAD (Nicklas et al., 1985, 1987; Heikkila et al, 1985; Ramsey et al., 1986; Mizuno et al., 1988).

4. Toxic and antioxidant compounds in Parkinson's disease

Oxidants, as hydrogen peroxide and superoxide radicals, are produced as by-products of oxidative phosphorylation into mitochondria, making these organelles the main site of ROS generation within the cells. In fact, mitochondria are a major source of ROS, with up to 2-3 % of all oxygen consumed by mitochondria being converted to hydrogen peroxide (Boveris et al., 1972). This is the normal condition and basal levels of ROS can be limited by the presence of efficient antioxidant defence systems, including the enzymatic antioxidants (superoxide dismutase, catalase, peroxidases, and heme oxygenase) and the non-enzymatic redox-regulating antioxidants (glutathione and vitamin C). However, in pathological neurodegenerative conditions, like in Parkinson's disease, where mitochondrial respiratory defects occur, the amount of ROS produced by the electron transport chain dramatically increases, abolishing the antioxidant protection systems (Parker et al., 1989). In studies on brain tissue in patients with PD, the activity of complex I is reduced in the substantia nigra, without any decrease in other brain regions. As shown by Haas et al. (Hass et al., 1995), the activity of complex I is reduced also in PD platelets of un-medicated patients. A decrease of coenzyme Q10 levels in platelets mitochondria, which is correlated with reduced complex I of respiratory chain, is reported in Shults et al. (Shults et al., 1997). In parkinsonian subjects platelets mitochondria were found to have lower levels of coenzyme Q10 than mitochondria from age/sex-matched controls. As shown in certain clinical studies, coenzyme Q10 appears to slow the progressive deterioration of function in PD (Shults et al., 2002). Coenzyme Q10 is necessary for the normal activity of the respiratory chain and transfers electrons from complexes I and II to III. It can be worthwhile to use coenzyme Q10 to restore the functions of the respiratory chain and scavenge ROS. Nevertheless, coenzyme Q10 protects primary dopaminergic neurons *in vitro* against cell death induced by MPTP (Gille et al., 2004), and seems that at least partially restores the function of complex I in the tissues of patients with PD (Shults et al., 1998; Storch et al., 2007). Moreover, it has antioxidant properties; it has been also shown to prevent peroxidation of membrane lipids and protect mitochondrial DNA from free oxygen radicals. Important results on the defects of complex I activity in the pathogenesis of PD are derived from studies with the toxin rotenone. Rotenone (Table 3) is a natural compound extracted from the roots of certain plants and has been used as an insecticide for vegetables. Rotenone rapidly crosses the blood-brain barrier due to its lipophilic structure, and rapidly crosses the biological membranes of mitochondria into the cells, in which the toxin reduces the activity of oxidative phosphorylation, by binding to PSST subunit of respiratory chain complex I (Schuler & Casida, 2001). It is known that rotenone is a highly specific inhibitor of complex I of the electrons transport chain. The possibility that rotenone and other pesticides are involved in the pathogenesis of PD stems from epidemiological studies (Gorell et al., 1998; Seidler et al., 1996). In fact, an atypical Parkinson's syndrome has developed in populations of the French West Indies, taking fruit and herbal tea containing insecticides (Caparros-Lefebvre & Elbaz, 1999). Pesticides and herbicides become highly suspect as potential PD triggers. A connection was long suspected between PD and rural living, including the drinking of contaminated well water or exposure to pesticides and herbicides (Hancock et al., 2008; Stephenson, 2000). Recently it was observed that high blood levels of homocysteine (Table 3) are present in patients with PD receiving L-dopa.

Agent	Structure
Homocysteine	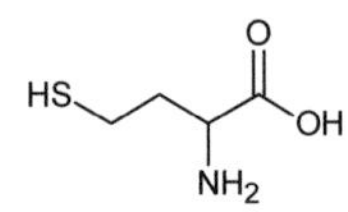
Rotenone	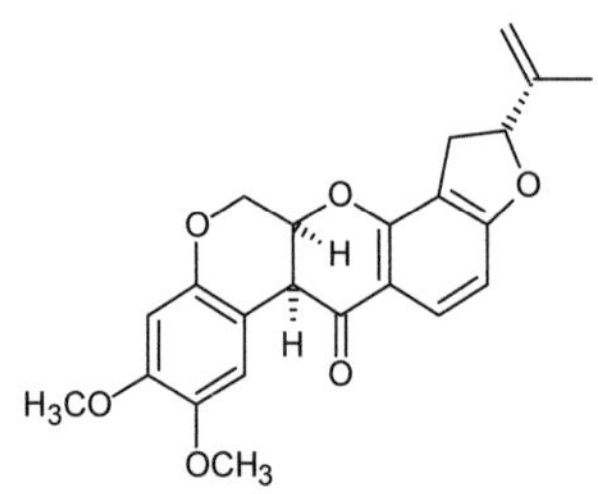

Table 3. Neurotoxic agents in Parkinsons's disease

On the other hand it is known that the increase in homocysteine is a risk factor for atherosclerosis, stroke, vascular disease, and dementia. There are many proposed mechanisms for toxicity of homocysteine in promoting neurodegenerative diseases such as of Parkinson's and Alzheimer's diseases (Postuma & Lang, 2004; Seshadri et al., 2002): free radicals formation, induction of inflammation, and altered vulnerability of complex I mitochondrial respiratory chain. The formation of homocysteine occurs from methionine which is converted to *S*-adenosylmethionine and then demethylated to *S*-adenosylhomocysteine, which forms homocysteine. Homocysteine itself is reused to form methionine by the action of two enzymes rate-limiting methylenetetrahydrofolate reductase (MTHFR) and betaine homocysteine methyltransferase (BHMT). Homocysteine can be metabolized to cysteine due to the cystathionine-betasintethase (CBS). The MTHFR requires cofactors such as vitamin B12 and folate, while the CBS requires vitamin B6. The administration of L-dopa urges COMT activities causing methylation of L-dopa to 3-O-methyl-dopa and, at the same time, the demethylation of *S*-adenosylmethionine to S-adenosylhomocysteine, which rapidly forms homocysteine. Therefore, since the demethylation of *S*-adenosylmethionine results in an increase of homocysteine, it is easy to understand why Parkinson's patients treated with L-dopa have higher levels of homocysteine. Consequently, any substance that can reduce blood levels of homocysteine should be administered to Parkinson's patients who require L-dopa: COMT inhibitors, vitamin B6, folate and vitamin B12. The toxicity of these compounds can be prevented with the administration of antioxidants. Complex I of respiratory chain is genetically coded for the ring-shaped mitochondrial DNA (mtDNA). A line of evidence, implicating mitochondria and mitochondrial genome (mtDNA) in PD pathogenesis, comes from "cybrid cells". While many proteins and enzymes of all electron transport chain complexes are coded from nuclear genes, 13 of them are coded in the small circular double-stranded mtDNA, located within the mitochondrial matrix. The human mitochondrial genome contains 37 genes (16,560 base pairs), including 13 that encode subunits of proteins of respiratory chain, and in particular 7 subunits of complex I. Mitochondrial genes exhibit a much higher mutation rate compared to nuclear genes and mtDNA is exposed to ROS generated during respiration. It is believed, therefore, that the oxidative damage to mitochondrial DNA and its mutation can play a role for mitochondrial dysfunction in PD. To determine if complex I is genetically abnormal, Swerdlow and colleagues (Swerdlow et al., 1996) devised an experiment with cybrid cells, generated to uncouple potential effects of a damaged mtDNA from effects of the nuclear DNA. These Swerdlow cybrid cells are hybrid cells which combine the nuclear genome from neuroblastoma cells with the mitochondrial genome from platelets of PD patients or healthy control subjects. Using these cybrid cells, Swerdlow and colleagues confirmed that PD mitochondria were less efficient in complex I activity (- 20%) associated with increased free radical production and apoptotic cell death (Gu et al., 1998; Swerdlow et al., 1996). Since only mtDNA is derived from the donor platelets, the Swerdlow experiment can be interpreted as a suggestion for mtDNA transmission of the mitochondrial defect. Besides, many authors suggest that alterations in processes of ubiquitination and degradation of proteins by the 26S proteasome can play a primary role in the PD pathogenesis (McNaught & Ienner, 2001; McNaught et al., 2001). Products of oxidative damage can contribute to substantia nigra degeneration in PD. The oxidized proteins can not be adequately ubiquitinated and recognized by the proteasomes and accumulated within the cells. The accumulation of ubiquitinated proteins and the loss of proteasomal activity can induce mitochondrial dependent apoptotic death of dopaminergic neurons in a manner similar to that occurring in the substantia nigra in PD. Although rare, some genetic cases of Parkinson's disease are linked to mutations in a synaptic protein called α-synuclein that was originally identified from smaller peptides isolated in amyloid-containing fractions of Alzheimer disease brains (Hong, 2005). The α-synuclein protein is another aggregating, fibril-forming protein that is a major component of the Lewy body lesions characteristic of PD as well as certain cases of Alzheimer (AD) and several other neurodegenerative conditions. α-Synuclein aggregates show evidence of nitration-based oxidative damage that might play a critical role in aggregate formation (Giasson et al., 2000). Recent studies have shown that the polyphenol curcumin (the active principle of turmeric *Curcuma longa*) can reduce the aggregation of α-synuclein, and its administration to cultured cells with α-synuclein aggregate formation results in fewer aggregates (Ono & Yamada, 2006; Pandey & Galvin, 2005). Also the pesticide rotenone leads to the presence of Lewy bodies with aggregation of α-synuclein (Sherer et al., 2003). The evidence that rotenone, a inhibitor of mitochondrial respiratory chain complex I, causes aggregation of Lewy bodies may means that mitochondrial dysfunction has a role in the development of these pathologic fibril-forming proteins in Parkinson's disease (Dawson & Dawson, 2003a). Rajeswary has shown that curcumin protects mouse brain from MPTP-induced neurotoxicity by virtue of its scavenger activity (Rajeswary, 2006). Moreover, curcumin has been shown to protect PC12 cells from MPP^+ by inducing bcl-2, a antiapoptotic protein, preventing the dissipation of membrane potential of mitochondria and reducing then ROS and iNOS levels (Chen et al., 2006). The importance of mitochondria in the neuroprotective effect of curcumin has been also emphasized by Mythri et al. (2007), who demonstrated that curcumin inhibits the formation of peroxynitrite responsible for the damage of respiratory chain complex I. Studies with humans and rodents have demonstrated that after oral administration curcumin is transformed to curcumin glucuronide and curcumin sulphate, not only in the liver (Rahaman et al., 2006) but also in the intestinal tract (Ireson et al., 2002). In these organs, curcumin is also reduced into dihydrocurcumin (DHC), tetrahydrocurcumin (THC), hexahydrocurcumin, octahydrocurcumin and hexahydrocurcuminol (Ireson et al., 2002; Rahaman et al., 2006); curcumin, DHC and THC can be further converted in glucuronide conjugates. It is important to note that curcumin and THC have anti-inflammatory activity; in humans and rodents curcumin inhibits the activity of cytochrome P450 enzymes, glutathione-transferase and UDP-glucuronosyl transferases (Basu et al., 2004; Hayeshi et al., 2007; Thapliyal & Maru, 2001). Moreover, it has been shown that a large number of polyphenolic antioxidants have a protective effect against the degeneration induced by high levels of ROS and RNS in cases of mitochondrial dysfunction. It has been proven that green tea polyphenols have a protective effect against 6-hydroxydopamine toxicity in SH-SY5Y cells (Guo et al., 2005). 6-Hydroxydopamine is a hydroxylated analogue of dopamine, extensively used in rodents. 6-Hydroxydopamine possess a high affinity for many membrane transporters of catecholamines and norepinephrine, allowing the drugs to freely enter both dopaminergic and noradrenergic neurons (Bovè et al., 2005). The efficacy of the green tea component epigallocatechin 3-gallate has been demonstrated in the MPTP mouse model of Parkinson's disease. It has been shown that in these treated rats there is both loss of dopaminergic neurons and attenuation of striatal dopamine levels (Choi et al., 2002). Choi et al. (2002) suggest that this protection is mediated by inhibition of NOS expression. Epidemiological evidence shows that two caps a day of green tea have a protective effect against the Parkinson's disease development (Chan et al., 1998). Another polyphenol used in the fight against Parkinson's disease is the oxyresveratrol, found in large amounts in mulberry wood, which has shown potent scavenger activity against ROS and RNS in glial cells exposed to hydrogen peroxide (Lorenz et al., 2003). In addition, in a study on 6-hydroxydopamine-treated neuroblastoma SH-SY5Y cells has been found that the oxyresveratrol drastically reduces the production of ROS and reduces also the apoptotic activity of caspase-3 caused by damaged mitochondria (Chao et al., 2008). Other important antioxidant is uric acid (Ames et al., 1981). Recent studies and epidemiological researches have shown a correlation between high levels of uric acid in serum and a lower incidence of Parkinson's disease (Annanmaki et al., 2007, Weisskopf et al., 2007; Winquist et al., 2010). It was also seen that the uric acid protects against the damage caused by free radicals on the mtDNA (Anderson & Harris, 2003), helping to maintain the integrity of the mitochondrial genome and prevent possible mutations. In addition, uric acid prevents the death of dopaminergic cells treated with rotenone and homocysteine; treatments that increase the production of ROS and act on mitochondrial membrane depolarization (Duan et al., 2002). Most likely uric acid neutralizes ROS through the Fenton reaction, thus providing dopaminergic neuroprotection. But we have to balance the benefits of dietary supplementation of uric acid on parkinsonism and the possible risk of developing gout and cardiovascular problems.

5. Acetyl-L-carnitine and other nutrients in age-dependent neurodegenerative diseases

A broad spectrum of both genetic and environmental factors has been suggested as contributing to the initiation and progression of PD. Among these, an important risk factor for the disease is the aging (Parris, 2000). It contributes to PD progression, perhaps because of accumulative oxidative damage and decrease of antioxidant capacity. Many evidences support the validity of the oxidative stress hypothesis, which suggests that lowered functional capacity in aged organisms is the result of an increased generation of reactive species. The increased levels of ROS and RNS can cause damage to intracellular macromolecules, as DNA, proteins and lipids and consequently impairing the function of vulnerable tissues and leading to the accumulation of altered gene products (Calabrese et al., 2006a). In addition, protein, lipid or glucose oxidation disrupts redox homeostasis and leads to accumulation of unfolded or misfolded proteins in the aging brain. For this reason Parkinson's and Alzheimer's diseases, having a common denominator, production of abnormal proteins, mitochondrial dysfunction and oxidative stress, are called "protein conformational diseases" (Calabrese et al., 2008). In particular, an unfolded protein response conformational disease is condition that arise from dysfunctional aggregation of proteins in non-native conformations. This is often associated with multiple metabolic derangements that result in the excessive production of ROS and oxidative stress (Zhang et al., 2006). Genetic studies have also revealed that aging can be controlled by changes in intracellular NAD/NADH ratio regulating sirtuins, a group of proteins linked to aging, metabolism and stress tolerance in several organisms. Consistently, the neuroprotective roles of dietary antioxidants including for example, curcumin, carnosine, resveratrol and acetyl-L-carnitine have been demonstrated through the activation of these redox-sensitive intracellular pathways. In particular, acetyl-L-carnitine has been proposed to have beneficial effects in preventing the loss of brain function which typically occurs during aging and neurodegenerative disorders. In fact, acetyl-L-carnitine treatment has been shown to prevent age-related changes in mitochondrial respiration and decrease oxidative stress biomarkers thorough the up-regulation of HO-1 (heme oxygenase-1), Hsp70 (heat shock protein 70) and superoxide dismutase-2 in senescent rats (Calabrese et al, 2006c). It acts through the activaction of transcription factor Nrf2, which after binding to the ARE (antioxidant responsive element) in the HO-1 gene, up-regulates both HO-1 and thioredoxin reductase (TrxR), thus counteracting pro-oxidant conditions. Heme oxygenase-1 is, in fact, a key enzyme in the prevention of brain damage (Calabrese et al., 2006; Maines, 1997; Mancuso, 2004). The neuroprotective effects of over-expressed HO-1 has been attributed to several factors such as: a) increased level of both cGMP and bcl-2 in neurons; b) inactivation of the pro-apoptotic transcription factor p53; c) increase in antioxidant sources, i.e. the iron sequestering protein, as ferritin (Panahian, 1999). Hsp70 is, instead, a member of the stress protein. Hsc70 (heat shock cognate, the constitutive form), Hsp70 (the inducible form, also referred to as Hsp72) and GRP-75 (a constitutively expressed glucose-regulated protein) are included in this family (Calabrese et al., 2006b; Yenari et al., 1999). Recently it has been demonstrated that overproduction of Hsp70 leads to protection in several models of nervous system injury (Fig. 3). Oxidative stress, which has been suggested to be involved in the pathogenesis of PD, may originate in glial cells (Jenner, 2003). This is supported by post-mortem studies demonstrating the capacity of oxidative stress and oxidizing toxin to induce nigral cell degeneration (Olanow et al., 1998). There is evidence to support that there are high levels of basal oxidative stress in the substantia nigra pars compacta in the normal brain and that this is increased in PD. The brain is therefore particularly sensitive to oxidative stress. This is due to several factors: a) the neurons are particularly enriched in polyunsaturated fatty acids, prime targets for oxidative attack (Kidd & Levine, 1985); b) the brain consumes a high share of the body's oxygen intake and consequently results in the oxyradical formation; c) the activity of the antioxidant enzymes catalase and peroxidase is low in the brain, instead the superoxide dismutase is active. They acquire superoxide oxyradical and convert it in hydrogen peroxide (H_2O_2).

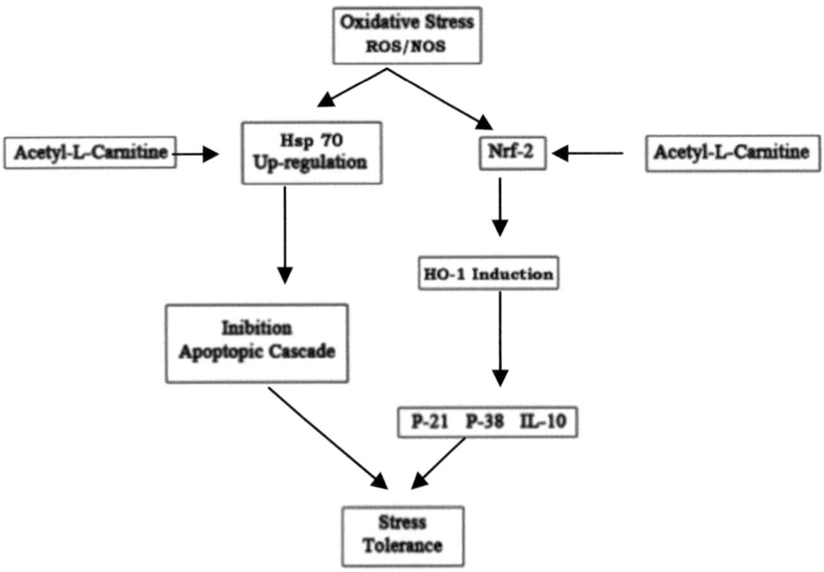

Fig. 3. The role of acetyl-L-carnitine in cell stress tolerance

In the absence of catalase and peroxidase, which normally would detoxify these peroxide products, that are done by glutathione peroxidase enzyme. This enzyme uses glutathione (GSH) as its essential cofactor, and when it is stimulated the brain's GSH reserves are more sensitive to depletion from oxidative attack (Kidd, 1997; Levine & Kidd 1985). As mentioned, the substantia nigra is particularly susceptible to oxidative stress and this is due to varied and many biochemical process that occur in it. It has a high content of dopamine and its metabolism and its "auto-oxidation" could be responsible for the high basal levels of oxidative stress. DA has a strong tendency to "auto-oxidation", generating reactive auto-metabolites, as 6-hydroxydopamine quinone and dopamine aminochrome, the formation of which can be accelerated by free (ionized) iron or by other redox-reactive elements such as copper, zinc or manganese (Pezzella, 1997; Youdim, 1989). Then, the degradation of dopamine by monoamine oxidase to produce H_2O_2 could increase the formation of oxidized glutathione (GS-SG), suggesting the presence of oxidative stress and impairment of the antioxidant system (Spina & Cohen, 1988). The H_2O_2 generated is also converted (by Fenton reaction), in the presence of the high levels of iron, in toxic hydroxyl radical which can damage DNA and other biomolecules (Youdim et al., 1989). It should be noted that an extremely high content of iron is concentrated in the substantia nigra zona compacta, and various iron-mediated reactions in substantia nigra would potentiate oxidative stress. For example ionized iron, or copper and zinc catalyze transformation of the protein α-synuclein into aggregated form, prominent component of the Lewy aggregates that develop in the SN of Parkinson's patients (Braak & Braak 2000; Paik et al., 2000). Moreover, important role of the iron is for dopamine-melanin, macromolecular material formed from the autoxidation of dopamine and normally scavenger of free radicals. When it is infiltrated with high levels of ionized iron it can drive Fenton reaction converting endogenous hydrogen peroxide to hydroxyl radical. The population of melanin-enriched, dopaminergic neurons found in the SN's zona compacta is the worst affected in PD. In the substantia nigra there are high levels of melanin and it could act as support matrix upon which ionized iron would catalyze oxyradical generation from available hydrogen peroxide or from neuromelanin itself (Youdim, et al., 1990).

6. Conclusion

Although the selective loss of DA neurons and the accumulation of α-synuclein are crucial in the development of PD, many evidences indicate that oxidative stress, and mitochondrial and proteasome dysfunctions have central role in this pathogenesis. Environmental factors, such as exposure to toxins, are also important in late-onset of the disease, whereas in early-onset PD, genetic factors assume predominant importance. Recently, the identification of several genes causing early-onset PD (such as α-synuclein; UCHLl, a ubiquitin carboxy-terminal hydrolase L1; parkin; DJ1, a parkin-associated protein involved with oxidative stress; PINK1, a putative serine threonine kinase) has yielded crucial insights into the possible pathogenic mechanisms (Dawson & Dawson, 2003b). The use of several neurotoxins to produce the clinical symptoms of PD both *in vitro* and *in vivo* has allowed to understand the molecular mechanism of disease. The functions of mitochondria make these subcellular organelles susceptible to oxidative damage, resulting in cell death by apoptosis and mtDNA mutations. In this context, the mitochondria represent, therefore, a highly promising target for the development of disease biomarkers by use of genetic and biochemical approaches.

The mitochondrial antioxidant/nutrient acetyl-L-carnitine, with its antioxidant energizing protective activities and with its trophic effects, at optimal doses, can be an effective and safe prevention strategy for PD, offering the possibility of new and innovative therapeutic strategies for this neurodegenerative disease. Acetyl-L-carnitine is a highly bioavailable molecule, it is thought to penetrate the brain barrier better than carnitine, and it is readily converted to carnitine as needed. Experimental evidences suggest that acetyl-L-carnitine boosts mitochondrial ATP production and helps to protect mitochondria against oxidative attack. This molecule is therefore of great interest for its wide clinical application in various neurological disorders, it has beneficial effects in preventing the loss of brain function which typically occurs during aging, and its neuroprotective benefits have been observed in the hippocampus, prefrontal cortex, substantia nigra and muscarinic receptor portions of the brain. These include antioxidant activity, improved mitochondrial energetics, stabilization of intracellular membranes and cholinergic neurotransmission. In particular, the most

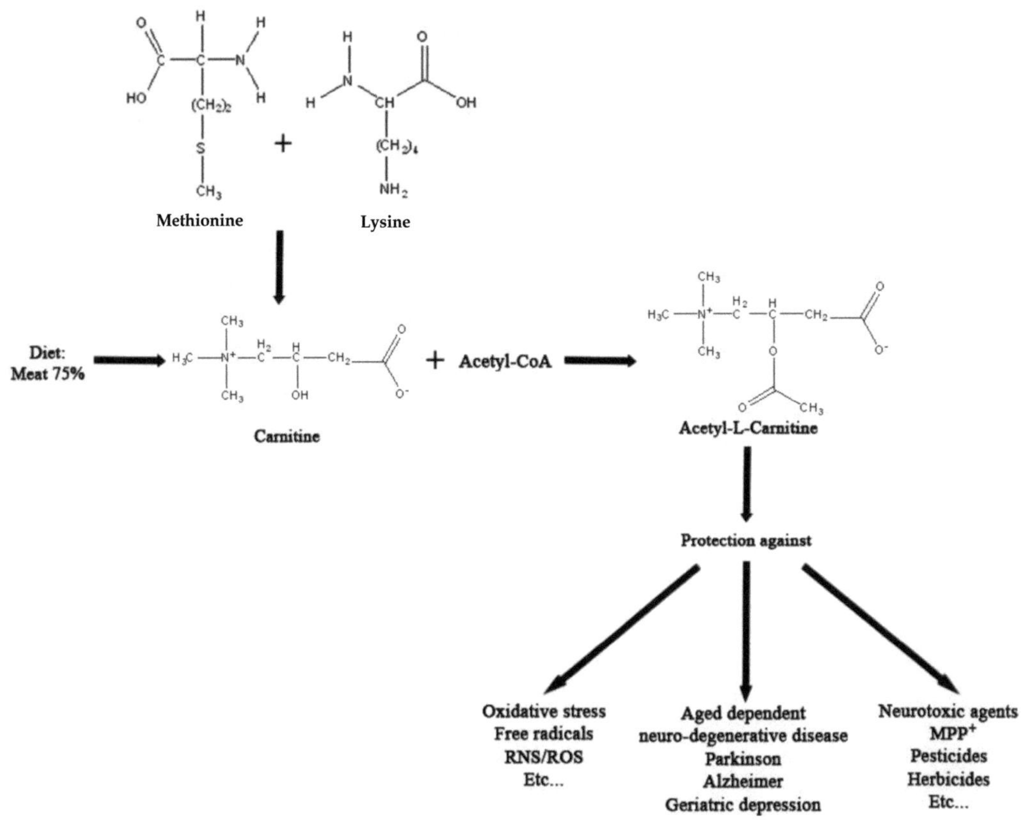

Fig. 4. Biosynthesis and physiological role of acetyl-L-carnitine

common function of acetyl-L-carnitine is the transport of fatty acids across the inner mitochondrial membrane, thereby being involved in the production of energy within the brain and in the maintenance of neuron and repairing of damages. Moreover, it has a variety of other neuronal effects. It increases protein kinase C (PKC) activity and reverse the age-related decline in the number of *N*-methyl-D-aspartate (NMDA) receptors on neuronal membranes. In addition, it is thought that it influences the cholinergic system acting as a cholinergic receptor agonist; it can also promote the synthesis and the release of acetylcholine and stimulates proteins and membrane phospholipids synthesis (Calabrese et al., 2005). Acetyl-L-carnitine can also increase the levels of neurotrophins such as nerve growth factor (NGF) and can reduce the energetic deficits in brain and phospholipids metabolism, probably because it aids mitochondrial functions (Mark et al., 2003). In fact, it increases mitochondrial biogenesis and decreases ROS production through the up-regulation of the PGC-1, as a possible underlying mechanism. In animal models, it partially protects the substantia nigra against 1-methyl-4-phenyl-pyridinium (MPP^+, active metabolite of MPTP) attack, by strengthening the dopaminergic transmission (Bodis-Wollner et al. 1991; Hongyu et. al., 2010; Sinicropi et al. 2010). In fact, brain histology reveals that acetyl-L-carnitine protects neurons in the substantia nigra, which otherwise have been devastated by MPTP attack. It has been well observed that long-term acetyl-L-carnitine administration in rats increases longevity and improves spatial learning, avoidance learning in aged rats, and long-term memory performance (Barnes et al., 1990; Ghiraldi et al., 1989;

Markowska et al., 1990). In summary, the protection provided by acetyl-L-carnitine offers the possibility of new therapeutic strategies for neurodegenerative diseases (including PD) which can share the same final neurotoxic pathway in mitochondria (Fig. 4).

7. Acknowledgment

This work was supported by grants from Ministero dell'Istruzione, dell'Università e della Ricerca (MIUR, Italy). The authors thank Biofutura Pharma s.p.a. (Sigma-Tau group) for their collaboration.

8. References

Albertini, P., Amenta, F., Bissoni, G., Cavallotti, C., Felici, L., Ferrante, F. & Garivaghi, G. (1989). Effect of acetyl-L-carnitine treatment on the density of muscarinic receptor in the brain of methylazomethanol-microencephalic rats. *Drugs Under Experimental & Clinical Research,* Vol.15, pp. 421-427, ISSN 0378-6501.

Anderson, R.F. & Harris, T.A. (2003). Dopamine and uric acid act as antioxidant in the repair of DNA radicals: implications in Parkinson's disease. *Free Radical Research,* Vol.37, No.10, (September 2003), pp. 1131-1136, ISSN 1029-2470.

Annanmaki, T., Muuronen A. & Murros, K. (2007). Low plasma uric acid level in Parkinson's disease. *Movement Disorders,* Vol.22, No.8, (June 2007), pp. 1133-1137, ISSN 0885-3185.

Barnes, C.A., Markowska, A.L., Ingram, D.K., Kametani, H., Spangler, E.L., Lemken, V.J. & Olton, D.S. (1990). Acetyl-L-carnitine 2: effects on learning and memory performance and aged rats in simple and complex mazes. *Neurobiology of Aging,* Vol.11, No.5, (September-October 1990), pp. 499-506, ISSN 0197-4580.

Basu, N.K., Ciotti, M., Hwang, M.S., Kole, L., Mitra, P.S., Cho, J.W. & Owens, I.S. (2004). Differential and special properties of the major human UGT1-encoded gastrointestinal UDP-glucuronosyltransferases enhance potential to control chemical uptake. *The Journal of Biological Chemistry,* Vol.279, No.4, (January 2004), pp. 1429-1414, ISSN 1083-351X.

Beal, M.F. (2003). Bioenergetic approachs for neuroprotection in Parkinson's disease. *Annals of Neurology,* Vol.53, No.S3, pp. S39-S48, ISSN 0364-5134.

Bloem, B.R., Irwin, I., Buruma, O.J.S., Haan, J., Roos, R.A.C., Tetrud, J.W. & Langston, J.W. (1990). The MPTP model: versatile contributions to the treatment of idiopathic Parkinson's disease. *Journal of Neurological Sciences,* Vol.97, No.2-3, (July 1990), pp. 273-293, ISSN 0022-510X.

Bodis-Wollner, I., Chung, E., Ghilardi, M.F., Glover, A., Onofrj, M., Pasik, P. & Samson, Y. (1991). Acetyl-levo-carnitine protects against MPTP-induced parkinsonism in primates. *Journal of Neural Transmission-Parkinson's Disease and Dementia Section,* Vol.3, No.1, pp. 63-72, ISSN 0936-3076.

Bovè, J., Prou, D., Perier, C. & Przedborski, S. (2005). Toxin-induced model of Parkinson's disease. *NeuroRx,* Vol.2, (July 2005), pp. 484-494, ISSN 1545-5351.

Boveris, A.; Oshino, N. & Chance, B. (1972). The cellular production of hydrogen peroxide. *Biochemical Journal,* Vol.128, No.3, pp. 617-630, ISSN 1470-8728.

Braak, H. & Braak, E. (2000) Pathoanatomy of Parkinson's disease. *Journal of Neurology,* Vol.247, No.S6 (June 2000), pp. 3-10, ISSN 0340-5354.

Braak, H., Del Tredici, K., Rub, U., de Vos, R.A.; Jansen Steur, E.N. & Braak, E. (2003). Staging of brain pathology related to sporadic Parkinson's disease. *Neurobiology of Aging*, Vol.24, No.2, (March-April 2003), pp. 197-211, ISSN 0197-4580.

Bremer, J. (1962). Carnitine in Intermediary Metabolism: The metabolism of fatty acid esters of carnitine by mitochondria. *The Journal of Biological Chemistry*, Vol.237, No.12, (December 1962), pp. 3628-3632, ISSN 1083-351X.

Broocks, D.R. (1999). Anticholinergic drugs used in Parkinson's disease. An overlooked class of drugs from a pharmacokinetic perspective. *Journal of Pharmacy and Pharmaceutical Sciences*, Vol.2, No.2, (May-August 1999), pp. 39-46, ISSN 1482-1826.

Calabrese, V., Ravagna, A., Colombrita, C., Scapagnini, G., Guagliano, E., Calvani, M., Butterfield, D.A. & Giuffrida Stella, A.M. (2005). Acetylcarnitine induces heme oxygenase in rat astrocytes and protects agonist oxidative stress: involvement of the transcription factor Nrf2. *Journal of Neuroscience Research*, Vol.79, No.4, (February 2005), pp. 509-521, ISSN 1097-4547.

Calabrese, V., Giuffrida Stella, A.M., Calvani, M. & Butterfield, D.A. (2006a) Acetylcarnitine and cellular stress response: roles in nutritional redox homeostasis and regulation of longevity genes. *Journal of Nutritional Biochemistry*, Vol.17, No.2, (February 2006), pp. 73-88, ISSN 0955-2863.

Calabrese, V., Butterfield, D.A., Scapagnini, G., Giuffrida Stella, A.M. & Maines, M.D. (2006b). Redox regulation of heat shock protein expression by signaling involving nitric oxide and carbon monoxide: relevance to brain aging, neurodegenerative disorders, and longevity. *Antioxidants & Redox Signaling*, Vol.8, No.3-4, (March-April 2006), pp. 444-477, ISSN 1557-7716.

Calabrese, V., Colombrita, C., Sultana, R., Scapagnani, G., Calvani, M., Butterfield, D.A. & Giuffrida Stella, A.M. (2006c). Redox modulation of heat shock protein expression by acetylcarnitine in aging brain: relationship to antioxidant status and mitochondrial function. *Antioxidants & Redox Signaling*, Vol.8, No.3-4, (March-April 2006), pp. 404-416, ISSN 1557-7716.

Calabrese, V., Cornelius, C., Mancuso, C., Pennisi, G., Calafato. S., Bellia, F., Bates, T.E., Giuffrida Stella, A.M., Schapira, T., Dinkova Kostova, A. & Rizzarelli, E. (2008). Cellular stress response: a novel target for chemoprevention and nutritional neuroprotection in aging, neurodegenerative disorders and longevity. *Neurochemical Research*, Vol.33, No. 12, (December 2008), pp. 2444-2471, ISSN 1573-6903.

Cancelli, I., Beltrame, M., Gigli, G.L. & Valente, M. (2009). Drugs with anticholinergic properties: Cognitive and neuropsychiatric side-effects in elderly patients. *Neurological Sciences*, Vol.30, No.2, (April 2009), pp. 87-92, ISSN 1590-3478.

Canesi, M., Zecchinelli, A.L., Pezzoli, G. & Antonini, A. (2008). Clinical experience of tolcapone in advances Parkinson's disease. *Neurological Sciences*, Vol.29, No.5, (December 2008) pp. S380–382, ISSN 1590-3478.

Caparros-Lefebvre, D. & Elbaz, A. (1999) Possible relation of atypical parkinsonism in the French West Indies with consumption of tropical plants: a case control study. Caribbean Parkinsonism Study Group. *The Lancet*, Vol.354, No.9175, (July 24, 1999), pp. 281-286, ISSN 0140-6736.

Casal, J., Elizan, T.S. & Yahr, M.D. (1998). Postencephalitic parkinsonism - a review. *Journal of Neural Transmission,* Vol.105, No. 6-7, (September 1998), pp. 645-676, ISSN 0300-9564.

Cavalli, A., Bolognesi, M.L., Minarini, A., Rosini, M., Tumiatti, V., Recanatini, M. & Melchiorre, C. (2008). Multi-target-Direct Ligands to Combat Neurodegenerative Disease. *Journal of Medicinal Chemistry,* Vol.51, No.3, (February 2008), pp. 347-372, ISSN 0022-2623.

Chan, D.K., Woo, J., Ho, S.C., Pang, C.P., Law, L.K., Ng, P.W., Hung, W.T., Kwok, T., Hui, E., Orr, K., Leung, M.F. & Kay, R. (1998). Genetic and environmental risk factors for Parkinson's disease in a Chinese population. *Journal of Neurolology, Neurosurgery, & Psychiatry,* Vol.65, No.5, (November 1998), pp. 781-784, ISSN 1468-330X.

Chao, J., Yu, M.S., Ho, Y.S., Wang, M. & Chahg, R.C.C. (2008) Dietary oxyresveratrol prevents parkinsonian mimetic 6-hydroxydopamine neurotoxicity. *Free Radical Biology and Medicine,* Vol.45, No.7, (October 2008), pp. 1019-1026, ISSN 0891-5849.

Chase, T.N. & Oh, J.D. (2000). Striatal dopamine- and glutamate-mediate dysregulation in experimental parkinsonism. *Trends in Neuroscience,* Vol.23, No.S10, (October 2000), pp. S86-S91, ISSN 0166-2236.

Chen, J., Tang, X.P, Zhi, J.L., Cui, Y., Yu, H.M., Tang, E.H., Sun, S.N., Feng, J.Q. & Chen, P.X. (2006) Curcumin protects PC12 cells against 1-methyl-4-phenylpyridinium ion-induced apoptosis by bcl-2 mitochondria-ROS-iNOS pathway. *Apoptosis,* Vol.11, No.6, (June 2006), pp.943-953, ISSN 1573-675X.

Choi J.Y., Park C.S., Kim D.J., Cho M.H., Jin B.K., Pie J.E. & Chung W.G. 2002. Prevention of nitric oxide-mediated 1-methyl-4-phenyl-1,2,3,6-tetrahydropyridine-induced Parkinson's disease in mice by tea phenolic epigallocatechin 3-gallate. *Neurotoxicology,* Vol.23, No.3, (September 2002), p. 367-374, ISSN 0161-813X.

Crag, S.J. (2006). Meaningful silence: How dopamine listens to the Ach pause. *Trends in Neuroscience,* Vol.29, No.3, (March 2006), pp. 125-131, ISSN 0166-2236.

Dawson, T.M., & Dawson V.L. (2003a) Molecular pathways of neurodegeneration in Parkinson's disease. *Science,* Vol.302, No.5646, (October 2003), pp. 819-822, ISSN 1095-9203.

Dawson, T.M., & Dawson, V.L. (2003b). Rare genetic mutation shed light on the pathogenesis of Parkinson disease. *The Journal of Clinical Investigation,* Vol.111, No.2, (January 2003), pp. 145-151, ISSN 0021-9738.

deRijk, M.C., Launer, L.J., Berger, K., Breteler, M.M., Dartigues, J.F., Baldereschi, M., Fratiglioni, L., Lobo, A., Martinez-Lage, J., Trenkwalder, C., & Hofman, A. (2000). Prevalence of Parkinson's disease in Europe: a collaborative study of population-based cohorts. *Neurology,* Vol.54, No.11, pp. S21–S23, ISSN 0028-3878.

Dexter, D.T., Holley, A.E., Flitter, W.D., Slater, TF, Wells, F.R., Daniel, S.E., Lees, A.J., Jenner, P. & Marsden, C.D. (1994). Increased levels of lipid hydroperoxides in the Parkinsonian substantia nigra: an HPLC and ESR study. *Movement Disorders,* Vol.9, No.1, pp. 92-97, ISSN 0885-3185.

Di Monte, D.A.; Lavasani, M. & Manning-Bog, A.B. (2002). Environmental factors in Parkinson's disease. *Neurotoxicology,* Vol.23, No.4-5, (October 2003), pp. 487-502, ISSN 0161-813X.

Duan, W., Ladenheim, B., Cutler, R.G., Kruman III, I.I., Cadet, J.L. & Mattson, M.P. (2002). Dietary folate deficiency and elevated homocysteine levels endanger dopaminergic neurons in models of Parkinson's disease. *Journal of Neurochemistry,* Vol.80, No.1, (January 2002), pp. 101-110, ISSN 1471-4159.

Encarnation, E.V. & Hauser, R.A. (2008). Levodopa-induced dyskinesias in Parkinson's disease: Etiology, impact on quality of life, and treatments. *European Neurology,* Vol.60, No.2, (July 2008), pp. 57-66, ISSN 0014-3022.

Fernandez, H.H. & Chen, J.J. (2007). Monoamine oxidase inhibitors: current and emerging agents for Parkinson disease. *Clinical Neuropharmacology,* Vol.30, No.3, (May-June 2007), pp. 150-168, ISSN 0362-5664.

Fonck, C. & Baudry, M. (2003) Rapid reduction of ATP synthesis and lack of free radical formation in rat brain synaptosomes and mitochondria. *Brain Research,* Vol.975, No.1-2, (June 2003), pp. 214-221, ISSN 0006-8993.

Fox, S.H. & Lang, A.E. (2008). Levodopa-related motor complications-phenomenology. *Movement disorders,* Vol.23 No.3, pp. S509-S514, ISSN 0885-3185.

Ghiraldi, O., Milano S., Ramanacci, M.T. & Angelucci, L. (1989). Long-term acetyl-L-carnitine preserves spatial learning in the senescent rat. *Progress in Neuro-Psychopharmacology and Biological Psychiatry,* Vol.13, No.1-2, pp. 237-245, ISSN 0278-5846.

Giasson, B..I, Duda, J.E., Murray, I.V., Chen, Q., Souza, J.M., Hurtig, H.I., Ischiropoulos, H., Trojanowski, J.Q. & Lee, V.M. (2000). Oxidative damage linked to neurodegeneration by selective alpha-synuclein nitration in synucleinopathy lesions. *Science,* Vol.290, No.5493, (November 2000), pp. 985–989, ISSN 1095-9203.

Gille, G., Hung, S.T., Reichmann, H. & Rausch, W.D. (2004). Oxidative stress to dopaminergic neurons as models of Parkinson's disease. *Annals of the New York Academy of Science,* Vol.1018, (June 2004), pp. 533-540, ISSN 00778923.

Gorell, J.M., Johnson, C.C., Rybicki, B.A., Peterson, E.L. & Richerdson, R.J. (1998) The risk of Parkinson's disease with exposure to pesticides, farming, well water, and rural living. *Neurology,* Vol.50, No.5, (May 1998), pp. 1346-1350, ISSN 0028-3878.

Gu, M., Cooper, J.M-, Taanmann, J.W. & Schapira A.H.V. (1998). Mitochondrial DNA transmission of the mitochondrial defect in Parkinson's disease. *Annals of Neurology,* Vol.44, No.2, (August 1998), pp. 177-186, ISSN 0364-5134.

Guo, S., Bezard, E & Zhao, B. (2005). Protective effect of green tea polyphenols on the SH-SY5Y cells against 6-OHDA induced apoptosis through ROS-NOS pathway. *Free Radical Biology and Medicine,* Vol.39, No.5, (September 2005), pp. 682-695, ISSN 0891-5849.

Haas, R.H., Nasirian, F., Nakano, K., Ward, D., Pay, M., Trojanowski, J.Q. & Lee, V.M. (1995). Low platelet mitochondrial complex I and complex II/III activity in early untreated Parkinson's disease. *Annals of Neurology,* Vol.37, No.6, (June 1995), pp. 714-722, ISSN 0364-5134.

Halliwell, B. (2006) Oxidative stress and neurodegeneration: where are we now? *Journal of Neurochemistry,* Vol.97, No.6, (June 2006), pp. 1634-1658, ISSN 1471-4159.

Hancock, D.B., Martin, E.R., Mayhew, G.M., Stajich, J.M., Jewett, R., Stacy, M.A., Scott, B.L., Vance, J.M., & Scott W.R., (2008). Pesticide exposure and risk of Parkinson's disease. A family –based case- control study. *BMC Neurology,* Vol.8, No.6, (March 2008), pp. 6-17, ISSN 1471-2377.

Hayeshi, R., Mutingwende, I., Mavengere, W., Masiyanise, V. & Mukanganyama, S. (2007). The inhibition of human glutathione S-transferase activity by plant polyphenolic compounds ellagic acid and curcumin. *Food and Chemical Toxicolology,* Vol.45, No.2, (February 2007), pp. 286-295, ISSN 0278-6915.

Hong, J.S. (2005). Role of inflammation in the pathogenesis of Parkinson's disease: Models, mechanisms, and therapeutic interventions. *Annals of the New York Academy of Science,* Vol.1053, (August 2005), pp. 151–152, ISSN 00778923.

Hongyu, Z., Haiqun, J., Jianghai, L., Ni, A., Bing,Y., Weili, S., Xuemin, W., Xin, L., Cheng, L. & Jiankang, L. (2010) Combined R-α-lipoic acid and acetyl-L-carnitine exerts efficient preventative effects in a cellular model of Parkinson's disease. *Journal of Cellular and Molecular Medicine,* Vol.14, No.1-2, (January-February 2010), pp. 215-225, ISSN 1582-1838.

Ireson, C.R., Jones, D.J., Orr, S., Coughtric, M.W., Boocock, D.J., Williams, M.L., Farmer, P.B., Steward, W.P. & Gescher, A.J. (2002). Metabolism of the cancer chemopreventive agent curcumin in human and rat intestine. *Cancer Epidemiology, Biomarkers & Prevention,* Vol.11, No.1, (January 2002), pp. 105-111, ISSN 1538-7755.

Jenner, P. (2003). Oxidative stress in Parkinson's disease. *Annals of Neurology,* Vol.53, No.3, pp. S26-S38, ISSN 0364-5134.

Jeulin , C., Soufir, J.C., Marson, J., Paquignon, M. & Dacheux, J.L. (1988). Acetylcarnitine and spermatozoa: relationship with epididymal maturation and motility in the boar and man. *Reproduction Nutrition Development,* Vol.28, No.5, pp. 1317-1327, ISSN 1297-9708.

Johnson, K.A., Conn, P.J. & Niswender, C.M. (2009), Glutamate receptors as therapeutic targets for Parkinson's disease. *CNS and Neurological Disorders- Drug Targets,* Vol.8, No.6, (December 2009), pp. 475-491, ISSN 1871-5273.

Kidd P.M. (1997). Gluthatione: systemic protectant against oxidative and free radical damage. *Alternative Medicine Review,* Vol.2, pp. 155-176, ISSN 1089-5159.

Kidd, P.M. & Levine, S.A. (1985). The biochemistry of free radicals, In: *Antioxidant Adaptation: Its Role in Free Radical Pathology,* S.A. Levine, P.M. Kidd, (Ed.) El Cerrito, ISBN 0961463007, CA: PMK

Kido, J., Tamai, I., Ohnari, A., Sai, Y., Kagami, T., Nezu, J., Nikaido, H., Hashimoto, N., Asano, M. & Tsuji, A. (2001). Functional relevance of carnitine transporter OCTN2 to brain distribution of L-carnitine and acetyl-L-carnitine across the blood-brain barrier. *Journal of Neurochemistry,* Vol.79, No. 5, (November 2001), pp. 959-969, ISSN 1471-4159.

Klaidman, L.K., Adams Jr., J.D., Leung, A.C., Kim, S.S. & Cadenas, E. (1993). Redox cycling of MPP^+ : evidence for a new mechanism involving hydride transfer with xanthine oxidase, aldehyde dehydrogenase, and lipoamide dehydrogenase. *Free Radical Biology and Medicine,* Vol.15, No.1, (July 1993), pp. 69-179, ISSN 0891-5849.

Lee, V. M. & Trojanowsky, J.Q. (2006). Mechanisms of Parkinson's disease linked to pathological alpha-synuclein: new targets for drug discovery. *Neuron,* Vol.52, No.1, (October 2006), pp. 33–38, ISSN 0896-6273.

Lees, A. (2005). Alternatives to levodopa in the initial treatment of early Parkinson's disease. *Drugs & Aging,* Vol.22, No.9, pp. 731-740, ISSN 1170-229X.

Levine, S.A. & Kidd, P.M. Antioxidant Adaptation: Its Role in Free Radical Pathology. San Leandro C.A. Biocurrents/Allergy Research group,1985

Liu, Y., Roghani, A. & Edwards R.H. (1992). Gene transfer of a reserpine-sensitive mechanism of resistance to *N*-methyl-4-phenylpyridinium. *Proceedings of the*

National Academy of Sciences of the United States of America. Vol.89, No.19, (October 1992), 9074-9078, ISSN 0027-8424.

Lorenz, P., Roychowdhury, M., Engelmann, M., Wolf, G. & Horn, T.F.W. (2003). Oxyresveratrol and resveratrol are potent antioxidant and free radical scavengers: effect on nitrosative and oxidative stress derived from microglial cells. *Nitric oxide – Biology and Chemistry.* Vol.9, No.2, (September), pp. 64-76, ISSN 1089-8603.

Maines, M.D. (1997). The heme oxygenase system: a regulator of second messenger gases. *Annuual Review of Pharmacolology and Toxicology,* Vol.37, (April 1997), pp. 517-554, ISSN 0362-1642.

Mancuso, C. (2004). Heme oxygenase and its products in the nervous system. *Antioxidants and Redox Signling,* Vol.6, No.5, (October 2004), pp. 878-887, ISSN 1523-0864.

Markowska, A.L., Ingram, D.K., Barnes, C.A., Spangler, E.L., Lemken, V.J., Kametani, H., Yee, W. & Olton, D.S. (1990). Acetyl-L-carnitine 1: effects on mortality; pathology and sensory-motor performance in aging rats. *Neurobiology of Aging,* Vol.11, No.5, (September-October 1990), pp. 491-498, ISSN 0197-4580.

Marquis, N.R. & Fritz, I.B. (1965). The distribution of carnitine, acetylcarnitine and acetyl transferase in rat tissues. *Journal of Biological Chemistry,* Vol.240, No.5, (May 1965), pp. 2193-2196, ISSN 1083-351X.

McDaniel, M.A., Maier, S.F., & Einstein, G.O. (2003). "Brain-Specific" Nutrients: A Memory Cure? *Nutrition,* Vol.19, No.11 (November 2003), pp. 957-975, ISSN 0899-9007.

McNaught, K.S. & Jenner, P. (2001). Proteasomal function is impaired in substantia nigra in Parkinson's disease. *Neuroscience Letters,* Vol.297, No.3, (January 2001), pp. 191-194, ISSN 0304-3940.

McNaught, K.S., Olanow, C.W., Halliwell, B., Isacson, O. & Jenner, P. (2001). Failure of the ubiquitin-proteasome system in Parkinson's disease. *Nature Review Neuroscience,* Vol.2, No.8, (August 2001), pp. 589-594, ISSN 1471-0048.

Metman, V.L., Del Dotto, P., van den Munckhog, P., Fang, J., Mouradian, M.M. & Chase, T.N. (1998). Amantadine as treatment for dyskinesias and motor fluctuations in Parkinson's disease. *Neurology,* Vol.50, No. 5, (May 1998), pp. 1323-1326 ISSN 0028-3878.

Mercuri, N.B. & Bernardi, G. (2005). The 'magic' of L-dopa: Why is the gold standard Parkinson's disease therapy? *Trends in Pharmacological Sciences,* Vol.26, No.7, (July 2005), pp. 341–344, ISSN 0165-6147.

Mizuno, Y., Saitoh, T. & Sone, N. (1987). Inhibition of mitochondrial alpha-ketoglutarate dehydrogenase by 1-methyl-4-phenylpyridinium ion. *Biochemical and Biophysical Research Communications,* Vol.143, No. 3, (March 1987), pp. 971-976, ISSN 0006-291X.

Mythri, R.B., Jagatha, B., Pradhan, N., Andersen, J. & Bharath, M.M. (2007). Mitochondrial complex I inhibition in Parkinson's disease; how can curcumin protect mitochondria? *Antioxidant and Redox Signaling,* Vol.9, No.3, (March 2007), pp. 399-408, ISSN 1523-0864.

Olanow C.W., Jenner P., Tatton N.A. & Tatton W.G. (1998). Neurodegeneration and Parkinson's disease, In *Parkinson's disease and movement disorders,* J. Jankovic, E. Tolosa, (Ed.), 67-103. Lippincott Williams & Wilkins , ISBN 0781778816, Baltimore.

Olanow, C.W., Jenner, P. & Youdim, M. Neurodegeneration and neuroprotection in Parkinson's disease. New York, NY: Academic Press: 1996.

Olanow, C.W. (2007). Pathogenesis of cell death in Parkinson's disease. *Movement Disorders,* Vol.22, No.S17, pp. S335-S342, ISSN 0885-3185.

Olanow, C.W., Stern, M.B. & Sethi, K. (2009). The scientific and clinical basis for the treatment of Parkinson disease. *Neurology,* Vol.72, No.21, (May 2009), pp. S1-S136, ISSN 0028-3878.

Ono, K. & Yamada, M. (2006). Antioxidant compounds have potent anti-fibrillogenic and fibril-destabilizing effects for alpha-synuclein fibrils *in vitro. Journal of Neurochemistry,* Vol.97, No.1, (April 2006), pp. 105-115, ISSN 1471-4159.

Paik, S.R., Shin, H.J. & Lee, J.H. (2000). Metal-catalyzed oxidation of alpha-synuclein in the presence of copper (II) and hydrogen peroxide. *Archives of Biochemistry and Biophysics,* Vol.378, pp. 269-277.

Panahian, N., Yoshiura, M. & Maines, M.D. (1999) Overexpression of heme oxygenase-1 is neuroprotective in a model of permanent middle cerebral artery occlusion in transgenic mice. *Journal of Neurochemistry,* Vol.72, No.3, (March 1999), pp. 1187-1203, ISSN 1471-4159.

Pandey, N. & Galvin, J.E. (2005) Curcumin prevents aggregation of alpha-synuclein. *Society for Neuroscience,* Vol.31, abs 1007.9.

Parker Jr., W.D., Boyson, S.J. & Parks, J.K. (1989). Abnormalities of the electron transport chain in idiopathic Parkinson's disease. *Annals of Neurology,* Vol.26, No.6, (December 1989), pp. 719-723, ISSN 0364-5134.

Parris, M.K. (2000). Parkinson's disease as multifactorial oxidative neurodegeneration: implications for integrative management. *Alternative Medicine Review,* Vol.5, pp. 502-545, ISSN 1089-5159.

Peeters, M., Maloteaux, J.M. & Hermans, E. (2003). Distinct effects of amantadine and memantine on dopaminergic transmission in the rat striatum. *Neuroscience Letters,* Vol.343, No.3, (June 2003), pp. 205-209, ISSN 0304-3940.

Perlmutter, D. BrainRecovery.com: Powerful therapy for challenging brain disorders. Naples, FL: The Perlmutter Health Center; www.brainrecovery.com; 2000.

Pettegrew, J.W., Levine, J. & McClure, R.J. (2000) Acetyl-L-carnitine physical-chemical, metabolic, and therapeutic properties: relevance for its mode of action in Alzheimer's disease and geriatric depression. *Molecular Psychiatry,* Vol.5, No.6, (November), pp. 616-632, ISSN 1476-5578.

Pezzella, A., d'Ischia, M., Napolitano, A., Misuraca, G. & Prota, G. (1997). Iron-mediated generation of the neurotoxin 6-hydroxydopamine quinone by reaction of fatty acid hydroperoxides with dopamine: as possible contributory mechanism for neuronal degeneration in Parkinson's disease. *Journal of Medicinal Chemistry,* Vol.40, No.14, (July 1997), pp. 2211-2216, ISSN 0022-2623.

Postuma, R.B. & Lang, A.E. (2004). Homocysteine and levodopa: should Parkinson disease patients receive preventive therapy? *Neurology,* Vol.63, No.5, (September 2004), pp. 886-891, ISSN 0028-3878.

Przedborski, S. & Vila, M. (2003). The 1-methyl-4-phenyl-1,2,3,6-tetrahydropyridine mouse model: a tool to explore the pathogenesis of Parkinson's disease. *Annals of the New York Academy of Sciences,* Vol.991, (June 2003), pp. 189-198 ISSN 00778923.

Rahaman, I., Biswas, S.K. & Kirkam, P.A. (2006). Regulation of inflammation and redox signalling by dietary polyphenols. *Biochemical Pharmacology,* Vol.72, No.11, (November 2006), pp. 1439-1452, ISSN 0006-2952.

Rajeswary, A. (2006). Curcumin protects mouse brain from oxidative stress caused by 1-methyl-4-phenyl-1,2,3,6-tetrahydropyridine. *European Review for Medical and Pharmacological Sciences,* Vol.10, No.4, pp. 157-161, ISSN 1128-3602.

Ramsay, R.R. & Singer, T.P. (1986) Energy-dependent uptake of N-methyl-4-phenylpyridinium, the neurotoxin metabolite of 1-methyl-4-phenyl-1,2,3,6-tetrahydropyridine, by mitochondria. *Journal of Biological Chemistry,* Vol.261, No.16, (June 1896), pp. 7585-7587, ISSN 1083-351X.

Ramsay, R.R., Krueger, M.J., Youngster, S.K., Gluck, M.R., Casida, J.E. & Singer T.P. (1991). Interaction of 1-methyl-4-phenylpyridinium ion (MPP) and its analogs with the rotenone/piericidin binding site of NADH dehydrogenase. *Journal of Neurochemistry,* Vol.56, No.4, (April 1991), pp. 1184-1190, ISSN 1471-4159.

Rao, K.V., Mawal, Y.R. & Qureshi I.A. (1997). Progressive decrease of cerebral cytochrome C oxidase activity in sparse-fur mice: role of acetyl-L-carnitine in restoring the ammonia-induced cerebral energy depletion. *Neuroscience Letters,* Vol.224, No.2, (March 1997), pp. 83-86, ISSN 0304-3940.

Sancher-Ramos, T.R., Overvik, E. & Ames, B.N. (1994). A marker of oxyradical-mediated DNA damage (8-hydroxy-2'-deoxyguanosine) is increased in nigro-striatum of Parkinson's disease brain. *Neurodegeneration,* Vol.3, pp. 197-201, ISSN 1068-719X.

Saunders CD. Parkinson's disease: a new hope. Boston MA: Harvard Health Publication; 2000.

Schapira, A.H.V. (2003). Neuroprotection in PD – a role for dopamine agonists? *Neurology,* Vol.61, No.6, (September 2003), pp. S34–S42, ISSN 0028-3878.

Schapira, A.H.V. (2008). Mitochondria in the aetiology and pathogenesis of Parkinson's disease. *The Lancet Neurology,* Vol.7, No.1, (January 2008), pp. 97-109, ISSN 1474-4422.

Schrag, A. (2005). Entacapone in the treatment of Parkinson's disease. *The Lancet Neurology,* Vol.4, No.6, (June 2005), pp. 366–370, ISSN 1474-4422.

Sculer, F. & Casida, J.E. (2001) Functional coupling of PSST and ND1 subunits in NADH: ubiquinone oxidoreductase ewstablished by photoaffinity labelling. *Biochimica and Biophysica Acta* Vol.1506, pp. 79-87, ISSN:0006-3002.

Seidler, A., Hellenbrand, W., Robra, B.P., Vieregge, P., Nischan, P., Joerg, J., Oertel, H., Ulm, G. & Schneider, E. (1996). Possible environmental, occupational, and other etiologic factors for Parkinson's disease: a case-control study in Germany. *Neurology,* Vol.46, No.5 (May 1996), pp. 1275-1284, ISSN 0028-3878.

Sherer, T.B., Kim, J.H., Betarber, R. & Greenamyre, J.T. (2003) Subcutaneous rotenone exposure causes highly selective dopaminergic degeneration and α-synuclein aggregation. *Experimental Neurology,* Vol.179, No.1, (January 2003), pp. 9-16, ISSN 0014-4886.

Shergill, J.K., Cammack, R., Cooper, C.E., Cooper, J.M., Mann, V.M. & Schapira, A.H.V. (1996). Detection of nitrosyl complexes in human substantia nigra in relation to Parkinson's disease. *Biochemical and Biophysical Research Communications,* Vol.228, No.2, (November 1996), pp. 298-303, ISSN 0006-291X.

Sesadri, S., Beiser, A., Selhub, J., Jacques, P.E., Rosenberg, I.H., D'Agostino, R.B., Wilson, P.W.F. & Wolf, P.A. (2002). Plasma homocysteine as a risk factor for dementia and Alzheimer disease. *New England Journal of Medicine,* Vol.346, No.7, (February 2002), pp. 476-483, ISSN 1533-4406.

Shults, C.W., Haas, R.H., Passov, D. & Beal, M.F. (1997). Coenzyme Q10 is reduced in mitochondria from parkinsonian patients. *Annals of Neurolology,* Vol.42, No.2, (August 1997), pp. 261-264, ISSN 0364-5134.

Shults, C.W., Beal, M.F., Fontaine, D., Nakano, K. & Haas, R.H. (1998). Absorption, tolerability, and effects on mitochondrial activity of oral coenzyme Q10 in parkinsonian patients. *Neurology,* Vol.50, No.3, (March 1998), pp. 793-795, ISSN 0028-3878.

Shults, C.W., Oakes, D., Kieburtz, K., Beal, M.F., Haas, R., Plumb, S., Juncos, J.L., Nutt, J., Shoulson, I., Carter, J., Kompoliti, K., Perlmutter, J.S., Reich, S., Stern, M., Watts, R.L., Kurlan, R., Molho, E, Harrison, M. & Lew, M. (2002). The Parkinson Study Group. Effects of coenzyme Q10 in early Parkinson's disease: evidence of slowing of the functional decline. *Archives of Neurolology,* Vol.59, No.10, (October 2002), pp. 1541-1550, ISSN 0375-8540.

Singh, N., Pillay, V. & Choonara, Y. E. (2007). Advances in the treatment of Parkinson's disease. *Progress in Neurobiology,* Vol.81, No.1, (January 2007), pp. 29–44, ISSN 0301-0082.

Sinicropi, M.S., Leone, F., Rovito, N. & Genchi, G. (2010). Behaviour of acetyl-L-carnitine injections (Nicetile® fiale) with different drugs used for combined therapy. *Advances in Therapy,* Vol.27, No.8, (August 2010), pp. 547-554, ISSN 0741-238X.

Spina M.B., & Cohen, G. (1988). Exposure of striatal synaptosomes to L-dopa increases levels of oxidized glutathione. *Journal of Pharmacology and Experimental Therapeutics,* Vol.247, No.2, (November 1988), pp. 502-507, ISSN 1521-0103.

Stephenson, J. (2000). Exposure to home pesticides linked to Parkinson's disease. *Journal of the American Medical Association.* Vol.283, No.23, (June 2000), pp. 3055-3056, ISSN 1538-3598.

Stoof, J.C., Booij, J. & Drukarch, B. (1992). Amantadine as a *N*-methyl-D-aspartic acid receptor antagonist: new possibilities for therapeutic application? *Clinical Neurology and Neurosurgery,* Vol.94, No.S1, pp. S4–S6, ISSN 0303-8467.

Storch, A., Jost, W.H., Vieregge, P., Spiegel, J., Greulich, W., Durner, J., Muller, T., Kupsch, A., Henningsen, H., Oertel, W.H., Fuchs, G., Kuhn, W., Niklowitz, P., Koch, R., Herting, B. & Reichmann, H. (2007). Randomized, double-blind, placebo-controlled trial on symptomatic effects on coenzyme Q(10) in Parkinson disease. *Archives of Neurology,* Vol.64, No.7, (July 2007), pp. 938-944, ISSN 0375-8540.

Swerdlow, R.H., Parks, J.K., Miller, S.W., Tuttle, J.B., Trimmer, P.A., Sheenam, J.P., Bennett, J.P., Davis, R.E. & Parker, W.D. (1996). Origin and functional consequences of the complex I defect in Parkinson's disease. *Annals of Neurology,* Vol.40, No.4, (October 1996), pp. 663-671, ISSN 0364-5134.

Thal, L.J., Carta, A., Clarke, W.R., Ferris, S.H., Friedland, R.P., Petersen, R.C., Pettegrew, J.W., Pfeiffer, E., Raskind, M.A., Sano, M., Tuszynski, M.H. & Wodson, R.F. (1996). A 1-year multicenter placebo-controlled study of acetyl-L-carnitine in patients with Alzheimer's disease. *Neurology,* Vol.47, No.3, (September 2007), pp. 705-711, ISSN 0028-3878.

Thapliyal, R. & Maru, G.B. (2001). Inhibition of P450 isoenzymes by curcumin *in vitro* and *in vivo. Food and Chemical Toxicolology,* Vol.39, No.6, (June 2001), pp. 541-547, ISSN 0278-6915.

Virmani, A. & Binienda, Z. (2004). Role of carnitine esters in brain neuropathology. *Molecular Aspects of Medicine,* Vol.25, No.5-6, (October-December 2004), pp. 533-549, ISSN 0098-2997.

Weisskopf, M.G., O'Reilly, E., Chen, H., Schwarzschild, M.A. & Ascherio, A. (2007). Plasma urate and risk of Parkinson' disease. *American Journal of Epidemiology,* Vol.166, No.5, (September 2007), pp. 561-567, ISSN 1476-6256.

Winquist, A., Steenland, K. & Shankar, A. (2010). Higher serum uric acid associated with decreased Parkinson's disease prevalence in a large community-based survey. *Movement disorders,* Vol.25, No.7, (May 2010), pp. 932-936, ISSN 0885-3185.

Wood-Kaczamar, A., Gandhi, S. & Wood, N.W. (2006). Understanding the molecular causes of Parkinson's disease. *Trends in Molecular Medicine,* Vol.12, No.11, (November 2006), pp. 521–528, ISSN 1471-4914.

Yenari, M.A., Giffard, R.G., Sapolosky, R.M. & Steinberg, G.K. (1999). The neuroprotective potential of heat shock protein 70 (HSP70). *Molecular Medicine Today,* Vol.5, No.12, (Dicember 1999), pp. 525-531, ISSN 1357-4310.

Youdim, M.B., Ben Schachar, D. & Riederer, P. (1989). Is Parkinson's disease a progressive siderosis of substantia nigra resulting in iron and melanin induced neurodegeneration? *Acta Neurologica Scandinavica,* Vol.80, No.S126, (November 1989), pp. 47-54, ISSN 1600-0404.

Youdim, M.B.H, Ben-Schachar, D. & Riederer, P. (1990). The role of monoamine oxidase, iron-melanin interaction, and intracellular calcium in Parkinson's disease. *Journal of Neural Transmission,*Vol.32, pp. S239-S248, ISSN 0300-9564.

Zhang, K. & Kaufman, R.J. (2006). The unfolded protein response: a stress signaling pathway critical for health and disease. *Neurology,* Vol.66, No.2, (January 2006), pp. S102-S109, ISSN 0028-3878.

20

Distribution and Regulation of the G Protein-Coupled Receptor Gpr88 in the Striatum: Relevance to Parkinson's Disease

Renaud Massart[1], Pierre Sokoloff[3] and Jorge Diaz[1,2]
[1] *INSERM UMR-894, Psychiatry and Neurosciences Center, Paris,*
[2]*Paris Descartes University, Faculty of Pharmacy / Laboratory of Neurobiology and Molecular Pharmacology (UMRs894 INSERM), Paris,*
[3]*Pierre Fabre Research Institute, Neurology and Psychiatry Department, Castres, France*

1. Introduction

The human basal ganglia constitutes a functional neural network located at the base of the forebrain. It receives most of its afferent inputs through the striatum, the major nucleus of the basal ganglia accomplishing fast neurotransmitter-mediated operations through somatotopically organized projections to the principal neuron cell type, the striatal GABAergic spiny projection neurons. This spiny projection neurons, which make up 95 % of the neuron population of striatum (Kemp & Powell 1971), receive excitatory glutamatergic inputs from all areas of the cortex and specific thalamic nuclei (Gerfen & Wilson 1996; Bolam et al., 2000; Voorn et al., 2004; Doig et al., 2010), and also modulatory dopaminergic inputs from the substantia nigra pars compacta (Smith & Kieval 2000; Utter. & Basso 2008). Spiny Projection Neurons include two major subpopulations giving rise to the direct striato-nigral pathway, and the indirect striato-pallidal pathway which communicates information to the basal ganglia output structures; the internal segment of the globus pallidus and the substantia nigra pars reticulata (Smith, Y. & Kieval 2000; Gerfen & Wilson 1996). Although the two neuron subpopulations are GABAergic, they differ in a number of properties including the expression of different complements of dopamine, Adenosine, NMDA and acetylcholine receptor subtypes as well as of peptide content; the direct striato-nigral pathway neurons coexpress substance P and dynorphin, whereas the indirect striato-pallidal pathway neurons express enkephalin (Gerfen et al., 1990, 1991; Reiner & Anderson 1990; Gerfen & Wilson 1996; Le Moine & Bloch, 1995).

Based on the fact that striatal medium-spiny neurons are the major input targets and the major projection neurons of striatum, it is thought that integration of neurotransmission in these neurons is an important determinant of the functional organization of the striatum. Thus, changes in neurotransmission on striatal spiny projection neurons have been involved in the regulation of voluntary movement, behavioral control, cognitive function and reward mechanisms. For instance, massive spiny projection neuron loss and major dopamine deficits in striatum lead to severe motor disorders, such as the excess of involuntary movements encountered in Huntington's disease and the rigidity and poverty of movements that typifies Parkinson's disease, respectively (Ross et al., 1997; Wolfgang & Stanley, 2003). Therefore, investigations addressed to characterize new receptor proteins displaying high densities and potential involvement in neurotransmission mechanisms within the striatum can provide new insight into the basal ganglia physiology and pathophysiology and also new clues for therapy of severe motor disorders.

A previous study reported a novel striatum-specific transcript, the strg/Gpr88, encoding an orphan G protein-coupled receptor of human and rodents (Mizushima et al., 2000). It display highest sequence homology with 5HT1D and β3 receptors. Since the original description, little data have been documented on the biological function (s) and the the cellular and subcellular distribution of the Gpr88 protein. Hence, the Gpr88 endogenous putative ligand, the detailed Gpr88 protein distribution and GPR88 functional roles are unknown. One approach to gain functional insights into this novel gene coding for an orphan receptor is the precise analysis of its spatial and temporal expression to provide information about the neural morphological substrates supporting Gpr88 functions in the striatal complex.

Hence, the present findings provide *in situ* hybridization and light-level immunohistochemical evidence for Gpr88 localization in the rat and monkey striatum and its subcellular distribution in striatal neurons by using a validated polyclonal antibody specifically recognizing Gpr88, (Massart et al 2009). We also describe morphological data on the spatiotemporal Gpr88 expression in the developing rat striatum, suggesting that both nigrostriatal and corticostriatal pathways control its normal striatal pattern of expression. Using treatments with l-DOPA and dopamine antagonists, in unilateral 6-hydroxydopamine- and cortical ibotenate-lesioned rats, we further demonstrated that striatal Gpr88 expression is modulated by dopamine- and glutamate-regulated mechanisms involving trans-synaptic influences of the corticostriatal pathway input activity.

2. Widespread Gpr88 expression within the striatal complex

Using *in situ* hybridization and immunohistochemistry approaches, we demonstrated that Gpr88 mRNA and protein expression are specially abundant within restricted basal telencephalic structures including the dorsal striatum, nucleus accumbens, and olfactory tubercle and also in the inferior olivary complex (Fig. 1).

2.1 All striatal GABAergic spiny projection neurons express Gpr88

Gpr88 is expressed throughout the two anatomical and functional patch/striosome-matrix compartments in the rat and monkey striatal complex (Figures 1F, 2A) with higher receptor expression in patch/striosome than in the surrounding matrix compartment. The prevalence of Gpr88 in the patch/striosome compartment and also within the dorsolateral striatal sector, indicates that Gpr88 may play a central role in the modulation of both limbic and motor cortical-basal ganglia circuits (Ragsdale & Graybiel; 1988; Graybiel A.M., 1995; Gerfen & Wilson, 1996). Immunofluorescent stainings and double labelling *in situ* hybridization experiments demonstrated that Gpr88 is present in all the spiny projection neurons of both the direct striato-nigral pathway and the indirect striato-pallidal pathway (Figure 2 C,D).

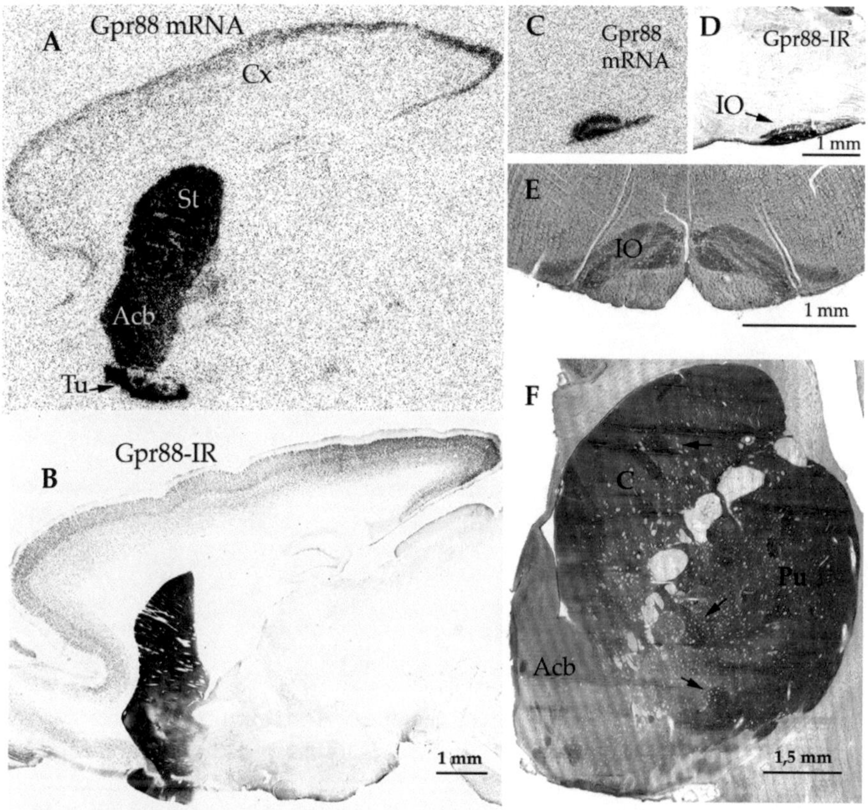

Fig. 1. Gpr88 distribution in the rat and the monkey brains. Both Gpr88 mRNA (A,C) and Gpr88 protein (B,D,E,F) are particularly concentrated throughout the striatum (St), nucleus accumbens (Acb), olfactory tubercle (Tu) and the inferior olive complex (IO) of the rat (A-E). Similar levels and distribution-pattern of Gpr88 immunorreactivity is detected in nucleus caudatus (C), putamen (Pu) and nucleus accumbens (Acb) of the monkey brain (F). Significant levels of Gpr88 are also present with a laminar distribution throughout the neocortex. Arrows in (F), point out small and intense Gpr88 stained areas corresponding to striosome striatal subcompartments. RT-QPCR data from rodents suggest that Gpr88 displays the highest expression levels compared to other known GPCRs of the striatum (Massart et al., 2007, 2008). The pattern of Gpr88 throughout the striatum of adult rats and monkeys is characterized by widespread distribution and regional differences (Figure 1), suggesting a central role of this orphan receptor in the modulation of sensorimotor related informations (Flaherty & Graybiel1994; Voorn et al., 2004). Although Gpr88 is prevalent in the striatal complex, we also detected moderate levels of both Gpr88 transcripts and protein throughout the cerebral neocortex (Figure 1A,B). Both signals display a similar non-homogeneous laminar distribution characterized by higher expression in the upper neocortical layers II-IV than in the lower layers V-VI. No Gpr88 expression was detected in the cortical layer I. Moreover, cortical Gpr88 expression represents about 20% of the GPR88 striatal expression, as assessed by different quantitive approaches including Western blot, immunohistochemistry and *in situ* hybridization. Double immuno-fluorescent labellings for Gpr88 and different neural cell-type specific markers have demonstrated that Gpr88 is an exclusive neuronal receptor of the brain, being absent from glial cells (Massart et al., 2009).

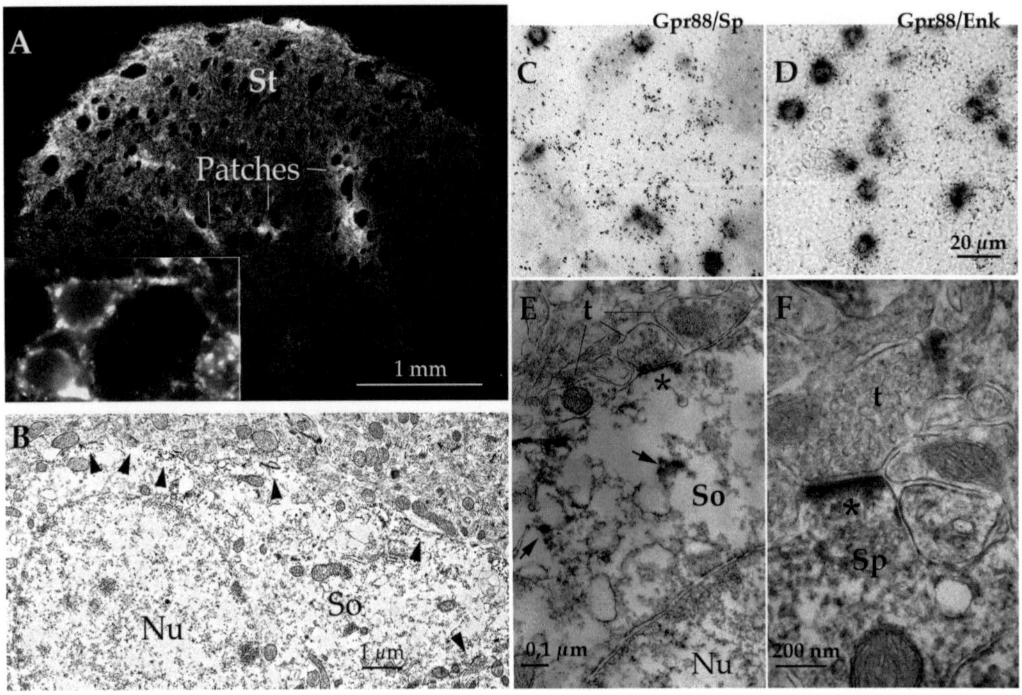

Fig. 2. Gpr88 distribution in the rat dorsal striatum. (A) The immunofluorescent Gpr88 signal is heterogeneously distributed within the dorsal striatum and characterized by its marked concentration in the striatal dorsolateral region and the patches compartments. The inset illustrates putative medium spiny neurons displaying intense Gpr88 labelling on the cell surface along the soma and dendrites. (C, D) double-labelling *in situ* hybridization indicates that all Substance P (dark-stained cells in C) and enkephalin (dark-stained cells in D) neurons, also express Gpr88 transcripts (detected by silver grain labellings). The distribution of the electron-dense immunoreactive reaction product, reflects the subcellular GPR88 presence in submembranous sites around the perikaryon (arrow-heads in B asterisk and arrows in E). The receptor is concentrated in symmetrical synapses in the cell body (asterisk in E) but also in asymmetrical synapses (asterisk in F) in dendritic spines (Sp). Note the absence of immunolabelling in synaptic contacts of two adjacent nerve terminals (t) in E. (Enk) Enkephalin, (Nu) Cell nucleus, (So) neuronal cell body, (Sp) Substance P in C, (Sp) dendritic spine in F.

Electron microscopic analysis of the Gpr88 immunolabelling in the rat dorsal striatum demonstrated a high proportion of electron dense Gpr88 positive dendritic spines, dendrite shafts and cell bodies (Figure 2 B,E,F) that are characteristic features of GABAergic spiny projection neurons (Somogyi et al., 1982; Bolam et al., 1983). However, no axonal or terminal Gpr88 immunolabeled profiles were observed. Likewise, globus pallidus and substantia nigra pars reticulata, two basal ganglia regions receiving the striato-pallidal and striato-nigral terminals respectively (Surmeier et al., 2007), lack Gpr88 immunoreactivity. All these morphological findings highlight a potential functional role for Gpr88 in synaptic events occurring on somatodendritic compartments and their integration in striato-nigral and striato-pallidal medium spiny neurons. Gpr88 immunoreactivity was often concentrated on discrete postsynaptic sub-membranous sites in a large proportion of asymmetrical (excitatory) synapses that generally receive glutamate as neurotransmitter (Bouyer et al., 1984; Bolam et al., 2000) and also on symmetrical (inhibitory) synapses which could be supplied by terminals originating from GABAergic aspiny or cholinergic interneurons or even by intrastriatal GABAergic axon-collaterals from medium-spiny projection neurons. Double immunofluorescent labellings in the same section demonstrated no association between Gpr88 immunoreactivity and tyrosine hydroxylase immunolabelled axon-terminals. In contrast, the Gpr88 immunoreactive signal was often juxtaposed to most vesicular glutamate transporter1 immunoreactive terminals, indicating that Gpr88 is preferentially located on synapses supplied by cortical inputs, rather than by vesicular glutamate transporter2 immunoreactive thalamic inputs contacting medium spiny neurons (Herzog et al., 2001; Kaneko & Fujiyama, 2002; Fremeau et al., 2004). Moreover, electron microscopy analysis demonstrates that Gpr88 immunoreactive signal is often present on the head of spines, where corticostriatal inputs mainly contact the dendritic tree of striatal spiny projection neurons (Bouyer et al., 1984; Dube et al., 1988; Ribak & Roberts 1990; Smith et al., 1994).

The preferential subcellular distribution of Gpr88 in striatal asymmetrical synapses of virtually all GABAergic projection neurons suggests a role for Gpr88 in the modulation of medium spiny neurons activity to cortical glutamatergic inputs and a potential role in the regulation of the flow of cortical information through the basal ganglia. Several lines of evidence indicate that cortical excitatory signals are modulated by dopaminergic synaptic contacts located on the neck of spines (Arbuthnott et al., 2000). Gpr88 location at specific synaptic sites, where corticostriatal and nigrostriatal afferents converge, further suggests involvement of Gpr88 in the modulation of both glutamatergic and dopaminergic signals received by the striatal medium spiny neurons.

3. Spatial and temporal Gpr88 expression in the developing rat striatum

To gain functional insights into striatal Gpr88 we have determined the profile of GPR88 expression in the prenatal and postnatal developing striatum of the rat by *in situ* hybridization and immunohistochemistry. Morphological data indicate that Gpr88 expression emerges with a homogeneous distribution, in the ventrolateral portion of the developing striatum at the embryonic day 16 (E16) of rat development (Figure 3A,B,C), a time when striatal neurons are both morphologically and functionally immature (van der Kooy & Fishell, 1987) and also when the patch-matrix striatal compartments, are not yet differentiated. The homogeneous Gpr88 mRNA distribution becomes heterogeneous when clusters of developing neurons displaying dense Gpr88 expression are seen throughout the dorsal and ventral striatal regions by the fetal stage E19-E20 (Figures 3D,E). Using double immunohistochemistry stained brain sections for Gpr88 and tyrosine hydroxylase, we confirmed that rich Gpr88 small areas strictly match the densely dopamine innervated striatal patch/striosome compartments (Gerfen et al., 1987). Levels of Gpr88 expression in patches compartments increase until the end of the first postnatal week and then decline in the second postnatal week with the ongoing development to eventually reach adult expression levels. Such developmental profile of Gpr88 expression in the prenatal and postnatal rat striatum suggests that the pattern of Gpr88 expression may be under the influence of afferent inputs reaching to the striatal primordia. This idea is based on the fact that the patchy-pattern profile of intense GPR88 expression in developing rat striatum closely matches the reported spatial and temporal development of the nigrostriatal dopamine afferents (Voorn et al., 1988), suggesting that the nigral dopamine inputs influence the patterning of striatal GPR88 expression. Such type of influence by the dopamine inputs has been demonstrated for the establishment of the pattern of opiate receptors expression in the embryonic patch compartment (van der Kooy & Fishell, 1992). The cortical projections are the second major afferent input to the striatum that may act in concert with nigral dopamine inputs to guide development of striatal subcompartment phenotypes. For instance, studies in the monkey have shown the patchy distribution of corticostriatal afferents before the day of birth (Goldman-Rakic, 1981). Moreover, organotypic assays involving co-cultures of the striatum with substantia nigra or cortex indicate that afferents from these structures have a prominent influence on the development of striatal patch/matrix compartments (Snyder-Keller & Costantini 1996; Snyder-Keller et al., 2001; Snyder-Keller, 2004). The mutual influence of dopaminergic and glutamatergic pathways within the developing striatum is probably important for the setting up of striatal neurotransmission circuits, as previously shown by dopamine manipulations that influence corticostriatal synaptic configurations (Meshul & Tan, 1994; Meshul et al., 1999; Meshul & Allen, 2000; Avila-Costa et al., 2005). These observations support the idea that cortical glutamatergic inputs and/or dopamine glutamate interactions may exert a control on Gpr88 expression in the developing medium spiny neurons.

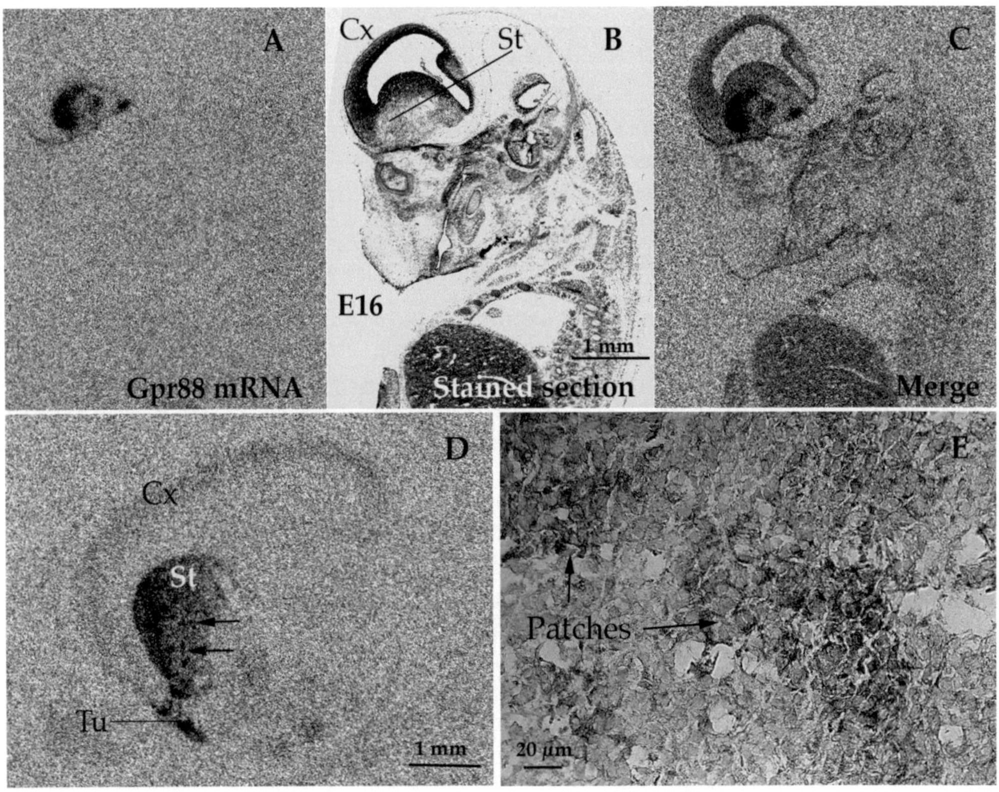

Fig. 3. Developmental profile of Gpr88 expression in the rat striatum. Gpr88 mRNA (A, D) and Gpr88-protein (E) expression in the developing striatum. (A) Homogeneous distribution of Gpr88 transcripts in the dorsolateral sector of differentiating striatum at E16. (D) Heterogeneous distribution of Gpr88-mRNA at E19. (F) Clusters of striatal developing neurons displaying dense Gpr88 immunoreactive signal (Gpr88-rich patches) at E20. (Cx) cortex, (St) striatum, (Tu) olfactory tubercle.

Although dopamine and glutamate afferents are the most likely candidates to modulate Gpr88 expression in developing medium-spiny projection neurons, other factors associated with nigral and cortical inputs may also play an important role in controlling Gpr88 expression within the striatal primordium. For instance, the nigrostriatal and corticostriatal pathways supply the striatum with brain-derived neurotrophic factor (BDNF) (Altar et al., 1997; Seroogy et al., 1994) which has been shown to influence survival, sprouting, and synaptogenesis in different neural systems (Hammond et al., 1999; Alsina et al., 2001; Mamounas et al., 2000). Moreover, studies in mature animals have shown that BDNF has profound effects on neurotransmission, activity-dependent synaptic remodeling, neurogenesis and receptors expression (Altar et al., 1997; Lessmann, 1998; Guillin et al., 2001; Tanaka et al., 2008; Taliaz, 2010). Rather than exclusive effects of either dopamine or glutamate on striatal Gpr88, continuous interplay among afferent signaling systems, including dopamine, glutamate and BDNF, is likely to refine the pattern expression of Gpr88 throughout the period of striatal development. Based on the spatiotemporal profile of GPR88 expression during striatal differentiation, we propose that the early receptor expression is modulated at least in part through a nigrostriatal and corticostriatal pathway dependent mechanisms. In support to the hypothesis of BDNF regulating Gpr88 expression during development, heterozygote BDNF-knockout mice have diminished Gpr88 mRNA levels in both the caude putamen and the shell of the nucleus accumbens (Massart et al., 2005).

4. Modulation of striatal Gpr88 expression by nigrostriatal and corticostriatal pathways in the rat in a model of Parkinson's disease

The demonstration of the regulation of striatal Gpr88 expression by nigrostriatal dopamine and cortical glutamate inputs was carried out in a rat model of Parkinson's disease (Schwarting & Huston 1996; Massart et al., 2009). Unilateral lesion of dopamine nigrostriatal pathway, caused by infusion of 6-OHDA in the medial forebrain bundle, produced a decrease in Gpr88 protein and mRNA expressions (Table 1). However, *in situ* hybridization analysis with double labelling showed that the effects of dopamine depletion were different in the two subpopulations of striatal medium spiny neurons. At the cellular level, 6-OHDA lesion induced a decrease in mRNA expression in striato-pallidal pathway neurons and inversely, a rise in striato-nigral projection neurons, in the dopamine depleted striatum (Table 1). Recently reported data (Heiman et al., 2008; Massart et al., 2009) showed that striatal Gpr88 mRNA expression is twice as high in striato-pallidal output neurons as in striato-nigral output neurons of rodents, the overall lesion-induced Gpr88 downregulation is consistent with the strong decrease in Gpr88 expression occurring in striato-pallidal pathway neurons, not compensated by the limited increase occurring in striato-nigral pathway neurons. These opposed variations are nearly completely reversed by a typical antiparkinsonian treatment with l-DOPA (Table 1).

Our finding revealed that D1 receptors, but not D2 receptors, activation exerts a positive influence on Gpr88 expression in the indirect striato-pallidal pathway of the dopamine-depleted hemisphere. On the contrary, D2 receptors stimulation controls Gpr88 expression in the direct striato-nigral pathway. This is rather surprising since D1 and D2 receptors are largely segregated to striatal neurons of the striato-nigral and striato-pallidal pathways, respectively (Gerfen et al., 1990; Le Moine & Bloch, 1995). In fact, in striato-pallidal medium spiny neurons harboring D2 receptors/Enk, in contrast to striato-nigral medium spiny

	Treatment	Gpr88 protein – immunohistochemistry		Gpr88 mRNA - *In situ* hybridization: Total mRNA		mRNA / SP+ cells		mRNA / ENK+ cells	
		Intact	Lesioned	Intact	Lesioned	Intact	Lesioned	Intact	Lesioned
6-OHDA lesion	Vehicle	107 ± 3.8	91 ± 2.9 *	69 ± 3.2	56 ± 1.4 *	22 ± 1.4	29 ± 1.9 ***	42 ± 2.1	31 ± 1.8 ***
	L- DOPA	99 ± 5.1	90 ± 4.6	73 ± 4.2	70 ± 3.7	22 ± 1.4	26 ± 1.7	40 ± 0.8	38 ± 1.3
	L-DOPA + SCH23390	108 ± 5.9	92 ± 5.6	76 ± 6.8	62 ± 3.2	23 ± 2.7	21 ± 1.6	43 ± 3.3	26 ± 4.3 ***
	L-DOPA + Haloperidol	100 ± 5.5	92 ± 6.1	74 ± 4.4	75 ± 3.0	37 ± 1.9 ***	26 ± 0.9	40 ± 1.4	39 ± 1.1
Ibotenate lesion	Vehicle	107 ± 3	83 ± 3 ***	89 ± 3.8	78 ± 1.9 ***	19 ± 0.5	17 ± 0.5	32 ± 0.9	23 ± 1.2 ***

Table 1. Effects on Gpr88 expression of dopamine depletion, induced by unilateral 6-OHDA infusion into the medial forebrain bundle, or of a bilateral lesion of the cortex induced by multiple infusions of ibotenate. All data are expressed as group mean ±SEM. The raw data for 6-OHDA (nigro-striatal) lesion were analysed by two-way ANOVA with lesion and treatment as independent variable and the Bonferroni test for multiple comparisons was applied in post hoc analysis to determine which values were significantly different. For data from ibotenate-induced lesion, the Student's unpaired two-tailed t-test was used to compare Ibotenate-injected vs. vehicle-injected rats. Alpha level level was set at 0.05. GraphPad 5 software (La Jolla, California, USA) was used to perform statistical analysis . * $P < 0.05$; ** $P < 0.01$; *** $P < 0.001$ vs. intact side (6-OHDA lesion) or intact, vehicle-infused animals (ibotenate lesion). See Massart et al. 2009 for details.

neurons containing D1 receptors/Sp, Gpr88 expression was downregulated by the 6-OHDA lesion and the reversion of this effect by l-DOPA was dependent on D1 receptor stimulation, as indicated by its blockade by the D1 receptor-selective antagonist SCH23390, but not by haloperidol, a D2 receptor-selective antagonist (Table 1). In parallel, in D1 receptor/Sp-expressing striato-nigral neurons, Gpr88 expression was upregulated by the lesion, in contrast to D2 receptor/Enk striato-pallidal output neurons. The reversion of this effect by l-DOPA was dependent of D2 receptors stimulation, as indicated by the absence of effects of SCH23390 (Table 1). Moreover, co-administration of l-DOPA and D2-receptor antagonist haloperidol raised Gpr88 expression in striato-nigral medium spiny neurons of the contralateral hemisphere (See Massart et al 2009; Taymans., 2005).

These results suggest that l-DOPA effects on Gpr88, in each of the two medium spiny neuron subsets, are not directly mediated by the respective dopamine receptor subtypes they express, but indirectly by dopamine receptor transmission through a different neurotransmitter afferent input to the medium spiny neurons. In particular l-DOPA and intrastriatal dopamine transmission can act as a neuromodulator of glutamate release in the dopamine depleted striatum (Jonkers et al., 2002; David et al., 2005; Stephens 2005). l-DOPA effects on Gpr88 expression in striato-pallidal pathway neurons are likely regulated through D1 receptor present on the soma and dendrites of excitatory corticostriatal projection neurons, leading to activation of the corticostriatal inputs. In contrast, l-DOPA/D2 receptors stimulation-induced Gpr88 decrease in striato-nigral neurons was probably mediated by reduced glutamate release from corticostriatal inputs by stimulation of presynaptic D2 receptors (Cepeda et al., 2001). Thus, l-DOPA-induced differential changes in Gpr88 levels on both striato-nigral and striato-pallidal medium spiny neurons, may be mediated through dopamine-induced influences in corticostriatal glutamatergic neurotransmission mechanisms, as previously suggested for the modulation of other striatal markers expressed in these neurons (Uhl et al., 1988; Salin et al., 1997; Zeng et al., 2000; Blandini et al., 2003; Robelet et al 2004; Carta et al., 2005).

In support to the above hypothesis, corticostriatal deafferentation, elicited by ibotenate infusions, induced a marked Gpr88 mRNA and protein down-regulation in striato-pallidal neurons without significantly affecting Gpr88 in striato-nigral neurons (Table 1). These data agree with the involvement of corticostriatal glutamatergic input in the effects of dopamine depletion induced Gpr88 changes in the striatal medium spiny projections neurons, and with a greater influence of cortical inputs on Gpr88 expression in the striato-pallidal pathway neurons.

5. Conclusions

Gpr88 is an important constituent of the basal ganglia, being one of the most abundant GPCR in this brain region. Although its function is unknown, detailed analysis of its gene expression in striatal spiny projection neurons suggests that Gpr88 has typical features of a GPCR in charge of transducing extracellular signals. First, it is expressed at the plasma membrane of striatal medium-spiny projection neurons, and probably exposed to the extracellular signals. Second, establishment of Gpr88 expression during development is concomitant with major dopaminergic and glutamatergic afferences reaching the embryonic striatum. Third, Gpr88 expression is enriched in the patch/striosome compartment, which suggests its involvement in the modulation of both limbic and motor cortical-basal ganglia circuits. Fourth, Gpr88 expression is influenced by modifications of cortical and nigral inputs to medium spiny neurons occurring in a situation modeling the pronounced loss of dopamine-producing neurons, occurring in Parkinson's disease.

Striato-nigral and striato-pallidal pathways neurons play an important role in integrating circuits of the basal ganglia/basal forebrain and finding on new proteins in these two major striatal output pathways, may contribute to a better understanding of certain pathophysiologic states (e.g., movement and psychiatric disorders). Hence, the rich and selective expression of GPR88 in the two striatal subpopulations medium-spiny projection neurons, directly receiving dopaminergic and glutamatergic inputs provides an anatomical basis for potential therapeutic applications, particularly in the striatum where modulation of glutamatergic and dopaminergic functions have important consequences for Parkinson's disease and its treatment.

6. References

Altar, C. A.; Cai, N.; Bliven, T.; Juhasz, M.; Conner, J. M.; Acheson, A. L.; Lindsay, R. M. & Wiegand, S. J. (1997) Anterograde transport of brain-derived neurotrophic factor and its role in the brain. *Nature*, Vol. 389, No. 6653, (February 1998), pp. 856-860, ISSN 0028-0836

Alsina, B.; Vu, T. & Cohen-Cory S. 2001. Visualizing synapse formation in arborizing optic axons in vivo: dynamics and modulation by BDNF. *Nat Neurosci., Vol.* 4, No. 11, (October 2001), pp. 1093-1101, ISSN 1097-6256

Arbuthnott, G. W.; Ingham, C. A. & Wickens, J. R. (2000). Dopamine and synaptic plasticity in the neostriatum. *J Anat.*, Vol. 196, No.4 , (August 2000), pp. 587-596 ISSN 0021-8782

Avila-Costa, M. R.; Colın-Barenque, L.; Aley-Medina, P.; Valdez, A. L.; Librado, J. L.; Martinez, E. F. & Fortoul, T. I. (2005). Bilateral increase of perforated synapses after unilateral dopamine depletion. *Int. J. Neurosci.*, Vol. 115, No. 1, (March 2005), pp. 79–86, ISSN 0020-7454

Blandini, F.; Fancellu, R.; Orzi, F.; Conti, G.; Greco, R.; Tassorelli, C. & Nappi G. (2003). Selective stimulation of striatal dopamine receptors of the D1 or D2-class causes opposite changes of fos expression in the rat cerebral cortex. Eur. *J. Neurosci.*, Vol. 17, No. 4, (February 2003), pp. 763-70, ISSN 0953-816X

Bolam, J. P.; Somogyi, P.; Takagi, H.; Fodor, I. & Smith, A. D. (1983). Localisation of substance P-like immunoreactivity in neurons and nerve terminals in the neostriatum of the rat: a correlated light and electron microscopic study. *J. Neurocytol.*, Vol. 12, No. 2, (April 1983), pp. 325-344, ISSN 0300-4864

Bolam, J. P.; Hanley, J. J.; Booth, P. A. C. & Bevan, M. D. (2000). Synaptic organisation of the basal ganglia. *J. Anat.*, Vol. 196, No. 4, (August 2000), pp. 527-542, ISSN 0021-8782

Bouyer, J. J.; Park D. H.; Joh, T. H. & Pickel V. M. (1984). Chemical and structural analysis of the relation between cortical inputs and tyrosine hydroxylase-containing terminals in rat neostriatum. *Brain Research*, Vol. 302, No. 2, (June 1984), pp. 267-275, ISSN 0006-8993

Carta, A. R.; Tronci, E.; Pinna, A. & Morelli M. (2005). Different responsiveness of striatonigral and striatopallidal neurons to L-DOPA after a subchronic intermittent L-DOPA treatment. *Eur. J. Neurosci.*, Vol. 21, No. 5, (April 2005), pp. 1196-204, ISSN 0953-816X

Cepeda, C.; Hurst, R. S.; Altemus, K. L.; Flores-Hernandez, J.; Calvert. C. R.; Jokel, E. S.; Grandy, D. K.; Low, M. J.; Rubinstein, M.; Ariano, M. A. & Levine, M. S. (2001). Facilitated glutamatergic transmission in the striatum of D2 dopamine receptor-deficient mice. *J. Neurophysiol.*, Vol. 85, No. 2, (February 2001), pp. 659–670, ISSN 0022-3077

David, H. N.; Ansseau, M. & Abraini, J. H. (2005). Dopamine–glutamate reciprocal modulation of release and motor responses in the rat caudate–putamen and nucleus accumbens of "intact" animals, *Brain Res. Rev.*, Vol. 50, No. 2, (November 2005), pp. 336–360, ISBN/ISSN (*no mentioned*)

Doig, N. M.; Moss, J. & Bolam, J. P. (2010). Cortical and Thalamic Innervation of Direct and Indirect Pathway Medium-Sized Spiny Neurons in Mouse. *J. Neurosci.*, Vol. 30, No. 44, (November 2010), pp.14610 –14618, ISSN 1529-2401 (Electronic), ISSN 0270-6474 (Linking)

Dube, L.; Smith, A. D. & Bolam, J. P. (1988) Identification of synaptic terminals of thalamic or cortical origin in contact with distinct medium-size spiny neurons in the rat neostriatum. *J. Comp. Neurol.*, Vol. 267, No. 4, (January 1988), pp. 455-471, ISSN 0021-9967

Flaherty, A. W. & Graybiel, A. M. (1994). Input-output organization of the sensorimotor striatum in the squirrel monkey. *J. Neurosci.*, Vol. 14, No. 2, (February 1994), pp. 599-610, ISSN 0270-6474

Fremeau, R. T.; Kam, K.; Qureshi, T.; Johnson, J.; Copenhagen, D. R.; Storm-Mathisen, J.; Chaudhry, F. A.; Nicoll, R. A. & Edwards, R. H. (2004). Vesicular glutamate transporters 1 and 2 target to functionally distinct synaptic release sites. *Science*, Vol. 304, No. 5678, (May 2004), pp. 1815-1819, ISSN 1095-9203 (Electronic), ISSN 0036-8075 (Linking)

Fujiyama, F.; Unzai, T.; Nakamura, K.; Nomura, S. & Kaneko, T. (2006). Difference in organization of corticostriatal and thalamostriatal synapses between patch and matrix compartments of rat neostriatum. *Eur. J. Neurosci.*, Vol. 24, No. 10, (December 2006), pp. 2813–2824, ISSN 0953-816X

Gerfen, C. R.; Herkenham, M. & Thibault J. (1987). The neostriatal mosaic: II. Patch- and matrix-directed mesostriatal dopaminergic and non-dopaminergic systems. *J Neurosci.*, Vol. 7, No. 12, (December 1987), pp. 3915-3934, ISSN 0270-6474

Gerfen, C. R.; Engber, T. M.; Mahan, L. C.; Susel, Z.; Chase, T. N.; Monsma, F. J. & Sibley, D. R. (1990). D1 and D2 dopamine receptor-regulated gene expression of striatonigral and striatopallidal neurons. *Science*, Vol. 250, No. 4986, (December 1990), pp. 1429-1432, ISSN 0036-8075

Gerfen, C. R.; McGinty, J. F. & Young, W. S. (1991). Dopamine differentially regulates dynorphin, substance P, and enkephalin expression in striatal neurons: in situ hybridisation histochemical analysis. *J. Neurosci.*, Vol. 11, No. 4, (April 1991), pp. 1016-1031, ISSN 0270-6474

Gerfen, C. R. & Wilson, C. (1996). The basal ganglia. In: *Handbook of chemical neuroanatomy. Integrated systems of the CNS, part III. Vol. 12*, Swanson, L. W., Björklund, A. & Hökfelt, T. (eds), pp. 371-468, Elsevier, ISBN 0-444-82451-0, Amsterdam, Netherlands

Gerfen, C. R. (2000). Molecular effects of dopamine on striatal-projection pathways. *Trends Neurosci.*, Vol. 23, No. 10 Suppl, (October 2000), pp. 64-70, ISSN 0166-2236

Goldman-Rakic P. S. (1981). Prenatal formation of cortical input and development of cytoarchitectonic compartments in the neostriatum of the rhesus monkey. *J Neurosci.*, Vol. 1, No. 7, (September 1981), pp. 721-735, ISSN 0270-6474

Graybiel, A. M. (1995). The basal ganglia. *Trends Neurosci.*, Vol. 18, No. 2, (February 1995), pp. 60-62, ISSN 0166-2236

Guillin, O.; Diaz, J.; Carroll, P.; Griffon, N.; Schwartz, J.-C. & Sokoloff, P. (2001). BDNF controls dopamine D3 receptor expression and triggers behavioral sensitisation. *Nature*, Vol. 411, No. 6833, (May 2001), pp. 86-89, ISSN 0028-0836

Hammond, E. N.; Tetzlaff, W.; Mestres, P. & Giehl, K. M. (1999). BDNF, but not NT-3, promotes long-term survival of axotomized adult rat corticospinal neurons in vivo. *Neuroreport*, Vol. 10, No. 12, (November 1999), pp. 2671-2675, ISSN 0959-4965

Heiman, M.; Schaefer, A.; Gong, S.; Peterson, J. D.; Day, M.; Ramsey, K. E.; Suarez-Farinas, M.; Schwarz, C.; Stephan, D. A.; Surmeier, D. J.; Greengard, P. & Heintz, N. (2008). A Translational Profiling Approach for the Molecular Characterization of CNS Cell Types. *Cell*, Vol. 135, No. 4, (November 2008), pp. 738–748, ISSN 1097-4172 (Electronic), ISSN 0092-8674 (Linking)

Herzog, E.; Bellenchi, G. C.; Gras, C.; Bernard, V.; Ravassard, P.; Bedet, C.; Gasnier, B.; Giros, B. & El Mestikawy, S. (2001). The existence of a second vesicular glutamate transporter specifies subpopulations of glutamatergic neurons. *J. Neurosci.*, Vol. 21, No. 22, (November 2001), pp. RC181, ISSN 1529-2401 (Electronic), ISSN 0270-6474 (Linking)

Jonkers, N.; Sarre, S.; Ebinger, G. & Michotte, Y. (2002). MK801 suppresses the L-DOPA-induced increase of glutamate in striatum of hemi-Parkinson rats. *Brain Res.*, Vol. 926, No. 1-2, (January 2002), pp. 149–155, ISSN 0006-8993

Kaneko, T. & Fujiyama, F. (2002). Complementary distribution of vesicular glutamate transporters in the central nervous system. *Neurosci. Res.*, Vol. 42, No. 4, (May 2002), pp. 243-250, ISSN 0168-0102

Kemp, J. M. & Powell, T.P. (1971). The structure of the caudate nucleus of the cat: light and electron microscopy. *Philos. Trans. R. Soc. Lond. B. Biol. Sci.,* Vol. 262, No. 845, (September 1971), pp. 383-401, ISSN 0962-8436

Le Moine, C. & Bloch, B. (1995). D1 and D2 dopamine receptor gene expression in the rat striatum: sensitive cRNA probes demonstrate prominent segregation of D1 and D2 mRNAs in distinct neuronal populations of the dorsal and ventral striatum. *J. Comp. Neurol.,* Vol. 355, No. 3, (May 1995), pp. 418-426, ISSN 0021-9967

Lessmann, V. (1998). Neurotrophin-dependent modulation of glutamatergic synaptic transmission in the mammalian CNS. *Gen Pharmacol.,* Vol. 31, No. 5, (November 1998), pp. 667-74, ISSN 0306-3623

Mamounas, L. A.; Altar, C. A.; Blue, M. E.; Kaplan, D. R.; Tessarollo, L. & Lyons, W. E. (2000). BDNF promotes the regenerative sprouting, but not survival, of injured serotonergic axons in the adult rat brain. *J Neurosci.,* Vol. 20, No. 2, (January 2000), pp. 771-782, ISSN 1529-2401 (Electronic), ISSN 0270-6474 (Linking)

Massart, R.; Diaz, J.; Griffon, N.; Vernier, P. & Sokoloff, P. (1995). Regional and cellular expression pattern of the striatum-specific orphan G protein-coupled receptor Gpr88. 7e Colloque de la Société des Neurosciences, France, May 2005

Massart, R.; Guilloux, J. P; Mignon, V.; Lauressergues, E.; Cussac, D.; Sokoloff, P. & Diaz, J. (2007). Complex regulation of the orphan G protein-coupled receptor GPR88 in the unilaterally 6-OHDA lesioned rat model of Parkinson's disease. 37th Annual Meeting of Neuroscience, San-Diego, USA, November 2007

Massart, R.; Guilloux, J. P.; Mignon, V.; Lauressergues, E.; Cussac, D.; Sokoloff, P. & Diaz, J. (2008) Striatal synaptic and cortical nuclear GPR88, a promising target for psychiatric and movement disorders. ECNP Workshop, Nice, France, Mars 2008

Massart, R.; Guilloux, J. P.; Mignon, V.; Sokoloff, P. & Diaz, J. (2009). Striatal Gpr88 expression is confined to the whole projection neuron population and is regulated by dopaminergic and glutamatergic afferents. *Eur J Neurosci.,* Vol. 30, No. 3, (August 2009), pp. 397-414, ISSN 1460-9568 (Electronic), ISSN 0953-816X (Linking)

Meshul, C. K. & Tan, S. E. (1994). Haloperidol-induced morphological alterations are associated with changes in calcium/calmodulin kinase II activity and glutamate immunoreactivity. *Synapse.,* Vol. 18, No. 3, (November 1994), pp. 205-217, ISSN 0887-4476

Meshul, C. K.; Emre, N.; Nakamura, C. M.; Allen, C.; Donohue, M. K. & Buckman, J. F. (1999). Time-dependent changes in striatal glutamate synapses following a 6-hydroxydopamine lesion. *Neuroscience.,* Vol. 88, No. 1, (March 1999), pp. 1-16, ISSN 0306-4522

Meshul, C. K. & Allen, C. (2000). Haloperidol reverses the changes in striatal glutamatergic immunolabeling following a 6-OHDA lesion. *Synapse,* Vol. 36, No. 2, (May 2000), pp. 129-142, ISSN 0887-4476

Mizushima, K.; Miyamoto, Y.; Tsukahara, F.; Hirai, M.; Sakaki, Y. & Ito, T. (2000). A novel G-protein-coupled receptor gene expressed in striatum. *Genomics,* Vol. 69, No. 3, (November 2000), pp. 314-321, ISSN 0888-7543

Ragsdale, C. W. & Graybiel, A. M. (1988). Fibers from the basolateral nucleus of the amygdala selectively innervate striosomes in the caudate nucleus of the cat. *J. Comp. Neurol.,* Vol. 269, No. 4, (March 1988), pp. 506-522, ISSN 0021-9967

Reiner, A. & Anderson, K. D. (1990). The patterns of neurotransmitter and neuropeptide co-occurrence among striatal projection neurons: conclusions based on recent findings. *Brain Res Rev.*, Vol. 15, No. 3, (September 1990), pp. 251-65, ISBN/ISSN (*no mentioned*)

Ribak, C. E. & Roberts, R. C. (1990). GABAergic synapses in the brain identified with antisera to GABA and its synthesizing enzyme, glutamate decarboxylase. *Journal of Electron Microscopy Technique*, Vol. 15, No. 1, (May 1990), pp. 34-48, ISSN 0741-0581

Robelet, S.; Melon, C.; Guillet, B.; Salin, P. & Kerkerian-Le Goff, L. (2004). Chronic l-DOPA treatment increases Extracellular glutamate levels and GLT1 expression in the basal ganglia in a rat model of Parkinson's disease. *Eur. J. Neurosci.*, Vol. 20, No. 5, (September 2004), pp. 1255–1266, ISSN 0953-816X

Ross, C. A.; Becher, M. W.; Colomer, V.; Engelender, S.; Wood J. D. & Sharp A. H. (1997). Huntington's disease and dentatorubral- allidoluysian atrophy: proteins, pathogenesis and pathology. *Brain Pathol.*, Vol. 7, No. 3, (July 1997), pp. 1003–1016, ISSN 1015-6305

Salin, P.; Dziewczapolski, G.; Gershanik, O. S.; Nieoullon, A. & Raisman-Vozari, R. (1997). Differential regional effects of long-term L-DOPA treatment on preproenkephalin and preprotachykinin gene expression in the striatum of 6-hydroxydopamine-lesioned rat. *Brain Res.Mol. Brain Res.*, Vol. 47, No. 1-2, (July 1997), pp. 311-321, ISSN 0169-328X

Schwarting, R. K. W. & Huston, J. P. (1996). Unilateral 6-hydroxydopamine lesions of meso-striatal dopamine neurons and their physiological sequelae. *Prog. Neurobiol.*, Vol. 49, No. 3, (June 1996), pp. 215-266, ISSN 0301-0082

Seroogy, K. B.; Lundgren, K. H.; Tran, T. M.; Guthrie, K. M.; Isackson, P. J. & Gall, C. M. (1994). Dopaminergic neurons in rat ventral midbrain express brain-derived neurotrophic factor and neurotrophin-3 mRNAs. *J Comp Neurol.*, Vol. 342, No. 3, (April 1994), pp. 321-334, ISSN 0021-9967

Smith, Y.; Bennett, B. D.; Bolam, J. P.; Parent, A. & Sadikot, A. F. (1994). Synaptic relationships between dopaminergic ,fferents and cortical or thalamic input in the sensorimotor territory of the striatum in monkey. *J. Comp. Neurol.*, Vol. 344, No. 1, (June 1994), pp. 1-19, ISSN 0021-9967

Smith, Y. & Kieval, J. Z. (2000) Anatomy of the dopamine system in the basal ganglia. *Trends Neurosci.*, 23, No. 10 Suppl, (October 2000), pp. 28-33, ISSN 0166-2236

Snyder-Keller, A. & Costantini, L. C. (1996). Glutamate receptor subtypes localize to patches in the developing striatum. *Brain Res Dev Brain Res.*, Vol. 94, No. 2, (July 1996), pp. 246-250, ISSN 0165-3806

Snyder-Keller, A.; Costantini, L. C. & Graber, D. J. (2001). Development of striatal patch/matrix organization in organotypic co-cultures of perinatal striatum, cortex and substantia nigra. *Neuroscience*, Vol. 103, No. 1, (April 2001), pp. 97-109, ISSN 0306-4522

Snyder-Keller, A. (2004). Pattern of corticostriatal innervation in organotypic cocultures is dependent on the age of the cortical tissue. *Exp Neurol.*, Vol. 185, No. 2, (January 2004), pp. 262-271, ISSN 0014-4886

Somogyi, P.; Priestley, J. V.; Cuello, A. C.; Smith, A. D. & Takagi, H. (1982). Synaptic connections of enkephalin-immunoreactive nerve terminals in the neostriatum: a correlated light and electron microscopic study. *J. Neurocytol.*, Vol. 11, No. 5, (October 1982), pp. 779-807, ISSN 0300-4864

Stephens, B.; Mueller, A. J.; Shering, A. F.; Hood, S. H.; Taggart, P.; Arbuthnott, G. W.; Bell, J. E.; Kilford, L.; Kingsbury, A. E.; Daniel, S. E. & Ingham, C.A. (2005). Evidence of a breakdown of corticostriatal connections in Parkinson's disease. *Neuroscience*, Vol. 132, No. 3, (April 2005), pp. 741-754, ISSN 0306-4522

Surmeier, D. J.; Ding, J.; Day, M.; Wang, Z. & Shen, W. (2007). D1 and D2 dopamine-receptor modulation of striatal glutamatergic signaling in striatal medium spiny neurons. *Trends Neurosci.*, Vol. 30, No.5 , (May 2007), pp. 228-235, ISSN 0166-2236

Taliaz, D .; Stall, N .; Dar, D. E. & Zangen. A. (2010). Knockdown of brain-derived neurotrophic factor in specific brain sites precipitates behaviors associated with depression and reduces neurogenesis. *Mol Psychiatry.*, Vol. 15, No. 1, (July 2009), pp. 80-92, ISSN 1476-5578 (Electronic), ISSN 1359-4184 (Linking)

Tanaka J.; Horiike Y.; Matsuzaki M.; Miyazaki, T.; Ellis-Davies G. C. & Kasai H. (2008). Protein synthesis and neurotrophin-dependent structural plasticity of single dendritic spines. *Science,* Vol. 319, No. 5870, (March 2008), pp. 1683-87, ISSN 1095-9203 (Electronic), 0036-8075 (Linking)

Taymans, J. M.; Kia, H. K.; Groenewegen, H. J.; Leysen, J.E. & Langlois, X. (2005). Bilateral control of brain activity by dopamine D1 receptors : evidence from induction patterns of regulator of G protein signalling 2 and c-fos mRNA in D1-challenged hemiparkinsonian rats. *Neuroscience,* Vol. 134, No. 2, (June 2005), pp. 643-56, ISSN 0306-4522

Uhl, G. R.; Navia, B. & Douglas, J. (1988). Differential expression of preproenkephalin and preprodynorphin mRNAs in striatal neurons: high levels of preproenkephalin expression depend on cerebral cortical afferents. *J. Neurosci.*, Vol. 8, No. 12, (December 1988), pp. 4755–4764, ISSN 0270-6474

Utter, A. A. & Basso, M. A. (2008). The basal ganglia: An overview of circuits and function. *Neuroscience and Biobehavioral Reviews*. Vol. 32, No. 3, (January 2008), pp. 333–342, ISSN 0149-7634

van der Kooy, D. & Fishell, G. (1987). Neuronal birthdate underlies the development of striatal compartments. *Brain Res.,* Vol. 401, No. 1, (January 1987), pp. 155-161, ISSN 0006-8993

van der Kooy, D. & Fishell, G. (1992). Embryonic lesions of the substantia nigra prevent the patchy expression of opiate receptors, but not the segregation of patch and matrix compartment neurons, in the developing rat striatum. *Brain Res Dev Brain Res.,* Vol. 66, No. 1, (March 1992), pp. 614-623, ISSN 0165-3806

Voorn, P.; Kalsbeek, A.; Jorritsma-Byham, B. & Groenewegen, H. J. (1988). The pre- and postnatal development of the dopaminergic cell groups in the ventral mesencephalon and the dopaminergic innervation of the striatum of the rat. *Neuroscience.,* Vol. 25, No. 3, (June 1988), pp. 857-887, ISSN 0306-4522

Voorn, P.; Vanderschuren, L. J.; Groenewegen, H. J.; Robbins, T.W. & Pennartz, C. M. A. (2004). Putting a spin on the dorsal-ventral divide of the striatum. *Trends Neurosci.,* Vol.27, No. 8, (August 2004), pp. 468-474, ISSN 0166-2236

Wolfgang, H. O. & Stanley, F. (2003) . Parkinsonism. In: *Movement Disorders. Neurological Disorders: Course and Treatment,* Second Edition, pp. 1021-1079, Elsevier Science, ISBN 978-0-12-125831-3, USA

Zeng, B. Y.; Pearce, R. K.; MacKenzie, G. M. & Jenner P. (2000). Alterations in preproenkephalin and adenosine-2a receptor mRNA, but not preprotachikinin mRNA correlate with occurrence of dyskinesia in normal monkeys chronically treated with L-DOPA. *Eur. J. Neurosci.,* Vol. 12, No. 3, (April 2000), pp. 1096-1104, ISSN 0953-816X

21

Human Lymphocytes and *Drosophila melanogaster*[1] as Model System to Study Oxidative Stress in Parkinson's Disease

Marlene Jimenez-Del-Rio and Carlos Velez-Pardo
School of Medicine, Medical Research Institute, Neuroscience Research Group, University of Antioquia, Medellin, Colombia

1. Introduction

Parkinson's disease (PD, OMIM entry #168600) is the most common progressive neurodegenerative disorder that not only affects a large group of individuals in Antioquia, Colombia (Pradilla et., 2003; Sanchez et al., 2004) but also affects other regions in the world. Actually, the prevalence of PD is between 0.1% and 0.3% in the general population and between 1% and 2% in persons 65 years of age or older (Alves et al., 2008). Moreover, the number of individuals with PD over age 50 has been projected between 8.7 and 9.3 million in Western countries by 2030 (Dorsey et al., 2007). PD is typified clinically by motor symptoms including bradykinesia, resting tremor, rigidity and gait posture abnormalities followed by postural instability and less frequent non-motor complication such as dementia, depression and autonomic dysfunction (Jancovic, 2008). Pathologically, the disorder is prominently characterized by progressive loss of 50–70% of dopaminergic neurons located in the substantia nigra, decrease of the neurotransmitter dopamine content in striatum (Forno, 1996), cytoplasmic inclusions of insoluble, aggregated proteins, including α-synuclein known as Lewy bodies (Cuervo et al., 2010), elevated levels and/or deposits of iron (Sian-Hülsmann et al., 2010) and selective neuronal vulnerability to oxidative stress (Wang & Michaelis, 2010). The cause of all cases of PD remains unknown. However, in the mid-1990s this situation changed with the identification of a mutation in the α-synuclein gene associated with autosomal dominant PD in Italian kindred (Polymeropoulos et al., 1997). Since then, more than 10 genes have been found either causal of the disease (e.g., *Parkin, DJ-1,* PTEN-induced putative kinase 1 (*PINK-1*), leucine rich region kinase 2 (*LRRK2*), *ATP13A2* (Xiromerisiou et al., 2010; Cookson, 2010; Hardy, 2010)) or as risk factor for PD (e.g. HLA region). Interestingly, the first gene that causes autosomal recessive

---

[1]***Drosophila melanogaster*** has misleadingly been known as the fruit fly. Strictly, "...real fruit flies,...attack unblemished fruit and in heavy infestations cause serious economic damage. In contrast, even if present in enormous numbers, *D. melanogaster* is innocuous and of no economic importance" (Green, MM. (2002). It really is not a fruit fly, *Genetics* 162: 1-3). It is therefore most adequate to name *Drosophila melanogaster* as just *Drosophila melanogaster* fly

juvenile Parkinsonism (AR-JP) was reported and named *parkin* in 1998 by Kitada and colleagues. AR-JP maps to the long arm of chromosome 6 (6q25.2-q27). The *parkin* gene is composed of 2,960 base pairs with a 1,395-base-pair open reading frame encoding for a protein of 465 amino acids with moderate similarity to ubiquitin at the amino terminus and a RING-finger motif at the carboxy terminus. The gene spans more than 500 kilobases and has 12 exons (Kitada et al., 1998). Subsequent studies have shown that *parkin* is a RING-finger-containing protein identified as an E3 protein-ubiquitin ligase (Shimura et al., 2000), which is an integral component of the cytoplasmic ubiquitin/ proteosomal degradation pathway (Betarbet et al., 2005). The reaction promoted by E3 ligases is the addition of a lysine-linked chain four or more ubiquitin molecules to the target protein, which is recognised by the subunits in the proteosome. Thus, mutation of the *parkin* gene could result in accumulation of misfolded proteins (Tanaka et al., 2001; Imai and Takahashi, 2004). Therefore, it is hypothesized that mutations in *parkin* gene, which result in loss of function, are unable to remove enough mutated or misfolded proteins leading to nigral neurodegeneration. Moreover, the Parkin protein may play a role in promoting autophagy of dysfunctional mitochondria following loss of mitochondrial membrane potential (Bueler, 2010).

Currently, AR-JP (OMIM entry #600116) is consider a distinct genetic entity characterised by early age at onset (<age 45), dystonia with parkinsonism and improvement of symptoms after sleep, slow disease progression, associated signs such as hyperflexia, dysautonomia, peripheral neuropathy and good response to low doses of L-DOPA (Zhang et al., 2001). Additionally, iron deposits are found in PD (Dexter et al., 1989; Sofic et al., 1991; Riederer et al., 1992; Griffiths et al., 1999) as well as in AR-JP (Takanashi et al., 2001). Why dopaminergic neurons in the substantia nigra are particularly vulnerable to the loss of parkin function and iron deposition is yet unknown. To date, the most common known form of hereditary Parkinsonism, i.e. AR-JP, diagnosed in Antioquia, Colombia is due to the *parkin* C212Y mutation. This mutation is a novel G to A transition in exon 6 at position 736 (G736A) of *parkin* gene. The C212Y mutation was identified in a genetic isolate community from two paisa family groups (PJF-1, PJF-3) by Pineda-Trujillo et al., (2001). Interestingly, the mutation was subsequently observed in a Spanish family, suggesting that it could have been taken to Antioquia by Spanish immigrants. Pineda-Trujillo et al., (2006) screened for the G736A mutation in additional Antioquian early onset PD cases and used haplotype analysis to investigate the relationship between Spanish and Antioquian G736A chromosomes. They confirmed the occurrence of an extensive founder effect in Antioquia. Thirteen individuals (10 homozygotes) from seven nuclear families were identified with the G736A mutation. Genealogical investigations demonstrated the existence of shared ancestors between six of these families four to five generations ago and no evidence of Spanish ancestry during this period. A second parkin mutation (a duplication of exon 3), was detected in the three G736A heterozygote carriers. Haplotype data exclude a recent common ancestry between the Spanish and Antioquian patients studied and are consistent with the introduction of the G736A mutation in Antioquia during early colonial times by about 16 generations ago. Further studies have also confirmed the presence of a GT insertion in exon 3 mutation among Paisa community previously identified in Spanish and French families with juvenile Parkinsonism (Pineda-Trujillo et al., 2001, 2009). Strikingly, the proteins that are reported to be related to familial PD such as PINK1, DJ-1, α-synuclein, LRRK2 and possibly parkin are either mitochondrial proteins or are associated with mitochondria. Interestingly, all those proteins are involved in pathways that elicit oxidative stress or free radical damage (Lin et al., 2009).

Free radials are defined as any atom or molecule that has one or more unpaired electrons in its outer shell such as anion superoxide radical ($\cdot O_2$), hydroxyl radical ($\cdot OH$), nitric oxide ($NO\cdot$) and their products (e.g. H_2O_2). Oxidative stress (OS) refers to a state in which free radicals are in excess of antioxidant defence mechanism (e. g. superoxide dismutase (SOD), glutathion peroxidase (GPx), catalase, vitamin C and E). As a result of this imbalance, the free radicals are capable of reacting with lipids, proteins, nucleic acids, and other molecules altering their structure and function. Accordingly, OS can lead to serious structural modifications in cells by excessive accumulation of oxidized products such as aldehydes and isoprostanes from lipid peroxidation, protein carbonyls from protein oxidation, and base adducts from DNA oxidation. Because the human brain is a high oxygen consumer organ, it is reasonable to assume that, under pathological conditions, it might be a target of permanent OS attack.

Over the last two decade, OS has been proposed to play a critical role in the pathogenesis of PD (Fahn and Cohen, 1992; Jenner & Olanow, 1996; Tsang & Chung, 2009). In fact, several markers of OS have been identified in post-mortem brain tissues including increased levels of DNA and RNA oxidation (e.g. 8-hydroxyl-2-deoxyguanosine and 8-hydroxyl deoxyguanosine), protein carbonyl levels, glycation and glycoxidation, lipid peroxidation and high iron concentration (Zhou et al., 2008). Moreover, given that iron and DA generate reactive oxygen species (ROS), they have been implicated in the OS observed in PD (Asanuma et al., 2004). Not surprisingly, lymphocytes have been used to test for oxidative stress (Battisti et al., 2008) and cell death (Calopa et al., 2010) in PD. For instance, Migliore et al., (2002) has demonstrated an increase in the incidence of spontaneous micronuclei, single strand breaks and oxidized purine bases in PD patients without treatment. These results clearly showed oxidative DNA damage demonstrable in lymphocytes. Moreover, we found that homozygote Cys212Tyr *parkin* mutation in AR-JP patients renders lymphocytes sensitive to dopamine, iron and hydrogen peroxide stimuli (Jimenez-Del-Rio et al., 2004). In agreement with these findings, Prigione and co-workers (2009) have shown increased oxidative stress in lymphocytes from untreated Parkinson's disease patients. Interestingly, Jiang et al., (2004) have shown that parkin protects human dopaminergic neuroblastoma cells against dopamine-induced cell death. Taken together these data suggest that analysis of DNA or lymphocytes response against oxidative stress might be used as an early marker of the OS status in PD patients.

Despite these evidences, there are still major unresolved issues in the understanding of the molecular and cellular biology of PD. Indeed, a complete picture of the precise molecular cascade leading to cell death in a single cellular model in this disorder is still lacking. Therefore, we have been interested in investigating the oxidative stress phenomenon and apoptosis signalling in lymphocytes and *Drosophila melanogaster*.

2. *In vitro* and *In vivo* models

2.1 Human lymphocytes resemble neuronal cells

The brain and the immune system are involved in functionally relevant cross-talk influencing one another's actions, whose main function is to maintain homeostasis. Therefore, to play such a role, lymphocytes are equipped with several biochemical systems that display comparable pathways to neural cells. This unusual characteristic makes lymphocytes an excellent *in vitro* model (Massaud et al., 1998; Kriesberg, 2011) to understand normal and abnormal function from gene to phenotype. Moreover, lymphocytes might provide the basis of biochemical and cytopathological mechanisms for preventive or therapeutic intervention. These cells thus appear to be particularly fascinating cell model for PD at least for three main reasons. First, lymphocytes express six homologous neurochemical systems (Table).

System	Protein Expression
1. Dopaminergic	Tyrosine hydroxylase & monoamine oxidase (Marino et al., 1999 & references within); dopamine transporter (Amenta et al., 2001; Marazziti et al., 2010); dopamine D2-, D3-, D4-, D5-like receptors (Ricci & Amenta, 1994; Ricci et al., 1995, 1997; Amenta et al., 1999; McKenna et al., 2002).
2. Serotonergic	Serotonin transporter (SERT, Faraj et al., 1991; Marazziti et al., 2010); serotonin receptors (Stefulj et al, 2000); tryptophan hydroxylase (Carrillo-Vico et al., 2004).
3. Cholinergic	Acetylcholine (Ach), muscarinic and nicotinic Ach receptors (mAChRs and nAChRs), choline acetyltransferase (ChAT), high affinity choline transporter and acetylcholinesterase (Kawashima & Fujii, 2004).
4. Glutamatergic	Ionotrophic glutamate receptors (Lombardi et al., 2001, 2004); group I metabotropic glutamate receptors (Miglio et al., 2005).
5. Adrenergic	β-2 adrenergic receptors (Sanders, 1998).
6. Gabaergic	γ-aminobutiric acid (GABA) receptors (Tillakaratne et al., 1995).

Table 1. Neuronal Molecular systems expressed in lymphocytes.

Second, lymphocytes express similar molecular death machinery leading to typical morphologic and biochemical features of apoptosis. Apoptosis is a type of programmed cell death initially defined by Kerr and co-workers in 1972 and recently refined by several others (Kerr et al., 1995; Xu & Shi, 2007; Kroemer et al., 2009). Apoptosis is originally a morphological phenomenon characterised by chromatin condensation and nuclear fragmentation, plasma membrane blebbing, cell shrinkage and preservation of organelles such as mitochondria. These characteristics can be recognised in lymphocytes under fluorescent microscopy (Fig. 1) or electron microscopy (Sakahira et al., 1999; Marini et al., 2001). Noticeably, what causes these morphological changes that we recognize as apoptosis occurs through multiple independent pathways that are initiated either from triggering events within the cell (i.e the "intrinsic pathway") or from outside the cell (i.e. the "extrinsic pathway"). The "intrinsic pathway" involves the release of mitochondrial proteins such as cytochrome C, second mitochondrial-derived activator of caspase/direct IAP-associated binding protein with low PI (Smac/DIABLO), apoptosis inducing factor (AIF) and Endonuclease G (Endo G). The "extrinsic pathway" involves Fas/FasL pathway, caspase-8 activation, bid degradation and releasing cytochrome C. Strikingly, both pathways converge on a common machinery of cell dismantling executed by a family of cysteine proteases known as Caspases. Indeed, caspases cleavage at aspartate residues of targeted proteins (Chowdhury et al., 2008). Particularly, caspase-3 degrades the inhibitor of caspase-activated DNase (ICAD/ DNA fragmentation Factor-45, DFF-45) protein releasing the caspase-activated DNase (CAD/ DFF-40) that result in DNA degradation ("DNA ladder pattern") from mouse T-cell lymphoma (Enari et al., 1998; Sakahira et al. 1998), Jurkat T cells (Liu et al, 1997) and HeLa cells (Halenbeck et al., 1998) under pro-apoptotic treatments. It is worth to mention that almost 18-years passed before an explanation could be drawn for one of the earliest well-recognized biochemical characteristics of apoptosis i.e. "DNA ladder pattern", from the time when Wyllie reported glucocorticoid-induced thymocytes apoptosis associated with endonuclease activation (Wyllie, 1980). Unquestionably, morphological and biochemical data have helped considerably to enlighten, yet unsettled, the mechanism of neural cell death in PD (Levy et al., 2009).

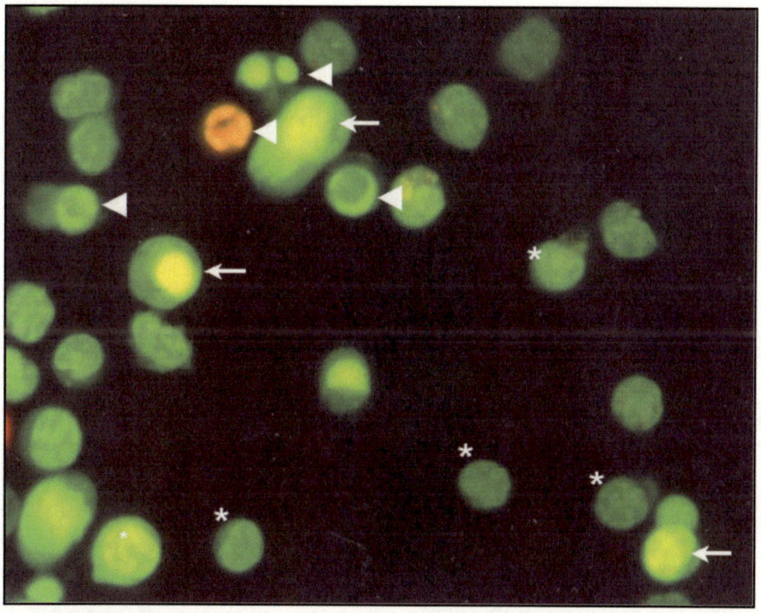

Fig. 1. **Human lymphocytes treated with xenobiotic paraquat, PQ for 24h.** Figure shows typical nuclear apoptotic morphology such as highly condensed chromatin (arrows) and nuclear fragmentation (arrowheads) from lymphocytes treated with PQ compared to normal nuclei (asterisk) stained with acridine orange/ ethidium bromide. A similar apoptotic morphology can be observed with dopamine, DA; 6-hydroxydopamine, 6-OHDA; 5,6 & 5,6 dihydroxydopamine, 5,6 & 5,7-DHT; rotenone, ROT. Jimenez-Del-Rio & Velez-Pardo, 2008. Reproduced with permission from Informa Healtcare UK Ltd.

Third, lymphocytes and neurons are post-mitotic cells, i.e. they become locked in a G_0 phase of the cell cycle. This is a remarkable biological feature to be cautiously considered when interpreting experimental data since evidence has accumulated that a cell division forced on a mature neuron leads to apoptosis rather than division (Herrup et al., 2004), but cell division is induced in lymphocytes. In other words, the use of cell lines instead of primary cultures could be confusing and /or misleading. For instance, NF-κB is a transcriptional factor composed of a p50/p65 heterodimer protein that upon activation binds to specific DNA sequences in target genes, designated as κB-elements. This factor is involved in both cell cycle-regulation and cell death processes. In dividing cells, NF-κB transcribes cyclin D1, which in association with cyclin-dependent kinases, CDK4 and CDK6, promotes G1/S phase transition through CDK-dependent phosphorilation of retinoblastoma protein (pRb), thereby releasing the transcription factor E2F, required from the activation of S phase-specific genes. Indeed, constitutive activation of NF-κB is intimately intertwined with cancer growth and metastasis (Prasad et al., 2010). On the other hand, the regulatory roles of NF-κB on apoptosis suggest that NF-κB is acting on the upstream pathways of apoptosis, either negatively or positively (Shishodia & Aggarwal, 2004; Qin et al., 2007). Noticeably, in non-dividing cells, these confounding matters connected with the role of NF-κB in apoptosis and cell-cycle control might not be an important issue given that NF-κB function can eventually be studied independently from the cell cycle function. Thus, G_0 represents not simply the absence of signals for mitosis but an active repression of the genes needed for mitosis.

2.1.1 Human lymphocytes as cellular model to study oxidative stress and apoptosis in PD.

Deciphering the Parkinson's disease cascade(s) is one of the ultimate research goals in the PD field not only because it offers the possibility to scrutinize a basic cellular machinery of response to different deleterious stimuli, but also because it brings the possibility to predict novel therapies. Accordingly, we postulated a unified molecular cascade model wherein H_2O_2 is definitely a paramount molecule involved in intracellular signalisation that induces neuronal loss in PD (Jimenez-Del-Rio & Velez-Pardo, 2000, 2004a & Fig. 2). Effectively, we were able to clarify the major signalling events by which DA (Jimenez-Del-Rio et al., 2004), monoamine related toxins (e.g. 6-OHDA; 5,6-DHT; 5,7-DHT: Jimenez-Del-Rio & Velez-Pardo, 2002), redox metals such as Fe^{2+}, Cu^{2+}, Mn^{2+}, Zn^{2+} (Jimenez-Del-Rio & Velez-Pardo, 2004b & Fig. 3) and H_2O_2 (Jimenez-Del-Rio & Velez-Pardo, 2006) might induced cell death in normal and/or mutated lymphocytes (e. g. C212Y in parkin) PD.

During the last few years, several reports have been published supporting our findings. Liang et al., (2007) have found that NF-κB contributes to 6-OHDA-induced apoptosis of nigral dopaminergic neurons through p53. Bernstein and co-worker (2011) have shown that 6-OHDA generated ROS induces DNA damage and p53- and PUMA-dependent cell death. Bilobalide, which is a constituent of *Ginkgo biloba* 761, inhibits 6-OHDA-induced activation of NF-κB and loss of dopaminergic neurons in rat substantia nigra (Li et al., 2008). Importantly, Aleyasin et al., (2004) have shown that acute inhibition of NF-κB via expression of a stable IκB mutant, down-regulation of the p65 NF-κB subunit by RNA interference (RNAi), or pharmacological NF-κB inhibitors significantly protected against DNA damage-induced neuronal death. NF-κB inhibition also reduced p53 transcripts and p53 activity as measured by the p53-inducible messages, Puma and Noxa, implicating the p53 tumor suppressor in the mechanism of NF-κB-mediated neuronal death. Takada et al. (2003) have shown that H_2O_2 activates NF-kappa B through tyrosine phosphorylation of IκBα and serine phosphorylation of p65 by IκBα kinase and Syk protein-tyrosine kinase. Prabhakaran et al., (2008) have shown that NF-κB induction and the activation of nitric oxide synthase through ROS represents a proximate mechanism for Mn-induced neurotoxicity. Therefore, we conclude that NF-κB, p53 and caspase-3 are crucial signalling molecules involved in H_2O_2-induced cell death. Based on this model, we predicted that molecules capable of generating

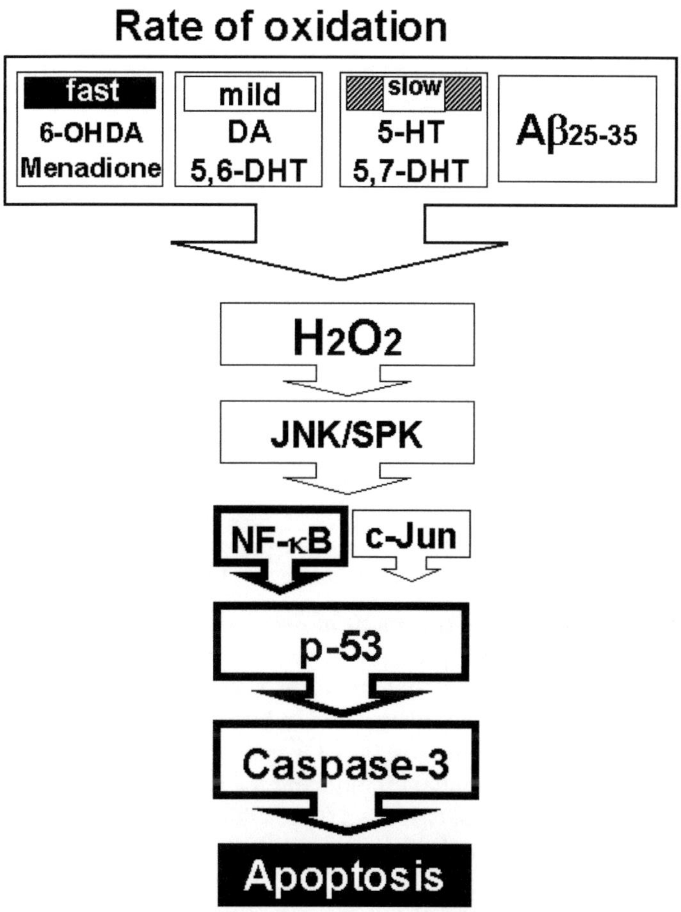

Fig. 2. **Schematic model of dopaminergic and serotonergic related toxins-induced apoptosis by an oxidative stress mechanism in PBL.** 6-OHDA; 5,6-& 5,7-DHT or protein fragment Aβ generate H_2O_2. This last compound might activates JNK/SAPK kinases pathway, which in turn activate in parallel both NF-κB and c-Jun transcription factors. NF-κB is able to activate the transcriptional factor p53 and subsequently it may activate the pro-apoptotic Bax protein, which induces cytochrome C release from mitochondria to activate the apoptosome complex leading to caspase-3 activation and apoptosis. Jimenez Del Rio and Velez-Pardo, 2002. Reproduced with permission from Elsevier.

H_2O_2 might induce a mechanism resembling the one depicted in Fig. 2. To further test our model, we used paraquat (PQ), also known as methyl viologen dichloride or 1,1′-dimethyl-4,4′-bipyridinium dichloride, and rotenone (ROT), a redox cycling herbicide and a mitochondrial complex I inhibitor as xenobiotic compound generally used to model PD (Bové et al., 2005). We concluded that both PQ-and ROT-induced time- and concentration-dependent apoptosis in lymphocytes which was mediated by anion superoxide radicals (O_2•)) / hydrogen peroxide, depolarization of mitochondria, caspase-3 activation, concomitantly with the nuclear translocation of transcription factors such as NF-κB, p53, c-Jun and nuclei fragmentation (Fig. 4-5, Jimenez-Del-Rio & Velez-Pardo, 2008; Avila-Gomez

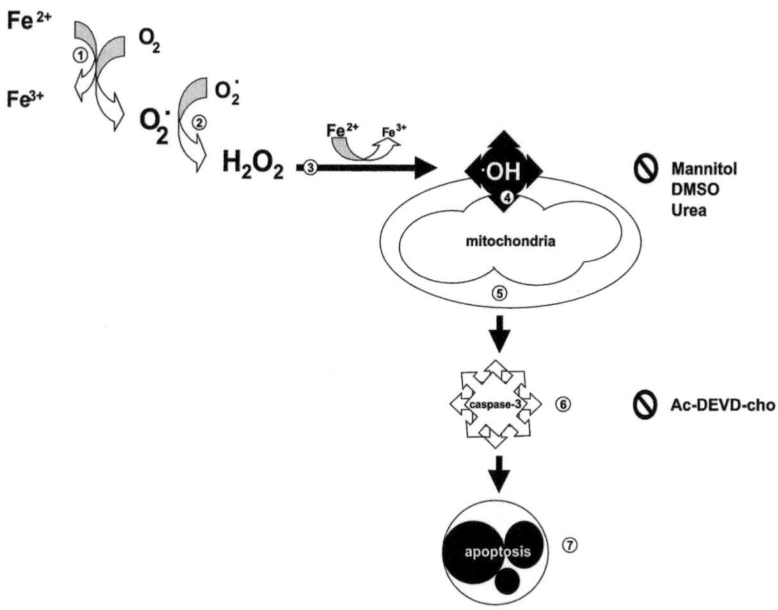

Fig. 3. **Schematic representation of the major molecular events induced by metals in lymphocytes.** Fe^{2+}-metal ions in the presence of molecular dioxygen (1) generate superoxide radicals (2), which dismutate either by enzymatic (e.g., superoxide dismutase, SOD) or spontaneously into H_2O_2 (3). This last compound in turn may react with Fe^{2+} to produce hydroxyl radicals (4) (OH·) by Fenton reaction. Over-production of (OH·) may alter the mitochondria transmembrane potential (5) inducing the liberation of different apoptogenic factors and subsequent activation of caspase-3 (6) resulting in disassembly and fragmentation of nuclear chromatin leading PBL to apoptosis (7). The symbol ( ) represents the inhibition (by indicated compound) of the critical steps of the molecular cascade leading to apoptosis by metal ions. Jimenez-Del-Rio & Velez-Pardo, 2004b. Reproduced with permission from Elsevier.

et al., 2010). Interestingly, Choi et al., (2010) have shown that JNK3 mediates PQ- and ROT-induced dopaminergic neuron death. Remarkably, the cell death routine depicted in Fig. 3 can be reversed by the action of cannabinoids (Jimenez-Del-Rio & Velez-Pardo, 2008), IGF-1 (Avila-Gomez et al., 2010) and glucose (Jimenez-Del-Rio & Velez-Pardo, 2008; Avila-Gomez et al., 2010). These data may provide innovating therapeutic strategies to intervene environmentally or genetically susceptible PD population to oxidative stress.

2.1.2 Alternative therapies for parkinson's diseases: a mechanistic igf-1, cannabinoids and glucose proposal

Based on recent progress in delineating the disease cascade and cell death process (Jenner & Olanow, 1998; Blum et al., 2001; Wirths et al., 2004; Jimenez-Del-Rio & Velez-Pardo; 2004a; Green & Kroemer, 2005; Przedborski, 2005; Jimenez-Del-Rio & Velez-Pardo, 2008; Avila-Gomez et al., 2010), discrete types of potentially disease modifying treatment could be administered for PD. In this regard, our data have highlighted the potential use of lymphocytes as a model to screen antioxidant strategies designed to remove (Fe^{2+})/(O_2·)/(H_2O_2)/(OH·), signalling inhibitors and/or restorative approaches as promising

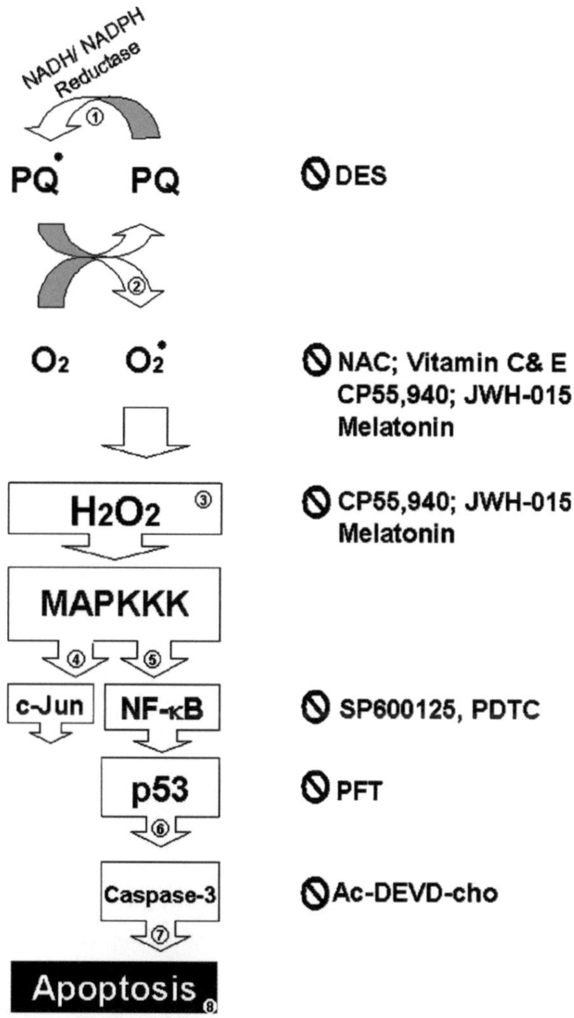

Fig. 4. **Schematic model of the major molecular events induced by PQ in lymphocytes.** PQ in the presence of NADH/NADPH reductases (1) is converted into monocationic radical compound which readily react with molecular dioxygen to generate superoxide radicals (2), which dismutase either by enzymatic (e.g. superoxide dismutase, SOD) or spontaneously into H_2O_2 (3) This last compound in turn may activate the mitogen-activated protein kinase kinase kinase (e.g. MEKK1) which can activate both c-Jun (4) via activation of MKK4/JNK, and NF-κB activation (5) via phosphorylation of the IκBa (i.e. the repressor of NF-κB) by the IKK complex. The NF-κB translocates into the nucleus and transcribes p53 protein (6). Consequently, this protein transcribes pro-apoptotic proteins (e.g. Bax) which are able to permeabilize mitochondria, thus, promoting the activation of caspase-3 (7) which signals chromatin fragmentation, typical of apoptotic morphology (8). The symbol ( ) represents the inhibition (by indicated compound) of the critical step of the molecular cascade leading to apoptosis by PQ. Jimenez Del Rio & Velez-Pardo, 2008. Reproduced with permission from Informa Healtcare UK Ltd.

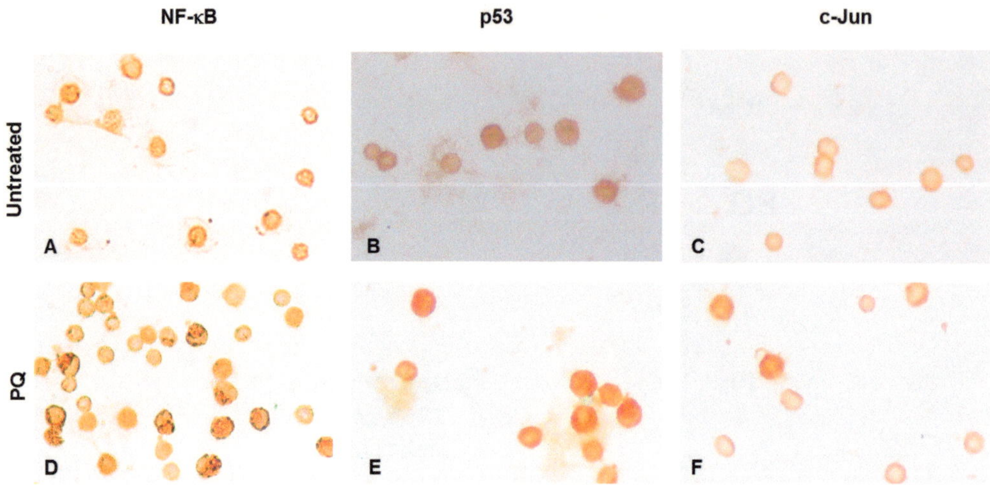

Fig. 5. PQ induces simultaneous activation of the transcription factors in lymphocytes. PBL cells were left untreated (A–C) or exposed to 1mMPQ (D–F) for 24 h. After this time of incubation, cells were stained with anti-NF-κB-p65 (A and D), anti-p53 (B and E) and anti-c-Jun (C and F) antibodies according to procedure described in Materials and methods. Notice that NF-κB, p53 and c-Jun positive-nuclei (dark brown color) reflect their nuclear translocation/activation and appear to correlate with the apoptotic nuclear morphology, i.e. condensed/fragmented nuclei when compared with untreated cells (A–C). Magnification 400 x (A–F). Jimenez-Del-Rio & Velez-Pardo, 2008. Reproduced with permission from Informa Healtcare UK Ltd.

therapy for PD. As depicted in Figs. 2-4, these mechanistic pathways may be of potential use for screening pharmacologically chemical libraries containing hundreds to thousands of compounds each that could modulate or control sensible molecules critical in cell fate (e. g., H_2O_2, NF-κB, p53, c-Jun, caspases). Recently, neurotrophic factors have come into focus as potential therapy in PD (Evans et al., 2008). One clue of its neuroprotective capability comes from the fact that IGF-1 is able to activate NF-κB against H_2O_2 oxidative stress (Heck et al., 1999). However, it has also been shown that NF-κB activation is involved in H_2O_2-induced apoptosis (Kutuk & Basaga, 2003). Therefore, the molecular mechanism(s) that explain the dual role of NF-κB as attenuator or promoter of apoptosis and the IGF-1's molecular mechanism of neuroprotection still remain to be established.

Taken advantage of the fact that human PBL express IGF-1 receptors (Tapson et al., 1988; Kooijman et al., 1992) and IGF-1 appears to be of potential therapeutic use against PD (Quesada et al., 2008), we were interested in the understanding of the molecular events that are thought to be downstream of IGF-1, in relation to the role played by NF-κB in survival and death-signalisation against PQ, ROT and H_2O_2 in lymphocytes, as a single cell model. We found that (100 nM) IGF-1 protects lymphocytes from (1 mM) PQ, (250 μM) ROT and (25, 50, 100μM) H_2O_2-induced apoptosis through NF-κB activation and p53 down regulation involving the phosphoinositide 3-kinase (PI-3K)–dependent pathway. Interestingly, IGF-1, PDTC (a NF-κB inhibitor) and pifithrin-α (PFT, a p53 inhibitor) were able to protect and rescue lymphocytes pre-exposed to PQ even when the three compounds were added up-to 6 h post-PQ exposure. Overall these observations suggest that survival and rescue of

lymphocytes from PQ and ROT toxicity is determined by p53 inactivation via IGF-1/ PI-3K pathway (Jimenez Del Rio & Velez-Pardo, 2008; Avila-Gomez et al., 2010).
Which molecular mechanism(s) explain the dual role of NF-κB as an attenuator or promoter of apoptosis? NF-κB has been reported to activate both pro-apoptotic genes such as p53 transcription factor (Wu & Lozano, 1994; Hellin et al., 1998; Jimenez Del Rio & Velez-Pardo, 2002; Velez-Pardo et al., 2002; Aleyasin et al., 2004), which in turn activates the expression of several genes that directly control or regulate the process of apoptosis such as Bax, which is a pro-apoptotic Bcl-2 protein family (Xiang et al., 1998), and anti-apoptotic genes such as Bcl-2, Bcl-X_L, X-linked inhibitor of apoptosis (Kairisalo et al., 2009). Therefore, one prevailing model proposes that when the molecular ratio of pro-survival (e.g. Bcl-2, Bcl-xL, Bcl-w) to pro-death Bcl-2 family members (e.g. Bax, Bad, Bak, Bid) is biased towards pro-death Bcl-2 family members either through changes in expression level, localization or activity, the outer mitochondrial membrane becomes permeable to apoptogenic proteins resulting in the activation of a cascade of effector caspases, such as caspase-3, that kill the cells by irreversible proteolysis of critical nuclear and cytoplasmic constituents. In this vein, our data suggest that IGF-1 might promote gene transcription of survival genes via NF-κB activation (Kane et al., 1999) and suppresses gene transcription of pro-apoptotic proteins through p53 inactivation. How then p53 turn-off could be related with IGF-1 citoprotection? One possible explanation for this phenomenon comes from the work by Ogawara and colleagues (2002) who showed that Akt enhances the ubiquitinization-promoting function of Mdm2 (murine double minute) by phosphorylation of S^{186}, which results in reduction of p53 protein. Furthermore, Feng and colleagues (2004) showed that PKB/Akt induces phosphorylation of Mdm2 at Ser^{166} and Ser^{188} resulting in Mdm2 protein stabilization. Based on this information and our data, it is reasonable to assume that p53 is modulated by IGF-1 through PI3K-Akt pathway. In fact, our findings reveal that p53 but not NF-κB is the critical transcription factor that may possibly balances the expression of pro-death proteins towards intracellular death decision under oxidative noxious stimuli (Lu, 2005). Therefore, an ideal natural or synthetic pharmacological compound would be one that efficiently function as an antioxidant (e.g. 17β-estradiol (Jimenez-Del-Rio & Velez-Pardo, 2001; vitamin E) and simultaneously act as a survival signalling molecule (e.g. IGF-1). To our surprise, the molecules exhibiting both features might come from the glandular hairs of *Cannabis sativa* or marijuana, actually known as cannabinoids.

2.1.2.1 Cannabinoids

Cannabinoids are a group of C_{21} terpenophenolic compounds (Elsohly & Slade, 2005), which exert their effects by binding to specific plasma membrane G-protein-couple receptors, termed CB1 (Matsuda et al., 1990) and CB2 (Munro et al., 1993) receptors. Activation of these receptors has been shown to trigger several $G_i/_o$-protein-mediated signalling pathways (Turu & Hunyady, 2010). Although, it is currently accepted that CB1 receptors are specially abundant in basal ganglia, hippocampus, cerebellum and cortical structures; and CB2 receptors are restricted to cell types related to the immune function such as spleen macrophages, tonsils, B cells and natural killer cells, monocytes, neutrophils, and T cells (Pazos et al., 2005), it has also been demonstrated the existence of CB2 receptors in purkinje cerebellar neurons (Skaper et al., 1996), microglia (Klegeris et al., 2003), oligodendrocytes (Molina-Holgado et al., 2002) and brainstem neurons (Van Sickle et al., 2005). Moreover, both receptors elicit similar signalling pathways such as inhibition of adenylate cyclase, stimulation of extracellular-signal-regulated kinase (Demuth & Molleman, 2006) and activation of phosphoinositide 3-kinase/PKB (Gomez Del Pulgar et al., 2000; 2002; Molina-Holgado et al., 2002; Sanchez MG et al., 2003). The physiological significance of these common characteristics is still unknown.

Cannabinoids have been proposed as potential therapeutic agents against PD (García-Arencibia et al., 2009) thanks to their involvement in control of cell death/ survival decision and in neuroprotection (van der Stelt & Di Marzo, 2005). However, the mechanism of both actions by cannabinoids is far from clear. Moreover, cannabinoids have been shown to function as antioxidant compounds via receptor-independent (Hampson et al., 1998; Chen et al., 2000; Marsicano et al., 2002) or receptor-dependent mechanisms (Nagayama et al., 1999; Kim et al., 2005) or both mechanisms (Kaplan et al., 2003). Although CB antagonists (v. gr. SR141716A) have been used to elucidate the neuroprotective mechanism of cannabinoids, they have not been conclusive (see Marsicano et al., 2002 versus Nagayama et al., 1999; Kim et al., 2005). Therefore, the molecular mechanism(s) of cannabinoids effect on cells is a complex and still controversial issue.

Despite intense investigation, the detailed intracellular mechanism(s) involved in cannabinoids survival effect remains to be elucidated. Because CB2 cannabinoid receptor is linked to activation of PI3K (Sanchez MG et al., 2003), and the non-classical cannabinoid (-)-CP55,940 (a CB1 and CB2 agonist) and JWH-015 (a CB2 agonist) are commercially available, we wanted to elucidate the molecular signalling downstream of CB2 receptor linked to the role played by NF-κB and p53 in survival and death-signalisation against oxidative stress stimuli. We found that both synthetic agonists protect and rescue PBL against $A\beta_{25-35}$- and PQ-induced apoptosis by receptor-independent and receptor-dependent pathway (Velez-Pardo & Jimenez-Del-Rio, 2006; Jimenez Del Rio & Velez-Pardo, 2008). In agreement with our previous observations with IGF-1, these results suggest that CP55,940 /(JWH-015) protective and rescue effect on PBL from noxious stimuli is determined by p53 inactivation.

Recently, we investigated the ability of CP55,940 and JWH-015 to scavenge reactive oxygen species and their effect on mitochondria permeability transition (MPT) in either a mitochondria-free superoxide anion generation system, intact rat brain mitochondria or in sub-mitochondrial particles (SMP) treated with PQ. Oxygen consumption, mitochondrial membrane potential ($\Delta\psi_m$) and MPT were determined as parameters of mitochondrial function. It was found that both cannabinoids effectively attenuate mitochondrial damage against PQ-induced oxidative stress by scavenging anion superoxide radical ($O_2^{\bullet -}$) and hydrogen peroxide (H_2O_2), maintaining $\Delta\psi_m$ and by avoiding Ca^{2+}-induced mitochondrial swelling (Velez-Pardo et al., 2010). Understanding the mechanistic action of cannabinoids on mitochondria might provide new insights into more effective therapeutic approaches for oxidative stress related disorders (Fig. 6). Further investigation is needed to classify cannabinoids molecules (Padgett, 2005; Thakur et al., 2005) with effective anti-oxidant from those with pro-oxidant actions.

2.1.2.2 Glucose

Glucose is a soluble sugar added to all cell culture media. In fact, glucose entry to the cell is facilitated by glucose transporters (GLUTs 1-13) (Manolescu et al., 2007) and depending on cell type, the amount of glucose in cell culture formulations ranges from 1 g/L (5.5 mM) to as high as 10 g/L (55 mM). This is an important consideration to take into account because the same processes that can affect cells and molecules *in vitro* can occur *in vivo*. Lymphocytes are ideal for learning about glucose metabolism and resistance against oxidative stress for several reasons. First, these cells express GLU-1 and GLU-3 transporter proteins

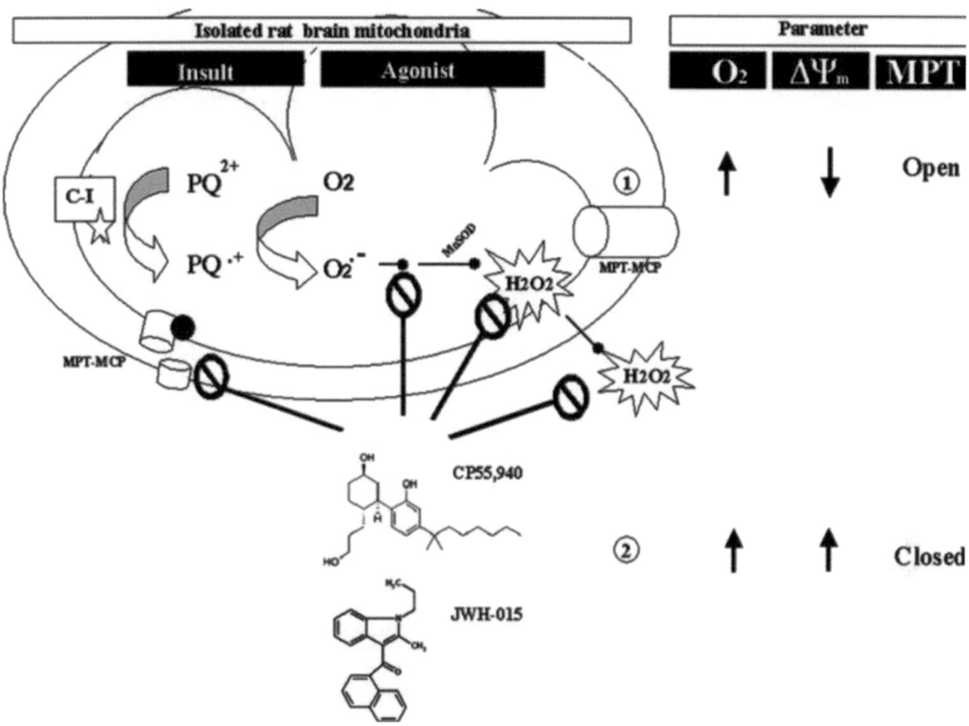

Fig. 6. **Scheme of proposed cannabinoid mechanism of action against Paraquat-induced mitochondrial oxidative stress.** High mitochondrial membrane potential ($\Delta\psi_m$) in intact rat brain mitochondria drives PQ compound into the mitochondrial matrix. Once inside, (1) PQ is reduced to the monocation radical PQ•- at complex I in the respiratory chain by electrons donated from NADH. PQ•- reacts rapidly with O_2 to produce superoxide (O_2•-), thereby consuming high amount of oxygen. In turn, the (O_2•-) is enzymatically dismutated by MnSOD into H_2O_2. Then, H_2O_2 induces mitochondrial permeability transition pore (MPT) and decreases $\Delta\psi_m$. Interestingly, when cannabinoids are present (2), they can remove both O_2•- and H_2O_2 thereby blocking further ROS signaling. Most interestingly, cannabinoids inhibit MPT probably through interactions with the cyclosporine A-binding cyclophilin-D protein (black circle). As a result, cannabinoids maintain the MPT-multiprotein complex (MPC) in a close-stated, high ($\Delta\psi$m) but O_2 consumption is still high. Taken in conjunction these actions, cannabinoids thus protect mitochondria from further damage. Velez-Pardo et al., 2010. Reproduced with permission from Springer Publishers Ltd.

(Piatkiewicz et al., 2007). Second, glucose metabolism in lymphocytes is a regulated process. Indeed, glucose can enter glycolytic, pentose phosphate and Krebs cycle pathways (Maciver et al., 2008). Therefore, these cells represent a remarkable non-neural cell model to understanding metabolic regulation of apoptosis and cell survival signaling against stressful stimuli.

Previously, we have demonstrated that PQ- and ROT-induce apoptosis in lymphocytes cultured in standard RPMI 1640 culture medium, which contains 11 mM glucose (11G), via a cascade of molecular events involving $O_2^{\cdot-}$ and H_2O_2, as prime death signals (Jimenez-De-Rio & Velez-Pardo, 2008; Avila-Gomez et al., 2010). Interestingly, by increasing the concentration of glucose to 55 mM (55G) in RPMI 1640 culture medium, it has been shown that glucose almost completely protected lymphocytes against PQ-and ROT-induced apoptotic cell death (Jimenez-De-Rio & Velez-Pardo, 2008; Avila-Gomez et al., 2010). These data thus suggest that the predominance of PQ- and ROT-induced oxidative stress damage may be adjusted by decreasing or increasing the concentration of glucose in the cell culture media. By using biochemical analysis and pharmacological inhibition, we found that 55G was effective in suppressing rotenone-induced apoptosis in lymphocytes via four acting pathways which involve the pentose phosphate pathway (PPP-II), glutathione pathway, SOD and CAT antioxidant system and PI3-K signalling. Moreover, it is shown for the first time that glucose induced lymphocyte survival by NF-κB activation and down-regulation of p53 and caspase-3 (Bonilla-Ramirez, L., Jimenez-De-Rio, M. & Velez-Pardo, C. (2011). Unpublished observations). Taken altogether these results suggest that antioxidants (e.g. cannabinoids), growth factors (e.g. IGF-1) and environmental factor (e.g. glucose) might regulate cell death in lymphocytes upon oxidative stress. Unfortunately, lymphocytes as *in vitro* model of PD do not provide information about executive functions (i.e. cognitive process), kinesthesia (i.e. physical movement) and/or diet-related to PD. To further study the effect of xenotoxicity, diet and movement alterations, we therefore turn out our attention to *Drosophila melanogaster*.

2.2 *Drosophila melanogaster*: an unexpected invertebrate in scene

During the last few years, *Drosophila melanogaster* has been recognized as a valuable model to study neurodegenerative diseases (Lu, 2009; Hirth, 2010), especially PD (Botella et al., 2009; Guo, 2010; Whitworth, 2011) for three main reasons. First, some genes implicated as causative of PD have at least one homolog in the fly (e.g. *parkin*, *DJ-1*, *PINK*::see htpp://superfly.ucsd.edu for further information). This unique feature has facilitated the functional interpretation of these genes in the human (Park et al., 2009; Bayersdorfer et al., 2010). Second, the expression of PD related genes in *Drosophila* can be performed by using the binary GAL-4-dependent upstream activating sequence (GAL4/UAS) system (Phelps & Brand, 1998), thus providing an excellent tool to express pathological proteins in the fly´s brain (e.g. α-synuclein, Feany & Bender, 2000). Third, the dopaminergic system of the fly is well characterised (Mao & Davis, 2009; White et al., 2010). Furthermore, comparable to the human condition, the *Drosophila* DA system is also involved in locomotor control (Riemensperger et al., 2011). Therefore, the similarity between the dopaminergic network, mode of drug action and behaviour in *D. melanogaster* and mammalian systems, has made the fly a very attractive model for anti-parkinsonism drug discovery (Whitworth et al., 2006). Additionally, *Drosophila* offers the power of rapid drug screening (Pendleton et al., 2002a; Faust et al., 2009). Amazingly, a variety of approaches have been used to model Parkinson's-like motor dysfunction in *Drosophila,* including specific genetic alterations (Feany & Bender, 2000; Pendleton et al., 2002b; Wang et al., 2007; Sang et al., 2007); pharmacological inhibition of crucial proteins in the dopamine system (Pendleton et al., 2002 a, b) or pharmacological insult (Coulom et al., 2004; Chaudhuri et al., 2007). Indeed, previous studies have demonstrated that paraquat (PQ) induces selective cell death of dopaminergic neurons (Chaudhuri et al., 2007) through interaction with complex I of the mitochondrial respiratory chain (Cocheme & Murphy, 2008) and oxidative stress (Bonilla et al., 2006). Therefore, on the understanding that the causes of PD are mainly oxidative stress and mitochondrial dysfunction, antioxidants, free radical scavengers, monoamine oxidase inhibitors, iron-chelators, and other such drugs are expected to be used. The study of antioxidants is becoming one of the most important subjects in PD research. Based on our *in vitro* data, we investigated the effect of cannabinoids and polyphenols, which are defined as a group of chemical substances present in plants, fruits and vegetables characterized by the presence of one or more than one phenol unit per molecule with several hydroxyl groups on aromatic rings, in *Drosophila melanogaster* against PQ-induced oxidative stress.

Recently, we have shown for the first time that CP55,940, a non-selective CB1/CB2 cannabinoid receptor agonist, significantly protects and rescues *Drosophila* against PQ toxicity via a receptor-independent mechanism (Fig. 7). Interestingly, CP55,940 restores the negative geotaxis activity (i.e., climbing capability) of the fly exposed to PQ. Moreover, *Drosophila* fed with (1–200 μM) SP600125, a specific inhibitor of the stress responsive Jun-N-terminal kinase (JNK) signalling, and 20 mM PQ increased survival percentage and movement function (i.e., climbing capability) when compared to flies only treated with PQ. Taken together our results suggest that exogenous antioxidant cannabinoids can protect against and rescue from locomotor dysfunction in wild type (Canton-S) *Drosophila* exposed to stress stimuli (Jimenez-Del-Rio et al., 2008). Therefore, cannabinoids may offer promising avenues for the design of molecules to prevent, delay, or ameliorate the treatment of population at high risk of suffering Parkinson disease.

Polyphenols are a group of chemical substances found in plants classified according to their chemical structural as (i) phenolic acids such as gallic (GA), caffeic (CA), coumaric (CouA), ferulic acid (FA), propyl gallate (PG); (ii) flavonoids, which are the largest group of polyphenols, and (iii) non-flavonoid polyphenols. Flavonoids involve anthocyanins and anthoxantins. The latter group is divided into flavonols, flavans, flavanols such as epicatechin (EC), epigallocatechin (EGC) and epigallocatechin-3-gallate (EGCG), flavones and isoflavones (D'Archivio et al., 2007). Numerous studies in the past decade have shown that polyphenols have *in vitro* and *in vivo* activity by preventing or reducing the deleterious effects of ROS associated with oxidative stress and neurodegeneration not only because of their strong antioxidant and metal-chelating properties (Sestili et al., 2002; Melidou et al., 2005; Perron & Brumaghim, 2009), but also because of their capability to induce intracellular signalling pathways associated with cell survival and gene expression (Ramassamy, 2006; Zaveri, 2006). We demonstrated for the first time that pure polyphenols GA, FA, CA, CouA, PG, EC, EGC, and EGCG protect, rescue and, most importantly, restore the impaired movement activity (i.e., climbing capability) induced by paraquat in *Drosophila melanogaster* (Fig. 8). We also showed for the first time that high concentrations of iron (e.g. 15 mM $FeSO_4$) were able to diminish fly survival and movement to a similar extent as (20 mM) paraquat treatment. Moreover, paraquat and iron synergistically affect both survival and locomotor function. Remarkably, propyl gallate and epigallocatechin gallate protected and maintained movement abilities in flies co-treated with paraquat and iron. Our findings indicate that pure polyphenols might be potent neuroprotective agents for the treatment of PD against stressful stimuli (Jimenez-Del-Rio et al., 2010).

It is generally accepted that the causes of PD are mainly oxidative stress, abnormal protein aggregation and mitochondrial dysfunction. Furthermore, substantial evidence suggests diet (Chen et al., 2007) and environmental risk factors such as pesticides (Dick et al., 2007) and heavy metals (Jones & Miller, 2008), in particular iron intake (Logroscino et al., 2008), as causative of PD. However, how genetic and environmental factors are related to the nutritional status of PD patients is still unknown. Moreover, it has not yet been definitively established whether the nutritional status of PD patients might contribute to the

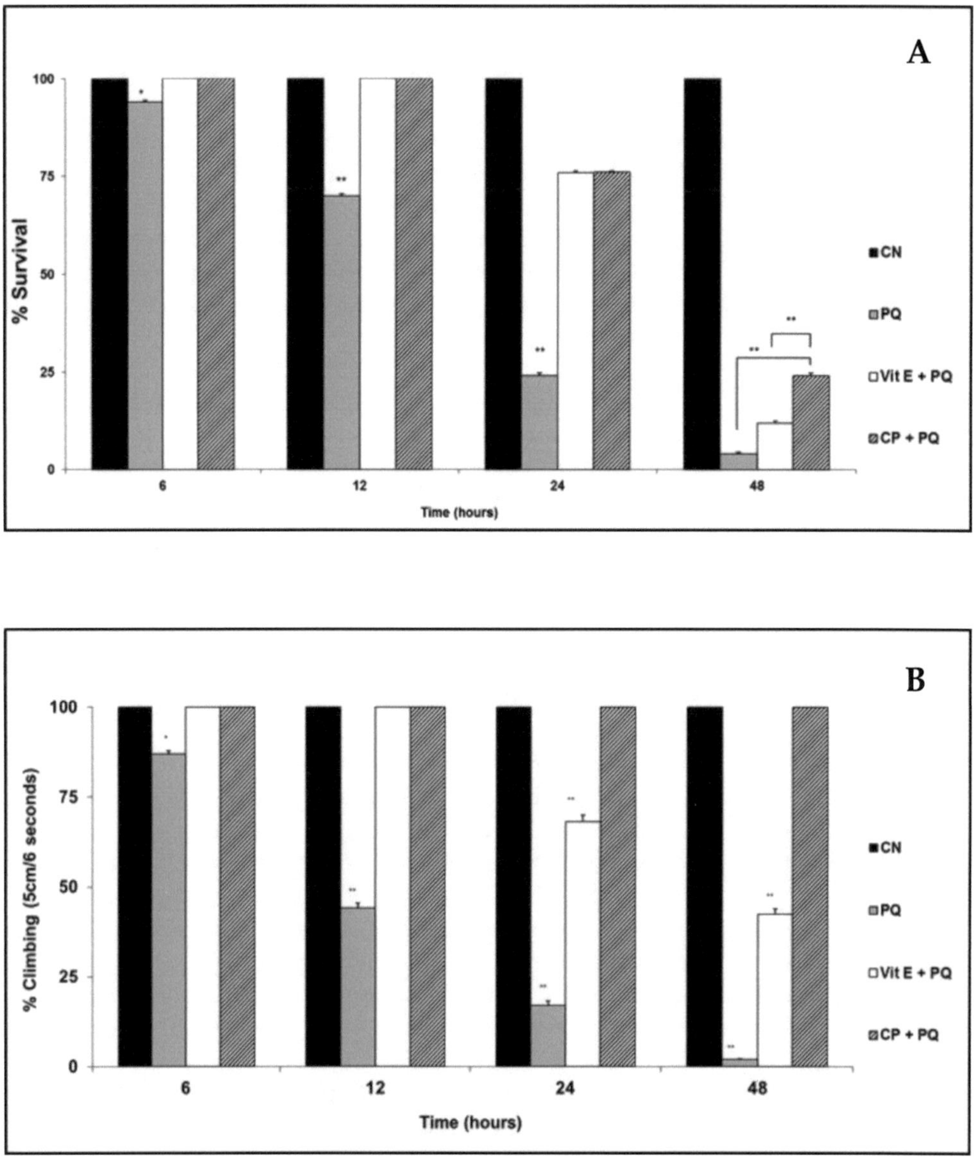

Fig. 7. **Protective effect of antioxidants in *Drosophila m.* exposed to paraquat**.
Female flies were pre-fed with either 1% glucose alone, 0.5 mM CP55,940 or 0.5 mM vitamin E with 1% glucose in dW for 72 h. Then, flies were left untreated (GLU) or treated with 20 mMparaquat (PQ; vit E + PQ; CP + PQ) for 6, 12, 24 and 48 h. (A) Survival rate (%) and (B) locomotion assay were recorded at the indicated time. *$p < 0.05$, **$p < 0.001$. Jimenez-Del-Rio et al., 2008. Reproduced with permission from Elsevier.

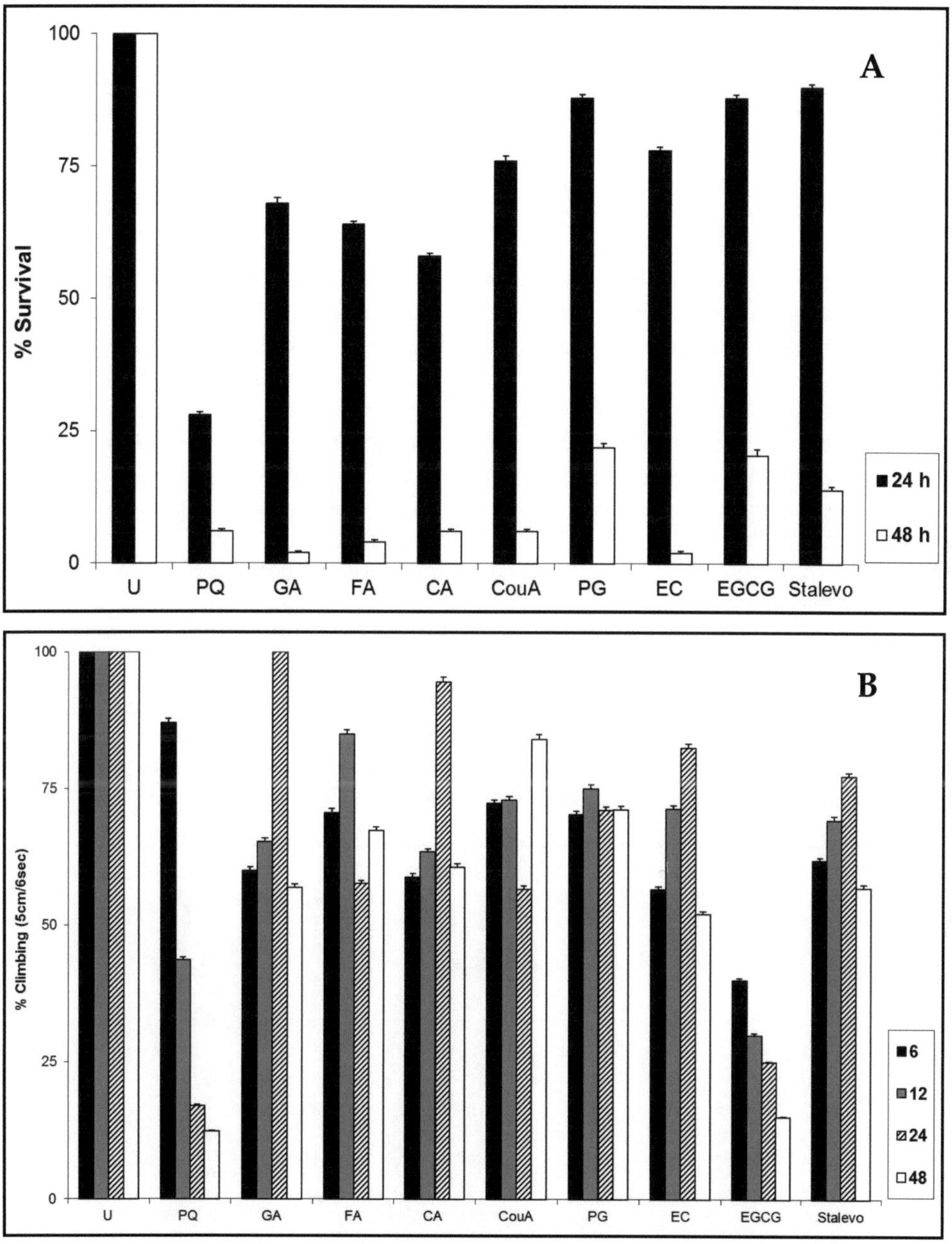

Fig. 8. **Protective effect of polyphenols in *D. melanogaster* exposed to paraquat.**
(A) Female flies were pre-fed with either 1% glucose alone or with 0.1 mM gallic acid (GA), ferulic acid (FA), caffeic acid (CA), coumaric acid (CouA), propyl gallate (PG), epicatecin (EC), epigallocatechin (EGC), epigallocatechin gallate (EGCG) polyphenols and 0.1 mg/ml Stalevo® with 1% glucose in distilled water (dW) for 72 h. Then, flies were left untreated (U) or treated with 20mM paraquat (PQ) for 24 and 48 h. Survival rate (%) and (**B**) locomotion assay were recorded at the indicated time. *$p<0.05$, ** $p<0.001$. Jimenez-Del-Rio et al., 2010. Reproduced with permission from Elsevier.

development of the disorder. Therefore, we investigated the effect of glucose in *Drosophila melanogaster* under oxidative stress stimuli.

We have shown that female *D. melanogaster* fed acutely with 20mM PQ in high concentration of glucose (e.g. 10%), as the sole energetic source, not only prolonged survival but also the locomotor activity remained unaltered when compared to fly fed with low concentration of glucose (e.g. 1%) and PQ over a period of 24-48 h (Fig. 9). Additionally, we found that polyphenols protect, rescue and restore the impaired movement activity in *Drosophila* induced by 20 mM PQ in 1% glucose for 24 h exposure (Fig. 8). We also showed that high concentrations of iron (e.g. 10-20 mM $FeSO_4$) were able to diminish fly survival and locomotor activity over a period of 120 h (5 days). Taken together these findings suggest that either glucose or polyphenols might modulate life span and movement capabilities in *D. melanogaster* exposed to PQ and iron in short time frame. Since there is compelling evidence that shows that the pre-clinical period of PD extends at least 20 years before the motor manifestations (Savica et al., 2010), it is necessary to establish a close parallel with the fly to better understand antioxidant therapy approaches over long period of time. Therefore, we studied the life span and locomotor activity (i.e. climbing capability) of *D. melanogaster* chronically exposed to increasing concentrations of PQ and iron alone or in combination upon 1% or 10% glucose feeding regimen for 15 days and determined whether polyphenols such as GA, PG, EC and EGCG affect the life span and locomotor activity of the fly exposed to PQ for 15 days. It is known that protein aggregation is associated to PD (Tan et al., 2009). Interestingly, high expression levels of the transcription GAL4 protein in *D. melanogaster* have been shown to result in reduced life span (Haywood et al., 2002). Therefore, by using *Ddc-GAL4 Drosophila melanogaster* line, we also investigated whether genetically altered *Ddc-GAL4* flies renders them sensitive to PQ-induced oxidative stress and whether glucose and polyphenols might modulate life span and/or locomotor activity in this line of *Drosophila melanogaster.*

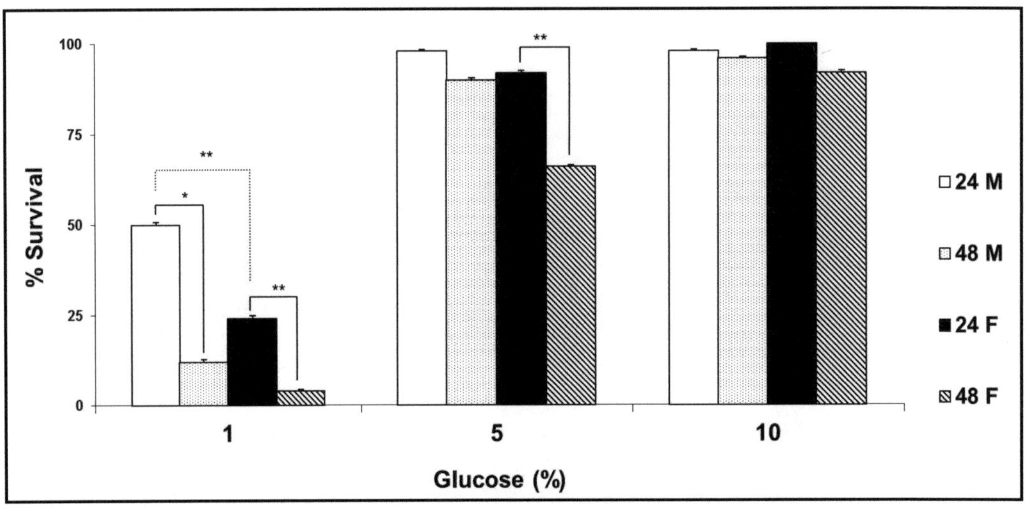

Fig. 9. **Effect of glucose concentration in *Drosophila m.* exposed to paraquat.**
Male (M) and female (F) were either pre-fed with 1, 5 or 10% glucose (GLU) in distilled water for 72 h. Then, flies were treated with 20 mM paraquat (PQ) for 24 and 48 h. Survival rate (%) weas recorded at the indicated time. $*p < 0.05$, $**p < 0.001$. Jimenez-Del-Rio et a., 2008. Reproduced with permission from Elsevier.

We found for the first time that polyphenols exposure prolong life span ($P<0.05$ by log-rang test) and restore locomotor activity (i.e., climbing capability, $P<0.05$ by χ^2 test) of *Drosophila melanogaster* chronically exposed to paraquat compared to flies treated with paraquat alone in 1% glucose (Fig. 10). We found that (10%) glucose partially prolongs life span and climbing in *Drosophila* exposed to iron, PQ or in combination, suggesting that both stimuli enhance a movement disorder in a concentration-dependent and temporal-related fashion. Moreover, chronic exposure of (1 mM) PQ/ (0.5 mM) iron synergistically affect both survival and locomotor function independently of the temporal order of the exposure to the toxicants, but the survival is modulated in a concentration and temporal fashion by glucose. This investigation is the first to report that *Ddc-GAL4* transgenic flies chronically fed with polyphenols increase life span ($P<0.05$ by log-rang test) and enhance movement abilities ($P<0.05$ by χ^2 test) compared to untreated *Ddc-GAL4* or treated with paraquat in 1% glucose. Our present findings support the notion that *Drosophila melanogaster* might be a suitable model to study genetic, environmental and nutritional factors as causal and/or modulators in the development of PD. Most importantly, according to our model, we have demonstrated for the first time chronic polyphenols exposure as potential therapeutic compounds in the treatment of PD. These findings altogether open new avenues for the screening, testing and development of novel antioxidant drugs against oxidative stress stimuli (Ortega-Arellano et al., 2011).

3. Conclusion

As noted by the Nobel Prize laureate Dr. S. Brenner (2002) "…choosing the right organism for one's research is as important as finding the right problems to work on…" In this regard, human peripheral blood lymphocytes and *Drosophila melanogaster* as model system are well validated and permit totally controlled experiments, are relatively low cost and ease to use, but most importantly, they resemble neuronal cells and clinical manifestation from PD patients, respectively. As any other model (e.g. animal or human tissue and cell lines), their limitation is your removal from the reality of the whole, integrated physiologic system. Despite this drawback, it turns out that their use in complex biologic investigations such as the one presented in this chapter, introduce lymphocytes and *Drosophila* as a unique opportunity to integrate oxidative stress, cell death, cell survival signalling and therapeutic pathways signalling in a single-cell and organism model.

Our present data support the notion that *Drosophila melanogaster* might be a suitable model to study genetic, environmental and nutritional factors as causal and/or modulators in the development of PD. Most importantly, according to our model, we have demonstrated for the first time that acute cannabinoids or chronic polyphenols exposure as potential therapeutic compounds in the treatment of PD.

These findings altogether open new avenues for the screening, testing, monitoring and development of novel antioxidant drugs against oxidative stress stimuli. Furthermore, based on our present findings, we propose that a combined therapy with antioxidant and high energetic agents should provide to pre-clinical genetically individuals at risk to suffer PD a means to delay or to prevent motor symptoms and/or frank PD-ARJP disorders, as those encounter in Antioquia, Colombia (Pineda-Trujillo et al., 2001, 2006, 2009). These data may contribute to a better understanding of the inherent nutritional status, genetic predisposition and environmental agents as causative factors of PD. However, further studies are needed to fully determine target selection and validation, pharmacology, measurement of efficacy

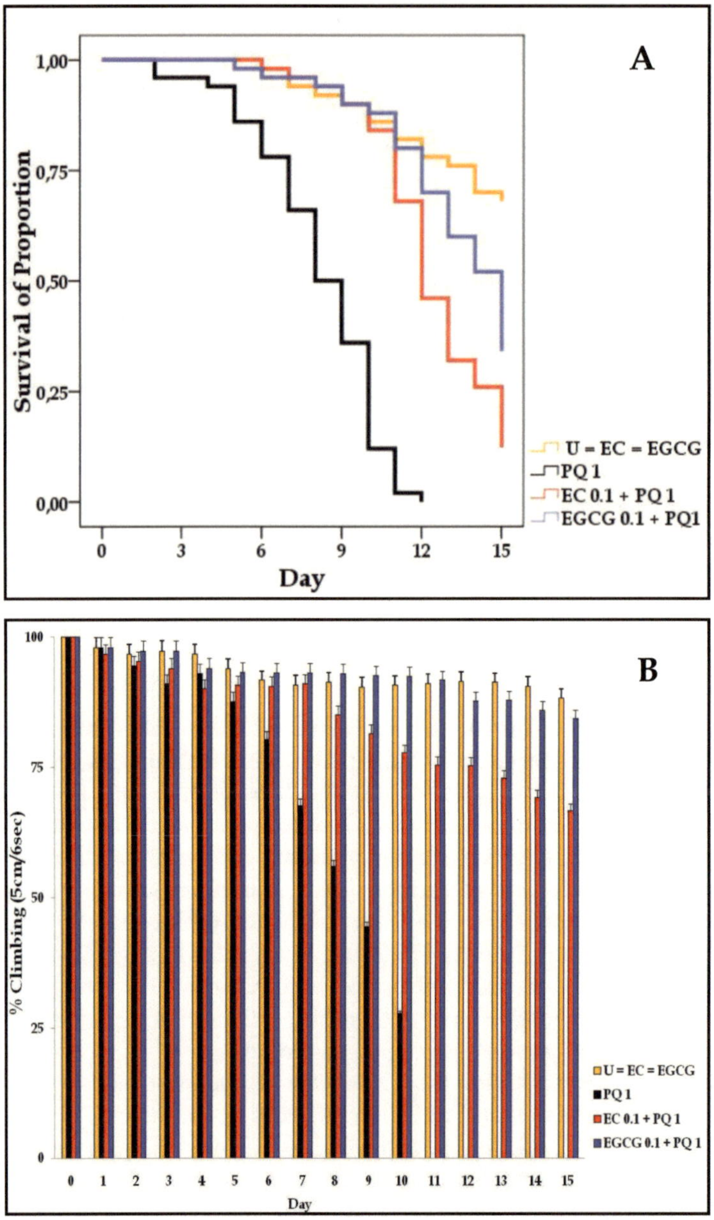

Fig. 10. **Survival (A) and locomotor activity (B) of *Drosophila melanogaster* in absence (0, gray bar) or presence of paraquat (1mM) alone (black bar) or in combination of polyphenols (epicathecin (EC, 0.1 mM, red bar) or epigallocathecin gallete, EGCG gallate (0.1 mM, blue bar) in 1% glucose.** Female flies (n= 50 per treatment) were treated as described in *Materials and Methods* section. The graphs show that the proportion of survival and climbing performance dramatically increased in flies exposed to polyphenols compared to PQ treatment alone. Statistical comparisons between treated flies with PQ and polyphenols and PQ alone showed (A) a $P<0.001$ by log-rank test and (B) a $P<0.05$ by χ^2 test. Ortega-Arellano et al., 2011. Reproduced with permission from Elsevier.

(Kieburtz & Ravina, 2007) and bioavailability (D'Archivio et al., 2010) of potential antioxidant molecules, particularly cannabinoids and polyphenols, before one can envision a preventive and effective neuroprotectant therapy against PD.

4. Acknowledgements

This work was supported by Colciencias grants #1115-343-19119 & #1115-408-20504; Programa Jovenes Investigadores from Colciencias #8790-018-2011; "Proyecto Investigaciones Enfermedades Neurodegenerativas" grants #8780, and "Programa de Sostenibilidad grants 2007/2008/2009/2010" to CV-P and MJ-Del-Rio.

5. References

Aleyasin, H., Cregan, SP., Lyirhiaro, G., O'Hare, MJ., Callaghan, SM., Slack, RS. & Park, DS. (2004). Nuclear factor-(kappa)B modulates the p53 response in neurons exposed to DNA damage, *J Neurosci* 24: 2963-2973.

Alves, G., Forsaa, EB., Pedersen, KF., Dreetz-Gjerstad, M. & Larsen, JP. (2008). Epidemiology of Parkinson's disease, *J Neurol* 255 Suppl 5:18-32.

Amenta, F., Bronzetti, E., Felici, L., Ricci, A. & Tayebati, SK. (1999). Dopamine D2-like receptors on human peripheral blood lymphocytes: a radioligand binding assay and immunocytochemical study, *J Auton Pharmacol* 19:151-159.

Amenta, F., Bronzetti, E., Cantalamessa, F., El-Assouad, D., Felici, L., Ricci, A. & Tayebati, SK. (2001). Identification of dopamine plasma membrane and vesicular transporters in human peripheral blood lymphocytes, *J Neuroimmunol* 117 (1-2):133-142.

Asanuma, M., Miyazaki, I., Diaz-Corrales, FJ. & Ogawa, N. (2004). Quinone formation as dopaminergic neuron-specific oxidative stress in the pathogenesis of sporadic Parkinson's disease and neurotoxin-induced parkinsonism, *Acta Med Okayama* 58: 221-233.

Avila-Gomez, I.C., Velez-Pardo, C. & Jimenez-Del-Rio, M. (2010). Effects of insulin-like growth factor-1 on rotenone-induced apoptosis in lymphocyte cells, *Basic Clin Pharmacol Toxicol* 106(1): 53-61.

Bayersdorfer, F., Voigt, A., Schneuwly, S. & Botella, JA. (2010). Dopamine-dependent neurodegeneration in Drosophila models of familial and sporadic Parkinson's disease, *Neurobiol Dis* 40(1):113-119.

Betarbet, R; Sherer, TB & Greenamyre, JT. (2005). Ubiquitin-proteasome system and Parkinson's disease, *Exp Neurol* 191 Suppl 1: S17-S27.

Battisti, C., Formichi, P., Radi, E. & Federico, A. (2008). Oxidative-stress-induced apoptosis in PBLs of two patients with Parkinson disease secondary to alpha-synuclein mutation, *J Neurol Sci* 267(1-2):120-124.

Bernstein, AI., Garrison, SP., Zambetti, GP. & O'Malley, KL. (2011). 6-OHDA generated ROS induces DNA damage and p53- and PUMA-dependent cell death, *Mol Neurodegener* 6(1):2.

Bonilla, E., Medina-Leendertz, S., Villalobos, V., Molero, L. & Bohórquez, A. (2006). Paraquat-induced oxidative stress in drosophila melanogaster: effects of melatonin, glutathione, serotonin, minocycline, lipoic acid and ascorbic acid, *Neurochem Res* 31(12):1425-1432.

Botella, JA., Bayersdorfer, F., Gmeiner, F. & Schneuwly, S. (2009). Modelling Parkinson's disease in Drosophila, *Neuromolecular Med* 11(4):268-280.

Bove, J., Prou, D., Perier, C. & Przedborski, S. (2005). Toxin-induced Models of Parkinson' disease, *NeuroRx* 2:484-494.

Blum, D., Torch, S., Lambeng, N., Nissou, M., Benabid, AL., Sadoul, R. & Verna, JM. (2001). Molecular pathways involved in the neurotoxicity of 6-OHDA, dopamine and MPTP: contribution to the apoptotic theory in Parkinson's disease, *Prog Neurobiol* 65:135-172.

Brenner, S. (2002). Nature's gift to science. Nobel lecture, December 8, (*www.nobelprize.com*).

Büeler, H. (2010). Mitochondrial dynamics, cell death and the pathogenesis of Parkinson's disease, *Apoptosis* 15(11):1336-1353.

Calopa, M., Bas, J., Callén, A. &, Mestre, M. (2010). Apoptosis of peripheral blood lymphocytes in Parkinson patients, *Neurobiol Dis* 38(1):1-7.

Carrillo-Vico, A., Calvo, JR., Abreu, P., Lardone, PJ., Garcia-Maurino, S., Reiter, RJ. & Guerrero, JM. (2004). Evidence of melatonin synthesis by human lymphocytes and its physiological significance: possible role as intracrine, autocrine, and/or paracrine substance, *FASEB J* 18: 537-539.

Cocheme, HM. & Murphy, MP. (2008). Complex I is the major site of mitochondrial superoxide production by paraquat, *J Biol Chem* 283: 1786–1798.

Cookson, MR. (2010). Unravelling the role of defective genes, *Prog Brain Res* 183:43-57.

Coulom, H. & Birman, S. (2004). Chronic exposure to rotenone models sporadic Parkinson's disease in Drosophila melanogaster, *J Neurosci* 24:10993–10998.

Chaudhuri, A., Bowling, K., Funderburk, C., Lawal, H., Inamdar, A., Wang, Z. & O'Donnell, JM. (2007). Interaction of genetic and environmental factors in a Drosophila parkinsonism model, *J Neurosci* 27:2457–2467.

Chen, Y. & Buck, J. (2000). Cannabinoids protect cells from oxidative cell death: a receptor-independent mechanism, *J Pharmacol Exp Ther* 293: 807-812.

Chen, H., O'Reilly, E., McCullough, ML., Rodriguez, C., Schwarzschild, MA., Calle, EE., Thun, MJ. & Ascherio, A. (2007). Consumption of dairy products and risk of Parkinson's disease, *Am J Epidemiol* 165(9):998-1006.

Choi, WS., Abel, G., Klintworth, H., Flavell, RA. & Xia, Z. (2010). JNK3 mediates paraquat- and rotenone-induced dopaminergic neuron death, *J Neuropathol Exp Neurol* 69(5):511-520.

Chowdhury, I., Tharakan, B. & Bhat, GK. Caspases- an update, *Comp Biochem Physiol B Biochem Mol Biol* 2008;151(1):10-27.

Cuervo, AM., Wong, ES. & Martinez-Vicente, M. (2010). Protein degradation, aggregation, and misfolding, *Mov Disord* 25 Suppl 1:S49-S54.

D'Archivio, M., Filesi, C., Di Benedetto, R., Gargiulo, R., Giovannini, C. & Masella, R. (2007). Polyphenols, dietary sources and bioavailability, *Ann Ist Super Sanita* 43(4):348-361.

D'Archivio, M., Filesi, C., Varì, R., Scazzocchio, B. & Masella R. (2010). Bioavailability of the polyphenols: status and controversies, *Int J Mol Sci* 11(4):1321-1342.

Demuth, DG. & Molleman, A. (2006). Cannabinoid signalling, *Life Sci* 78: 549-563.

Dexter, DT., Wells, FR., Lees, AJ., Agid, F., Agid, Y., Jenner, P. & Marsden, CD. (1989). Increased nigral iron content and alterations in other metal ions occurring in brain in Parkinson's disease, *J Neurochem* 52:1830-1836.

Dick, FD., De Palma, G., Ahmadi, A., Scott, NW., Prescott, GJ., Bennett, J., Semple, S., Dick, S., Counsell, C., Mozzoni, P., Haites, N., Wettinger, SB., Mutti, A., Otelea, M., Seaton, A., Soderkvist, P., Felice A, & Geoparkinson study group. (2007). Environmental risk factors for Parkinson's disease and parkinsonism: the Geoparkinson study, *Occup Environ Med* 64:666–672.

Dorsey, ER., Constantinescu, R., Thompson, JP., Biglan, KM., Holloway, RG., Kieburtz, K., Marshall, FJ., Ravina, BM., Schifitto, G., Siderowf, A. & Tanner CM. (2007). Projected number of people with Parkinson disease in the most populous nations, 2005 through 2030, *Neurology* 68(5):384-386.

Elsohly, MA. & Slade, D. (2005). Chemical constituents of marijuana: the complex mixture of natural cannabinoids, *Life Sci* 78: 539-548.

Enari, M., Sakahira, H., Yokoyama, H., Okawa, K., Iwamatsu, A. & Nagata, S. (1998). A caspase-activated DNase that degrades DNA during apoptosis, and its inhibitor ICAD. *Nature* 391: 43-50. Erratum in: *Nature* 1998; 393:396.

Evans, JR. & Barker, RA. (2008). Neurotrophic factors as a therapeutic target for Parkinson's disease, *Expert Opin Ther Targets* 12(4):437-447.

Fahn, S. & Cohen, G. (1992). The oxidant stress hypothesis in Parkinson's disease: evidence supporting it, *Ann Neurol* 32: 804-812.

Faraj, BA., Olkowski, ZL. & Jackson, RT. (1991). Binding of [3H]-dopamine to human lymphocytes: possible relationship to neurotransmitter uptake sites, *Pharmacology* 42:135-141.

Faust, K., Gehrke, S., Yang, Y., Yang, L., Beal, MF. & Lu, B. (2009). Neuroprotective effects of compounds with antioxidant and anti-inflammatory properties in a Drosophila model of Parkinson's disease, *BMC Neurosci* 10:109.

Feany, MB. & Bender, WW. (2000). A Drosophila model of Parkinson's disease, *Nature* 404:394–398.

Feng, J., Tamaskovic, R., Yang, Z., Brazil, DP., Merlo, A., Hes, D. & Hemmings, BA. (2004). Stabilization of Mdm2 via decreased ubiquitination is mediated by protein Kinase/Akt-dependent phosphorylation. *J Biol Chem* 279: 35510-35517.

Forno, LS. (1996). Neuropathology of Parkinson's disease, *J Neuropathol Exp Neurol* 55:259-272.

García-Arencibia, M., García, C. & Fernández-Ruiz, J. (2009). Cannabinoids and Parkinson's disease, *CNS Neurol Disord Drug Targets* 8(6):432-439.

Gomez Del Pulgar, T., Velasco, G. & Guzman, M. (2000). The CB 1 cannabinoid receptor is coupled to the activation of protein kinase B/Akt, *Biochem J* 347: 369-373.

Gomez Del Pulgar, T., de Ceballos, ML., Guzman, M. & Velasco, G. (2002). Cannabinoids protect astrocytes from ceramide-induced apoptosis through the phosphatidylinositol 3-kinase/protein kinase B pathway, *J Biol Chem* 277: 36527-36533.

Guo, M. (2010). What have we learned from Drosophila models of Parkinson's disease? *Prog Brain Res* 184:3-16.

Griffiths, PD., Dobson, BR., Jones, GR. & Clarke, DT. (1999). Iron in the basal ganglia in Parkinson's disease. An in vitro study using extended X-ray absorption fine structure and cryo-electron microscopy, *Brain* 122 (Pt 4):667-673.

Halenbeck, R., MacDonald, H., Roulston, A., Chen, TT., Conroy, L. & Williams, LT. (1998). CPAN, a human nuclease regulated by the caspase-sensitive inhibitor DFF45, *Curr Biol* 8: 537-540.

Hampson, AJ., Grimaldi, M., Axelrod, J. & Wink, D. (1998). Cannabidiol and (-) Delta9-tetrahydrocannabinol are neuroprotective antioxidants, *Proc Natl Acad Sci USA* 95: 8268-8273.

Hardy, J. (2010). Genetic analysis of pathways to Parkinson disease, *Neuron* 68(2):201-206.

Haywood, A.F.M., Saunders, LD. & Staveley, BE. (2002). Dopa decarboxylase (Ddc)-GAL4 dramatically reduces life span, *Dros Inf Serv* 85: 42-45.

Heck, S., Lezoualc'h, F., Engert, S. & Behl, C. (1999). Insulin-like growth factor-1-mediated neuroprotection against oxidative stress is associated with activation of nuclear factor κB, *J Biol Chem* 274:9828–9835.

Herrup, K., Neve, R., Ackerman, SL & Copani, A. (2004). Divide and die: cell cycle events as triggers of nerve cell death, *J Neurosci* 24:9232-9239.

Hirth, F. (2010). Drosophila melanogaster in the study of human neurodegeneration, *CNS Neurol Disord Drug Targets* 9(4):504-523.

Imai, Y., Soda, M. & Takahashi, R. (2000). Parkin suppresses unfolded protein stress-induced cell death through its E3 ubiquitin-protein ligase activity, *J Biol Chem* 275: 35661-35664.

Jankovic, J. (2008). Parkinson's disease: clinical features and diagnosis, *J Neurol Neurosurg Psychiatry* 79(4):368-376.

Jenner, P. & Olanow, W. (1996). Oxidative stress and the pathogenesis of Parkinson´s disease. *Neurology* 47 (Suppl. 3):S161-S170.

Jenner, P. & Olanow, CW. (1998). Understanding cell death in Parkinson's disease. *Ann Neurol.* 44 (3 Suppl 1):S72-S84.

Jiang, H., Ren, Y., Zhao, J. & Feng, J. (2004). Parkin protects human dopaminergic neuroblastoma cells against dopamine-induced apoptosis, *Human Mol Genet* 13:1745–1754.

Jimenez-Del-Rio, M. & Velez-Pardo, C. (2000). Molecular mechanism of monoamine toxicity in Parkinson's disease: A hypothetical cell death model, *Medic Hypotheses* 54: 269-274.

Jimenez-Del-Rio, M & Velez-Pardo, C. (2001). 17β-Estradiol protects lymphocytes against dopamine and iron-induced apoptosis by a genomic-independent mechanism Implication in Parkinson's disease, *Gen Pharmacol* 35: 1– 9.

Jimenez-Del-Rio, M. & Velez-Pardo, C. (2002). Monoamine neurotoxin-induced apoptosis in lymphocytes by a common mechanism: involvement of hydrogen peroxide (H_2O_2), caspase-3, and nuclear factor kappa-B (NF-κB), p53, c-Jun transcription factor, *Biochem Pharmacol* 63: 677-688.

Jimenez-Del-Rio, M., Moreno, S., Garcia-Ospina, G., Buritica, O., Uribe, CS., Lopera, F. & Velez-Pardo, C. (2004). Autosomal recessive juvenile parkinsonism Cys212Tyr mutation in parkin renders lymphocytes susceptible to dopamine and iron-mediated apoptosis, *Mov Disord* 19: 324-330.

Jimenez-Del-Rio, M. & Velez-Pardo, C. (2004a). The hydrogen peroxide and its importance in the Alzheimer's and Parkinson's disease, Current Medical Chemistry- Central Nervous System Agents 4: 279-285.

Jimenez-Del-Rio, M. & Velez-Pardo, C. (2004b). Transition metals-induced apoptosis in lymphocytes via hydroxyl radical generation, mitochondria dysfunction and caspase-3 activation: an *in vitro* model for neurodegeneration, *Arch Medic Res* 35:185-193.

Jimenez-Del-Rio, M. & Velez-Pardo, C. (2006). Insulin-like growth factor-1 prevents $A\beta_{[25-35]}$ /(H_2O_2)-induced apoptosis in lymphocytes by reciprocal NF-κB activation and p53 inhibition via PI3K-dependent pathway. *Growth Factors* 24: 67-78.

Jimenez-Del-Rio, M. & Velez-Pardo, C. (2008). Paraquat induces apoptosis in human lymphocytes: Protective and rescue effects of glucose, cannabinoids and Insulin-like growth factor-1, *Growth Factors* 26(1): 49-60.

Jimenez-Del-Rio, M., Daza-Restrepo, A. & Velez-Pardo, C. (2008). The cannabinoid CP55, 940 prolongs survival and improves locomotor activity in Drosophila melanogaster against paraquat: implications in Parkinson's disease, *Neurosci Res* 61:404–411.

Jimenez-Del-Rio, M., Guzman-Martinez, C. & Velez-Pardo, C. (2010). The effects of polyphenols on survival and locomotor activity in Drosophila melanogaster exposed to iron and paraquat, *Neurochem Res* 35(2):227-238.

Jones, DC. & Miller, GW. (2008). The effects of environmental neurotoxicants on the dopaminergic system: a possible role in drug addiction, *Biochem Pharmacol* 76:569–581.

Kairisalo, M., Korhonen, L., Blomgren, K. & Lindholm, D. (2007). X-linked inhibitor of apoptosis protein increases mitochondrial antioxidants through NF-kappaB activation, *Biochem Biophys Res Commun* 364(1):138-144.

Kane, LP., Shapiro, VS., Stokoe, D. & Weiss, A. (1999). Induction of NF-kappaB by the Akt/PKB kinase. *Curr Biol.* 9: 601-604.

Kawashima, K. & Fujii, T. (2004). Expression of non-neuronal acetylcholine in lymphocytes and its contribution to the regulation to the regulation of immune function, *Frontiers Biosci* 9:2063-2085.

Kerr, JFR., Wyllie, AH. & Currie, AR. (1972). Apoptosis: a basic biological phenomenon with wide ranging implications in tissue kinetics, *Br J Cancer* 26: 239-257.

Kerr, JFR., Gobe, GC., Winterford, CM. & Harmon, BV. Anatomical methods in cell death. In: Schwartz, LM. & Osborne, BA; editors. *Methods in cell biology: cell death.* New York: Academic Press; 1995; pp. 1–27.

Kim, SH., Won, SJ., Mao, XO., Jin, K. & Greenberg, DA. (2005). Involvement of protein kinase A in cannabinoid receptor-mediated protection from oxidative neuronal injury, *J Pharmacol Exp Ther* 313: 88-94.

Kitada, T., Asakawa, S., Hattori, N., Matsumine, H., Yamamura, Y., Minoshima, S., Yokochi, M., Mizuno, Y. & Shimizu, N. (1998). Mutations in the parkin gene cause autosomal recessive juvenile parkinsonism, *Nature* 392:605-608.

Kooijman, R., Willems, M., DeCarla, HJC., Rijkers, GT., Schuurmans, ALG., Van Buul-Offers, SC., Heijnen, CJ. & Zegers, BJM. (1992). Expression of type I insulin-like growth factor receptors on human peripheral blood mononuclear cells, *Endocrinol* 131: 2244-2250.

Kutuk, O. & Basaga, H. (2003). Aspirin prevents apoptosis and NFkappaB activation induced by H_2O_2 in HeLa cells, *Free Radic Res* 37:1267–1276.

Kaplan, BL., Rockwell, CE. & Kaminski, NE. (2003). Evidence for cannabinoid receptor-dependent and -independent mechanisms of action in leukocytes, *J Pharmacol Exp Ther* 306(3):1077-1085.

Kieburtz, K. & Ravina, B. (2007). Why hasn't neuroprotection worked in Parkinson's disease? Nat Clin Pract Neurol 3(5):240-241.

Kriesberg, N. (2011). Animals as models. (http://ori.dhhs.gov/education/products/ncstate/models.htm, available in April, 2011).

Klegeris, A., Bissonnette, CJ. & McGeer, PL. (2003). Reduction of human monocytic cell neurotoxicity and cytokine secretion by ligands of the cannabinoid-type CB2 receptor. *Br J Pharmacol*. 139: 775-786.

Kroemer, G., Galluzzi, L., Vandenabeele, P., Abrams, J., Alnemri, ES., Baehrecke, EH., Blagosklonny, MV., El-Deiry, WS., Golstein, P., Green, DR., Hengartner, M., Knight, RA., Kumar, S., Lipton, SA., Malorni, W., Nuñez, G., Peter, ME., Tschopp, J., Yuan, J., Piacentini, M., Zhivotovsky, B., Melino, G. & Nomenclature Committee on Cell Death 2009. (2009. Classification of cell death: recommendations of the Nomenclature Committee on Cell Death 2009, *Cell Death Differ* 16(1):3-11.

Levy, OA., Malagelada, C. & Greene, LA. (2009). Cell death pathways in Parkinson's disease: proximal triggers, distal effectors, and final steps, *Apoptosis* 14(4):478-500.

Liang, ZQ., Li, YL., Zhao, XL., Han, R., Wang, XX., Wang, Y., Chase, TN., Bennett, MC. & Qin, ZH. (2007). NF-κB contributes to 6-hydroxydopamine-induced apoptosis of nigral dopaminergic neurons through p53. *Brain Res* 1145:190-203.

Li, LY., Zhao, XL., Fei, XF., Gu, ZL., Qin, ZH. & Liang, ZQ. (2008). Bilobalide inhibits 6-OHDA-induced activation of NF-kappaB and loss of dopaminergic neurons in rat substantia nigra, *Acta Pharmacol Sin* 29(5):539-547.

Lin, TK., Liou, CW., Chen, SD., Chuang, YC., Tiao, MM., Wang, PW., Chen, JB. & Chuang, JH. (2009). Mitochondrial dysfunction and biogenesis in the pathogenesis of Parkinson's disease, *Chang Gung Med J* 32(6):589-599.

Liu, X., Zou, H., Slaughter, C. & Wang, X. (1997). DFF, a heterodimeric protein that functions downstream of caspase-3 to trigger DNA fragmentation during apoptosis, *Cell*. 89:175-184.

Logroscino, G., Gao, X., Chen, H., Wing A. & Ascherio, A. (2008). Dietary iron intake and risk of Parkinson's disease, *Am J Epidemiol* 168(12):1381-1388.

Lombardi, G., Dianzani, C., Miglio, G., Canonico, PL. & Fantozzi, R. (2001). Characterization of ionotropic glutamate receptors in human lymphocytes, *Br J Pharmacol* 133: 936-944.

Lombardi, G., Miglio, G., Dianzani, C., Mesturini, R., Varsaldi, F., Chiocchetti, A., Dianzani, U., Fantozzi, R. (2004). Glutamate modulation of human lymphocyte growth: in vitro studies, *Biochem Biophys Res Commun*. 28; 318: 496-502.

Lu, Y. (2005). p53: a heavily dictated dictator of life and death, *Curr Opin Genet Dev* 15: 27-33.

Lu, B. (2009). Recent advances in using Drosophila to model neurodegenerative diseases, *Apoptosis* 14(8):1008-1020.

Maciver, NJ., Jacobs, SR., Wieman, HL., Wofford, JA., Coloff, JL. & Rathmell, JC. (2008). Glucose metabolism in lymphocytes is a regulated process with significant effects on immune cell function and survival, *J. Leukoc. Biol*. 84,949-957.

Manolescu, AR., Witkowska, K., Kinnaird, A., Cessford T., Cheeseman, C. (2007). Facilitated hexose transporters: new perspectives on form and function, *Physiology (Bethesda)* 22, 234-240.

Mao, Z. & Davis, RL. (2009). Eight different types of dopaminergic neurons innervate the Drosophila mushroom body neuropil: anatomical and physiological heterogeneity, *Front Neural Circuits* 3:5.

Marazziti, D., Consoli, G., Masala, I., Catena Dell'Osso, M. & Baroni, S. (2010). Latest advancements on serotonin and dopamine transporters in lymphocytes, *Mini Rev Med Chem* 10(1):32-40.

Marini, M., Frabetti, F., Canaider, S., Dini, L., Falcieri, E. & Poirier, GG. (2001). Modulation of caspase-3 activity by zinc ions and by the cell redox state, *Exp Cell Res* 266:323-332.

Marino, F., Cosentino, M., Bombelli, R., Ferrari, M., Lecchini, S. & Frigo, G. (1999). Endogenous catecholamine synthesis, metabolism, storage, and uptake in human peripheral blood mononuclear cells, *Exp Hematol* 27:489-495.

Marsicano, G., Moosmann, B., Hermann, H., Lutz, B. & Behl, C. (2002). Neuroprotective properties of cannabinoids against oxidative stress: role of the cannabinoid receptor CB1, *J Neurochem* 80: 448-456.

Massoud, TF., Hademenos, GJ., Young, WL., Gao, E., Pile-Spellman, J., Viñuela, F. (1998). Principles and philosophy of modeling in biomedical research,*FASEB J* 12(3):275-285.

Matsuda, LA., Lolait, SJ., Brownstein, M., Young, A. & Bonner, TI. (1990). Structure of a cannabinoid receptor and functional expression of the cloned cDNA, *Nature* 346: 561-564.

Melidou, M., Riganakos, K. & Galaris, D. (2005). Protection against nuclear DNA damage offered by flavonoids in cells exposed to hydrogen peroxide: the role of iron chelation, *Free Radic Biol Med* 39:1591–1600.

Miglio, G., Varsaldi, F., Dianzani, C., Fantozzi, R. & Lombardi, G. (2005). Stimulation of group I metabotropic glutamate receptors evokes calcium signals and c-jun and c-fos gene expression in human T cells, *Biochem Pharmacol* 70:189-199.

Migliore, L., Petrozzi, L., Lucetti, C., Gambaccini, G., Bernardini, S., Scarpato, R., Trippi, F., Barale, R., Frenzilli, G., Rodilla, V. & Bonuccelli, U. (2002). Oxidative damage and cytogenetic analysis in leukocytes of Parkinson's disease patients, *Neurology* 58: 1809-1815.

Miyashita, T. & Reed, JC. (1995). Tumor suppressor p53 is a direct transcriptional activator of the human bax gene, *Cell* 80: 293–299.

Molina-Holgado, E., Vela, J.M., Arevalo-Martin, A., Almazan, G., Molina-Holgado, F., Borrell, J. & Guaza, C. (2002). Cannabionoids promote oligodendrocyte progenitor survival: involvement of cannabinoid receptors and phospahatidylinositol-3 kinase/Akt signaling, *J Neurosc* 22: 9742-9753.

Munro, S., Thomas, KL. & Abu-Shaar, M. (1993). Molecular characterization of a peripheral receptor for cannabinoids, *Nature* 365: 61-65.

McKenna, F., McLaughlin, PJ., Lewis, BJ., Sibbring, GC., Cummerson, JA., Bowen-Jones, D. & Moots, RJ. (2002). Dopamine receptor expression on human T- and B-lymphocytes, monocytes, neutrophils, eosinophils and NK cells: a flow cytometric study, *J Neuroimmunol.* 132 (1-2):34-40.

Nagayama, T., Sinor, AD., Simon, RP., Chen, J., Graham, SH., Jin, K. & Greenberg, DA. (1999). Cannabinoids and neuroprotection in global and focal cerebral ischemia and in neuronal cultures, *J Neurosci* 19: 2987-2995.

Ogawara, Y., Kishishita, S., Obata, T., Isazawa, Y., Suzuki, T., Tanaka, K., Masuyama, N. & Gotoh, Y. (2002). Akt enhances Mdm2-mediated Ubiquitination and degradation of p53, *J Biol Chem* 277: 21843-21850.

Ortega-Arellano, HF., Jimenez-Del-Rio, M. & Velez-Pardo, C. (2011). Life span and locomotor activity modification by glucose and polyphenols in *Drosophila melanogaster* chronically exposed to oxidative stress-stimuli: Implications in Parkinson's disease, *Neurochem Res* 36: 1073-1086.

Padgett, LW. (2005). Recent developments cannabinoid ligands, *Life Sci* 77: 1767-1798.

Pendleton, RG., Parvez, F., Sayed, M., Hillman, R. (2002a). Effects of pharmacological agents upon a transgenic model of Parkinson's disease in Drosophila melanogaster, *J Pharmacol Exp Ther* 300:91–96.

Pendleton, RG., Rasheed, A., Sardina, T., Tully, T. & Hillman, R. (2002b). Effects of tyrosine hydroxylase mutants on locomotor activity in Drosophila: a study in functional genomics, *Behav Genet* 32: 89–94.

Park, J., Kim, Y., Chung, J. (2009). Mitochondrial dysfunction and Parkinson's disease genes: insights from Drosophila, *Dis Model Mech* 2(7-8):336-340.

Pazos, MR., Nunez, E., Benito, C., Tolon, RM. & Romero, J. (2005). Functional neuroanatomy of the endocannabinoid system, *Pharmacol Biochem Behav* 81:239-247.

Perron, NR. & Brumaghim, JL. (2009). A review of the antioxidant mechanisms of polyphenol compounds related to iron binding, *Cell Biochem Biophys* 53:75–100.

Phelps, CB. & Brand, AH. (1998). Ectopic gene expression in Drosophila using GAL4 system, *Methods* 14(4):367-379.

Piatkiewicz, P., Czech, A. & Tatoń, J. (2007). Glucose transport in human peripheral blood lymphocytes influenced by type 2 diabetes mellitus, *Arch. Immunol. Ther. Exp. (Warsz)* 55,119-126.

Pineda-Trujillo, N., Carvajal-Carmona, LG., Buritica, O., Moreno, S., Uribe, C., Pineda, D., Toro, M., Garcia, F., Arias, W., Bedoya, G., Lopera, F. & Ruiz-Linares, A. (2001). A novel Cys212Tyr founder mutation in parkin and allelic heterogeneity of juvenile Parkinsonism in a population from North West Colombia, *Neurosci Lett* 298: 87-90.

Pineda-Trujillo, N., Apergi, M., Moreno, S., Arias, W., Lesage, S., Franco, A., Sepulveda-Falla, D., Cano, D., Buritica, O., Pineda, D., Uribe, CS., de Yebenes, JG., Lees, AJ., Brice, A., Bedoya, G., Lopera, F. & Ruiz-Linares, A. (2006). A genetic cluster of early onset Parkinson's disease in a Colombian population, *Am J Med Genet B Neuropsychiatr Genet* 141B(8):885-888.

Pineda-Trujillo, N., Dulcey-Cepeda, A., Arias-Pérez, W., Moreno-Masmela, S., Saldarriaga-Henao, A., Sepúlveda-Falla, D., Bedoya-Berrío, G., Lopera-Restrepo F. & Ruiz-Linares, A. (2009). Una mutación en el gen *PARK2* causa enfermedad de Parkinson juvenil en una extensa familia colombiana, *IATREIA* 22(2): 122-131.

Polymeropoulos, MH., Lavedan, C., Leroy, E., Ide, SE., Dehejia, A., Dutra, A., Pike, B., Root, H., Rubenstein, J., Boyer, R., Stenroos, ES., Chandrasekharappa, S., Athanassiadou, A., Papapetropoulos, T., Johnson, WG., Lazzarini, AM., Duvoisin, RC., Di Iorio G., Golbe LI. & Nussbaum, RL. (1997). Mutation in the alpha-synuclein gene identified in families with Parkinson's disease, *Science* 27; 276:2045-2047.

Prabhakaran, K., Ghosh, D., Chapman, GD. & Gunasekar, PG. (2008). Molecular mechanism of manganese exposure-induced dopaminergic toxicity, *Brain Res Bull* 76(4):361-367.

Pradilla, AG., Vesga, ABE., León-Sarmiento, FE; GENECO. (2003). [National neuroepidemiological study in Colombia (EPINEURO)], *Rev Panam Salud Publica* 14(2):104-11.

Prasad, S., Ravindran, J. & Aggarwal, BB. (2010). NF-kappaB and cancer: how intimate is this relationship, *Mol Cell Biochem* 336(1-2):25-37.

Przedborski, S. (2005). Pathogenesis of nigral cell death in Parkinson's disease, *Parkinsonism Relat Disord* 11 Suppl 1:S3-S7.

Prigione, A., Isaias, IU., Galbussera, A., Brighina, L., Begni, B., Andreoni, S., Pezzoli, G., Antonini, A., Ferrarese, C. (2009). Increased oxidative stress in lymphocytes from untreated Parkinson's disease patients, *Parkinsonism Relat Disord* 15(4):327-328.

Qin, ZH., Tao, LY. & Chen, X. (2007). Dual roles of NF-kappaB in cell survival and implications of NF-kappaB inhibitors in neuroprotective therapy, *Acta Pharmacol Sin* 28(12):1859-72.

Quesada, A., Lee, BY. & Micevych, PE. (2008). PI3 kinase/Akt activation mediates estrogen and IGF-1 nigral DA neuronal neuroprotection against a unilateral rat model of Parkinson's disease, *Dev Neurobiol* 68(5):632-644.

Ramassamy, C. (2006). Emerging role of polyphenolic compounds in the treatment of neurodegenerative diseases: a review of their intracellular targets, *Eur J Pharmacol* 545:51–64.

Ricci, A. & Amenta, F. (1994). Dopamine D5 receptors in human peripheral blood lymphocytes: a radioligand binding study, *J Neuroimmunol* 53: 1-7.

Ricci, A., Veglio, F. & Amenta, F. (1995). Radioligand binding characterization of putative dopamine D3 receptor in human peripheral blood lymphocytes with {3H} 7OH-DPAT, *J Neuroimmunol* 58: 139-144.

Ricci, A., Bronzetti, E., Felici, L., Tayebati, SK. & Amenta, F. (1997). Dopamine D4 receptor in human peripheral blood lymphocytes: a radioligand binding assay study, *Neurosci Lett* 229: 130-134.

Riederer, P., Dirr, A., Goetz, M., Sofic, E., Jellinger, K. & Youdim, MB. (1992). Distribution of iron in different brain regions and subcellular compartments in Parkinson's disease, *Ann Neurol* 32 Suppl: S101-S104.

Riemensperger, T., Isabel, G., Coulom, H., Neuser, K., Seugnet, L., Kume, K., Iché-Torres, M., Cassar, M., Strauss, R., Preat, T., Hirsh, J. & Birman, S. (2011). Behavioral consequences of dopamine deficiency in the Drosophila central nervous system, *Proc Natl Acad Sci U S A* 108(2):834-839.

Sanchez, MG., Ruiz-Llorente, L., Sanchez, AM. & Diaz-Leviada, I. (2003). Activation of phosphoinositide 3-kinase/PKB pathway by CB(1) and CB(2) cannabinoid receptors expressed in prostate PC-3 cells. Involvement in Raf-1 stimulation and NGF induction, *Cell Signal* 15: 851-859.

Sanchez, JL., Buritica-Henao, O., Pineda Salazar, DA., Ribe, CS. & Palacio-Baena, LG. (2004). Prevalence of Parkinson´s disease and Parkinsonism in a Colombian population using the capture recapture methods. *Int J Neurosci* 113:175-182.

Sanders, VM. (1998). The role of norepinephrine and beta-2 adrenergic receptor stimulation in the modulation of Th1, Th2, and B lymphocyte function, *Adv Exp Med Biol* 437:269-278.

Sang, TK., Chang, HY., Lawless, GM., Ratnaparkhi, A., Mee, L., Ackerson, LC., Maidment, NT., Krantz, DE. & Jackson, GR. (2007). A Drosophila model of mutant human parkin-induced toxicity demonstrates selective loss of dopaminergic neurons and dependence on cellular dopamine, *J Neurosci* 27:981–992.

Sakahira, H., Enari, M. & Nagata, S. (1998). Cleavage of CAD inhibitor in CAD activation and DNA degradation during apoptosis, *Nature* 391: 96-99.

Sakahira, H., Enari, M., Ohsawa, Y., Uchiyama, Y. & Nagata, S. (1999). Apoptotic nuclear morphological change without DNA fragmentation, *Curr Biol* 9: 543-546.

Savica, R., Rocca, WA. & Ahlskog, JE. (2010). When does Parkinson disease start? *Arch Neurol* 67(7):798-801.

Sestili, P., Diamantini, G., Bedini, A., Cerioni, L., Tommasini, I., Tarzia, G. & Cantoni, O. (2002). Plant-derived phenolic compounds prevent the DNA single-strand breakage and cytotoxicity induced by tertbutylhydroperoxide via an iron-chelating mechanism, *Biochem J* 364(Pt 1):121–128.

Sian-Hülsmann, J., Mandel, S., Youdim, HMB. & Riederer, P. (2010). The Relevance of iron in the pathogenesis of Parkinson's Disease, *J Neurochem* doi: 10.1111/j.1471-4159.2010.07132.x.

Sofic, E., Paulus, W., Jellinger, K., Riederer, P. & Youdim, MB. (1991). Selective increase of iron in substantia nigra zona compacta of parkinsonian brains, *J Neurochem*. 56: 978-982.

Shishodia, S. & Aggarwal, BB. (2004). Nuclear factor kB: a friend or a foe in cancer? *Biochem Pharmacol* 68: 1071-1080.

Shimura, H., Hattori, N., Kubo, S., Mizuno, Y., Asakawa, S., Minoshima, S., Shimizu, N., Iwai, K., Chiba, T., Tanaka, K. & Suzuki, T. (2000). Familial Parkinson disease gene product, parkin is an ubiquitin-protein ligase, *Nat Genet* 25:302-305.

Skaper, SD., Buriani, A., Dal Toso, R., Petrelli, L., Romanello, S., Facci, L. & Leon, A. (1996). The Aliamide palmitoylethanolamine and cannabinoids, but not anandamide, are protective in a delayed postglutamate paradigm of exocitotoxic death in cerebellar granule neurons, *Proc Natl Acad Sci USA* 93: 3984-3989.

Stefulj, J., Jernej, B., Cicin-Sain, L., Rinner, I. & Schauenstein K. (2000). mRNA expression of serotonin receptors in cells of the immune tissues of the rat, *Brain Behav Immun* 14(3):219-224.

Tan, JM., Wong, ES. & Lim, KL. (2009). Protein misfolding and aggregation in Parkinson's disease, *Antioxid Redox Signal* 11(9):2119-2134.

Takada, Y., Mukhopadhyay, A., Kundu, GC., Mahabeleshwar, GH., Singh, S. & Aggarwal, BB. (2003). Hydrogen peroxide activates NF-kappa B through tyrosine hosphorylation of I kappa B alpha and serine phosphorylation of p65: evidence for the involvement of I kappa B alpha kinase and Syk protein-tyrosine kinase, *J Biol Chem* 278: 24233-24241.

Takanashi, M., Mochizuchi, H., Yokomizo, K., Hattori, N., Mori, H., Yamamura, Y. & Mizuno, Y. (2001). Iron accumulation in the substantia nigra of autosomal recessive juvenile parkinsonism (ARJP), *Parkinsonism Relat Disord* 7: 311–314.

Tanaka, K., Suzuki, T., Chiba, T., Shimura, H., Hattori, N. & Mizuno, Y. (2001). Parkin is linked to the ubiquitin pathway, *J Mol Med* 79: 482-494.

Tapson, VF., Schenetzler, B., Pilch, PF., Center, DM. & Berman, JS. (1988). Structural and functional characterization of the human T lymphocyte receptor for insulin-like growth factor I in vitro, *J Clin Invest* 82: 950-957.

Tillakaratne, NJ., Medina-Kauwe, L. & Gibson, KM. (1995). Gamma Aminobutyric acid (GABA) metabolism in mammalian neural and non-neural tissues, *Comp Biochem Physiol A Physiol* 112(2):247-263.

Thakur, GA., Duclos, RI Jr. & Makriyannis, A. (2005). Natural cannabinoids: Templates for drug discovery, *Life Sci* 78: 454-466.

Tsang, AH. & Chung, KK. (2009). Oxidative and nitrosative stress in Parkinson's disease, *Biochim Biophys Acta* 1792(7):643-650.

Turu, G. & Hunyady, L. (2010). Signal transduction of the CB1 cannabinoid receptor, *J Mol Endocrinol* 44(2):75-85.

Van der Stelt, M. & Di Marzo, V. (2005). Cannabinoid receptors and their role in neuroprotection, *Neuromolecular Med.* 7(1-2):37-50.

Van Sickle, MD., Duncan, M., Kingsley, PJ., Mouihate, A., Urbani, P., Mackie, K., Stella, N., Makriyannis, A., Piomelli, D., Davison, JS., Marnett, LJ., Di Marzo, V., Pittman, QJ., Patel, KD. & Sharkey, KA. (2005). Identification and functional characterization of brainstem cannabinoid CB2 receptors, *Science* 310:329-332.

Velez-Pardo, C. & Jimenez-Del-Rio, M. (2006). Avoidance of Aβ[25-35] /(H_2O_2)-induced apoptosis in lymphocytes by the cannabinoid agonists CP55,940 and JWH-015 via receptor-independent and PI3K-dependent mechanisms: Role of NF-κB and p53, *Medicinal Chemistry* 2: 471-479.

Velez-Pardo, C., Jimenez-Del-Rio, M., Lores-Arnaiz, S. & Bustamante, J. (2010). Protective effects of the synthetic cannabinoids CP55,940 and JWH-015 on rat brain mitochondria upon paraquat exposure, *Neurochemical Research* 35:1323–1332.

Wang, C., Lu, R., Ouyang, X., Ho, M.W., Chia, W., Yu, F., & Lim, K.L. (2007). Drosophila overexpressing parkin R275W mutant exhibits dopaminergic neuron degeneration and mitochondrial abnormalities, *J Neurosci* 27:8563–8570.

White, KE., Humphrey, DM., Hirth, F. (2010). The dopaminergic system in the aging brain of Drosophila, *Front Neurosci* 4:205.

Wu, H; Lozano, G. (1994). NF-κB activation of p53, *J Biol Chem* 269: 20067–20074.

Wyllie, AH. (1980). Glucocorticoid-induced thymocytes apoptosis associated with endogenous endonuclease activation, *Nature* 284: 555-556.

Wang, C., Lu, R., Ouyang, X., Ho, M.W., Chia, W., Yu, F., & Lim, K.L. (2007). Drosophila overexpressing parkin R275W mutant exhibits dopaminergic neuron degeneration and mitochondrial abnormalities, *J Neurosci* 27:8563–8570.

Wang, X. & Michaelis, EK. (2010) Selective neuronal vulnerability to oxidative stress in the brain, *Front Aging Neurosci* 2:12.

Whitworth, AJ., Wes, PD. & Pallanck, LJ. (2006). Drosophila models pioneer a new approach to drug discovery for Parkinson's disease, *Drug Discov Today* 11(3-4):119-126.

Whitworth, AJ. (2011). Drosophila models of Parkinson's disease, *Adv Genet* 73:1-50.

Xiang, H., Kinoshita, Y., Knudson, CM., Korsmeyer, SJ., Schwartzkroin, PA. & Morrison, RS. (1998). Bax involvement in p53-mediated neuronal cell death, *J Neurosci* 18(4):1363-1373.

Xiromerisiou, G., Dardiotis, E., Tsimourtou, V., Kountra, PM., Paterakis, KN., Kapsalaki, EZ., Fountas, KN. & Hadjigeorgiou, GM. (2010). Genetic basis of Parkinson disease, *Neurosurg Focus* 28(1):E7.

Xu, G. & Shi, Y. (2007). Apoptosis signaling pathways and lymphocyte homeostasis, *Cell Res* 17(9):759-771.

Zaveri, NT. (2006). Green tea and its polyphenolic catechins: medicinal uses in cancer and noncancer applications, *Life Sci* 78:2073–2080.

Zhang, Y., Dawson, VL. & Dawson, TM. (2001). Parkin: clinical aspects and neurobiology, *Clin Neurosci Res* 1: 467– 482.

Zhou, C., Huang, Y., Przedborski, S. (2008). Oxidative stress in Parkinson's disease: a mechanism of pathogenic and therapeutic significance, *Ann N Y Acad Sci* 1147:93–104.

22

Inflammation in Parkinson's Disease: Causes and Consequences

Louise M. Collins, André Toulouse and Yvonne M. Nolan
Department of Anatomy and Neuroscience, University College Cork
Ireland

1. Introduction

Parkinson's disease (PD) is the second most common progressive neurodegenerative disorder after Alzheimer's disease (AD) with a prevalence of 0.5-1% among persons older than 65 years of age (Toulouse & Sullivan, 2008). The incidence increases to 2.6% in persons aged 85 and older, and has a mean age of onset of 55 years. Statistics released in 1990 from a unique global study carried out by the World Health Organisation, suggest that there are approximately 4 million PD patients worldwide. However, despite intensive research, the aetiology of this neurodegenerative disease still remains unclear and despite substantial efforts, a cure remains elusive. This, coupled with the increasing aging demographics, makes the importance of research into PD imperative, and the development of novel drug treatments a primary aim, both for economic and humanitarian purposes. The disease is a chronic, progressive neurodegenerative motor disorder, resulting in the selective loss of dopaminergic (DA) neurons within the substantia nigra (SN) pars compacta (pc) of the midbrain. As the disease progresses there is gradual circuitry degeneration within the nigrostriatal pathway, producing motor, cognitive and psychiatric symptoms (Braak et al., 2003). Lewy bodies are classified as the focal pathological hallmark of PD and their presence is necessary for the *post-mortem* diagnosis of the disease. They are not unique to PD however and are also found in other diseases such as dementia with Lewy Bodies and diffuse Lewy Body disease (Braak et al., 2003). PD can be further characterised by the presence of an accumulation of activated microglia within the SNpc (McGeer et al., 1988).

PD exists in many forms and can be classified into both familial and idiopathic (also referred to as sporadic) forms, with epidemiological studies indicating approximately 5-10% of cases as being familial, and 90-95% as idiopathic (Tomiyama et al., 2008). Familial PD can be transmitted in an autosomal dominant (AD-PD) or recessive fashion (AR-PD). The study of genetic forms of PD has led to a better understanding of the underlying molecular mechanisms occurring during the disease progression. To date, six genes (SNCA, LRRK2, PRKN, DJ-1, PINK1 and ATP13A2) have been implicated in familial forms of PD (Bekris et al., 2010). In contrast to idiopathic PD, the genetic forms of this disease display a significantly younger age of onset and a shorter disease duration (Pankratz & Foroud, 2007). Despite this, patients with the autosomal dominant form of the disease have similar clinical and pathological features to those with idiopathic PD. In idiopathic PD, environmental factors such as toxins, free radicals and inflammation have been considered the most likely candidates as causative agents. For example, pesticides can induce oxidative stress (an increased production of activated oxygen species such as superoxide anions and hydroxyl radicals) which leads to lipid peroxidation, DNA damage and mitochondrial dysfunction (Dick, 2006; Jenner, 2003). Moreover, there is evidence to suggest that the oxidative stress that occurs at a basal level in the SNpc is increased during PD (Jenner, 2003). The involvement of inflammation in the progression of PD has been well documented and is generally typified by an accumulation of activated microglia in damaged regions of the brain (Gao & Hong, 2008; Long-Smith et al., 2009). Initial evidence stems from a *post-mortem* study over twenty years ago, which demonstrated the presence of activated microglia and T-lymphocytes in the SNpc of a PD patient (McGeer et al., 1988). Since then, an abundance of studies have supported a role for neuroinflammation and activated microglia in the pathology of PD (Banati et al., 1998; Hirsch & Hunot, 2009; Imamura et al., 2003; McGeer & McGeer, 2004; Orr et al., 2002). Activated microglia are predominantly found in the SNpc in the vicinity of degenerating DA neurons in *post-mortem* PD brains, but have also been detected in the hippocampus, transentorhinal cortex, cingulate cortex and temporal cortex, where neuronal loss is also prevalent (Banati et al., 1998; Imamura et al., 2003; McGeer et al., 1988; Sawada et al., 2006). The presence of activated microglia in rat brains lesioned with 6-hydroxydopamine (6-OHDA), a neurotoxin used to model PD, has been reported by numerous groups (Akiyama & McGeer, 1989; Crotty et al., 2008; Depino et al., 2003; He et al., 2001). Further evidence implicating inflammation in PD comes from studies that report an increase in the expression of the pro-inflammatory cytokines, interleukin (IL)-1β, tumour necrosis factor-α (TNF-α) and IL-6 in PD patients compared with healthy subjects (Boka et al., 1994; Dobbs et al., 1999; Mogi et al., 1994a; Mogi et al., 1994b). Enzymes associated with inflammation, such as inducible nitric oxide synthase (iNOS) and cyclooxygenase-2 (COX-2), have also been identified *post-mortem* in PD brains (Hunot et al., 1996; Knott et al., 2000).

2. Neuroinflammation in Parkinson's disease

2.1 Microglia

Microglia are the resident immune-competent cells of the central nervous system (CNS). They monitor the brain for invading pathogens and immune insults and are capable of stimulating an adaptive immune response (Garden & Moller, 2006). Pio del Rio-Hortega first ignited interest in microglia in the early 20th century when he identified them as a separate glial entity (del Rio Hortega, 1932), providing a complete and comprehensive framework of their involvement in brain pathology (Raivich et al., 1999). There are currently two proposed subsets of microglia residing within the CNS. There are the "*resting*" microglia found ramified throughout the brain parenchyma and mostly a permanent population, and the perivascular microglia, which are periodically replaced by bone-marrow derived elements and are strategically located in the basal lamina of brain capillaries and the choroid plexus (Santambrogio et al., 2001). These two subsets differ in their expression of leucocyte common antigen, CD45, which is high ($CD45^{high}$) in perivascular and low ($CD45^{low}$) in parenchymal microglia (Sedgwick et al., 1991). The production of microglia is complex. There is an initial production of microglia during development, a constant turnover of microglia during adulthood and throughout senescence, and an up-regulated production of microglia in response to pathological conditions. Furthermore, each of these stages is likely to be governed by diverse mechanisms. The origin of microglia remains contentious, but the majority of the neuroscience community support the premise that they are derived from mesodermal precursor cells of hematopoietic lineage (Barron, 1995; Cuadros & Navascues, 1998) due to their expression of macrophage antigens, such as F4/80, Fc receptor (FcR) and macrophage-1 antigen (MAC-1) (Carson et al., 1998). Mesodermal precursor cells infiltrate the brain during embryonic and early postnatal phases of development and have the potential to differentiate into macrophages, dendritic cells (DCs) and granulocytes (Santambrogio et al., 2001). Factors which govern and propel this invasion are not widely understood but are believed to involve cell surface bound molecules and components of the extracellular matrix (Cuadros & Navascues, 1998). As with the origin of microglia, the mechanism of microglial renewal *in situ* remains controversial. This prolonged controversy to unequivocally differentiate activated endogenous microglia from those of infiltrating blood monocytes is due to a lack of distinguishable cell surface or enzymatic markers (Ransohoff & Cardona, 2010). In addition, the prevailing technique of lethally irradiated chimeras to examine this appears to be fraught with confounding factors. Ajami et al., (2007) utilised chimeric animals obtained through parabiosis, which does not require experimental manipulation, and found that microglial homeostasis is maintained independently of bone-marrow derived precursors. They also reported that mature resident microglia are capable of focal self-renewal and microgliosis in response to insult or injury (Ajami et al., 2007).

Within the healthy adult brain microglia reside as a ubiquitously distributed quiescent cell population, representing 10-20% of non-neuronal cells within the CNS parenchyma. They are functionally related to peripheral tissue macrophages and other cells of the monocyte lineage, but differ in their down-regulated expression of a number of cytoplasmic molecules (Perry, 1998). Historically referred to as *"resting"* microglia, which discriminates them morphologically from their active amoeboid form found during insult to the CNS, they are characterised by a small rod-shaped somata and numerous elongated, highly ramified processes. Through their protrusions, they are in direct contact with astrocytes, neuronal cell bodies and blood vessels, suggesting that they dynamically interact with a variety of neural elements (Nimmerjahn et al., 2005). As immune effector cells of the CNS, they are extremely receptive to subtle change in their microenvironment, rapidly undergoing morphological as well as functional transformations (Ladeby et al., 2005). Although research in recent years has greatly advanced our knowledge of activated microglia, little has been established concerning the function of the microglia residing in the unperturbed CNS. This is due in part to the exceedingly complex predicament many have faced while trying to culture *"resting"* microglia *in vitro*. The removal and dissociation of cells from CNS tissue, either by mechanical or proteolytic means inevitably leads to some level of activation (Garden & Moller, 2006). Many have observed microglial cells *in vitro* exhibiting an amoeboid morphology in a non-pathogenic environment. Eder and co-workers exposed murine microglia to astrocyte-conditioned medium and noted a dramatic transformation in morphology from a *"resting"* ramified appearance to *"active"* amoeboid microglia. within a few hours of treatment. As well as this, they observed a down-regulation in macrophage surface molecules such as major-histocompatibility complex (MHC) class-II, and the adhesion molecules leucocyte function-associated antigen-1 (LFA-1) and intercellular adhesion molecule-1 (ICAM-1) (Eder et al., 1999). Well-established histological approaches have allowed *"resting"* microglia to be examined *in situ*, capturing them in a "freeze-frame picture" at the time of being placed in fixative but this approach also has limitations and thus may obscure potentially important dynamic processes (Davalos et al., 2005). Advances in multi-photon *in vivo* microscopy however, have shed some light on the function of *"resting"* microglia *in situ*. By examining the behaviours of eGFP-expressing parenchymal microglia in heterozygous CX_3CR1-mice, it was revealed that microglial processes are incessantly palpating their microenvironment. The protrusions extend and retract rapidly and dynamically, reaching up to several micrometres in length over intervals of seconds to minutes (Davalos et al., 2005; Nimmerjahn et al., 2005). It was postulated that their high motility serves as a "housekeeping" function allowing them to effectively manage the brain milieu and to clear the parenchyma of accumulated metabolic products and deteriorated tissue components (Nimmerjahn et al., 2005). Indeed it has been estimated that they are capable of probing the entire volume of the brain every 4-5 hours. The highly ramified form of microglia covers 30-40μm in diameter and though their processes are in close proximity, they are not in direct contact, suggesting that each cell occupies its own exclusive patrol territory (McGeer & McGeer, 2007; Raivich et al., 1999). As such, they are now more appropriately termed *"surveillant"* microglia to properly describe their rapid and continuous monitoring of the surrounding vicinity (Ransohoff & Cardona, 2010).

"Surveillant" ramified microglia respond to activating stimuli with a rapid morphological transformation into *"active"* amoeboid microglia (Nakajima & Kohsaka, 2001). Activated microglia are found in the brain under almost all pathological conditions and are involved in tissue repair, amplification of inflammatory effects, neuronal degeneration and the phagocytosis of dead cells and cellular debris (Davalos et al., 2005). Microglia express a perplexing array of cell surface receptors such as complement receptor 3 and MHC class I and II, whose up-regulation is concomitant with activation of microglia (Nakajima & Kohsaka, 2001). These receptors play a pivotal role in enabling microglia to detect subtle changes in their microenvironment, triggering them to extend their processes to the surrounding area of insult, and to engulf damaged cells via phagocytosis (Davalos et al., 2005). In addition, microglia are considered the main antigen presenting cell (APC) population within the CNS, as both *in vivo* and *in vitro* studies have demonstrated their capacity for antigen presentation in response to a variety of CNS pathological conditions (Graeber & Streit, 2010). Activation of microglia and the consequent up-regulation of MHC class II, CD40 and ICAM-1 stimulate T cell proliferation and the production of IL-2, IFNγ and IL-4. However, the ability of endogenous microglia to act as APCs has been brought into question, with many postulating that it may be the role of perivascular macrophages or invading DCs (Perry, 1998). Today, growing evidence suggests that DCs do in fact participate in the regulation of T-cell responses (Teo & Wong, 2010). Microglia in common with other cells of the myeloid lineage also have the ability to secrete immunomodulatory molecules such as cytokines, chemokines, neurotrophins, reactive oxygen and nitrogen species, which communicate signals to surrounding cells to regulate the innate immune response (Garden & Moller, 2006). Cytokines, such as ILs, IFNs and TNFα/β are low-molecular weight proteins that are usually classified as pro- or anti-inflammatory, and microglia express receptors for these cytokines in an autocrine feedback loop that is critical for down-regulating inflammation and restoration of homeostasis. In the brain, it has been reported that cytokines function in growth promotion, inhibition and proliferation of astrocytes and oligodendrocytes (Hanisch, 2002), modulation of neurotransmitter release (Zalcman et al., 1994) long-term potentiation (Nolan et al., 2005) behavioural impairments such as memory impairment (Yirmiya et al., 2002) anhedonia (Konsman et al., 2002) and anxiety (Anisman & Merali, 1999).

2.2 Activated microglia in Parkinson's disease

The first evidence for a role of inflammation in PD came from McGeer and colleagues who observed activated microglia and T cells in the *post-mortem* SNpc of a PD patient (McGeer et al., 1988). We now know from a multitude of studies that microglial activation and consequent neuroinflammatory processes play a role in PD (Hirsch & Hunot, 2009). Whereas mild activation of microglia has apparent beneficial effects, chronic microglial activation in response to neuronal damage, as is evident in PD, results in the death of otherwise viable cells. Activation of microglia either directly via a toxin, pathogen or endogenous protein or indirectly from dying neurons may be both long-lived and self-propelling due to positive feedback from degenerating neurons even after the initial insult has ceased (Gao & Hong, 2008). This repetitive cycle of neurotoxic activation of microglia in response to neuronal damage is referred to as *reactive microgliosis* (Block et al., 2007) and is a feature of several brain pathologies (Carson et al., 1998). DA neurons in the SNpc are particularly susceptible to microglial-mediated neurotoxicity due to the high densities of microglia present (Kim et al., 2000). Thus, microglial activation and hence neuroinflammation, may be propagated and potentially amplify the destruction of neurons in PD (Gao & Hong, 2008). Substances which are produced by dying DA neurons and can activate microglia include α-synuclein-aggregates (Zhang et al., 2005), neuromelanin (Wilms et al., 2003), adenosine triphosphate (ATP) (Davalos et al., 2005) and matrix metalloproteinase-3 (MMP-3) (Kim et al., 2007; Kim et al., 2005).

Aggregated α-synuclein, the major constituent of Lewy bodies in PD, has been reported to be surrounded by activated microglia or inflammatory mediators (McGeer et al., 1988; Yamada et al., 1992). It has also been shown to activate microglia in primary mesencephalic cultures, which in turn amplify α-synuclein-mediated neurotoxicity (Zhang et al., 2005). The phagocytosis of extracellular aggregated α-synuclein and activation of NADPH-oxidase is essential to further activate microglia and propel DA neurodegeneration (Zhang et al., 2005). Neuromelanin, a neuro-pigment released from stressed DA neurons has been shown to induce microglial activation (Wilms et al., 2003) through proteasomal inhibition (Kim et al., 2006). Its accumulation in human SNpc correlates with age progression, and extra neural melanin has been found in close proximity to activated microglial cells in patients suffering from juvenile idiopathic and methyl-4-phenyl-2,3-dihydropyridine (MPTP)-induced Parkinsonism (Wilms et al., 2007). Supplementation of microglial cultures with human neuromelanin *in vitro* has been shown to induce chemotactic effects and stimulate the release of TNFα, IL-6 and NO (Wilms et al., 2003). Thus, the release of neuromelanin can augment microglial activation and contribute to a self-perpetuating cycle of neuronal degeneration and chronic inflammation (Kim et al., 2006). Extracellular ATP, a purinergic neurotransmitter, was initially described as an activator of microglial cells in 1993 (Kettenmann et al., 1993). The effects of ATP released from damaged neurons are mediated through its signalling with purinergic receptors, namely the metabotropic G-protein coupled P2Y receptors and the ligand gated ionotropic P2X receptors, both of which are expressed on microglia (Butt, 2011). Upon stimulation, activated microglia migrate along a chemotactic gradient to the site of injury or inflammation, facilitated by the release of pro-migratory factors such as extracellular ATP, UTP and members of the chemokine family from damaged cells. ATP then interacts with P2 receptors on microglia to stimulate the release of TNFα, IL-1β, iNOS and NO. Experiments by Kim *et al* have identified a pivotal role for the protease MMP-3 in DA neuronal activity (Kim et al., 2005). MPP^+-stressed primary mesencephalic DA neurons induce and release active MMP-3, which is toxic to DA neurons. It has been reported that primary microglial cultures treated with catalytically active recombinant MMP-3 stimulated microglial activation, superoxide generation and enhanced DA neuronal cell death while MPTP-treated MMP-3$^{-/-}$ mice attenuated microglial activation, superoxide generation and DA degeneration (Kim et al., 2007).

Stimulation with the glycolipid endotoxin lipopolysaccharide (LPS) is currently one of the most common methods for activating microglia *in vitro*. LPS interacts with Toll-like receptor (TLR) 4, one of a family of pathogen recognition receptors (PPRs) responsive to microbial signals. Microglia have been reported to express 9 of the 12 TLRs (Jack et al., 2005). LPS-stimulated microglia release inflammatory cytokines (IL-1β, IL-1 receptor antagonist (IL-1RA), IL-6, IL-8, IL-10, IL-12, IL-18, macrophage colony stimulating factor), chemokines (macrophage inflammatory protein (MIP)-1α, MIP-1β, TNF-α, TNF-β, monocyte chemoattractant protein-1 (MCP-1), RANTES), and prostaglandins (Kim & de Vellis, 2005; Nakamura, 2002), as well as stimulating an increase in myristoylated alanine-rich C kinase substrate (MARCKS), MARCKS-related protein, protein kinase-C, iNOS and NO production (Garden & Moller, 2006). Cytokines produced by LPS-stimulated microglia can potentiate microglial activation through autocrine signalling to create a self-propagating cycle of expression. Pro-inflammatory cytokines IL-1β, TNFα, IL-2 and IL-6 are constitutively expressed at basal levels in PD patients as evidenced in *post-mortem*, serum and cerebrospinal fluid *in vivo* (Boka et al., 1994; Dobbs et al., 1999; Mogi et al., 1994a; Mogi et al., 1994b; Stypula et al., 1996). Moreover, the death signalling receptor TNF receptor type-1 (TNFR-1) is expressed on DA neurons in human SNpc (Boka et al., 1994; Mogi et al., 2000).

Animal studies support an involvement of pro-inflammatory cytokines in the DA neuronal degeneration evident in PD. For example, induction of chronic expression of IL-1β in adult rat SNpc using a recombinant adenovirus resulted in DA neuronal cell death after three weeks (Ferrari et al., 2006). Another study using neutralising antibodies to IL-1β and TNF-α showed that approximately 50% of LPS-induced DA neuronal cell death in primary cultures of rat midbrain was mediated by the production of these two cytokines (Gayle et al., 2002).

It has been postulated that microglia are maintained in a quiescent state by numerous micro-environmental inhibitory influences, many of which are produced by neurons. Hence, microglial activation during pathological insult may be due to a "*switching-off*" of these inhibitory neuronal signals (Ransohoff & Cardona, 2010). One such neuron-cell inhibitory signalling mechanism is the direct cell-to-cell interactions between neuronal-CD200 (OX2) and its receptor CD200R, expressed on microglia. The CD200-CD200R interaction is essential for maintaining microglial homeostasis in the unperturbed CNS. A down-regulation of CD200 expression has been observed in neurons exposed to inflammatory conditions, and inhibition of CD200 causes microglial activation (Lyons et al., 2007). Therefore, there is a direct neuronal mechanism for regulating microglial activity, and loss of this interaction during neuronal cell degeneration may stimulate up-regulation of CD200, facilitating microglial activation. Recent evidence has implicated an impairment of CD200-CD200R interaction as a contributing factor in PD neurodegeneration (Wang et al., 2011). Blockade of CD200R selectively and significantly enhanced DA neuronal cell susceptibility to rotenone and iron-induced neurotoxicity in mesencephalic neuron-glia co-cultures. This was coupled with elevated microglial activation and superoxide generation and a decrease in CD200 expression on DA neurons. Microglia have also been shown to receive inhibitory inputs from a neuronal membrane-tethered chemokine CX_3CL1, through its receptor CX_3CR1. Removal of this inhibition also unleashed microglial activity (Shan et al., 2011). Other inhibitory signals exist between CD22-CD45, CD172A-CD47 and ICAM5-LFA-1 (Ransohoff & Perry, 2009).

3. Systemic inflammation and Parkinson's disease

It has been proposed that in chronic neurodegenerative diseases like PD, systemic infections and inflammation can exacerbate symptoms and promote neurodegeneration (Perry et al., 2007). A systemic response includes the liver acute phase response and the behavioural and metabolic components that induce sickness behaviour (Ferrari & Tarelli, 2011; Perry et al., 2007). Specifically, peripheral monocytes, macrophages and Kupffer cells express TLRs and PPRs, which innately recognise specific pathogen-associated molecular patterns (PAMPs) associated with invading pathogens (Dantzer, 2009). A prototypical PAMP, LPS, is specifically recognised by TLR4, which results in the production of pro-inflammatory cytokines IL-1α, IL-1β. Through autocrine signalling these cytokines induce self-synthesis and the synthesis of further cytokines (Dantzer, 2009) inducing general inflammation. Compromise of the blood-brain barrier (BBB) which is observed in neurological disorders, stimulates peripheral leucocytes and systemic inflammatory mediators such as cytokines, to migrate into the brain parenchyma where they induce the activation of microglia and the subsequent release of more cytokines (Ferrari & Tarelli, 2011). For example, peripheral TNFα can stimulate microglia to secrete chronically elevated pro-inflammatory mediators, which in turn can induce chronic self-perpetuating neuroinflammation, resulting in a slow and progressive loss of DA neurons in the SNpc (Qin et al., 2007). The brain recognises cytokines as molecular signals of sickness and induces symptoms of malaise, lassitude, fatigue, anhedonia, apathy, numbness, coldness, and reduced appetite and body temperature (Dantzer, 2009; Perry et al., 2007). To reinforce this theory, it has been demonstrated that a systemic inflammatory challenge in an animal with chronic neurodegeneration exhibits exaggerated brain inflammation, sickness behaviour and an increase in acute neurodegeneration (Perry et al., 2007). This emerging *"two-hit hypothesis"* in the aetiology of neurodegenerative diseases such as PD, suggests that the disease is multifactorial and a consequence of *"multiple-hits"* involving diverse inflammatory stimuli (Di Monte, 2003). Infectious agents may comprise the first *"hit"*, therefore sensitising the brain to subsequent *"hits"*, which may not have been pathogenic in the absence of an already *"primed"* system (Jang et al., 2009a). In this instance, microglia in the aged or diseased brain are said to be *"primed"* and can evoke an exaggerated response contributing to disease progression (Perry et al., 2007).

Clinical and epidemiological reports suggest a correlation between systemic inflammatory events, chronic neuroinflammation and the aetiology and progressive nature of PD (Ferrari & Tarelli, 2011; Long-Smith et al., 2009; Perry, 2010). Postulated risk factors implicated in idiopathic PD include age, genetic predisposition, bacterial or viral infections, neuronal injury such as traumatic brain injury or stroke, and environmental toxins (Koprich et al., 2008; Tansey & Goldberg, 2010). Associations were first established towards the end of the first world war (1924-1918) when the H1N1 influenza-A pandemic was coupled with a dramatic increase in post-encephalitic Parkinsonism (PEP) (also referred to as *"sleeping sickness"* or von Economo encephalitis) (Jang et al., 2009a; Rail et al., 1981; Tansey et al., 2007). People born during this time were at a 2-3 fold increased risk of developing PD, with PEP implicated in 50% of all Parkinsonism cases (Jang et al., 2009a; Tansey et al., 2007). PEP shares cardinal symptomatology with idiopathic PD including rigidity and bradykinesia but a lack of Lewy body formation (Jang et al., 2009a). Moreover, Takahashi et al., 1995 demonstrated that the H1N1 virus preferentially targets the SNpc, the primary site of pathology in PD (Takahashi et al., 1995). It has also been shown that exposure to the highly pathogenic neurotropic H5N1 influenza virus increases susceptibility to developing PD with an observed onset of post-influenzal encephalopathies (Jang et al., 2009b). Other viruses associated with secondary Parkinsonism include coxsackie virus (Poser et al., 1969; Walters, 1960), Japanese encephalitis B (Ogata et al., 1997), St. Louis virus (Pranzatelli et al., 1994), west Nile virus (Robinson et al., 2003) and HIV (Tse et al., 2004). Infection with Japanese-encephalitis virus (JEV), which occurs predominantly in India, China and Southeast Asia, for a prolonged period is likely to induce PEP (Ogata et al., 2000; Shoji et al., 1993; Tansey et al., 2007). People with JEV have similar neuropathological and locomotor symptoms to patients with idiopathic PD (Tansey et al., 2007), and the virus has previously been used to create a pre-clinical model of PD in rats (Ogata et al., 1997). This group demonstrated that in Fisher rats infected with JEV, there was marked gliosis and DA neuronal loss in the SNpc similar to that seen in PD, and bradykinesia which could be reversed with L-DOPA and monoamine oxidase (MAO) inhibitors. More recently, in a cohort of 60 JEV patients, transient-type Parkinsonian features were observed in 16 patients, with 19 displaying Parkinsonism with additional dystonia (Misra & Kalita, 2010).

Oxidative stress, through the generation of reactive oxygen species (ROS) is a key regulator of the neuroinflammatory process, with the underlying purpose of removing the cause of inflammation. Progressive neurodegenerative diseases like PD however, are associated with an overproduction of ROS causing neuronal oxidative damage as well as microglial activation, which subsequently leads to the generation of more ROS (Block & Hong, 2005). Moreover, oxidative stress preferentially affects DA neurons in the SNpc, which are particularly vulnerable as they operate under high oxidant conditions due to reduced levels of the anti-oxidant glutathione (Misra & Kalita, 2010; Sian et al., 1994). Accordingly, it has been postulated that pre-exposure to environmental toxins such as heavy metals, organophosphate compounds, neurotoxins, and pesticides like paraquat and rotenone which can induce oxidative stress and the generation of free radicals, increases the susceptibility to the development of PD in later life (Calne & Langston, 1983; Jang et al., 2009a). Pathological and clinical evidence has also identified the involvement of the gastrointestinal tract in enhancing susceptibility to idiopathic Parkinsonism, with *Helicobacter pylori* infection proposed as a potential trigger in disease progression (Tansey & Goldberg, 2010; Weller et al., 2005). Indeed, polymorphisms in the nucleotide-binding oligiomerisation domain 2 (NOD2) gene associated with Crohn's disease, a chronic inflammatory bowel disease, have been shown to be over-represented in patients with idiopathic PD (Bialecka et al., 2007).

Evidence now suggests that a disruption in neurovascular homeostasis with increased BBB permeability due to factors secreted by activated glia is associated with neuroinflammation in age-related neurodegenerative diseases. Activated glia have an up-regulated expression of cellular adhesion molecules and the subsequent induction of chemokine gradients direct peripheral leucocytes to the site of inflammation (Chung et al., 2010; Stone et al., 2009). Indeed, positron emission tomography (PET) and histological studies of PD patients as well as MPTP and LPS-induced models of PD reveal a pathogenic link between neuroinflammation, increased BBB permeability and the consequent infiltration of systemic inflammatory molecules, and DA neuronal death (Chung et al., 2010). PD patients have a reported dysfunction in the BBB transporter system (Kortekaas et al., 2005) and blood vessels in the midbrain (Faucheux et al., 1999). Increased levels of vascular endothelial growth factor (VEGF) and pigment epithelium-derived factor have been demonstrated in PD patients and in the MPTP model (Yasuda et al., 2007). A report from a study using animals provides evidence that nigral injection of VEGF to mice disrupted the BBB permeability and induced DA neuronal death in the ventral mesencephalon (VM) (X. Chen et al., 2008). In another study, systemic injection of high concentrations of LPS to rats caused functional breakdown of the BBB resulting in granulocyte infiltration and activation of parenchymal microglia. The subsequent infiltration of immune cells contributed to the degeneration of DA neurons in the SNpc (Brochard et al., 2009).

Assessment of serum obtained from PD subjects corroborates the involvement of systemic inflammation in PD (Hirsch & Hunot, 2009). Increased levels of $CD4^+$ have been reported in the serum of patients with PD, suggesting peripheral activation of lymphocytes (Bas et al., 2001; Fiszer et al., 1994; Hirsch & Hunot, 2009). Infiltrating cytotoxic $CD4^+$ and $CD8^+$ T cells, but not B cells, have been observed in the inflamed SNpc of *post-mortem* PD human specimens and in the MPTP-induced mouse model of PD during the course of neurodegeneration (Brochard et al., 2009; Ferrari & Tarelli, 2011; Stone et al., 2009). In support of a role for systemic immune cells in the degeneration of nigral DA neurons, $CD4^{-/-}$ mice have been shown to be resistant to MPTP-induced neurotoxicity in the SN (Brochard et al., 2009). Amplified TNFα, IL-2, IL-6 and RANTES (Brodacki et al., 2008; Dobbs et al., 1999; Rentzos et al., 2007; Stypula et al., 1996) levels have also been detected in serum obtained from PD patients. Increases in serum cytokines may serve as a therapeutic marker for PD as a blood sample study of men with high plasma concentrations of IL-6 revealed an increased risk of developing PD (H. Chen et al., 2008). In a cohort of 46 PD patients, increased serum levels of soluble TNFR-1, which modulates TNFα activity were detected, which is in agreement with studies showing elevated TNFR-1 in the SNpc of PD brains (Mogi et al., 2000), although this was not associated with clinical parameters. Another group however, has demonstrated that LPS-induced increase of MCP-1, RANTES, MIP-1α, IL-8, IL-6 and IFNγ levels secreted by peripheral blood mononuclear cells significantly correlated with the severity of PD symptoms (Reale et al., 2009). Systemic low level of inflammation induced by a non-toxic dose of LPS has been shown to increase the severity of nigral DA neuronal cell loss in response to a subsequent low-dose of 6-OHDA in the rat model of PD (Koprich et al., 2008), while chronic systemic IL-1β also exacerbated neurodegeneration and microglial activation in the SN of 6-OHDA-treated rats (Pott Godoy et al., 2008). These data support the role of primed microglia, in the *"two-hit hypothesis"*.

Evidence now suggests that prenatal infections may be a risk factor for the development of PD in later life. Brains from postnatal day (P) 21 rat pups born to dams that were intraperitoneally injected with LPS at the gestation window of vulnerability (embryonic day (E) 10.5), displayed reduced numbers of tyrosine hydroxylase (TH) immunoreactive cells in the SN and ventral tegmental area. This apparent DA neuronal loss was associated with reduced striatal dopamine and an increase in TNFα in the striatum and mesencephalon. The loss of TH^+ cells was still observed 33 days post- injection (Ling et al., 2002). It has thus been suggested that prenatal infections such as bacterial vaginosis (BV) in humans may be potential risk factors for PD. Indeed, during pregnancy, levels of LPS and TNFα are elevated in the chorioamniotic environment of women with BV, which may hinder typical DA neuron development (Ling et al., 2002). One group has reported loss of DA neurons up to 16 months post prenatal exposure of rats to LPS, which corresponds to the mean age in humans at which PD symptoms are first observed. Thus, prenatal exposure of rats to LPS has been suggested as a potential model of PD as it induces a slow, protracted loss of nigral DA neurons (Carvey et al., 2003). Further validation for this model was demonstrated by significant dopamine and serotonin reductions observed in the frontal cortex, nucleus accumbens, striatum, amygdala, hippocampus and hypothalamus, comparable to the neurochemical alterations evident in PD subjects (Wang et al., 2009). In a study to examine the effect of systemic inflammation on the progression of PD, prenatally LPS-exposed rats were subjected to a moderate dose of 6-OHDA at four-months. The data revealed that both prenatal LPS exposure and postnatal 6-OHDA-treatment produced significant DA neuron loss. However, the combined effect was additive and not synergistic. This may have been due to the young age of the animal or the toxin used (Ling et al., 2004). This model was subsequently investigated but with prenatally LPS-exposed rats treated with rotenone rather than 6-OHDA postnatally. The combined effects of LPS and rotenone produced a synergistic TH^+ cell loss in the SN relative to controls, which was associated with increased striatal-dopamine activity, TNFα and increased reactive microglia (Ling et al., 2004).

4. Inflammation in animal models of Parkinson's disease

4.1 MPTP model

The MPTP model of PD has been extensively used to elucidate the basal ganglia response to nigrostriatal deficits as well as to examine the validity of novel drug treatments for PD. The MPTP neurotoxin was initially discovered during the 1980s in humans intoxicated with a by-product of an illicit drug synthesis scheme who presented with symptoms manifesting as severe Parkinsonism (Langston et al., 1983; Langston & Ballard, 1983). *Post-mortem* analysis, ranging between 3-16 years post-MPTP administration, revealed selective DA neurodegeneration and gliosis, with microglial clustering occurring around nerve cells (Langston et al., 1999). It was subsequently postulated that activated microglia might perpetuate DA neuronal degeneration after a primary insult of environmental or genetic origin (Hirsch et al., 2003). Currently, MPTP administration is the most universally used agent for reproducing PD pathologies. It is primarily used in murine and non-human primate models of PD but less frequently in rats, as rat DA neurons are elusively resistant to MPTP-toxicity and are incapable of recapitulating analogous symptoms (Przedborski & Vila, 2003). Motor-impairment symptoms of PD such as bradykinesia, tremor at rest, gait disturbances, postural instability and rigidity have all been observed in MPTP-treated primate models (Bove et al., 2005). While MPTP can mimic a wide range of PD-like symptoms it does not manifest one of the pathological hallmarks of PD, namely the formation of Lewy body-like inclusions, nor can it induce sustained motor impairments. MPTP is highly lipophilic and can easily infiltrate the BBB where it is spontaneously oxidised to an active form, 1-methyl-4-phenyl-2,3-dihydropyridium ($1\text{-}MPP^+$) by MAO-B in glial cells. $1\text{-}MPP^+$ is released into the extracellular space where it is taken up by DA neurons via the DA transporter (DAT) (Przedborski & Vila, 2003). Here, it accumulates in the mitochondrial complex and is involved in potently inhibiting mitochondrial complex-1 of the electron transfer chain, leading to an increased production of ROS such as O_2^- and a decrease in ATP. In addition, $1\text{-}MPP^+$ can bind to vesicular monoamine transporter-2, enabling its translocation into the synaptic vesicles where it stimulates the extrusion of synaptic DA. This excess DA is auto-metabolised resulting in a burst of ROS such as hydrogen peroxide (H_2O_2) and superoxide radicals (O_2^-). Accumulation of ROS subsequently causes oxidative degradation of DNA, lipids and proteins resulting in the demise of nigral neurons. This MPTP-induced burst of ROS is generated by microglial

NADPH, therefore, activated microglia have been shown to play an essential role in MPTP-induce neurotoxicity (Gao et al., 2003; Wu et al., 2003). Moreover, cytosolic DA oxidation can be catalysed by COX-2, which has been shown to be up-regulated in nigral DA neurons in both MPTP-treated mice, rats and in human *post-mortem* samples (Teismann & Ferger, 2001; Teismann et al., 2003).

In an effort to examine a potential role for glia in DA neuronal degeneration, focus was initially placed on deciphering the temporal relationship between DA neurodegeneration and glial activation in MPTP-induced PD murine models. Significant depletion of DA fibres and activated astroglia in the striatum was observed 24-48 hours and 48 hours post-MPTP-administration, respectively (O'Callaghan et al., 1990). The duration of astroglia activation was directly dependent on the extent of DA neuronal damage, and was sustained for the duration of MPTP-administration. It was subsequently reported that microglial activation was observed in the striatum 48 hours post-MPTP administration (Francis et al., 1995), while further studies elucidated that activated microglia were present in the SNpc 24 hours post MPTP and that activation was sustained for 14 days (Czlonkowska et al., 1996; Kohutnicka et al., 1998). Other groups pinpoint microglial activation in the SN of mice as early as 12 hours and peaking at 24 hours post-MPTP-administration (Dehmer et al., 2000; Liberatore et al., 1999). It has since been reported that activated amoeboid microglia have been observed in the SN of monkeys years after systemic MPTP-injection (McGeer et al., 2003). A further study has implicated a role for cytokines and chemokines in the acute MPTP mouse model of PD by demonstrating that real-time PCR detected elevated mRNA expression of TNFα, MCP-1 and IL-1α in the mouse striatum 2-4 hours post MPTP-administration (Sriram et al., 2006). However, ablation of TNFα or TNFR-1 did not affect chronic MPTP-induced nigral DA neuronal cell degeneration in mice (Ferger et al., 2004; Leng et al., 2005).

4.2 6-OHDA model

6-OHDA is a hydroxylated analogue of DA, which is actively taken up into DA neurons via DAT expressed on the nerve terminals. It is directly toxic to DA neurons and is used to model PD in rodents. However, since it is unable to cross the BBB, it must be stereotaxically injected into the SN, which results in a widespread and almost immediate destruction of DA neurons (Stanic et al., 2003). The standard delivery method of 6-OHDA is unilateral injection into either the VM, the medial forebrain bundle or the striatum, avoiding areas containing noradrenergic neurons as 6-OHDA can be taken up via the noradrenaline transporter (Deumens et al., 2002). Striatal lesions result in destruction of the nigral DA neuronal terminals leading to a dying back mechanism whereby the cell bodies in the SN are affected secondarily and progressively (Kirik et al., 1998; Sauer & Oertel, 1994). This creates a therapeutic window of opportunity whereby potential neuroprotective strategies can be evaluated. Loss of TH^{+}-immunoreactive cells are detectable as early as 24 hours post-6-OHDA lesion in the striatum, peaking in the third week post-lesion. However, loss of TH^{+} cells in the SN does not appear until the second week post-lesion (Blandini et al., 2007). Behavioural testing such as drug-induced rotations can then be performed to assess the anti-Parkinsonian abilities of potential therapies. While the 6-OHDA-lesion model remains one of the most popular animal models of PD to date, like the MPTP model, it fails to encapsulate all the hallmarks of PD pathology, particularly a lack of Lewy body formation. Secondly, PD is a chronic disorder potentially lasting 1-2 decades, so the 6-OHDA-model is in fact regarded as an acute model of PD. As in the MPTP-induced animal model of PD, activated microglia have been observed in the SN and nigrostriatal tract of 6-OHDA-lesioned rats (Akiyama & McGeer, 1989; Depino et al., 2003; He et al., 2001). Microglial activation was initially observed 1-day post 6-OHDA-lesion but appeared transient in nature (Akiyama & McGeer, 1989). We have observed a significant increase in the number of activated microglia, indicated by MHC class II in the SNpc of 6-OHDA-lesioned rats at 10-28 days post lesion (Crotty et al., 2008). Pro-inflammatory cytokines have also been implicated as neurotoxic mediators of 6-OHDA-induced DA neuronal death; blockade of the soluble form of the TNF-α receptor but not the transmembrane form was found to attenuate the death of DA neurons in 6-OHDA-lesioned rats (McCoy et al., 2006). We have previously demonstrated that conditioned-medium (CM) obtained from LPS-stimulated rat glial-enriched cortical cultures can induce loss of DA neurons in primary VM cultures and that this effect can be exacerbated by 6-OHDA treatment. IL-1β released from activated microglia in the CM mediated this effect as blockade of IL-1R1 with IL-1RA attenuated the CM-induced DA neuronal toxicity (Long-Smith et al., 2010).

4.3 LPS model

LPS is one of the main constitutes of gram-negative bacteria and is used as a tool to mimic general infection as it is a potent stimulator of immune cells. Intranigral injection of LPS in rats has been shown to manifest Parkinsonism-like symptoms, such as the selective loss of DA neurons in the SN (Arimoto et al., 2006; Castano et al., 1998; Herrera et al., 2000). Thus the LPS model has served as a valuable tool in deciphering the role of glial cells, especially microglia, in the DA neurodegeneration process and has been described by many as the neuroinflammatory model of PD. LPS binds to the serum LPS-binding protein (LBP), which facilitates binding to the CD14 receptor expressed on microglia. The LBP can then dissociate and allow the LPS-CD14 complex to bind to TLR4, resulting in a cascade of intracellular signalling. The adapter protein myeloid differentiation factor 88 (myD88) attaches to TLR4 and interacts with IL-1 receptor-associated kinase (IRAK), which phosphorylates, activating TNF-R-associated factor-6 (TRAF6). The mitogen-activated protein kinases (MAPK) p38 and c-Jun N-terminal kinase (JNK) are activated downstream of this, leading to the up-regulation of transcription factors such as nuclear-factor-κB (NF-κB). This up-regulation results in the production of pro-inflammatory cytokines (McGettrick & O'Neill, 2010).
Intranigral injection of LPS in rats has been shown to result in a significant decrease of DA levels in the striatum, microglial activation and a time and LPS-dose-dependent degeneration of DA neurons in the SN (Castano et al., 1998). In this study, microglial activation was observed at 6 hours and peaked at 1-2 days post LPS injection, while DA neuronal degeneration persisted up to at least 21 days after intranigral injection of LPS demonstrating that LPS-induced microglial activation can induce progressive degeneration of nigral DA neurons. Furthermore, it has been reported that prenatal exposure of LPS to rats results in sustained microglial activation and the development of fewer than normal nigral DA neurons (Ling et al., 2006). Systemic administration of LPS has also been found to induce progressive degeneration of nigral DA neurons in rats (Qin et al., 2007). It had previously been suggested that LPS-mediated DA neuronal toxicity required the presence of glia (Bronstein et al., 1995) and indeed a subsequent study reported that a single intranigral injection of LPS induced selective DA neuronal degeneration up to one year post injection (Herrera et al., 2000). Thus, unlike MPTP and 6-OHDA, LPS is not a direct toxin but rather causes indirect death of DA neurons by activating microglia, inducing an inflammatory

reaction and subsequent DA neuronal death. Studies on rat mesencephalic cultures suggest that DA neurons are twice as sensitive to LPS as non-DA neurons and that the toxicity of LPS occurs via microglial activation (Bronstein et al., 1995; Gayle et al., 2002). Although many *in vitro* studies have supported an involvement of NO in microglial-mediated DA neuronal death after LPS-treatment (Chao et al., 1992; Gibbons & Dragunow, 2006), others have suggested that NO is not involved (Castano et al., 1998; Gayle et al., 2002). The pro-inflammatory cytokines IL-1β and TNF-α are thought to be involved in LPS-mediated toxicity (Gayle et al., 2002). In support of a role for LPS-induced pro-inflammatory cytokines in DA neurotoxicity, we have shown that IL-1β in CM released from LPS-stimulated microglia significantly reduces the percentage of DA neurons in embryonic rat neuronal-enriched cultures that IL-1R1 is expressed on these DA neurons, and that blockade of IL-1R1 prevented the CM-induced DA neuronal death (Long-Smith et al., 2010). Furthermore, blockade of the soluble form of the TNF-α receptor has been reported to reduce microglial activation in the *in vivo* LPS model of PD (McCoy et al., 2006). Also, Ling and co-workers found that the decreased numbers of nigral DA neurons in rats after prenatal exposure to LPS, was accompanied by elevated levels of TNF-α in the striatum (Ling et al., 2004).

5. Neuroinflammatory diagnostic tools for Parkinson's disease

Microglial responsiveness to injury and neurodegenerative disease suggests that it may serve as a marker for the diagnosis and progression of disease pathology in PD. There is a current drive to develop non-invasive imaging tools to assess and quantify the dynamics of activated microglia in neurodegenerative diseases like PD. Advances in this technology, especially for identification of microglial biomarkers at the early stages of disease, would have important implications for PD diagnosis, assessment of progression, and therapy. Currently, the best-studied imaging paradigm for microglial activation is the radiolabelled translocator protein (TSPO) ligand using PET (Dolle et al., 2009). This line of research initially started when a correlation was observed between increased binding of Ro5-4864 (a benzodiazepine) and PK11195 (an isoquinoline) to receptors on the surface of mitochondria primarily localised in glial cells (Arlicot et al., 2008; Chauveau et al., 2008). These receptors were originally referred to as peripheral type benzodiazepine receptors and were increased in activated microglia (Park et al., 1996; Stephenson et al., 1995). The nomenclature has since been changed to TSPO as further research elucidated that these receptors are expressed throughout the brain and body (Papadopoulos et al., 2006). Gene-expression analysis in brains of rodents, primates and humans have illustrated that TSPO expression is nearly absent in parenchyma-microglia (Winkeler et al., 2010) but is elevated in many neurodegenerative disorders including, stroke, AD, PD, multiple sclerosis, Huntington's disease and amyotrophic lateral sclerosis, (Arlicot et al., 2008) thus emphasising the involvement of microglial activation and neuroinflammation in these diseases. TSPOs are the prototypical biomarkers of neuroinflammatory changes in a variety of CNS disorders and have therefore been proposed as potential diagnostic targets for *in vivo* imaging (Arlicot et al., 2008; Chauveau et al., 2008).

Currently, functional PET and single photon emission tomography (SPECT), in conjunction with ligands for TSPO, can detect microglial activation *in vivo*. Examples of radiolabelled TSPO ligands include [^{11}C]Ro5-4864 and [^{11}C](*R*)-PK11195 (1-(2-chlorophenyl)-N-methyl-N-(1-methylpropyl)-3 isoquinoline carboxamide) (Chauveau et al., 2008). In PD subjects, PET imaging revealed microglial activation in the pons, basal ganglia, and frontal and temporal cortical areas. Longitudinal studies of these patients revealed stable [^{11}C](*R*)-PK11195 binding potential (BP; a parameter that mixes receptor density with ligand affinity), indicative of early activation of microglia in PD pathology (Gerhard et al., 2006; Winkeler et al., 2010). However, the [^{11}C](*R*)-PK11195 tracer is limited, as it is incapable of distinguishing between phenotypic differences, and thus possibly functional differences of microglia. To overcome this, a PET tracer for the dopamine-transporter, [^{11}C]CFT, has been used in conjunction with [^{11}C](*R*)-PK11195 to examine the viability of the presynaptic DA neurons (Ouchi et al., 2009). This study of 10 drug-naïve PD patients, demonstrated changes in microglial activity in conjunction with DAT density which were investigated using PET imaging with [^{11}C](*R*)-PK11195 and [^{11}C]CFT tracers. Subjects underwent magnetic resonance imaging (MRI) prior to PET measurement to define the regions of interest, which would allow for the evaluation of microglial activation in parallel with presynaptic neuronal degeneration *in vivo*. Elevated midbrain [^{11}C](*R*)-PK11195 BP levels were significantly inversely correlated with [^{11}C]CFT BP localised in the putamen. The elevated [^{11}C](*R*)-PK11195 BP also correlated with motor impairment. A follow-up 4-year scan revealed increased microglial activation spread over the extrastriatal region (Ouchi et al., 2009). PET imaging and *post-mortem* analysis of the brain of a rat lesioned with 6-OHDA revealed reduced [^{11}C]CFT BP in the striatum, indicative of DA degeneration, while [^{11}C](*R*)-PK11195 BP was markedly increased in the striatum and SNpc. *Post-mortem* immunohistochemical analysis corroborated this finding by showing activated microglia in the striatum and SNpc at 4 weeks post-lesion (Cicchetti et al., 2002). Alternative SPECT imaging biomarkers for TSPO such as [^{123}I]CLINDE (2-(4'iodophenyl)-3-(N,N-diethyl)-imidazo[1,2-a]pyridine-3-acetamide) have been examined *in vivo* and also pose as potential image-guided diagnostic tools for microglial activation in neurodegenerative diseases like PD (Arlicot et al., 2008).

6. Immunomodulatory therapies

As the wealth of evidence continues to accumulate regarding the role of microglial activation in the pathogenesis of PD, a large number of inhibitory drugs have been investigated. The use of broad spectrum steroidal and non-steroidal anti-inflammatory drugs, specific microglial inhibitors or anti-inflammatory cytokines have not only helped decipher the role of microglial activation in neuroinflammation in PD but also indicated that inhibiting the specific processes involved in microglial activation may be a therapeutic avenue for PD.

The glucocorticoids are well known for their broad range of anti-inflammatory effects and have long been used in clinical settings for the treatment of brain inflammation (Castano et al., 2002). Microglial cells express the glucocorticoid receptor which is involved in the regulation of the transcription factors NF-κB and activator protein-1 (AP-1) (Scheinman et al., 1995) which in turn are key regulators of pro-inflammatory cytokine expression (Nadeau & Rivest, 2003). Of particular interest, the synthetic steroid dexamethasone was shown to provide neuroprotection against LPS or MPTP-induced toxicity in rodent models. In both models, the delivery of dexamethasone prevented the activation of microglia usually associated with neurodegeneration (Castano et al., 2002; Kurkowska-Jastrzebska et al., 2004). However, the severe side-effects associated with glucocorticoid use prevent any long-term usage in neuroprotective therapies for PD. Large scale epidemiological studies have shown that the chronic use of non-steroidal anti-inflammatory drugs (NSAID) such as aspirin or ibuprofen could provide some level of protection against PD (Chen et al., 2005; Chen et al., 2003). Other studies suggest that the role of NSAIDs in decreasing the risk of PD is extremely limited (Hancock et al., 2007; Hernan et al., 2006). A recent meta-analysis of studies published between 1966 and 2008 showed that while NSAIDs as a class do not modify the risk of developing PD, the chronic intake of ibuprofen may have a beneficial effect (Gagne & Power, 2010; Gao et al., 2011; Samii et al., 2009). Ibuprofen possibly mediates this effect via its inhibition of COX activity to inhibit the production of pro-inflammatory lipid mediator prostaglandins (Mitchell et al., 1993). Some of the beneficial effects observed could also be mediated via other mechanisms associated with NSAIDs such as inactivation of the pro-inflammatory nuclear receptor NF-κB (Grilli et al., 1996; Kopp & Ghosh, 1994), activation of peroxisome proliferator-activated receptor gamma (PPARγ), a nuclear factor mediating anti-inflammatory effects in microglia (Bernardo et al., 2005) or activation of the Rho kinase pathway (Zhou et al., 2003). Results from animal models of PD demonstrate that aspirin and indomethacin have both been shown to prevent MPTP-induced loss of striatal dopamine in the mouse (Aubin et al., 1998; Kurkowska-Jastrzebska et al., 2002). The NSAID Celecoxib reversed striatal DA neuronal fibre and nigral DA neuronal cell loss in 6-OHDA-treated rats (Sanchez-Pernaute et al., 2004) while aspirin has been shown to prevent 6-OHDA-induced striatal dopamine depletion (Di Matteo et al., 2006).

Other neuroimmunomodulatory strategies include the use of the second generation tetracycline analogue, minocycline. It has been shown to inhibit microglial activation and prevent iNOS and NADPH oxidase generation as well as IL-1β up-regulation (Du et al., 2001). It is a lipophilic molecule which easily crosses the BBB and is reported to have anti-inflammatory and neuroprotective activities (Kim & Suh, 2009). Some studies in experimental models of PD have shown that it is neuroprotective against MPTP-, LPS, or 6-OHDA induced neurodegeneration (Du et al., 2001; He et al., 2001; Tomas-Camardiel et al., 2004; Wu et al., 2002) while others showed that it exacerbated the deleterious effects of MPTP in rodents and non-human primates (Diguet et al., 2004; Yang et al., 2003). While the reason for the discrepancies is unknown, differences between the various studies include doses and timing of intervention and may reflect the dual role of microglia in inflammation. Despite these contradictory results, a phase II randomized double-blind futility clinical trial was set-up. Results after 12 and 18 months suggest that minocycline is well tolerated and does not negatively impact on symptomatic treatment. It is therefore currently recommended for phase III clinical trials to assess its long-term effect on disease progression (NINDS-NET-PD-Investigators, 2006, 2008).

In addition to the role of glial-associated innate immunity, an adaptive immune response may also be involved in triggering cell death in DA neurons. Manipulating this adaptive response mediated by T cells could be a successful approach for neuroprotection. This immuno-intervention aims at redirecting the harmful T cell response towards an anti-inflammatory and protective immune response by means of an antigen-based immunisation. Preclinical results using glatiramer acetate (a random amino acid polymer composed of alanine, glutamine, lysine and tyrosine amino acids) as the immunisation agent showed that this approach could be successful. Glatiramer-acetate primed T cells transferred to MPTP-treated mice were shown to reach the brain where they suppressed microglial activation and provided neuroprotection to the nigrostriatal neurons by inducing the neurotrophic factor glial cell-derived neurotrophic factor (GDNF). Furthermore, specific depletion of the donor T cells abrogated this neuroprotective effect confirming that the effect is donor T cell dependent (Benner et al., 2004). Interestingly, the donor T cells were shown to secrete high levels of anti-inflammatory cytokines IL-4, IL-10 and TGFβ (Benner et al., 2004). As glatiramer acetate has already been shown to be safe and tolerable in clinical trial and has had significant reduction effects on disability in multiple sclerosis patients (Comi et al., 2011), it represents a very attractive possibility. Interestingly, another neuropeptide, vasoactive intestinal peptide, has been reported to prevent MPTP-induced loss of nigral DA neurons and striatal DA fibres in the mouse while also down-regulating IL-1β and TNF-α expression and iNOS generation (Delgado & Ganea, 2003).

Alternatively, the delivery of anti-inflammatory cytokines such as IL-10 could be considered as an anti-inflammatory therapeutic strategy for PD. Pre-treatment of mesencephalic neuroglial cultures with IL-10 inhibited LPS-stimulated microglial activation and degeneration of DA neurons (Qian et al., 2006). Similar neuroprotective effects were observed *in vivo* after chronic infusion of IL-10 into the SNpc of rats that were challenged with LPS (Arimoto et al., 2006). More recently, gene therapy approaches have been developed to deliver IL-10 into the rat SNpc, and have proved effective in attenuating the neuronal loss and behavioural deficits in the 6-OHDA rat model of PD (Johnston et al., 2008). Furthermore, the blockade of pro-inflammatory cytokines should be considered as a potential therapeutic avenue. Blocking the soluble TNF signalling by delivery of a dominant-negative form has been shown to promote neuronal survival and reduce the behavioural deficits in the hemi-Parkinsonian rat model of PD (McCoy et al., 2006; McCoy et al., 2008). While these pre-clinical results are interesting, the availability of a broad spectrum of compounds acting on TNF signalling makes this molecule a very attractive target. Etanercept and Infliximab are a new generation of engineered inhibitors of TNF that are broadly used for the treatment of rheumatoid arthritis and other peripheral inflammatory diseases. Their use in CNS diseases is however limited by their general inability to cross the BBB (Tweedie et al., 2007). While direct intrastriatal delivery or long-term gene transfer as illustrated above are possibilities, other inhibitors of TNF synthesis may prove useful such as the infamous antiemetic compound thalidomide. Thalidomide is a sedative, immunosuppressive and anti-inflammatory drug that has teratogenic effects (Smithells & Newman, 1992) and inhibits the synthesis of TNF-α (Sampaio et al., 1991). Thalidomide was shown to protect nigrostriatal neurons and prevent striatal DA depletion in the early stages of MPTP-induced neurodegeneration (Boireau et al., 1997; Ferger et al., 2004).

PPARγ has been shown to exert anti-inflammatory functions in both the periphery and the CNS where it is detected in glial and neuronal cells. Following activation by its naturally occurring ligands eicosanoids and prostaglandin J2, it regulates the expression of pro-inflammatory molecules such as iNOS, COX-2 and, indirectly, of broad array of cytokines through its interactions with the transcription factor NF-κB (Chaturvedi & Beal, 2008; Chung et al., 2008). Pioglitazone and rosiglitazone are two synthetic agonists of PPARγ that are approved for the treatment of type II diabetes. In the CNS they exhibit neuroprotective effects in models of neurodegenerative disorders, including PD, by preventing inflammation, oxidative damage and apoptosis (Chaturvedi & Beal, 2008). Specifically, pioglitazone prevents MPTP-induced activation of microglia and DA neuronal cell loss in murine SNpc *in vivo* (Dehmer et al., 2004). This has been shown to occur through inhibition of MAO-B, the enzyme responsible for conversion of MPTP to its toxic metabolite MPP+ (Quinn et al., 2008). When pioglitazone was administered to rats that were also injected intrastriatally with LPS, the resultant LPS-induced microglial activation and DA degeneration was attenuated (Hunter et al., 2007). Recently, the neuroprotective effects of rosiglitazone have been shown in the MPTP mouse model of PD; chronic administration of the drug prevented behavioural deficits, DA neuronal loss and microglial activation in the SNpc *in vivo* (Schintu et al., 2009).

As mentioned above, NF-κB plays an important role in the regulation of chronic diseases through the promotion of inflammation and of cell survival. Activation of NF-κB requires the activity of the IκB kinase (IKK) complex (Kim et al., 2006). Activated NF-κB has been detected in neurons and activated microglia in the SN of PD patients and MPTP-treated animals suggesting that some of the pro-inflammatory mechanisms regulated by the NF-κB pathways may play an important role in the pathogenesis of PD (Ghosh et al., 2007; Hunot et al., 1997). Recent studies have shown that blockade of NF-κB activity either directly or through IκB can inhibit components of the inflammatory pathways in microglia namely, the oxidative stress pathway and the production of pro-inflammatory cytokines (Anrather et al., 2006; Gauss et al., 2007). Selective inhibition of NF-κB activity by a peptide blocking the IKK complex prevented DA neuronal loss in MPTP-treated mice and suppressed microglial activation (Ghosh et al., 2007). Finally, a selective pharmacological IKKβ inhibitor has demonstrated neuroprotective properties in LPS- and MPTP-induced models of PD. Treatment with this compound prevented neuronal damage in a process dependant on the presence of microglia. Particularly, it prevented the activation of microglial oxidative pathways and the release of pro-inflammatory cytokines by specific blockade of the NF-κB signalling pathway (Zhang et al., 2010).

7. Conclusion

The death of dopaminergic neurons in the SNpc is the key pathology of PD. Therefore, it is imperative that research is undertaken, not only in areas which could provide protective strategies for the remaining neurons, or which involve dopaminergic neuronal cell replacement therapies, but also into understanding the fundamental mechanisms by which these cells die. Although the precise role of inflammation in the pathogenesis of PD remains unclear, an array of evidence from the clinic and from animal models now points to its substantial involvement in this debilitating disease.

8. Acknowledgment

The authors thank Declan Conroy and Aoife Nolan for technical assistance.

9. References

Ajami, B., Bennett, J.L., Krieger, C., Tetzlaff, W. & Rossi, F.M. (2007). Local self-renewal can sustain CNS microglia maintenance and function throughout adult life. *Nat Neurosci*, Vol.10, No.12, pp. 1538-1543

Akiyama, H. & McGeer, P.L. (1989). Microglial response to 6-hydroxydopamine-induced substantia nigra lesions. *Brain Res*, Vol.489, No.2, pp. 247-253

Anisman, H. & Merali, Z. (1999). Anhedonic and anxiogenic effects of cytokine exposure. *Adv Exp Med Biol*, Vol.461, No., pp. 199-233

Anrather, J., Racchumi, G. & Iadecola, C. (2006). NF-kappaB regulates phagocytic NADPH oxidase by inducing the expression of gp91phox. *J Biol Chem,* Vol.281, No.9, pp. 5657-5667

Arimoto, T., Choi, D.Y., Lu, X., Liu, M., Nguyen, X.V., Zheng, N., Stewart, C.A., Kim, H.C. & Bing, G. (2006). Interleukin-10 protects against inflammation-mediated degeneration of dopaminergic neurons in substantia nigra. *Neurobiol Aging,* Vol.28, No.6, pp. 894-906

Arlicot, N., Katsifis, A., Garreau, L., Mattner, F., Vergote, J., Duval, S., Kousignian, I., Bodard, S., Guilloteau, D. & Chalon, S. (2008). Evaluation of CLINDE as potent translocator protein (18 kDa) SPECT radiotracer reflecting the degree of neuroinflammation in a rat model of microglial activation. *Eur J Nucl Med Mol Imaging,* Vol.35, No.12, pp. 2203-2211

Aubin, N., Curet, O., Deffois, A. & Carter, C. (1998). Aspirin and salicylate protect against MPTP-induced dopamine depletion in mice. *J Neurochem,* Vol.71, No.4, pp. 1635-1642

Banati, R.B., Daniel, S.E. & Blunt, S.B. (1998). Glial pathology but absence of apoptotic nigral neurons in long-standing Parkinson's disease. *Mov Disord,* Vol.13, No.2, pp. 221-227

Barron, K.D. (1995). The microglial cell. A historical review. *J Neurol Sci,* Vol.134 Suppl, No., pp. 57-68

Bas, J., Calopa, M., Mestre, M., Mollevi, D.G., Cutillas, B., Ambrosio, S. & Buendia, E. (2001). Lymphocyte populations in Parkinson's disease and in rat models of parkinsonism. *J Neuroimmunol,* Vol.113, No.1, pp. 146-152

Bekris, L.M., Mata, I.F. & Zabetian, C.P. (2010). The genetics of Parkinson disease. *J Geriatr Psychiatry Neurol,* Vol.23, No.4, pp. 228-242

Benner, E.J., Mosley, R.L., Destache, C.J., Lewis, T.B., Jackson-Lewis, V., Gorantla, S., Nemachek, C., Green, S.R., Przedborski, S. & Gendelman, H.E. (2004). Therapeutic immunization protects dopaminergic neurons in a mouse model of Parkinson's disease. *Proc Natl Acad Sci U S A,* Vol.101, No.25, pp. 9435-9440

Bernardo, A., Ajmone-Cat, M.A., Gasparini, L., Ongini, E. & Minghetti, L. (2005). Nuclear receptor peroxisome proliferator-activated receptor-gamma is activated in rat microglial cells by the anti-inflammatory drug HCT1026, a derivative of flurbiprofen. *J Neurochem,* Vol.92, No.4, pp. 895-903

Bialecka, M., Kurzawski, M., Klodowska-Duda, G., Opala, G., Juzwiak, S., Kurzawski, G., Tan, E.K. & Drozdzik, M. (2007). CARD15 variants in patients with sporadic Parkinson's disease. *Neurosci Res,* Vol.57, No.3, pp. 473-476

Blandini, F., Levandis, G., Bazzini, E., Nappi, G. & Armentero, M.T. (2007). Time-course of nigrostriatal damage, basal ganglia metabolic changes and behavioural alterations following intrastriatal injection of 6-hydroxydopamine in the rat: new clues from an old model. *Eur J Neurosci,* Vol.25, No.2, pp. 397-405

Block, M.L. & Hong, J.S. (2005). Microglia and inflammation-mediated neurodegeneration: multiple triggers with a common mechanism. *Prog Neurobiol,* Vol.76, No.2, pp. 77-98

Block, M.L., Zecca, L. & Hong, J.S. (2007). Microglia-mediated neurotoxicity: uncovering the molecular mechanisms. *Nat Rev Neurosci,* Vol.8, No.1, pp. 57-69

Boireau, A., Bordier, F., Dubedat, P., Peny, C. & Imperato, A. (1997). Thalidomide reduces MPTP-induced decrease in striatal dopamine levels in mice. *Neurosci Lett,* Vol.234, No.2-3, pp. 123-126

Boka, G., Anglade, P., Wallach, D., Javoy-Agid, F., Agid, Y. & Hirsch, E.C. (1994). Immunocytochemical analysis of tumor necrosis factor and its receptors in Parkinson's disease. *Neurosci Lett,* Vol.172, No.1-2, pp. 151-154

Bove, J., Prou, D., Perier, C. & Przedborski, S. (2005). Toxin-induced models of Parkinson's disease. *NeuroRx,* Vol.2, No.3, pp. 484-494

Braak, H., Del Tredici, K., Rub, U., de Vos, R.A., Jansen Steur, E.N. & Braak, E. (2003). Staging of brain pathology related to sporadic Parkinson's disease. *Neurobiol Aging,* Vol.24, No.2, pp. 197-211

Brochard, V., Combadiere, B., Prigent, A., Laouar, Y., Perrin, A., Beray-Berthat, V., Bonduelle, O., Alvarez-Fischer, D., Callebert, J., Launay, J.M., Duyckaerts, C., Flavell, R.A., Hirsch, E.C. & Hunot, S. (2009). Infiltration of CD4+ lymphocytes into the brain contributes to neurodegeneration in a mouse model of Parkinson disease. *J Clin Invest,* Vol.119, No.1, pp. 182-192

Brodacki, B., Staszewski, J., Toczylowska, B., Kozlowska, E., Drela, N., Chalimoniuk, M. & Stepien, A. (2008). Serum interleukin (IL-2, IL-10, IL-6, IL-4), TNFalpha, and INFgamma concentrations are elevated in patients with atypical and idiopathic parkinsonism. *Neurosci Lett,* Vol.441, No.2, pp. 158-162

Bronstein, D.M., Perez-Otano, I., Sun, V., Mullis Sawin, S.B., Chan, J., Wu, G.C., Hudson, P.M., Kong, L.Y., Hong, J.S. & McMillian, M.K. (1995). Glia-dependent neurotoxicity and neuroprotection in mesencephalic cultures. *Brain Res,* Vol.704, No.1, pp. 112-116

Butt, A.M. (2011). ATP: A ubiquitous gliotransmitter integrating neuron-glial networks. *Semin Cell Dev Biol,* Vol.22, No.2, pp. 205-213

Calne, D.B. & Langston, J.W. (1983). Aetiology of Parkinson's disease. *Lancet,* Vol.2, No.8365-66, pp. 1457-1459

Carson, M.J., Reilly, C.R., Sutcliffe, J.G. & Lo, D. (1998). Mature microglia resemble immature antigen-presenting cells. *Glia,* Vol.22, No.1, pp. 72-85

Carvey, P.M., Chang, Q., Lipton, J.W. & Ling, Z. (2003). Prenatal exposure to the bacteriotoxin lipopolysaccharide leads to long-term losses of dopamine neurons in offspring: a potential, new model of Parkinson's disease. *Front Biosci,* Vol.8, No., pp. s826-837

Castano, A., Herrera, A.J., Cano, J. & Machado, A. (1998). Lipopolysaccharide intranigral injection induces inflammatory reaction and damage in nigrostriatal dopaminergic system. *J Neurochem,* Vol.70, No.4, pp. 1584-1592

Castano, A., Herrera, A.J., Cano, J. & Machado, A. (2002). The degenerative effect of a single intranigral injection of LPS on the dopaminergic system is prevented by dexamethasone, and not mimicked by rh-TNF-alpha, IL-1beta and IFN-gamma. *J Neurochem,* Vol.81, No.1, pp. 150-157

Chao, C.C., Hu, S., Molitor, T.W., Shaskan, E.G. & Peterson, P.K. (1992). Activated microglia mediate neuronal cell injury via a nitric oxide mechanism. *J Immunol,* Vol.149, No.8, pp. 2736-2741

Chaturvedi, R.K. & Beal, M.F. (2008). PPAR: a therapeutic target in Parkinson's disease. *J Neurochem,* Vol.106, No.2, pp. 506-518

Chauveau, F., Boutin, H., Van Camp, N., Dolle, F. & Tavitian, B. (2008). Nuclear imaging of neuroinflammation: a comprehensive review of [11C]PK11195 challengers. *Eur J Nucl Med Mol Imaging,* Vol.35, No.12, pp. 2304-2319

Chen, H., Jacobs, E., Schwarzschild, M.A., McCullough, M.L., Calle, E.E., Thun, M.J. & Ascherio, A. (2005). Nonsteroidal antiinflammatory drug use and the risk for Parkinson's disease. *Ann Neurol,* Vol.58, No.6, pp. 963-967

Chen, H., O'Reilly, E.J., Schwarzschild, M.A. & Ascherio, A. (2008). Peripheral inflammatory biomarkers and risk of Parkinson's disease. *Am J Epidemiol,* Vol.167, No.1, pp. 90-95

Chen, H., Zhang, S.M., Hernan, M.A., Schwarzschild, M.A., Willett, W.C., Colditz, G.A., Speizer, F.E. & Ascherio, A. (2003). Nonsteroidal anti-inflammatory drugs and the risk of Parkinson disease. *Arch Neurol,* Vol.60, No.8, pp. 1059-1064

Chen, X., Lan, X., Roche, I., Liu, R. & Geiger, J.D. (2008). Caffeine protects against MPTP-induced blood-brain barrier dysfunction in mouse striatum. *J Neurochem,* Vol.107, No.4, pp. 1147-1157

Chung, J.H., Seo, A.Y., Chung, S.W., Kim, M.K., Leeuwenburgh, C., Yu, B.P. & Chung, H.Y. (2008). Molecular mechanism of PPAR in the regulation of age-related inflammation. *Ageing Res Rev,* Vol.7, No.2, pp. 126-136

Chung, Y.C., Ko, H.W., Bok, E., Park, E.S., Huh, S.H., Nam, J.H. & Jin, B.K. (2010). The role of neuroinflammation on the pathogenesis of Parkinson's disease. *BMB Rep,* Vol.43, No.4, pp. 225-232

Cicchetti, F., Brownell, A.L., Williams, K., Chen, Y.I., Livni, E. & Isacson, O. (2002). Neuroinflammation of the nigrostriatal pathway during progressive 6-OHDA dopamine degeneration in rats monitored by immunohistochemistry and PET imaging. *Eur J Neurosci,* Vol.15, No.6, pp. 991-998

Comi, G., Cohen, J.A., Arnold, D.L., Wynn, D. & Filippi, M. (2011). Phase III dose-comparison study of glatiramer acetate for multiple sclerosis. *Ann Neurol,* Vol.69, No.1, pp. 75-82

Crotty, S., Fitzgerald, P., Tuohy, E., Harris, D.M., Fisher, A., Mandel, A., Bolton, A.E., Sullivan, A.M. & Nolan, Y. (2008). Neuroprotective effects of novel phosphatidylglycerol-based phospholipids in the 6-hydroxydopamine model of Parkinson's disease. *Eur J Neurosci,* Vol.27, No.2, pp. 294-300

Cuadros, M.A. & Navascues, J. (1998). The origin and differentiation of microglial cells during development. *Prog Neurobiol,* Vol.56, No.2, pp. 173-189

Czlonkowska, A., Kohutnicka, M., Kurkowska-Jastrzebska, I. & Czlonkowski, A. (1996). Microglial reaction in MPTP (1-methyl-4-phenyl-1,2,3,6-tetrahydropyridine) induced Parkinson's disease mice model. *Neurodegeneration,* Vol.5, No.2, pp. 137-143

Dantzer, R. (2009). Cytokine, sickness behavior, and depression. *Immunol Allergy Clin North Am,* Vol.29, No.2, pp. 247-264

Davalos, D., Grutzendler, J., Yang, G., Kim, J.V., Zuo, Y., Jung, S., Littman, D.R., Dustin, M.L. & Gan, W.B. (2005). ATP mediates rapid microglial response to local brain injury in vivo. *Nat Neurosci,* Vol.8, No.6, pp. 752-758

Dehmer, T., Heneka, M.T., Sastre, M., Dichgans, J. & Schulz, J.B. (2004). Protection by pioglitazone in the MPTP model of Parkinson's disease correlates with I kappa B alpha induction and block of NF kappa B and iNOS activation. *J Neurochem,* Vol.88, No.2, pp. 494-501

Dehmer, T., Lindenau, J., Haid, S., Dichgans, J. & Schulz, J.B. (2000). Deficiency of inducible nitric oxide synthase protects against MPTP toxicity in vivo. *J Neurochem,* Vol.74, No.5, pp. 2213-2216

del Rio Hortega, P. (1932). *Microglia.* In: Penfield, W. (Ed.), Cytology and cellular pathology of the nervous system. Hoeber, New York, pp. 481-534.

Delgado, M. & Ganea, D. (2003). Neuroprotective effect of vasoactive intestinal peptide (VIP) in a mouse model of Parkinson's disease by blocking microglial activation. *FASEB J,* Vol.17, No.8, pp. 944-946

Depino, A.M., Earl, C., Kaczmarczyk, E., Ferrari, C., Besedovsky, H., del Rey, A., Pitossi, F.J. & Oertel, W.H. (2003). Microglial activation with atypical proinflammatory cytokine expression in a rat model of Parkinson's disease. *Eur J Neurosci,* Vol.18, No.10, pp. 2731-2742

Deumens, R., Blokland, A. & Prickaerts, J. (2002). Modeling Parkinson's disease in rats: an evaluation of 6-OHDA lesions of the nigrostriatal pathway. *Exp Neurol,* Vol.175, No.2, pp. 303-317

Di Matteo, V., Pierucci, M., Di Giovanni, G., Di Santo, A., Poggi, A., Benigno, A. & Esposito, E. (2006). Aspirin protects striatal dopaminergic neurons from neurotoxin-induced degeneration: an in vivo microdialysis study. *Brain Res,* Vol.1095, No.1, pp. 167-177

Di Monte, D.A. (2003). The environment and Parkinson's disease: is the nigrostriatal system preferentially targeted by neurotoxins? *Lancet Neurol,* Vol.2, No.9, pp. 531-538

Dick, F.D. (2006). Parkinson's disease and pesticide exposures. *Br Med Bull,* Vol.79-80, No.1, pp. 219-231

Diguet, E., Fernagut, P.O., Wei, X., Du, Y., Rouland, R., Gross, C., Bezard, E. & Tison, F. (2004). Deleterious effects of minocycline in animal models of Parkinson's disease and Huntington's disease. *Eur J Neurosci,* Vol.19, No.12, pp. 3266-3276

Dobbs, R.J., Charlett, A., Purkiss, A.G., Dobbs, S.M., Weller, C. & Peterson, D.W. (1999). Association of circulating TNF-alpha and IL-6 with ageing and parkinsonism. *Acta Neurol Scand,* Vol.100, No.1, pp. 34-41

Dolle, F., Luus, C., Reynolds, A. & Kassiou, M. (2009). Radiolabelled molecules for imaging the translocator protein (18 kDa) using positron emission tomography. *Curr Med Chem,* Vol.16, No.22, pp. 2899-2923

Du, Y., Ma, Z., Lin, S., Dodel, R.C., Gao, F., Bales, K.R., Triarhou, L.C., Chernet, E., Perry, K.W., Nelson, D.L., Luecke, S., Phebus, L.A., Bymaster, F.P. & Paul, S.M. (2001). Minocycline prevents nigrostriatal dopaminergic neurodegeneration in the MPTP model of Parkinson's disease. *Proc Natl Acad Sci U S A,* Vol.98, No.25, pp. 14669-14674

Eder, C., Schilling, T., Heinemann, U., Haas, D., Hailer, N. & Nitsch, R. (1999). Morphological, immunophenotypical and electrophysiological properties of resting microglia in vitro. *Eur J Neurosci,* Vol.11, No.12, pp. 4251-4261

Faucheux, B.A., Bonnet, A.M., Agid, Y. & Hirsch, E.C. (1999). Blood vessels change in the mesencephalon of patients with Parkinson's disease. *Lancet,* Vol.353, No.9157, pp. 981-982

Ferger, B., Leng, A., Mura, A., Hengerer, B. & Feldon, J. (2004). Genetic ablation of tumor necrosis factor-alpha (TNF-alpha) and pharmacological inhibition of TNF-synthesis attenuates MPTP toxicity in mouse striatum. *J Neurochem,* Vol.89, No.4, pp. 822-833

Ferrari, C.C., Pott Godoy, M.C., Tarelli, R., Chertoff, M., Depino, A.M. & Pitossi, F.J. (2006). Progressive neurodegeneration and motor disabilities induced by chronic expression of IL-1beta in the substantia nigra. *Neurobiol Dis,* Vol.24, No.1, pp. 183-193

Ferrari, C.C. & Tarelli, R. (2011). Parkinson's disease and systemic inflammation. *Parkinsons Dis,* Vol.2011, No., pp. 436813

Fiszer, U., Mix, E., Fredrikson, S., Kostulas, V., Olsson, T. & Link, H. (1994). gamma delta+ T cells are increased in patients with Parkinson's disease. *J Neurol Sci,* Vol.121, No.1, pp. 39-45

Francis, J.W., Von Visger, J., Markelonis, G.J. & Oh, T.H. (1995). Neuroglial responses to the dopaminergic neurotoxicant 1-methyl-4-phenyl-1,2,3,6-tetrahydropyridine in mouse striatum. *Neurotoxicol Teratol,* Vol.17, No.1, pp. 7-12

Gagne, J.J. & Power, M.C. (2010). Anti-inflammatory drugs and risk of Parkinson disease: a meta-analysis. *Neurology,* Vol.74, No.12, pp. 995-1002

Gao, H.M. & Hong, J.S. (2008). Why neurodegenerative diseases are progressive: uncontrolled inflammation drives disease progression. *Trends Immunol,* Vol.29, No.8, pp. 357-365

Gao, H.M., Liu, B., Zhang, W. & Hong, J.S. (2003). Critical role of microglial NADPH oxidase-derived free radicals in the in vitro MPTP model of Parkinson's disease. *FASEB J,* Vol.17, No.13, pp. 1954-1956

Gao, X., Chen, H., Schwarzschild, M.A. & Ascherio, A. (2011). Use of ibuprofen and risk of Parkinson disease. *Neurology,* Vol.76, No.10, pp. 863-869

Garden, G.A. & Moller, T. (2006). Microglia biology in health and disease. *J Neuroimmune Pharmacol,* Vol.1, No.2, pp. 127-137

Gauss, K.A., Nelson-Overton, L.K., Siemsen, D.W., Gao, Y., DeLeo, F.R. & Quinn, M.T. (2007). Role of NF-kappaB in transcriptional regulation of the phagocyte NADPH oxidase by tumor necrosis factor-alpha. *J Leukoc Biol,* Vol.82, No.3, pp. 729-741

Gayle, D.A., Ling, Z., Tong, C., Landers, T., Lipton, J.W. & Carvey, P.M. (2002). Lipopolysaccharide (LPS)-induced dopamine cell loss in culture: roles of tumor necrosis factor-alpha, interleukin-1beta, and nitric oxide. *Brain Res Dev Brain Res,* Vol.133, No.1, pp. 27-35

Gerhard, A., Pavese, N., Hotton, G., Turkheimer, F., Es, M., Hammers, A., Eggert, K., Oertel, W., Banati, R.B. & Brooks, D.J. (2006). In vivo imaging of microglial activation with [11C](R)-PK11195 PET in idiopathic Parkinson's disease. *Neurobiol Dis,* Vol.21, No.2, pp. 404-412

Ghosh, A., Roy, A., Liu, X., Kordower, J.H., Mufson, E.J., Hartley, D.M., Ghosh, S., Mosley, R.L., Gendelman, H.E. & Pahan, K. (2007). Selective inhibition of NF-kappaB activation prevents dopaminergic neuronal loss in a mouse model of Parkinson's disease. *Proc Natl Acad Sci U S A,* Vol.104, No.47, pp. 18754-18759

Gibbons, H.M. & Dragunow, M. (2006). Microglia induce neural cell death via a proximity-dependent mechanism involving nitric oxide. *Brain Res,* Vol.1084, No.1, pp. 1-15

Graeber, M.B. & Streit, W.J. (2010). Microglia: biology and pathology. *Acta Neuropathol,* Vol.119, No.1, pp. 89-105

Grilli, M., Pizzi, M., Memo, M. & Spano, P. (1996). Neuroprotection by aspirin and sodium salicylate through blockade of NF-kappaB activation. *Science,* Vol.274, No.5291, pp. 1383-1385

Hancock, D.B., Martin, E.R., Stajich, J.M., Jewett, R., Stacy, M.A., Scott, B.L., Vance, J.M. & Scott, W.K. (2007). Smoking, caffeine, and nonsteroidal anti-inflammatory drugs in families with Parkinson disease. *Arch Neurol,* Vol.64, No.4, pp. 576-580

Hanisch, U.K. (2002). Microglia as a source and target of cytokines. *Glia,* Vol.40, No.2, pp. 140-155

He, Y., Appel, S. & Le, W. (2001). Minocycline inhibits microglial activation and protects nigral cells after 6-hydroxydopamine injection into mouse striatum. *Brain Res,* Vol.909, No.1-2, pp. 187-193

Hernan, M.A., Logroscino, G. & Garcia Rodriguez, L.A. (2006). Nonsteroidal anti-inflammatory drugs and the incidence of Parkinson disease. *Neurology,* Vol.66, No.7, pp. 1097-1099

Herrera, A.J., Castano, A., Venero, J.L., Cano, J. & Machado, A. (2000). The single intranigral injection of LPS as a new model for studying the selective effects of inflammatory reactions on dopaminergic system. *Neurobiol Dis,* Vol.7, No.4, pp. 429-447

Hirsch, E.C., Hoglinger, G., Rousselet, E., Breidert, T., Parain, K., Feger, J., Ruberg, M., Prigent, A., Cohen-Salmon, C. & Launay, J.M. (2003). Animal models of Parkinson's disease in rodents induced by toxins: an update. *J Neural Transm Suppl,* Vol.65, No., pp. 89-100

Hirsch, E.C. & Hunot, S. (2009). Neuroinflammation in Parkinson's disease: a target for neuroprotection? *Lancet Neurol,* Vol.8, No.4, pp. 382-397

Hunot, S., Boissiere, F., Faucheux, B., Brugg, B., Mouatt-Prigent, A., Agid, Y. & Hirsch, E.C. (1996). Nitric oxide synthase and neuronal vulnerability in Parkinson's disease. *Neuroscience,* Vol.72, No.2, pp. 355-363

Hunot, S., Brugg, B., Ricard, D., Michel, P.P., Muriel, M.P., Ruberg, M., Faucheux, B.A., Agid, Y. & Hirsch, E.C. (1997). Nuclear translocation of NF-kappaB is increased in dopaminergic neurons of patients with parkinson disease. *Proc Natl Acad Sci U S A,* Vol.94, No.14, pp. 7531-7536

Hunter, R.L., Dragicevic, N., Seifert, K., Choi, D.Y., Liu, M., Kim, H.C., Cass, W.A., Sullivan, P.G. & Bing, G. (2007). Inflammation induces mitochondrial dysfunction and dopaminergic neurodegeneration in the nigrostriatal system. *J Neurochem,* Vol.100, No.5, pp. 1375-1386

Imamura, K., Hishikawa, N., Sawada, M., Nagatsu, T., Yoshida, M. & Hashizume, Y. (2003). Distribution of major histocompatibility complex class II-positive microglia and cytokine profile of Parkinson's disease brains. *Acta Neuropathol,* Vol.106, No.6, pp. 518-526

Jack, C.S., Arbour, N., Manusow, J., Montgrain, V., Blain, M., McCrea, E., Shapiro, A. & Antel, J.P. (2005). TLR signaling tailors innate immune responses in human microglia and astrocytes. *J Immunol,* Vol.175, No.7, pp. 4320-4330

Jang, H., Boltz, D., Sturm-Ramirez, K., Shepherd, K.R., Jiao, Y., Webster, R. & Smeyne, R.J. (2009b). Highly pathogenic H5N1 influenza virus can enter the central nervous system and induce neuroinflammation and neurodegeneration. *Proc Natl Acad Sci U S A,* Vol.106, No.33, pp. 14063-14068

Jang, H., Boltz, D.A., Webster, R.G. & Smeyne, R.J. (2009a). Viral parkinsonism. *Biochim Biophys Acta,* Vol.1792, No.7, pp. 714-721

Jenner, P. (2003). Oxidative stress in Parkinson's disease. *Ann Neurol,* Vol.53 Suppl 3, No., pp. S26-36; discussion S36-28

Johnston, L.C., Su, X., Maguire-Zeiss, K., Horovitz, K., Ankoudinova, I., Guschin, D., Hadaczek, P., Federoff, H.J., Bankiewicz, K. & Forsayeth, J. (2008). Human interleukin-10 gene transfer is protective in a rat model of Parkinson's disease. *Mol Ther,* Vol.16, No.8, pp. 1392-1399

Kettenmann, H., Banati, R. & Walz, W. (1993). Electrophysiological behavior of microglia. *Glia,* Vol.7, No.1, pp. 93-101

Kim, H.J., Hawke, N. & Baldwin, A.S. (2006). NF-kappaB and IKK as therapeutic targets in cancer. *Cell Death Differ,* Vol.13, No.5, pp. 738-747

Kim, H.S. & Suh, Y.H. (2009). Minocycline and neurodegenerative diseases. *Behav Brain Res,* Vol.196, No.2, pp. 168-179

Kim, S.U. & de Vellis, J. (2005). Microglia in health and disease. *J Neurosci Res,* Vol.81, No.3, pp. 302-313

Kim, W.G., Mohney, R.P., Wilson, B., Jeohn, G.H., Liu, B. & Hong, J.S. (2000). Regional difference in susceptibility to lipopolysaccharide-induced neurotoxicity in the rat brain: role of microglia. *J Neurosci,* Vol.20, No.16, pp. 6309-6316

Kim, Y.S., Choi, D.H., Block, M.L., Lorenzl, S., Yang, L., Kim, Y.J., Sugama, S., Cho, B.P., Hwang, O., Browne, S.E., Kim, S.Y., Hong, J.S., Beal, M.F. & Joh, T.H. (2007). A pivotal role of matrix metalloproteinase-3 activity in dopaminergic neuronal degeneration via microglial activation. *FASEB J,* Vol.21, No.1, pp. 179-187

Kim, Y.S., Kim, S.S., Cho, J.J., Choi, D.H., Hwang, O., Shin, D.H., Chun, H.S., Beal, M.F. & Joh, T.H. (2005). Matrix metalloproteinase-3: a novel signaling proteinase from apoptotic neuronal cells that activates microglia. *J Neurosci,* Vol.25, No.14, pp. 3701-3711

Kirik, D., Rosenblad, C. & Bjorklund, A. (1998). Characterization of behavioral and neurodegenerative changes following partial lesions of the nigrostriatal dopamine system induced by intrastriatal 6-hydroxydopamine in the rat. *Exp Neurol,* Vol.152, No.2, pp. 259-277

Knott, C., Stern, G. & Wilkin, G.P. (2000). Inflammatory regulators in Parkinson's disease: iNOS, lipocortin-1, and cyclooxygenases-1 and -2. *Mol Cell Neurosci,* Vol.16, No.6, pp. 724-739

Kohutnicka, M., Lewandowska, E., Kurkowska-Jastrzebska, I., Czlonkowski, A. & Czlonkowska, A. (1998). Microglial and astrocytic involvement in a murine model of Parkinson's disease induced by 1-methyl-4-phenyl-1,2,3,6-tetrahydropyridine (MPTP). *Immunopharmacology,* Vol.39, No.3, pp. 167-180

Konsman, J.P., Parnet, P. & Dantzer, R. (2002). Cytokine-induced sickness behaviour: mechanisms and implications. *Trends Neurosci,* Vol.25, No.3, pp. 154-159

Kopp, E. & Ghosh, S. (1994). Inhibition of NF-kappa B by sodium salicylate and aspirin. *Science,* Vol.265, No.5174, pp. 956-959

Koprich, J.B., Reske-Nielsen, C., Mithal, P. & Isacson, O. (2008). Neuroinflammation mediated by IL-1beta increases susceptibility of dopamine neurons to degeneration in an animal model of Parkinson's disease. *J Neuroinflammation,* Vol.5, No., pp. 8

Kortekaas, R., Leenders, K.L., van Oostrom, J.C., Vaalburg, W., Bart, J., Willemsen, A.T. & Hendrikse, N.H. (2005). Blood-brain barrier dysfunction in parkinsonian midbrain in vivo. *Ann Neurol,* Vol.57, No.2, pp. 176-179

Kurkowska-Jastrzebska, I., Babiuch, M., Joniec, I., Przybylkowski, A., Czlonkowski, A. & Czlonkowska, A. (2002). Indomethacin protects against neurodegeneration caused by MPTP intoxication in mice. *Int Immunopharmacol,* Vol.2, No.8, pp. 1213-1218

Kurkowska-Jastrzebska, I., Litwin, T., Joniec, I., Ciesielska, A., Przybylkowski, A., Czlonkowski, A. & Czlonkowska, A. (2004). Dexamethasone protects against dopaminergic neurons damage in a mouse model of Parkinson's disease. *Int Immunopharmacol,* Vol.4, No.10-11, pp. 1307-1318

Ladeby, R., Wirenfeldt, M., Garcia-Ovejero, D., Fenger, C., Dissing-Olesen, L., Dalmau, I. & Finsen, B. (2005). Microglial cell population dynamics in the injured adult central nervous system. *Brain Res Brain Res Rev,* Vol.48, No.2, pp. 196-206

Langston, J.W., Ballard, P., Tetrud, J.W. & Irwin, I. (1983). Chronic Parkinsonism in humans due to a product of meperidine-analog synthesis. *Science,* Vol.219, No.4587, pp. 979-980

Langston, J.W. & Ballard, P.A., Jr. (1983). Parkinson's disease in a chemist working with 1-methyl-4-phenyl-1,2,5,6-tetrahydropyridine. *N Engl J Med,* Vol.309, No.5, pp. 310

Langston, J.W., Forno, L.S., Tetrud, J., Reeves, A.G., Kaplan, J.A. & Karluk, D. (1999). Evidence of active nerve cell degeneration in the substantia nigra of humans years after 1-methyl-4-phenyl-1,2,3,6-tetrahydropyridine exposure. *Ann Neurol,* Vol.46, No.4, pp. 598-605

Leng, A., Mura, A., Feldon, J. & Ferger, B. (2005). Tumor necrosis factor-alpha receptor ablation in a chronic MPTP mouse model of Parkinson's disease. *Neurosci Lett,* Vol.375, No.2, pp. 107-111

Liberatore, G.T., Jackson-Lewis, V., Vukosavic, S., Mandir, A.S., Vila, M., McAuliffe, W.G., Dawson, V.L., Dawson, T.M. & Przedborski, S. (1999). Inducible nitric oxide synthase stimulates dopaminergic neurodegeneration in the MPTP model of Parkinson disease. *Nat Med,* Vol.5, No.12, pp. 1403-1409

Ling, Z., Gayle, D.A., Ma, S.Y., Lipton, J.W., Tong, C.W., Hong, J.S. & Carvey, P.M. (2002). In utero bacterial endotoxin exposure causes loss of tyrosine hydroxylase neurons in the postnatal rat midbrain. *Mov Disord,* Vol.17, No.1, pp. 116-124

Ling, Z., Zhu, Y., Tong, C., Snyder, J.A., Lipton, J.W. & Carvey, P.M. (2006). Progressive dopamine neuron loss following supra-nigral lipopolysaccharide (LPS) infusion into rats exposed to LPS prenatally. *Exp Neurol,* Vol.199, No.2, pp. 499-512

Ling, Z.D., Chang, Q., Lipton, J.W., Tong, C.W., Landers, T.M. & Carvey, P.M. (2004). Combined toxicity of prenatal bacterial endotoxin exposure and postnatal 6-hydroxydopamine in the adult rat midbrain. *Neuroscience,* Vol.124, No.3, pp. 619-628

Long-Smith, C.M., Collins, L., Toulouse, A., Sullivan, A.M. & Nolan, Y.M. (2010). Interleukin-1beta contributes to dopaminergic neuronal death induced by lipopolysaccharide-stimulated rat glia in vitro. *J Neuroimmunol,* Vol.226, No.1-2, pp. 20-26

Long-Smith, C.M., Sullivan, A.M. & Nolan, Y.M. (2009). The influence of microglia on the pathogenesis of Parkinson's disease. *Prog Neurobiol,* Vol.89, No.3, pp. 277-287

Lyons, A., Downer, E.J., Crotty, S., Nolan, Y.M., Mills, K.H. & Lynch, M.A. (2007). CD200 ligand receptor interaction modulates microglial activation in vivo and in vitro: a role for IL-4. *J Neurosci,* Vol.27, No.31, pp. 8309-8313

McCoy, M.K., Martinez, T.N., Ruhn, K.A., Szymkowski, D.E., Smith, C.G., Botterman, B.R., Tansey, K.E. & Tansey, M.G. (2006). Blocking soluble tumor necrosis factor signaling with dominant-negative tumor necrosis factor inhibitor attenuates loss of dopaminergic neurons in models of Parkinson's disease. *J Neurosci,* Vol.26, No.37, pp. 9365-9375

McCoy, M.K., Ruhn, K.A., Martinez, T.N., McAlpine, F.E., Blesch, A. & Tansey, M.G. (2008). Intranigral lentiviral delivery of dominant-negative TNF attenuates neurodegeneration and behavioral deficits in hemiparkinsonian rats. *Mol Ther,* Vol.16, No.9, pp. 1572-1579

McGeer, E.G. & McGeer, P.L. (2007). The role of anti-inflammatory agents in Parkinson's disease. *CNS Drugs,* Vol.21, No.10, pp. 789-797

McGeer, P.L., Itagaki, S., Boyes, B.E. & McGeer, E.G. (1988). Reactive microglia are positive for HLA-DR in the substantia nigra of Parkinson's and Alzheimer's disease brains. *Neurology,* Vol.38, No.8, pp. 1285-1291

McGeer, P.L. & McGeer, E.G. (2004). Inflammation and the degenerative diseases of aging. *Ann N Y Acad Sci,* Vol.1035, No., pp. 104-116

McGeer, P.L., Schwab, C., Parent, A. & Doudet, D. (2003). Presence of reactive microglia in monkey substantia nigra years after 1-methyl-4-phenyl-1,2,3,6-tetrahydropyridine administration. *Ann Neurol,* Vol.54, No.5, pp. 599-604

McGettrick, A.F. & O'Neill, L.A. (2010). Regulators of TLR4 signaling by endotoxins. *Subcell Biochem,* Vol.53, No.1, pp. 153-171

Misra, U.K. & Kalita, J. (2010). Overview: Japanese encephalitis. *Prog Neurobiol,* Vol.91, No.2, pp. 108-120

Mitchell, J.A., Akarasereenont, P., Thiemermann, C., Flower, R.J. & Vane, J.R. (1993). Selectivity of nonsteroidal antiinflammatory drugs as inhibitors of constitutive and inducible cyclooxygenase. *Proc Natl Acad Sci U S A,* Vol.90, No.24, pp. 11693-11697

Mogi, M., Harada, M., Kondo, T., Riederer, P., Inagaki, H., Minami, M. & Nagatsu, T. (1994a). Interleukin-1 beta, interleukin-6, epidermal growth factor and transforming growth factor-alpha are elevated in the brain from parkinsonian patients. *Neurosci Lett,* Vol.180, No.2, pp. 147-150

Mogi, M., Harada, M., Riederer, P., Narabayashi, H., Fujita, K. & Nagatsu, T. (1994b). Tumor necrosis factor-alpha (TNF-alpha) increases both in the brain and in the cerebrospinal fluid from parkinsonian patients. *Neurosci Lett,* Vol.165, No.1-2, pp. 208-210

Mogi, M., Togari, A., Kondo, T., Mizuno, Y., Komure, O., Kuno, S., Ichinose, H. & Nagatsu, T. (2000). Caspase activities and tumor necrosis factor receptor R1 (p55) level are elevated in the substantia nigra from parkinsonian brain. *J Neural Transm,* Vol.107, No.3, pp. 335-341

Nadeau, S. & Rivest, S. (2003). Glucocorticoids play a fundamental role in protecting the brain during innate immune response. *J Neurosci,* Vol.23, No.13, pp. 5536-5544

Nakajima, K. & Kohsaka, S. (2001). Microglia: activation and their significance in the central nervous system. *J Biochem,* Vol.130, No.2, pp. 169-175

Nakamura, Y. (2002). Regulating factors for microglial activation. *Biol Pharm Bull,* Vol.25, No.8, pp. 945-953

Nimmerjahn, A., Kirchhoff, F. & Helmchen, F. (2005). Resting microglial cells are highly dynamic surveillants of brain parenchyma in vivo. *Science,* Vol.308, No.5726, pp. 1314-1318

NINDS-NET-PD-Investigators. (2006). A randomized, double-blind, futility clinical trial of creatine and minocycline in early Parkinson disease. *Neurology,* Vol.66, No.5, pp. 664-671

NINDS-NET-PD-Investigators. (2008). A pilot clinical trial of creatine and minocycline in early Parkinson disease: 18-month results. *Clin Neuropharmacol,* Vol.31, No.3, pp. 141-150

Nolan, Y., Maher, F.O., Martin, D.S., Clarke, R.M., Brady, M.T., Bolton, A.E., Mills, K.H. & Lynch, M.A. (2005). Role of interleukin-4 in regulation of age-related inflammatory changes in the hippocampus. *J Biol Chem,* Vol.280, No.10, pp. 9354-9362

O'Callaghan, J.P., Miller, D.B. & Reinhard, J.F., Jr. (1990). Characterization of the origins of astrocyte response to injury using the dopaminergic neurotoxicant, 1-methyl-4-phenyl-1,2,3,6-tetrahydropyridine. *Brain Res,* Vol.521, No.1-2, pp. 73-80

Ogata, A., Tashiro, K., Nukuzuma, S., Nagashima, K. & Hall, W.W. (1997). A rat model of Parkinson's disease induced by Japanese encephalitis virus. *J Neurovirol,* Vol.3, No.2, pp. 141-147

Ogata, A., Tashiro, K. & Pradhan, S. (2000). Parkinsonism due to predominant involvement of substantia nigra in Japanese encephalitis. *Neurology,* Vol.55, No.4, pp. 602

Orr, C.F., Rowe, D.B. & Halliday, G.M. (2002). An inflammatory review of Parkinson's disease. *Prog Neurobiol,* Vol.68, No.5, pp. 325-340

Ouchi, Y., Yagi, S., Yokokura, M. & Sakamoto, M. (2009). Neuroinflammation in the living brain of Parkinson's disease. *Parkinsonism Relat Disord,* Vol.15 Suppl 3, No., pp. S200-204

Pankratz, N. & Foroud, T. (2007). Genetics of Parkinson disease. *Genet Med,* Vol.9, No.12, pp. 801-811

Papadopoulos, V., Baraldi, M., Guilarte, T.R., Knudsen, T.B., Lacapere, J.J., Lindemann, P., Norenberg, M.D., Nutt, D., Weizman, A., Zhang, M.R. & Gavish, M. (2006). Translocator protein (18kDa): new nomenclature for the peripheral-type benzodiazepine receptor based on its structure and molecular function. *Trends Pharmacol Sci,* Vol.27, No.8, pp. 402-409

Park, C.H., Carboni, E., Wood, P.L. & Gee, K.W. (1996). Characterization of peripheral benzodiazepine type sites in a cultured murine BV-2 microglial cell line. *Glia,* Vol.16, No.1, pp. 65-70

Perry, V.H. (1998). A revised view of the central nervous system microenvironment and major histocompatibility complex class II antigen presentation. *J Neuroimmunol,* Vol.90, No.2, pp. 113-121

Perry, V.H. (2010). Contribution of systemic inflammation to chronic neurodegeneration. *Acta Neuropathol,* Vol.120, No.3, pp. 277-286

Perry, V.H., Cunningham, C. & Holmes, C. (2007). Systemic infections and inflammation affect chronic neurodegeneration. *Nat Rev Immunol,* Vol.7, No.2, pp. 161-167

Poser, C.M., Huntley, C.J. & Poland, J.D. (1969). Para-encephalitic parkinsonism. Report of an acute case due to coxsackie virus type B 2 and re-examination of the etiologic concepts of postencephalitic parkinsonism. *Acta Neurol Scand,* Vol.45, No.2, pp. 199-215

Pott Godoy, M.C., Tarelli, R., Ferrari, C.C., Sarchi, M.I. & Pitossi, F.J. (2008). Central and systemic IL-1 exacerbates neurodegeneration and motor symptoms in a model of Parkinson's disease. *Brain,* Vol.131, No.Pt 7, pp. 1880-1894

Pranzatelli, M.R., Mott, S.H., Pavlakis, S.G., Conry, J.A. & Tate, E.D. (1994). Clinical spectrum of secondary parkinsonism in childhood: a reversible disorder. *Pediatr Neurol,* Vol.10, No.2, pp. 131-140

Przedborski, S. & Vila, M. (2003). The 1-methyl-4-phenyl-1,2,3,6-tetrahydropyridine mouse model: a tool to explore the pathogenesis of Parkinson's disease. *Ann N Y Acad Sci,* Vol.991, No., pp. 189-198

Qian, L., Hong, J.S. & Flood, P.M. (2006). Role of microglia in inflammation-mediated degeneration of dopaminergic neurons: neuroprotective effect of interleukin 10. *J Neural Transm Suppl,* Vol., No.70, pp. 367-371

Qin, L., Wu, X., Block, M.L., Liu, Y., Breese, G.R., Hong, J.S., Knapp, D.J. & Crews, F.T. (2007). Systemic LPS causes chronic neuroinflammation and progressive neurodegeneration. *Glia,* Vol.55, No.5, pp. 453-462

Quinn, L.P., Crook, B., Hows, M.E., Vidgeon-Hart, M., Chapman, H., Upton, N., Medhurst, A.D. & Virley, D.J. (2008). The PPARgamma agonist pioglitazone is effective in the MPTP mouse model of Parkinson's disease through inhibition of monoamine oxidase B. *Br J Pharmacol,* Vol.154, No.1, pp. 226-233

Rail, D., Scholtz, C. & Swash, M. (1981). Post-encephalitic Parkinsonism: current experience. *J Neurol Neurosurg Psychiatry,* Vol.44, No.8, pp. 670-676

Raivich, G., Bohatschek, M., Kloss, C.U., Werner, A., Jones, L.L. & Kreutzberg, G.W. (1999). Neuroglial activation repertoire in the injured brain: graded response, molecular mechanisms and cues to physiological function. *Brain Res Brain Res Rev,* Vol.30, No.1, pp. 77-105

Ransohoff, R.M. & Cardona, A.E. (2010). The myeloid cells of the central nervous system parenchyma. *Nature,* Vol.468, No.7321, pp. 253-262

Ransohoff, R.M. & Perry, V.H. (2009). Microglial physiology: unique stimuli, specialized responses. *Annu Rev Immunol,* Vol.27, No., pp. 119-145

Reale, M., Iarlori, C., Thomas, A., Gambi, D., Perfetti, B., Di Nicola, M. & Onofrj, M. (2009). Peripheral cytokines profile in Parkinson's disease. *Brain Behav Immun,* Vol.23, No.1, pp. 55-63

Rentzos, M., Nikolaou, C., Andreadou, E., Paraskevas, G.P., Rombos, A., Zoga, M., Tsoutsou, A., Boufidou, F., Kapaki, E. & Vassilopoulos, D. (2007). Circulating interleukin-15 and RANTES chemokine in Parkinson's disease. *Acta Neurol Scand,* Vol.116, No.6, pp. 374-379

Robinson, R.L., Shahida, S., Madan, N., Rao, S. & Khardori, N. (2003). Transient parkinsonism in West Nile virus encephalitis. *Am J Med,* Vol.115, No.3, pp. 252-253

Samii, A., Etminan, M., Wiens, M.O. & Jafari, S. (2009). NSAID use and the risk of Parkinson's disease: systematic review and meta-analysis of observational studies. *Drugs Aging,* Vol.26, No.9, pp. 769-779

Sampaio, E.P., Sarno, E.N., Galilly, R., Cohn, Z.A. & Kaplan, G. (1991). Thalidomide selectively inhibits tumor necrosis factor alpha production by stimulated human monocytes. *J Exp Med,* Vol.173, No.3, pp. 699-703

Sanchez-Pernaute, R., Ferree, A., Cooper, O., Yu, M., Brownell, A.L. & Isacson, O. (2004). Selective COX-2 inhibition prevents progressive dopamine neuron degeneration in a rat model of Parkinson's disease. *J Neuroinflammation,* Vol.1, No.1, pp. 6

Santambrogio, L., Belyanskaya, S.L., Fischer, F.R., Cipriani, B., Brosnan, C.F., Ricciardi-Castagnoli, P., Stern, L.J., Strominger, J.L. & Riese, R. (2001). Developmental plasticity of CNS microglia. *Proc Natl Acad Sci U S A,* Vol.98, No.11, pp. 6295-6300

Sauer, H. & Oertel, W.H. (1994). Progressive degeneration of nigrostriatal dopamine neurons following intrastriatal terminal lesions with 6-hydroxydopamine: a combined retrograde tracing and immunocytochemical study in the rat. *Neuroscience,* Vol.59, No.2, pp. 401-415

Sawada, M., Imamura, K. & Nagatsu, T. (2006). Role of cytokines in inflammatory process in Parkinson's disease. *J Neural Transm Suppl,* Vol., No.70, pp. 373-381

Scheinman, R.I., Gualberto, A., Jewell, C.M., Cidlowski, J.A. & Baldwin, A.S., Jr. (1995). Characterization of mechanisms involved in transrepression of NF-kappa B by activated glucocorticoid receptors. *Mol Cell Biol,* Vol.15, No.2, pp. 943-953

Schintu, N., Frau, L., Ibba, M., Caboni, P., Garau, A., Carboni, E. & Carta, A.R. (2009). PPAR-gamma-mediated neuroprotection in a chronic mouse model of Parkinson's disease. *Eur J Neurosci,* Vol.29, No.5, pp. 954-963

Sedgwick, J.D., Schwender, S., Imrich, H., Dorries, R., Butcher, G.W. & ter Meulen, V. (1991). Isolation and direct characterization of resident microglial cells from the normal and inflamed central nervous system. *Proc Natl Acad Sci U S A,* Vol.88, No.16, pp. 7438-7442

Shan, S., Hong-Min, T., Yi, F., Jun-Peng, G., Yue, F., Yan-Hong, T., Yun-Ke, Y., Wen-Wei, L., Xiang-Yu, W., Jun, M., Guo-Hua, W., Ya-Ling, H., Hua-Wei, L. & Ding-Fang, C. (2011). NEW evidences for fractalkine/CX3CL1 involved in substantia nigral microglial activation and behavioral changes in a rat model of Parkinson's disease. *Neurobiol Aging,* Vol.32, No.3, pp. 443-458

Shoji, H., Watanabe, M., Itoh, S., Kuwahara, H. & Hattori, F. (1993). Japanese encephalitis and parkinsonism. *J Neurol,* Vol.240, No.1, pp. 59-60

Sian, J., Dexter, D.T., Lees, A.J., Daniel, S., Agid, Y., Javoy-Agid, F., Jenner, P. & Marsden, C.D. (1994). Alterations in glutathione levels in Parkinson's disease and other neurodegenerative disorders affecting basal ganglia. *Ann Neurol,* Vol.36, No.3, pp. 348-355

Smithells, R.W. & Newman, C.G. (1992). Recognition of thalidomide defects. *J Med Genet,* Vol.29, No.10, pp. 716-723

Sriram, K., Matheson, J.M., Benkovic, S.A., Miller, D.B., Luster, M.I. & O'Callaghan, J.P. (2006). Deficiency of TNF receptors suppresses microglial activation and alters the susceptibility of brain regions to MPTP-induced neurotoxicity: role of TNF-alpha. *FASEB J,* Vol.20, No.6, pp. 670-682

Stanic, D., Finkelstein, D.I., Bourke, D.W., Drago, J. & Horne, M.K. (2003). Timecourse of striatal re-innervation following lesions of dopaminergic SNpc neurons of the rat. *Eur J Neurosci,* Vol.18, No.5, pp. 1175-1188

Stephenson, D.T., Schober, D.A., Smalstig, E.B., Mincy, R.E., Gehlert, D.R. & Clemens, J.A. (1995). Peripheral benzodiazepine receptors are colocalized with activated microglia following transient global forebrain ischemia in the rat. *J Neurosci,* Vol.15, No.7 Pt 2, pp. 5263-5274

Stone, D.K., Reynolds, A.D., Mosley, R.L. & Gendelman, H.E. (2009). Innate and adaptive immunity for the pathobiology of Parkinson's disease. *Antioxid Redox Signal,* Vol.11, No.9, pp. 2151-2166

Stypula, G., Kunert-Radek, J., Stepien, H., Zylinska, K. & Pawlikowski, M. (1996). Evaluation of interleukins, ACTH, cortisol and prolactin concentrations in the blood of patients with parkinson's disease. *Neuroimmunomodulation,* Vol.3, No.2-3, pp. 131-134

Takahashi, M., Yamada, T., Nakajima, S., Nakajima, K., Yamamoto, T. & Okada, H. (1995). The substantia nigra is a major target for neurovirulent influenza A virus. *J Exp Med,* Vol.181, No.6, pp. 2161-2169

Tansey, M.G. & Goldberg, M.S. (2010). Neuroinflammation in Parkinson's disease: its role in neuronal death and implications for therapeutic intervention. *Neurobiol Dis,* Vol.37, No.3, pp. 510-518

Tansey, M.G., McCoy, M.K. & Frank-Cannon, T.C. (2007). Neuroinflammatory mechanisms in Parkinson's disease: potential environmental triggers, pathways, and targets for early therapeutic intervention. *Exp Neurol,* Vol.208, No.1, pp. 1-25

Teismann, P. & Ferger, B. (2001). Inhibition of the cyclooxygenase isoenzymes COX-1 and COX-2 provide neuroprotection in the MPTP-mouse model of Parkinson's disease. *Synapse,* Vol.39, No.2, pp. 167-174

Teismann, P., Tieu, K., Choi, D.K., Wu, D.C., Naini, A., Hunot, S., Vila, M., Jackson-Lewis, V. & Przedborski, S. (2003). Cyclooxygenase-2 is instrumental in Parkinson's disease neurodegeneration. *Proc Natl Acad Sci U S A,* Vol.100, No.9, pp. 5473-5478

Teo, B.H. & Wong, S.H. (2010). MHC class II-associated invariant chain (Ii) modulates dendritic cells-derived microvesicles (DCMV)-mediated activation of microglia. *Biochem Biophys Res Commun,* Vol.400, No.4, pp. 673-678

Tomas-Camardiel, M., Rite, I., Herrera, A.J., de Pablos, R.M., Cano, J., Machado, A. & Venero, J.L. (2004). Minocycline reduces the lipopolysaccharide-induced inflammatory reaction, peroxynitrite-mediated nitration of proteins, disruption of the blood-brain barrier, and damage in the nigral dopaminergic system. *Neurobiol Dis,* Vol.16, No.1, pp. 190-201

Tomiyama, H., Mizuta, I., Li, Y., Funayama, M., Yoshino, H., Li, L., Murata, M., Yamamoto, M., Kubo, S., Mizuno, Y., Toda, T. & Hattori, N. (2008). LRRK2 P755L variant in sporadic Parkinson's disease. *J Hum Genet,* Vol.53, No.11-12, pp. 1012-1015

Toulouse, A. & Sullivan, A.M. (2008). Progress in Parkinson's disease-where do we stand? *Prog Neurobiol,* Vol.85, No.4, pp. 376-392

Tse, W., Cersosimo, M.G., Gracies, J.M., Morgello, S., Olanow, C.W. & Koller, W. (2004). Movement disorders and AIDS: a review. *Parkinsonism Relat Disord,* Vol.10, No.6, pp. 323-334

Tweedie, D., Sambamurti, K. & Greig, N.H. (2007). TNF-alpha inhibition as a treatment strategy for neurodegenerative disorders: new drug candidates and targets. *Curr Alzheimer Res,* Vol.4, No.4, pp. 378-385

Walters, J.H. (1960). Postencephalitic Parkinson syndrome after meningoencephalitis due to coxsackie virus group B, type 2. *New England Journal of Medicine,* Vol.263, No.15, pp. 744-747

Wang, S., Yan, J.Y., Lo, Y.K., Carvey, P.M. & Ling, Z. (2009). Dopaminergic and serotoninergic deficiencies in young adult rats prenatally exposed to the bacterial lipopolysaccharide. *Brain Res,* Vol.1265, No., pp. 196-204

Wang, X.J., Zhang, S., Yan, Z.Q., Zhao, Y.X., Zhou, H.Y., Wang, Y., Lu, G.Q. & Zhang, J.D. (2011). Impaired CD200-CD200R-mediated microglia silencing enhances midbrain dopaminergic neurodegeneration: Roles of aging, superoxide, NADPH oxidase, and p38 MAPK. *Free Radic Biol Med,* Vol.50, No.9, pp. 1094-1106

Weller, C., Oxlade, N., Dobbs, S.M., Dobbs, R.J., Charlett, A. & Bjarnason, I.T. (2005). Role of inflammation in gastrointestinal tract in aetiology and pathogenesis of idiopathic parkinsonism. *FEMS Immunol Med Microbiol,* Vol.44, No.2, pp. 129-135

Wilms, H., Rosenstiel, P., Sievers, J., Deuschl, G., Zecca, L. & Lucius, R. (2003). Activation of microglia by human neuromelanin is NF-kappaB dependent and involves p38 mitogen-activated protein kinase: implications for Parkinson's disease. *FASEB J,* Vol.17, No.3, pp. 500-502

Wilms, H., Zecca, L., Rosenstiel, P., Sievers, J., Deuschl, G. & Lucius, R. (2007). Inflammation in Parkinson's diseases and other neurodegenerative diseases: cause and therapeutic implications. *Curr Pharm Des,* Vol.13, No.18, pp. 1925-1928

Winkeler, A., Boisgard, R., Martin, A. & Tavitian, B. (2010). Radioisotopic imaging of neuroinflammation. *J Nucl Med,* Vol.51, No.1, pp. 1-4

Wu, D.C., Jackson-Lewis, V., Vila, M., Tieu, K., Teismann, P., Vadseth, C., Choi, D.K., Ischiropoulos, H. & Przedborski, S. (2002). Blockade of microglial activation is neuroprotective in the 1-methyl-4-phenyl-1,2,3,6-tetrahydropyridine mouse model of Parkinson disease. *J Neurosci,* Vol.22, No.5, pp. 1763-1771

Wu, D.C., Teismann, P., Tieu, K., Vila, M., Jackson-Lewis, V., Ischiropoulos, H. & Przedborski, S. (2003). NADPH oxidase mediates oxidative stress in the 1-methyl-4-phenyl-1,2,3,6-tetrahydropyridine model of Parkinson's disease. *Proc Natl Acad Sci U S A,* Vol.100, No.10, pp. 6145-6150

Yamada, T., McGeer, P.L. & McGeer, E.G. (1992). Lewy bodies in Parkinson's disease are recognized by antibodies to complement proteins. *Acta Neuropathol,* Vol.84, No.1, pp. 100-104

Yang, L., Sugama, S., Chirichigno, J.W., Gregorio, J., Lorenzl, S., Shin, D.H., Browne, S.E., Shimizu, Y., Joh, T.H., Beal, M.F. & Albers, D.S. (2003). Minocycline enhances MPTP toxicity to dopaminergic neurons. *J Neurosci Res,* Vol.74, No.2, pp. 278-285

Yasuda, T., Fukuda-Tani, M., Nihira, T., Wada, K., Hattori, N., Mizuno, Y. & Mochizuki, H. (2007). Correlation between levels of pigment epithelium-derived factor and vascular endothelial growth factor in the striatum of patients with Parkinson's disease. *Exp Neurol,* Vol.206, No.2, pp. 308-317

Yirmiya, R., Winocur, G. & Goshen, I. (2002). Brain interleukin-1 is involved in spatial memory and passive avoidance conditioning. *Neurobiol Learn Mem,* Vol.78, No.2, pp. 379-389

Zalcman, S., Green-Johnson, J.M., Murray, L., Nance, D.M., Dyck, D., Anisman, H. & Greenberg, A.H. (1994). Cytokine-specific central monoamine alterations induced by interleukin-1, -2 and -6. *Brain Res,* Vol.643, No.1-2, pp. 40-49

Zhang, F., Qian, L., Flood, P.M., Shi, J.S., Hong, J.S. & Gao, H.M. (2010). Inhibition of IkappaB kinase-beta protects dopamine neurons against lipopolysaccharide-induced neurotoxicity. *J Pharmacol Exp Ther,* Vol.333, No.3, pp. 822-833

Zhang, W., Wang, T., Pei, Z., Miller, D.S., Wu, X., Block, M.L., Wilson, B., Zhou, Y., Hong, J.S. & Zhang, J. (2005). Aggregated alpha-synuclein activates microglia: a process leading to disease progression in Parkinson's disease. *FASEB J*, Vol.19, No.6, pp. 533-542

Zhou, Y., Su, Y., Li, B., Liu, F., Ryder, J.W., Wu, X., Gonzalez-DeWhitt, P.A., Gelfanova, V., Hale, J.E., May, P.C., Paul, S.M. & Ni, B. (2003). Nonsteroidal anti-inflammatory drugs can lower amyloidogenic Abeta42 by inhibiting Rho. *Science*, Vol.302, No.5648, pp. 1215-1217

23

Neurotensin as Modulator of Basal Ganglia-Thalamocortical Motor Circuit – Emerging Evidence for Neurotensin NTS_1 Receptor as a Potential Target in Parkinson's Disease

Luca Ferraro[1], Tiziana Antonelli[1], Sarah Beggiato[1], Maria Cristina Tomasini[1], Antonio Steardo[1], Kjell Fuxe[2] and Sergio Tanganelli[1]

[1]*Department of Clinical and Experimental Medicine, Section of Pharmacology, University of Ferrara, Italy and IRET Foundation, Ozzano Emilia, Bologna*

[2]*Department of Neuroscience, Karolinska Institute, Stockholm*

[1]*Italy*

[2]*Sweden*

1. Introduction

This chapter is focused on the putative role of neurotensin in the development of Parkinson's disease, a neurodegenerative disorder mainly characterized by a progressive loss of nigrostriatal dopaminergic neurons (Schimpff et al., 2001). Although a direct causal role of neurotensin in Parkinson's disease has not yet clearly demonstrated, some convincing animal and human studies support the potential role of the peptide in the etiopathogenesis of this motor disorder. Special emphasis is placed on the significance that neurotensin plays on basal ganglia neuroplasticity and neurodegeneration. This is mainly supported by recent findings clearly demonstrating that neurotensin enhances glutamate excitotoxicity in mesencephalic dopamine neurons and that neurotensin receptors are involved in the modulation of NMDA-induced excitotoxicity (Antonelli et al., 2002; 2004). Through these mechanisms neurotensin could contribute to the development and/or the progression of neurodegenerative disorders. The possible use of neurotensin receptor antagonists, in combination with conventional therapy, in the treatment of Parkinson's disease, is also discussed.

2. Basal ganglia

In Parkinson's disease, the degeneration of dopaminergic neurons in the substantia nigra pars compacta and the consequent striatal dopamine deficiency lead to a cascade of functional modifications in the activity of the basal ganglia-thalamocortical motor circuit, responsible for the motor disturbances characteristic of the pathology (Silkis, 2001). The basal ganglia are a collective group of structures, which include the neostriatum (caudate nucleus and putamen), the external and internal parts of the globus pallidus, the subthalamic nucleus, the substantia nigra pars reticulata and the substantia nigra pars compacta.

From a simplistic point of view, motor information coming from glutamatergic neurons located in several areas of the cerebral cortex, reach the striatum, which represents the primary input nucleus of the basal ganglia. These information, processed in the striatum, are transmitted by the so called "direct" and "indirect" pathways, to the main output nuclei of the basal ganglia (substantia nigra pars reticulata and the internal part of the globus pallidus; Fig. 1). The "indirect pathway" encompasses a trisynaptic link including *i)* GABAergic/enkephalinergic neurons, which connect the striatum to the external part of the globus pallidus; *ii)* the external part of the globus pallidus GABAergic neurons projecting to subthalamic nucleus and *iii)* glutamatergic subthalamic nucleus neurons, which project to the basal ganglia output structures (internal part of the globus pallidus/substantia nigra pars reticulata) and send collaterals to external part of the globus pallidus (Gerfen, 1992). On the other hand, the "direct" monosynaptic pathway consists of GABAergic neurons which directly connect the striatum to the main basal ganglia output structures (substantia nigra pars reticulata and the internal part of the globus pallidus). Outputs from these nuclei consist of inhibitory GABAergic neurons projecting to the ventral-anterior and ventrolateral nuclei of the thalamus which, through excitatory glutamatergic fibers, project back to the prefrontal and motor cortices. The differences in neuronal connectivity between the "direct" and "indirect" pathways show dissimilar functional consequences: the stimulation of the "direct pathway" inhibits substantia nigra pars reticulata and the internal part of the globus pallidus activity, thus leading to a disinhibition of thalamocortical neurons and a consequent facilitation of motor initiation. On the contrary, the stimulation of the "indirect pathway" produces motor inhibition. In spite of the model of the "direct" and "indirect" pathways is an oversimplification of the basal ganglia organization, it still represents the cornerstone for modern research on the basal ganglia functions (for review, Smith and Villalba, 2008).

Dopamine released by terminals of neurons located in substantia nigra pars compacta markedly affects the functional activity of the striatum. In the striatum dopamine D_1 and D_2 receptor subtypes are respectively expressed on the "direct" and "indirect" striatonigral pathways and modulate motor information (Gerfen, 2003). Although the degree of this anatomical separation of D_1 and D_2 receptors has been for a time a controversial topic, recent studies, using transgenic mice have confirmed that dopamine receptor subtypes have mainly a different expression on separate populations of GABAergic medium-spiny projection neurons (Wang et al., 2006; Galvan and Wichmann, 2008). Due to the different location of its receptor subtypes, striatal dopamine physiologically activates the "direct pathway" (D_1 receptors) and inhibits the "indirect pathway" (D_2), leading to an increase of thalamocortical motor drive (*see* above). In addition, striatal glutamate release from corticostriatal glutamatergic terminals is tonically inhibited by dopaminergic input coming from the substantia nigra pars compacta and activating dopamine D_2 heteroreceptors (Bamford et al., 2004). In this synaptic arrangement, dopamine depletion within the striatum not only removes tonic dopamine inhibitory control over corticostriatal glutamatergic drive, but also induces an imbalance between the "direct" and the "indirect" pathways (Fig. 1). In particular, this deficit produces an overactivity of the GABAergic projections from the striatum to the external part of the globus pallidus, leading to an excessive inhibition of thalamocortical and brainstem motor systems. From a pathological point of view, the hyperactivity of striatopallidal GABAergic neurons is considered one of the anomaly responsible for generation of motor parkinsonian symptoms. Pharmacological interventions

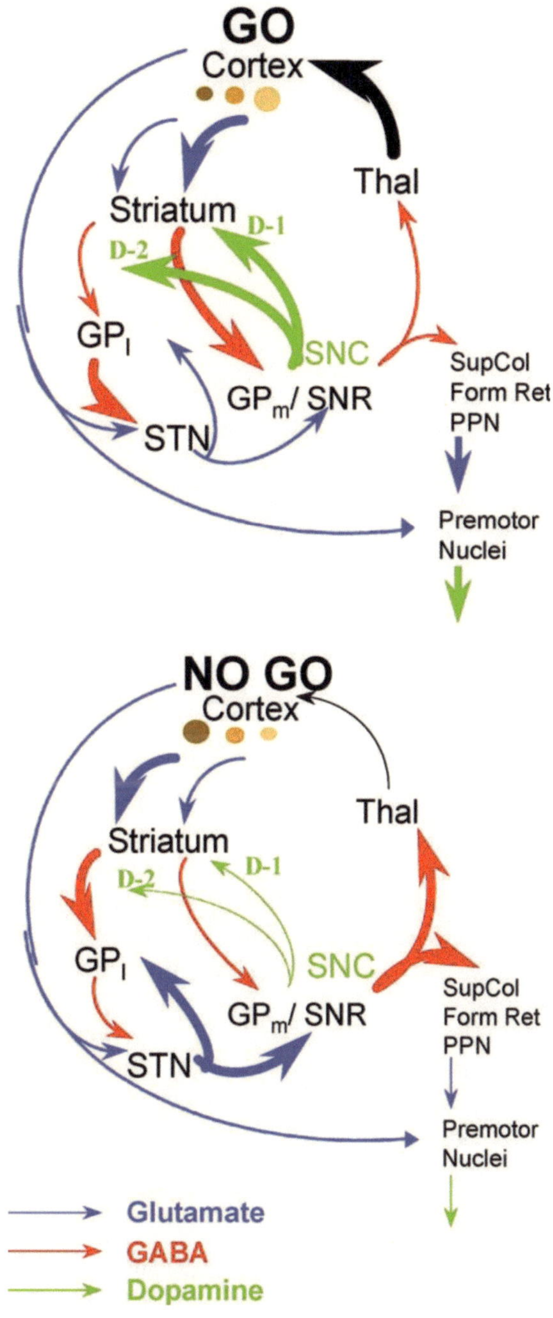

Fig. 1. The changes in the activity of basal ganglia circuits in normal state ('GO') vs Parkinson's Disease ('NO GO') are indicated. Heavy arrows, high activity; thin arrows, low activity. Abbreviations used: GP$_l$, globus pallidus, lateral; GP$_m$, globus pallidus, medial; SNC, Substantia nigra, zona compacta; SNR,Substantia nigra, zona reticulata; SupCol, Superior colliculus; Form Ret, formatio retucularis; PPN, Pedunculo pontine nucleus (from Tanganelli et al., 2004).

that can compensate for loss of dopamine and suppress the expression of motor symptoms in the pre-motor stages of Parkinson's disease are represented by the reduction of: *i)* the excitatory corticostriatal inputs that excite striatal output neurons of the "indirect pathway" or *ii)* the overactivity of striato-pallidal GABAergic neurons. The use of selective D_2 receptor agonist, A_{2A} adenosine receptor antagonism, blockade of GABA receptors in the external part of the globus pallidus or reduction of the excitatory NMDA receptor-mediated corticostriatal inputs, impinging upon striatal output neurons of the "indirect pathway", can be helpful for slowing progression of Parkinson's disease symptoms.

3. Neurotensin and its receptors

Neuropeptides represent undoubtedly one of the most common signaling molecules in the central nervous system. Accumulating evidence have implicated a vast number of neuropeptides and their receptors in the control of a wide range of physiological functions and pathological events, including neurodegenerative disorders.

Like all neuropeptides, neurotensin, an endogenous 13 amino acid peptide (Figure 2), is synthesized as part of a larger inactive precursor (Proneurotensin/neuromedin N).

Neurotensin tridecapeptide

pGlu-Leu-Tyr-Glu-Asn-Lys-Pro-Arg-Arg-Pro-Tyr-Ile-Leu-OH

Fig. 2. Sequence of neurotensin (modified from Ferraro et al., 2009).

The precursor molecule, a highly conserved polypeptide of 169-170 amino acid, contains one copy each of neurotensin and neuromedin N near the C-terminus and undergoes a differential tissue-specific cleavage at its four dibasic sites by proprotein convertases. Pro-neurotensin/neuromedin N may therefore be processed to generate different sets of peptides. Four biologically active products of Pro-neurotensin/neuromedin N processing have been described: neurotensin, neuromedin N, large neurotensin and large neuromedin N (Kitabgi, 2010). In the brain, Pro-neurotensin/neuromedin N processing mainly depends on proprotein convertase 2 activity and leads to high amounts of neurotensin and neuromedin N and small quantities of large neurotensin and large neuromedin N (Kitabgi, 2010). Using radioimmunoassay techniques, it has been demonstrated that the regional distribution of neurotensin and neuromedin N in brain tissues is, generally, the same. However, marked differences in the ratio of neurotensin over neuromedin N have been observed in different brain areas, being neurotensin generally more abundant in dopaminergic region such as substantia nigra pars compacta and ventral tegmental area.

Once processed as an active peptide in neurons, neurotensin is stored in dense core vesicles. The physiological inactivation of neurotensin is operated by endopeptidases belonging to the family of metallopeptidases, which act on primary cleavage sites in the peptide sequence: Arg8-Arg9, Pro10-Tyr11 and Tyr11-Ile12 bonds. Another mechanism that produces an inactivation of neurotensin transmission is the process of neurotensin internalization.

Neurotensin is widely expressed in nerve cells, fibers and terminals (Uhl, 1982; Emson et al., 1985) and exhibits diverse biological actions in the regulation of central nervous system functions of mammals, including man. The peptide is also highly expressed in the periphery, where it mainly acts as a modulator of the gastrointestinal and cardiovascular systems (Wang and Evers, 1999). Neurotensin was originally isolated and sequenced from bovine hypothalamus (Carraway and Leeman, 1973). Subsequent anatomical and functional studies have provided evidence that, in the brain, neurotensin behaves as neurotransmitter and/or neuromodulator (Nemeroff and Cain, 1985; Mendez et al., 1997). Neurotensin is released by neurons through sodium and calcium-dependent mechanisms. Once released, neurotensin produces its biological effects by interacting with three different receptor subtypes (NTS_1, NTS_2 and NTS_3/sortilin). The large distribution in the central nervous system of this family of membrane receptors explains the wide range of physiologic and pathologic effects mediated by the neuropeptide (Barroso et al., 2000). NTS_1 and NTS_2 receptors belong to the family of G-protein-coupled receptors with seven transmembrane domains, which share 60% homology. The NTS_1 receptor displays a high affinity for neurotensin, while NTS_2 receptor has a substantially lower affinity for the peptide and a high affinity to levocabastine, a histamine H_1 receptor antagonist (Chalon et al., 1996; Vincent et al., 1999). NTS_3/sortilin receptor is a single transmembrane protein located in intracellular vesicles of neurons and glia and appears involved in cell sorting and in tropism in cancer cells (Nouel et al., 1999; Mazella et al., 1998). NTS_1 receptor is coupled to a variety of signaling cascades, including production of inositol phosphates through activation of phospholipase C, formation of cAMP and cGMP, and induction of mitogen-activated protein kinase phosphorylation. Autoradiographic ligand binding, in situ hybridization, and immunohistochemical studies have yielded abundant information on the distribution of NTS_1 receptors in mammalian brain. NTS_1 receptors are markedly expressed in brain regions rich in dopamine cell bodies, such as the substantia nigra pars reticulata and pars compacta, the ventral tegmental area, and in projection areas of both nigrostriatal and mesocorticolimbic dopaminergic pathways, such as striatum, nucleus accumbens and frontal cortex (Palacios and Kuhar, 1981; Goulet et al., 1999; Boudin et al., 1998; Binder et al., 2001). In the striatum and nucleus accumbens, NTS_1 receptors are co-localized at post-synaptic level with dopamine D_2 receptors and, although in low density, at the pre-synaptic levels too (Pickel et al., 2001; Delle Donne et al., 2004). This receptor co-distribution together with the demonstration that neurotensin is localized within the nigrostriatal and mesolimbic dopamine neurons explain the role that the neuropeptide plays in the modulation of dopamine neurotransmission (Jennes et al., 1982). It is worth noting that in the striatum, NTS_1 receptors are significantly located on cortical glutamatergic terminals as well as on the striatopallidal GABA neurons (Boudin et al., 1996; Alexander and Leeman, 1998; Tanji et al., 1999). Finally, in the globus pallidus, neurotensin receptors (NTS_1 and NTS_2) exist in different neurons and are located both pre-synaptically and post-synaptically (Fassio et al., 2000; Sarret et al., 2003) thus regulating (mainly NTS_1 receptors), both pallidal glutamatergic and GABAergic transmission (Chen et al., 2004; 2006). Such distribution of NTS_1 receptors justifies the modulation that neurotensin exerts on the mesolimbic, mesocortical and nigrostriatal dopamine neurons, as well as on glutamatergic and GABAergic neurones (Deutch and Zahm, 1992; Fuxe et al., 1992 a,b; Rostene et al., 1992; Binder et al., 2001; Dobner et al., 2003; Petrie et al., 2005). Most of the central and peripheral functions controlled by NTS_1 receptors have been elucidated by the use of the non-peptide neurotensin antagonist SR48692, which preferentially binds NTS_1 receptors (Gully et al., 1993; Rostene et al., 1997).

4. Neurotensin levels, neurotensin binding sites and Parkinson's disease

The high concentrations of neurotensin in brain regions associated with dopaminergic cell bodies and projections, such as the striatum, substantia nigra, ventral tegmental area and globus pallidus (for a review, see Binder et al., 2001) indicate that neurotensin and dopamine are closely linked. In particular, the influence of neurotensin on nigrostriatal and mesocorticolimbic dopaminergic systems suggests that neurotensin may play a relevant role in dopamine-associated pathologies, such as some neurodegenerative disorders and neuropsychiatric diseases (Rostene et al., 1992; Lambert et al., 1995; St-Gelais et al., 2006).

In the following part of this section, data obtained from human and animal studies providing the existence of relationships between neurotensin and neurodegenerative disorders, will be shortly summarized.

Numerous studies have tried to determine whether, in humans, changes in the neurotensinergic system could be associated to Parkinson's disease. In an early study, high levels of neurotensin-like immunoreactivity were detected in lumbar cerebrospinal fluid from Parkinson's disease patients, whilst no significant changes in neurotensin content were observed (Emson et al., 1985). Successively, Fernandez et al. (1995, 1996) found that in post-mortem samples from basal ganglia of Parkinson's disease patients there were changes in the levels of different neuropeptides. In particular, substantia nigra neurotensin levels were two-fold higher in Parkinson's disease patients than in healthy subjects. It is worth noting that in incidental Lewy body disease, which is considered as a pre-symptomatic phase of Parkinson's disease, neurotensin levels tended to increase as in parkinsonian patients, even if this increase was not statistically significant (Fearnley and Lees, 1991). Similarly, in 6-hydroxydopamine-lesioned rats or in 1-methyl-4-phenyl-1,2,3,6-tetrahydropyridine-treated monkeys, two well-characterized animal models of Parkinson's disease, an increase in striatal and globus pallidus neurotensin levels was found, and such an enhancement was not modified by L-dopa treatment. In view of the above results, the authors suggested that changes in neurotensin levels and other neuropeptides may be considered as an early component of an integral part of the pathology rather than a secondary biochemical alteration resulting from loss of the nigrostriatal pathway or a drug-induced event. However, in contrast to the above results, in a previous study, Taylor et al. (1992) showed that substantia nigra neurotensin levels were unchanged following 6-hydroxydopamine lesion, but increased by a prolonged treatment with L-dopa. The authors concluded that changes in neurotensin levels appear to be only a secondary event, due to dopamine neuron loss in combination with protracted drug therapy. Despite these contrasting results, the hypothesis that an enhancement of neurotensin levels, associated to an activation of NTS_1 receptor located on the nigral dopamine neurons, contributes to the degeneration of these dopamine cells in Parkinson's disease, is supported by other animals studies. In particular, these findings indicate that a neurotensin-induced increase in both striatal and cortical endogenous glutamate release, is significantly coupled to an enhancement of neuronal excitotoxicity, which can contribute to nigral dopamine cell loss. In addition, it has been demonstrated that the neuropeptide increases the energy demands due to an increased firing rate in the dopamine cells. These enhancements are, at least in part, caused by a reduction of the D_2 autoreceptor signaling via an antagonistic NTS_1/D_2 receptor interaction (Fuxe et al., 1992a). These neurochemical and morphological results will be carefully described in the subsequent sections (5 and 6).

Besides the changes in neurotensin levels, biochemical and histological investigations in post-mortem brain tissues of parkinsonian patients have shown a significant reduction of neurotensin-binding sites in several specific brain areas of the basal ganglia as respect to healthy subjects (Chinaglia et al. 1990; Fernandez et al., 1994). In particular, Chinaglia et al. (1990), using a receptor autoradiography technique, compared the distribution of neurotensin receptors in post-mortem brain tissues from parkinsonian patients, with that found in patients affected by progressive supranuclear palsy and-in age-matched controls. Significant decreases in neurotensin receptor density were found in the substantia nigra, caudate nucleus, putamen and globus pallidus of both groups of patients in comparison to healthy subjects. In addition, a significant decrement of neurotensin receptor density was found in the ventral tegmental area, nucleus accumbens and dorsal part of caudate in patients with Parkinson's disease as regards to patients with progressive supranuclear palsy, indicating differential involvement of neurotensin receptor alterations in these two neurological disorders. Interestingly, in this cohort of Parkinson's disease patients, the reduction of striatal neurotensin binding sites was lower than the decrease of dopamine content in this nucleus, suggesting only a partial localization of neurotensin receptors on nigrostriatal dopaminergic projections. Using in situ hybridization, it has been possible to more specifically illustrate that NTS_1 receptor mRNA levels were decreased in the substantia nigra of patients with parkinsonism (Yamada and Richelson, 1995). These human results were confirmed in 1-methyl-4-phenyl-1,2,3,6-tetrahydropyridine-treated monkeys, where a decrease in the number of neurotensin-binding sites in the striatum and substantia nigra was found (Goulet et al., 1999; Tanji et al., 1999). The reduction of NTS_1 receptors in the substantia nigra of parkinsonian patients might be related to the loss of the nigrostriatal dopaminergic neurons. In contrast, the interpretation of the decrease in neurotensin-binding sites observed in the striatum of Parkinson's disease patients is certainly more difficult since, at present, the results concerning the pre-synaptic or the post-synaptic localization of striatal neurotensin receptors are still contradictory (Quirion et al., 1985; Cadet, 1991). However, it may be suggested that the decrease in striatal neurotensin-binding sites may reflect the loss of neurotensin receptors not only on dopaminergic nigrostriatal terminals but also on striatal GABAergic medium spiny neurons.

Taken together, the above mentioned studies from Parkinson's disease patients suggest a significant relationship between the alteration of neurotensinergic system and Parkinson's disease. On the basis of these findings, Schimpff et al. (2001) evaluated whether plasma neurotensin concentrations in parkinsonian patients could be considered as a marker in diagnosis and severity of this motor disorder. The results emerging from this study showed that the plasma neurotensin concentrations were significantly higher in Parkinson's disease patients than in healthy controls. Accordingly, neurotensin concentration in the plasma of untreated patients was higher than that observed in treated patients. It is worth noting that these findings were compatible with the enhancement of neurotensin levels detected in post-mortem brain tissues from parkinsonian patients and data obtained from animal studies. Thus, the authors concluded that in addition to the diagnostic criteria for Parkinson's disease "*measurement of extracted plasma neurotensin concentrations in patients with Parkinson may prove useful as an index in diagnosis*".

In summary, it can be concluded that the increase in striatal and nigral neurotensin tissue concentrations, as well as in cerebrospinal fluid and plasma levels may be due either to a loss of dopamine neurons and/or to a dysregulation of neurotensin transmission on striatal output, favoring the striatopallidal GABAergic pathway. Further work is needed to better understand the role of neurotensin in the pathophysiology of Parkinson's disease.

5. Striatal neurotensin and Parkinson's disease: neurochemical animal studies

5.1 Neurotensin modulation of pre- and post-synaptic D_2 receptors. Relevance for the control of striatopallidal GABAergic projections

As stated above, the motor deficits that characterize Parkinson's disease are associated to an imbalance on the functional activity of the "direct"–"indirect" circuits in favor of the "indirect pathway", *i.e.* reduced activity in the "direct pathway" and/or increased activity in the "indirect pathway" (Obeso et al., 2000; 2008). Several lines of evidence indicate that neurotensin is co-localized and co-distributed with dopamine neurons of the basal ganglia, including the somatodendritic complex and axon terminals of various neuronal elements in the substantia nigra and striatum. This close anatomical relationship, reinforces functional findings demonstrating the existence of reciprocal modulations between neurotensinergic and dopaminergic systems in these brain areas (Hökfelt et al., 1984; Nemeroff and Cain, 1985; Blaha et al., 1990; Castel et al., 1994; Tanganelli et al., 1994; Rostène et al., 1997; Werkman et al., 2000). Intensive animal studies have well documented that neurotensin, in addition to its direct excitatory effects on dopamine neurons, significantly modulates D_2 auto- and hetero-receptors functions through the activation of its high-affinity NTS_1 receptor (Kalivas and Duffy, 1990; Werkman et al., 2000; Binder et al., 2001). The regulation of dopaminergic transmission, especially at the level of nigrostriatal and mesocorticolimbic dopamine pathways, by neurotensin (Kitabgy et al., 1989; Deutch and Zahm, 1992) is mainly due to an antagonistic action of the activated NTS_1 receptor on D_2 receptor recognition and signaling. In the striatum, neurotensin has been shown to reduce the affinity of D_2 agonist binding sites and their transduction signals through a receptor-receptor interaction at both pre- and post-synaptic levels (Agnati et al., 1983; von Euler and Fuxe 1987; Shibata et al., 1987; Da-Silva et al., 1989; Fuxe et al., 1992 a,b). In particular, neurotensin by increasing the Kd value of D_2 receptor agonist binding, significantly decreases the affinity of D_2 receptors for endogenous dopamine and dopamine receptor agonists. The neurotensin-induced reduction of D_2 receptor agonist affinity has been demonstrated both in sections and in membrane preparations. The presence at the cellular level of NTS_1 and D_2 receptors in the same axon terminals and dendrites (Delle Donne et al., 2004), together with the demonstrated antagonistic intramembrane NTS_1/D_2 receptor–receptor interactions using biochemical radioligand binding analysis in striatal membranes (Agnati et al., 1983; von Euler and Fuxe 1987; Tanganelli et al., 1989; Fuxe et al., 1992b; Li et al., 1995; Diaz-Cabiale et al., 2002; Antonelli et al., 2007), give indirect evidence for the existence of NTS_1/D_2 receptor heteromerization. By using intrastriatal monoprobe microdialysis and measuring dopamine release from striatal terminals, in vivo evidence has been obtained that the neurotensin/D_2 antagonistic receptor–receptor interaction exists at the pre-junctional level in striatal dopamine transmission. This study demonstrate that, as expected, intrastriatal perfusion with the preferential dopamine D_2 receptor agonist pergolide decreased local dopamine outflow, an effect which reflects a stimulation of terminal D_2 auto-receptors causing the inhibition of striatal dopamine outflow. Interestingly, when neurotensin was co-perfused at a low nanomolar threshold concentration, together with pergolide, the inhibitory effect of the preferential dopamine D_2 receptor agonist on dopamine release is fully abolished as measured in the striatum of awake unrestrained rats. This provides a functional in vivo correlate to the binding results indicating the existence of antagonistic neurotensin/D_2 receptor–receptor interactions previously shown in neostriatal membranes and sections. A possible direct interaction between D_2 and NTS_1 receptors with the formation of heteromers has also been considered by Jomphe et al. (2006) as one of the possible, but not the exclusive, mechanisms underlying the functional control of striatal dopamine D_2-mediated transmission by neurotensin.

Biochemical and functional evidence suggests the existence of an antagonistic NTS_1/D_2 receptor-receptor interaction in rat neostriatum also at the post-synaptic level (Fuxe et al., 1992a; Ferraro et al., 1997). Post-synaptic D_2 receptors in the neostriatum exist predominantly on medium sized GABAergic neurons of the "indirect pathway", which project to the globus pallidus and exert an inhibitory influence on striopallidal GABA transmission (Reid et al., 1990; Ferre' et al., 1993). Converging evidence suggests that the behavioural catalepsy associated with blockade of striatal D_2 receptors is mediated by increased striopallidal GABA transmission, which leads to a decrease in thalamocortical motor drive (Drew et al., 1990; Osborne et al., 1994). Neurochemical findings, obtained employing in vivo dual-probe microdialysis technique, whereby one probe was implanted into the striatum and the other into the ipsilateral globus pallidus, demonstrated that intrastriatal perfusion with D_2 agonists inhibits striopallidal GABA release (Reid et al., 1990; Ferre' et al., 1993). On the contrary, D_2 receptor antagonists enhance striopallidal GABA release (Drew et al., 1990). Interestingly, intrastriatal co-perfusion of neurotensin, at a concentration by itself ineffective on pallidal extracellular GABA levels, in combination with pergolide, fully antagonizes the inhibitory effects of the preferential D_2 agonist on pallidal GABA release. The presence in the perfusate medium of the selective neurotensin receptor antagonist SR48692 removes the antagonistic effect of neurotensin, thus restoring the pergolide-induced inhibition of pallidal GABA levels. It is worth noting that higher concentrations of neurotensin, via a direct activation of NTS_1 receptor subtypes, significantly increase pallidal GABA outflow. SR48692 fully counteracts the facilitatory effects of neurotensin, indicating the involvement of NTS_1 receptors located on striopallidal GABAergic neurons in this effect. In view of the evidence showing that behavioural catalepsy in rodents and akinesia in humans are mediated by an increased striopallidal GABA transmission (Scheel-Kruger, 1986; Drew et al., 1990; Osborne et al., 1994), these findings suggest that the cataleptic profile of neurotensin (Shibata et al., 1987; Da-Silva et al., 1989) may be explained by its ability to influence neurotransmission in the "indirect pathway". In particular, the cataleptic action of neurotensin may be in part related to an enhancement of endogenous neurotensin signalling and in part to a reduction of post-synaptic D_2 receptors affinity. The existence of this intramembrane antagonistic neurotensin/D_2 receptor interaction is also supported by the finding that haloperidol-induced catalepsy is associated with an increase in pallidal GABA release (Drew et al., 1990; Osborne et al., 1994). Briefly, neurotensin-induced increase of pallidal GABA release and the consequent activation of striopallidal GABA transmission, may represent the neurochemical substrate to explain the behavioural data indicating that the activation of striatal NTS_1 receptors reduces motor activity (Poncelet et al., 1994).

5.2 Neurotensin modulation of striatal pre- and post-synaptic D_2 receptors. Functional consequences on the activity of the "indirect pathway"

As previously reported, in the "indirect pathway" the striatopallidal GABAergic projection corresponds to the first neuron of the trisynaptic connection that projects to the substantia nigra pars reticulata. The GABAergic projection from the globus pallidus to the subthalamic nucleus represents the second neuron whereas the subthalamic nucleus glutamatergic cells projecting terminals to the substantia nigra pars reticulata and collaterals to the internal part of the globus pallidus, the third one. Thus, changes in the activation of striatopallidal GABA neurons lead to modifications of the activity of subthalamic nucleus glutamate neurons and consequent variations in substantia nigra pars reticulata and pallidal glutamate release. In view of the above data and to analyze the functional relevance of striatal NTS_1 receptor activation on the activity of the "indirect pathway", a dual-probe microdialysis analysis was planed. One probe was implanted into the striatum and the other one in the ipsilateral globus pallidus of the awake rat; the effects of neurotensin on striatal and pallidal glutamate levels were then measured. In this part of the present section the results coming from these microdialysis studies, will be summarized.

5.2.1 Effects of striatal NTS_1 receptor activation on pallidal glutamate levels

Extracellular pallidal glutamate levels are mainly derived from the collaterals of the subthalamic nucleus-substantia nigra pars reticulata neurons (*see* above). Intrastriatal infusion with a high concentration of neurotensin increases striatal and pallidal glutamate as well as pallidal GABA levels (*see* also the above section). All these effects are counteracted by the local perfusion with the NTS_1 receptor antagonist SR48692. Thus, the intrastriatal neurotensin-induced increase of pallidal glutamate levels may be related to a direct activation of somatodendritic NTS_1 receptors located on the striatopallidal GABA neurons or to the antagonistic NTS_1/D_2 receptor-receptor interaction. The demonstration that the striatal neurotensin-induced increase in pallidal glutamate levels is counteracted by the intrapallidal perfusion of the $GABA_A$ receptor antagonist (-)-bicuculline, suggests that this effect is mediated via the activation of striatopallidal neurons. In fact, it seems likely that the stimulation of striatal NTS_1 receptors, by increasing striatopallidal GABA release, reduces the activity of GABAergic neurons projecting from the globus pallidus to the subthalamic nucleus, thus increasing pallidal glutamatergic transmission. In other words, this sequence of GABA-mediated inhibitory modulations induces a disinhibition of the excitatory glutamatergic subthalamic nucleus-substantia nigra pars reticulata efferents which send axon collaterals to the globus pallidus (Alexander and Crutcher, 1990). The intrapallidal (-)-bicuculline perfusion was employed since previous studies demonstrated the role of $GABA_A$ receptor activation in regulating the pallidal output system toward the subthalamic nucleus (Kita, 1992; Amalric et al., 1994). Accordingly, an electrophysiological study (Soltis et al., 1994) demonstrated that the infusion of bicuculline into subthalamic nucleus increased the firing rate of pallidal neurons.

5.2.2 Effects of NTS1 receptor activation on striatal glutamate levels

Extracellular striatal glutamate levels are derived in part, from the terminals of cortical and thalamic afferents (Sirinathsinghji and Heavens, 1989; Parent and Hazrati, 1995). As previously stated, intrastriatal perfusion with neurotensin at a high concentration increases striatal glutamate levels and this effect is fully counteracted by SR48692. Immunohistochemical studies have shown that in the striatum and nucleus accumbens, NTS_1 receptors and dopamine D_2 receptors are expressed on axon terminals, including the glutamatergic ones (Delle Donne et al., 2004). In this context, it seems possible that at least two mechanisms might underlay the neurotensin-mediated enhancement of striatal glutamate release. The first one may be related to a direct activation of local NTS_1 receptors expressed on striatal glutamate terminals. The second mechanism implies that the formation of a NTS_1/D_2 heteromeric receptor complex mainly located on the plasma membrane of striatal glutamate terminals, antagonizes the inhibitory D_2 receptor mediated signaling (*see* above) on the glutamate terminals, leading to an increase of glutamate release. The presence of a functional antagonistic pre-synaptic NTS_1/D_2 interaction on glutamatergic striatal terminals has been demonstrated since a threshold concentration of neurotensin counteracts the D_2 agonist quinpirole-induced inhibition of K^+-evoked striatal glutamate levels.

5.3 Neurochemical studies: concluding remarks

The analysis of all the above microdialysis results suggests that the over-activity of striatopallidal GABA pathway is under the control of NTS_1 receptors located both on medium size spiny striatal GABAergic neurons and on striatal glutamatergic terminals. The mechanisms involved in this control are mainly associated to a direct activation of NTS_1 receptor homomer or to an antagonistic NTS_1/D_2 receptor-receptor interaction (Figure 3). Based on these molecular mechanisms, it might be suggested that the activation of NTS_1 receptors suppresses the inhibitory control mediated by nigrostriatal dopaminergic neurons on striatopallidal GABAergic neurons and enhances the excitatory cortico-striatal glutamatergic signaling. The final consequence of these combined opposite modulations is the hyperactivity of the striatopallidal GABAergic neurons of the "indirect pathway" which is considered one of the anomaly responsible for generation of motor parkinsonian symptoms (*see* section 2). Thus, neurotensin receptor antagonists, by counteracting the neurotensin-induced hyperactivity of striatopallidal GABAergic neurons, could be useful to reduce motor symptoms in Parkinson's disease patients.

6. Neurotensin and Parkinson's disease: biochemical and morphological analyses in neuronal cell cultures

The substantial elevation in extracellular glutamate accompanied by an excessive activation of excitatory amino acid receptors generates neuronal cell death (Sonsalla et al., 1998). Glutamate has been one of the major focus of research into the excitotoxic basis of neurodegenerative diseases (Choi, 1988; Meldrum and Garthwaite, 1990). In vivo and in vitro studies have shown that neurotensin significantly increases endogenous glutamate outflow in discrete rat brain regions, such as the striatum, globus pallidus, frontal cortex, substantia nigra and parabrachial nucleus-ventrobasal thalamus (Sanz et al., 1993; Saleh, 1997; Ferraro et al., 1998, 2000, 2001). These findings suggest that neurotensin may play a relevant role in reinforcing the effects exerted by glutamate on a variety of central nervous system functions. In particular, the observations that neurotensin amplifies glutamate levels and antagonizes the dopamine D_2 receptor-mediated inhibition of dopamine transmission in the basal ganglia (Fuxe et al., 1992 a,b), indicate that neurotensin may contribute to enhance the firing rate and energy demands in the nerve cells. In this context, as illustrated in section 4, a putative role of neurotensin in the development of Parkinson's disease, has been suggested (Fernandez et al., 1995, 1996; Tanji et al., 1999; Schimpff et al., 2001).
In this paragraph, the effects of neurotensin in modulating the glutamate-induced neurodegenerative effects in cultured rat mesencephalic dopaminergic (Antonelli et al., 2002) and cortical (Antonelli et al., 2004) neurons will be shortly summarized.

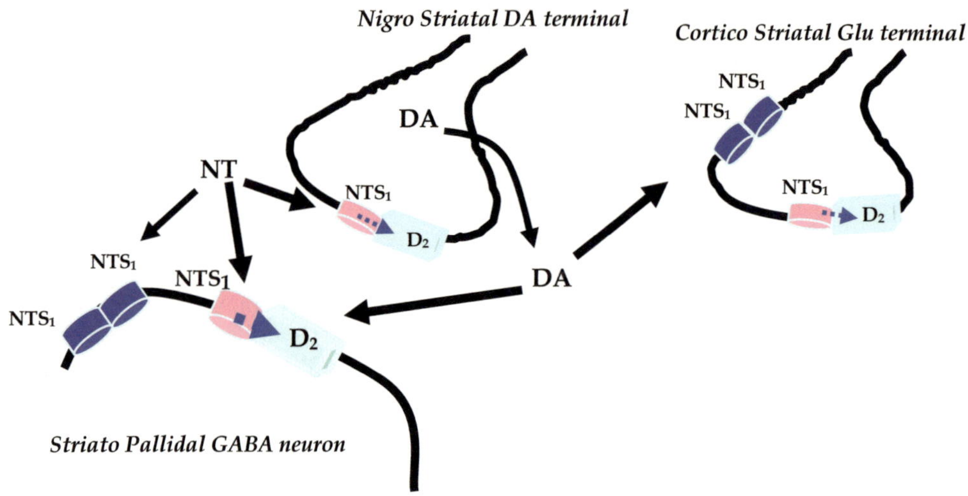

Fig. 3. Schematic representation of the pre-and postjunctional neurotensin (NT) receptor (NTS_1) and dopamine (DA) D_2 receptor interactions in the striatum taking place in NTS_1/D_2 heteromers in balance with excitatory NT receptor homomers (Modified from Ferraro et al., 2008).

6.1 Effects of neurotensin on glutamate-induced excitotoxicity in primary cultures of mesencephalic neurons

Biochemical and morphological approaches (Antonelli et al., 2002), provided evidence that the neurotoxic effects of glutamate on primary cultures of mesencephalic neurons are exacerbated by neurotensin.

Mesencephalic cell cultures, which contain dopaminergic neurons, express glutamate receptors (Meltzer et al., 1997; Yung, 1998; Mateu et al., 2000) as well as functional neurotensin receptors (Nalivaiko et al., 1998; Nouel et al., 1999). Thus, this in vitro preparation represents a suitable model for testing the influence of neurotensin on glutamate-induced neurotoxicity. Measurement of [^{3}H]dopamine uptake in mesencephalic cell cultures has been proved a reliable parameter with which to evaluate the metabolic and structural integrity of the dopaminergic neurons in culture (Mount et al., 1989; Antonelli et al., 2002). In particular, in mesencephalic cell cultures intoxicated with glutamate, a reduction of [^{3}H]dopamine uptake, is observed. The exposure of cells to neurotensin exacerbates the glutamate-induced neurotoxicity, causing a further reduction of [^{3}H]dopamine uptake. Similar results were also obtained by evaluating the vulnerability of the mesencephalic cells to glutamate using tyrosine hydroxylase immunoreactivity. The tyrosine hydroxylase-immunoreactive cell count allows to quantify dopamine cell survival or loss of phenotype (Bowenkamp et al., 1996). As shown in Figure 4, the enhancing action of neurotensin on glutamate-induced toxicity in dopaminergic neurons has also been demonstrated by the increased disappearance of tyrosine hydroxylase-immunoreactive neurons pretreated with glutamate and neurotensin in combination. The selective neurotensin receptor antagonist SR48692 counteractes the above-mentioned effects of neurotensin, indicating that NTS_1 receptor was mainly involved in the neurotensin-induced

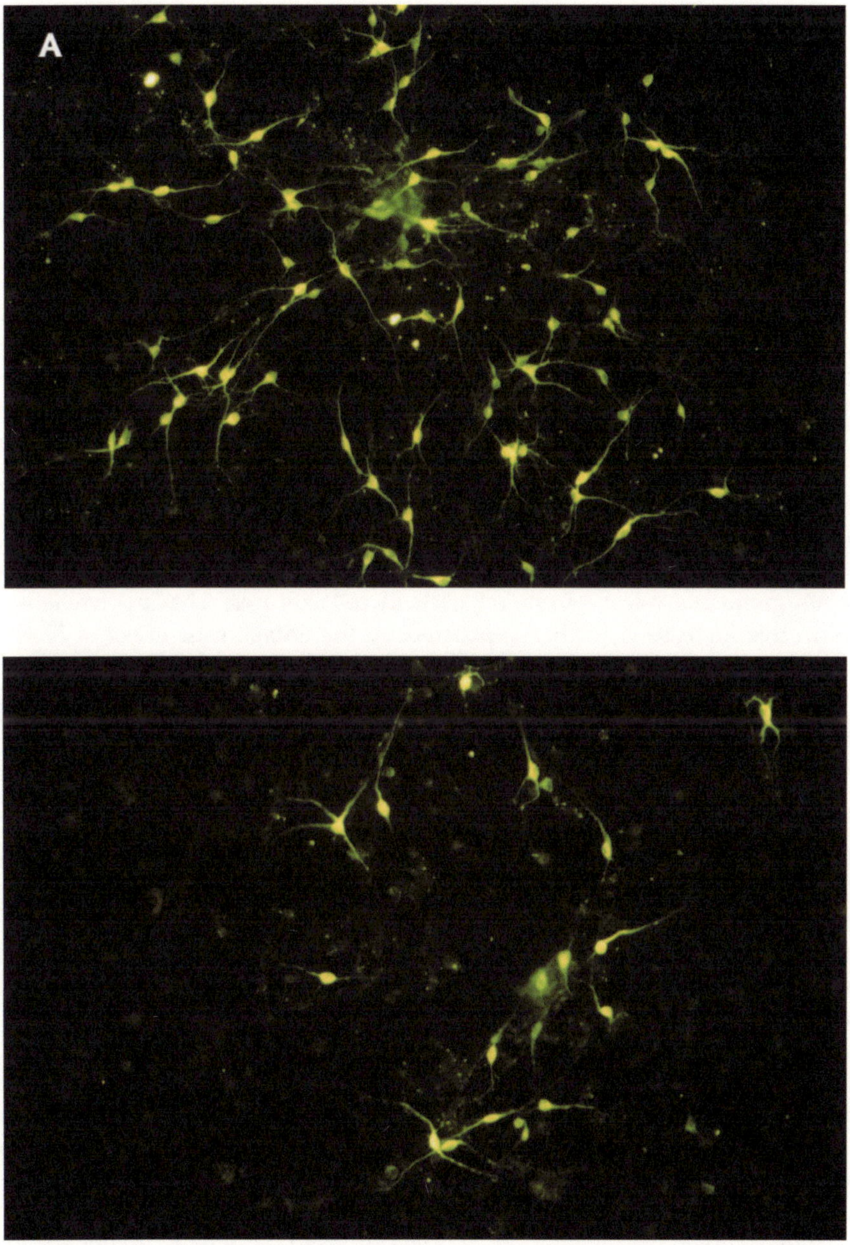

Fig. 4. Representative photomicrographs of tyrosine hydroxylase-immunoreactive mesencephalic cells in culture. **A** (control) shows a typical culture of tyrosine hydroxylase-immunoreactive neurons, with long processes and network. **B** shows a field of tyrosine hydroxylase-immunoreactive neurons exposed to 100 μM glutamate for 10 min, in which there is an evident neuronal loss (from Antonelli et al., 2002).

enhancement of glutamate injury. Since NTS_1 receptors are coupled to phospholipase C (Cathala and Paupardin-Tritsch, 1997; Trudeau, 2000), the effect of the combination of neurotensin with glutamate on [^{3}H]dopamine uptake was also evaluated in the presence of the specific protein kinase C inhibitor calphostin C (Kobayashi et al., 1989). The neurotensin-induced enhancement of glutamate neurotoxicity is completely prevented by calphostin C. Thus, it seems possible that the nigral NTS_1 receptors located on dopamine cells (Nalivaiko et al., 1998) enhance glutamate receptor subtype signaling through a protein kinase C activation. This finding suggests that neurotensin-mediated rise of glutamate excitotoxicity could be mediated by phosphorylation(s) of receptor-associated protein(s) involved in receptor signaling and/or trafficking.

6.2 Effects of neurotensin in modulating the neuronal activity of NMDA receptor in primary cortical cell cultures of rat

Evidence has been accumulated that the excessive activation of glutamate receptors, particularly NMDA receptors, may contribute to the neuronal cell death associated with chronic neurodegenerative disorders including Parkinson's disease and Alzheimer's disease. In this paragraph, the evidence for a functional role of NTS_1 receptors in modulating the neuronal activity of NMDA receptor in cortical glutamatergic nerve cells, will be discussed.

Accordingly to the above in vivo and in vitro experiments, neurotensin increases basal endogenous glutamate release from rat cortical cell cultures. The involvement of NTS_1 receptors in this increase is further supported by the antagonistic effect of SR48692. The exposure of cortical cell cultures to NMDA induces a concentration-dependent increase in endogenous extracellular glutamate levels, an increase that is enhanced in the presence of a sub-threshold concentration of neurotensin. These results indicate that NTS_1 receptor activation enhances the NMDA-receptor signaling and suggest the existence of facilitatory NTS_1/NMDA interactions at the membrane level. The lack of a neurotensin-mediated enhancement of glutamate outflow in the presence of NMDA receptor blockade further supports the hypothesis that neurotensin is a modulator of NMDA receptor function. Morphological analysis strengths the above hypothesis since neurotensin, in threshold concentration, enhances the glutamate-induced increase in the number of the apoptotic cells and such an effect is counteracted by SR48692 (Antonelli et al., 2004). A direct facilitatory NTS_1/NMDA interaction may therefore produce plastic changes in glutamate transmission and, if excessive, produce increases in glutamate-induced excitotoxicity. Under physiological conditions such a postulated NTS_1/NMDA heteromeric complex may modulate metaplasticity which is another main mode of homeostatic plasticity (*see* Perez-Otano and Ehlers, 2005), which serves to establish that receptor plasticity may exist in a proper working range, avoiding *e.g.* a dramatic NMDA receptor internalization and downregulation.

At the present, several mechanisms possibly underlying the demonstrated synergistic NTS_1/NMDA receptor interactions can be hypothesized: *i)* both receptors are known to produce an increase in intracellular Ca^{++} levels and their co-activation may therefore lead to a rapid and robust rise of intracellular Ca^{++} levels; *ii)* synergistic NTS_1/NMDA effect may involve a protein kinase C mediated phosphorylation of the NMDA receptors. It is worth noting that the inhibition of the protein kinase C by calphostin C suppresses the NTS_1-mediated enhancement of NMDA-induced increases of extracellular glutamate levels. (Antonelli et al., 2004). This finding assumes a particular relevance in view of the demonstration that protein kinase C is likely to be an important regulator of neuronal NMDA receptors in vivo. The activation of protein kinase C increases NMDA channel opening rate and a rapid delivery of functional NMDA receptors to the cell surface. Thus, regulation of neuronal NMDA receptors by protein kinases plays a critical role in synaptic transmission and synaptic plasticity of NMDA receptors. Since phospholipase C–protein kinase C–inositol triphosphate pathway is the major signal transduction of NTS_1 receptors, it may be suggested that the existence of a neurotensin-mediated potentiation of NMDA receptors involves the activation of protein kinase C. Similarly to the above hypothesis, it has been demonstrated that mGluR1 activation potentiates NMDA receptors by an activation of protein kinase C (Skeberdis et al., 2001; Matsuyama et al., 2002); *iii)* it also seems possible that NTS_1 receptor by forming a receptor heteromer with the NMDA receptor (NTS_1/NMDA heteromer) may contribute to enhance NMDA receptor signalling and its surface expression; *iv)* a recent paper reported that neurotensin receptor agonists robustly increased extracellular concentrations of glycine in the rat prefrontal cortex (Li et al., 2010). It is well known that normal NMDA receptor function depends on not only the binding of glutamate to the receptor but also the binding of glycine to an allosteric site on this receptor. Thus, it could be suggested that neurotensin modulates NMDA receptor functions by modulating allosteric glycine activity.

Taken together, the results obtained in mesencephalic and cortical cell cultures suggest that neurotensin receptor antagonists, by counteracting the neurotensin-induced amplification of glutamate excitotoxicity could display neuroprotective properties.

7. Neurotensin receptor blockade in an animal model of Parkinson's disease

The postulated neuroprotective properties of neurotensin receptor antagonists are also supported by experiments (Ferraro et al., 2008) carried out in a rat model of Parkinson's disease [unilateral nigral 6-hydroxydopamine induced lesion of the nigrostriatal DA pathway, hemiparkinson model]. In this study, behavioural and biochemical experiments have been performed in control animals and in 6-hydroxydopamine unilaterally lesioned rats chronically treated with saline or with the NTS_1 receptor antagonist SR48692 from one-week before until one-week after the lesion. A conventional behavioural assessment using apomorphine-induced rotation was performed to quantify the unilateral nigrostriatal lesion-induced motor asymmetry after ipsilateral 6-hydroxydopamine injection. As expected, in 6-hydroxydopamine-lesioned rats, but not in control rats, the apomorphine injection produced a controlateral turning behaviour that significantly and progressively increased from week 1 to the 3rd week following the lesion. However, interestingly, in the SR48692-treated group, but not in the vehicle-treated group, the apomorphine-induced rotational behaviour is significantly reduced at each time of evaluation (day 7, 14 and 21 post lesion). Moreover, whereas the treatment stopped 2 weeks before, the effect of the compound remains significant. This finding suggests that systemic administration of NTS_1 antagonist decreased the functional consequence of a partial dopaminergic lesion induced by intranigral application of the neurotoxin 6-hydroxydopamine in the rat.

In view of the above behavioural findings, neurochemical experiments have been carried out in control animals and in rats chronically treated with SR48692 or its vehicle from one-week before until one week after the 6-hydroxydopamine injection. In particular, the responsivity to a challenge with NMDA has been assessed. The results obtained from this study demonstrate that in 6-hydroxydopamine-lesioned control and vehicle-treated rats,

intrastriatal perfusion with NMDA induced a slight increase in glutamate extracellular levels that was significantly lower than that observed in sham-operated animals. Interestingly, in 6-hydroxydopamine-lesioned rats chronically treated with SR48692, the effect of intrastriatal perfusion of NMDA induced an increase in glutamate extracellular levels that was significantly higher with respect to that obtained in the group of 6-hydroxydopamine lesioned rats but still lower to that observed in control rats.
These neurochemical results are in line with previous microdialysis data indicating that dopamine denervation is associated with a reduction of the enhancement of striatal glutamate transmission induced by a high micromolar NMDA concentration. Since it has been demonstrated that endogenous dopamine in the striatum facilitates strong excitatory inputs, the reduction of NMDA-stimulated glutamate levels in lesioned-animals could imply a loss of facilitatory dopamine receptor mediated signals. In this view, the observation that in rats chronically treated with SR48692 the excitatory response to a NMDA stimulus on the striatal glutamatergic transmission is partially restored may support a protective action of the NTS1 antagonist against 6-hydroxydopamine-induced dopamine neuron degeneration.

8. Conclusion

Parkinson's disease is associated to a progressive loss of nigrostriatal dopaminergic neurons. The decrease of dopamine levels in the striatum of parkinsonian patients is responsible for the main motor disturbances characteristic of the disease such as akinesia, muscular rigidity and tremor. The strict interactions between the tridecapeptide neurotensin and the dopaminergic systems lead to hypothesize that the peptide could be involved in some aspects of Parkinson's disease. In this context, the present chapter discusses the putative role of neurotensin in the development and symptoms of Parkinson's disease.
Human studies provide evidence that in the basal ganglia of Parkinson's disease patients there is an increase in neurotensin levels. These changes might be an integral part of the pathology rather than a consequence of the dopamine neuron degeneration. In addition, neurotensin receptor binding sites, especially in the nigrostriatal dopamine system, are reduced in brains of Parkinson's disease patients and in the basal ganglia of hemiparkinsonian rats. This is probably a result of the ongoing degeneration of nigral dopamine cells in which the peptide actively participates.
Based on neurochemical and morphological animals studies, the hypothesis is now introduced that the activation of NTS_1 receptors by enhancing glutamate release and by amplifying the NMDA-mediated glutamate signalling contributes to the degeneration of dopaminergic neurons in Parkinson's disease. In addition, the reduction of the D_2 autoreceptor signaling due to the antagonistic NTS_1/D_2 receptor-receptor interaction, by enhancing the firing rate of dopamine neurons and energy demand may further contribute to this degeneration.
The neurochemical studies have also clearly demonstrated that increased striatal neurotensin levels, by leading to an over-activity to the "indirect pathway" in the basal ganglia, could also play a role in motor Parkinson's disease symptoms.
In closing, in view of the presented results, it could be suggested that NTS_1 antagonists, in combination with conventional drug treatments, may provide a possible novel therapeutic approach for the treatment of neurodegenerative pathologies, especially Parkinson's disease. This hypothesis is supported by studies demonstrating the putative neuroprotective

effects of the neurotensin receptor antagonist SR48692 (systemically administered) in an in vivo animal model of Parkinson's disease. However, Mesnage et al. (2004) in an exploratory study reported that SR48692 could not improve parkinsonian motor disability. However, in this paper the authors reported that the lack of efficacy of NTS_1 receptor antagonists could be attributed to the low dose used, as demonstrated by the absence of adverse events observed in any of the patients tested. In fact, it was concluded that further studies with higher doses of neurotensin receptor antagonists are needed.

Taken together, the reported findings prompt to continue these preclinical studies in order to better understand the role of neurotensin in Parkinson's disease development and symptoms.

9. Acknowledgement

This work has been supported by grants from Sanofi-Aventis and University of Ferrara (Fondo di Ateneo per la Ricerca Scientifica).

The authors thank Dr. Jacqueline Fournier (Sanofi-Aventis) for her excellent scientific support during the research development.

10. References

Agnati, LF.; Fuxe, K.; Benfenati, F. & Battistini, N. (1983). Neurotensin in vitro markedly reduces the affinity in subcortical limbic [3H]N-propylnorapomorphine binding sites. *Acta Physiol. Scan.* 119, (December 1983), pp. 459-461, ISSN 0001-6772.

Alexander, GE. & Crutcher, M. (1990). Functional architecture of basal ganglia circuits: neuronal substrates of parallel processing. *Trends Neurosci.* 13, (July 1990), pp. 266-271, ISSN 0166-2236.

Alexander, MJ. & Leeman, SE. (1998). Widespread expression in adult rat forebrain of mRNA encoding high-affinity neurotensin receptor. *J. Comp. Neurol.* 402, (December 1998), pp. 475-500, ISSN 0021-9967.

Amalric, M.; Farin, D.; Dormont, JF. & Schmied, A. (1994). GABA-receptor activation in the globus pallidus and entopeduncular nucleus: opposite effects on reaction time performance in the cat. *Exp. Brain Res.* 102, pp.244-258, ISSN 0014-4819.

Antonelli, T.; Tomasini, MC.; Finetti, S.; Giardino, L.; Calzà, L.; Fuxe, K.; Soubriè, P.; Tanganelli, S. & Ferraro, L. (2002). Neurotensin enhances Glutamate excitotoxicity in mesencephalic neurons. *J. Neurosci. Res.* 70, (December 2002), pp. 766-773, ISSN 0360-4012.

Antonelli, T., Ferraro, L.; Fuxe, K.; Finetti, S.; Fournier, J.; Tanganelli, S.; De Mattei, M. & Tomasini, M. C. (2004). Neurotensin enhances endogenous extracellular glutamate levels in primariy cultures of rat cortical neurons. Involment of neurotensin receptor in NMDA induced excitotoxicity. *Cerebral Cortex* 1, (April 2004), pp. 466-473, ISSN 1047-3211.

Antonelli, T.; Tomasini, MC.; Fuxe, K.; Agnati, LF.; Tanganelli, S. & Ferraro, L. (2007) Receptor-receptor interactions as studied with microdialysis. Focus on NTR/D2 interactions in the basal ganglia. *J. Neural Transm.* 114, (January 2007), pp. 105-13. ISSN 0300-9564.

Bamford, NS.; Robinson, S.; Palmiter, RD.; Joyce, JA.; Moore, C. & Meshul, CK. (2004) Dopamine modulates release from corticostriatal terminals. *J. Neurosci.* 24, (October 2004), pp. 9541-9552, ISSN 0270-6474.

Barroso, S.; Richard, F.; Nicolas-Etheve, D.; Reversat, JL.; Bernassau, JM.; Kitabgi, P. & Labbè-Julliè, C. (2000). Identification of residues involved in neurotensin binding and modelling of the agonist binding site in neurotensin receptor 1. *J. Biol. Chem.* 275, (January 2000), pp. 328-336, ISSN 0021-9258.

Binder, EB.; Kinkead, B.; Owens, MJ. & Nemeroff, CB. (2001). Neurotensin and dopamine interactions. *Pharmacol. Rev.* 53, (December 2001), pp. 453-486, ISSN 0031-6997.

Blaha, CD.; Coury, A.; Fibiger, HC. & Phillips, AG. (1990). Effects of neurotensin on DA release and metabolism in the rat striatum and nucleus accumbens: cross-validation using in vivo voltammetry and microdialysis. *Neuroscience* 34, pp. 699-705, ISSN 0306-4522.

Boudin, H.; Pélaprat, D.; Rostène, W. & Beaudet, A. (1996). Cellular distribution of neurotensin receptors in rat brain: immunohistochemical study using an antipeptide antibody against the cloned high affinity receptor, *J. Comp. Neurol.* 373, (September 1996), pp. 76–89, ISSN 0021-9967.

Boudin, H.; Pelaprat, D.; Rostène, W.; Pickel, VM. & Beaudet, A. (1998). Correlative ultrastructural distribution of neurotensin receptor proteins and binding sites in the rat substantia nigra. *J. Neurosci.* 18, (October 1998), pp.8473-8484, ISSN 0270-6474.

Bowenkamp, KE.; David, D.; Lapchak, PL.; Henry, MA.; Granholm, AC.; Hoffer, BJ. & Mahalik, TJ. (1996). 6-hydroxydopamine induces the loss of the dopaminergic phenotype in substantia nigra neurons of the rat. A possible mechanism for restoration of the nigrostriatal circuit mediated by glial cell line-derived neurotrophic factor. *Exp. Brain Res.* 111, (September 1996), pp.1-7, ISSN 0014-4819.

Cadet, JL.; Kujirai, K. & Przedborski, S. (1991). Bilateral modulation of [3H]neurotensin binding by unilateral intrastriatal 6-hydroxydopamine injections: evidence from a receptor autoradiographic study. *Brain Res.* 564, (November 1991), pp. 37-44, ISSN 0006-8993.

Carraway, R. & Leeman, SE. (1973). The isolation of a new hypotensive peptide, neurotensin, from bovine hypothalami. *J. Biol. Chem.* 248, (October 1973), pp.6854-6861, ISSN 0021-9258.

Castel, MN.; Morino, P.; Nylander, I.; Terenius, L. & HöKfelt, T. (1994) Differential dopaminergic regulation of the neurotensin striatonigral and striatopallidal pathways in the rat. *Eur. J. Pharmacol.* 262, (September 1994), pp.1-10, ISSN 0014-2999.

Cathala, L. & Paupardin-Tritsch, D. (1997). Neurotensin inhibition of the hyperpolarization-activated cation current (Ih) in the rat substantia nigra pars compacta implicates the protein kinase C pathway. *J. Physiol.* 503, (August 1997), pp.87-97, ISSN 0022-3751.

Chalon, P.; Vita, N.; Kaghad, M.; Guillemot, M.; Bonnin, J. & Delpech, B. (1996). Molecular cloning of a levocabastine-sensitive neurotensin binding site. *FEBS Lett.* 386, (May 1996), pp. 91–94, ISSN 0014-5793.

Chen, L.; Yung, KK. & Yung, WH. (2004). Neurotensin depolarizes globus pallidus neurons in rats via neurotensin type-1 receptor. *Neuroscience* 125, pp.853-859, ISSN 0306-4522.

Chen, L.; Yung, KK. & Yung, WH. (2006). Neurotensin selectively facilitates glutamatergic transmission in globus pallidus. *Neuroscience* 141, (September 2006), pp.1871-1878, ISSN 0306-4522 .

Chinaglia, G.; Probst, A. & Palacios, JM. (1990). Neurotensin receptors in Parkinson's disease and progressive supranuclear palsy: an autoradiographic study in basal ganglia. *Neuroscience* 39, pp.351-360, 0306-4522.

Choi, DW. (1988). Glutamate neurotoxicity and diseases of the nervous system. *Neuron* 1, (October 1988), pp.623-34. ISSN 0896-6273.

Da-Silva, SL.; Brandäo, ML. & Tomaz, C. (1989) Behavioral effects of neurotensin applied to periventricular structures of rats. *Braz. J. Med. Biol. Res.* 22, pp.711-715, ISSN 0100-879X.

Delle Donne, KT.; Chan , J.; Boudin, H.; Pélaprat, D.; Rostène, W. & Pickel, VM. (2004). Electron microscopic dual labeling of high-affinity neurotensin and dopamine D2 receptors in the rat nucleus accumbens shell. *Synapse*. 52, (June 2004), pp.176-187, ISSN 0887-4476.

Dobner, PR.; Deutch, AY. & Fadel, J. (2003). Neurotensin: dual roles in psychostimulant and antipsychotic drug responses. *Life Sci.* 73,(June 2003), pp.801-811. Rev, ISSN 0024-3205.

Deutch, AY. & Zahm, DS. (1992). The current status of neurotensin-dopamine interactions: issues and speculations. *Ann. N.Y. Acad. Sci.* 668, pp.232-252, ISSN 0077-8923.

Diaz-Cabiale, Z., Fuxe, K.; Narvaez, JA.; Finetti, S.; Antonelli, T.; Tanganelli, S. & Ferraro, L. (2002). Neurotensin-induced modulation of dopamine D2 receptors and their function in rat striatum: Counteraction by NTR1-lik receptor antagonist. *Neuroreport* 13, (May 2002), pp.763-766, ISSN 0959-4965.

Drew, KL.; O'Connor, WT.; Kehr, J. & Ungerstedt, U. (1990). Regional specific effects of clozapine and haloperidol on GABA and dopamine release in rat basal ganglia. *Eur. J. Pharm.* 187, (October 1990), pp. 385-397, ISSN 0014-2999

Emson, PC.; Horsfield, PM.; Goedert, M.; Rossor, MN. & Hawkes, CH. (1985). Neurotensin in human brain: regional distribution and effects of neurological illness. *Brain Res.* 347, (November 1985), pp.239-244 ISSN 0006-8993.

Fassio, A.; Evans, G.; Grisshammer, R.; Bolam, JP.; Mimmack, M. & Emson, PC. (2000). Distribution of the neurotensin receptor NTS1 in the rat CNS studied using an amino-terminal directed antibody. *Neuropharmacology* 39, (June 2000), pp. 1430–1442, ISSN 0028-3908.

Fearnley, JM. & Lees, AJ. (1991). Ageing and Parkinson's disease: substantia nigra regional selectivity. *Brain* 114, (October 1991), pp. 2283-2301, ISSN 0006-8950.

Fernandez, A.; De Ceballos, ML. & Jenner, P. (1994). Neurotensin, substance P, delta and mu opioid receptors are decreased in basal ganglia of Parkinson's disease patients. *Neuroscience* 61, (July 1994), pp.73-79, ISSN 0306-4522.

Fernandez, A.; Jenner, P.; Marsden, CD. & De Ceballos, ML. (1995). Characterization of neurotensin-like immunoreactivity in human basal ganglia: increased neurotensin levels in substantia nigra in Parkinson's disease. *Peptides*. 16, pp.339-346, ISSN 0196-9781.

Fernandez, A.; De Ceballos, ML.; Rose, S.; Jenner, P. & Marsden, CD. (1996) Alterations in peptide levels in Parkinson's disease and incidental Lewy body disease. *Brain* 119 (Pt 3), (June 1996), pp.823-830, ISSN 0006-8950.

Ferraro. L.; O'Connor, WT.; Antonelli, T.; Fuxe, K. & Tanganelli, S. (1997). Differential effects of intrastriatal neurotensin(1–13) and neurotensin(8–13) on striatal dopamine and pallidal GABA release. A dual-probe microdialysis study in the awake rat. *Eur. J. Neurosci.* 9, (September 1997), pp.1838-1846, ISSN 0953-816X.

Ferraro, L.; Tomasini, MC.; Siniscalchi, A.; Fuxe, K.; Tanganelli, S. & Antonelli, T. (2000). Neurotensin increases endogenous glutamate release in rat cortical slices. *Life Sci.* 66, pp.927-936, ISSN 0024-3205.

Ferraro, L.; Tomasini, MC.; Fernandez, M.; Bebe, BW.; O'Connor, WT.; Fuxe, K.; Glennon, JC.; Tanganelli, S & Antonelli, T. (2001). Nigral neurotensin receptor regulation of nigral glutamate and nigroventral thalamic GABA transmission: a dual-probe microdialysis study in intact conscious rat brain. *Neuroscience* 102, pp.113-120, ISSN 0306-4522.

Ferraro, L.; Tomasini, MC.; Mazza, R.; Fuxe, K.; Fournier, J.; Tanganelli, S. & Antonelli, T. (2008). Neurotensin receptors as modulators of glutamatergic transmission. *Brain Res. Rev.* 58 (August 2008) pp.365-373, ISSN 0165-0173.

Ferraro L, Tomasini MC, Beggiato S, Guerrini R, Salvadori S, Fuxe K, Calzà L, Tanganelli S, Antonelli T. Emerging evidence for neurotensin receptor 1 antagonists as novel pharmaceutics in neurodegenerative disorders. *Mini Rev Med Chem.* 9 (October 2009), pp. 1429-1438, ISSN: 1389-5575 (Print).

Ferrè, S.; O'Connor, WT.; Fuxe, K. & Ungerstedt, U. (1993). The striopallidal neuron: a main locus for adenosine-dopamine interactions in the brain. *J. Neurosci.* 13, (December 1993) pp.5402–5406, ISSN 0270-6474.

Fuxe, K.; von Euler, G.; Agnati, LF.; Merlo Pich, E.; O'Connor, WT.; Tanganelli, S.; Li, XM.; Tinner, B.; Cintra, A.; Carani, C. & Benfenati, F. (1992a). Intramembrane interactions between neurotensin receptors and dopamine D2 receptors as a major mechanism for the neuroleptic-like action of neurotensin. *Ann. N.Y. Acad. Sci.* 668, pp.186-204, ISSN 0077-8923.

Fuxe, K.; O'Connor, WT.; Antonelli, T.; Osborne, PG.; Tanganelli, S.; Agnati, LF. & Ungerstedt, U. (1992b). Evidence for a substrate of neuronal plasticity based on pre- and postsynaptic neurotensin-dopamine receptor interactions in the neostriatum. *Proc. Natl. Acad. Sci.* 89, (June 1992), pp.5591-5595, ISSN 0027-8424.

Galvan, A. & Wichmann T. (2008). Phatophisiology of Parkinsonism. *Clinical Neurophysiol.* 119, (July 2008), pp.1459-1474. Rew, ISSN 1388-2457.

Gerfen, CR. (1992). The neostriatal mosaic: multiple levels of compartmental organization in the basal ganglia. *Ann. Rev. Neurosci.* 15, pp.285-320, ISSN 0147-006X.

Gerfen, CR. (2003). D1 dopamine receptor supersensitivity in the dopamine-depleted striatum animal model of Parkinson's disease. *Neuroscientist* 9, (December 2003), pp.455-62, ISSN 1073-8584.

Goulet, M.; Morissette, M. & Grondin, R. (1999). Neurotensin receptors and dopamine transporters: effects of MPTP lesioning and chronic dopaminergic treatments in monkeys. *Synapse* 32, (June 1999), pp.153-64, ISSN 0887-4476.

Gully, D.; Canton, M.; Boidegrain, R.; Jeanjean, F.; Molimard, JC.; Poncelet, M.; Gueudet, C.; Heaulme, M.; Leyris, A.; Brouard, A.; Pelaprat, D.; Labbe-Jullie, C.; Mazella, J.; Soubrie, P.; Maffrand, JP.; Rostene, W.; Kitbagi, P. & Le Fur, G. (1993) Biochemical and pharmacological profile of a potent and selective nonpeptide antagonist of the neurotensin receptor. *Proc. Natl. Acad. Sci.* 90, (January 1993), pp.65–69, ISSN 0027-8424.

Kalivas, PW. & Duffy, P. (1990). Effect of acute and daily neurotensin and enkephalin treatments on extracellular dopamine in the nucleus accumbens. *J. Neurosci.* 10, (September 1990), pp.2940-2949, ISSN 0270-6474.

Kita, H. (1992). Responses of globus pallidus neurons to cortical stimulation: intracellular study in the rat. *Brain Res.* 589, (August 1992), pp.84-90, ISSN 0006-8993.

Kitabgi, P.; Herve, D.; Studler, JM.; Tramu, G.; Rostene, W. & Tassin, JP. (1989). Neurotensin/dopamine interactions. *Encephale* 15, (January-February 1989), pp.91–94, ISSN 0013-7006.

Kitabgi, P. (2010). Neurotensin and neuromedin N are differentially processed from a common precursor by prohormone convertases in tissues and cell lines. *Results Probl. Cell Differ.* 50, pp.50:85-96.

Kobayashi, E.; Nakano, H.; Morimoto, M. & Tamaoki, T. (1989). Calphostin C (UCN-1028C), a novel microbial compound, is a highly potent and specific inhibitor of protein kinase C. *Biochem. Biophys. Res. Commun.* 159, (March 1989), pp.548-553, ISSN 0006-291X.

Hökfelt, T.; Everitt, BJ.; Theodorsson-Norheim, E. & Goldstein, M. (1984). Occurrence of neurotensinlike immunoreactivity in subpopulations of hypothalamic, mesencephalic, and medullary catecholamine neurons. *J. Comp. Neurol.* 222, (February 1984), pp.543-59, ISSN 0021-9967.

Jennes, L.; Stumpf, WE. & Kalivas, PW. (1982). Neurotensin: Topographical distribution in rat brain by immunohistochemistry. *J. Comp. Neurol.* 210, (September 1982), pp.211-224, ISSN 0021-9967.

Jomphe, C.; Lemelin, PL.; Okano, H. & Trudeau, LE. (2006). Bidirectional regulation of dopamine D2 and neurotensin NTS1 receptors in dopamine neurons. *Eur. J. Neurosci.* 24, (November 2006), pp.2789-2800, ISSN 0953-816X.

Lambert, PD.; Gross, R.; Nemeroff, CB. & Kilts, CD., (1995). Anatomy and mechanisms of neurotensin–dopamine interactions in the central nervous system. *Ann. N. Y. Acad. Sci.* 757, (May 1995), pp. 377–389, ISSN 0077-8923.

Li, X M.; Ferraro, L.; Tanganelli, S.; O'Connor, WT.; Hasselrot, U.; Ungerstedt, U. & Fuxe, K. (1995). Neurotensin peptides antagonistically regulate postsynaptic dopamine D2 receptor in rat nucleus accumbens: a receptor binding and microdialysis study. *J. Neural Transm. [Gen Sect]*, 102, pp.125-137, ISSN 0300-9564.

Li, Z.; Boules ,M.; Williams, K.; Peris, J. & Richelson, E. (2010) The novel neurotensin analog NT69L blocks phencyclidine (PCP)-induced increases in locomotor activity and

PCP-induced increases in monoamine and amino acids levels in the medial prefrontal cortex. *Brain Res.*, 1311, (January 2010), pp. 28-36, ISSN 0006-8993.

Mateu, G.; Privat, A.; Thibault. J. & Vignon, J. (2000). Modulation of glutamate neurotoxicity on mesencephalic dopaminergic neurons in primary cultures by the presence of striatal target cells. *Int. J. Dev. Neurosci.* 18, (October 2000), pp.607–613, ISSN 0736-5748.

Matsuyama, S.; Higashi, H.; Maeda, H.; Greengard, P. & Nishi, A. (2002). Neurotensin regulates DARPP-32 thr34 phosphorylation in neostriatal neurons by activation of dopamine D1-type receptors. *J. Neurochem.* 81, (April 2002), pp.325-334, ISSN 0022-3042.

Mazella, J.; Zsurger, N.; Navarro, V.; Chabry, J.; Kaghad, M. & Caput, D. (1998) The 100-kDa neurotensin receptor is gp95/sortilin, a non-G-protein-coupled receptor, *J. Biol. Chem.* 273, (October 1998), pp.26273–26276, ISSN 0021-9258.

Meldrum, B. & Garthwaite, J. (1990). Excitatory amino acid neurotoxicity and neurodegenerative disease. *Trends Pharmacol. Sci.* 11, (September 1990) pp.379-387, ISSN 0165-6147.

Meltzer, LT.; Christoffersen, CL. & Serpa, KA. (1997). Modulation of dopamine neuronal activity by glutamate receptor subtypes. *Neurosci. Biobehav.* 21, (July 1997), pp.511-518. ISSN 0149-7634.

Mendez, M.; Souaze, F.; Nagano, M.; Kelly, PA.; Rostene, W. & Forgez, P. (1997). High affinity neurotensin receptor mRNA distribution in rat brain and peripheral tissues. Analysis by quantitative RT-PCR. *J. Mol. Neurosci.* 9, (October 1997), pp.93–102, ISSN 0895-8696.

Mesnage, V.; Houeto, JL.; Bonnet, AM.; Clavier, I.; Arnulf, I.; Cattelin, F.; Le Fur, G.; Damier, P.; Welter, ML. & Agid Y. (2004). Neurokinin B, neurotensin and Cannabinoid receptor antagonists and Parkinson disease. *Clin. Neuropharmacol.* 27, (May-June 2004), pp.108-110, ISSN 0362-5664.

Mount, H.; Welner, S.; Quirion, R. & Boksa, P. (1989). Glutamate stimulation of3H]dopamine release from dissociated cell cultures of rat ventral mesencephalon. *J Neurochem* 52, (april 1989) pp.1300–1310, ISSN 0022-3042.

Nalivaiko, E.; Michaud, JC.; Soubrié, P. & Le Fur, G. (1998). Electrophysiological evidence for putative subtypes of neurotensin receptors in guinea-pig mesencephalic dopaminergic neurons. *Neuroscience* 86, (October 1998), pp.799-811, ISSN 0306-4522.

Nemeroff, CB. & Cain, ST. (1985). Neurotensin-dopamine interactions in the CNS. *Trends Pharmacol. Sci.* 6, pp.201-205. ISSN 0165-6147.

Nouel, D.; Sarret, P.; Vincent, JP.; Mazella, J. & Beaudet, A. (1999). Pharmacological, molecular and functional characterization of glial neurotensin receptors. *Neuroscience* 94, pp.1189-1197, ISSN 0306-4522.

Obeso, JA.; Linazasoro, G.; Guridi, J.; Ramos, E. & Rodriguez-Oroz, MC. (2000). High frequency stimulation of the subthalamic nucleus and levodopa induced dyskinesias in Parkinson's disease. *J. Neurol. Neurosurg. Psychiatry* 68, (January 2000), pp.122-3, ISSN 0022-3050.

Obeso, JA.; Marin, C.; Rodriguez-Oroz, C.; Blesa, J.; Benitez-Temiño, B.; Mena-Segovia. J.; Rodríguez, M. & Olanow. CW. (2008). The basal ganglia in Parkinson's disease: current concepts and unexplained observations. *Ann Neurol.* 64 Suppl2, (December 2008), S30-46, ISSN 0364-5134.

Osborne, PG.; O'Connor, WT.; Beck, O. & Ungerstedt, U. (1994). Acute vs chronic haloperidol; Relationship between tolerance to catalepsy and caudate and accumbens DA, GABA and Acetylcholine release. *Brain Res.* 643, (January 1994), pp.20–30, ISSN 0006-8993.

Palacios, JM. & Kuhar, MJ. (1981).Neurotensin receptors are located on dopamine-containing neurones in rat midbrain. *Nature.* 294, (December 1981), pp.587-589, ISSN 0028-0836.

Parent, A. & Hazrati, LN. (1995). Functional anatomy of the basal ganglia. I. The cortico-basal ganglia-thalamo-cortical loop. *Brain Res Brain Res Rev* 20, (January 1995), pp.91–127, ISSN 0165-0173.

Perez-Otano, I. & Ehlers, M.D. (2005). Homeostatic plasticity and NMDA receptor trafficking. *Trends Neurosci.* 28, (May 2005), pp. 229-238, ISSN 0165-6147.

Petrie, Ak.; Schmidt, D.; Busber, M.; Fadel, J.; Carraway, RE. & Deutch, A. (2005) Neurotensin activates GABAergic interneurons in the prefrontal cortex. *J. Neurosci.* 25, (February 2005), pp.1629-1636, ISSN 0270-6474.

Poncelet, M.; Gueudet, C.; Gully, D.; Soubriè, P. & Le Fur, G. (1994) Turning behavior induced by intrastriatal injection of neurotensin in mice: sensitivity to non-peptide neurotensin antagonists. *Naunyn Schmiedeberg's Arch. Pharmacol.* 349, (January 1994), pp.57-60, ISSN 0028-1298.

Pickel, VM.; Chan, J.; Delle Donne, KT.; Boudin, H.; Pélaprat, D. & Rosténe, W. (2001). High-affinity neurotensin receptors in the rat nucleus accumbens: subcellular targeting and relation to endogenous ligand. *J. Comp. Neurol.* 435, (June 2001), pp.142-155, ISSN 0021-9967.

Quirion, R.; Chiueh, CC.; Everist, HD. & Pert, A. (1985). Comparative localization of neurotensin receptors on nigrostriatal and mesolimbic dopaminergic terminals, *Brain Res.* 327, (February 1985), pp.385–389, ISSN 0006-8993.

Reid, MS.; O'Connor, WT.; Herrera-Marschitz, M. & Ungerstedt, U. (1990). The effect of intranigral GABA and dynorphin A injections on striatal dopamine and GABA release: evidence that dopamine provides inhibitory regulation of striatal GABA neurons via D2 type receptors. *Brain Res.* 519, (June 1990), pp.255–260, ISSN 0006-8993.

Rostene, W.; Brouard, A.; Dana, C.; Masuo, Y.; Agid, F.; Vial, M.; Lhiaubet, AM. Rostene, W. & Pelaprat, D. (1992). Interaction between neurotensin and dopamine in the brain. Morphofunctional and clinical evidence. *Ann. N.Y. Acad. of Sci.* 668, pp. 217–231, ISSN 0077-8923.

Rostene, W.; Azzi, M.; Boudin, H.; Lepee, I.; Souaze, F.; Mendez-Ubach, M.; Betancur, C. & Gully, D. (1997). Use of nonpeptide antagonists to explore the physiological roles of neurotensin. Focus on brain neurotensin/dopamine interactions. *Ann. N.Y. Acad. Sci.* 814,(April 1997), pp.125-141, ISSN 0077-8923.

Saleh, TM.; Kombian, SB.; Zidichouski, JA. & Pittman, QJ. (1997). Cholecystokinin and neurotensin inversely modulate excitatory synaptic transmission in the parabrachial nucleus in vitro. *Neuroscience* 77, (March 1997), pp. 23-35, ISSN 0306-4522.

Sanz, B.; Exposito, I. & Mora, F. (1993). Effects of neurotensin on the release of glutamic acid in the prefrontal cortex and striatum of the rat. *Neuroreport* 4, (September 1993), pp.1194-1196, ISSN 0959-4965.

Sarret, P.; Perron, A.; Stroh, T. & Beaudet, A. (2003). Immunohistochemical distribution of NTS2 neurotensin receptors in the rat central nervous system. *J. Comp. Neurol.* 461, (July 2003), pp.520–538, ISSN 0021-9967 .

Scheel-Krüger, J. (1986). Dopamine-GABA interactions: evidence that GABA transmits, modulates and mediates dopaminergic functions in the basal ganglia and the limbic system. *Acta Neurol. Scand. Suppl.* 107, pp.1-54, ISSN 0065-1427.

Shibata, K.; Yamada, K. & Furukawa, T. (1987). Possible neuronal mechanisms involved in neurotensin-induced catalepsy in mice. *Psychopharmacology (Berl).* 91, pp.288-292, ISSN 0033-3158.

Schimpff , RM.; Avard, C.; Fénelon, G.; Lhiaubet, AM.; Tennezé, L.; Vidailhet, M. & Rostène, W. (2001). Increased plasma neurotensin concentrations in patients with Parkinson's disease .*J Neurol Neurosurg. Psychiatry* 70, (June 2001), pp.784–786, ISSN 0022-3050.

Silkis, I. (2001). The cortico-basal ganglia-thalamocortical circuit with synaptic plasticity. II. Mechanism of synergistic modulation of thalamic activity via the direct and indirect pathways through the basal ganglia. *Biosystems.* 59, (January 2001), pp.7-14, ISSN 0303-2647.

Sirinathsinghji, DJS. & Heavens, RP. (1989). Stimulation of GABA release from the rat neostriatum and globus pallidus in vivo by corticotropinreleasing factor. *Neurosci. Lett.* 100, (May 1989), pp. 203–209, ISSN 0304-3940.

Skeberdis, VA.; Lan, J.; Opitz, T.; Zheng, X.; Bennett, MV. & Zukin, RS. (2001). mGluR1-mediated potentiation of NMDA receptors involves a rise in intracellular calcium and activation of protein kinase C. *Neuropharmacology* 40, (June 2001), pp.856-865, ISSN 0028-3908.

Smith, Y. & Villalba, R. (2008). Striatal and extrastriatal dopamine in the basal ganglia: an overview of its anatomical organization in normal and Parkinsonian brains. *Mov Disord.* 23 Suppl (3), S534-547, ISSN 0885-3185.

Soltis, RP.; Anderson, LA.; Walters, JR. & Kelland, MD. (1994). A role for non-NMDA excitatory amino acid receptors in regulating the basal activity of rat globus pallidus neurons and their activation by the subthalamic nucleus. *Brain Res.* 666, (December 1994), pp.21-30, ISSN 0006-8993.

Sonsalla, PK.; Albers, DS. & Zeevalk, GD. (1998). Role of glutamate in neurodegeneration of dopamine neurons in several animal models of parkinsonism. *Amino Acids.* 14, pp.69-74, ISSN 0939-4451.

St-Gelais, F.; Jomphe, C. & Trudeau, LE. (2006). The role of neurotensin in central nervous system pathophysiology: what is the evidence? *J. Psychiatry Neurosci.* 31, (July 2006), pp. 229-245, ISSN 1180-4882.

Tanganelli, S.; von Euler, G.; Fuxe, K.; Agnati, LF. & Ungerstedt, U. (1989). Neurotensin counteracts apomorphine-induced inhibition of dopamine release as studied by microdialysis in rat neostriatum. *Brain Res.* 502, (November 1989), pp.319-324, ISSN 0006-8993.

Tanganelli, S.; O'Connor, WT.; Ferraro, L.; Bianchi, C.; Beani, L.; Ungerstedt, U. & Fuxe, K. (1994). Facilitation of GABA release by neurotensin is associated with a reduction of dopamine release in rat nucleus accumbens. *Neuroscience* 60, (June 1994), pp.649-657, ISSN 0306-4522.

Tanganelli, S.; Sandager Nielsen, K.; Ferraro, L.; Antonelli, T.; Kehr, J.; Franco, R.; Ferré, S.; Agnati, LF.; Fuxe, K. & Scheel-Krüger, J. (2004). Striatal plasticity at the network level. Focus on adenosine A2A and D2 interactions in models of Parkinson's Disease. *Parkinsonism Relat. Disord.* 10, (July 2004), pp.273-80, ISSN 1353-8020.

Tanji, H.; Araki, T.; Fujihara, K. (1999). Alteration of neurotensin receptors in MPTP-treated mice. *Peptides* 20, pp.803-807, ISSN 0196-9781.

Taylor, MD.; De Ceballos, ML.; Rose, S.; Jenner, P. & Marsden, CD. (1992). Effects of a unilateral 6-hydroxydopamine lesion and prolonged L-3,4-dihydroxyphenylalanine treatment on peptidergic systems in rat basal ganglia. *Eur. J. Pharmacol.* 219, (August 1992), pp.183-192, ISSN 0014-2999 .

Trudeau, LE. (2000). Neurotensin regulates intracellular calcium in ventral tegmental area astrocytes: evidence for the involvement of multiple receptors. *Neuroscience* 97, pp.293-302, ISSN 0306-4522.

Uhl, GR. (1982). Distribution of neurotensin and its receptor in the central nervous system. *Ann. N. Y. Acad. Sci.* 400, pp.132-49, ISSN 0077-8923.

Vincent, J.P.; Mazella, J. & Kitabgi, P. (1999). Neurotensin and neurotensin receptors. *Trends Pharmacol. Sci.* 20, (July 1999) pp.302-309, ISSN 0165-6147.

Von Euler, G. & Fuxe, K. (1987). Neurotensin reduces the affinity of D2 receptors in rat striatal membranes. *Acta Physiol. Scand.* 131, (December 1987), pp.625-626, ISSN 0001-6772.

Wang, Z.; Kai, L.; Day, M.; Ronesi, J.; Yin, HH. & Ding, J. (2006). Dopaminergic control of corticostriatal long-term synaptic depression in medium spiny neurons is mediated by cholinergic interneurons. *Neuron* 50, (May 2006), pp.443–452, ISSN 0896-6273.

Wang, XM. & Evers, BM. (1999). Characterization of early developmental pattern of expression of neurotensin/neuromedin N gene in foregut and midgut. *Dig. Dis. Sci.* 44, (January 1999), pp.33-40, ISSN 0163-2116.

Werkman, TR.; Kruse, CG.; Nievelstein, H., Long, SK. & Wadman, WJ. (2000). Neurotensin attenuates the quinpirole-induced inhibition of the firing rate of dopamine neurons in the rat substantia nigra pars compacta and the ventral tegmental area. *Neuroscience* 95, pp.417-423, ISSN 0306-4522.

Yamada, M. & Richelson, E. (1995). Heterogeneity of melanized neurons expressing neurotensin receptor messenger RNA in the substantia nigra and the nucleus paranigralis of control and Parkinson's disease brain. *Neuroscience* 64, (January 1995), pp.405-417, ISSN 0306-4522.

Yung, KK. (1998). Localization of ionotropic and metabotropic glutamate receptors in distinct neuronal elements of the rat substantia nigra. *Neurochem. Int.* 33, (December 1998), pp.313–326, ISSN 0197-0186.

24

Application of Embryonic Stem Cells in Parkinson's Disease

Hassan Niknejad
Nanomedicine and Tissue Engineering Research Center, Shahid Beheshti University of Medical Sciences, Tehran, Iran

1. Introduction

The nervous system is a stimulating target for regenerative medicine. Parkinson's disease (PD), which afflicts over a 1 million people in the US, is a chronic neurodegenerative disorder characterized by the degeneration and death of midbrain neurons that produce the neurotransmitter dopamine (DA), resulting in tremors at rest, an inability to initiate or complete routine movements, muscle rigidity, postural instability, and lack of facial expression. Although the etiology of idiopathic PD is not known, several predisposing factors for the dopaminergic depletion associated with the disease have been suggested, including programmed cell death, viral infection, and environmental toxins.

DA neurons, in the substantia nigra pars compacta, play a prominent role in the control of many brain functions, such as voluntary movements and many behavioral processes (Maxwell & Li, 2005). These neurons can be identified via the expression of some specific transcription factors, including Engrailed 1 (EN1), PITX3, NURR1, and LMX1b, which are also very important in the development of DA neurons (Smidt et al., 2003).

2. Current therapeutic strategies for PD

2.1 Drug therapy and DBS

Current established therapeutic strategies for PD patients comprise drug treatments such as L-dopa (a precursor of dopamine), DA agonists, enzyme inhibitors and deep brain stimulation in the thalamus, subthalamic nucleus and globus pallidus (Figure 1). However, these treatments are effective in early stage and can temporarily ameliorate symptoms and cannot cure the disease. Therefore, there is a need for novel therapeutic approaches which one of them is to regenerate the damaged tissue. Since direct regeneration of brain tissues is difficult to achieve, an alternate supply of neural cells is required in order to attain any therapeutic goal. Cell replacement therapy (neurotransplantation) has been suggested to have a great potential for restorative therapy in PD (Freed et al., 2001; Hagell & Brundin, 2001; Olanow et al., 2003).

2.2 Cell replacement therapy

2.2.1 Foetal mesencephalic tissue

Transplantation of human foetal ventral mesencephalic tissues into the putamen or caudate nucleus of PD patients has been adopted as a potentially curative cell replacement therapy

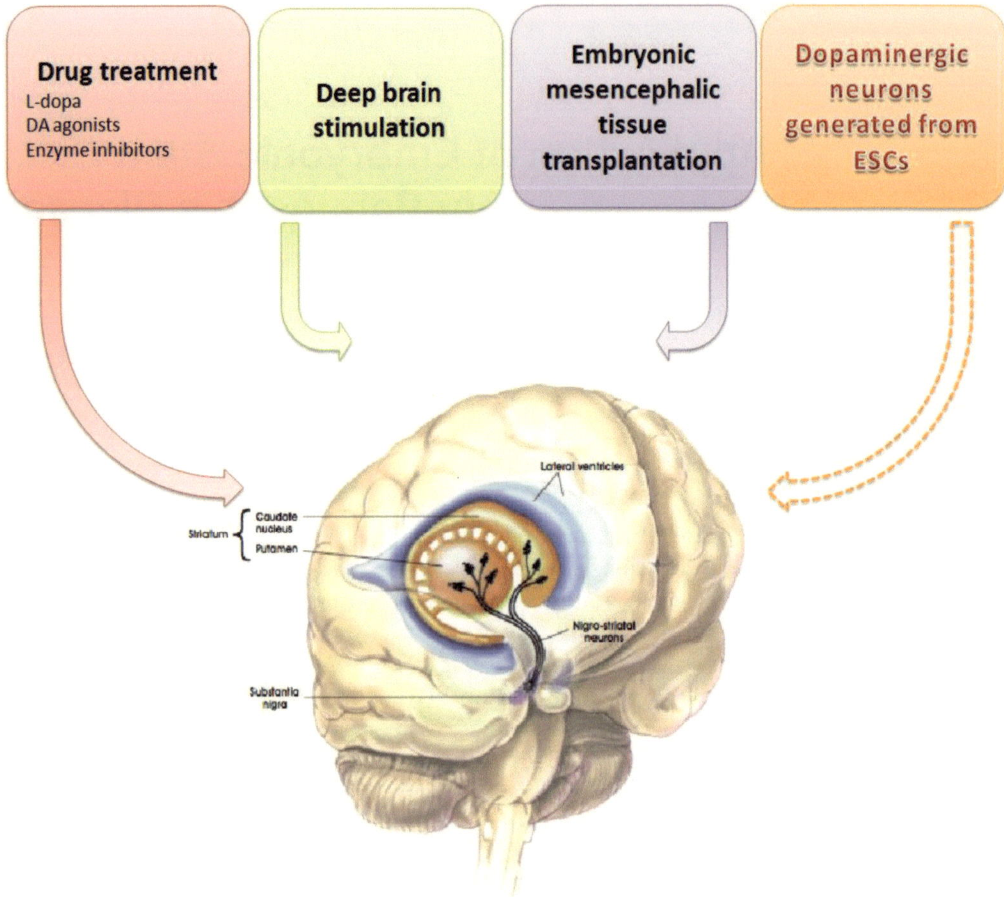

Fig. 1. In the normal brain, DA neurons located in the substantia nigra send their axons to the striatum (i.e. the putamen and caudate nucleus). In the PD brain, the main pathology leading to motor symptoms is a degeneration of these neurons causing a loss of DA in the striatum. Drug treatment, deep brain stimulation and embryonic mesencephalic tissue transplantation are current therapeutic approaches for PD. Transplantation of DA neurons generated from embryonic stem cells has been suggested to restore striatal dopaminergic innervation thereby alleviating PD symptoms.

with long term survival of grafted cells (Kordower et al., 2008a; Li et al., 2008; Mendez et al., 2008). A bulk of experimental and clinical studies have shown functional efficacy of grafting of embryonic mesencephalic tissue into the striatum and a biological mechanism underlying the observed improvement. In spite of promising results of foetal mesencephalic cells transplantation, so far numerous unresolved problems remain to be addressed, such as ethical and religious questions and logistics of acquiring foetal tissues, graft-induced off-medication dyskinesias in up to 56% of transplanted patients (Freed et al., 2001; Hagell et al., 2002; Olanow et al., 2003) and inadequate foetal tissues for transplantation (since treatment of a single PD patient requires DA neurons from six to ten human aborted foetuses). To bypass these difficulties, neurons with a DA phenotype generated from embryonic stem cells (ESCs) could be employed as a practical and effective alternative for foetal brain tissues for transplantation.

2.2.2 Embryonic stem cells

ESCs, derived from the inner cell mass of early post-fertilization blastocysts, are capable of unlimited cell expansion *in vitro* while maintaining their pluripotency. These characteristics of ESCs make them an excellent source of functional differentiated cells for cell replacement therapy of neurodegenerative medicine such as PD, provided that reliable means of inducing differentiation to specific cell types can be achieved. After differentiation, ESCs-derived neurons have to work at least similar to those in embryonic mesencephalic transplantations. Therefore, these neurons have to achieve the following requirements to improve PD markedly after grafting: (i) release DA and exhibit the molecular, morphological and electrophysiological properties of midbrain DA neurons (Mendez et al., 2005; ,Isacson et al., 2003); (ii) reverse motor deficits in animal models resembling the symptoms in patients; (iii) enable 100000 or more grafted DA neurons to survive long term in each human putamen (Hagell & Brundin, 2001); (iv) re-establish a dense terminal network throughout the striatum; and (v) become functionally integrated into host neural circuitries (Piccini et al., 2000).

Two basic strategies can be employed to use ESCs as a cell source for cell replacement therapy: they can be used without any previous in vitro differentiation based on the hypothesis that regional microenvironment is the best inductive cue to obtain the required cell type. An alternative strategy would be to partly or totally differentiate ESCs into the desired cells based on the hypothesis that the host tissue-derived inductive cues are not sufficient to achieve this and to avoid tumor formation at the same time.

Although it has been reported that transplantation of undifferentiated ESCs into the midbrain parkinsonian rats resulted in dopaminergic differentiation of these cells, high rate of differentiated cells were serotonergic neurons (a relation of 2:1 of dopaminergic to serotonergic neurons). Due to this fact that serotonergic neurons in grafts are responsible for off-medication dyskinesias in clinical transplantation studies (Carlsson et al., 2007), it is rather unlikely that the resulting cell composition is well suited for successful transplantation. A more limiting issue was that 20% of the grafted animals had to be sacrificed before the defined study endpoint because of teratoma formation. Although several strategies have been employed to reduce the risk of tumor formation (Chung et al., 2006; Li et al., 1998; Schuldiner et al., 2003), the use of undifferentiated ESCs remains an unsafe strategy.

3. In vitro neural differentiation of ESCs

The in vitro differentiation of ESCs toward dopaminergic neurons has followed different culture protocols in the presence of various combinations of growth factors and signaling molecules. By studying these signaling molecules present in the midbrain microenvironment during development and in the adult, and which key regulatory transcription factors the cells express, protocols for controlling *ex vivo* dopaminergic neurons differentiation can be achieved.

3.1 The major signaling molecules

Retinoic acid (RA) is one of the most important signaling molecules that promote neuralization in embryos and later in development (Bain et al., 1996; Guan et al., 2001; Diez del Corral & Storey, 2004). All-trans RA, which can bind to both RAR subtypes, is commonly employed to induce neuronal differentiation *in vitro*. RA induces a pan-neuronal differentiation and the cell population obtained after application of this differentiation factor is relatively heterogeneous (Carpenter et al., 2001, Schuldiner et al., 2000). Takahashi *et al* showed that cells cultured with RA and fetal bovine serum (FBS) expressed markers for GABAergic, dopaminergic, and cholinergic neuronal phenotypes at low levels (Takahashi et al., 1999).

Wnt3a is another signaling molecule recently shown to play a key role in regulating neurogenesis in the adult brain. *In vivo* expression of a Wnt3a inhibitor reduced neurogenesis in the adult hippocampus. By contrast, Wnt3 overexpression *in vivo* and *in vitro* increased neuronal differentiation (Lie et al., 2005). However, Wnt3's overexpression *in vitro* resulted in a mixed culture of glia and neurons. Also, it is yet to be determined whether Wnt signaling induces a specific neuronal phenotype or serves as a nonspecific, pan-neuronal signal.

BMP is another inhibitory signal found within neural differentiation. It has been shown that the overexpression of the BMP antagonist Noggin increased neural differentiation in neurosphere culture (Setoguchi et al., 2004). BMP signaling activation in undifferentiated cells can result in extraembryonic endoderm committed cells and epidermogenesis. In addition, it has been reported that BMP4 can induce mesodermal differentiation. Noggin is a well characterized BMP2 and BMP4 antagonist and has been shown as neural inducer in *Xenopus* embryos (Niknejad et al., 2010). Since ESCs are pluripotent and susceptible to give rise to all three germ layers, blocking BMP signaling using its antagonist noggin can induce neuronal differentiation by its inhibitory effects on the mesodermal, endodermal, and epidermal fate of ESCs (Gerrard et al., 2005). In addition, inhibiting Notch and BMP-2 signaling may synergistically enhance neuronal differentiation more than suppressing either alone.

However, using these signaling molecules solely result in the mixed population of neural cells, indicating that there are most likely other signals found within the *in vivo* microenvironment that work in conjunction with each other to ensure a neuronal cell fate commitment.

3.2 Current protocols for DA differentiation

Numerous methods have been employed to differentiate mouse and human ESCs into neural cells. Mouse ESCs can be induced into neural progenitors by several methods, such as the use of retinoic acid (RA) treatment of embryoid body (EB) (Bain et al., 1995; Wichterle et al., 2002), a multistep-induction and selection culture (Lee et al., 2000), an adherent monoculture system in serum-free medium (Ying et al., 2003), and a co-culture with stromal cell types (Kawasaki et al., 2000, Barberi et al., 2003). Human ESCs can be induced into the neural lineages using similar methodologies: through the formation of EBs in suspension (Zhang et al., 2006), an adherent monoculture system (Benzing et al., 2006), with co-culture (Ueno et al., 2006) and through spontaneous differentiation of human ESCs (Zhang et al., 2001, Reubinoff et al., 2001). Each of these protocols has its pros and cons. In the following part, the most used procedures for neural differentiation of ESCs will be described.

3.2.1 Embryoid body formation

The well-studied system for neuronal differentiation of ESCs involves the formation of three-dimensional structures called embryoid bodies (EBs) that, to a limited extent, simulates embryonic development *in vivo* (Itskovitz-Eldor et al., 2000). EBs are spontaneously generated when ESCs are cultured in suspension cultures without LIF or serum, in either non-adhesive dishes or hanging drops. The cells in EB begin to differentiate into a heterogeneous

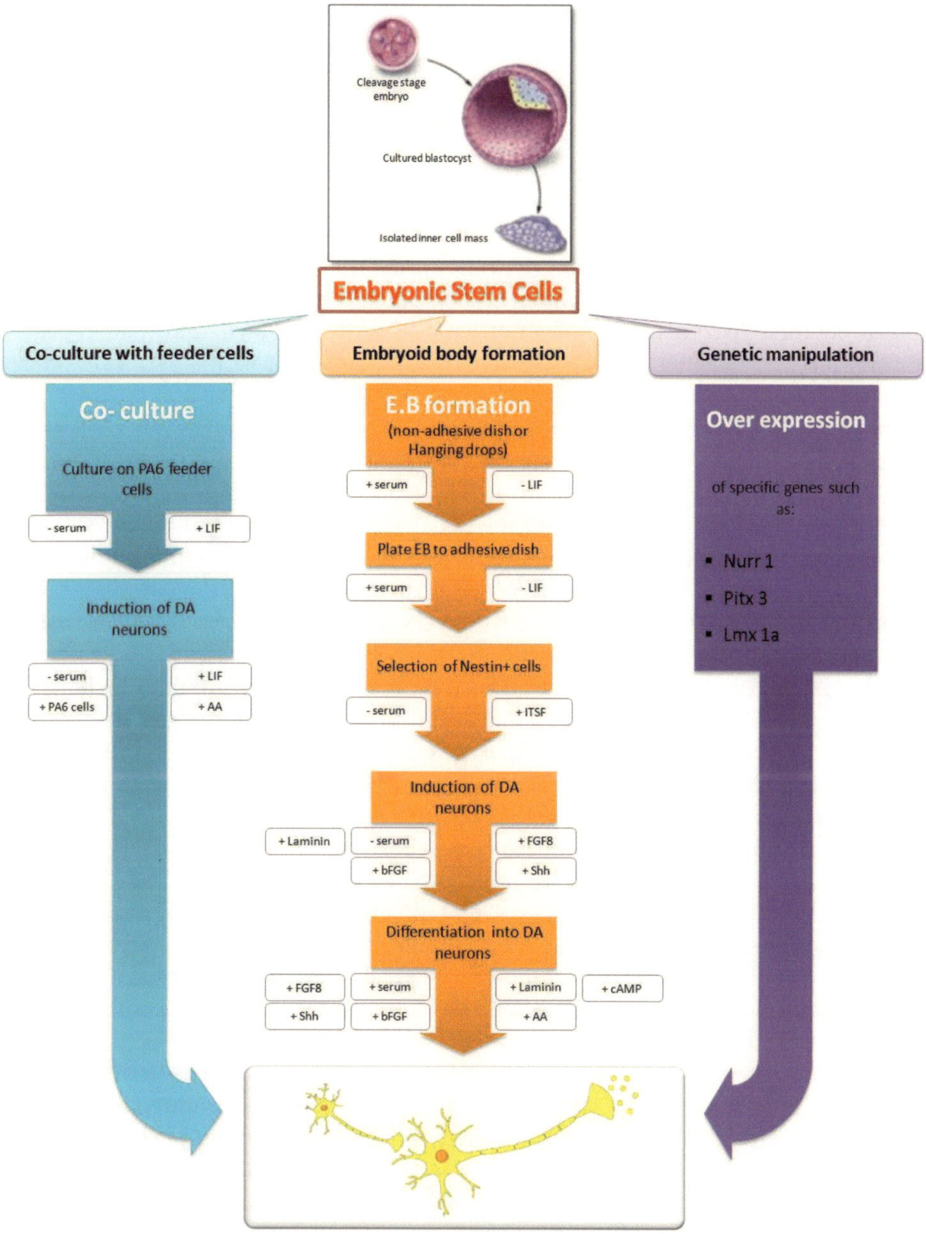

Fig. 2. Schemata depicting steps of three protocols by which ESCs are induced to adopt the DA Lineage.

population of progenitor cells that can form all cell types from the three germ layers, such as skeletal muscle, cardiac, hematopoietic and neuron-like cells. Therefore, spontaneous differentiation of EBs yields only a small fraction of cells with neural lineages. By using different morphogens and growth factors during EB formation, a higher fraction of neural cells can be produced (Figure 2).

After transfer of EBs from a low attachment plate into a normal adhesion plate, the EBs form neuroepithelial cells that organize into neural tube like rosettes. After dissociation of neuroepithelial cells and addition of neural differentiation medium, which consists of BDNF, GDNF, AMP, and ascorbic acid, DA differentiation begins 3–4 weeks after the initial treatment of ESCs (Yan et al., 2005).

EB formation method is still commonly used with the addition of the other supplementary to media such as growth factors. Bain *et al* were the first to show that RA can induce neural differentiation in EBs derived from mouse ESCs, i.e. a high proportion of the resulting cells expressed neuronal markers and had neuronal properties (Bain et al., 1995). In this work, EBs were cultured with RA for 4 days and then plated on laminin-coated dishes. The cells expressed neuronal markers beta-tubulin III and NF-M as well as neural-related genes such as transmitter synthesizing genes glutamic acid decarboxylase (GAD), TH, transmitter receptor subunits GluRs, and a cytoskeletal subunit, NF-L.

RA applied to ESCs can induce concentration-dependent differentiation of neural cells. Okada *et al* tested the effects of different concentrations of RA on the neural differentiation of mouse ESCs (Okada et al., 2004). Lower RA levels (10^{-8}M) were found to induce neural progenitor cells from ESCs, indicated by the high protein expression of the neural precursor marker nestin and low expression of neuronal and glial markers beta-tubulin III and GFAP, respectively. In contrast, high levels of RA (2 X 10^{-6} M) decreased the expression of nestin while increasing beta-tubulin III and GFAP levels. These results are consistent with other studies demonstrating differentiation of neural progenitors at high RA concentrations (Wichterle., 2002, Bain et al., 1996). RA also directs neural differentiation in human ESCs derived-EB cultures (Guan et al., 2001). The addition of RA and nerve growth-factor (NGF) increased the rate of neuronal cells that formed within human ESC-derived EBs (Schuldiner et al., 2001). However, RA is a strong teratogen and should therefore be used at lower doses to prevent toxicity.

One strategy to direct mouse and human ESCs into "midbrain dopaminergic" neurons is through formation of EBs, followed by the combined addition of Shh and FGF-8 and at a later stage ascorbic acid (AA) (Lee et al., 2000). Using this method, 34% of the resulting beta-tubulin III positive neurons derived from mouse ESCs were TH positive. To shorten induction protocol time, Lau *et al* cultured EBs in KO DMEM supplemented with EGF, FGF-2, and ascorbic acid (Lau et al., 2006). After 3 days, EBs were plated on gelatin-coated dishes and cultured with DMEM/F12 containing EGF, FGF-8, Shh, and ascorbic acid. Cells were subsequently cultured in Neurobasal medium with ascorbic acid. This method generated approximately 40% DA neurons, characterized by their expression of dopamine transporter DAT in 14 days. This chemically defined system for ESCs derivation of DA neurons may be advantageous compared to the co-culturing method, which will be discussed in the next part, as it reduces exposure to animal-derived components and allows for easier determination of factors that influence cell fate.

Another strategy to obtain "midbrain dopaminergic" neurons is the growth of EBs in a conditioned medium with a human hepatocarcinoma cell line followed by conventional serum- free culture in a medium containing bFGF (Schulz et al., 2004, Schulz et al., 2003), or by co-culturing them with telomerase-immortalized fetal midbrain astrocytes (Roy et al., 2006). EBs plated on tissue culture dishes and in the presence of serum-free ITSF medium showed induced differentiation toward dopaminergic precursors within 10 days. In the next step, the cells were transferred to polyornithine/laminin-coated dishes and exposed to a new medium supplemented with FGF2 and Shh (Roy et al., 2006). Withdrawal of these factors, but the addition of BDNF, GDNF, and FBS, yields dopaminergic neurons that are TH positive. The majority of TH positive cells expressed simultaneously G-protein gated inwardly rectifying potassium channel type 2 (Sonntag et al., 2007), which is almost exclusively expressed in the membrane of DA neurons projecting to the dorsolateral putamen, and are functionally linked to dopamine D2 and GABAB receptors (Sonntag et al., 2007).

3.2.2 Co-culture with feeder cells

Another important strategy to enhance the differentiation toward neuron lineage is co-culture of ESCs with stromal cell lines such as PA6 (Kawasaki et al., 2000) and MS5 (Barberi et al., 2003). This effect of PA6 cells has been named the inductive factor stromal cell-derived inducing activity (SDIA) (Mizusekiet et al., 2003; Kawasaki et al., 2000). After screening various cell lines, Kawasaki *et al* found that PA6 stromal cells derived from mouse skull bone marrow is a potent inducer of neural differentiation from ESCs (Figure 2). In contrast to EB formation protocol, this method does not require growth in serum, the formation of EBs, or the selection of neural precursor cells. In this method, ESCs were co-cultured without serum on PA6 cells for 8 days in differentiation medium and for an additional 6-12 days in G-MEM supplemented with N2 and other components. Ninety-two percent of the colonies contained differentiated neurons positive for neural markers NCAM, nestin, and beta-tubulin III and MAP2 and only less than 2% of the colonies were positive for mesodermal and glial markers.

Co-culturing with stromal cell lines with some modifications has become a common strategy to differentiate ESCs into neural cells. In comparison to EB formation protocol, this method has fewer steps and is relatively easier and more reproducible for the generation of neural precursors and neuronal subtypes (Figure 2). Due to the risk of contamination with animal-derived components (Martin et al., 2005), some alternative approaches were recently developed to use instead of stromal feeders. Human amniotic membrane, the innermost layer of placenta has been used as an alternative (Ueno et al., 2006; Niknejad et al., 2008). This approach involves the co-culture of matrix layers of human amniotic membrane with human ESCs for neural induction. Fifteen days after culturing on amniotic membrane, human ESCs produced a population of cells that were greater than 85% nestin positive, and many of these formed rosette-like clusters. While this method eliminates the introduction of animal-derived products, identification of the factors involved in the regulation of neural differentiation, and overcoming inherent limitations in the scale up of processes involving cell co-cultures, need to be further addressed.

Kitajima *et al* devised a co-culture method for producing neurospheres using PA6 stromal cells (Kitajima et al., 2005). To induce neural spheres, ESCs were differentiated on PA6 stroma for 7 days, detached, dissociated, and cultured in growth medium with FGF-2 and EGF. The resulting neurospheres expressed multiple neural markers such as nestin, MAP2 and GFAP, indicative of a heterogeneous population of neural progenitors, mature neurons, and glial cells. Co-culture with PA6 cells for 0-13 days progressively increased the number of spheres generated in a time-dependent manner until day 11. The resulting neurospheres could be further propagated when switched to a serum-free culture and then differentiated into all three neural types. By changing the time of co-culture with PA6 cells, it was also possible to induce different proportions of neuronal and glial precursor cells. This system thus enabled the production of large numbers of spheres without utilizing EB formation.

Also, using MS5 instead of PA6 stromal cells efficiently induced neural differentiation of mouse ES cells, and the resulting cells were able to differentiate into more neuronal types (GABAergic, sertonergic, dopaminergic and cholinergic neurons) (Barberi et al., 2003).
Yue *et al* showed that primate ESCs can differentiate into dopaminergic neurons by coculture of ESCs with sertoli cells. Neurons that had been differentiated on sertoli cells were positive for Pax2, En1, and AADC; midbrain related markers and negative for dopamine-β-hydroxylase, a marker of noradrenergic neurons and could release dopamine *in vitro* when depolarized by KCL (Yue et al., 2006).

3.2.3 Genetic manipulation

At this time, EB formation protocol and co-culture with feeder cells typically lead to a mixed population of cell types. Moreover, to effectively use this approaches *in vitro* the dose, order of addition, and time of exposure to growth factors are all important parameters that must be optimized. This is a difficult task since many of the signals involved in regulating neuronal differentiation are only now being elucidated. It seems transfection of key genes such as important transcription factors (using conventional DNA delivery, lentiviral and adenoviral vectors, and homologous recombination) to ESCs is capable of inducing a specific neural lineage and can potentially increase the homogeneity of differentiated cells (Figure 2).
To enhance TH expression in neural stem cells, Sakurada *et al* used a retrovirus to overexpress Nurr1, a transcription factor belonging to the nuclear receptor super family that is expressed in midbrain DA neurons. This approach induced TH expression in nearly all infected cells *in vitro*. However, infected cells did not express detectable levels of DOPA, the dopamine precursor whose production is catalyzed by TH, and functional production of DOPA was only detected when the cells were differentiated with retinoic acid. Even though the resulting population uniformly expressed TH, the frequency of neuronal markers within these TH positive cells was still low (Sakurada et al., 1999). These results implicate a need for additional manipulations to increase neuronal maturation and the functional production of dopamine.
Similar results were observed in neural stem cells derived from E13/E14 rat foetal brain tissue, in which Nurr1 overexpression led to an increase in TH expression (Kim et al., 2003). However, infected cells did not mature. Park *et al* used retroviral vectors that co-expressed Nurr1 and a second transcription factor to force neuronal differentiation. They examined the bHLH transcription factors Mash1, Ngn1, Ngn2 and NeuroD1, all known to induce neuronal differentiation (Kageyama& Nakanishi, 1997), and they reported that the induction of TH expression depended on which bHLH transcription was co-expressed with Nurr1. Ngn1, Ngn2 and NeuroD1 decreased the Nurr1-induced expression of TH, whereas Mash1 overexpression not only maintained expression but also increased the fraction of cells that expressed the neuronal marker Map2ab. Importantly, they showed that the combined expression of Mash1 and Nurr1 yielded neurons with electrophysiological properties similar to those of mature DA neurons (Park et al., 2006a).
Furthermore, Park *et al* showed that when grafted into Parkinsonian rats, cells co-expressing Nurr1 and Mash1 reversed behavioral deficits. Intriguingly, a retrovirus encoding Shh, the anti-apoptotic protein Bcl-xl, and Nurr1 produced functionally mature dopaminergic neurons similar to the Mash1 vector studies (Park et al., 2006b). These studies demonstrate the potency of genetic manipulation and highlight the fact that significant additional work

will be needed to explore whether extracellular signal combinations can achieve similar results.

In addition to its role in directing differentiation towards a DA phenotype, Nurr1 synergizes with Pitx3 to promote terminal maturation of midbrain DA neurons from both mouse and human ESCs (Martinat et al., 2006). Lentiviral vectors carrying Nurr1, Pitx3, Lmx1b, or En1 were introduced at the neural precursor stage after induction into EBs from mouse ESCs. The combined transduction of Nurr1 and Pitx3 dramatically induced the expression of the late marker DAT (dopamine transporter), but not TH. Only Nurr1 alone induced expression of TH.

The two predominant methods developed on mouse cells, transfection of mouse ESCs with specific factors such as Nurr-1 and Lmx1a as well as co-cultures with stromal cells, have been translated to human ESCs to direct DA neuron differentiation. Similar results were found after human ES cells were transduced with lentiviral vectors carrying both Nurr1 and Pitx3 at the neural precursor stage as well as co-cultured with stromal cells (Martinat et al., 2006). Nurr1 and Pitx3 together promoted the maturation of midbrain DA neurons and led to an increase in TH positive cells. In electrophysiological analysis, differentiated human ESCs displayed basic neuronal characteristics such as action potentials, burst firing, and miniature spontaneous excitatory postsynaptic currents. Transplantation of these cells into a mouse model of PD improved some motor ability 6 weeks post-transplantation; however, there was limited maturation of the engrafted human ES-derived cells, as assessed by low expression of TH

4. ESCs in PD: hype or hope

Despite all of the advantages of ESCs for cell replacement therapy, some pitfalls must be overcome before ESCs are used therapeutically for PD. The major limitation is ethical issues concerning to their embryonic origin. Human embryos are most often destroyed as the stem cells are harvested. Hence the question: Can we intentionally kill a developing human being at this stage to expand scientific knowledge and potentially provide medical benefit to others? As a result, some regulations limit funding of research to the initial set of derived human ESCs, strictly withholding support for the study and derivation of new stem cells lines. However, creating new stem lines by deriving human ESCs from single blastomeres (Klimanskaya et al., 2006), without destroying the embryo was a promising result to bypass the ethical problem of ESCs.

The other challenge in employing ESCs for developmental biology research and their possible application in cell replacement therapy is to direct their wide differentiation potential into specific neural cell lineages. The most important concern of the mentioned protocols of ESCs differentiation toward specific neural lineages is the nonspecific generation of cell populations derived from the three germ layers in the total cell population. In all protocols, the presence of mesodermal- and endodermal-originated cell lineages is unavoidable, which is undesirable for further application in regenerative medicine. Hence, understanding the coordination and roles of intrinsic factors with extrinsic factors will be a critical step to direct ESCs differentiation into dopaminergic neuronal cells.

In addition to mesodermal and endodermal lineages, current protocols result in heterogonous population of glia and neural cells, such as serotonergic, GABAergic and noradrenergic. To date, it is uncertain which of these ingredients are of positive or negative impact on the clinical effectiveness of the transplants. For example in transplantation of foetal mesencephalon which is a mixture of all neural cell types homing to the foetal midbrain, containing serotonergic neurons might be responsible for dyskinetic side effects. On the other hand, it has been shown that foetal midbrain-derived astrocytes have beneficial effects on in vitro differentiation of ESCs into DA neurons. Transplanting a mixture of dopaminergic precursors/neurons and midbrain-specific astrocytes might thus be more effective than a purified DA cell source. No information is available on the effect of GABAergic or noradrenergic neurons also present in midbrain transplants. Therefore, further studies will be required to investigate the effects of the other constituents of neural cells other than DA neurons on dopaminergic differentiation of ESCs and after grafting in the animal model of PD.

As mentioned, current differentiation protocols rely on the use of animal products (e.g. PA6 is a mouse stromal cell line) and thus carry the potential to induce disease transmission through contamination with bacteria, viruses or other infectious agents, such as those responsible for transmissible spongiform encephalopathy. Therefore, animal products should, where possible, be replaced by components of human origin and defined and feeder-free conditions should be developed for differentiation of ESCs into dopaminergic neurons if the cells are going to be implanted in patients.

The other unresolved problem is whether the grafts will be affected by the PD process. The results of foetal mesencephalic tissue transplantations provide evidence that PD pathology might propagate from host to graft (Kordower et al., 2008a; Li et al., 2008; Brundin et al., 2008, Kordower et al., 2008b). However, it seems that at least one decade is required for the development of Lewy bodies (LBs) in the grafted cells (Kordower et al., 2008a; Mendez et al., 2008). This issue should be noticed in the animal model of PD.

Rejection of grafts is an important issue in cell replacement therapy, particularly for ESCs which are transplanted as an allograft. Although immune responses to brain allografts are moderate and survival can be obtained even without immunosuppression (Freed et al., 2001), most investigators prefer to use immunosuppressive agents for 6 to 12 months after transplantation (Brundin etal., 2000, Mendez et al., 2005; Olanow et al., 2003). Another way to keep away from immune reactions after transplantation is the using of therapeutic cloning. It has been shown that genetically identical ESCs derived DA neurons, generated by transfer of autologous nuclei from fibroblasts, improve functional deficits without immune reaction in PD mice (Tabar et al. 2008). However, it should be evaluated whether genetically modified cells would be acceptable in a clinical protocol.

Tumor formation remains another obstacle concerning the transplantation of ESCs that has to be eliminated before human ESCs can be safely applied in PD. Because life expectancy is almost normal in PD patients, even a minor risk of tumor formation associated with cell replacement therapy is unacceptable in this disorder. To improve safety, it might be necessary to engineer ESCs with regulated suicide genes or to use cell sorting to eliminate cells that could give rise to tumors.

In the end, on the basis of the available experimental data, ESCs are promising source for the cell replacement therapy. Although much more studies will be required to overcome the mentioned challenging issues, it seems it is now possible to start defining a road map including the main steps towards clinical application of ESCs in PD.

5. Acknowledgment

Author would like to thank Prof. H. Peirovi, Prof M. Jorjani, Prof. A. Ahamdiani, B.J. Nooshin and Dr. Tina Deihim for their critical comments.

6. References

Bain G, Kitchens D, Yao M, Huettner JE & Gottlieb DI. (1995). Embryonic stem cells express neuronal properties *in vitro. Dev Biol*, 168, pp. 342-57

Bain G., Ray W. J., Yao M. & Gottlieb DI. (1996). Retinoic acid promotes neural and represses mesodermal gene expression in mouse embryonic stem cells in culture. *Biochem Biophys Res Commun*, 223, pp. 691-4

Barberi T, Klivenyi P, Calingasan NY, Lee H, Kawamata H, Loonam K., Perrier AL, Bruses J, Rubio ME, Topf N, Tabar V, Harrison NL, Beal MF, Moore MA & Studer L. (2003). Neural subtype specification of fertilization and nuclear transfer embryonic stem cells and application in parkinsonian mice. *Nat Biotechnol*, 21, pp. 1200-7

Benzing C, Segschneider M, Leinhaas A, Itskovitz-Eldor J & Brustle O. (2006). Neuralconversion of human em bryonic stem cell colonies in the presence of fibroblast growth factor-2. *Neuroreport*, 17, pp. 1675-81

Brundin P, Pogarell O, Hagell P, Piccini P, Widner H, Schrag A, Kupsch A, Crabb L, Odin P, Gustavii B, Björklund A, Brooks DJ, Marsden CD, Oertel WH, Quinn NP, Rehncrona S & Lindvall O. (2000). Bilateral caudate and putamen grafts of embryonic mesencephalic tissue treated with lazaroids in Parkinson's disease. *Brain*, 123, 1380–1390

Carlsson T, Carta M, Winkler C, Bjorklund A & Kirik D. (2007). Serotonin neuron transplants exacerbate L-DOPA-induced dyskinesias in a rat model of Parkinson's disease. *J Neurosci*, 27, pp. 8011–8022

Carpenter MK, Inokuma MS, Denham J, Mujtaba T, Chiu CP & Rao MS. (2001). Enrichment of neurons and neural precursors from human embryonic stem cells. *Exp Neurol*, 172, pp. 383–397

Chung S, Shin BS, Hedlund E, Pruszak J, Ferree A, Kang UJ, Isacson O & Kim KS. (2006). Genetic selection of sox1GFPexpressing neural precursors removes residual tumorigenic pluripotent stem cells and attenuates tumor formation after transplantation. *J Neurochem*, 97, pp. 1467–1480

Diez del Corral, R. & Storey K. G. (2004). Opposing FGF and retinoid pathways: a signalling switch that controls differentiation and patterning onset in the extending vertebrate body axis. *Bioessays*, 26, pp. 857-69

Freed CR, Greene PE, Breeze RE, Tsai WY, Du Mouchel W, Kao R, Dillon S, Winfield H, Culver S, Trojanowski JQ, Eidelberg D & Fahn S. (2001). Transplantation of embryonic dopamine neurons for severe Parkinson's disease. *N Engl J Med*, 344, pp. 710–719

Gerrard L, Rodgers L & Cui W. (2005). Differentiation of human embryonic stem cells to neural lineages in adherent culture by blocking bone morphogenetic protein signaling. *Stem Cells*, 23(9), pp. 1234-41

Guan K., Chang H, Rolletschek A & Wobus AM. (2001). Embryonic stem cell derived neurogenesis. Retinoic acid induction and lineage selection of neuronal cells. *Cell Tissue Res*, 305, pp. 171-6

Hagell P & Brundin P. (2001). Cell survival and clinical outcome following intrastriatal transplantation in Parkinson disease. *J Neuropathol Exp Neurol*, 60, pp.741–752

Hagell P, Piccini P, Bjorklund A, Brundin P, Rehncrona S, Widner H, Crabb L, Pavese N, Oertel WH, Quinn N, Brooks DJ & Lindvall O. (2002). Dyskinesias following neural transplantation in Parkinson's disease. *Nat Neurosci*, 5, pp. 627–628

Isacson O. Bjorklund LM &Schumacher JM. (2003). Toward full restoration of synaptic and terminal function of the dopaminergic system in Parkinson's disease by stem cells. *Ann Neurol*, 53 (Suppl. 3), pp. S135–S146

Itskovitz-Eldor J, Schuldiner M, Karsenti D, Eden A, Yanuka O, Amit M, Soreq H & Benvenisty N. (2000). Differentiation of human embryonic stem cells into embryoid bodies compromising the three embryonic germ layers. *Mol Med*, 6 pp. 88 –95

Kageyama R & Nakanishi S. (1997). Helix-loop-helix factors in growth and differentiation of the vertebrate nervous system. *Curr Opin Genet Dev*, 7, pp.659-65

Kawasaki H, Mizuseki K, Nishikawa S, Kaneko S, Kuwana Y, Nakanishi S, Nishikawa SI & Sasai Y. (2000). Induction of midbrain dopaminergic neurons from ES cells by stromal cell-derived inducing activity. *Neuron*, 28, pp. 31-40

Kim JY, Koh HC, Lee JY, Chang MY, Kim YC, Chung HY, Son H, Lee YS, Studer L, McKay R & Lee SH. (2003). Dopaminergic neuronal differentiation from rat embryonic neural precursors by Nurr1 overexpression. *J Neurochem*, 85, pp. 1443-54

Kitajima H, Yoshimura S, Kokuzawa J, Kato M, Iwama T, Motohashi T, Kunisada T & Sakai N. (2005). Culture method for the induction of neurospheres from mouse embryonic stem cells by coculture with PA6 stromal cells. *J Neurosci Res*, 80, pp. 467-74

Klimanskaya I, Chung Y, Becker S, Lu SJ & Lanza R. (2006). Human embryonic stem cell lines derived from single blastomeres. *Nature*, 444, pp. 481-5

Kordower JH, Chu Y, Hauser RA, Freeman TB & Olanow CW. (2008a). Lewy body like pathology in long-term embryonic nigral transplants in Parkinson's disease. *Nat Med*, 14, pp. 504–6

Kordower JH Chu Y, Hauser RA, Olanow CW & Freeman TB. (2008b). Transplanted dopaminergic neurons develop PD pathologic changes: a second case report. *Mov Disord*, 23, pp. 2303–2306

Lau T, Adam S & Schloss P. (2006). Rapid and efficient differentiation of dopaminergic neurons from mouse embryonic stem cells. *Neuroreport*, 17, pp. 975-9

Lee SH, Lumelsky N, Studer L, Auerbach JM & McKay RD. (2000). Efficient generation of midbrain and hindbrain neurons from mouse embryonic stem cells. *Nat Biotechnol*, 18, pp. 675-9

Li JY, Englund E, Holton JL, Soulet D, Hagell P, Lees AJ, Lashley T, Quinn NP, Rehncrona S, Björklund A, Widner H, Revesz T, Lindvall O & Brundin P. (2008). Lewy bodies in grafted neurons in subjects with Parkinson's disease suggest host-to-graft disease propagation. *Nat Med*, 14, pp. 501–3

Li M, Pevny L, Lovell-Badge R & Smith A. (1998). Generation of purified neural precursors from embryonic stem cells by lineage selection. *Curr Biol*, 8, pp. 971–974

Lie DC, Colamarino SA, Song HJ, Desire L, Mira H, Consiglio A, Lein ES, Jessberger S, H. Lansford, Dearie AR & Gage FH. (2005). Wnt signalling regulates adult hippocampal neurogenesis. *Nature*, 437, pp. 1370-5

Maxwell SL & Li M. (2005). Midbrain dopaminergic development in vivo and in vitro from embryonic stem cells. *J Anat*, 207, pp. 209 –218

Martin MJ, Muotri A, Gage F & Varki A. (2005). Human embryonic stem cells express an immunogenic nonhuman sialic acid. *Nat Med*, 11, pp. 228-32

Martinat C, Bacci JJ, Leete T, Kim J, Vanti WB, Newman AH, Cha JH, Gether U, Wang H & Abeliovich A. (2006) Cooperative transcription activation by Nurr1 and Pitx3 induces embryonic stem cell maturation to the midbrain dopamine neuron phenotype. *Proc Natl Acad Sci U S A*, 103, pp. 2874-9

Mendez, I, Sanchez-Pernaute R, Cooper O, Viñuela A, Ferrari D, Björklund L, Dagher A & Isacson O. (2005). Cell type analysis of functional fetal dopamine cell suspension transplants in the striatum and substantia nigra of patients with Parkinson's disease. *Brain*, 128, pp. 1498–1510

Mendez I, Vinuela A, Astradsson A, Mukhida K, Hallett P, Robertson H, Tierney T, Holness R, Dagher A, Trojanowski JQ & Isacson O. (2008). Dopamine neurons implanted into people with Parkinson's disease survive without pathology for 14 years. *Nat Med*, 14, pp. 507–9

Mizuseki K, Sakamoto T, Watanabe K, Muguruma K, Ikeya M, Nishiyama A, Arakawa A, Suemori H, Nakatsuji N, Kawasaki H, Murakami F & Sasai Y. (2003).Generation of neural crest-derived peripheral neurons and floor plate cells from mouse and primate embryonic stem cells. *Proc Natl Acad Sci U S A*, 100, pp. 5828–5833

Niknejad H, Peirovi H, Jorjani M, Ahmadiani A, Ghanavi J & Seifalian AM. (2008). Properties of the amniotic membrane for potential use in tissue engineering. *Eur Cell Mater*, 15, pp. 88-99

Niknejad H, Peirovi H, Ahmadiani A, Ghanavi J & Jorjani M. (2010). Differentiation factors that influence neuronal markers expression in vitro from human amniotic epithelial cells. *Eur Cell Mater*, 19, pp. 22-9

Okada Y, Shimazaki T, Sobue G & Okano H. (2004) Retinoic-acid-concentration-dependent acquisition of neural cell identity during *in vitro* differentiation of mouse embryonic stem cells. *Dev Biol*, 275, pp.124-42

Olanow CW, Goetz CG, Kordower JH, Stoessl AJ, Sossi V, Brin MF, Shannon KM, Nauert GM, Perl DP, Godbold J & Freeman TB. (2003). A double-blind controlled trial of bilateral fetal nigral transplantation in Parkinson's disease. *Ann Neurol*, 54, pp. 403–414

Park CH, Kang JS, Kim JS, Chung S, Koh JY, Yoon EH, Jo AY, Chang MY, Koh HC, Hwang S, Suh- Kim H, Lee YS, Kim KS & Lee SH. (2006a). Differential actions of the proneural genes encoding Mash1 and neurogenins in Nurr1- induced dopamine neuron differentiation. *J Cell Sci*, 119, pp. 2310-20

Park CH, Kang JS, Shin YH, Chang MY, Chung S, Koh HC, Zhu MH, Oh SB, Lee YS, Panagiotakos G, Tabar V, Studer L & Lee SH. (2006b). Acquisition of *in vitro* and *in vivo* functionality of Nurr1-induced dopamine neurons. *Faseb J*,20, pp. 2553-5

Piccini P, Lindvall O, Björklund A, Brundin P, Hagell P, Ceravolo R, Oertel W, Quinn N, Samuel M, Rehncrona S, Widner H & Brooks DJ. (2000). Delayed recovery of movement-related cortical function in Parkinson's disease after striatal dopaminergic grafts. *Ann Neurol*, 48, pp. 689–695

Reubinoff BE, Itsykson P, Turetsky T, Pera MF, Reinhartz E, Itzik A & Ben-Hur T. (2001). Neural progenitors from human embryonic stem cells. *Nat Biotechnol*, 19, pp. 1134-40

Roy NS, Cleren C, Singh SK, Yang L, Beal MF & Goldman SA. (2006). Functional engraftment of human ES cell-derived dopaminergic neurons enriched by coculture with telomerase-immortalized midbrain astrocytes. *Nat Med*,12, pp. 1259 -1268

Sakurada K, Ohshima-Sakurada M, Palmer TD & Gage FH. (1999). Nurr1, an orphan nuclear receptor, is a transcriptional activator of endogenous tyrosine hydroxylase in neural progenitor cells derived from the adult brain. *Development*, 126, pp. 4017-26

Schuldiner M, Eiges R, Eden A, Yanuka O, Itskovitz-Eldor J, Goldstein RS & Benvenisty N. (2001). Induced neuronal differentiation of human embryonic stem cells. *Brain Res*, 913, pp.201-5

Schuldiner M, Itskovitz-Eldor J & Benvenisty N. (2003). Selective ablation of human embryonic stem cells expressing a ''suicide'' gene. *Stem Cells*, 21, pp. 257–265

Schuldiner M, Yanuka O, Itskovitz-Eldor J, Melton DA & Benvenisty N. (2000). Effects of eight growth factors on the differentiation of cells derived from human embryonic stem cells. *Proc Natl Acad Sci U S A*, 97, pp. 11307–11312

Schulz TC, Noggle SA, Palmarini GM, Weiler DA, Lyons IG, Pensa KA, Meedeniya AC, Davidson BP, Lambert NA & Condie BG. (2004). Differentiation of human embryonic stem cells to dopaminergic neurons in serum-free suspension culture. *STEM CELLS*, 22:1218 -1238.

Schulz TC, Palmarini GM, Noggle SA, Weiler DA, Mitalipova MM & Condie BG. (2003). Directed neuronal differentiation of human embryonic stem cells. *BMC Neurosci*, 4, pp.27

Setoguchi T., Nakashima K, Takizawa T, Yanagisawa M, Ochiai W, Okabe M, Yone K, Komiya S & Taga T. (2004). Treatment of spinal cord injury by transplantation of fetal neural precursor cells engineered to express BMP inhibitor. *Exp Neurol*, 189, pp. 33-44

Smidt MP, Smits SM & Burbach JP. (2003) Molecular mechanisms underlying midbrain dopamine neuron development and function. *Eur J Pharmacol*, 480, pp. 75- 88

Sonntag KC, Pruszak J, Yoshizaki T, van Arensbergen J, Sanchez-Pernaute R & Isacson O. (2007). Enhanced yield of neuroepithelial precursors and midbrain-like dopaminergic neurons from human embryonic stem cells using the bone morphogenic protein antagonist noggin. *STEM CELLS*, 25, pp. 411- 418

Tabar V. Tomishima M, Panagiotakos G, Wakayama S, Menon J, Chan B, Mizutani E, Al-Shamy G, Ohta H, Wakayama T, & Studer L. (2008). Therapeutic cloning in individual parkinsonian mice. *Nat Med*, 14, pp. 379–381

Takahashi J., Palmer T D & Gage FH. (1999). Retinoic acid and neurotrophins collaborate to regulate neurogenesis in adultderived neural stem cell cultures. *J neurobiol*, 38, pp. 65-81

Ueno M, Matsumura M, Watanabe K, Nakamura T, Osakada F, Takahashi M, Kawasaki H, Kinoshita S & Sasai Y. (2006). Neural conversion of ES cells by an inductive activity on human amniotic membrane matrix. *Proc Natl Acad Sci U S A*, 103, pp. 9554-9

Wichterle H, Lieberam I, Porter JA& Jessell TM. (2002). Directed differentiation of embryonic stem cells into motor neurons. *Cell*, 110, pp. 385-97

Yan Y, Yang D, Zarnowska ED, Du Z, Werbel B, Valliere C, Pearce RA, Thomson JA & Zhang SC. (2005). Directed differentiation of dopaminergic neuronal subtypes from human embryonic stem cells. *STEM CELLS*, 23 pp.781–790

Ying QL, Stavridis M, Griffiths D, Li M & Smith A. (2003). Conversion of embryonic stem cells into neuroectodermal precursors in adherent monoculture. *Nat Biotechnol*, 21, pp. 183-6

Yue F, Cui L, Johkura K, Ogiwara N & Sasaki K. (2006). Induction of midbrain dopaminergic neurons from primate embryonic stem cells by coculture with sertoli cells. *Stem Cells*, 24(7), pp. 1695-706.

Zhang SC, Wernig M, Duncan ID, Brustle O. & Thomson JA. (2001). *In vitro* differentiation of transplantable neural precursors from human embryonic stem cells. *Nat Biotechnol*, 19, pp. 1129-33

Zhang X, Cai J., Klueber KM, Guo Z, Lu C, Winstead WI, Qiu M & Roisen FJ. (2006). Role of transcription factors in motoneuron differentiation of adult human olfactory neuroepithelial-derived progenitors. *Stem Cells*, 24, pp. 434-42

25

The Role of the Neuropeptide Substance P in the Pathogenesis of Parkinson's Disease

Emma Thornton and Robert Vink
University of Adelaide
Australia

1. Introduction

Parkinson's disease (PD) was first described by James Parkinson in 1815 as "shaking palsy syndrome". Today, it is the second most common neurodegenerative disorder, with a lifetime risk of 1 in 45 of developing the debilitating disease and currently affecting 1% of the population over the age of 65 (G. Alves, et al., 2008).

PD is characterized by a slow and progressive loss of the pigmented dopaminergic neurons of the substantia nigra pars compacta (SNc). This loss of dopaminergic neurons is often accompanied by a loss of the noradrenergic pigmented neurons of the locus ceruleus, and in the later stages of the disease, both the cholinergic neurons of the nucleus basalis of Meynert and the serotoninergic neurons of the dorsal raphe nucleus may also degenerate (Marey-Semper, et al., 1995). In remaining DA neurons proteinaceous cytoplasmic inclusions called Lewy bodies (LBs) are found. They are filamentous in nature and predominantly contain alpha-synuclein and ubiquitin proteins (Bennett, 2005). Although LBs are also found in other diseases, such as diffuse Lewy body dementia and incidental Lewy body disease, they are considered to be the pathological hallmark of PD (Greenfields, 1992).

The dopaminergic neurons of the SNc are part of the basal ganglia (BG), an integral part of the brain that ensures smooth execution of movement. Accordingly motor symptoms such as resting tremor, bradykinesia, akinesia, rigidity and postural instability are most common. Degeneration of dopaminergic neurons is slow, with progressive loss of about 5% per year (Blum, et al., 2001), suggesting that a therapy could halt or slow down the progression of the disease, but to date no known neuroprotective therapy exists. Instead, current treatment involves managing patients' symptoms. Normally this treatment is L-DOPA, the precursor to DA. The rationale for this therapy is to restore DA levels to near normal and therefore restore normal function of the basal ganglia for a period of time. Unfortunately, following prolonged use many patients fail to maintain a good response and often experience "wearing off" effects, which is a reduction in the length of time that L-DOPA effectively alleviates symptoms (Krasnova, et al., 2000). Furthermore, motor complications like dyskinesia, or involuntary movements, occur in approximately 50-80% of PD patients who have been on L-DOPA for more than 5-10 years. These side effects are often more debilitating than the original motor deficits (Chen, et al., 2004).

In addition to the loss of dopaminergic neurons, there is also a reduction in the expression of the neuropeptide, substance P (SP), an important neurotransmitter in the BG, which is essential for proper execution of function. However, this loss of SP has been observed in animal and human studies under conditions that represented end-stage PD. We suggest that this late loss of SP content is an event secondary to dopamine neuronal death. In the early phase of the disease, we propose that SP expression may actually be increased, and that this increase in SP may contribute to dopaminergic cell death through its effects on inflammatory processes and blood brain barrier (BBB) dysfunction. This review critically analyses the evidence that SP contributes to the pathogenesis of PD.

2. The basal ganglia

The BG is a group of nuclei located within the midbrain whose primary function is the smooth execution of movement. Apart from the substantia nigra, which also contains the pars reticulta (SNr), the BG nuclei include the striatum (caudate/putamen), the globus pallidus, both internal (GPi) and external segments (GPe), and the subthalamic nucleus (STN). Although the thalamus is not strictly part of the BG, it is fundamental to its function. In order for the BG to function correctly, it requires the two main signalling pathways, the direct and indirect pathway, to act in concert.

The direct signalling pathway involves an excitatory glutamatergic signal being sent from the cortex to striatal GABAergic projection neurons that project to the GPi and SNr resulting in inhibition of these nuclei. These nuclei also send inhibitory GABAergic signals, the inhibition of GPi/SNr neurons results in decreased inhibitory output to the thalamus. Consequently, the activity of thalamic neurons are increased causing excitatory glutamatergic signals to be sent back to the cortex, reinforcing cortical activity. The direct pathway therefore provides positive feedback for the cortex to allow movement (Silkis, 2001). Alternatively, the indirect pathway involves an excitatory signal being sent from the cortex to striatal inhibitory GABAergic neurons that project to the GPe, resulting in increased inhibition of the GPe neurons. As these neurons send an inhibitory GABAergic signal to the STN, the inhibition of these neurons leads to increased glutamatergic excitatory output from the STN. Subsequently, the STN sends excitatory signals to the inhibitory GPi and SNr neurons increasing their inhibitory output to the thalamus ensuring inhibition of the thalamic neurons and thus inhibition of cortical activity. The indirect pathway is therefore involved in negative feedback to the cortex and inhibition of the posture keeping the limb there (Sil'kis, 2002). These signalling pathways are kept in balance to ensure the almost simultaneous inhibition of the original position and initiation of the new required movement.

The direct and indirect signalling pathways are kept in balance by the dopaminergic input from the SNc to the striatum, known as the nigrostriatal pathway. The striatal GABAergic projection neurons express both DA receptors, namely D1 and D2 (Yelnik, 2002), although there are higher numbers of D1 receptors on the projections neurons involved in the direct pathway and D2 receptors for the indirect pathway (Aizman, et al., 2000). Through binding to D1 receptors, DA increases cAMP production, thereby reinforcing the activity of the direct pathway. In contrast, when DA binds to D2 receptors, cAMP production is reduced, creating a reversal of the activity of the nuclei within the indirect pathway and a decrease in its activity. As the indirect pathway is involved in negative feedback to the cortex, DA causes increased activity of the cortical neurons and reinforcement of cortical activity (van der Stelt and Di Marzo, 2003). Thus, the release of striatal DA within the nigrostriatal pathway of the BG allows fine-tuning of movement control and smooth execution of movement.

2.1 Basal ganglia function in Parkinson's disease

The initial loss of dopaminergic neurons in early PD does not decrease striatal DA activity due to pre- and post-synaptic compensatory responses of the dopaminergic system. These include upregulation of D1 and D2 dopamine receptor expression, which have a lower threshold for activation than normal, and an increase in activity of the surviving dopaminergic neurons (Deumens, et al., 2002). These compensatory mechanisms are able to sustain normal activity until approximately 50% of DA neurons and 80% of the total striatal DA is lost. Once this threshold level of striatal DA is reached, the direct and indirect signalling pathways become imbalanced producing a subsequent increase in the indirect signalling pathway and a decrease in the direct signalling pathway (Contreras-Vidal and Stelmach, 1996, Wardas, et al., 2003). Although these pathways also control the limbic system, the deficiency of DA in PD is heterogenous and DA is predominantly lost in the putamen area of the striatum, which is mainly involved in motor function of the BG. Therefore, PD is a hypokinetic disorder where the decreased activity of the direct pathway and increased activity of the indirect pathway results in a lack of movement as the common symptom (Silkis, 2001).

The BG does not only contain classical neurotransmitters such as glutamate, GABA and DA, but it also involves neuropeptides such as SP, neurokinin A (NKA) and the opioids enkephalin and dynorphin that act together for the fine-tuning of BG pathways (Graybiel, 1990, Hauber, 1998). These neurotransmitters can be segregated into the two pathways, with SP, NKA and dynorphin located in the GABAergic projection neurons of the direct pathway, whereas enkephalin is found within the striatal GABAergic projections neurons of the indirect pathway. Accordingly, in PD the change in activity of signalling pathways creates abnormal levels of these neurotransmitters. Changes in SP may be particularly important with respect to PD.

3. Substance P

Substance P was first discovered in 1934 by Gaddum and Schild, as the active principle in a stable dry powder. In 1936, Von Euler suggested the peptidergic nature of SP as its activity was stopped following digestion with trypsin, although later it was discovered that the degradation of SP was due to chymotrypsin as SP is trypsin-resistant (Leeman and Ferguson, 2000). Consequently it became part of the tachykinin family of which NKA and neurokinin B (NKB) are also members. Tachykinins are located in capsaicin-sensitive neurons, also known as primary sensory neurons, within the CNS, peripheral tissue and non-neuronal cells including endothelial cells and inflammatory cells (Hokfelt, et al., 2001). Within the brain there is a heterogeneous distribution of SP, with higher levels found in the grey matter. The highest concentration of SP is actually found within the SN (Ribeiro-da-Silva and Hokfelt, 2000), where SP immunoreactivity in the SNc is 25% higher than that in the SNr (Sutoo, et al., 1999). Also, within the BG SP expression is high within the internal segment of the globus pallidus.

Tachykinins share a common terminal sequence, Phe-X-Gly-Leu-Met-NH2, where X is Phe or Val (Harrison and Geppetti, 2001, Saria, 1999). This sequence is essential for their biological activity and thus there is a certain amount of cross reactivity amongst the tachykinin receptors and their ligands (Gerard, et al., 1991, Khawaja and Rogers, 1996). Each tachykinin has varying affinities for the tachykinin receptors, with SP having the greatest affinity for the tachykinin NK1 receptor (NK_1), NKA to NK_2 and NKB to NK_3 tachykinin receptors.

Tachykinin receptors have a rhodopsin-like membrane structure comprising of 7 hydrophobic transmembrane domains connected by extra- and intracellular loops and coupled to G-proteins (Harrison and Geppetti, 2001). NK_1 and NK_3 receptors are mainly found in the CNS, but are also present in peripheral tissues (Otsuka and Yoshioka, 1993). Throughout the brain, greatest NK_1 receptor immunoreactivity is found in the striatum, nucleus accumbens, hippocampus, hypothalamus and the raphe nuclei (Harrison and Geppetti, 2001), whereas NK_3 receptors are most abundant in the cortex and on glial cells (Yip and Chahl, 2000). In contrast, NK_2 receptors are widely distributed in the peripheral nervous system (PNS) especially in the smooth muscle of the respiratory, gastrointestinal and urinary tracts (Maggi, 1995).

SP binds to the hydrophobic ligand-binding pocket within the extracellular loops of the NK_1 receptor causing rapid internalisation of the ligand and its receptor (Harrison and Geppetti, 2001). Ligand binding stimulates the activity of adenylate cyclase and the conversion of adenosine triphosphate (ATP) to adenosine monophosphate, which inturn activates phospholipase C_B (PLC_B) (Saria, 1999). Activation of PLC_B results in an increased turnover of intracellular inositol 1,4,5-triphosphate and a subsequent elevation of intracellular calcium (Ca^{2+}) (Gerard, et al., 1991). The NK_1 receptor has a 5′ untranslated region containing a cyclic AMP (cAMP) binding protein that responds to elevated levels of cAMP and Ca^{2+} by increasing gene transcription of SP (Saria, 1999). This creates a positive feedback loop for SP production and release. Conversely, SP may also block potassium channels causing membrane depolarisation and/or activate NK_1 autoreceptors to inhibit its own release (Harrison and Geppetti, 2001).

SP is synthesized from the preprotachykinin (PPT)-A gene, which also encodes NKA, neuropeptide K (NPK) and neuropeptide Y (NPY), the latter two being elongated versions of NKA (Hokfelt, et al., 2001). Alternative splicing of the PPT-A gene results in 3 distinct mRNAs: α-PPT-A, β-PPT-A and γ-PPT-A. Although all 3 PPT-A mRNAs encode for SP (Harrison and Geppetti, 2001), α-PPT-A mRNA is the main isoform of mRNA in the brain, whereas α- and γ-PPT-A mRNA are primarily expressed within the periphery (Severini, et al., 2002). NKB is encoded by the PPT-B gene and like PPT-A gene is conserved amongst species (Hoyle, 1998).

Synthesis of SP occurs within ribosomes in cell bodies of the dorsal root ganglia before it is packaged into large dense core vesicles with processing enzymes called convertases, which cleave at Lys-Arg, Arg-Arg or Arg-Lys bonds to release the active form of SP (Severini, et al., 2002). When stimulated, SP-containing vesicles undergo retrograde axonal transport to the terminal endings in both the CNS and PNS, where they undergo final enzymatic processing and post-translational enzymatic modifications such as C-terminal amidation (Hokfelt, et al., 2000). As previously mentioned, SP release is triggered by a small rise in intracellular Ca^{2+}, which will increase the pH within the vesicle resulting in alkinisation and release of SP by exocytosis (Otsuka and Yoshioka, 1993). NK_1 receptors are also synthesized and then anterogradely transported along axons to peripheral and perhaps central terminals. Thus, upon release SP can activate the postsynaptic NK_1 receptors (Malcangio and Bowery, 1999).

3.1 Substance P regulation of basal ganglia function

Substance P is important in regulating the function of the SN and BG (Bell, et al., 1998, Maubach, et al., 2001) where it acts as an excitatory neurotransmitter (Napier, et al., 1995). Like in other areas of the brain, SP is released in the BG due to an elevation in Ca^{2+} (Otsuka and Yoshioka, 1993). Once released, it may bind to NK_1 receptors located on striatal interneurons to increase the firing rate and depolarise membrane potentials causing the release of other BG neurotransmitters such as GABA, glutamate and acetylcholine (Aosaki and Kawaguchi, 1996, Bailey, et al., 2004, Kemel, et al., 2002).

It is now known that NK_1 receptors are also located on 90% of DA neurons in the SNc (L-W. Chen, et al., 2004). However, earlier studies reported that there was an absence of NK_1 receptors in the SN and a mismatch between SP and NK_1 in this region (Humpel and Saria, 1993). This mismatch in the expression and binding of SP in the SN was subsequently thought to be due to the rapid internalisation of the SP/NK_1 complex following SP binding resulting in NK_1 being mainly located intracellularly (Levesque, et al., 2007). Accordingly, through binding to NK_1 receptors on dopaminergic neurons, SP can directly cause the release of DA within the striatum (Galarraga, et al., 1999, Orosz and Bennett, 1990, Reid, et al., 1990a, Reid, et al., 1990b). Moreover, as DA receptors are located on SP-containing striatal projection neurons, DA or DA agonists can potentiate SP release within the SN (Humpel and Saria, 1993). Therefore, SP and DA within the BG are modulated through a positive feedback mechanism. Accordingly, an injection of SP into the BG induces behavioural effects such as sniffing, rearing, grooming and increased motor activity in rats by promoting striatal DA release (Saria, 1999). However in PD, the loss of striatal DA interrupts this positive feedback mechanism and therefore a reduction in striatal SP gene transcription and SP protein content within the SN has been observed.

3.2 Substance P expression in Parkinson's disease

Post-mortem immunohistochemical studies have shown that there is a loss of SP content in the striatum and SN in PD brains (De Ceballos and Lopez-Lozano, 1999, Mauborgne, et al., 1983, Nisbet, et al., 1995, Sivam, 1991, Tenovuo, et al., 1984). Along with this loss of SP, there is also a significant deficit of NK_1 receptors in the putamen and GP of PD patients compared to aged matched controls (Fernandez, et al., 1994). Moreover, in a case of idiopathic PD, where the person died shortly after diagnosis from an unrelated cause, LBs were observed in surviving SP-containing neurons of the pedunculopontine tegmental nucleus, suggesting that these SP neurons were affected early in PD (Gai, et al., 1991).

Decrease in SP has also been extensively studied in the 6-OHDA rodent and MPTP non-human primate models of PD. Like in human PD, there is a decrease in SP content in the SN and striatum in these animal models (Bannon, et al., 1995, Schwarting and Huston, 1996). However, in a study by Orosz and Bennet in 1990 using the 6-OHDA rat model of PD, it was shown that although there was a decline in SP-immunoreactivity and SP mRNA in tissue levels of the SN, there was a rise in SP-immunoreactivity in the extracellular space of the SN. Subsequently, it was suggested that this rise was a compensatory mechanisms for the loss of intracellular SP (Orosz and Bennett, 1990). This was the first study to show an increase in extracellular SP during PD. Due to the tissue loss of SP, 6-OHDA animals were given replacement SP treatment into either the lateral ventricle or directly into the SN restoring striatal DA content (Krasnova, et al., 2000). Additionally, pre-treatment with SP assisted the recovery from a 6-OHDA lesion. The authors suggested that this was due to prolonged changes in SP release that helped to negate the tissue loss of SP caused by 6-OHDA (Nikolaus, et al., 1997). Thus basal levels of SP are fundamental for proper function.

In the non-human primate MPTP model of PD, which represents the model most similar to human PD, it was shown that there was a reduction in striatal SP gene expression and that this deficiency in SP correlated with the degree of motor symptoms present (Wade and Schneider, 2001). However when primates were treated with L-DOPA the decrease in SP gene expression was reversed (Herrero, et al., 1995).

It is important to note that these studies have all been undertaken in post-mortem tissue or in models that replicate the end stage of the disease. Therefore, the SP changes observed may be a secondary effect due to the loss of DA input into the striatum and the activation of the direct pathway. Indeed, research in our laboratory has shown that SP may actually be increased in the early stages of PD. In nigrostriatal organotypic cell culture, 6-OHDA treatment caused an immediate and prolonged elevation in SP content that was significantly correlated with lactate dehydrogenase content, a marker of cell death. Furthermore, the 6-OHDA induced cell death was prevented by treatment with an NK_1 receptor antagonist (Thornton, et al., 2010).

Subsequent *in vivo* studies using the rodent striatal 6-OHDA model also measured SP content in the striatum and SN at days 3 and 7 following lesioning using an enzyme-linked immunosorbent assay (ELISA) method, which determines SP content from a standardized amount of protein (Figure 1). Despite the difference in SP content between the hemispheres in sham (control) animals, there was an apparent increase in SP content in the contralateral (left) and ipsilateral (right) striatum at both 3 and 7 days following 6-OHDA administration. However, SP content was not elevated within the SN until day 7 following 6-OHDA striatal lesions. Dopaminergic neuronal loss as assessed by tyrosine hydroxylase immunoreactivity was also not apparent at day 3 but had begun by day 7 and was significant by day 14 post-lesion. Nonetheless, a small loss of striatal DA terminals was observed by day 3. These results suggest that increased SP expression may contribute to the loss of dopaminergic terminals and neurons, however dopaminergic cell loss must also have initiated an increase in SP content within the SN. Furthermore, as the majority of dopaminergic degeneration occurs from day 7 to 14, the rise in SP content may act to potentiate this cell loss.

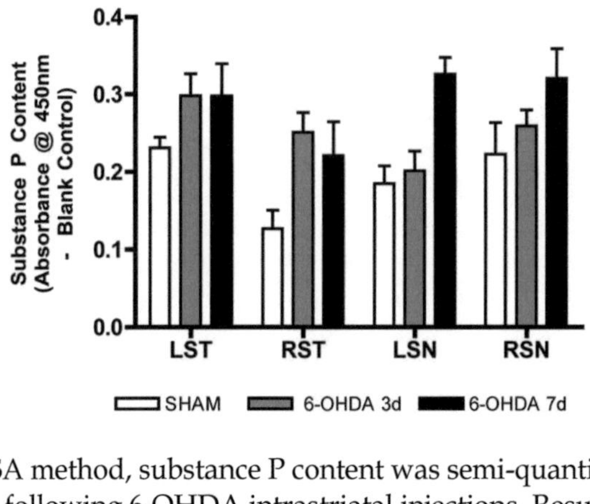

Fig. 1. Using an ELISA method, substance P content was semi-quantified within the striatum and substantia nigra following 6-OHDA intrastriatal injections. Results are displayed as mean+SEM (n=5/group).

Substance P has been associated with cell loss and functional deficits in other brain pathologies such as traumatic brain injury and stroke (Donkin, et al., 2009, R. J. Turner, et al., 2006). This detrimental effect of SP was credited to its ability to induce BBB breakdown and the subsequent genesis of cerebral oedema (R. Turner and Vink, 2007). Although cerebral oedema does not occur in PD, a decrease in BBB integrity has recently been linked to dopaminergic cell loss and the progression of PD (Bartels, et al., 2008, Kortekaas, et al., 2005). Moreover, SP has been shown to play an integral role in the inflammatory response within both the peripheral and central nervous systems (R.V. Alves, et al., 1999). Recently, neuroinflammation has also received much interest for its potential role in DA degeneration and disease progression. We therefore hypothesize that SP may be involved in dopaminergic cell death in early PD by promoting neuroinflammation and BBB dysfunction.

4. Potential role for substance P in dopaminergic degeneration in PD

4.1 Inflammatory processes

Two of the main inflammatory cells within the brain are microglia and astrocytes. Resting microglia are important for maintaining cellular homeostasis, and once activated are involved in the removal of cellular debris (Mosley, et al., 2006, Rock and Peterson, 2006). However, activated microglia produce proinflammatory trophic factors and cytokines such as interleukin-1 (IL-1), IL-2, IL-6 and tumour necrosis factor-α (TNF-α), all of which are potentially cytotoxic (Blum, et al., 2001). Chronic activation of microglia and therefore prolonged expression of cytokines can be especially damaging to neurons. Indeed, activated microglia have been observed in post-mortem PD tissue and in experimental models long after the induction of PD (Depino, et al., 2003, Marinova-Mutafchieva, et al., 2009, McGeer and McGeer, 2008). Moreover, in human cases and animal models of PD a rise in these proinflammatory factors and cytokines has been demonstrated in the SN, striatum and cerebrospinal fluid (CSF) (Jenner and Olanow, 1998, Liu and Hong, 2003).

Activated microglia can also generate reactive oxygen species (ROS) such as hydrogen peroxide and superoxide (O_2^-) through activation of NADPH oxidase (Wu, et al., 2003). Under normal conditions this is important for the microglial role in brain immune surveillance and ability to kill foreign organisms that enter the brain. However, excessive production of ROS can result in oxidative damage to proteins, lipids and DNA, resulting in dopaminergic cell death (reviewed by (Mosley, et al., 2006)). In addition, microglia contain inducible NOS (iNOS), enabling the secretion of nitric oxide (NO). NO can react with ROS to form reactive nitrogen species (RNS) such as peroxynitrite ($ONOO^-$), which is more stable than O^{2-} and can cross cell membranes and thus can be more damaging to cells than ROS. Indeed, by-products of oxidative damage are found in the SN of PD brains at post-mortem (Marsden and Olanow, 1998).

Usually, the SN contains large numbers of microglia compared to other areas of the brain. This is consistent with dopaminergic neurons already being in a state of oxidative stress due to the production of ROS during normal DA metabolism, making these neurons particularly vulnerable to insults (Berretta, et al., 2005, Liu and Hong, 2003, Olanow, et al., 2004). Moreover, oxidative damage by ROS and RNS is exacerbated in PD due to a deficiency of glutathione and superoxide dismutase, two of the main antioxidant enzymes that scavenge ROS, RNS and reduce H_2O_2 to its non-reactive state (Canals, et al., 2001).

Apart from causing damage to cellular structures, RNS and ROS may also cause mitochondrial dysfunction. In PD, a 30 to 40% decrease in complex I (NADH dehydrogenase) activity of the electron transport chain (ETC) is observed in mitochondria within the SN (Blum, et al., 2001, Squire, et al., 2003). The ETC, through oxidative phosphorylation, produces ATP, an important energy source for cell organelles, enzymes and transport systems. Thus, mitochondrial dysfunction causes a bioenergetic deficit that leads to membrane depolarisation, disruption of Ca^{2+} homeostasis and further production of free radicals and ROS (Shults, 2004). Specifically, a reduction in ATP causes impairment of the mitochondrial membrane potential, and subsequent opening of the mitochondrial permeability transition pore. Pore opening stimulates the release of mitochondrial proteins, such as cytochrome c and apoptosis-inducing factor, that trigger apoptosis (Rego and Oliveira, 2003). Consistent with this, DA neurons are thought to die via apoptotic cell death cascades in PD (Olanow and Tatton, 1999).

With the loss of ATP production, there is also a consequential loss of the magnesium blockade of N-methyl-D-aspartate (NMDA) receptors, resulting in elevated levels of glutamate and NO (Q. Chen, et al., 1996). Dopaminergic neurons in the SN are rich in functional NMDA glutamate receptors and therefore affected by any change in glutamate levels (Olanow and Tatton, 1999). Glutamate, an excitatory amino acid, causes an increase in intracellular Ca^{2+} resulting in FR production, mitochondrial damage and activation of degradative enzymes. These enzymes, including proteases, endonucleases and phospholipases, result in degradation of plasma membranes, the cytoskeleton and nuclear material and subsequent cell death. This deleterious cascade of events, known as glutamate excitotoxicity, is also a major contributor to cell loss in PD (Beal, 1992).

Notably, production of ROS and RNS during inflammation and mitochondrial dysfunction are critically linked since activation of microglia can lead to mitochondrial dysfunction, and vice versa (Di Filippo, et al., 2010). The combined effects of these disease mechanisms in dopaminergic degeneration are further reinforced in experimental models of PD as the complex 1 inhibitor rotenone causes DA degeneration and microglial activation following either systemic or intracerebral administration (Gao, et al., 2003). Additionally, MPTP and 6-OHDA models also demonstrate both mitochondrial dysfunction and an exacerbated inflammatory response (Blum, et al., 2001, Chung, et al., 2010a).

Activation of microglia is not only a vicious cycle whereby the degeneration of neurons stimulates further microglial activation (Raivich, et al., 1999), it may also precede DA degeneration (Wojtera, et al., 2005). Activated microglia may prematurely phagocytose damaged DA neurons that may not have gone on to degenerate as evidence by the fact that phagocytotic CD68 positive microglia are observed prior to caspase-3 positive apoptotic DA neurons in the 6-OHDA model of PD (Marinova-Mutafchieva, et al., 2009).

The astrocytic response in PD has received less attention than microglia for its potential role in the pathogenesis of PD. Nevertheless, in all animal models of PD, there is an increase in glial fibrillary acidic protein immunoreactivity in both the striatum and SN, with the presence of reactive, hypertrophic astrocytes (Depino, et al., 2003, Takagi, et al., 2007). Furthermore, a 30% increase in these reactive astrocytes within the SN was seen in PD tissue at post-mortem (Wu, et al., 2003). However, activation of astrocytes may be both beneficial, through secretion of neurotrophic substances such as glial derived nerve factor and brain derived nerve factor, and detrimental through secretion of pro-inflammatory cytokines (Brahmachari, et al., 2006, Hirsch, 2000). These cytokines stimulate the activation of additional microglia or astrocytes, thereby further exacerbating the inflammatory response and tissue damage previously described for microglia (Chauhan, et al., 2008, Raivich, et al., 1999). In reactive astrocytes, myeloperoxidase produces RNS and damage to DA neurons (Choi, et al., 2005). However, the presence of astrocytes may be also beneficial as the density of astrocytes is low in the SNc compared to the ventral tegmental area, an area much less susceptible to DA damage in clinical and experimental models of PD. Nonetheless, reactive astrocytes are thought to contribute to disease progression, although their exact role remains controversial (Chung, et al., 2010b).

The CNS immune response in PD can result in apoptosis of neurons by causing mitochondrial dysfunction and production of cytokines. An increase in cytokines, especially TNFα, can initiate apoptosis through binding at the tumour necrosis factor-α receptor 1 (TNFαR1), a known cell death receptor located on dopaminergic cell bodies in the SN (Mladenovic, et al., 2004).

4.1.1 Substance P and inflammation

Substance P and its NK_1 receptor have long been known to be important mediators of CNS inflammation (Harrison and Geppetti, 2001, Martin, et al., 1992). SP binding at NK_1 receptors expressed on microglia and astrocytes may directly result in the activation of these glial cells in the CNS (Mantyh, et al., 1989, Marriott, 2004). SP can also cause the indirect activation of astrocytes and microglia through its ability to promote cytokine and NO production, as they are able to modulate the activation of each other during the inflammatory response (Brahmachari, et al., 2006, Rodrigues, et al., 2001). Furthermore, pro-inflammatory cytokine production, for example, Il-1β can upregulate the expression of NK_1 receptors on glial cells (Guo, et al., 2004). Due to its ability to modulate the inflammatory response, SP may play a critical role in inflammation-induced damage. Indeed, in bacterial diseases of the CNS, SP/NK_1 interactions exacerbate the glial immune responses through both initiating and progressing the subsequent inflammation (Chauhan, et al., 2008).

In vitro studies also have increased our understanding of the signal transduction pathways induced by SP in microglia and astrocytes and resulting in pro-inflammatory cytokine production. SP can stimulate the secretion of TNF-α from microglia and astrocytes following treatment with the endotoxin lipopolysaccharide (LPS) (Luber-Narod, et al., 1994). The presence of NK_1 receptors could not be demonstrated on microglia, therefore suggesting that this effect was mediated via the SP induced release of IL-1 from astrocytes, causing TNF-α release from both glial cell populations. However, the authors concede that their methods may have not have detected NK_1 receptors. Subsequent studies have shown functional NK_1 receptors expressed on murine microglia *in vitro* (Rasley, et al., 2002). The production of pro-inflammatory cytokines from glial cells has been shown to occur following the translocation of NF-κβ. SP by binding to NK_1 activated the NF-κβ pathway stimulating cytokine production (Lieb, et al., 1997). Moreover, SP has also been shown to induce IL-6 production by activating p39 MAPK pathway (Fiebich, et al., 2000).

The role of inflammation in dopaminergic cell loss is further confirmed by the efficacy of anti-inflammatory agents in PD as they have been shown to slow down disease progression (Qian, et al., 2010). A meta-analysis of peer reviewed data between 1966 and 2008 indicated NSAIDs may be slightly protective in PD through their ability to halt the pro-inflammatory response, prevent cyclooxygenase activity and scavenge ROS and RNS (Samii, et al., 2009). Furthermore, Minocycline, a microglial inhibitor, has advanced to phase III clinical trials (Tansey and Goldberg, 2010). These promising results suggest that inhibiting SP signalling through antagonism of the NK_1 receptor may reduce the inflammatory response in PD, thus offering a novel therapeutic target to slow the progression of PD.

4.2 Blood brain barrier dysfunction

Recently, BBB dysfunction has been implicated in the pathophysiology of PD. In clinical PD, p-glycoprotein function, a marker of BBB integrity, was reduced suggesting a loss of barrier integrity (Bartels, 2008; Kortekaas 2005). The authors suggested that this loss of barrier function may contribute to the progression of PD. In the SN the BBB is known to be weaker than in other brain regions and consequently is easily disrupted (Ionov, 2008). Notably, dopaminergic neurons demonstrate a greater vulnerability to barrier breakdown. In a study by Rite and collegues (2007), intracerebral injection of vascular endothelium growth factor (VEGF) into the SN and striatum caused BBB breakdown as assessed by fluorescently tagged FITC-albumin infiltration. This resulted in dopaminergic terminal degeneration and apoptotic markers, caspase-3 and TUNEL expression in DA neurons. In contrast, injection of VEGF into the hippocampus caused no apparent apoptosis of hippocampal neurons (Rite, et al., 2007).

A correlation between BBB breakdown, the astrocytic and microglial response and dopaminergic degeneration has been previously described (Tomas-Camardiel, et al., 2004). In experimental models of PD, barrier dysfunction has been reported in MPTP, 6-OHDA and rotenone models of PD (Carvey, et al., 2005, Chao, et al., 2009, Ravenstijn, et al., 2008) and has also been observed in our own studies (unpublished). Further evidence for the BBB and CNS inflammation contributing to dopaminergic cell death is that mesenchymal stem cell (MSC) transplantation was found to be protective to DA neurons in the MPTP model of PD (Chao, et al., 2009). MSC transplantation reduced microglial activation and restored BBB function as reflected in reduced FITC-labelled albumin leakage, and returned expression of tight junction proteins, claudin 1 and 5 expression back to basal levels. The authors attributed this beneficial effect of MSCs expression of TGF-β1, which has an anti-inflammatory effect.

BBB dysfunction may also result in damage to DA neurons by allowing the influx of peripheral immune cells, such as blood borne macrophages, T-lymphocytes and leukocytes into the brain (Hunot, et al., 1999, Kortekaas, et al., 2005). Similar to CNS immune cells, peripheral immune cells secrete cytokines following the translocation of transcription factor NF-κβ. Accordingly, PD patients challenged with LPS had significantly exacerbated release of cytokines / chemokines from peripheral borne macrophage cells as compared to healthy controls (Reale, et al., 2009). Blood inflammatory cells such as neutrophils may also infiltrate through the disrupted BBB and activate microglia. Indeed, increased neutrophil infiltration, greater BBB permeability and decreased astrocyte numbers in SNc are thought to contribute to selective DA degeneration (Ji, et al., 2008). Furthermore, a study by Brochard and colleagues has shown that peripheral immune cells such as CD4+ T leukocytes are involved in MPTP induced cell death in mice while CD4+ null mice have reduced DA degeneration (Brochard, et al., 2009).

Thus, the infiltration and production of pro-inflammatory cytokines by peripheral cells can activate resident brain immune cells such as microglia. Therefore, not only do peripheral immune cells directly injure dopaminergic neurons, they can also indirectly activate microglia and astrocytes to further exacerbate inflammatory and cell death cascades. These results suggest that peripheral cytokine production and infiltration across the BBB may contribute to PD pathogenesis.

4.2.1 Substance P and blood brain barrier dysfunction

Along with its known role in modulating the peripheral immune response, SP is an important regulator of BBB integrity and can potentiate barrier breakdown through neurogenic inflammation. Neurogenic inflammation is a neurally elicited local inflammatory response characterised by vasodilation, protein extravasation and tissue swelling, which can be induced by certain types of injury or infection (Vink, et al., 2003). It is caused by a release of calcitonin-gene related peptide (CGRP) and SP from primary sensory nerve fibers surrounding blood vessels with subsequent activation of NK_1 receptors on endothelial cells (Lever, et al., 2003). CGRP, the most potent vasodilator, increases blood flow, bringing cytokines and inflammatory mediators to the area (Woie, et al., 1993), whereas SP binding to NK_1 receptors increases vessel permeability, leading to plasma extravasation and BBB breakdown (Hokfelt, et al., 2001). Neurogenic inflammation has been well described in the periphery but has also recently been reported to occur in the CNS (Nimmo, et al., 2004, R. Turner and Vink, 2007).

Another mechanism whereby SP may affect BBB permeability is through histamine. SP instigates the release of histamine from mast cells, to further increase vessel permeability and extravasation (R.V. Alves, et al., 1999). Thus, SP plays a central role in mediating extravascular migration of inflammatory cells into inflamed tissue (Harrison and Geppetti, 2001). Interestingly in PD, patients demonstrate elevated plasma histamine levels (Coelho, et al., 1991) and intranigral injection of histamine results in DA cell death and glial cell activation (Vizuete, et al., 2000).

5. Conclusion

We conclude that SP may be involved in the pathogenesis of PD, particularly in relation to inflammation and BBB breakdown. We suggest that the reported loss of SP expression in PD may be a secondary effect due to the decrease in striatal dopamine and therefore the loss of the SP/dopaminergic positive feedback mechanism. In contrast, SP may actually be increased within the BG *early* in PD and induce nigral BBB breakdown through neurogenic inflammation, as well as contribute to local inflammatory responses. Therefore, treatment with a NK_1 receptor antagonist may be a novel neuroprotective agent to slow the progression of PD.

6. References

Aizman, O., Brismar, H., Uhlen, P., Zettergren, E., Levey, A. I., Forssberg, H., Greengard, P.&Aperia, A., (2000). Anatomical and physiological evidence for D1 and D2 dopamine receptor colocalization in neostriatal neurons. *Nat Neurosci*. Vol. 3, No. 3, (Mar, 2000), pp. (226-30).

Alves, G., Forsaa, E. B., Pedersen, K. F., Dreetz Gjerstad, M.&Larsen, J. P., (2008). Epidemiology of Parkinson's disease. *J Neurol*. Vol. 255 Suppl 5, No., (Sep, 2008), pp. (18-32).

Alves, R. V., Campos, M. M., Santos, A. R. S.&Calixto, J. B., (1999). Receptor subtypes involved in tachykinin-mediated edema formation. *Peptides*. Vol. 20, No., 1999), pp. (921-927).

Aosaki, T.&Kawaguchi, Y., (1996). Actions of substance P on rat neostriatal neurons in vitro. *J Neurosci*. Vol. 16, No. 16, (Aug 15, 1996), pp. (5141-53).

Bailey, C. P., Maubach, K. A.&Jones, R. S., (2004). Neurokinin-1 receptors in the rat nucleus tractus solitarius: pre- and postsynaptic modulation of glutamate and GABA release. *Neuroscience*. Vol. 127, No. 2, 2004), pp. (467-79).

Bannon, M. J., Brownschidle, L. A., Tian, Y., Whitty, C. J., Poosch, M. S., D'sa, C.&Moody, C. A., (1995). Neurokinin-3 receptors modulate dopamine cell function and alter the effects of 6-hydroxydopamine. *Brain Res.* Vol. 695, No., 1995), pp. (19-24).

Bartels, A. L., Willemsen, A. T., Kortekaas, R., de Jong, B. M., de Vries, R., de Klerk, O., van Oostrom, J. C., Portman, A.&Leenders, K. L., (2008). Decreased blood-brain barrier P-glycoprotein function in the progression of Parkinson's disease, PSP and MSA. *J Neural Transm.* Vol. 115, No. 7, (Jul, 2008), pp. (1001-9).

Beal, M. F., (1992). Mechanisms of excitotoxicity in neurologic diseases. *Faseb J.* Vol. 6, No. 15, (Dec, 1992), pp. (3338-44).

Bell, M. I., Richardson, P. J.&Lee, K., (1998). Characterization of the mechanism of action of tachykinins in rat striatal cholinergic interneurons. *Neuroscience.* Vol. 87, No. 3, (Dec, 1998), pp. (649-58).

Bennett, M. C., (2005). The role of alpha-synuclein in neurodegenerative diseases. *Pharmacol Ther.* Vol. 105, No. 3, (Mar, 2005), pp. (311-31).

Berretta, N., Freestone, P. S., Guatteo, E., Castro, D. D., Geracitano, R., Bernardi, G., Mercuri, N. B.&Lipski, J., (2005). Acute Effects of 6-Hydroxydopamine on Dopaminergic Neurons of the Rat Substantia Nigra Pars Compacta In Vitro. *Neurotoxicology.* Vol., No., (May 9, 2005), pp.).

Blum, D., Torch, S., Lambeng, N., Nissou, M., Benabid, A. L., Sadoul, R.&Verna, J. M., (2001). Molecular pathways involved in the neurotoxicity of 6-OHDA, dopamine and MPTP: contribution to the apoptotic theory in Parkinson's disease. *Prog Neurobiol.* Vol. 65, No. 2, (Oct, 2001), pp. (135-72).

Brahmachari, S., Fung, Y. K.&Pahan, K., (2006). Induction of glial fibrillary acidic protein expression in astrocytes by nitric oxide. *J Neurosci.* Vol. 26, No. 18, (May 3, 2006), pp. (4930-9).

Brochard, V., Combadiere, B., Prigent, A., Laouar, Y., Perrin, A., Beray-Berthat, V., Bonduelle, O., Alvarez-Fischer, D., Callebert, J., Launay, J. M., Duyckaerts, C., Flavell, R. A., Hirsch, E. C.&Hunot, S., (2009). Infiltration of CD4+ lymphocytes into the brain contributes to neurodegeneration in a mouse model of Parkinson disease. *J Clin Invest.* Vol. 119, No. 1, (Jan, 2009), pp. (182-92).

Canals, S., Casarejos, M. J., de Bernardo, S., Rodriguez-Martin, E.&Mena, M. A., (2001). Glutathione depletion switches nitric oxide neurotrophic effects to cell death in midbrain cultures: implications for Parkinson's disease. *J Neurochem.* Vol. 79, No. 6, (Dec, 2001), pp. (1183-95).

Carvey, P. M., Zhao, C. H., Hendey, B., Lum, H., Trachtenberg, J., Desai, B. S., Synder, J., Zhu, Y. G.&Ling, Z. D., (2005). 6-hydroxydopamine-induced alteration in blood-brain barrier permeability. *Eur J Neurosci.* Vol. 22, No., 2005), pp. (1158-1168.).

Chao, Y. X., He, B. P.&Tay, S. S., (2009). Mesenchymal stem cell transplantation attenuates blood brain barrier damage and neuroinflammation and protects dopaminergic neurons against MPTP toxicity in the substantia nigra in a model of Parkinson's disease. *J Neuroimmunol.* Vol. 216, No. 1-2, (Nov 30, 2009), pp. (39-50).

Chauhan, V. S., Sterka, D. G., Jr., Gray, D. L., Bost, K. L.&Marriott, I., (2008). Neurogenic exacerbation of microglial and astrocyte responses to Neisseria meningitidis and Borrelia burgdorferi. *J Immunol.* Vol. 180, No. 12, (Jun 15, 2008), pp. (8241-9).

Chen, L.-W., Yung, K. K. L.&Chan, Y. S., (2004). Neurokinin peptides and neurokinin receptors as potential therapeutic intervention targets of basal ganglia in the prevention and treatment of Parkinson's disease. *Current Drug Targets*. Vol. 5, No., 2004), pp. (1-10).

Chen, Q., Veenman, C. L.&Reiner, A., (1996). Cellular expression of ionotropic glutamate receptor subunits on specific striatal neuron types and its implication for striatal vulnerability in glutamate receptor-mediated excitotoxicity. *Neuroscience*. Vol. 73, No. 3, (Aug, 1996), pp. (715-31).

Choi, D. K., Pennathur, S., Perier, C., Tieu, K., Teismann, P., Wu, D. C., Jackson-Lewis, V., Vila, M., Vonsattel, J. P., Heinecke, J. W.&Przedborski, S., (2005). Ablation of the inflammatory enzyme myeloperoxidase mitigates features of Parkinson's disease in mice. *J Neurosci*. Vol. 25, No. 28, (Jul 13, 2005), pp. (6594-600).

Chung, Y. C., Kim, S. R.&Jin, B. K., (2010a). Paroxetine prevents loss of nigrostriatal dopaminergic neurons by inhibiting brain inflammation and oxidative stress in an experimental model of Parkinson's disease. *J Immunol*. Vol. 185, No. 2, (Jul 15, 2010a), pp. (1230-7).

Chung, Y. C., Ko, H. W., Bok, E., Park, E. S., Huh, S. H., Nam, J. H.&Jin, B. K., (2010b). The role of neuroinflammation on the pathogenesis of Parkinson's disease. *BMB Rep*. Vol. 43, No. 4, (Apr, 2010b), pp. (225-32).

Coelho, M. H., Silva, I. J., Azevedo, M. S.&Manso, C. F., (1991). Decrease in blood histamine in drug-treated parkinsonian patients. *Mol Chem Neuropathol*. Vol. 14, No. 2, (Apr, 1991), pp. (77-85).

Contreras-Vidal, J. L.&Stelmach, G. E., (1996). Mini Review: Effects of Parkinsonism on motor control. *Life Sciences*. Vol. 58, No. 3, 1996), pp. (165-176).

De Ceballos, M. L.&Lopez-Lozano, J. J., (1999). Subgroups of parkinsonian patients differentiated by pertidergic immunostaining of caudate nuclues biopsies. *Peptides*. Vol. 20, No., 1999), pp. (249-257).

Depino, A. M., Earl, C., Kaczmarczyk, E., Ferrari, C., Besedovsky, H., del Rey, A., Pitossi, F. J.&Oertel, W. H., (2003). Microglial activation with atypical proinflammatory cytokine expression in a rat model of Parkinson's disease. *Eur J Neurosci*. Vol. 18, No. 10, (Nov, 2003), pp. (2731-42).

Deumens, R., Blokland, A.&Prickaerts, J., (2002). Modeling Parkinson's disease in rats: an evaluation of 6-OHDA lesions of the nigrostriatal pathway. *Exp Neurol*. Vol. 175, No. 2, (Jun, 2002), pp. (303-17).

Di Filippo, M., Chiasserini, D., Tozzi, A., Picconi, B.&Calabresi, P., (2010). Mitochondria and the link between neuroinflammation and neurodegeneration. *J Alzheimers Dis*. Vol. 20 Suppl 2, No., 2010), pp. (S369-79).

Donkin, J. J., Nimmo, A. J., Cernak, I., Blumbergs, P. C.&Vink, R., (2009). Substance P is associated with the development of brain edema and functional deficits after traumatic brain injury. *J Cereb Blood Flow Metab*. Vol. In press, No., 2009), pp.).

Fernandez, A., de Ceballos, M. L., Jenner, P.&Marsden, C. D., (1994). Neurotensin, substance P, delta and mu opioid receptors are decreased in basal ganglia of Parkinson's disease patients. *Neuroscience*. Vol. 61, No. 1, (Jul, 1994), pp. (73-9).

Fiebich, B. L., Schleicher, S., Butcher, R. D., Craig, A.&Lieb, K., (2000). The neuropeptide substance P activates p38 mitogen-activated protein kinase resulting in IL-6 expression independently from NF-kappa B. *J Immunol*. Vol. 165, No. 10, (Nov 15, 2000), pp. (5606-11).

Gai, W. P., Halliday, G. M., Blumbergs, P. C., Geffen, L. B.&Blessing, W. W., (1991). Substance P-containing neurons in the mesopontine tegmentum are severely affected in Parkinson's disease. *Brain*. Vol. 114 (Pt 5), No., (Oct, 1991), pp. (2253-67).

Galarraga, E., Hernandez-Lopez, S., Tapia, D., Reyes, A.&Bargas, J., (1999). Action of substance P (neurokinin-1) receptor activation on rat neostriatal projection neurons. *Synapse*. Vol. 33, No. 1, (Jul, 1999), pp. (26-35).

Gao, H. M., Liu, B.&Hong, J. S., (2003). Critical role for microglial NADPH oxidase in rotenone-induced degeneration of dopaminergic neurons. *J Neurosci*. Vol. 23, No. 15, (Jul 16, 2003), pp. (6181-7).

Gerard, N. P., Garraway, L. A., Eddy, J., R.L., Shows, T. B., Iijima, H., Paquet, J.-L.&Gerard, C., (1991). Human substance P receptor(NK-1): Organisation of the gene, chromosome localization, and functional expression of cDNA clones. *Biochemistry*. Vol. 30, No. 44, 1991), pp. (10640-10646).

Graybiel, A. M., (1990). Neurotransmitters and neuromodulators in the basal ganglia. *TINS*. Vol. 13, No. 7, 1990), pp. (244-254).

Guo, C. J., Douglas, S. D., Gao, Z., Wolf, B. A., Grinspan, J., Lai, J. P., Riedel, E.&Ho, W. Z., (2004). Interleukin-1beta upregulates functional expression of neurokinin-1 receptor (NK-1R) via NF-kappaB in astrocytes. *Glia*. Vol. 48, No. 3, (Nov 15, 2004), pp. (259-66).

Harrison, S.&Geppetti, P., (2001). Review: Substance P. *The International Journal of Biochemistry & Cell Biology*. Vol. 33, No., 2001), pp. (555-576).

Hauber, W., (1998). Involvement of basal ganglia transmitter systems in movement initiation. *Prog Neurobiol*. Vol. 56, No. 5, (Dec, 1998), pp. (507-40).

Herrero, M.-T., Augood, S. J., Hirsch, E. C., Javoy-Agid, F., Luquin, M. R., Agid, Y., Obeso, J. A.&Emson, P. C., (1995). Effects of L-DOPA on preproenkephalin and preprotachykinin gene expression in the MPTP-treated monkey striatum. *Neurosci*. Vol. 68, No. 4, 1995), pp. (1189-1198).

Hirsch, E. C., (2000). Glial cells and Parkinson's disease. *J Neurol*. Vol. 247 Suppl 2, No., (Apr, 2000), pp. (II58-62).

Hokfelt, T., Broberger, C., Xu, Z.-Q. D., Sergeyev, V., Ubink, R.&Diez, M., (2000). Neuropeptides- an overview. *Neuropharmacology*. Vol. 39, No., 2000), pp. (1337-1356).

Hokfelt, T., Pernow, B.&Wahren, J., (2001). Substance P: a pioneer amongst neuropeptides. *J of Internal Medicine*. Vol. 249, No., 2001), pp. (27-40).

Hoyle, C. H., (1998). Neuropeptide families: evolutionary perspectives. *Regul Pept*. Vol. 73, No. 1, (Jan 2, 1998), pp. (1-33).

Humpel, C.&Saria, A., (1993). Intranigral injection of selective neurokinin-1 and neurokinin-3 but not neurokinin-2 receptor agonists biphasically modulate striatal dopamine metabolism but not striatal preprotachykinin-A mRNA in the rat. *Neurosci Lett*. Vol. 157, No. 2, (Jul 23, 1993), pp. (223-6).

Hunot, S., Dugas, N., Faucheux, B., Hartmann, A., Tardieu, M., Debre, P., Agid, Y., Dugas, B.&Hirsch, E. C., (1999). FcepsilonRII/CD23 is expressed in Parkinson's disease and induces, in vitro, production of nitric oxide and tumor necrosis factor-alpha in glial cells. *J Neurosci*. Vol. 19, No. 9, (May 1, 1999), pp. (3440-7).

Ionov, I. D., (2008). Self-amplification of nigral degeneration in Parkinson's disease: a hypothesis. *Int J Neurosci*. Vol. 118, No. 12, (Dec, 2008), pp. (1763-80).

Jenner, P.&Olanow, C. W., (1998). Understanding cell death in Parkinson's disease. *Ann Neurol*. Vol. 44, No. 3 Suppl 1, (Sep, 1998), pp. (S72-84).

Ji, K. A., Eu, M. Y., Kang, S. H., Gwag, B. J., Jou, I.&Joe, E. H., (2008). Differential neutrophil infiltration contributes to regional differences in brain inflammation in the substantia nigra pars compacta and cortex. *Glia*. Vol. 56, No. 10, (Aug 1, 2008), pp. (1039-47).

Kemel, M. L., Perez, S., Godeheu, G., Soubrie, P.&Glowinski, J., (2002). Facilitation by endogenous tachykinins of the NMDA-evoked release of acetylcholine after acute and chronic suppression of dopaminergic transmission in the matrix of the rat striatum. *J Neurosci*. Vol. 22, No. 5, (Mar 1, 2002), pp. (1929-36).

Khawaja, A. M.&Rogers, D. F., (1996). Tachykinins: receptor to effector. *Int J Biochem Cell Biol*. Vol. 28, No. 7, 1996), pp. (721-738).

Kortekaas, R., Leenders, K. L., van Oostrom, J. C., Vaalburg, W., Bart, J., Willemsen, A. T.&Hendrikse, N. H., (2005). Blood-brain barrier dysfunction in parkinsonian midbrain in vivo. *Ann Neurol*. Vol. 57, No. 2, (Feb, 2005), pp. (176-9).

Krasnova, I. N., Bychkov, E. R., Lioudyno, V. I., Zubareva, O. E.&Dambinova, S. A., (2000). Intracerebroventricular administration of Substance P increases dopamine content in the brain of 6-hydroxydopamine-lesioned rats. *Neurosci*. Vol. 95, No. 1, 2000), pp. (113-117).

Leeman, S. E.&Ferguson, S. L., (2000). Substance P: an historical perspective. *Neuropeptides*. Vol. 34, No. 5, 2000), pp. (249-254).

Lever, I. J., Grant, A. D., Pezet, S., Gerard, N. P., Brain, S. D.&Malcangio, M., (2003). Basal and activity-induced release of substance P from primary afferent fibers in NK_1 receptor knockout mice: evidence for negative feedback. *Neuropharmacology*. Vol. 45, No. 8, 2003), pp. (1101-1110).

Levesque, M., Wallman, M. J., Parent, R., Sik, A.&Parent, A., (2007). Neurokinin-1 and neurokinin-3 receptors in primate substantia nigra. *Neurosci Res*. Vol. 57, No. 3, (Mar, 2007), pp. (362-71).

Lieb, K., Fiebich, B. L., Berger, M., Bauer, J.&Schulze-Osthoff, K., (1997). The neuropeptide substance P activates transcription factor NF-kappa B and kappa B-dependent gene expression in human astrocytoma cells. *J Immunol*. Vol. 159, No. 10, (Nov 15, 1997), pp. (4952-8).

Liu, B.&Hong, J. S., (2003). Role of microglia in inflammation-mediated neurodegenerative diseases: mechanisms and strategies for therapeutic intervention. *J Pharmacol Exp Ther*. Vol. 304, No. 1, (Jan, 2003), pp. (1-7).

Luber-Narod, J., Kage, R.&Leeman, S. E., (1994). Substance P enhances the secretion of tumor necrosis factor-alpha from neuroglial cells stimulated with lipopolysaccharide. *J Immunol*. Vol. 152, No. 2, (Jan 15, 1994), pp. (819-24).

Maggi, C. A., (1995). The mammalian tachykinin receptors. *Gen Pharmac*. Vol. 26, No. 5, 1995), pp. (911-944).

Malcangio, M.&Bowery, N. G., (1999). Peptide autoreceptors: does an autoreceptor exist for substance P. *TiPS*. Vol. 20, No., 1999), pp. (405-407).

Mantyh, P. W., Johnson, D. J., Boehmer, C. G., Catton, M. D., Vinters, H. V., Maggio, J. E., Too, H. P.&Vigna, S. R., (1989). Substance P receptor binding sites are expressed by glia in vivo after neuronal injury. *Proc Natl Acad Sci U S A*. Vol. 86, No. 13, (Jul, 1989), pp. (5193-7).

Marey-Semper, I., Gelman, M.&Levi-Strauss, M., (1995). A selective toxicity toward cultured mesencephalic dopaminergic neurons is induced by the synergistic effects of energetic metabolism impairment and NMDA receptor activation. *J Neurosci*. Vol. 15, No. 9, 1995), pp. (5912-5918).

Marinova-Mutafchieva, L., Sadeghian, M., Broom, L., Davis, J. B., Medhurst, A. D.&Dexter, D. T., (2009). Relationship between microglial activation and dopaminergic neuronal loss in the substantia nigra: a time course study in a 6-hydroxydopamine model of Parkinson's disease. *J Neurochem*. Vol. 110, No. 3, (Aug, 2009), pp. (966-75).

Marriott, I., (2004). The role of tachykinins in central nervous system inflammatory responses. *Front Biosci*. Vol. 9, No., (Sep 1, 2004), pp. (2153-65).

Marsden, C. D.&Olanow, C. W., (1998). The causes of Parkinson's disease are being unraveled and rational neuroprotective therapy is close to reality. *Ann Neurol*. Vol. 44, No. 3 Suppl 1, (Sep, 1998), pp. (S189-96).

Martin, F. C., Charles, A. C., Sanderson, M. J.&Merrill, J. E., (1992). Substance P stimulates IL-1 production by astrocytes via intracellular calcium. *Brain Res*. Vol. 599, No. 1, (Dec 18, 1992), pp. (13-8).

Maubach, K. A., Martin, K., Smith, D. W., Hewson, L., Frankshun, R. A., Harrison, T.&Seabrook, G. R., (2001). Substance P stimulates inhibitory synaptic transmission in the guinea pig basolateral amygdala in vitro. *Neuropharmacology*. Vol. 40, No. 6, (May, 2001), pp. (806-17).

Mauborgne, A., Javoy-Agid, F., Legrand, J. C., Agid, Y.&Cesselin, F., (1983). Decrease of substance P-like immunoreactivity in the substantia nigra and pallidum of parkinsonian brains. *Brain Res*. Vol. 268, No. 1, (May 23, 1983), pp. (167-70).

McGeer, P. L.&McGeer, E. G., (2008). Glial reactions in Parkinson's disease. *Mov Disord*. Vol. 23, No. 4, (Mar 15, 2008), pp. (474-83).

Mladenovic, A., Perovic, M., Raicevic, N., Kanazir, S., Rakic, L.&Ruzdijic, S., (2004). 6-Hydroxydopamine increases the level of TNFalpha and bax mRNA in the striatum and induces apoptosis of dopaminergic neurons in hemiparkinsonian rats. *Brain Res*. Vol. 996, No. 2, (Jan 23, 2004), pp. (237-45).

Mosley, R. L., Benner, E. J., Kadiu, I., Thomas, M., Boska, M. D., Hasan, K., Laurie, C.&Gendelman, H. E., (2006). Neuroinflammation, Oxidative Stress and the Pathogenesis of Parkinson's Disease. *Clin Neurosci Res*. Vol. 6, No. 5, (Dec 6, 2006), pp. (261-281).

Napier, T. C., Mitrovic, I., Churchill, L., Klitenick, M. A., Lu, X. Y.&Kalivas, P. W., (1995). Substance P in the ventral pallidum: projection from the ventral striatum, and electrophysiological and behavioral consequences of pallidal substance P. *Neuroscience*. Vol. 69, No. 1, (Nov, 1995), pp. (59-70).

Nikolaus, S., Huston, J. P., Korber, B., Thiel, C.&Schwarting, R. K. W., (1997). Pretreatment with neurokinin substance P but not with cholecystokinin-8S can alleviate functional deficits of partial nigrostriatal 6-hydoxydopamine lesion. *Peptides*. Vol. 18, No. 8, 1997), pp. (1161-1168).

Nimmo, A. J., Cernak, I., Heath, D. L., Hu, X., Bennett, C. J.&Vink, R., (2004). Neurogenic inflammation is associated with development of edema and functional deficits following traumatic brain injury in rats. *Neuropeptides*. Vol. 38, No. 1, (Feb, 2004), pp. (40-7).

Nisbet, A. P., Foster, O. J., Kingsbury, A., Eve, D. J., Daniel, S. E., Marsden, C. D.&Lees, A. J., (1995). Preproenkephalin and preprotachykinin messenger RNA expression in normal human basal ganglia and in Parkinson's disease. *Neuroscience*. Vol. 66, No. 2, (May, 1995), pp. (361-76).

Olanow, C. W.&Tatton, W. G., (1999). Etiology and pathogenesis of Parkinson's disease. *Annu Rev Neurosci*. Vol. 22, No., 1999), pp. (123-144).

Olanow, C. W., Agid, Y., Mizuno, Y., Albanese, A., Bonucelli, U., Damier, P., De Yebenes, J., Gershanik, O., Guttman, M., Grandas, F., Hallet, M., Hornykiewicz, O., Jenner, P., Katzenschlager, R., Langston, W. J., LeWitt, P., Melamed, E., Mena, M. A., Michel, P. P., Mytilineou, C., Obeso, J. A., Poewe, W., Quinn, N., Raisman-Vozari, R., Rajput, A. H., Rascol, O., Sampaio, C.&Stocchi, F., (2004). Levodopa in the treatment of Parkinson's disease: current controversies. *Movement Disorders*. Vol. 19, No. 9, 2004), pp. (997-1005).

Orosz, D.&Bennett, J. P., Jr., (1990). Baseline and apomorphine-induced extracellular levels of nigral substance P are increased in an animal model of Parkinson's disease. *Eur J Pharmacol*. Vol. 182, No. 3, (Jul 17, 1990), pp. (509-14).

Otsuka, M.&Yoshioka, K., (1993). Neurotransmitter functions of mammalian tachykinins. *Physiol Rev*. Vol. 73, No. 2, (Apr, 1993), pp. (229-308).

Qian, L., Flood, P. M.&Hong, J. S., (2010). Neuroinflammation is a key player in Parkinson's disease and a prime target for therapy. *J Neural Transm*. Vol. 117, No. 8, (Aug, 2010), pp. (971-9).

Raivich, G., Bohatschek, M., Kloss, C. U., Werner, A., Jones, L. L.&Kreutzberg, G. W., (1999). Neuroglial activation repertoire in the injured brain: graded response, molecular mechanisms and cues to physiological function. *Brain Res Brain Res Rev*. Vol. 30, No. 1, (Jul, 1999), pp. (77-105).

Rasley, A., Bost, K. L., Olson, J. K., Miller, S. D.&Marriott, I., (2002). Expression of functional NK-1 receptors in murine microglia. *Glia*. Vol. 37, No. 3, (Mar 1, 2002), pp. (258-67).

Ravenstijn, P. G., Merlini, M., Hameetman, M., Murray, T. K., Ward, M. A., Lewis, H., Ball, G., Mottart, C., de Ville de Goyet, C., Lemarchand, T., van Belle, K., O'Neill, M. J., Danhof, M.&de Lange, E. C., (2008). The exploration of rotenone as a toxin for inducing Parkinson's disease in rats, for application in BBB transport and PK-PD experiments. *J Pharmacol Toxicol Methods*. Vol. 57, No. 2, (Mar-Apr, 2008), pp. (114-30).

Reale, M., Iarlori, C., Thomas, A., Gambi, D., Perfetti, B., Di Nicola, M.&Onofrj, M., (2009). Peripheral cytokines profile in Parkinson's disease. *Brain Behav Immun*. Vol. 23, No. 1, (Jan, 2009), pp. (55-63).

Rego, A. C.&Oliveira, C. R., (2003). Mitochondrial dysfunction and reactive oxygen species in excitotoxicity and apoptosis: implications for the pathogenesis of neurodegenerative diseases. *Neurochem Res*. Vol. 28, No. 10, (Oct, 2003), pp. (1563-74).

Reid, M. S., Herrera-Marschitz, M., Hokfelt, T., Lindefors, N., Persson, H.&Ungerstedt, U., (1990a). Striatonigral GABA, dynorphin, substance P and neurokinin A modulation of nigrostriatal dopamine release: evidence for direct regulatory mechanisms. *Exp Brain Res*. Vol. 82, No. 2, 1990a), pp. (293-303).

Reid, M. S., Herrera-Marschitz, M., Hokfelt, T., Ohlin, M., Valentino, K. L.&Ungerstedt, U., (1990b). Effects of intranigral substance P and neurokinin A on striatal dopamine release--I. Interactions with substance P antagonists. *Neuroscience*. Vol. 36, No. 3, 1990b), pp. (643-58).

Ribeiro-da-Silva, A.&Hokfelt, T., (2000). Neuroanatomical localisation of Substance P in the CNS and sensory neurons. *Neuropeptides*. Vol. 34, No. 5, 2000), pp. (256-271).

Rite, I., Machado, A., Cano, J.&Venero, J. L., (2007). Blood-brain barrier disruption induces in vivo degeneration of nigral dopaminergic neurons. *J Neurochem*. Vol. 101, No. 6, (Jun, 2007), pp. (1567-82).

Rock, R. B.&Peterson, P. K., (2006). Microglia as a pharmacological target in infectious and inflammatory diseases of the brain. *J Neuroimmune Pharmacol*. Vol. 1, No. 2, (Jun, 2006), pp. (117-26).

Rodrigues, R. W. P., Gomide, V. C.&Chadi, G., (2001). Astroglial and microglial reaction after partial nigrostriatal degeneration induced by the striatal injection of different doses of 6-hydroxydopamine. *International Journal of Neuroscience*. Vol. 109, No., 2001), pp. (91-126).

Samii, A., Etminan, M., Wiens, M. O.&Jafari, S., (2009). NSAID use and the risk of Parkinson's disease: systematic review and meta-analysis of observational studies. *Drugs Aging*. Vol. 26, No. 9, 2009), pp. (769-79).

Saria, A., (1999). The tachykinin NK_1 receptor in the brain: pharmacology and putative functions. *Eur J of Pharmacol*. Vol. 375, No., 1999), pp. (51-60).

Schwarting, R. K.&Huston, J. P., (1996). Unilateral 6-hydroxydopamine lesions of meso-striatal dopamine neurons and their physiological sequelae. *Prog Neurobiol*. Vol. 49, No. 3, (Jun, 1996), pp. (215-66).

Severini, C., Improta, G., Falconieri-Erspamer, G., Salvadori, S.&Erspamer, V., (2002). The tachykinin peptide family. *Pharmacol Rev*. Vol. 54, No., 2002), pp. (385-322).

Shults, C. W., (2004). Mitochondrial dysfunction and possible treatments in Parkinson's disease-a review. *Mitochondrion*. Vol. 4, No. 5-6, (Sep, 2004), pp. (641-8).

Sil'kis, I. G., (2002). A possible mechanism for the dopamine-evoked synergistic disinhibition of thalamic neurons via the "direct" and "indirect" pathways in the basal ganglia. *Neurosci Behav Physiol*. Vol. 32, No. 3, (May-Jun, 2002), pp. (205-12).

Silkis, I., (2001). The cortico-basal ganglia-thalamocortical circuit with synaptic plasticity. II. Mechanism of synergistic modulation of thalamic activity via the direct and indirect pathways through the basal ganglia. *Biosystems*. Vol. 59, No. 1, (Jan, 2001), pp. (7-14).

Sivam, S. P., (1991). Dopamine dependent decrease in enkephalin and substance P levels in basal ganglia regions of postmortem Parkinsonian brains. *Neuropeptides*. Vol. 18, No., 1991), pp. (201-207).

Sutoo, D., Yabe, K.&Akiyama, K., (1999). Quantitative imaging of substance P in the human brain using a brain mapping analyzer. *Neurosci Res*. Vol. 35, No., 1999), pp. (339-346).

Takagi, S., Hayakawa, N., Kimoto, H., Kato, H.&Araki, T., (2007). Damage to oligodendrocytes in the striatum after MPTP neurotoxicity in mice. *J Neural Transm*. Vol. 114, No. 12, 2007), pp. (1553-7).

Tansey, M. G.&Goldberg, M. S., (2010). Neuroinflammation in Parkinson's disease: its role in neuronal death and implications for therapeutic intervention. *Neurobiol Dis*. Vol. 37, No. 3, (Mar, 2010), pp. (510-8).

Tenovuo, O., Rinne, U. K.&Viljanen, M. K., (1984). Substance P immunoreactivity in the post-mortem parkinsonian brain. *Brain Res.* Vol. 303, No. 1, (Jun 11, 1984), pp. (113-6).

Thornton, E., Tran, T. T.&Vink, R., (2010). A substance P mediated pathway contributes to 6-hydroxydopamine induced cell death. *Neurosci Lett.* Vol. 481, No. 1, (Aug 30, 2010), pp. (64-7).

Tomas-Camardiel, M., Rite, I., Herrera, A. J., de Pablos, R. M., Cano, J., Machado, A.&Venero, J. L., (2004). Minocycline reduces the lipopolysaccharide-induced inflammatory reaction, peroxynitrite-mediated nitration of proteins, disruption of the blood-brain barrier, and damage in the nigral dopaminergic system. *Neurobiol Dis.* Vol. 16, No. 1, (Jun, 2004), pp. (190-201).

Turner, R.&Vink, R., (2007). Inhibition of neurogenic inflammation as a novel treatment for ischemic stroke. *Drug News Perspect.* Vol. 20, No. 4, (May, 2007), pp. (221-6).

Turner, R. J., Blumbergs, P. C., Sims, N. R., Helps, S. C., Rodgers, K. M.&Vink, R., (2006). Increased substance P immunoreactivity and edema formation following reversible ischemic stroke. *Acta Neurochir Suppl.* Vol. 96, No., 2006), pp. (263-6).

van der Stelt, M.&Di Marzo, V., (2003). The endocannabinoid system in the basal ganglia and in the mesolimbic reward system: implications for neurological and psychiatric disorders. *Eur J Pharmacol.* Vol. 480, No. 1-3, (Nov 7, 2003), pp. (133-50).

Vink, R., Young, A., Bennett, C. J., Hu, X., Connor, C. O., Cernak, I.&Nimmo, A. J., (2003). Neuropeptide release influences brain edema formation after diffuse traumatic brain injury. *Acta Neurochir Suppl.* Vol. 86, No., 2003), pp. (257-60).

Vizuete, M. L., Merino, M., Venero, J. L., Santiago, M., Cano, J.&Machado, A., (2000). Histamine infusion induces a selective dopaminergic neuronal death along with an inflammatory reaction in rat substantia nigra. *J Neurochem.* Vol. 75, No. 2, (Aug, 2000), pp. (540-52).

Wade, T. V.&Schneider, J. S., (2001). Expression of striatal preprotachykinin mRNA in symptomatic and asymptomatic 1-methyl-4-phenyl-1,2,3,6-tetrahydropyridine-exposed monkeys is related to parkinsonian motor signs. *J Neurosci.* Vol. 21, No. 13, (Jul 1, 2001), pp. (4901-7).

Wardas, J., Peitraszek, M., Wolfarth, S.&Ossowska, K., (2003). The role of metabotropic glutamate receptors in regulation of striatal proenkephalin expression: Implications for the therapy of Parkinson's disease. *Neurosci.* Vol. 122, No., 2003), pp. (747-756).

Woie, K., Koller, M. E., Heyeraas, K. J.&Reed, R. K., (1993). Neurogenic inflammation in rat trachea is accompanied by increased negativity of interstitial fluid pressure. *Circ Res.* Vol. 73, No. 5, (Nov, 1993), pp. (839-45).

Wojtera, M., Sikorska, B., Sobow, T.&Liberski, P. P., (2005). Microglial cells in neurodegenerative disorders. *Folia Neuropathol.* Vol. 43, No. 4, 2005), pp. (311-21).

Wu, D. C., Teismann, P., Tieu, K., Vila, M., Jackson-Lewis, V., Ischiropoulos, H.&Przedborski, S., (2003). NADPH oxidase mediates oxidative stress in the 1-methyl-4-phenyl-1,2,3,6-tetrahydropyridine model of Parkinson's disease. *Proc Natl Acad Sci U S A.* Vol. 100, No. 10, (May 13, 2003), pp. (6145-50).

Yelnik, J., (2002). Functional anatomy of the basal ganglia. *Mov Disord.* Vol. 17 Suppl 3, No., 2002), pp. (S15-21).

Yip, J.&Chahl, L. A., (2000). Localization of tachykinin receptors and fos-like immunoreactivity induced by substance P in guinea pig brain. *Clinical and Experimental Pharmacology and Physiology*. Vol. 27, No., 2000), pp. (943-946).

26

Noradrenergic Mechanisms in Parkinson's Disease and L-DOPA-Induced Dyskinesia: Hypothesis and Evidences from Behavioural and Biochemical Studies

Amal Alachkar
University of Aleppo
Syria

1. Introduction

The key pathological characteristic of Parkinson's disease PD is the degeneration of dopaminergic neurons in the substantia nigra pars compacta SNc that project to the striatum (Barolin and Horykiewicz 1967). The depletion of dopamine leads to abnormalities of the transmission in striatal projections to the lateral or medial segments of the globus pallidus, or to the substantia nigra reticulata SNr (Brotchie et al, 1993; Albin et al., 1989). It is well known, however, that in PD, besides dopaminergic degeneration, a considerable loss of noradrenergic neurons, as well as, a decrease of noradrenaline levels in several brain regions occurs (Hornykiewicz & Kish 1987).

Interestingly, the neural loss in PD in Locus coreleus is greater than that of dopamine in the substantia nigra (Zarow et al., 2003).

The influence of noradrenergic neurotransmission on dopamine-mediated behaviour has been the focus of several studies over the last four decades, and has confirmed the importance of the relationship between dopaminergic and noradrenergic pathways in the control of locomotor activity. The progressive neurodegeneration of the main noradrenergic nucleus - the locus coeruleus LC - might influence not only the progression of Parkinson's disease but also the response to dopaminergic replacement. Furthermore, additional evidences support the notion that noradrenaline deficit might be relevant for the pathogenesis of long-term complications of L-DOPA treatment such as the wearing-off phenomenon and dyskinesias (Bezard et al., 2001; Obeso et al., 2000; Marsden and Parkes, 1976).

However, in spite of the bulk of data on the influence of the alterations of noradrenergic transmission on locomotor behaviour, much of these data is conflicting and not conclusive. Therefore, definitive conclusions, as to the specific role of the noradrenergic system in the generation of symptoms of Parkinson's disease and L-DOPA-induced dyskinesia LID, cannot yet be drawn.

Based on a number of behavioural studies, demonstrating the alleviation of dyskinesia by α_2 adrenergic receptor antagonists, in addition to other biochemical studies, this chapter aims to test the hypothesis that the noradrenergic system plays a role in the neural mechanisms underlying Parkinson's disease and L-DOPA-induced dyskinesia.
The model presented here suggests that the degeneration of noradrenergic neurons contributes to the pathophysiology and symptomatology of PD, and that the remaining intact noradrenergic neurons exert a compensatory mechanism in PD. Furthermore, we suggest a role for L-DOPA metabolites in the mechanism of LID; this role might be mediated through the activation of α_2 adrenoceptors.
Our data and other studies presented in this chapter demonstrate a potential role for noradrenergic system in Parkinson's disease and LID.

2. Parkinson's disease and L-DOPA-induced dyskinesia

Parkinson's disease is a progressive hypokinetic neurodegenerative disorder, characterised by bradykinesia, rigidity, tremor, akinesia, and abnormal posture. Non-motor symptoms such as cognitive decline, depression, sleep disturbances and autonomic and sensorimotor dysfunction also occur (Marsden, 1990, Remy et al., 2005; Schapira, 2008). The key pathological characteristic of Parkinson's disease is the degeneration of dopaminergic neurons in the substantia nigra that project to the striatum (Barolin and Horykiewicz 1967).
Dopamine neurons degenerate with advancing age more than other neuronal systems in the brain (Fearnley & Lees, 1991). Neurons in the SNc and VTA are lost at a rate of 1% per year in parkinsonian patients compared to 0.5% per year in non-parkinsonian subjects (Scherman et al, 1989). Parkinsonian symptoms become apparent when striatal dopamine levels fall by about 70% (Altar and Marien, 1989). Post-mortem studies show substantial depletion of dopamine in the putamen. In caudal parts of the putamen, dopamine content is less than 1% of control levels, whereas the dopamine content of the caudate nucleus is relatively well preserved i.e. 40% of control levels (Hornykiewicz, 1973; Kish et al, 1988). The degeneration of cells in the SNc is accompanied by the presence of eosinophilic intraneuronal, cytoplasmic inclusions called Lewy bodies, which are characterised by a central core and peripheral halo (McGeer et al, 1988; Quinn et al, 1989). Lewy bodies show immunoreactivity for tubulin and ubiquitin (Jellinger, 1990).
The loss of dopaminergic neurons in the substantia nigra pars compacta, which results in a reduction in the level of dopamine in the striatum, leads to alterations in the activity of striatal output nuclei. This results in changes in the other nuclei basal ganglia, which can be summarized as following: (a) Degeneration of the nigrostriatal pathway, (b) the underactivity of the GABA/dynorphin striato-medial pallidal/SNr nigral pathway, (c) the overactivity of the GABA/enkephalin striato-lateral-pallidal pathway, (d) the overactivity of the subthalamic nucleus, (e) the overactivity of the GABA medial pallidal/SNr (output regions of the basal ganglia) -thalamic projection (Brotchie et al, 1993). The overactivity of basal ganglia output results in increased inhibition of excitatory glutamatergic projections from the thalamus to the cortex. Cortical motor outputs are, thus, underactive leading to the movement paucity in Parkinson's disease (Albin et al., 1989).

Although the predominant pathology of PD is the loss of dopaminergic cells in the substantia nigra, however, there is also degeneration of other neurotransmission systems, such as cholinergic, noradrenergic, serotoninergic and peptidergic brainstem nuclei (Jellinger, 1991).

Some of these alterations in neurotransmitters occur before the appearance of parkinsonian symptoms (Bezard et al, 2001). Noradrenaline (NA) is particularly implicated in certain symptoms of Parkinson's disease. Biochemical analysis revealed that 40-80% of the brain's content of NA is depleted in PD (Agid, et al., 1987; Gerlach et al, 1994).

Current strategies for the treatment of PD still depend largely on the replacement of lost dopamine. Levodopa, a precursor of dopamine, has proved very successful as an antiparkinsonian agent (Cotzias et al 1967). L-DOPA can cross the blood-brain barrier and is converted to dopamine by aromatic amino acid decarboxylase, presumably in the striatum at the synaptic sites of surviving nigrostriatal cells (Melamed et al 1984). However, due to the massive degeneration of nigrostriatal terminals, it is unlikely that the majority of dopamine synthesis occurs in nigrostriatal terminals (Snyder & Zigmond, 1990). Within the striatum, 5-HT terminals, striatal interneurons and glial cells also contain aromatic amino acid decarboxylase, and these sites may play a role in the conversion of L-DOPA to dopamine in the degenerated striatum (Opacka-Juffry, 1995; Mura et al, 1995).

Initially, L-DOPA is successful in reversing parkinsonian symptoms, akinesia, rigidity and tremor. However, as treatment progresses, the effectiveness of L-DOPA treatment decreases and dyskinesia, fluctuations in mobility and freezing episodes, occur (Marsden & Parkes, 1976; Mouradian et al, 1991). With the progress of treatment, the dose of L-DOPA required to induce dyskinesia gradually decreases and the dose of L-DOPA required to alleviate parkinsonian symptoms is increased, thereby, resulting in the development of a narrow therapeutic window (Mouradian et al, 1988).

The mechanism, underlying L-DOPA-induced dyskinesia, is still far from being fully understood. The fact, that dyskinesia results from prolonged replacement of dopamine, suggests that it arises through the overactivity of dopaminergic mechanisms. Similarities in the choreic dyskinesia seen among various brain disorders, i.e. L-DOPA-induced dyskinesia, tardive dyskinesia and hemiballism, has led to the suggestion of a common mechanism for all dyskinesia (Crossman (review) 1990).

According to the most acceptable model, L-DOPA-induced dyskinesia is associated with an imbalance of basal ganglia circuitry in favour of the direct pathway. Data obtained from animal models of PD have implicated a relative underactivity of the indirect pathway, and overactivity of the direct pathway. The net effect of the overactive GABAergic projection in the direct and indirect pathways and the underactive glutamatergic projection of the STN, will lead to the cumulative inhibitory effects on the output nuclei of the basal ganglia. This, in turn, leads to the decrease of the inhibition of thalamocortical neurons and overactivation of cortical motor areas.

- PD.: Decreased activity in the dopaminergic nigrostriatal pathway, Overactivity of the GABA striato-lateral-pallidal pathway, Overactivity of the subthalamic nucleus, Overactivity of the regions of the basal ganglia that project to non-basal ganglia motor regions, i.e., the medial pallidal segment and the SNr (Blandini et al, 2000).

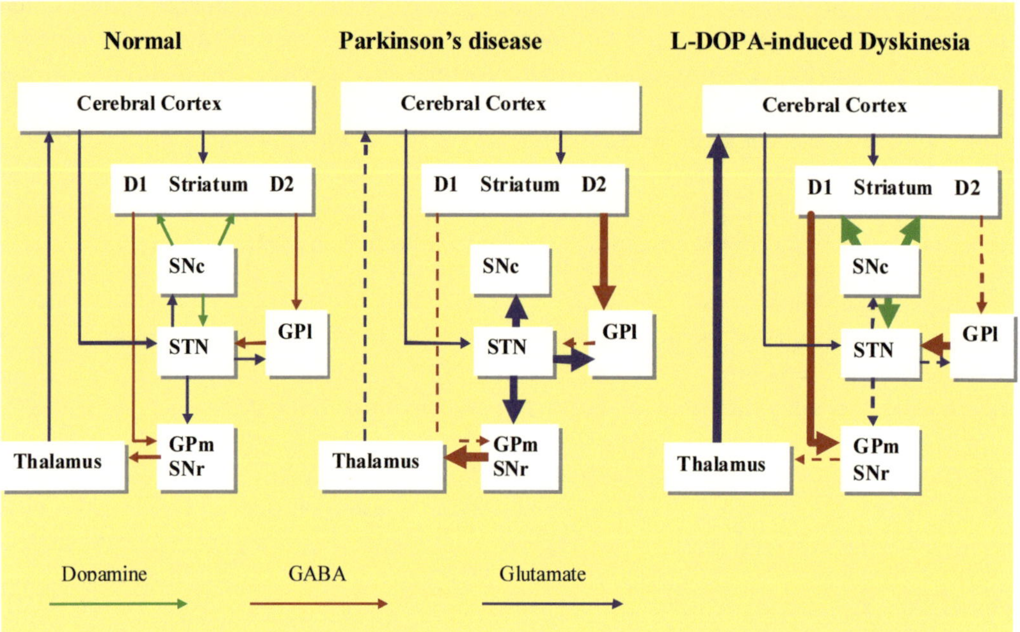

Fig. 1. **Diagram illustrating the changes in the organisation of the basal ganglia in Parkinson's disease and L-DOPA-induced Dyskinesia.**

- LID: Increased activity in the dopaminergic nigrostriatal pathway, Underactivity of the GABA striato-lateral-pallidal pathway, Underactivity of the subthalamic nucleus, Underactivity of the regions of the basal ganglia that project to non-basal ganglia motor regions, i.e., the medial pallidal segment and the SNr.

3. Noradrenergic system

The main noradrenergic system is the locus coeruleus LC (A6-cell group), in which about 45% of brain noradrenergic cells are present.

The total estimated number of noradrenergic neurons in the LC of the normal young adult human brain ranges from 45,000 to 60,000 (Baker et al, 1989; , German et al., 1988). The vast majority (90%) of LC efferent projections remain ipsilateral (Ader et al., 1980; Mason & Fibiger, 1979; Room et al., 1981). There are two types of LC axonal terminals: regular synaptic terminals, and varicosities that are believed to cause an extra-synaptic release of noradrenaline, which then may diffuse over a distance (Aoki, 1992; Beaudet & Descarries, 1978; Koda et al., 1978; Parnavelas & Papadopoulos, 1989).

The main projections of the LC are to the neocortex, where LC neurons project to all layers of the neocortex, although the density of fibres varies according to the cortical regions and the species (Morrison et al, 1979; Morrison et al, 1982). The LC also sends efferents to the hippocampus, amygdala, septum, thalamus and hypothalamus. Morphologically different types of neurons in the locus coeruleus project to different regions of the CNS (Loughlin, et al, 1986), and the axons of LC neurons are extensively ramified, as one axon may branch up to 100,000 times (Moore & Bloom, 1979). Noradrenaline may co-exist with other neurotransmitters and modulators, and the type of modulators co-existing with NA depends, in part, on species. For instance, noradrenergic neurons have been reported to have immunoreactive staining for enkephalin in cats, vasopressin in rats, and neuropeptide Y (NPY) in rats and humans (Caffe et al, 1985).

The firing activity of noradrenergic neurons in the LC is regulated by somatodendritic autoreceptors of the α_2- adrenergic subtype. These receptors are believed to decrease the firing rate of NA neurons primarily through an increase in potassium conductance.

The firing rate of LC cells is influenced by behavioural activity and sensory input and seems to relate closely to arousal and sleep-waking cycles (Astone -Jones et al, 1991). The LC cells are completely inactive during rapid-eye-movement (REM) sleep (Aston-Jones & Bloom, 1981). The changes in cell firing in sleep-waking cycles suggest a contribution of LC to the mechanisms controlling sleep-waking states (Foote et al, 1980; Mallick, 2002).

Numbers of LC cells and the concentration of brain noradrenaline decline with age in normal brain respectively by 25% and 50% between the fourth and ninth decades of life (Mann, 1983; Mann et al, 1983).

4. Noradrenaline functions

Electrophysiological and behavioural studies have revealed an important role for noradrenaline in attention, arousal and waking (Grant and Redmond 1984; Kumar, 2003). There is an increase in the activity of the LC in rats and primates during high awareness, whereas the activity is decreased during grooming, feeding and sleeping (Grant and Redmond 1984). Furthermore, the α_2 adrenoceptor agonist clonidine increases the total duration of sleep and significantly reduces the duration of REM sleep. In contrast, yohimbine, an α_2 adrenoceptor antagonist, reverses the effects of clonidine (Autret et al, 1977).

Noradrenaline has also been implicated in controlling feeding behaviour (Goldman et al, 1985). Injection of noradrenaline or the α_2 receptor agonist clonidine into the area of the paraventricular nucleus (PVN), caused a potent feeding response in satiated animals, an effect probably mediated via α_2 adrenoceptors located postsynaptically (Weiss &Leibowitz, 1985; Goldman et al, 1985). Further studies have suggested that feeding behaviour is stimulated by low levels of clonidine, and decreased by further production of noradrenaline (Bungo et al, 1999).

The noradrenaline system has also been implicated in anxiety-related behaviours since α_2 agonists are of clinical benefit in treating some types of anxiety (Hoehen-Saric et al, 1981; Crespi, 2009), while α_2 antagonists elicit intense anxiety (Charney et al, 1983; Graeff, 1994). However, it is not clear whether these effects are mediated through pre-or postsynaptic adrenoceptors. A study by Tanak et al., has suggested that the increased release of noradrenaline in the locus coeruleus is, in part, involved in the frustration of anxiety and/or fear in animals exposed to stress (Tanaka et al, 2000). On the other hand, genetic studies on α_{2a} adrenoceptor knock-out mice suggest that α_{2a} may play a protective role in some types of depression and anxiety (Schramm et al, 2001).

Noradrenaline is also involved in cognitive processes such as memory, learning and selective attention (Franowicz, & Arnsten, 1998; Franowicz et al, 2002; Gibbs & Summers, 2002; Marrs et al, 2005; Timofeeva & Levin, 2008). In Alzheimer Type Dementia (ATD), both the concentration of noradrenaline and the noradrenaline transporters sites are significantly decreased in a number of brain regions including the Locus coeruleus, cingulate gyrus, putamen, hypothalamus, medial thalamic nucleus, and raphe area (Arai et al, 1984; Tejani et al, 1993).

Evidence has accumulated suggesting that noradrenaline is also involved in controlling body temperature (Lin et al, 1981, Sallinen et al, 1997), endocrine secretion (Endroczi et al, 1978; Valet et al, 1989; Ruffolo et al, 1991), and sexual behaviour (Morales et al, 1987; Guiliano & Rampin, 1997).

5. Noradrenaline in the basal ganglia

The synthesis of noradrenaline (Glowinski & Iverson, 1966) and its release (Coyle & Henry, 1973) was initially demonstrated in the striatum. Later studies revealed that the striatum receives little noradrenergic projection from the locus coeruleus and has low levels of dopamine β-hydroxylase (Swanson & Hartman, 1975). Nevertheless, the striatum shows high levels of α_2 adrenoceptor gene expression (mRNA) (Scheinin et al, 1994) and high radioligand binding to α_{2C} adrenoceptors (Uhlen et al, 1997). Noradrenergic terminals and uptake sites have also been demonstrated in the SNc (Fuxe, 1965), subthalamic nucleus (Carpenter et al, 1981b; Parent & Hazrati, 1995; Belujon et al, 2007) and the SNr (Gehlert et al, 1993).

The precise role of noradrenaline in the basal ganglia is not yet clear. However, the noradrenergic inputs to the basal ganglia appear to have a modulatory effect on other neurotransmitters in different structures of the basal ganglia.

Noradrenaline derived from the LC may induce an inhibition of striatal neurons trans-synaptically activated by nigral stimulation (Fujimoto et al, 1981). It has been shown that the α_2 antagonist yohimbine increases the synthesis and release of dopamine in the striatum, while the agonist clonidine can reverse this effect (Anden and Grabowska, 1976). α_2 presynaptic heteroreceptors also seem to regulate the release of amino acid neurotransmitters such as glutamic acid, aspartic acid, GABA as evaluated with synaptosoms (Bristow and Bennett, 1988, Kamisaki, et al, 1992, Bickler and Hansen, 1996, Pralong and Magistretti, 1995). Immunocytochemical studies reveal that 94% of spiny GABAergic neurons in the striatum contain α_{2C} adrenergic receptors (Holmberg et al, 1999), which are negatively coupled to adenylyl cyclase (Zhang et al, 1999). These α_{2C} receptors are thought to play a regulatory role on the direct and indirect pathways of the basal ganglia by modulating GABA transmission. Recent studies on α_2 receptor knock-out mice indicate that α_{2a} and α_{2C} adrenoceptors are located on different neurons in the striatum, and that striatal GABA release is mediated by the activation of α_{2C} but not α_{2a} adrenoceptor (Zhang & Ordway, 2003). These authors suggest that the effect of α_{2C} on GABA release might be mediated by dopamine.

In the basal ganglia, α adrenoceptors are mainly found in the striatum, globus pallodus, substantia nigra pars compacta SNc and substantia nigra pars reticulata SNr (Unnerstall et al, 1984; Boyajian et al, 1987; Uhlen et al, 1997; Winzer-Srhan et al, 1997).

Noradrenergic pathways might have a significant role in regulating basal ganglia function and thus motor activity by modulating the spontaneous activity of the STN neurons. Accordingly, noradrenaline has been reported to induce stimulation of the firing rate of a neuronal subpopulation of the subthalamic nucleus, and this stimulation was suggested to be mediated through the activation of α_1 adrenoceptors (Arcos et al, 2003).

The modulation of dopamine neurone firing by the noradrenergic system of the locus coeruleus in the rat has provided further evidence for the role of noradrenaline in regulating the activity of the basal ganglia. Interestingly, noradrenaline has been reported to evoke excitation followed by inhibition of the electrical activity of dopaminergic cells (Grenhoff et al, 1993; Grenhoff et al, 1995).

The SNr represents, with medial segment of globus pallidus, the main output regions of the basal ganglia and therefore, plays a crucial role in movement initiation. The GABAergic neurons in the substantia nigra are spontaneously active and the modulation of their activity would significantly influence the basal ganglia functions. Indeed, there is evidence supporting the regulatory action of noradrenaline upon the neurons of the SNr. Noradrenaline has been demonstrated to increase the tonic firing of principal cells in the SNr (Berretta et al, 2000). On the other hand, we demonstrated the stimulatory effects of both the activation and blockade of α_2 adrenergic receptors on the release of GABA from slices of the SNr. (Alachkar et al, 2006).

6. Noradrenaline- dopamine interaction

The interaction between dopamine and noradrenaline systems has been demonstrated, previously, in the brain. Dopamine, for instance, has long been demonstrated to have stimulatory actions upon noradrenergic neurons in the locus coeruleus (Persson and Waldeck, 1970). On the other hand, noradrenaline has been shown to reduce the spontaneous firing of dopaminergic neurons in the SNc (White & Wang, 1984), although, other workers have reported excitatory responses of the SNc to the stimulation of the locus coeruleus (Grenhoff, 1993). Other studies have provided evidences for the mutual inhibition of dopaminergic and noradrenergic systems (Persson & Waldeck, 1970; Guiard et al, 2008). A number of studies indicate, interestingly, that dopamine is co-released with noradrenaline from noradrenergic neurons in the locus coeruleus (Anden et al, 1973; Devoto et al, 2001).

On the other hand, dopamine may activate α_2 adrenoceptors in more than a region in the brain (Segawa et al, 1998; Cornil et al, 2002; Alachkar et al, 2010a). It is well documented that a molecular relationship exists, at the level of the amino acid sequence, between α_2 and dopamine D2 receptors, in that D2 dopamine receptors are more closely related to α_2 adrenoceptors than to D1 dopaminergic receptors (Harrison et al, 1991).

NA was found to act as a D1 dopaminergic agonist (Kubrusly et al., 2007), and mimic the effect of DA on the DA D2 receptor (Onali et al., 1985). Furthermore, it was demonstrated that NA binds to the human DA D4 receptor with high affinity (Lanau et al., 1997; Newman-Tancredi et al., 1997) and 10% of total D2-like receptors are of the DA D4 receptor located in the caudate putamen (Tarazi et al., 1997).

α_2 adrenoceptor mRNA, type A and C, is present in high levels in the striatum and locus coeruleus (Nicholas et al, 1993; Scheinin et al, 1994, our unpublished results), with receptors binding located in the striatum, and SNr (Rosin et al, 1996; Lee et al, 1998a,b).

The presence of noradrenaline uptake sites in the SNr (Gehlert et al, 1995; Strazielle et al, 1999) indicates noradrenaline release in this nucleus.

The NA could affect the activity of the SNr through their direct noradrenergic projections and their indirect influence by the action of SNc and other parts of basal ganglia.

7. Noradrenaline in Parkinson's disease

In Parkinson's disease, a significant loss of noradrenergic cells of the locus coeruleus and the noradrenergic pathways occurs, in addition to the degeneration of the nigrostriatal dopaminergic pathway, (Hornykiewicz & Kish 1987; Zarow et al., 2003). Moreover, there is a considerable decrease in NA levels in a number of brain structures including the hypothalamus, cerebral cortex, substantia nigra and caudate nucleus in patients with this disease (Fahn et al, 1971; Rinne & Sonninen, 1973; Kish et al, 1984). The significance of the loss of LC cells to Parkinson's disease is still largley unknown. It is possible that noradrenergic depletion contributes to the degeneration of other brain nuclei. Postmortem studies have revealed that the symptoms of depression and dementia in PD were associated with a significant loss of noradrenergic neurons in the LC and NA depletion in the cortex (Zweig et al., 1993; Bosboom et al., 2004; Remy et al., 2005; Ridderinkhof et al., 2004; Ramos and Arnsten, 2007). LC-noradrenergic neurotransmitter system may be involved in the pathogenesis of non-motor symptoms in PD. A decrease in α_2 receptor density in the prefrontal cortex has also been shown in animal models of Parkinson's disease (Mavridis et al, 1991). Administration of α_2-adrenergic agonist was demonstrated to improve the cognitive impairments in PD patients (Remy et al., 2005; Riekkinen and Riekkinen, 1999).

The great extent to which LC cell loss occurs in PD is emphasized by the study by Zarow et al. who, interestingly, demonstrated that the greatest loss of neurons in PD was found in the LC (83.2%). The degree of cell loss in the LC seemed to be even more extensive than that observed in the substantia nigra (77.8% loss) (Zarow et al. 2003). Significant depletions (>80%) of noradrenaline in the substantia nigra pars compacta and reticulata, of postmortem PD brains have also been described (Taquet et al., 1982).

The NA depletion in the LC was proved to decrease DA release in the striatum (Lategan et al., 1990; Lategan et al., 1992). Furthermore, clinical studies have indicated that some motor symptoms of PD are likely to result from noradrenergic lesions (Grimbergen et al., 2009). These findings suggest the implication of the LC-noradrenergic system in the pathophysiology of PD.

Experimental data suggest that the LC noradrenaline system may have a neuroprotective role on dopaminergic SN neurons (Gesi et al, 2000). For instance, noradrenaline depletion significantly increased MPTP- as well as methylamphetamine-induced striatal dopamine depletion in mice and monkeys (Forani et al, 1995, Marien et al 1993; Archer and Fredriksson, 2006; Nishi et al., 1991). Furthermore, lesions of LC by 6-OHDA in MPTP treated monkeys produced a more significant depletion and greater loss of substantia nigra cell compared to normal controls, and impaired the recovery which usually occurs from the parkinsonian manifestations induced by MPTP (Mavridis et al, 1991; Bing et al, 1994). A potentiation of parkinsonian symptoms following locus coeruleus noradrenaline depletion has been reported in 6-OHDA-lesioned rats (Srinivasan & Schmidt, 2003).

The mechanism by which the locus coeruleus may protect dopaminergic neurons is still unknown. The activation of α_2 adrenoceptors by clonidine, α_2 agonist, has been demonstrated to suppress MPTP-induced reduction of striatal dopamine and tyrosine hydroxylase activity in mice (Bristow and Bennett, 1988; Fornai et al, 1995).

Noradrenaline may exert its neuroprotective effects by facilitating the release of trophic factors, such as the nerve growth factor NGF; this was suggested to occur through an action on β-adrenoceptors on the glial cells (Mochetti et al, 1989). Noradrenaline may suppress the formation of toxic MPP^+ from MPTP by inhibiting the production of glial monoamine oxidase B in the substantia nigra (Stone and Ariano, 1989). Interestingly, the administration of L-threo-3, 4 dihydroxyphenylserine (L-threo-DOPS) an immediate precursor of noradrenaline, seems to alleviate parkinsonian symptoms (Narabayashi et al, 1984). Although L-threo DOPS causes an increase in dopamine as well as noradrenaline levels, its anti-parkinsonian action was inhibited by adrenoceptor antagonists and dopamine β-hydroxylase inhibitors. The α_2 adrenoceptor antagonist R47 243 has been found to reverse some parkinsonian signs in a monkey in which MPTP's effects had been progressive, by a mechanism that is still unknown (Colpaert et al, 1991). On the other hand, blockade of α_2 adrenoceptors counteracted to some extent the development of parkinsonian symptoms and neurochemical alterations in the rotenone model of Parkinson's disease (Alam et al, 2009). In addition Belujon et al have provided behavioral and electrophysiological evidence for the noradrenergic modulation of subthalamic nucleus activity in intact and 6-hydroxydopamine-lesioned rats. The authors have shown that the firing of STN neurons is controlled by noradrenergic system through the activation of α_1- and α_2 adrenergic receptors (Belujon et al, 2007).

Firing activity of LC-noradrenergic neurons was demonstrated to increase in rats after the SNc lesion (Guiard et al, 2008; Wang et al., 2009), which may imply an overactivity of LC-noradrenergic neurons and enhanced influence of LC in rats with SNc lesion.

On the other hand, lesions of the LC in rat models of PD caused further hyperactivity of SNr neurons implying that LC-noradrenergic system may play a role in decreasing the activity of the output regions of the basal ganglia (wang et al, 2010). Intact noradrenergic neurons of the LC were believed to play a crucial role in the compensational mechanism after the dopaminergic depletion in the SNc (Gesi et al., 2000; Rommelfanger and Weinshenker, 2007).

8. Noradrenaline and L-DOPA-induced dyskinesia

Progressive neurodegeneration of the noradrenergic neurons in the locus coeruleus was suggested to influence the response to dopaminergic replacement (Cotzias et al., 1967), and the pathogenesis of long-term complications of L-DOPA treatment (Bezard et al., 2001; Marsden and Parkes, 1976; Obeso et al., 2000).

The involvement of noradrenergic transmission in L-DOPA-induced dyskinesia has been the focus of several investigations. This was based on the well documented interaction between dopaminergic and noradrenergic system. Early studies on reserpine-treated rats revealed that the hyperkinesia induced by L-DOPA was mediated via activation of the noradrenergic system (Anden et al, 1969; Stromber & Svensson, 1971). A number of studies substantiated evidence that the noradrenergic system may have a modulatory effect on L-DOPA-induced dyskinesia. Gomez-Mancilla and Bedard (1993) investigated the effects of several agents acting on the noradrenergic system in the brain on L-DOPA-induced dyskinesia. They reported that the α_2 adrenergic receptor antagonist, yohimbine, decreased L-DOPA-induced dyskinesia without reducing the anti-parkinsonian action of L-DOPA, in MPTP-treated monkeys. Further studies have reported that the reduction of dyskinesia can be mediated by blocking the actions of α_2 adrenergic receptors, shown using a number of α_2 antagonists (Henry et al 1999, Fox et al 2001; Grondin et al, 2000; Rascol, 2001, Savola et al, 2003; Dekundy et al, 2007). The mechanism by which α_2 antagonists can alleviate L-DOPA-induced dyskinesia is unknown; however, activation of α_2 adrenoceptors on the striatal output neuron terminals has been suggested to reduce GABA release and inhibition of the lateral segment of the globus pallidus (GPl) in the indirect pathway (Henry et al, 1999). Therefore, blockade at these sites may up-regulate the inhibitory striatopallidal connections and reduce STN inhibition and dyskinesia. The other explanation for the effect of α_2 adrenoceptor antagonists in reducing L-DOPA-induced dyskinesia may be the blockade of the action of noradrenaline synthesised from levodopa on α_{2c} receptors in the basal ganglia (Fox et al, 2001). There is evidence that local administration of NA into the lesioned striatum can induce dyskinetic movements in rats in a similar manner to intrastriatal L-DOPA treatment (Buck & Ferger, 2009).

On the other hand, noradrenaline synthesized from exogenous L-DOPA administered in Parkinson's disease therapy may, in part, be involved in the locomotor activity produced by L-DOPA (Dolphin et al, 1976). This implies that at least some symptoms of LID are mediated through the activation of the noradrenergic system. Therefore, the therapeutic actions of α_2 antagonists may be correlated with this noradrenergic disruption in Parkinson's disease and LID.

Fox et al., have reported that α_2 antagonism reduces L-DOPA-induced dyskinesia but did not affect apomorphine-induced dyskinesia suggesting that L-DOPA-induced dyskinesia but not dopamine agonist-induced dyskinesia, involves activation of adrenoceptors (Fox et al, 2001). The authors suggested that the pharmacological characteristics of the neural mechanisms underlying levodopa-induced dyskinesia and dopamine agonist-induced dyskinesia in parkinsonism are distinct, at least with respect to the involvement of α_2 adrenoceptors.

9. Noradrenergic mechanisms in PD and LID: A theory

9.1 Parkinson's disease PD

We present here a model to explain the mechanism by which noradrenergic system may modulate the activity of the basal ganglia in PD.This model attempts to answer the question of whether noradrenergic abnormalities reflect a response to, or the cause of, the PD. Our scenario is based on the discussion above and most importantly the following three observations:

- Certain evidences support the belief that LC lesion may exacerbate the abnormal activity of basal ganglia in PD, resulting in a further overactivity of the SNr neurons. This implies that LC-noradrenergic system may play a role in decreasing the activity of the output regions of the basal ganglia in PD (wang et al, 2010).
- Further evidence indicates that the firing activity of LC-noradrenergic neurons increases after the SNc lesion (Guiard et al, 2008; Wang et al., 2009), which may imply an overactivity of LC-noradrenergic neurons; and enhanced influence of LC in PD.
- Several studies have described the anti-parkinsonian effects of the blockade of α_2 inhibitory receptors. Although the site of action of these receptors is not known for certain, the data of other several studies conform to a model where alpha-2 antagonists produce their effects in the SNr by interacting with GABAergic transmission.

According to our model, changes in Parkinson's disease that occur in noradrenergic transmission contribute to the mechanism of PD, and partially compensate for the degeneration of the dopaminergic system.

Based on the discussion above, we propose that in Parkinson's disease, the degeneration of 83% of LC neurons and depletion of noradrenaline exacerbate the Parkinsonian symptoms through increasing the overactivity of the substantia nigra pars reticulata. On the other hand, the destruction of the dopamine-containing cells in the SNc results in a decrease in the inhibition, by dopamine, on the firing of the locus coeruleus and therefore, the remaining intact noradrenergic neurons of the LC are deemed to play a crucial role in the compensational mechanism after the dopaminergic depletion in the SNc (Gesi et al., 2000; Rommelfanger and Weinshenker, 2007). Noradrenaline released from overactive remaining LC neurons is thought to act as an inhibitory transmitter on α_2 adrenoceptors located on the GABAergic striatal projecting neurons, and on the neurons of SNr. This would decrease the firing rate and the activity of the inhibitory GABAergic projection of SNr (which is overactive in PD) to the motor regions of the thalamus, and hence alleviate Parkinsonian symptoms. Accordingly, noradrenaline may contribute to the pathological and the compensational mechanisms in Parkinson's disease. The prevalence of one of these two contradictory effects of noradrenergic system depends mainly on the extent of the degeneration of LC cells. The greater degeneration of LC noradrenergic neurons indicates more extensive abnormalities of the basal ganglia and overactivity of SNr, and thus further potentiation of the Parkinsonian symptoms.

9.2 L-DOPA-induced dyskinesia LID

Administration of L-DOPA with an AADC inhibitor, NSD1015, produced hyperlocomotor activity in reserpine-treated rats (Alachkar et al, 2010b). It seems likely that L-DOPA, or one or more of its metabolites not formed via routes involving direct decarboxylation of L-DOPA, are responsible for the generation of hyperkinesia. Significantly, α_2 receptor antagonist, rauwolscine, reduced centre vertical movement induced by L-DOPA and NSD1015 and shifted the time-course response curve to the left, (i.e. it caused earlier onset of L-DOPA and NSD1015 action). Thus, the behavioural effect of L-DOPA and NSD1015 given together is exerted, at least, in part, by the noradrenergic system.

The prediction, arising from studies on the behavioural effects of L-DOPA, is that manipulation of α_2 or/and dopamine receptors by L-DOPA or its metabolites may result in hyperlocomotor activity. This prediction was tested in a study by radioligand binding in membranes prepared from cell lines expressing α_2 and dopaminergic receptors (Alachkar et al, 2010a). We reported that 3-MT bound to α_{2a} receptors with high affinity compared to α_{2C} adrenoceptors and dopaminergic receptors. The finding in the same study that dopamine bound to α_2 adrenoceptors with relatively high affinities, provides evidence confirming previous reports on the direct activation of α_2 adrenoceptors by dopamine (Cornil et al, 2002; Zhang et al, 1999).

A mechanism underlying the hyperkinesia induced by L-DOPA following the inhibition of central decarboxylase was suggested. According to these results, L-DOPA is metabolised in two steps leading to the formation of 3-MT, which will cause hyperkinesia (Nakazato & Akiyama, 2002; Nakazato, 2002), possibly through interaction with D1, or α_{2a} adrenoceptors (Alachkar et al, 2010a). The reduction of vertical hyperlocomotor activity by rauwolscine supports that 3-MT interacts with α_2 adrenoceptors (Alachkar et al, 2010b).

In Parkinson's disease, there is a decrease in the activity (Gjedde et al., 1993; Kuwabara et al., 1995) and expression (Ichinose et al., 1994) of the enzyme aromatic amino acid decarboxylase AADC. Interestingly, treatment with L-DOPA produces a further decrease in AADC (Tanaka et al., 1973; Fisher et al, 2000) and an increase of COMT (Liu et al, 2000; Zhao et al, 2001). In view of these observations, we propose that following long-term treatment with L-DOPA, the major portion of exogenous L-DOPA will not be metabolised to dopamine, instead a large portion of L-DOPA will be methylated to 3,O, methyldopa. 3-O-methyldopa has a longer half-life than L-DOPA itself (15 hours vs ½ hour) (Kuruma et al, 1971; Cedarbaum, 1987) and, consequently, 3,O,methyldopa formed from exogenous L-DOPA accumulates in the plasma and the brain to be subsequently metabolised slowly (Kuruma et al, 1971). The decarboxylation of 3,O,methyldopa leads to the formation of 3-MT. The significance of methoxy groups in the production of abnormal induced movements was the focus of very early studies (Ericsson et al, 1971). A number of early studies suggested that the occupation of the meta position by a OCH_3 group in the absence of similar groups at the para position caused hyperkinesias in rats (Hornykiewicz, 1966) and induced abnormal movements (Huntington chorea) in humans (Ericsson & Wertman, 1971). More recent studies have confirmed these early finding, as 3-MT was demonstrated to induce hyperactivity in rats (Nakazato & Akiyama, 2002; Nakazato, 2002). As a result, 3-MT seems to be the candidate metabolite to induce dyskinesia following long term treatment with L-DOPA in Parkinson's disease.

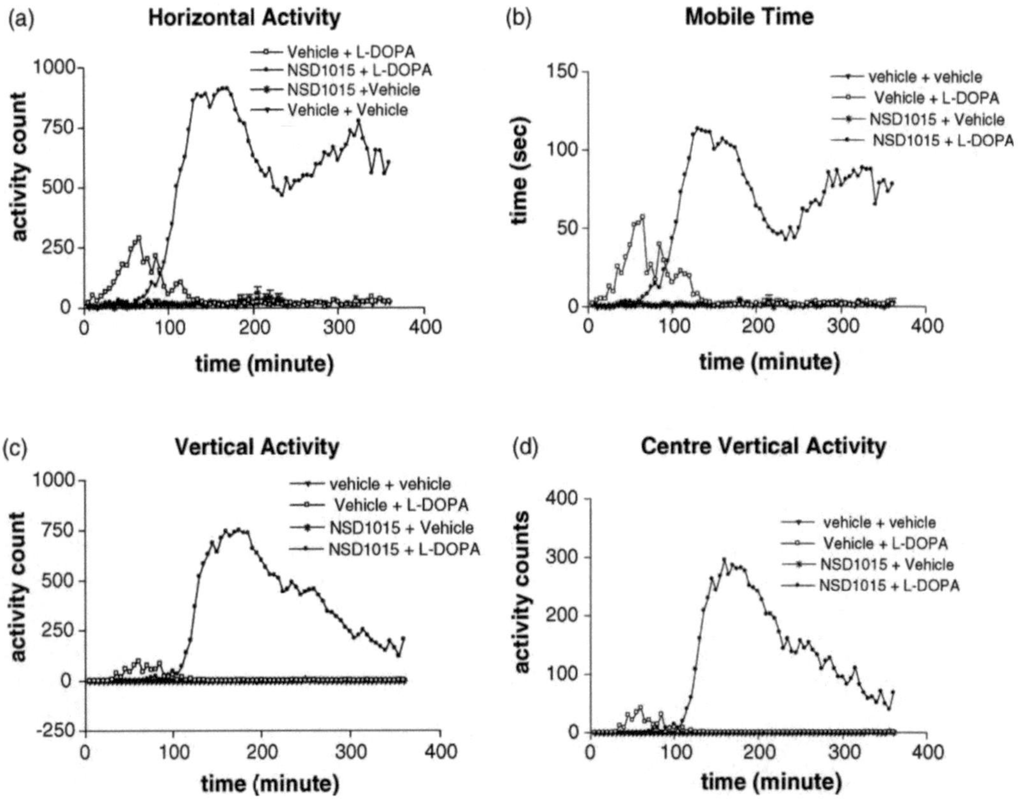

Fig. 2. **Effect of NSD1015 on the stimulant action of L-DOPA on locomotor activity.**

3-MT was found to bind to α_{2a} adrenoceptors with relatively high affinity (Alachkar et al, 2010a). The pharmacological experiments to determine whether 3-MT acts as an agonist or antagonist at α_{2a} adrenoceptors have not yet been undertaken. However, the similarities in the chemical structures between 3-MT and other catecholamines such as α-methylnoradrenaline and epinephrine, which are known to activate α_2 adrenoceptors, suggest that 3-MT may act as an agonist at these receptors. According to the present scenario, a high concentration of 3,O,methyldopa, and hence 3-MT will occur in Parkinson's disease and following long-term treatment with L-DOPA. The 3-MT will then bind to α_{2a} receptors located presynaptically on the locus coeruleus terminals in the SNr. This hypothesis is supported by the finding of Mela et al. (2007) who demonstrated an increase in extracellular GABA release after administration of L-DOPA in dyskinetic rats in the substantia nigra pars reticulata (Mela et al., 2007).

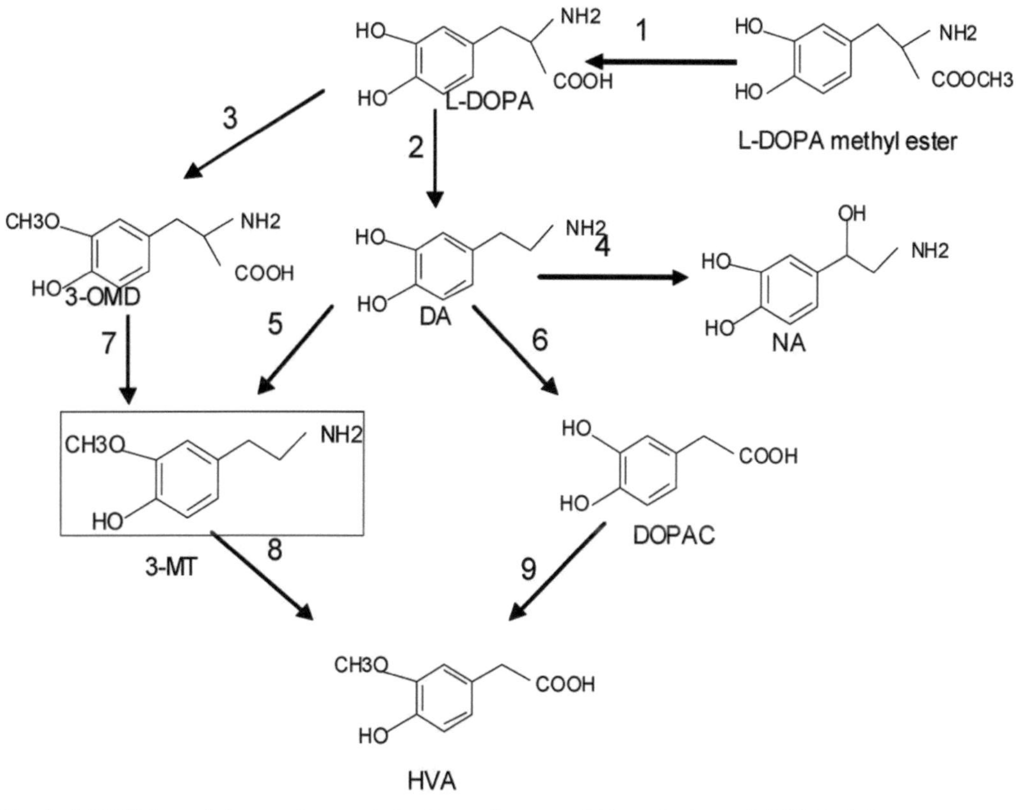

Fig. 3. **l-DOPA and dopamine metabolic pathways.** Abbreviations: l-DOPA, l-3,4-dihydroxyphenylalanine; DA dopamine; NA noradrenaline; 3-OMD 3-O-methyldopa; 3-MT 3-methoxytyramine; DOPAC dihydroxyphenylacetic acid; HVA homovanilic acid. (1) Esterase or hydrolase; (2) aromatic amino acid decarboxylase AADC; (3) catechol O-methyl transferase COMT; (4) dopamine _-hydroxylase BDH; (5) COMT; (6) monoamine oxidase MAO; (7) unknown; (8) MAO; (9) COMT (Alachkar et al, 2010a).

The activation of α_2 inhibitory autoreceptors would result in an inhibition of noradrenaline release from these terminals and, therefore, a decrease in the inhibitory tone on GABA release from striato-nigral projection to the SNr. This leads to the increase of the activity of the GABAergic direct pathway, resulting in an increase of the inhibition of the output regions of the basal ganglia, counteracting the underactivity of this structure, which is the key pathological mechanism of LID. Thus, the abnormalities in noradrenergic transmission may contribute to, or facilitate, the development of LID.

Previous experimental studies have demonstrated that α_2 adrenoceptor antagonists such as yohimbine reduce L-DOPA-induced dyskinesia in rodent (Lundblad et al., 2002; Dekundy et al., 2007) as well as primate models (Gomez-Mancilla and Bedard, 1993). Moreover, some α_2 adrenoceptor antagonists like idazoxan and fipamezole have shown antidyskinetic efficacy without compromising the anti-parkinsonian action of L-DOPA in monkey studies (Grondin et al., 2000; Fox et al., 2001; Savola et al., 2003) and clinical trials.

A series of behavioural studies have demonstrated the therapeutic benefits of non-selective α_2 antagonists in reducing LID in animal models of Parkinson's disease (Henry et al, 1999; Gomez-mancilla & Bedard, 1993). The anti-dyskinetic effects of the α_{2a} selective antagonist fipamezole in non-human primate model of PD have been demonstrated (Savola et al, 2003). It was suggested in this study that in LID, the activation of α_2 adrenoceptors that regulate the activity of the direct pathway, by L-DOPA or its metabolites, may facilitate LID (Savola et al, 2003). Although the exact site of α_2 adrenoceptor antagonist was not determined in the study by Savola et al, the authors have reached a similar conclusion by suggesting the involvement of the direct pathway in the mechanism of α_2 adrenoceptor antagonists.

According to the previous discussion, the anti-dyskinetic effect of α_2 adrenoceptors can be simply explained by the blockade, by the antagonist, of the effect of 3-MT at the inhibitory presynaptic α_{2a} in the terminals of locus coeruleus projection to the substantia nigra, resulting in facilitation of noradrenaline release. Noradrenaline, subsequently, exerts an inhibitory action on the GABAergic projection in the direct pathway, counteracting the overactivity of this pathway.

10. Conclusion

In conclusion, the discussions presented in this review demonstrate a potential role for noradrenergic system in Parkinson's disease and LID. Several lines of evidence suggest that the noradrenergic system regulates the activity of the direct pathway of the basal ganglia, through presynaptic α_2 receptors located in the SNr, and the indirect pathway through pre- and postsynaptic α_2 in the striatum, and α_2 and α_2 in the subthalamic nucleus. The model presented here suggests that the degeneration of noradrenergic neurons contributes to the pathophysiology and symptomatology of PD, and that the remaining intact noradrenergic neurons exert a compensatory mechanism in PD. Furthermore, we suggest a role for L-DOPA metabolites in the mechanism of LID; this role might be mediated through the activation of α_2 adrenoceptors. According to this model, the anti-dyskinesic action of α_2 antagonists might be mediated by the blockade of α_{2a} adrenoceptors located in the terminals of locus coeruleus projection to the SNr.

11. References

Ader, J.P., P. Room, F. Postema, J. Korf, Bilaterally diverging axon collaterals and contralateral projections from rat locus coeruleus neurons, demonstrated by fluorescent retrograde double labeling and norepinephrine metabolism, J. Neural Transm. 49 (1980) 207–208. ISSN: 0300-9564

Agid, Y., F. Javoy-Agid, M. Ruberg (1987). "Biochemistry of neurotransmitters in Parkinson's disease In: Marsden CD, Fahn S, eds. Movement Disorders. New York: Buttersworth & Co. 1987;166-230.

Alachkar, A., Brotchie, J. M., Jones, O. (2006). "alpha2-Adrenoceptor-mediated modulation of the release of GABA and noradrenaline in the rat substantia nigra pars reticulata." Neurosci Lett 395(2): 138-42. ISSN: 0304-3940

Alachkar, A., Brotchie, J. M., Jones, O. (2010a) "Binding of dopamine and 3-methoxytyramine as l-DOPA metabolites to human alpha(2)-adrenergic and dopaminergic receptors." Neurosci Res 67(3): 245-9. ISSN: 1872-8111

Alachkar, A., Brotchie, J. M., Jones, O. (2010b) "Locomotor response to L-DOPA in reserpine-treated rats following central inhibition of aromatic L-amino acid decarboxylase: further evidence for non-dopaminergic actions of L-DOPA and its metabolites." Neurosci Res 68(1): 44-50. ISSN: 1872-8111

Alam, M., W. Danysz, Schmidt, W. J. Dekundy, A. (2009). "Effects of glutamate and alpha2-noradrenergic receptor antagonists on the development of neurotoxicity produced by chronic rotenone in rats." Toxicol Appl Pharmacol 240(2): 198-207. ISSN: 1096-0333

Albin, R. L., J. W. Aldridge, A. B.Young, S.Gilman (1989). "Feline subthalamic nucleus neurons contain glutamate-like but not GABA-like or glycine-like immunoreactivity." Brain Res 491(1): 185-8. ISSN: 0006-8993

Altar, C. A. and M. R. Marien (1989). "Preservation of dopamine release in the denervated striatum." Neurosci Lett 96(3): 329-34. ISSN: 0304-3940

Anden, N. and M. Grabowska (1976). "Pharmacological evidence for a stimulation of dopamine neurons by noradrenaline neurons in the brain." Eur J Pharmacol 39(2): 275-82. ISSN: 0014-2999

Anden, N. E., A. Carlsson, J. Haggendal, (1969). "Adrenergic mechanisms." Annu Rev Pharmacol 9: 119-34. ISSN: 0066-4251

Anden, N. E., C. V. Atack, T. H. Svensson, (1973). "Release of dopamine from central noradrenaline and dopamine nerves induced by a dopamine-beta-hydroxylase inhibitor." J Neural Transm 34(2): 93-100. ISSN: 0300-9564

Aoki, C., Beta-adrenergic receptors: astrocytic localization in the adult visual cortex and their relation to catecholamine axon terminals as revealed by electron microscopic immunocytochemistry, J. Neurosci. 12 (1992) 781–792. ISSN: 0270-6474

Arai, H., K. Kosaka, R. izuka (1984). "Changes of biogenic amines and their metabolites in postmortem brains from patients with Alzheimer-type dementia." J Neurochem 43(2): 388-93. ISSN: 0022-3042

Archer, T., Fredriksson, A., 2006. Influence of noradrenaline denervation on MPTP-induced deficits in mice. J.Neural Transm. 113, 1119–1129. ISSN: 0300-9564

Arcos, D., A. Sierra, A. Nunez, G. Flores, J. Aceves, J. A. Arias-Montano (2003). "Noradrenaline increases the firing rate of a subpopulation of rat subthalamic neurons through the activation of alpha1-adrenoceptors." Neuropharmacology 45(8): 1070-9. ISSN: 0028-3908

Aston-Jones, G. and F. E. Bloom (1981). "Activity of norepinephrine-containing locus coeruleus neurons in behaving rats anticipates fluctuations in the sleep-waking cycle." J Neurosci 1(8): 876-86. ISSN: 0270-6474

Aston-Jones, G., C. Chiang, T. Alexinsky (1991). "Discharge of noradrenergic locus coeruleus neurons in behaving rats and monkeys suggests a role in vigilance." Prog Brain Res 88: 501-20. ISSN: 0079-6123

Autret, A., M. Minz, T. Beillevaire, H. P. Cathala, H. Schmitt (1977). "Effect of clonidine on sleep patterns in man." Eur J Clin Pharmacol 12(5): 319-22. ISSN: 0031-6970

Baker, K.G., I. Tork, J.P. Hornung, P. Halasz, The human locus coeruleus complex: an immunohistochemical and three dimensional reconstruction study, Exp. Brain Res. 77 (1989) 257– 270. ISSN: 0014-4819

Barolin, G. S. and O. Hornykiewicz (1967). "[On the diagnostic value of homovanillic acid in the cerebrospinal fluid]." Wien Klin Wochenschr 79(44): 815-8. ISSN: 0043-5325

Beaudet, A., L. Descarries, The monoamine innervation of rat cerebral cortex: synaptic and nonsynaptic axon terminals, Neuroscience 3 (1978) 851–860. ISSN: 0306-4522

Belujon, P., Bezard, E.,Taupignon,A., Bioulac, B., Benazzouz,A., 2007. Noradrenergic modulation of subthalamic nucleus activity: behavioral and electrophysiological evidence in intact and 6-hydroxydopamine-lesioned rats. J. Neurosci. 27, 9595–9606. ISSN: 1529-2401

Berretta, N., G. Bernardi, N. B. Mercuri (2000). "Alpha(1)-adrenoceptor-mediated excitation of substantia nigra pars reticulata neurons." Neuroscience 98(3): 599-604. ISSN: 0306-4522

Bezard, E., P. Ravenscroft, C. E. Gross, A. R. Crossman, J. M. Brotchie (2001). "Upregulation of striatal preproenkephalin gene expression occurs before the appearance of parkinsonian signs in 1-methyl-4-phenyl- 1,2,3,6-tetrahydropyridine monkeys." Neurobiol Dis 8(2): 343-50. ISSN: 0969-9961

Bickler, P. E. and B. M. Hansen (1996). "Alpha 2-adrenergic agonists reduce glutamate release and glutamate receptor-mediated calcium changes in hippocampal slices during hypoxia." Neuropharmacology 35(6): 679-87. ISSN: 0028-3908

Bing, G., Y. Zhang, Y. Watanabe, B. S. McEwen, E. A. Stone (1994). "Locus coeruleus lesions potentiate neurotoxic effects of MPTP in dopaminergic neurons of the substantia nigra." Brain Res 668(1-2): 261-5. ISSN: 0006-8993

Bosboom, J., Stoffers, D., Wolters, E., 2004. Cognitive dysfunction and dementia in Parkinson's disease. J. Neural Transm. 111, 1303–1315. ISSN: 0300-9564

Boyajian, C. L., S. E. Loughlin, F. M. Leslie (1987). "Anatomical evidence for alpha-2 adrenoceptor heterogeneity: differential autoradiographic distributions of [3H]rauwolscine and [3H]idazoxan in rat brain." J Pharmacol Exp Ther 241(3): 1079-91. ISSN: 0022-3565

Bristow, L. J. and G. W. Bennett (1988). "Biphasic effects of intra-accumbens histamine administration on spontaneous motor activity in the rat; a role for central histamine receptors." Br J Pharmacol 95(4): 1292-302. ISSN: 0007-1188

Brotchie, J., A. Crossman, I. Mitchell, S. Duty, C. Carroll, A. Cooper, B. Henry, N. Hughes, Y. Maneuf (1993). "Chemical signalling in the globus pallidus in parkinsonism." Prog Brain Res 99: 125-39. ISSN: 0079-6123

Buck, K. and B. Ferger (2009). "Comparison of intrastriatal administration of noradrenaline and l-DOPA on dyskinetic movements: a bilateral reverse in vivo microdialysis study in 6-hydroxydopamine-lesioned rats." Neuroscience 159(1): 16-20. ISSN: 0306-4522

Bungo, T., M. Shimojo, Y.Masuda, Y. H. Choi, D. M. Denbow, M. Furuse (1999). "Induction of food intake by a noradrenergic system using clonidine and fusaric acid in the neonatal chick." Brain Res 826(2): 313-6. ISSN: 0006-8993

Caffe, A. R., F. W. van Leeuwen, R. M. Buijs, G. J. de Vries, M. Geffard, (1985). "Coexistence of vasopressin, neurophysin and noradrenaline immunoreactivity in medium-sized cells of the locus coeruleus and subcoeruleus in the rat." Brain Res 338(1): 160-4. ISSN: 0006-8993

Carpenter, M. B., S. C. Carleton, J. T. Keller, P. Conte (1981). "Connections of the subthalamic nucleus in the monkey." Brain Res 224(1): 1-29. ISSN: 0006-8993

Cedarbaum, J. M. (1987). "Clinical pharmacokinetics of anti-parkinsonian drugs." Clin Pharmacokinet 13(3): 141-78. ISSN: 0312-5963

Charney, D. S., G. R. Heninger, D. E., Redmond, Jr. (1983). "Yohimbine induced anxiety and increased noradrenergic function in humans: effects of diazepam and clonidine." Life Sci 33(1): 19-29. ISSN: 0024-3205

Colpaert, F. C., A. D. Degryse, H. V. Van Craenendonck (1991). "Effects of an alpha 2 antagonist in a 20-year-old Java monkey with MPTP-induced parkinsonian signs." Brain Res Bull 26(4): 627-31. ISSN: 0361-9230

Cornil, C. A., J. Balthazart, P.Motte, L. Massotte, V. Seutin, (2002). "Dopamine activates noradrenergic receptors in the preoptic area." J Neurosci 22(21): 9320-30. ISSN: 1529-2401

Cotzias, G. C., M. H. Van Woert, L. M. Schiffer (1967). "Aromatic amino acids and modification of parkinsonism." N Engl J Med 276(7): 374-9. ISSN: 0028-4793

Coyle, J. T. and D. Henry (1973). "Catecholamines in fetal and newborn rat brain." J Neurochem 21(1): 61-7. ISSN: 0022-3042

Crespi, F. (2009). "Anxiolytics antagonize yohimbine-induced central noradrenergic activity: a concomitant in vivo voltammetry-electrophysiology model of anxiety." J Neurosci Methods 180(1): 97-105. ISSN: 1872-678X

Crossman, A. R. (1990). "A hypothesis on the pathophysiological mechanisms that underlie levodopa- or dopamine agonist-induced dyskinesia in Parkinson's disease: implications for future strategies in treatment." Mov Disord 5(2): 100-8. ISSN: 0885-3185

Dekundy A, Lundblad M, Danysz W, Cenci MA (2007) Modulation of L-DOPA-induced abnormal involuntary movements by clinically tested compounds: further validation of the rat dyskinesia model. Behav Brain Res 179(1):76–89. ISSN: 0166-4328

Devoto, P., G. Flore, L.Pira, M. Diana, L. Gessa, (2002). "Co-release of noradrenaline and dopamine in the prefrontal cortex after acute morphine and during morphine withdrawal." Psychopharmacology (Berl) 160(2): 220-4. ISSN: 0033-3158

Dolphin, A., P. Jenner, C. D. Marsden (1976). "Noradrenaline synthesis from L-DOPA in rodents and its relationship to motor activity." Pharmacol Biochem Behav 5(4): 431-9. ISSN: 0091-3057

Endroczi, E., I. Marton, Z. Radnai, J. Biro (1978). "Effect of the depletion on brain noradrenaline on the plasma FSH and growth hormone levels in ovariectomized rats." Acta Endocrinol (Copenh) 87(1): 55-60. ISSN: 0001-5598

Ericsson, A. D. and B. G. Wertman (1971). "Sensitivity studies of L-dopa metabolites in reserpinized rats and their clinical significance." Neurology 21(11): 1129-33. ISSN: 0028-3878

Ericsson, A. D., B. G. Wertman, K. M. Duffy (1971). "Reversal of the reserpine syndrome with L-dopa metabolites in reserpinized rats." Neurology 21(10): 1023-9. ISSN: 0028-3878

Fahn, S., L. R. Libsch, R. W. Cutler (1971). "Monoamines in the human neostriatum: topographic distribution in normals and in Parkinson's disease and their role in akinesia, rigidity, chorea, and tremor." J Neurol Sci 14(4): 427-55. ISSN: 0022-510X

Fearnley JM, Lees AJ. 1991. Ageing and Parkinson's disease: Substantia nigra regional selectivity. Brain 114:2283–2301.

Fisher, A., C. S. Biggs, O. Eradiri, M. S. Starr (2000). "Dual effects of L-3,4-dihydroxyphenylalanine on aromatic L-amino acid decarboxylase, dopamine release and motor stimulation in the reserpine-treated rat: evidence that behaviour is dopamine independent." Neuroscience 95(1): 97-111. ISSN: 0306-4522

Foote, S. L., G. Aston-Jones, F. E. Bloom (1980). "Impulse activity of locus coeruleus neurons in awake rats and monkeys is a function of sensory stimulation and arousal." Proc Natl Acad Sci U S A 77(5): 3033-7. ISSN: 0027-8424

Fornai, F., L. Bassi, et al. (1995). "Norepinephrine loss exacerbates methamphetamine-induced striatal dopamine depletion in mice." Eur J Pharmacol 283(1-3): 99-102. ISSN: 0014-2999

Fox, S. H., B. Henry, M. P. Hill, D. Peggs, A. R. Crossman, J. M. Brotchie, (2001). "Neural mechanisms underlying peak-dose dyskinesia induced by levodopa and apomorphine are distinct: evidence from the effects of the alpha(2) adrenoceptor antagonist idazoxan." Mov Disord 16(4): 642-50. ISSN: 0885-3185

Franowicz, J. S. and A. F. Arnsten (1998). "The alpha-2a noradrenergic agonist, guanfacine, improves delayed response performance in young adult rhesus monkeys." Psychopharmacology (Berl) 136(1): 8-14. ISSN: 0033-3158

Franowicz, J. S., L. E. Kessler, C. M. Borja, B. K. Kobilka, L. E. Limbird, Arnsten, A. F. (2002). "Mutation of the alpha2A-adrenoceptor impairs working memory performance and annuls cognitive enhancement by guanfacine." J Neurosci 22(19): 8771-7. ISSN: 1529-2401

Fujimoto, S., M. Sasa, S. Takaori (1981). "Inhibition from locus coeruleus of caudate neurons activated by nigral stimulation." Brain Res Bull 6(3): 267-74. ISSN: 0361-9230

Fuxe, K. (1965). "Evidence for the Existence of Monoamine Neurons in the Central Nervous System. Iv. Distribution of Monoamine Nerve Terminals in the Central Nervous System." Acta Physiol Scand 64: SUPPL 247:37+. ISSN: 0302-2994

Gehlert, D. R., S. L. Gackenheimer, D. W. Robertson (1993). "Localization of rat brain binding sites for [3H]tomoxetine, an enantiomerically pure ligand for norepinephrine reuptake sites." Neurosci Lett 157(2): 203-6. ISSN: 0304-3940

Gerlach, M., D. Ben-Shachar, P. Riederer, M. B. Youdim (1994). "Altered brain metabolism of iron as a cause of neurodegenerative diseases?" J Neurochem 63(3): 793-807. ISSN: 0022-3042

German, D.C., B.S. Walker, K. Manaye, W.K. Smith, D.J. Woodward, A.J. North, The human locus coeruleus: computer reconstruction of cellular distribution, J. Neurosci. 8 (1988) 1776– 1788. ISSN: 0270-6474

Gesi M, Soldani P, Giorgi FS, Santinami A, Bonaccorsi I, Fornai F. The role of the locus coeruleus in the development of Parkinson's disease. Neurosci Biobehav Rev 2000;24:655–68. ISSN: 0149-7634

Gibbs, M. E. and R. J. Summers (2002). "Role of adrenoceptor subtypes in memory consolidation." Prog Neurobiol 67(5): 345-91. ISSN: 0301-0082

Gjedde, A., G. C. Leger, P. Cumming, Y. Yasuhara, A. C. Evans, M. Guttman, H. Kuwabara (1993). "Striatal L-dopa decarboxylase activity in Parkinson's disease in vivo: implications for the regulation of dopamine synthesis." J Neurochem 61(4): 1538-41. ISSN: 0022-3042

Glowinski, J. and L. Iversen (1966). "Regional studies of catecholamines in the rat brain. 3. Subcellullar distribution of endogenous and exogenous catecholamines in various brain regions." Biochem Pharmacol 15(7): 977-87. ISSN: 0006-2952

Goldman, C. K., L. Marino, S. F. Leibowitz (1985). "Postsynaptic alpha 2-noradrenergic receptors mediate feeding induced by paraventricular nucleus injection of norepinephrine and clonidine." Eur J Pharmacol 115(1): 11-9. ISSN: 0014-2999

Gomez-Mancilla, B. and P. J. Bedard (1993). "Effect of nondopaminergic drugs on L-dopa-induced dyskinesias in MPTP-treated monkeys." Clin Neuropharmacol 16(5): 418-27. ISSN: 0362-5664

Graeff, F. G. (1994). "Neuroanatomy and neurotransmitter regulation of defensive behaviors and related emotions in mammals." Braz J Med Biol Res 27(4): 811-29. ISSN: 0100-879X

Grant, S. J. and D. E. Redmond, Jr. (1984). "Neuronal activity of the locus ceruleus in awake Macaca arctoides." Exp Neurol 84(3): 701-8. ISSN: 0014-4886

Grenhoff, J., M. Nisell, S. Ferre, G. Aston-Jones, T. H. Svensson (1993). "Noradrenergic modulation of midbrain dopamine cell firing elicited by stimulation of the locus coeruleus in the rat." J Neural Transm Gen Sect 93(1): 11-25. ISSN: 0300-9564

Grenhoff, J., R. A. North, S. W. Johnson (1995). "Alpha 1-adrenergic effects on dopamine neurons recorded intracellularly in the rat midbrain slice." Eur J Neurosci 7(8): 1707-13. ISSN: 0953-816X

Grimbergen, Y., Langston, J., Roos, R., Bloem, B., 2009. Postural instability in Parkinson's disease: the adrenergic hypothesis and the locus coeruleus. Expert. Rev. Neurother. 9, 279–290. ISSN: 1744-8360

Grondin, R., A. Hadj Tahar, V. D. Doan, P. Ladure, P. J. Bedard (2000). "Noradrenoceptor antagonism with idazoxan improves L-dopa-induced dyskinesias in MPTP monkeys." Naunyn Schmiedebergs Arch Pharmacol 361(2): 181-6. ISSN: 0028-1298

Guiard, B. P., M. El Mansari, P. Blier (2008) "Cross-talk between dopaminergic and noradrenergic systems in the rat ventral tegmental area, locus ceruleus, and dorsal hippocampus." Mol Pharmacol 74(5): 1463-75. ISSN: 1521-0111

Guiard, B. P., M. El Mansari, Z. Merali, P. Blier (2008) "Functional interactions between dopamine, serotonin and norepinephrine neurons: an in-vivo electrophysiological study in rats with monoaminergic lesions." Int J Neuropsychopharmacol 11(5): 625-39. ISSN: 1461-1457

Guiliano, F., O. Rampin, G. Benoit, A. Jardin (1997). "[The peripheral pharmacology of erection]." Prog Urol 7(1): 24-33. ISSN: 1166-7087

Harrison, J. K., D. D. D'Angelo, D. D. D'Angelo, D. W. Zeng, K. R. Lynch, (1991). "Pharmacological characterization of rat alpha 2-adrenergic receptors." Mol Pharmacol 40(3): 407-12. ISSN: 0026-895X

Henry, B., S. H. Fox, D. Peggs, A. R. Crossman, J. M. Brotchie, (1999b). "The alpha2-adrenergic receptor antagonist idazoxan reduces dyskinesia and enhances antiparkinsonian actions of L-dopa in the MPTP-lesioned primate model of Parkinson's disease." Mov Disord 14(5): 744-53. ISSN: 0885-3185

Hoehn-Saric, R., A. F. Merchant, M. L. Keyser, V. K. Smith (1981). "Effects of clonidine on anxiety disorders." Arch Gen Psychiatry 38(11): 1278-82. ISSN: 0003-990X

Holmberg, M., M. Scheinin, H. Kurose, R. Miettinen (1999). "Adrenergic alpha2C-receptors reside in rat striatal GABAergic projection neurons: comparison of radioligand binding and immunohistochemistry." Neuroscience 93(4): 1323-33. ISSN: 0306-4522

Hornykiewicz, O. (1966). "Dopamine (3-hydroxytyramine) and brain function." Pharmacol Rev 18(2): 925-64. ISSN: 0031-6997

Hornykiewicz, O. (1973). "Parkinson's disease: from brain homogenate to treatment." Fed Proc 32(2): 183-90. ISSN: 0014-9446

Hornykiewicz, O. and S. J. Kish (1987). "Biochemical pathophysiology of Parkinson's disease." Adv Neurol 45: 19-34. ISSN: 0091-3952

Ichinose, H., T. Ohye, K. Fujita, F. Pantucek, K.Lange, P. Riederer, T. Nagatsu, (1994). "Quantification of mRNA of tyrosine hydroxylase and aromatic L-amino acid decarboxylase in the substantia nigra in Parkinson's disease and schizophrenia." J Neural Transm Park Dis Dement Sect 8(1-2): 149-58. ISSN: 0936-3076

Jellinger, K. (1990). "New developments in the pathology of Parkinson's disease." Adv Neurol 53: 1-16. ISSN: 0091-3952

Jellinger, K. A. (1991). "Pathology of Parkinson's disease. Changes other than the nigrostriatal pathway." Mol Chem Neuropathol 14(3): 153-97. ISSN: 1044-7393

Kamisaki, Y., T. Hamada, K. Maeda, M. Ishimura, T. Itoh, (1993). "Presynaptic alpha 2 adrenoceptors inhibit glutamate release from rat spinal cord synaptosomes." J Neurochem 60(2): 522-6. ISSN: 0022-3042

Kish, S. J., K. S. Shannak, A. H. Rajput, J. J. Gilbert, O. Hornykiewicz (1984). "Cerebellar norepinephrine in patients with Parkinson's disease and control subjects." Arch Neurol 41(6): 612-4. ISSN: 0003-9942

Kish, S. J., K. Shannak, O. Hornykiewicz (1988). "Uneven pattern of dopamine loss in the striatum of patients with idiopathic Parkinson's disease. Pathophysiologic and clinical implications." N Engl J Med 318(14): 876-80. ISSN: 0028-4793

Koda, L.Y., J.A. Schulman, F.E. Bloom, Ultrastructural identification of noradrenergic terminals in rat hippocampus: unilateral destruction of the locus coeruleus with 6-hydroxydopamine, Brain Res. 145 (1978) 190–195. ISSN: 0006-8993

Kubrusly RC, Ventura AL, de Melo Reis RA, Serra GC, Yamasaki EN, Gardino PF, de Mello MC, de Mello FG (2007) Norepinephrine acts as D1-dopaminergic agonist in the embryonic avian retina: late expression of beta1-adrenergic receptor shifts norepinephrine specificity in the adult tissue. Neurochem Int 50(1):211–218. ISSN: 0197-0186

Kumar, V. M. (2003). "Role of noradrenergic fibers of the preoptic area in regulating sleep." J Chem Neuroanat 26(2): 87-93. ISSN: 0891-0618

Kuruma, I., G. Bartholini, R. Tissot, A. Pletscher (1971). "The metabolism of L-3-O-methyldopa, a precursor of dopa in man." Clin Pharmacol Ther 12(4): 678-82. ISSN: 0009-9236

Kuwabara, H., P. Cumming, Y. Yasuhara, G. C. Leger, M. Guttman, M. Diksic, A. C. Evans, A. Gjedde, (1995). "Regional striatal DOPA transport and decarboxylase activity in Parkinson's disease." J Nucl Med 36(7): 1226-31. ISSN: 0161-5505

Lanau F, Zenner MT, Civelli O, Hartman DS (1997) Epinephrine and norepinephrine act as potent agonists at the recombinant human dopamine D4 receptor. J Neurochem 68(2):804–812. ISSN: 0022-3042

Lategan, A., Marien, M., Colpaert, F., 1990. Effects of locus coeruleus lesions on the release of endogenous dopamine in the rat nucleus accumbens and caudate nucleus as determined by intracerebral microdialysis. Brain Res. 523, 134–138. ISSN: 0006-8993

Lategan, A., Marien, M., Colpaert, F., 1992. Suppression of nigrostriatal and mesolimbic dopamine release in vivo following noradrenaline depletion by DSP-4: a microdialysis study. Life Sci. 50, 995–999. ISSN: 0024-3205

Lee, A., A. E. Wissekerke, D. L. Rosin, K. R. Lynch (1998a). "Localization of alpha2C-adrenergic receptor immunoreactivity in catecholaminergic neurons in the rat central nervous system." Neuroscience 84(4): 1085-96. ISSN: 0306-4522

Lee, A., D. L. Rosin, E. J. Van Bockstaele (1998b). "alpha2A-adrenergic receptors in the rat nucleus locus coeruleus: subcellular localization in catecholaminergic dendrites, astrocytes, and presynaptic axon terminals." Brain Res 795(1-2): 157-69. ISSN: 0006-8993

Lin, M. T., J. J. Jou, W. C. Ko (1981). "Effects of intracerebroventricular injection of clonidine on metabolic, respiratory, vasomotor and temperature responses in the rabbit." Naunyn Schmiedebergs Arch Pharmacol 315(3): 195-201. ISSN: 0028-1298

Liu, X. X., K. Wilson, C. G. Charlton (2000). "Effects of L-dopa treatment on methylation in mouse brain: implications for the side effects of L-dopa." Life Sci 66(23): 2277-88. ISSN: 0024-3205

Loughlin, S. E., S. L. Foote, F. E. Bloom (1986). "Efferent projections of nucleus locus coeruleus: topographic organization of cells of origin demonstrated by three-dimensional reconstruction." Neuroscience 18(2): 291-306. ISSN: 0306-4522

Lundblad M, Andersson M, Winkler C, Kirik D, Wierup N, Cenci MA. Pharmacological validation of behavioural measures of akinesia and dyskinesia in a rat model of Parkinson's disease. Eur J Neurosci 2002;15:120–32. ISSN: 0953-816X

Mallick, B. N., S. Majumdar, M. Faisal, V. Yadav, V. Madan, D. Pal (2002). "Role of norepinephrine in the regulation of rapid eye movement sleep." J Biosci 27(5): 539-51. ISSN: 0250-5991

Mann, D., The locus coeruleus and its possible role in ageing and degenerative disease of the human central nervous system, Mech. Ageing Dev. 23 (1983) 73– 94. ISSN: 0047-6374

Mann, D.M., P.O. Yates, J. Hawkes, The pathology of the human locus ceruleus, Clin. Neuropathol. 2 (1983) 1 -7. ISSN: 0722-5091

Marien, M., M. Briley, F. Colpaert (1993). "Noradrenaline depletion exacerbates MPTP-induced striatal dopamine loss in mice." Eur J Pharmacol 236(3): 487-9. ISSN: 0014-2999

Marrs, W., Kuperman, J., Avedian, T., Roth, R. H., Jentsch, J. D. (2005). "Alpha-2 adrenoceptor activation inhibits phencyclidine-induced deficits of spatial working memory in rats." Neuropsychopharmacology 30(8): 1500-10. ISSN: 0893-133X

Marsden, C. D. (1990). "Parkinson's disease." Lancet 335(8695): 948-52. ISSN: 0140-6736

Marsden, C. D. and J. D. Parkes (1976). ""On-off" effects in patients with Parkinson's disease on chronic levodopa therapy." Lancet 1(7954): 292-6. ISSN: 0140-6736

Mason, S.T., H.C. Fibiger, Regional topography within noradrenergic locus coeruleus as revealed by retrograde transport of horseradish peroxidase, J. Comp. Neurol. 187 (1979) 703– 724. ISSN: 0021-9967

Mavridis, M., F.C. Colpaert, M.J. Millan, Differential modulation of (+)-amphetamine-induced rotation in unilateral substantia nigra-lesioned rats by alpha 1 as compared to alpha 2 agonists and antagonists, Brain Res. 562 (1991) 216–224. ISSN: 0006-8993

McGeer, P. L., S. Itagaki, B. E. Boyes, E. G. McGeer (1988). "Reactive microglia are positive for HLA-DR in the substantia nigra of Parkinson's and Alzheimer's disease brains." Neurology 38(8): 1285-91. ISSN: 0028-3878

Melamed, E., F. Hefti, V. Bitton, M. Globus (1984). "Suppression of L-dopa-induced circling in rats with nigral lesions by blockade of central dopa-decarboxylase: implications for mechanism of action of L-dopa in parkinsonism." Neurology 34(12): 1566-70. ISSN: 0028-3878

Mocchetti, I., M. A. De Bernardi, A. M. Szekely, H. Alho, G. Brooker, E. Costa, (1989). "Regulation of nerve growth factor biosynthesis by beta-adrenergic receptor activation in astrocytoma cells: a potential role of c-Fos protein." Proc Natl Acad Sci U S A 86(10): 3891-5. ISSN: 0027-8424

Moore, R. Y. and F. E. Bloom (1979). "Central catecholamine neuron systems: anatomy and physiology of the norepinephrine and epinephrine systems." Annu Rev Neurosci 2: 113-68. ISSN: 0147-006X

Morales, A., M. Condra, J. A. Owen, D. H. Surridge, J. Fenemore, C. Harris, (1987). "Is yohimbine effective in the treatment of organic impotence? Results of a controlled trial." J Urol 137(6): 1168-72. ISSN: 0022-5347

Morrison, J. H., M. E. Molliver, R. Grzanna, J. T. Coyle (1979). "Noradrenergic innervation patterns in three regions of medial cortex: an immunofluorescence characterization." Brain Res Bull 4(6): 849-57. ISSN: 0361-9230

Morrison, J. H., S. L. Foote, D. O'Connor, F. E. Bloom (1982). "Laminar, tangential and regional organization of the noradrenergic innervation of monkey cortex: dopamine-beta-hydroxylase immunohistochemistry." Brain Res Bull 9(1-6): 309-19. ISSN: 0361-9230

Mouradian, M. M., I. J. Heuser, F. Baronti, M. Giuffra, K. Conant, L. Davis, T. Chase, T. N. (1991). "Comparison of the clinical pharmacology of (-)NPA and levodopa in Parkinson's disease." J Neurol Neurosurg Psychiatry 54(5): 401-5. ISSN: 0022-3050

Mouradian, M. M., J. L. Juncos, G. Fabbrini, J. Schlegel, J. J. Bartko, T. N. Chase, (1988). "Motor fluctuations in Parkinson's disease: central pathophysiological mechanisms, Part II." Ann Neurol 24(3): 372-8. ISSN: 0364-5134

Mura, A., D. Jackson, M. S. Manley, S. J. Young, P. M. Groves (1995). "Aromatic L-amino acid decarboxylase immunoreactive cells in the rat striatum: a possible site for the conversion of exogenous L-DOPA to dopamine." Brain Res 704(1): 51-60. ISSN: 0006-8993

Nakazato, T. (2002). "The medial prefrontal cortex mediates 3-methoxytyramine-induced behavioural changes in rat." Eur J Pharmacol 442(1-2): 73-9. ISSN: 0014-2999

Nakazato, T. and A. Akiyama (2002). "Behavioral activity and stereotypy in rats induced by L-DOPA metabolites: a possible role in the adverse effects of chronic L-DOPA treatment of Parkinson's disease." Brain Res 930(1-2): 134-42. ISSN: 0006-8993

Narabayashi, H., T. Kondo, T. Nagatsu, A. Hayashi, T. Suzuki, (1984). "DL-threo-3,4-dihydroxyphenylserine for freezing symptom in parkinsonism." Adv Neurol 40: 497-502. ISSN: 0091-3952

Newman-Tancredi A, Audinot-Bouchez V, Gobert A, Millan MJ (1997) Noradrenaline and adrenaline are high affinity agonists at dopamine D4 receptors. Eur J Pharmacol 319(2–3):379–383. ISSN: 0014-2999

Nicholas, A. P., V. Pieribone, T. Hokfelt (1993). "Distributions of mRNAs for alpha-2 adrenergic receptor subtypes in rat brain: an in situ hybridization study." J Comp Neurol 328(4): 575-94. ISSN: 0021-9967

Nishi, K., Kondo, T., Narabayashi, H., 1991. Destruction of norepinephrine terminals in 1-methyl-4-phenyl-1236-tetrahydropyridine (MPTP)-treated mice reduces locomotor activity induced by L-DOPA. Neurosci. Lett. 123, 244–247. ISSN: 0304-3940

Obeso JA, Olanow CW, Nutt JG. Levodopa motor complications in Parkinson's disease. Trends Neurosci 2000; 23:S2–7. ISSN: 0166-2236

Onali P, Olianas MC, Gessa GL (1985) Characterization of dopamine receptors mediating inhibition of adenylate cyclase activity in rat striatum. Mol Pharmacol 28(2):138–145. ISSN: 0026-895X

Opacka-Juffry, J. and D. J. Brooks (1995). "L-dihydroxyphenylalanine and its decarboxylase: new ideas on their neuroregulatory roles." Mov Disord 10(3): 241-9. ISSN: 0885-3185

Parent, A. and L. N. Hazrati (1995). "Functional anatomy of the basal ganglia. II. The place of subthalamic nucleus and external pallidum in basal ganglia circuitry." Brain Res Brain Res Rev 20(1): 128-54. PMID: 7711765

Parnavelas, J.G., G.C. Papadopoulos, The monoaminergic innervations of the cerebral cortex is not diffuse and nonspecific, Trends Neurosci. 12 (1989) 315– 319. ISSN: 0166-2236

Persson, T. and B. Waldeck (1970). "Further studies on the possible interaction between dopamine and noradrenaline containing neurons in the brain." Eur J Pharmacol 11(3): 315-20. ISSN: 0014-2999

Pralong, E. and P. J. Magistretti (1995). "Noradrenaline increases K-conductance and reduces glutamatergic transmission in the mouse entorhinal cortex by activation of alpha 2-adrenoreceptors." Eur J Neurosci 7(12): 2370-8. ISSN: 0953-816X

Quinn, N. P., P. Luthert, M. Honavar, C. D. Marsden (1989). "Pure akinesia due to lewy body Parkinson's disease: a case with pathology." Mov Disord 4(1): 85-9. ISSN: 0885-3185

Ramos, B., Arnsten, A., 2007. Adrenergic pharmacology and cognition: focus on the prefrontal cortex. Pharmacol. Ther. 113, 523–536. ISSN: 0163-7258

Rascol, O., I. Arnulf, H. Peyro-Saint Paul, C. Brefel-Courbon, M. Vidailhet, C. Thalamas, A. M. Bonnet, S. Descombes, B. Bejjani, N. Fabre, J. L. Montastruc, Y. Agid (2001). "Idazoxan, an alpha-2 antagonist, and L-DOPA-induced dyskinesias in patients with Parkinson's disease." Mov Disord 16(4): 708-13. ISSN: 0885-3185

Remy, P., Doder, M., Lees, A., Turjanski, N., Brooks, D., 2005. Depression in Parkinson's disease: loss of dopamine and noradrenaline innervation in the limbic system. Brain 128, 1314–1322. ISSN: 1460-2156

Ridderinkhof, K., Ullsperger, M., Crone, E., Nieuwenhuis, S., 2004. The role of the medial frontal cortex in cognitive control. Science 306, 443–447. ISSN: 1095-9203

Riekkinen, M., Riekkinen, P.J., 1999. Alpha2-adrenergic agonist clonidine for improving spatial working memory in Parkinson's disease. J. Clin. Psychopharmacol. 19, 444–449. ISSN: 0271-0749

Rinne, U. K. and V. Sonninen (1973). "Brain catecholamines and their metabolites in Parkinsonian patients. Treatment with levodopa alone or combined with a decarboxylase inhibitor." Arch Neurol 28(2): 107-10. ISSN: 0003-9942

Rollema, H., (1992). "Indole-N-methylation of beta-carbolines: the brain's bioactivation route to toxins in Parkinson's disease?" Ann N Y Acad Sci 648: 263-5. ISSN: 0077-8923

Rommelfanger KS, Weinshenker D (2007) Norepinephrine: The redheaded stepchild of Parkinson's disease. Biochem Pharmacol 74(2):177–190. ISSN: 0006-2952

Room, P., F. Postema, J. Korf, Divergent axon collaterals of rat locus coeruleus neurons: demonstration by a fluorescent double labeling technique, Brain Res. 221 (1981) 219– 230. ISSN: 0006-8993

Rosin, D. L., E. M. Talley, A.Lee, R. L. Stornetta, B. D. Gaylinn, P. G. Guyenet, K. R. Lynch (1996). "Distribution of alpha 2C-adrenergic receptor-like immunoreactivity in the rat central nervous system." J Comp Neurol 372(1): 135-65. ISSN: 0021-9967

Ruffolo, R. R., Jr., A. J. Nichols, Hieble (1991). "Metabolic regulation by alpha 1- and alpha 2-adrenoceptors." Life Sci 49(3): 171-83. ISSN: 0024-3205

Sallinen, J., R. E. Link, A. Haapalinna, T. Viitamaa, M. Kulatunga, B. Sjoholm, E. Macdonald, M. Pelto-Huikko, T. Leino, G. S. Barsh, B. K. Kobilka, M. Scheinin (1997). "Genetic alteration of alpha 2C-adrenoceptor expression in mice: influence on locomotor, hypothermic, and neurochemical effects of dexmedetomidine, a subtype-nonselective alpha 2-adrenoceptor agonist." Mol Pharmacol 51(1): 36-46. ISSN: 0026-895X

Savola, J. M., M. Hill, M. Engstrom, H. Merivuori, S. Wurster, S. G. McGuire, S. H. Fox, A. R. Crossman, J. M. Brotchie (2003). "Fipamezole (JP-1730) is a potent alpha2 adrenergic receptor antagonist that reduces levodopa-induced dyskinesia in the MPTP-lesioned primate model of Parkinson's disease." Mov Disord 18(8): 872-83. ISSN: 0885-3185

Schapira, A., 2008. Progress in Parkinson's disease. Eur. J. Neurol. 15, 1. ISSN: 1468-1331

Scheinin, M., J. W. Lomasney, D. M. Hayden-Hixson, U. B. Schambra, M. G. Caron, R. J. Lefkowitz, R. T. Fremeau, Jr. (1994). "Distribution of alpha 2-adrenergic receptor subtype gene expression in rat brain." Brain Res Mol Brain Res 21(1-2): 133-49. ISSN: 0169-328X

Scherman, D., C. Desnos, F. Darchen, P. Pollak, F. Javoy-Agid, Y. Agid (1989). "Striatal dopamine deficiency in Parkinson's disease: role of aging." Ann Neurol 26(4): 551-7. ISSN: 0364-5134

Schramm, N. L., M. P. McDonald, L. E. Limbird (2001). "The alpha(2a)-adrenergic receptor plays a protective role in mouse behavioral models of depression and anxiety." J Neurosci 21(13): 4875-82. ISSN: 1529-2401

Segawa, T., H. Ito, Inoue, K. Wada, H. Minatoguchi, S.Fujiwara, H. (1998). "Dopamine releases endothelium-derived relaxing factor via alpha 2-adrenoceptors in canine vessels: comparisons between femoral arteries and veins." Clin Exp Pharmacol Physiol 25(9): 669-75. ISSN: 0305-1870

Snyder, G. L. and M. J. Zigmond (1990). "The effects of L-dopa on in vitro dopamine release from striatum." Brain Res 508(2): 181-7. ISSN: 0006-8993

Srinivasan, J. and W. J. Schmidt (2003). "Potentiation of parkinsonian symptoms by depletion of locus coeruleus noradrenaline in 6-hydroxydopamine-induced partial degeneration of substantia nigra in rats." Eur J Neurosci 17(12): 2586-92. ISSN: 0953-816X

Stone, E. A. and M. A. Ariano (1989). "Are glial cells targets of the central noradrenergic system? A review of the evidence." Brain Res Brain Res Rev 14(4): 297-309. PMID: 2560410

Strazielle, C., R. Lalonde, C. Hebert, T. A. Reader (1999). "Regional brain distribution of noradrenaline uptake sites, and of alpha1-alpha2- and beta-adrenergic receptors in PCD mutant mice: a quantitative autoradiographic study." Neuroscience 94(1): 287-304. ISSN: 0306-4522

Stromberg, U. and T. H. Svensson (1971). "L-DOPA induced effects on motor activity in mice after inhibition of dopamine-beta-hydroxylase." Psychopharmacologia 19(1): 53-60. ISSN: 0033-3158

Swanson, L. W. and B. K. Hartman (1975). "The central adrenergic system. An immunofluorescence study of the location of cell bodies and their efferent connections in the rat utilizing dopamine-beta-hydroxylase as a marker." J Comp Neurol 163(4): 467-505. ISSN: 0021-9967

Tanaka, M., M. Yoshida, H. Emoto, H. Ishii (2000). "Noradrenaline systems in the hypothalamus, amygdala and locus coeruleus are involved in the provocation of anxiety: basic studies." Eur J Pharmacol 405(1-3): 397-406. ISSN: 0014-2999

Tanaka, M., T. Oshima, S. Hayashi, C. Ishibashi, S. Kobayashi (1973). "Enhancement of the pharmacological action of 3,4-dihydroxy-L-phenylalanine(L-dopa) and reduction of dopa decarboxylase activity in rat liver after chronic treatment with L-dopa." Eur J Pharmacol 22(3): 360-2. ISSN: 0014-2999

Taquet, H., F. Javoy-Agid, F. Cesselin, M. Hamon, J.C. Legrand, Y. Agid, Microtopography of methionine-enkephalin, dopamine and noradrenaline in the ventral mesencephalon of human control and Parkinsonian brains, Brain Res. 235 (1982) 303–314. ISSN: 0006-8993

Tarazi FI, Kula NS, Baldessarini RJ (1997) Regional distribution of dopamine D4 receptors in rat forebrain. Neuroreport 8(16): 3423–3426. ISSN: 0959-4965

Tejani-Butt, S. M., Yang, J., Zaffar, H. (1993). "Norepinephrine transporter sites are decreased in the locus coeruleus in Alzheimer's disease." Brain Res 631(1): 147-50. ISSN: 0006-8993

Timofeeva, O. A. & Levin E. D. (2008). "Idazoxan blocks the nicotine-induced reversal of the memory impairment caused by the NMDA glutamate receptor antagonist dizocilpine." Pharmacol Biochem Behav 90(3): 372-81. ISSN: 0091-3057

Uhlen, S., J. Lindblom, A. Johnson, J. E. Wikberg (1997). "Autoradiographic studies of central alpha 2A- and alpha 2C-adrenoceptors in the rat using [3H]MK912 and subtype-selective drugs." Brain Res 770(1-2): 261-6. ISSN: 0006-8993

Unnerstall, J. R., T. A. Kopajtic, M. J. Kuhar (1984). "Distribution of alpha 2 agonist binding sites in the rat and human central nervous system: analysis of some functional, anatomic correlates of the pharmacologic effects of clonidine and related adrenergic agents." Brain Res 319(1): 69-101. ISSN: 0006-8993

Valet, P., M. Taouis, M. A. Tran, P. Montastruc, M. Lafontan, M. Berlan (1989). "Lipomobilizing effects of procaterol and yohimbine in the conscious dog:

comparison of endocrinological, metabolic and cardiovascular effects." Br J Pharmacol 97(1): 229-39. ISSN: 0007-1188

Wang, T., Zhang, Q.J., Liu, J., Wu, Z.H., Wang, S., 2009. Firing activity of locus coeruleus noradrenergic neurons increases in a rodent model of Parkinsonism. Neurosci. Bull. 25, 15–20. ISSN: 1673-7067

Wang, Y., Q. J. Zhang, Liu, J. Ali, U. Gui, Z. H. Hui, Y. P. Chen, L. Wu, Z. H. Li, Q. (2010). "Noradrenergic lesion of the locus coeruleus increases apomorphine-induced circling behavior and the firing activity of substantia nigra pars reticulata neurons in a rat model of Parkinson's disease." Brain Res 1310: 189-99. 1872-6240

Weiss, G. F. and S. F. Leibowitz (1985). "Efferent projections from the paraventricular nucleus mediating alpha 2-noradrenergic feeding." Brain Res 347(2): 225-38. ISSN: 0006-8993

White, F. J. and R. Y. Wang (1984). "A10 dopamine neurons: role of autoreceptors in determining firing rate and sensitivity to dopamine agonists." Life Sci 34(12): 1161-70. ISSN: 0024-3205

Winzer-Serhan, U. H., H. K. Raymon, R. S. Broide, Y. Chen, F. M. Leslie (1997). "Expression of alpha 2 adrenoceptors during rat brain development--I. Alpha 2A messenger RNA expression." Neuroscience 76(1): 241-60. ISSN: 0306-4522

Zarow, C., S.A. Lyness, J.A. Mortimer, H.C. Chui, Neuronal loss is greater in the locus coeruleus than nucleus basalis and substantia nigra in Alzheimer and Parkinson diseases, Arch. Neurol. 60 (2003) 337–341. ISSN: 0003-9942

Zhang, W. and G. A. Ordway (2003). "The alpha(2C)-adrenoceptor modulates GABA release in mouse striatum." Brain Res Mol Brain Res 112(1-2): 24-32. ISSN: 0169-328X

Zhang, W., V. Klimek, J. T. Farley, M. Y. Zhu, G. A. Ordway (1999). "alpha2C adrenoceptors inhibit adenylyl cyclase in mouse striatum: potential activation by dopamine." J Pharmacol Exp Ther 289(3): 1286-92. ISSN: 0022-3565

Zhao, W. Q., L. Latinwo, X. X. Liu, E. S. Lee, N. Lamango, C. G. Charlton (2001). "L-dopa upregulates the expression and activities of methionine adenosyl transferase and catechol-O-methyltransferase." Exp Neurol 171(1): 127-38. ISSN: 0014-4886

Zweig, R., Cardillo, J., Cohen, M., Giere, S., Hedreen, J., 1993. The locus ceruleus and dementia in Parkinson's disease. Neurology 43, 986–991. ISSN: 0028-3878

27

Mitochondrial Haplogroups Associated with Japanese Parkinson's Patients

Shigeru Takasaki
Toyo University, Izumino 1-1-1, Ora-gun Itakuracho, Gunma, Japan

1. Introduction

Mitochondria are essential cytoplasmic organelles generating cellular energy in the form of adenosine triphosphate by oxidative phosphorylation. Most cells contain hundreds of mitochondria, each of which has several mitochondrial DNA (mtDNA) copies, so each cell contains thousands of mtDNA copies. mtDNA has a very high mutation rate, and when a mutation occurs the cell initially contains a mixture of wild-type and mutant mtDNAs, a situation known as heteroplasmy. If the percentage of mutant mtDNA increases enough that the cell's ATP production falls below the level needed for normal cell function, disease symptoms appear and become progressively worse. A wide variety of diseases—such as Parkinson's disease (PD), Alzheimer's disease (AD), and cancer—are reportedly linked to mitochondrial dysfunction, and it is clear that mitochondrial diseases encompass an extraordinary assemblage of clinical problems (Wallace 1999; Vila and Przedborski 2003; Taylor and Turnbull 2005).

Although mtDNA mutations have been reported to be related both to a wide variety of diseases and aging (Lin *et al.* 1992; Schoffner *et al.* 1993; Kosel *et al.* 1994; Mayr-Wohlfart *et al.* 1996; Schnopp *et al.* 1996; Simon *et al.* 2000; Tanaka *et al.* 2002; Dawson and Dawson 2003; Ross *et al.* 2003; Lustbader *et al.* 2004; Niemi *et al.* 2005; Alexe *et al.* 2007; Fuku *et al.* 2007; Chinnery *et al.* 2008; Kim *et al.* 2008; Maruszak *et al.* 2008; Feder *et al.* 2008), there are few reports regarding the relations between all mtDNA mutations and either disease patients or centenarians. The previous reports have also focused on mutations causing amino acid replacements in mitochondrial proteins and, although mitochondrial functions can of course be affected directly by amino acid replacements, they can also be affected indirectly by mutations in mtDNA control regions. It is therefore important to examine the relations between all mtDNA mutations and disease patients or centenarians.

In the article reported here the relations between Japanese PD patients and their mitochondrial single nucleotide polymorphism (mtSNP) frequencies were analyzed using a method based on radial basis function (RBF) networks (Poggio and Girosi 1990; Wu and McLarty 2000) and a modified method based on RBF network predictions (Takasaki 2009). In addition, the relations between the haplogroups of the PD patients and those of the other four classes of people (centenarians, AD patients, T2D patients, and healthy non-obese young males) are also described using the same analysis method. The results described here are quite different from those reported previously (Saxena *et al.* 2006; Alexe *et al.* 2007; Fuku *et al.* 2007; Bilal *et al.* 2008).

2. Materials and methods

2.1 mtSNPs

We used complete mtDNA sequences available in GiiB Human Mitochondrial Genome Polymorphism Database (http://mtsnp.tmig.or.jp/mtsnp). The mtSNPs used were those in 96 Japanese PD patients (43 males and 53 females), 96 Japanese centenarians (30 males and 66 females), 96 Japanese AD patients (20 males and 76 females), 96 Japanese type 2 diabetes (T2D) patients (54 males and 42 females), and 96 Japanese healthy non-obese young males (Tanaka *et al.* 2004).

2.2 RBF-based method of mtSNP classification

A RBF network is an artificial network used in supervised learning problems such as regression, classification, and time series prediction. In supervised learning a function is inferred from examples (training set) that a teacher supplies. The elements in the training set are paired values of the independent (input) variable and dependent (output) variable.

The RBF network shown in Fig. 1 was learned from the training set as the mtSNPs of the PD patients were regarded as correct and the mtSNPs of other four classes of people (centenarians, AD patients, T2D patients, and healthy non-obese young males) were regarded as incorrect. Similarly, in the mtSNP classification for the centenarians the mtSNPs of the centenarians are regarded as correct and those of the other four classes are regarded as incorrect. The mtSNPs of the AD patients, T2D patients, and healthy non-obese young males were also classified this way.

The mitochondrial genome sequences of the PD patients were partitioned into two sets: training data comprising the sequences of 64 of the PD patients, and validation data comprising the sequences of the other 32 PD patients. The training and validation steps are described in detail elsewhere (Takasaki *et al.* 2006).

2.3 Modified classification method based on probabilities predicted by the RBF network

Since a RBF network can predict the probabilities that persons with certain mtSNPs belong to certain classes (e.g., PD patients, centenarians, AD patients, T2D patients, or healthy non-obese young males), these predicted probabilities are used to identify mtSNP features. By examining the relations between individual mtSNPs and the persons with high predicted probabilities of belonging to one of these classes, we are able to identify other mtSNPs useful for distinguishing between the members in different classes. A modified classification method based on the probabilities predicted by the RBF network was thus carried out in the following way (Takasaki 2009).

1. Select the analysis target class (i.e., PD patients, centenarians, AD patients, T2D patients, or healthy non-obese young males).
2. Rank individuals according to their predicted probabilities of belonging to the target class.
3. Either select individuals whose probabilities are greater than a certain value or select the desired number of individuals from the top, and set them as a modified cluster.

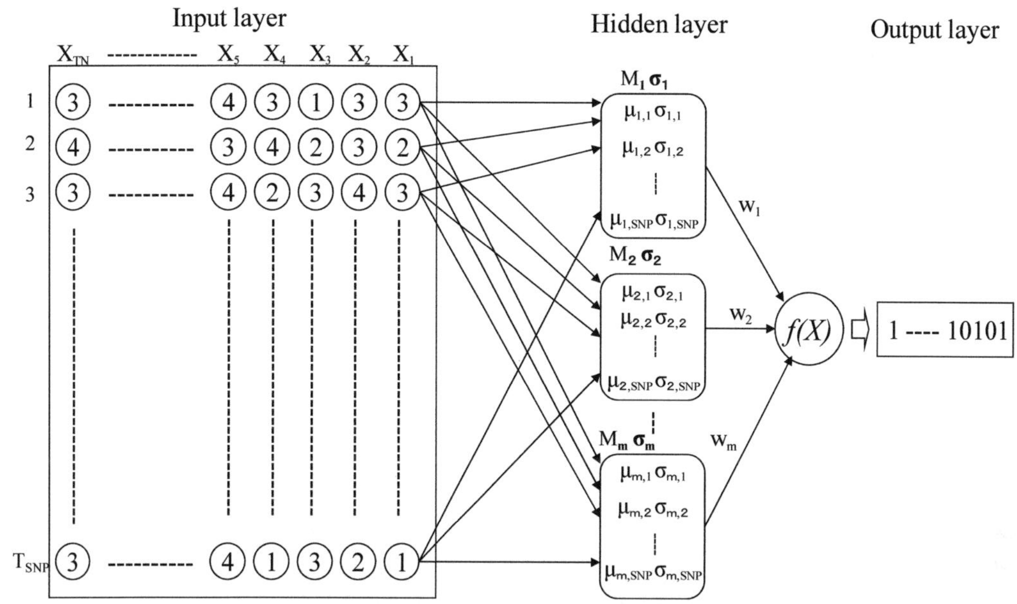

Fig. 1. RBF network representation of the relations between individual mtSNPs and the PD patients. The input layer is the set of mtSNP sequences represented numerically (A, G, C, and T are converted to 1, 2, 3, and 4). The hidden layer classifies the input vectors into several clusters depending on the similarities of individual input vectors. The output layer is determined depending on which analysis is carried out. In the case of PD patients, 1 corresponds to PD patients and 0 corresponds to other four classes of people. In the case of centenarians, 1 corresponds to centenarians and 0 corresponds to other four classes of people. The AD patients, T2D patients, and healthy non-obese young males are also carried out in similar way. X_i : *i*-th input vector, *TN* : maximum number of vectors (in this example, *TN*=320 (64x5)), T_{SNP} : maximum number of mtSNPs (in this example, T_{SNP} =562), M_m: the location vector, *m*: the number of basis functions, μ: basis function, σ: standard deviation, w_i: *i*-th weighting variable, *f(X)*: weighted sum function.

3. Results and discussion

3.1 Associations between haplogroups and the mtSNPs of the PD patients

When the mtSNPs of the PD patients were classified by the RBF-based method described above, ten mtSNP clusters were obtained. The average predicted probabilities of these clusters for becoming the PD patients were respectively 63%, 62.5%, 52.9%, 30%, 29.4%, 15.4%, 7.7%, 4.3%, 3.4% and 0%. Then the 15 individuals with the highest probabilities of becoming PD patients were selected using the modified classification method, and their nucleotide distributions at individual mtDNA positions were examined. After that, the relations between Asian/Japanese haplogroups and the mtSNPs for the PD patients were examined (Herrnstadt *et al.* 2002; Kong *et al.* 2003; Tanaka *et al.* 2004). The associations between the haplogroups and mtSNPs for the PD patients are shown in Fig. 2. The features of associations for the PD patients were L3-M-M7b2 (33%), L3-M-G2a (27%), L3-N-B4e (13%), B5b (13%), and N9a (7%).

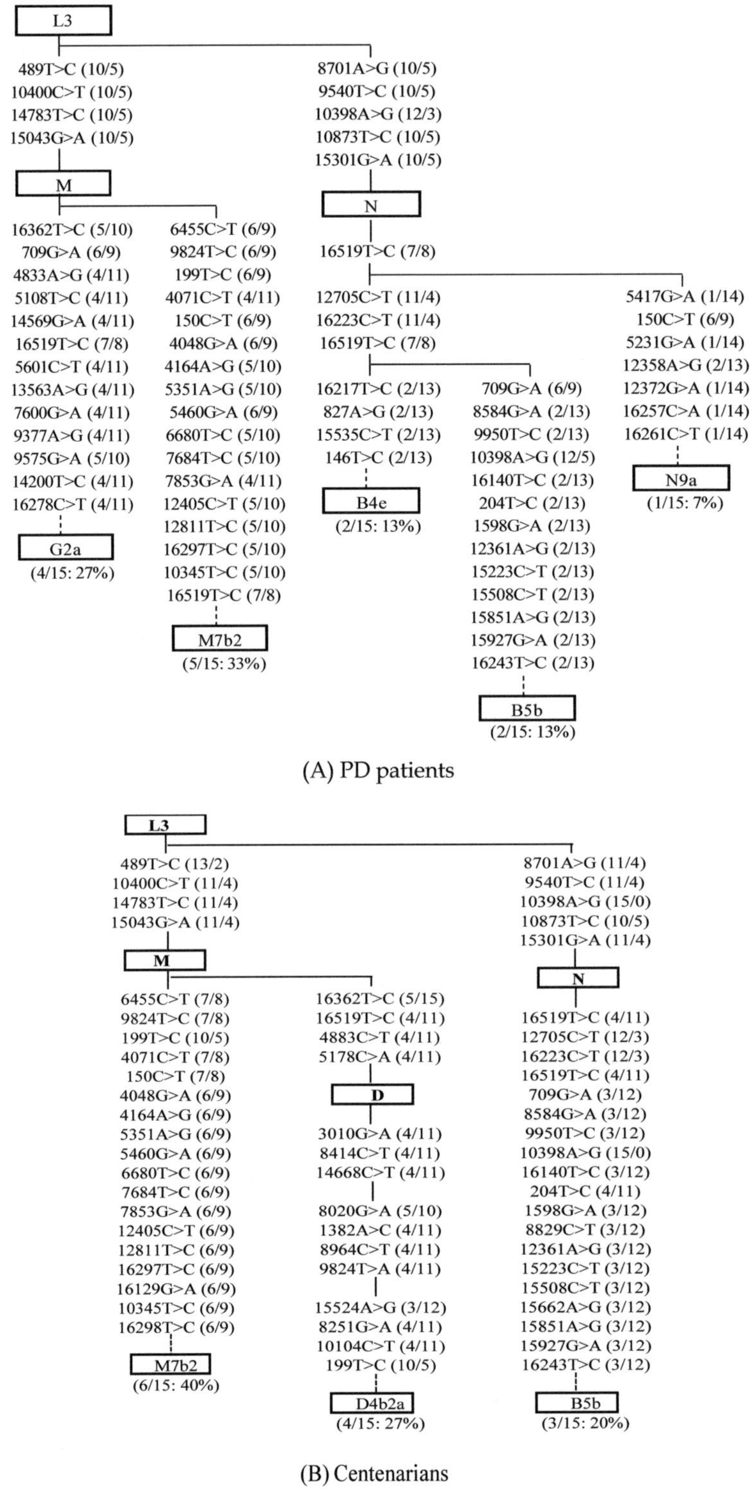
L3
489T>C (10/5)
10400C>T (10/5)
14783T>C (10/5)
15043G>A (10/5)
M
16362T>C (5/10)
709G>A (6/9)
4833A>G (4/11)
5108T>C (4/11)
14569G>A (4/11)
16519T>C (7/8)
5601C>T (4/11)
13563A>G (4/11)
7600G>A (4/11)
9377A>G (4/11)
9575G>A (5/10)
14200T>C (4/11)
16278C>T (4/11)
G2a
(4/15: 27%)
6455C>T (6/9)
9824T>C (6/9)
199T>C (6/9)
4071C>T (4/11)
150C>T (6/9)
4048G>A (6/9)
4164A>G (5/10)
5351A>G (5/10)
5460G>A (6/9)
6680T>C (5/10)
7684T>C (5/10)
7853G>A (4/11)
12405C>T (5/10)
12811T>C (5/10)
16297T>C (5/10)
10345T>C (5/10)
16519T>C (7/8)
M7b2
(5/15: 33%)
8701A>G (10/5)
9540T>C (10/5)
10398A>G (12/3)
10873T>C (10/5)
15301G>A (10/5)
N
16519T>C (7/8)
12705C>T (11/4)
16223C>T (11/4)
16519T>C (7/8)
16217T>C (2/13)
827A>G (2/13)
15535C>T (2/13)
146T>C (2/13)
B4e
(2/15: 13%)
709G>A (6/9)
8584G>A (2/13)
9950T>C (2/13)
10398A>G (12/5)
16140T>C (2/13)
204T>C (2/13)
1598G>A (2/13)
12361A>G (2/13)
15223C>T (2/13)
15508C>T (2/13)
15851A>G (2/13)
15927G>A (2/13)
16243T>C (2/13)
B5b
(2/15: 13%)
5417G>A (1/14)
150C>T (6/9)
5231G>A (1/14)
12358A>G (2/13)
12372G>A (1/14)
16257C>A (1/14)
16261C>T (1/14)
N9a
(1/15: 7%)
(A) PD patients
L3
489T>C (13/2)
10400C>T (11/4)
14783T>C (11/4)
15043G>A (11/4)
M
6455C>T (7/8)
9824T>C (7/8)
199T>C (10/5)
4071C>T (7/8)
150C>T (7/8)
4048G>A (6/9)
4164A>G (6/9)
5351A>G (6/9)
5460G>A (6/9)
6680T>C (6/9)
7684T>C (6/9)
7853G>A (6/9)
12405C>T (6/9)
12811T>C (6/9)
16297T>C (6/9)
16129G>A (6/9)
10345T>C (6/9)
16298T>C (6/9)
M7b2
(6/15: 40%)
16362T>C (5/15)
16519T>C (4/11)
4883C>T (4/11)
5178C>A (4/11)
D
3010G>A (4/11)
8414C>T (4/11)
14668C>T (4/11)
8020G>A (5/10)
1382A>C (4/11)
8964C>T (4/11)
9824T>A (4/11)
15524A>G (3/12)
8251G>A (4/11)
10104C>T (4/11)
199T>C (10/5)
D4b2a
(4/15: 27%)
8701A>G (11/4)
9540T>C (11/4)
10398A>G (15/0)
10873T>C (10/5)
15301G>A (11/4)
N
16519T>C (4/11)
12705C>T (12/3)
16223C>T (12/3)
16519T>C (4/11)
709G>A (3/12)
8584G>A (3/12)
9950T>C (3/12)
10398A>G (15/0)
16140T>C (3/12)
204T>C (4/11)
1598G>A (3/12)
8829C>T (3/12)
12361A>G (3/12)
15223C>T (3/12)
15508C>T (3/12)
15662A>G (3/12)
15851A>G (3/12)
15927G>A (3/12)
16243T>C (3/12)
B5b
(3/15: 20%)
(B) Centenarians

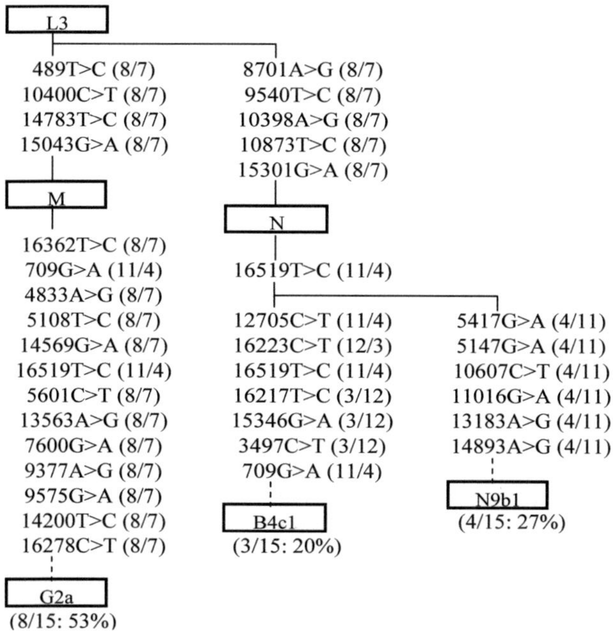

(C) AD patients

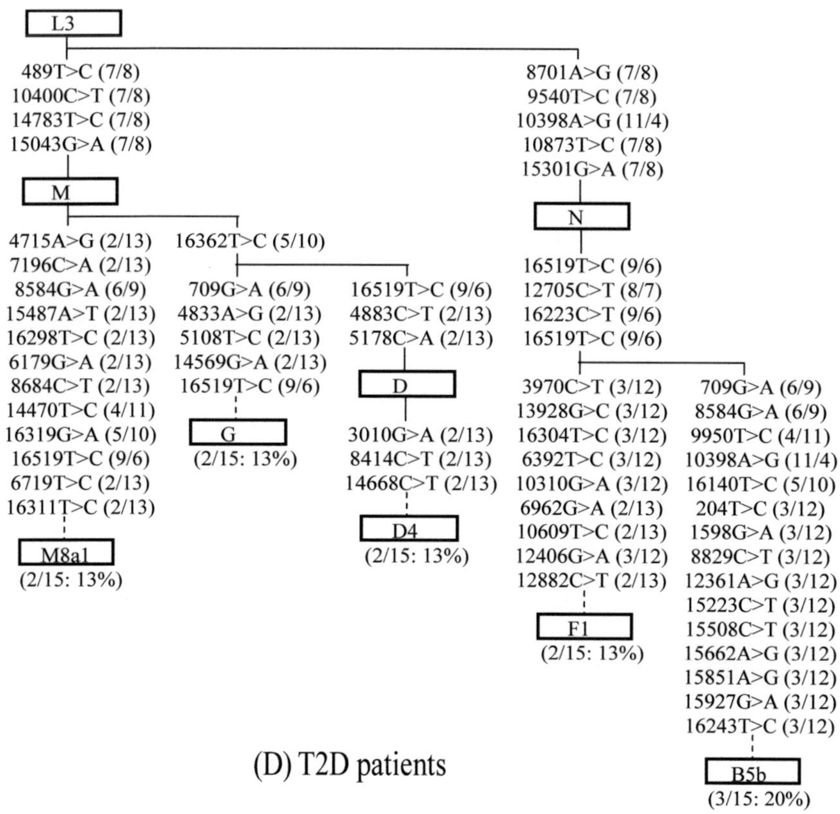

(D) T2D patients

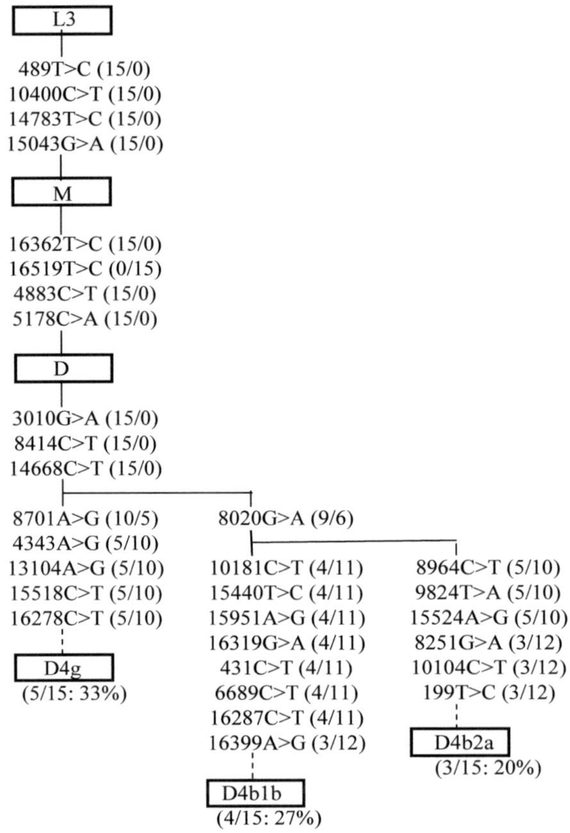

(E) Non-obese young males

Fig. 2. Associations between haplogroups and the mtSNPs of the 15 persons with the highest probabilities of becoming PD patients. This description of associations is based on the phylogenetic tree for macrohaplogroups M and N described in Tanaka *et al.* [26]. The locus of mtDNA polymorphism (*mmm*), the normal nucleotide (rCRS) at the position *mmm* (N_N), the mtDNA mutation at that position (N_M), the number of the mtDNA mutations at *mmm* in individual clusters (*Y*), and the number of the normal nucleotides at *mmm* in individual clusters (*X*) are expressed as $mmmN_N>N_M$ *(Y/X)*. For example, 489T>C (10/5) indicates the mtDNA locus (489), the normal nucleotide at that position (T), the mutation at that position (C), the number of mutations (10), and the number of the normal nucleotides in the cluster (5). (B) Centenarians, (C) AD patients, (D) T2D patients, (E) Non-obese young males.

To compare the mitochondrial haplogroups of the PD patients with those of other classes of people, we used the same modified method to examine the relations between the other four classes (i.e., centenarians, AD patients, T2D patients, and non-obese young males) and their mtSNPs. The associations between the haplogroups and mtSNPs for four classes of Japanese people are shown in Fig. 2 B to E. The centenarians were associated haplogroups L3-M-M7b2 (40%), L3-M-D-D4b2a (27%), and L3-N-B5b (20%); the AD patients were associated haplogroups L3-M-G2a (53%), L3-N-B4c1 (20%), and N9b1 (27%); the T2D patients were associated haplogroups L3-M-D-D4 (13%), L3-M-M8a1 (13%), G (13%), L3-N-B5b (20%), and F1 (13%); and the healthy non-obese young males were associated haplogroups L3-M-D-D4g

(33%), D4b2a (20%), and D4b1b (27%). The relations among the haplogroups for these five classes of people are listed in Table 1.

Classification consideration	PD patients	Centenarians	AD patients	T2D patients	Non-obese males
15 persons from the top				M8a1 (13%)	
	M7b2 (33%)	M7b2 (40%)			
				G (13%)	
	G2a (27%)		G2a (53%)		
				D4 (13%)	
					D4b1b (27%)
					D4b2a (20%)
		D4b2a (27%)			
					D4g (33%)
	B4e (13%)				
	B5b (13%)	B5b (20%)		B5b (20%)	
			B4c1 (20%)		
	N9a (7%)				
			N9b1 (27%)		
				F1 (13%)	
Persons whose probabilities are greater than 50%				M8a1 (4%)	
	M7a1a (19%)				
	M7b2 (14%)	M7b2 (13%)			
				G (11%)	
			G1 (9%)		
	G1a (14%)				
	G2a (11%)		G2a (17%)		
			D4 (19%)	D4 (47%)	
		D4a (15%)			
					D4b1b (24%)
					D4b2 (35%)
		D4b2a (9%)			
		D4b2b (16%)			
					D4g (29%)
				D5a (6%)	
	B4e (5%)				
			B4c1 (11%)		
	B5b (5%)	B5b (7%)		B5b (6%)	
	N9a (16%)		N9a (4%)		
			N9b1 (9%)	N9b1 (6%)	
			F1 (11%)	F1 (6%)	

Table 1. The relations among the haplogroups for five classes of people

In Table 1 we see that the haplogroup Mb2 was common in PD patients and centenarians, G2a was common in PD patients and AD patients; and B5b was common in PD patients, centenarians, and T2D patients. The haplogroups of the PD patients are therefore different from those of the other four classes of people. The results are therefore considered new findings.

Then individuals whose probabilities of becoming PD patients were greater than 50% were selected, and the nucleotide distributions of those 37 persons were examined. The associations between haplogroups and the mtSNPs of those PD patients are shown in Fig. 3. Individuals whose probabilities of becoming PD patients were greater than 50% were classified into more haplogroups than were the 15 persons most likely to become PD patients. The ratios of the haplogroups M7b2, G2a, B4e, B5b and N9a for the 15 persons most likely to become PD patients were respectively changed from 33% to 14%, 27% to 11%, 13%

to 5%, 13% to 5%, and 7% to 16%, and new haplogroups M7a1a (19%) and G1a (14%) were classified for the persons whose probabilities were greater than 50%. The other four classes of people were also examined for the persons whose probabilities were greater than 50%. The selected numbers of the four classes were 55 for centenarians, 47 for AD patients, 47 for T2D patients, and 17 for healthy non-obese young males. The associations between the haplogroups and mtSNPs for four classes of people are shown in Fig. 3 B to E. The centenarians were associated haplogroups L3-M-M7b2 (13%), L3-M-D-D4a (15%), D4b2a (9%), D4b2b (16%), and L3-N-B5b (7%); the AD patients were associated haplogroups L3-M-G1 (9%), G2a (17%), L3-M-D-D4 (19%), L3-N-F1 (11%), B4c1 (11%), N9a (4%), and N9b1 (9%); the T2D patients were associated haplogroups L3-M-M8a1 (4%), G (11%), L3-M-D-D4 (47%), D5a (6%), L3-N-F1 (6%), B5b (6%), and N9b1 (6%); and the healthy non-obese young males were associated haplogorups L3-M-D-D4g (29%), D4b1b (24%), and D4b2 (35%). The relations among the haplogroups of the selected persons for the five classes of people are also listed in Table 1, where one sees that the individual classes of people were classified into more haplogroups when the mtSNP analysis was based on the persons whose probabilities were greater than 50% than they were when the analysis was based on the highest 15 persons from the top.

3.2 Comparison with previous works for T2D patients and Centenarians

Although there is no report regarding the relations between mtSNP haplogroups and PD patients but there were a few studies concerning the relations between mtSNP haplogroups and T2D patients or centenarians, the differences between previous works and the work reported here are discussed based on the mtSNP haplogroups obtained.

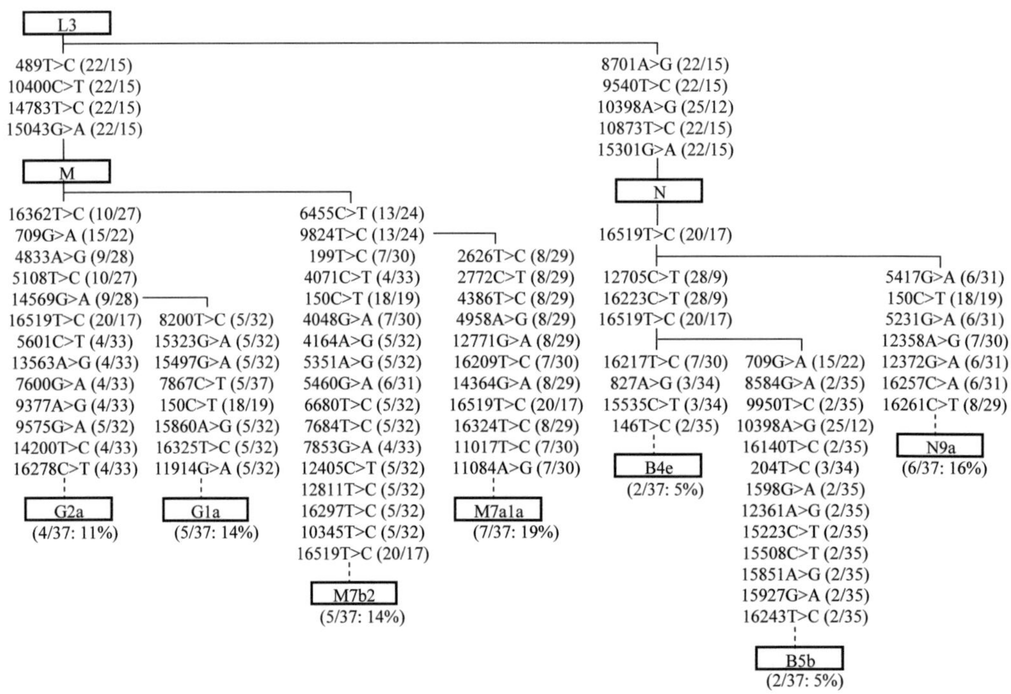

(A) PD patients

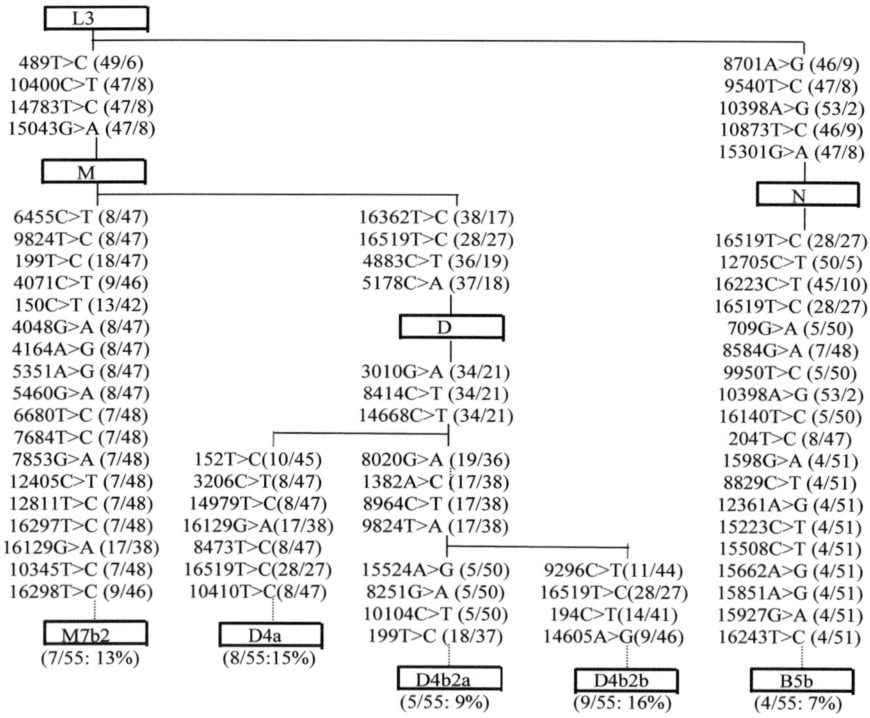

(B) Centenarians

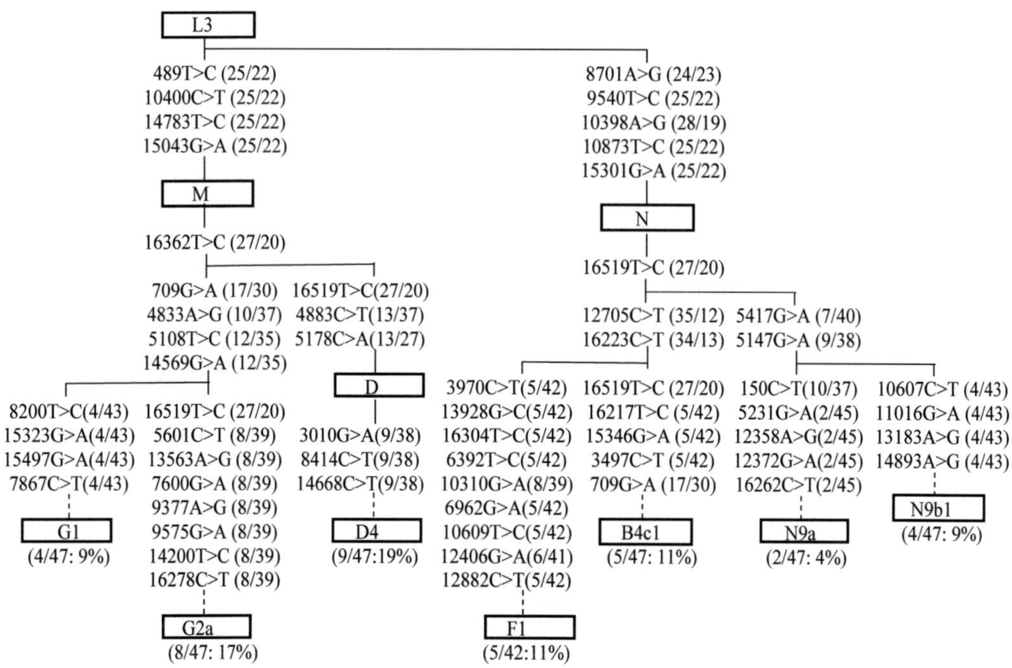

(C) AD patients

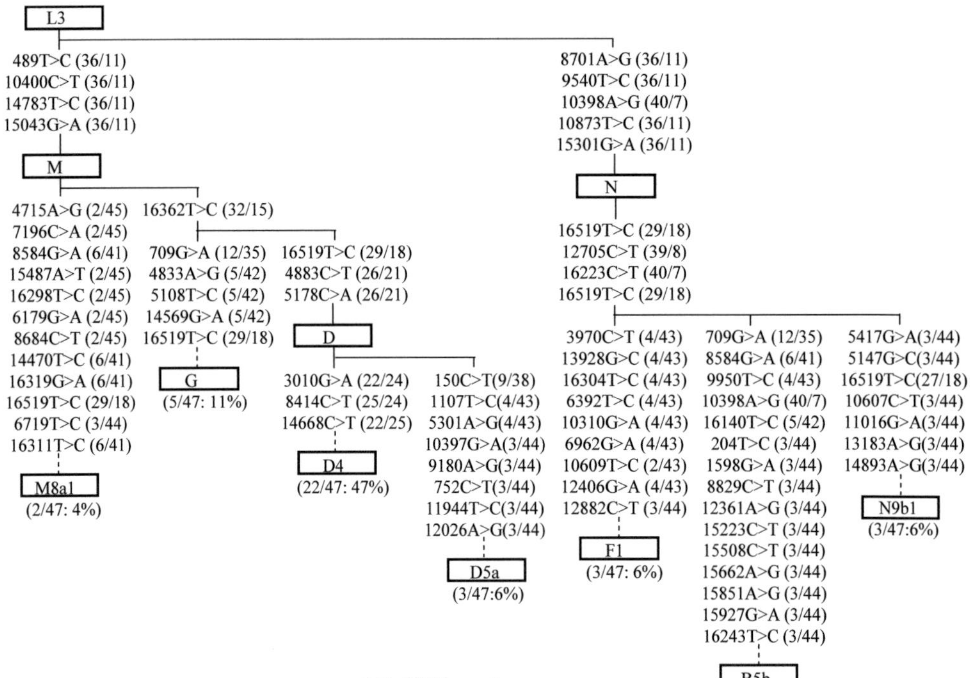

(D) T2D patients

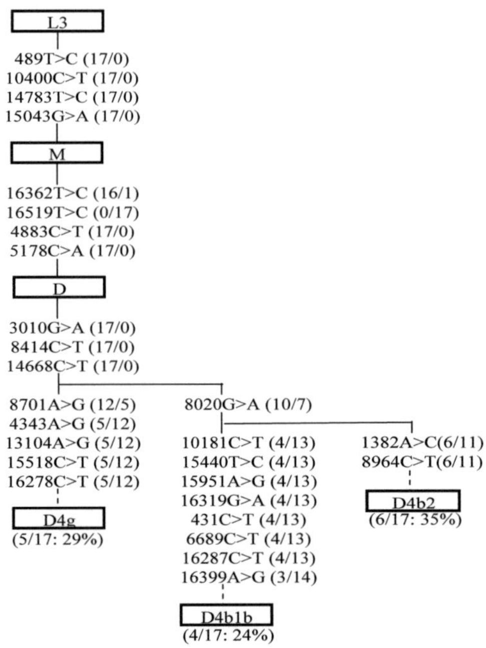

(E) Non-obese young males

Fig. 3. Associations between haplogroups and the mtSNPs of the persons whose probabilities of becoming PD patients are greater than 50%. (B) Centenarians, (C) AD patients, (D) T2D patients, (E) Non-obese young males.

Fuku et al. (2007) reported that the mitochondrial haplogroup F in Japanese individuals had a significantly increased risk of type 2 diabetes mellitus (T2DM) (odds ratio 1.53, P=0.0032) using hospital based sampling data for large-scale association study (Fuku et al., 2007). They indicated that there were three mtSNPs in the haplogroup F - 3970C>T, 13928G>C, and 10310G>A. In the present analysis, the risk of T2D patients for the haplogroup F1 was approximately 13% (Fig. 2D). Other haplogroups related to the risk of T2D patients were B5b (20%), M8a1 (13%), D4 (13%) and G (13%) (Fig. 2D and Table 2). There were therefore big differences between the analyses of Fuku et al. (2007) and the results reported here. The significantly increased risk of T2DM was the haplogroup F in Fuku et al. (2007), whereas that of the results obtained was the haplogroup B5b. Although Fuku et al. (2007) indicated that the haplogroup F was the increased risk of T2DM, the F has four sub-haplogroups F1, F2, F3, and F4. In the work reported here, the only haplogroup F1 was obtained by the modified clustering method. The haplogroup F by Fuku et al. (2007) was characterized by three mtSNPs—3970C>T, 13928G>C, and 10310G>A, whereas the haplogroup F1 by the proposed method was featured by many mtSNPs—3970C>T, 13928G>C, 16304T>C, 6392T>C, 10310G>A, 6962G>A, 10609T>C, 12406G>A, and 12882C>T (Tanaka et al., 2004) (Fig. 2D). Furthermore, as Saxena et al. (2006) reported that there was no evidence of association between common mtDNA polymorphism and type 2 diabetes mellitus, the results obtained may indicate new findings for T2D patients (Saxena et al., 2006).

In addition, Alexe et al. (2007) reported the associations between Asian haplogroups and the longevity of Japanese people using the same GiiB data (Alexe et al., 2007). They showed the enrichment of longevity phenotype in mtDNA haplogroups D4b2b, D4a, and D5 in the Japanese population using statistical techniques (t-test and P-value). However, the results here showed that the haplogroups M7b2, D4b2a, and B5b were associated with Japanese centenarians. There is therefore no common haplogroup in both methods. Alexe et al. (2007) showed that the haplogroup D5 was characterized by mtSNPs 11944T>C, 12026A>G, 1107T>C, 5301A>G, 10397A>G, and 752C>T, whereas there was no frequency in the corresponding mtSNPs in the present analysis. Although they reported that the centenarian enrichment was not found in the haplogroup D4b2a, the present results showed that the corresponding D4b2a was characterized by many mtSNPs with a frequency of 27% (Fig. 2B). Although Alexe et al. (2007) described that there was no haplogroup having mtSNPs significantly enriched in centenarians other than D mega-group in M macrohaplogroup, the present analysis indicated that the haplogroup M7b2 was characterized by many mtSNPs (Fig. 2B and 3B). They also reported that there was no enrichment haplogroup for centenarians in macrohaplogroup N, whereas the haplogroup B5b obtained by the proposed method also had many mtSNPs enriched in centenarians (Figs. 2B and 3B).

Bilal et al. (2008) reported the haplogroup D4a was a marker for extreme longevity in Japan by analyzing the complete mtDNA sequences from 112 Japanese semi-supercentenarians (aged over 105 years old) combined with previously published data (Bilal et al., 2008). These semi-supercentenarians were also examined using the proposed method. Since the predicted probabilities of individual clusters for the semi-supercentenarians were lower than those of the centenarians, 43 individuals with predicted probabilities over 46% (the average is 54%) were selected. The obtained results were the haplogroups D4a (30%), B4c1a (14%), M7b2 (12%), F1 (9%), M1 (7%) and B5b (2%) shown in Fig. 4. As the highest haplogroup was D4a, this was the same as the marker described by Bilal et al. (2008). However, there are other haplogroups indicating the characteristics of semi-supercentenarians. This means that other haplogroups also have the possibilities of becoming semi-supercentenarians. The common haplogroups between the centenarians and semi-supercentenarians were M7b2 and B5b.

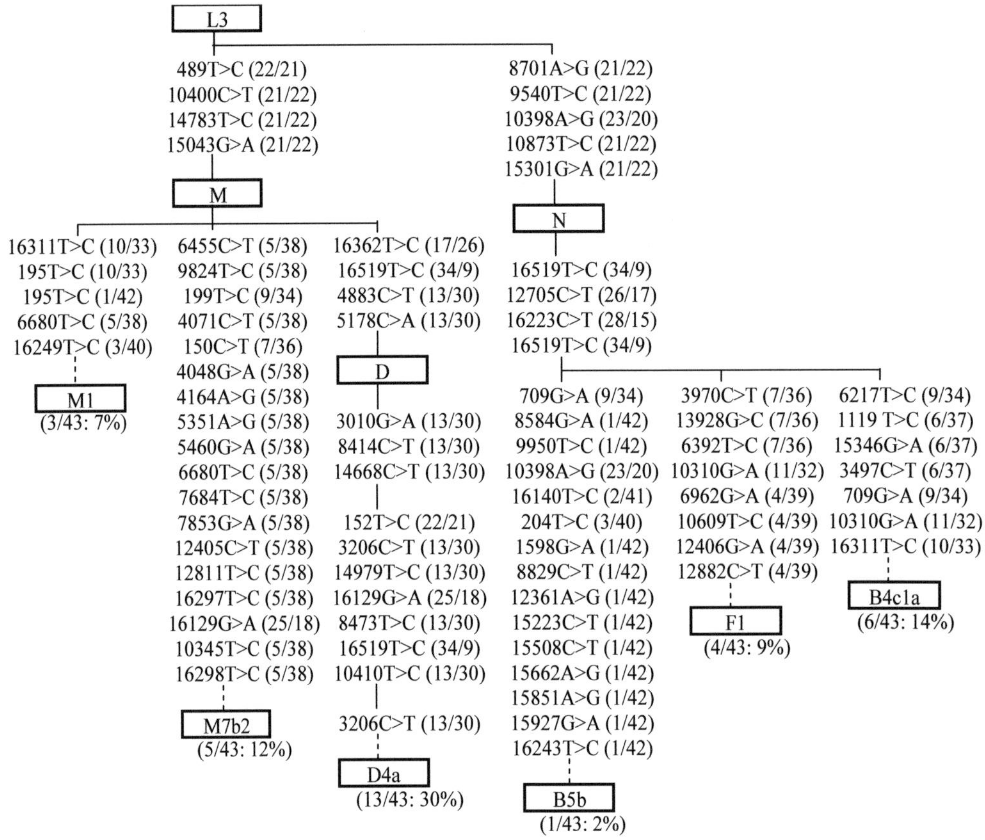

Fig. 4. Associations between Asian/Japanese haplogroups and mtSNPs of semi-supercentenarians.

3.3 Differences between statistical technique and the modified RBF method

Although the haplogroups of the PD patients were obtained by the modified RBF method, there are clear differences between the previously reported statistical technique and the method described here. As the previously reported methods analyzed the relations between mtSNPs and Japanese PD patients, centenarians, AD patients, T2D patients, or semi-supercentenarians using standard statistical techniques (Alexe et al., 2007; Fuku et al., 2007; Bilal et al., 2008), they could not indicate mutual relations among the other classes of people—centenarians, AD patients, T2D patients and healthy non-obese young males. On the other hand, the proposed method was able to show differences and mutual relations among these classes of people. In addition, the prediction probabilities of associations between mtSNPs and these classes of people cannot be obtained by the statistical techniques used in the previous methods, whereas the method proposed is able to compute them based on learning mtSNPs of individual classes.

It is considered that the relations among individual mtSNPs for these classes of people should be analyzed as mutual mtSNP connections in the entire mtSNPs. A learning method, a RBF network, was therefore adopted for extracting individual characteristics from the entire mtSNPs, although the previous methods used standard statistical techniques.

	Statistical technique	Proposed method
Technique	Relative relations between target and normal data	Supervised learning (RBF) by using correct and incorrect data
Analysis position	Each locus of mtDNA polymorphisms (independent position)	Entire loci of mtDNA polymorphisms (succesive positions)
Input (required data)	Target (individual cases) and control (normal data)	Correct (individual cases) and incorrect (others except correct)
Output (results)	Odds ratio or relative risk	Clusters with predictions
Analysis	Check odds ratio or relative risk at each position	Check individuals in clusters based on prediction probabilities

Table 2. Differences between the statistical technique and the proposed (modified RBF) method

The differences between standard statistical technique and the proposed method are listed in Table 2. In the statistical technique, the analysis of odds ratios or relative risks is based on the relative relations between target and control data at each polymorphic mtDNA locus. In the modified RBF method, on the other hand, clusters indicating predicted probabilities are examined on the basis of the RBF using correct and incorrect data for the entire polymorphic mtDNA loci. The statistical technique determines characteristics of haplogroups using independent mtDNA polymorphisms that indicate high odds ratios, whereas the modified RBF method determines them by checking individuals with high predicted probabilities. This means that the statistical technique uses the results of independent mutation positions, whereas the modified RBF method uses the results of entire mutation positions. As there are the differences between the two methods, which method is better depends on future research. Furthermore, the method described here may have possibilities for use in the initial diagnosis of various diseases or longevity on the basis of the individual predicted probabilities.

4. Acknowledgement

I thank Dr. Y. Kawamura for his encouragement and technical support.

5. References

Alexe, G., Fuku, N., Bilal, E., Ueno, H., Nishigaki, Y., Fujita, Y., Ito, M., Arai, Y., Hirose, N., Bhanot, G., and Tanaka, M. (2007). Enrichment of longevity phenotype in mtDNA haplogroups D4b2b, D4a, and D4 in the Japanese population, Hum. Genet. 121: 347 - 356.

Bilal, E., Rabadan, R., Alexe, G., Fuku, N., Ueno, H., Nishigaki, Y., Fujita, Y., Ito, M., Arai, Y., Hirose, N., Ruckenstein, A., Bhanot, G., and Tanaka, M. (2008). Mitochondrial DNA Haplogroup D4a Is a Marker for Extreme Longevity in Japan, PLoS ONE 3(6): e2421.

Chinnery, P.F., Mowbray, C., Patel, S.K., Elson, J.L., Sampson, M., Hitman, G.A., McCarthy, M.I., Hattersley,A.T., and Walker, M. (2008). Mitochondrial DNA haplogroups and type 2 diabetes: a study of 897 cases and 1010 controls, J Med Genet. 44: e80.

Dawson, T.M., and Dawson, V.L. (2003). Molecular Pathway of Neurodegeneration in Parkinson's Disease, Science 302: 819 - 822.

Fuku, N., Park, K.S., Yamada, Y., Nishigaki, Y., Cho, Y.M., Matsuo, H., Segawa, T., Watanabe, S., Kato, K., Yokoi, K., Nozawa, Y., Lee, K.H., and Tanaka M. (2007). Mitochondrial Haplogroup N9a Confers Resistance against Type 2 diabetes in Asians, Am J Hum Genet. 80: 407 - 415.

Feder, J., Blech, I., Ovadia, O., Amar, S., Wainstein, J., Raz, I., Dadon, S., Arking, D.E., Glaser, B., and Mishmar, D. (2008). Differences in mtDNA haplogroup distribution among 3 Jewish populations alter susceptibility to T2DM complications, BMC Genomics 9: 198.

Herrnstad, C., Elson, J.L., Fahy, E., Preston, G., Turnbull, D.M., Anderson, C., Ghosh, S.S., Olefsky, J.M., Beal, M.F., Davis, R.E., and Howell, N. (2002). Reduced-median-network Analysis of complete mitochondrial DNA coding-region sequences for major African, Asian and European haplogroups, Am J Hum Genet. 70: 1152 - 1171.

Kim, W., Yoo, T.K., Shin, D.J., Rho, H.W., Jin, H.J., Kim, E.T., and Bae, Y.S. (2008). Mitochondrial haplogroup analysis reveals no association between the common genetic lineages and prostate cancer in the Korean population, PLoS ONE 3: e2211.

Kosel, S., Egensperger, R., Mehraein, P., and Graeber, M.B. (1994). No association of mutations at nucleotide 5460 of mitochondrial NADH dehydrogenase with Alzheimer's disease, Biochem. Biophy. Res. Comm. 203: 745 - 749.

Kong, Q.P., Yao, Y.G., Sun, C., Bandelt, H.J., Zhu, C.L., and Zhang, Y.P. (2003). Phylogeny of East Asian mitochondrial DNA lineages inferred from complete sequences, Am J Hum Genet. 73: 671 - 676.

Lin, F., Lin, R., Wisniewski, H.M., Hwang, Y., Grundke-Iqbal, I., Healy-Louie, G., and Iqbal, K. (1992). Detection of point mutations in codon 331 of mitochondrial NADH dehydrogenase subunit 2 in Alzheimer's brains, Biochem. Biophy. Res. Comm. 182: 238 - 246.

Lustbader, J.W., Cirilli, M., Lin, C., Xu, H.W., Takuma, K., Wang, N., Caspersen, C., Chen, X., Pollak, S., Chaney, M., Trinchese, F., Liu, S., Gunn-Moore, F., Lue, L.F., Walker, D.G., Kuppusamy, P., Zewier, Z.L., Arancio, O., Stern, D., Yan, S.S., and Wu, H. (2004). ABAB DirectlyLinks Aβ to Mitochondrial Toxicity in Alzheimer's Disease, Science 304: 448 - 452.

Mayr-Wohlfart, U., Paulus, C., and Rodel, G. (1996). Mitochondrial DNA mutations in multiple sclerosis patients with severe optic involvement, Acta Neurol. Scand. 94: 167 - 171.

Maruszak, A., Canter, J.A., Styczynska, M., Zekanowski, C., and Barcikowska, M. (2008). Mitochondrial haplogroup H and Alzheimer's disease - Is there a connection?, Neurobiol Aging, doi: 10.1016.

Niemi, A.K., Moilanen, J.S., Tanaka M., Hervonen, A., Hurme, M., Lehtimaki, T., Arai, Y., Hirose, N., and Majamaa, K. A. (2005). A combination of three common inherited mitochondrial DNA polymorphisms promotes longevity in Finnish and Japanese subjects, Eur. J Hum. Genet. 13: 166 - 170.

Poggio, T., and Girosi, F. (1990). Networks for approximation and learning, Proc. of IEEE 78: 1481-1497.

Ross, O.A., MaCormack, R., Maxwell, L.D., Duguid, R.A., Quinn, D.J., Barnett, Y.A., Rea, I.M., El-Agnaf, O.M., Gibson, J.M., Wallace, A., Middleton, D., and Curran, M.D. (2003). mt4216C variant in linkage with the mtDNA TJ cluster may confer a susceptibility to mitochondrial dysfunction resulting in an increased risk of Parkinson's disease in Irish, Exp Gerontol. 38: 397 - 405.

Saxena, R., de Bakker, PIW., Singer, K., Mootha, V., Burtt, N., Hirschhorn, J.N., Gaudet, D., Isomaa, B., Daly, M.J., Groop, L., Ardlie, K.G., and Altshuler, D. (2006). Comprehensive Association Testing of Common Mitochondrial DNA Variation in Metabolic Disease, Am J Hum Genet. 79: 54 - 61.

Schoffner, J.M., Brown, M.D., Torroni, A., Lott, M.T., Cabell, M.F., Miorra, S.S., Beal, M.F., Yang, C.C., Gearing, M., Salvo, R., Watts, R.L., Juncos, J.L., Hansen, L.A., Crain, B.J., Fayad, M., Reckord, C.L., and Wallace, D.C. (1993). Mitochondrial DNA variants observed in Alzheimer disease and Parkinson disease Patients, Genomics 17: 171 - 184.

Schnopp, N.M., Kosel, S., Egensperger, R., and Graeber, M.B. (1996). Regional heterogeneity of mtDNA hetroplasmy in parkinsonian brain, Clin Neuropathol. 15: 348 - 352.

Simon, D.K., Mayeux, R., Marder, K., Kowall, N.W., Beal, M.F., and Jons, D.R. (2000). Mitochondrial DNA mutations in complex I and tRNA genes in Parkinson's disease, Neurology 54: 703 - 709.

Tanaka, M., Fuku, N., Takeyasu, T Guo, L.J., Hirose, R., Kurata, M., Borgeld, H.J., Yamada, Y., Maruyama, W., Arai, Y., Hirose, N., Oshida, Y., Sato, Y., Hattori, N., Mizuno, Y., Iwata, S., and Yagi, K. (2002). Golden Mean to Longevity: Rareness of Mitochondrial Cytochrome b Varianats in Centenarians But Not in Patients With Parkinson's Disease, J. Neuro. Res. 70: 347 - 355.

Tanaka, M., Cabrera, V.M., Gonzalez, A.M., Larruga, J.M., Takeyasu, T., Fuku, N., Guo, L.J., Hirose, R., Fujita, Y., Kurata, M., Shinoda, K., Umetsu, K., Yamada, Y., Oshida, Y., Sato, Y., Hattori, N., Mizuno, Y., Arai, Y., Hirose, N., Ohta, S., Ogawa, O., Tanaka, Y., Kawamori, R., Shamoto-Nagai, M., Maruyama, W., Shimokata, H., Suzuki, R., and Shimodaira, H. (2004). Mitochondrial genome variation in Eastern Asia and the peopling of Japan, Genome Research 14: 1832 - 1850.

Takasaki, S., Kawamura, Y., and Konagaya, A. (2006). Selecting effective siRNA sequences by using radial basis function network and decision tree learning, BMC Bioinformatics 7: s5-s22, doi: 10.1186/147-2105-7-s5-s22.

Takasaki S (2009) Mitochondrial haplogroups associated with Japanese centenarians, Alzheimer's patients, Parkinson's patients, type 2 diabetic patients and healthy non-obese young males. J. Genetics and Genomics. 36: 425-434.

Taylor, R.W., and Turnbull, D.M. (2005). Mitochondrial DNA Mutations in Human Disease, Nature Rev. Genetics 6: 389 - 402.

Vila, M., and Przedborski, S. (2003). Targeting Programmed Cell Death Neurodegenerative Diseases, Nature Rev. Neuro. 4: 1 - 11.

Wallace, D.C. (1999). Mitochondrial Diseases in Man and Mouse, Science 283: 1482 - 1488.

Wu. C.H., and McLarty, J.W. (2000). Neural Networks and Genome Informatics. Elsevier Science Ltd., NY.

28

Role of ^{123}I-Metaiodobenzylguanidine Myocardial Scintigraphy in Parkinsonian Disorders

Masahiko Suzuki
Department of Neurology, The Jikei University School of Medicine, Aoto Hospital, Tokyo, Japan

1. Introduction

Parkinson's disease (PD) is a relatively common neurological disorder in the elderly. However, only 76% of patients considered clinically to have PD are confirmed to have PD after postmortem examination (Hughes et al., 1993). The most common atypical form of parkinsonism is multiple system atrophy (MSA) (Hughes et al., 1994). MSA is clinically characterized by a combination of parkinsonian, autonomic, pyramidal and/or cerebellar symptoms and signs. The differential diagnosis of disorders with parkinsonism is very important because prognosis and treatment options differ substantially (Wenning et al., 1997). However, although the diagnoses of PD and MSA are based on current clinical criteria (Gelb et al., 1999; Gilman et al., 1999), they continue to lack sufficient specificity (Hughes et al., 1992; Litvan et al., 1997), particularly early in the disease course (Osaki et al., 2002).

Extrapyramidal signs in dementia with Lewy bodies (DLB) resemble those seen in PD, although less rest tremor and left/right asymmetry, but more severe rigidity, favors a diagnosis of DLB. The subtle differences in the nature of extrapyramidal signs between DLB and PD may be of limited help in clinically differentiating the two disorders. This is particularly true in the early disease stages because the sensitivity of the clinical diagnosis of DLB based on the consensus criteria of the DLB International Workshop was 0.22 compared with 0.83 based on a neuropathological diagnosis (McKeith et al., 1996).

The clinical features of PD and autosomal recessive juvenile parkinsonism (AR-JP) are also similar. Thus, it may be difficult to differentiate these two disorders. Neuropathological studies in AR-JP have revealed selective degeneration with gliosis of the pigmented neurons of the substantia nigra and locus ceruleus, but generally no Lewy bodies (Takahashi et al., 1994; Mori et al., 1998; Paviour et al., 2004), suggesting that the pathological findings and disease process of AR-JP differ from those of PD.

Metaiodobenzylguanidine (MIBG) is a physiological analogue of noradrenaline (norepinephrine) (Wieland et al., 1981) and ^{123}I-MIBG myocardial scintigraphy has been used to evaluate postganglionic cardiac sympathetic innervation in parkinsonian disorders (Braune et al., 1999; Orimo et al., 1999; Druschky et al., 2000; Taki et al., 2000; Suzuki et al., 2005). ^{123}I-MIBG myocardial scintigraphy can be performed safely and is clinically used to estimate local myocardial sympathetic nerve damage in PD (Braune et al., 1998; Orimo et al., 1999; Takatsu et al., 2000a). Myocardial innervation imaging using ^{123}I-MIBG has also

emerged as a useful method to confirm or exclude the presence of PD (Jost et al., 2010). Thus, ^{123}I-MIBG scintigraphy is the only method that can distinguish with a high degree of sensitivity and specificity between parkinsonian disorders and PD.
In the present study, we evaluated ^{123}I-MIBG myocardial scintigraphy in patients with PD, DLB, AR-JP, and MSA in order to enhance the differentiation of PD from these other neurological diseases that mimic PD.

2. Material and methods

2.1 Patients

A total of 74 subjects were enrolled prospectively based on the criteria outlined below for PD (n = 36), DLB (n = 6), MSA (n = 14), AR-JP (n = 2), and normal control groups (NC; n = 16). There was no significant difference in age between patients with parkinsonism and NC (P = 0.25), and none of the enrolled subjects had clinical evidence of diabetes mellitus or cardiovascular disease. Cases were excluded if no relevant clinical information was provided. In addition, none of the participating subjects were taking drugs that might interfere with ^{123}I-MIBG uptake (Solanki et al., 1992; Wafelman et al., 1994; Braune et al., 2001).
The diagnosis of probable DLB was made based on the criteria of DLB adopted by the International National Workshop on DLB (McKeith et al., 1996). Six patients with DLB had early recurrent visual hallucinations and delusions unrelated to therapy, marked fluctuations in alertness, progressive cognitive decline, and spontaneous motor features of parkinsonism. These psychiatric symptoms became worse with administration of anticholinergic agents and dopamine agonists.
Thirty-six patients with idiopathic PD (Hoehn and Yahr (HY) stage 1, 8 patients; HY 2, 22 patients; HY 3, 6 patients) showed two or more of the following cardinal features of PD: rest tremor, bradykinesia, muscular rigidity, loss of postural reflexes, and unilateral symptoms; thus fulfilling standard diagnostic criteria 6. All PD patients had a good or excellent initial response to levodopa treatment.
Fourteen patients presented with probable MSA according to the criteria reported by Gilman and colleagues (Gilman et al., 1999); all showed extrapyramidal symptoms and corticospinal dysfunction, sporadic adult-onset, and rapid disease progression without dementia. These patients tended to be unresponsive to levodopa or dopamine agonist therapy.
The study included two patients with AR-JP. Both had consanguineous parents and were only first generation. Their clinical features included early-onset (in the 20s) and levodopa-responsive parkinsonism, diurnal fluctuation, and slow progression of the disease. The disease presented initially with dystonic posture of the legs followed by a gradual development of parkinsonism. Their parkinsonian symptoms were responsive to levodopa, although a gradual decline in the efficacy was noted. The parkinsonian triad was mild, and the tremor was usually fine and postural. The levodopa efficacy was sufficient and the clinical course was benign; however, both showed a clear wearing-off phenomenon.

2.2 ^{123}I-MIBG myocardial scintigraphy

^{123}I-MIBG myocardial scintigraphy was performed in all subjects using an intravenous injection of 111 MBq ^{123}I-MIBG (Daiichi Radioisotope Laboratories Co, Tokyo, Japan). Single positron emission computed tomographic and planar images of the chest were obtained after 30 minutes for early images and after 4 hours for delayed images, using a triple-headed gamma camera (MULTI SPECT III, Siemens, IL, USA) equipped with low-energy and high-resolution collimators. The photopeak of ^{123}I was centered at 159 keV with a 20% energy window. For the anterior planar image, the data was acquired for 4 minutes with a 256 x 256 matrix for image acquisition. The organ uptake of ^{123}I-MIBG was determined by setting the region of interest (ROI) on the anterior view. An ROI was drawn in the left ventricle of the heart and an angular ROI was also set in the upper mediastinum in early imaging, with the same also used for the delayed imaging. The heart to mediastinum ratio (H/M ratio) represented the average counts per pixel in the heart (H) and mediastinum (M).

2.3 Statistical analysis

All data are expressed as mean ± standard deviations. Differences in continuous variables were examined for statistical significance using Student's t-test. A *P* value less than 0.01 was considered to denote a significant difference. All tests were performed with the STATA 8.0 software program (STATA Corporation, College Station, TX). The AR-JP group was excluded from the analysis because of the small number of subjects.

3. Results

The normal mean values of the H/M ratio in 16 NC were 2.04 (SD 0.18) (range; 1.86-2.55) in the early phase and 2.12 (0.15) (1.91-2.43) in the delayed phase (Table 1). The mean H/M ratio in the early/delayed phase was 1.25 (0.11) (1.11-1.37)/1.18 (0.12) (1.01-1.39) in patients with DLB, 1.45 (0.19) (1.13-1.79)/1.36 (0.22) (1.03-1.99) in those with PD, and 1.88 (0.27) (1.46-2.34)/1.88 (0.40) (1.33-2.47) in those with MSA, respectively. In patients with DLB, the H/M ratio in the early/delayed phases was significantly lower than in MSA and NC groups. In patients with PD, the H/M ratio in the early/delayed phases was also significantly lower than that in MSA and NC groups. In the early phase, the mean value of H/M ratio in patients with DLB was significantly lower than that in patients with PD. However, the H/M ratio in the delayed phase for patients with DLB was lower than that in PD patients, although the difference was not significant (P = 0.015) (Table 1). Overall, there was no significant difference in the early/delayed H/M ratio between the MSA and NC groups (P = 0.077, P = 0.054, respectively). In the two patients with AR-JP, the H/M ratios in the early/delayed phases were preserved within the same range (1.99/2.13, 2.00/2.10, respectively) as the mean value of H/M ratio in NC (Figure 1).

Diagnosis	n (M/F)	Age (years)	H/M ratio		WR (%)
			Early image	Delayed image	
DLB	6 (5/1)	68 ± 8	1.3 ± 0.1*†¶	1.2 ± 0.1*†	39 ± 5
PD	36 (24/12)	64 ± 9	1.5 ± 0.2*†	1.4 ± 0.2*†	42 ± 6
MSA	14 (8/6)	63 ± 8	1.9 ± 0.3 ns	1.9 ± 0.4 ns	35 ± 7 ns
NC	16 (11/5)	64 ± 9	2.0 ± 0.2	2.1 ± 0.2	35 ± 4

Data are mean±SD. *P < 0.001, compared with normal control subjects; ns, not significant, compared with normal control subjects; †P < 0.001, compared with MSA; ¶P < 0.004, compared with PD. DLB, dementia with Lewy bodies; PD, Parkinson's disease; MSA, multiple system atrophy; NC, normal control subjects; M, male; F, female; H/M ratio, heart to mediastinum ratio.

Table 1. Subjects' background and data summary

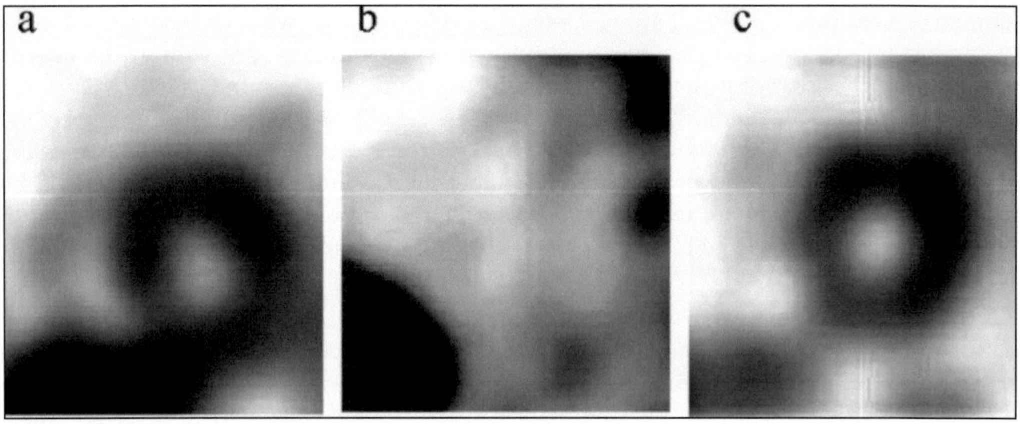

Fig. 1. Short-axis views of ^{123}I-MIBG myocardial scintigraphy

Short-axis views in the early phase of single-photon emission computed tomography of iodine-123–labeled metaiodobenzylguanidine (^{123}I-MIBG) myocardial scintigraphy in a 62-year-old man with autosomal recessive juvenile parkinsonism (a), a 58-year-old man with idiopathic Parkinson's disease (Hoehn and Yahr Stage II, b), and a healthy 62-year-old man (c).

4. Discussion

The major findings of the present study were that 1) ^{123}I-MIBG uptake of the myocardium was significantly lower in patients with Lewy body disease (LBD) including PD and DLB than in controls, 2) the mean values of both the early and delayed H/M ratios in patients with DLB were significantly lower than those in patients with PD, and 3) the mean values of H/M ratios in the early and delayed phases in patients with MSA and AR-JP were well within the range of healthy control subjects.

Decreased cardiac uptake of ^{123}I-IMIBG has been reported in LBD (Yoshita et al., 2001; Watanabe et al., 2001; Nagayama et al., 2005; Suzuki et al., 2006; Suzuki et al., 2007), and a role for postganglionic cardiac sympathetic nerves in PD was demonstrated (Orimo et al., 2001). Thus, reduced uptake of ^{123}I-MIBG is considered to reflect lesions in postganglionic cardiac sympathetic neurons in PD. Lower amounts of cardiac ^{123}I-MIBG uptake were also reported in DLB, even in the early disease stage (Watanabe et al., 2001; Yoshita et al., 2001; Suzuki et al., 2006). These studies suggested that uptake of ^{123}I-MIBG reflects myocardial sympathetic nerve function and that lowered myocardial ^{123}I-MIBG uptake could reflect a disturbance of the postganglionic cardiac sympathetic nerves. In this context, the present study indicated marked reduction of ^{123}I-MIBG uptake in DLB, indicating impairment of the cardiac sympathetic nervous system in this disorder and possible lesions in the postganglionic cardiac sympathetic neurons in DLB, as in PD (Suzuki et al., 2006). These observations might indeed reflect actual cardiac sympathetic denervation, which precedes the neuronal loss in the sympathetic ganglia (Orimo et al., 2005). Cardiac uptake of 6-^{18}F fluorodopamine on positron emission tomography, which can also assess cardiac sympathetic innervation, was decreased in patients with PD (Goldstein et al., 1997; Goldstein et al., 2000), supporting that cardiac sympathetic denervation occurs in LBD.

Decreased cardiac uptake of MIBG has been reported even in the early stages of PD, which suggests early involvement of the cardiac sympathetic nerves. To investigate this proposal,

Orimo et al. (2007) immunohistochemically examined heart tissues, the sympathetic ganglia, and the medulla oblongata at the level of the dorsal vagal nucleus in 20 patients with incidental Lewy body disease (ILBD), which is thought to represent a presymptomatic stage of PD, and 10 control subjects, using antibodies against TH and NF. TH- and NF-immunoreactive nerve fibers of fascicles in the epicardium were well preserved in 10 of the 20 patients with ILBD and in all control subjects. In contrast, TH-immunoreactive nerve fibers had almost entirely disappeared in 6 patients and were moderately decreased in 4 of the 20 patients with ILBD. In addition, none of these ILBD patients showed neuronal loss in the dorsal vagal nucleus or sympathetic ganglia (Orimo et al., 2007). These findings suggested that degeneration of the cardiac sympathetic nerve begins even in the presymptomatic stage of PD, when neuronal loss in the dorsal vagal nucleus is not yet evident.

The present study also revealed relatively preserved cardiac ^{123}I-MIBG uptake in MSA, consistent with previous studies (Yoshita et al., 1998; Nagayama et al., 2005). Taki et al. (2004) previously reported preserved ^{123}I-MIBG uptake in MSA, suggesting that central and preganglionic neurons are predominantly affected, while postganglionic sympathetic neurons are usually spared. Thus, cardiac ^{123}I-MIBG uptake could be unimpaired, indicating the significance of ^{123}I-MIBG imaging as a discriminator between PD and MSA (Yoshita et al., 1998; Braune et al., 1999; Orimo et al., 1999; Druschky et al., 2000; Takatsu et al.; 2000a, 2000b). Postmortem studies demonstrated that postganglionic cardiac sympathetic nerve fibers are markedly decreased in all PD patients, but not necessarily in those with MSA, providing substantial evidence of discrepant ^{123}I-MIBG uptake between PD and MSA (Orimo et al., 2001, 2002). Recent myocardial innervation imaging with ^{123}I-MIBG scintigraphy also demonstrated a high sensitivity for PD detection and adequate specificity for discriminating between PD and MSA (Köllensperger et al., 2007; Chung et al., 2009; Fröhlich et al., 2010). However, Nagayama et al. (2010) recently suggested that MSA cannot consistently be distinguished from PD based on ^{123}I-MIBG myocardial scintigraphy. Their study clearly showed that cardiac MIBG uptake is not always preserved in patients with MSA and that approximately 30% of patients with MSA showed decreased MIBG uptake without any correlation to disease duration or severity. The precise mechanisms underlying low cardiac MIBG uptake in MSA patients remain unclear. The same authors also reported an autopsied patient with MSA showing low cardiac MIBG uptake with an incidental LB pathology in addition to a typical MSA pathology (Nagayama et al, 2008). Therefore, the presence of LB pathology may be a suitable explanation for the low myocardial MIBG uptake observed in patients with MSA. The second consensus statement on the diagnosis of MSA gave no advice about the usefulness and reliability of MIBG scintigraphy scanning in the workup of suspected patients with MSA (Gilman et al., 2008), while the Quality Standards Subcommittee of the American Academy of Neurology found insufficient evidence to recommend MIBG cardiac imaging for differentiating PD from MSA (Suchowersky et al., 2006).

In contrast, myocardial uptake of ^{123}I-MIBG in AR-JP was normal in our study (Suzuki et al., 2005). The H/M ratios in the early and delayed phases in two patients were well within the range for healthy control subjects. These findings might explain the tendency for cardiac sympathetic function to be normal in patients with AR-JP. The pathological background of PD is a systemic distribution of Lewy bodies and Lewy neuritis, spreading to the peripheral autonomic nervous system, including the cardiac plexus (Wakabayashi et al., 1997; Iwanaga et al., 1999). Thus, although the present study included only two patients with AR-JP, it indicated that cardiac sympathetic nerve denervation occurs in PD, and thus accounted for the decrease in cardiac uptake of ^{123}I-MIBG in PD patients and not in those with AR-JP. In this regard, quantification of cardiac ^{123}I-MIBG uptake is considered a valuable tool to identify patients with PD and to distinguish them from patients with other parkinsonian syndromes, including AR-JP (Braune et al., 1999; Orimo et al., 1999; Druschky et al., 2000; Taki et al., 2000). However, a recent study of PD patients showed a low myocardial ^{123}I-MIBG uptake in one patient with PARK2 mutation and autonomic dysfunction, while early-phase MIBG uptake was normal in all other patients free of autonomic dysfunction (Yoritaka et al., 2011). Similar to the above study, a low uptake of ^{123}I-MIBG was reported in 1 of 4 patients with PARK2 mutations, with disease duration of 12 years and ill-defined autonomic dysfunction (Quattrone et al., 2008). In addition, 3 patients in the above study who had low ^{123}I-MIBG uptake were slightly older than the other patients. Incidentally, Estorch et al. (1995) reported that the uptake of ^{123}I-MIBG decreases with age, suggesting that aging could affect patients with PARK2 mutations. Decreased myocardial uptake of ^{123}I-MIBG is also considered to indicate the presence of α-synuclein aggregates in the axons of PD patients (Orimo et al., 2008), while the H/M ratio of patients with PARK2 mutations was reported to be within the range of the normal controls (Suzuki et al., 2005). Moreover, postmortem examination of patients with PARK2 mutations showed well preserved tyrosine hydroxylase immunoreactive nerve fibers in the epicardium (Orimo et al., 2005), suggesting normal functioning myocardial sympathetic nerve terminals in patients with PARK2 mutations. MIBG scintigraphy might be a marker for α-synuclein in patients with PARK2 mutations; however, there are no pathological reports on the presence of Lewy bodies in patients with PARK2 mutations with low MIBG uptake (Yoritaka et al., 2011).

5. Conclusion

The results of the present study indicated that inclusion of ^{123}I-MIBG myocardial scintigraphy in the clinical assessment can potentially increase the chance of correctly distinguishing LBD from the other parkinsonian syndromes. Our study also indicated a difficulty in the differential diagnosis of PD from DLB by ^{123}I-MIBG findings alone. In comparison with PD, mild degeneration of the cardiac sympathetic nervous system may occur in patients with MSA. Finally, abnormalities of ^{123}I-MIBG uptake in genetically identified cases of AR-JP are rare and inconsistent findings. Together, our findings support the conclusions of previous studies that ^{123}I-MIBG myocardial scintigraphy is a potentially useful tool for the differential diagnosis of LBD based on the decreased ^{123}I-MIBG uptake in cardiac postganglionic sympathetic nerve fibers.

6. References

Braune, S., Reinhardt, M. & Bathmann, J. (1998). Impaired cardiac uptake of meta-123I iodobenzylguanidine in Parkinson's disease with autonomic failure. *Acta Neurologica Scandinavia* Vol. 97, pp. 307-314, ISSN 0001-6314

Braune, S., Reinhardt, M. & Schnitzer, R. (1999). Cardiac uptake of ^{123}I-MIBG separates Parkinson's disease from multiple system atrophy. *Neurology* Vol. 53, pp. 1020-1025, ISSN 0028-3878

Braune, S. (2001). The role of cardiac metaiodobenzylguanidine uptake in the differential diagnosis of parkinsonian syndromes. *Clinical Autonomic Research* Vol. 11, pp. 351-355, ISSN 0959-9851

Chung, E.J., Lee, W.Y. & Yoon, W.T. (2009). MIBG scintigraphy for differentiating Parkinson's disease with autonomic dysfunction from Parkinsonism-predominant multiple system atrophy. *Movement Disorders* Vol. 24, pp. 1650-1655, ISSN 1531-8257

Druschky, A., Hilz, M.J. & Platsch, G. (2000). Differentiation of Parkinson's disease and multiple system atrophy in early disease stages by means of I-123-MIBG-spect. *Journal of Neurological Sciences* Vol. 175, pp. 3-12, ISSN 0022-510X

Estorch, M., Carrio, I. & Berna, L. (1995). Myocardial iodine-labeled metaiodobenzylguanidine 123 uptake relates to age. *Journal of Nuclear Cardiology* Vol. 2, pp. 126-132, ISSN 1071-3581

Fröhlich, I., Pilloy, W. & Vaillant, M. (2010). Myocardial MIBG scintigraphy: a useful clinical tool? : A retrospective study in 50 parkinsonian patients. *Neurological Sciences* Vol. 31, pp. 403-406, ISSN 1590-3478

Gelb, D.J., Oliver, E. & Gilman, S. (1999). Diagnostic criteria for Parkinson disease. *Archives of Neurol* Vol. 56, pp. 33-39, ISSN 0003-9942

Gilman, S., Low, P.A. & Quinn, N. (1999). Consensus statement on the diagnosis of multiple system atrophy. *Journal of Neurological Sciences,* Vol. 163, pp. 94-98, ISSN 0022-510X

Gilman, S., Wenning, G.K. & Low, P.A. (2008). Second consensus statement on the diagnosis of multiple system atrophy. *Neurology,* Vol. 71, pp. 670-676, ISSN 1526-632X

Goldstein, D.S., Holmes, C. & Cannon, R.O. III. (1997). Sympathetic cardioneuropathy in dysautonomias. *New England Journal of Medicine,* Vol.336, pp. 696-702, ISSN 0028-4793

Goldstein, D.S., Holmes, C. & Li, S-T. (2000). Cardiac sympathetic denervation in Parkinson disease. *Annals of Internal Medicine,* Vol.133, pp. 338-347, ISSN 0003-4819

Hughes, A.J., Daniel, S.E. & Kilford, L. (1992). Accuracy of clinical diagnosis of idiopathic Parkinson's disease: A clinico-pathological study of 100 cases. *Journal of Neurology, Neurosurgery, and Psychiatry,* Vol. 55, pp. 181-184, ISSN 0022-3050

Hughes, A.J., Daniel, S.E. & Blankson, S. (1993). A clinicopathologic study of 100 cases of Parkinson's disease. *Archives of Neurology,* Vol.50, pp. 140-148, ISSN 0003-9942

Iwanaga, K., Wakabayashi, K. & Yoshimoto, M. (1999). Lewy body-type degeneration in cardiac plexus in Parkinson's and incidental Lewy body diseases, *Neurology,* Vol. 52, pp. 1269-1271, ISSN 0028-3878

Jost, W.H., Del Tredici, K., & Landvogt, C. (2010). Importance of ^{123}I-metaiodobenzylguanidine scintigraphy/single photon emission computed tomography for diagnosis and differential diagnostics of Parkinson syndromes. *Neurodegenerative Diseases* Vol. 7, pp. 341-347, ISSN 1660-2862

Köllensperger, M., Seppi, K. & Liener, C. (2007). Diffusion weighted imaging best discriminates PD from MSA-P: A comparison with tilt table testing and heart MIBG scintigraphy. *Movement Disorders,* Vol. 22, pp. 1771-1776, ISSN 0885-3185

Litvan, I., Goetz, C.G. & Jankovic, J. (1997). What is the accuracy of the clinical diagnosis of multiple system atrophy? A clinicopathologic study. *Archives of Neurology,* Vol. 54, pp. 937-944, ISSN 0003-9942

McKeith, I.G., Galasko, D. & Kosaka, K. (1996). Consensus guidelines for the clinical and pathologic diagnosis of dementia with Lewy bodies (DLB): Report of the consortium on DLB international workshop. *Neurology,* Vol. 47, pp. 1113-1124, ISSN 0028-3878

Mori, H., Kondo, T., & Yokochi, M. (1998). Pathologic and biochemical studies of juvenile parkinsonism linked to chromosome 6q. *Neurology,* Vol. 51, pp. 890-892, ISSN 0028-3878

Nagayama, H., Hamamoto, M. & Ueda, M. (2005). Reliability of MIBG myocardial scintigraphy in the diagnosis of Parkinson's disease. *Journal of Neurology, Neurosurgery and Psychiatry,* Vol. 76, pp. 249-251, ISSN 0022-3050

Nagayama, H., Yamazaki, M. & Ueda, M. (2008). Low myocardial MIBG uptake in multiple system atrophy with incidental Lewy body pathology: an autopsy case report. *Movement Disorders,* Vol. 23, pp. 1055–1057, ISSN 1531-8257

Nagayama, H., Ueda, M. & Yamazaki, M. (2010). Abnormal cardiac ^{123}I-meta-iodobenzylguanidine uptake in multiple system atrophy. *Movement Disorders,* Vol. 25, pp. 1744-1747, ISSN 1531-8257

Orimo, S., Ozawa, E. & Oka, T. (2001). Different histopathology accounting for a decrease in myocardial MIBG uptake in PD and MSA. *Neurology,* Vol. 57, pp. 1140-1141, ISSN 0028-3878

Orimo, S., Ozawa, E. & Nakade, S. (1999). ^{123}I-metaiodobenzylguanidine myocardial scintigraphy in Parkinson's disease. *Journal of Neurology, Neurosurgery, and Psychiatry,* Vol. 67, pp. 189-194, ISSN 0022-3050

Orimo, S., Oka, T. & Miura, H. (2002). Sympathetic cardiac denervation in Parkinson's disease and pure autonomic failure but not in multiple system atrophy. *Journal of Neurology, Neurosurgery, and Psychiatry,* Vol. 73, pp. 776-777, ISSN 0022-3050

Orimo, S., Amino, T. & Itoh, Y. (2005). Cardiac sympathetic denervation precedes neuronal loss in the sympathetic ganglia in Lewy body disease. *Acta Neuropathologica (Berlin)* Vol. 109, pp. 583-588, ISSN 0001-6322

Orimo, S., Takahashi, A, & Uchihara, T. (2007). Degeneration of cardiac sympathetic nerve begins in the early disease process of Parkinson's disease. *Brain Pathology,* Vol. 17, pp. 24-30, ISSN 1015-6305

Orimo, S,. Uchihara, T. & Nakamura, A. (2008). Axonal α-synuclein aggregates herald centripetal degeneration of cardiac sympathetic nerve in Parkinson's disease. *Brain,* Vol. 131, pp. 642-650, ISSN 1460-2156

Osaki, Y., Wenning, G.K. & Daniel, S.E. (2002). Do published criteria improve clinical diagnostic accuracy in multiple system atrophy? *Neurology,* Vol. 59, pp. 1486-1491, ISSN 0028-3878

Paviour, D.C., Surtees, R.A. & Lees, A.J. (2004). Diagnostic considerations in juvenile parkinsonism. *Movement Disorders,* Vol. 19, pp. 123-135, ISSN 0885-3185

Quattrone, A., Bagnato, A. & Annesi, G. (2008). Myocardial ^{123}metaiodobenzylguanidine uptake in genetic Parkinson's disease. *Movement Disorders* Vol. 23, pp. 21-27, ISSN 1531-8257

Solanki, K.K., Bomanji, J. & Moyes, J. (1992). A pharmacological guide to medicines which interfere with the biodistribution of radiolabelled meta-iodobenzylguanidine (MIBG). *Nuclear Medicine Communications,* Vol.13, pp. 513-521, ISSN 0143-3636

Suchowersky, O., Reich, S. & Perlmutter, J. (2006). Practice parameter: diagnosis and prognosis of new onset Parkinson disease (an evidence-based review): report of the Quality Standards Subcommittee of the American Academy of Neurology. *Neurology,* Vol. 66, pp. 968-975, ISSN 1526-632X

Suzuki, M., Hattori, N. & Orimo, S. (2005). Preserved myocardial ^{123}I-metaiodobenzylguanidine uptake in autosomal recessive juvenile parkinsonism: First case report. *Movement Disorders,* Vol.20, pp. 634-636, ISSN 0885-3185

Suzuki, M., Kurita, A. & Hashimoto, M. (2006). Impaired myocardial ^{123}I-metaiodobenzylguanidine uptake in Lewy body disease: Comparison between dementia with Lewy bodies and Parkinson's disease. *Journal of Neurological Sciences,* Vol. 240, pp. 15-19, ISSN 0022-510X

Suzuki, M., Urashima, M. & Oka., H. (2007). Cardiac sympathetic denervation in bradykinesia-dominant Parkinson's disease. *Neuroreport,* Vol.18, pp. 1867-1870, ISSN 0959-4965

Takahashi, H., Ohama, E. & Suzuki, S. (1994). Familial juvenile parkinsonism: Clinical and pathologic study in a family. *Neurology,* Vol. 44, pp. 437-441, ISSN 0028-3878

Takatsu, H., Nishida, H. & Matsuo, H. (2000a). Cardiac sympathetic denervation from the early stage of Parkinson's disease: Clinical and experimental studies with radiolabeled MIBG. *Journal of Nuclear Medicine,* Vol. 41, pp. 71-77, ISSN 0161-5505

Takatsu, H., Nagashima, K. & Murase, M. (2000b). Differentiating Parkinson disease from multiple-system atrophy by measuring cardiac iodine-123 metaiodobenzylguanidine accumulation. *Journal of the American Medical Association,* Vol. 284, pp. 44-45, ISSN 0098-7484

Taki, J., Nakajima, K. & Hwang, E.H. (2000). Peripheral sympathetic dysfunction in patients with Parkinson's disease without autonomic failure is heart selective and disease specific. *European Journal of Nuclear Medicine,* Vol. 27, pp. 566-573, ISSN 0340-6997

Taki, J., Yoshita, M. & Yamada, M. (2004). Significance of ^{123}I-MIBG scintigraphy as a pathophysiological indicator in the assessment of Parkinson's disease and related disorders: It can be a specific marker for Lewy body disease. *Annals of Nuclear Medicine,* Vol. 18, pp. 453-461, ISSN 0914-7187

Wafelman, A.R., Hoefnagel, C.A. & Maes, R.A. (1994). Radioiodinated metaiodobenzylguanidine: A review of its biodistribution and pharmacokinetics, drug interactions, cytotoxicity and dosimetry. *European Journal of Nuclear Medicine,* Vol. 21, pp. 545-559, ISSN 0340-6997

Wakabayashi, K. & Takahashi, H. (1997). Neuropathology of autonomic nervous system in Parkinson's disease. *European Neurology,* Vol. 38, Suppl 2:2-7, ISSN 0014-3022

Watanabe, H., Ieda, T. & Katayama, T. (2001). Cardiac ^{123}I-meta-iodobenzylguanidine (MIBG) uptake in dementia with Lewy bodies: Comparison with Alzheimer's disease. *Journal of Neurology, Neurosurgery, and Psychiatry,* Vol. 70, pp.781-783, ISSN 0022-3050

Wenning, G.K., Tison, F. & Ben Shlomo, Y. (1997). Multiple system atrophy: A review of 203 pathologically proven cases. *Movement Disorders,* Vol. 12, pp. 133-147, ISSN 0885-3185

Wieland, D.M., Brown, L.E. & Rogers, W.L. (1981). Myocardial imaging with a radioiodinated norepinephrine storage analog. *Journal of Nuclear Medicine,* Vol. 22, pp. 22-31, ISSN 0161-5505

Yoshita, M. (1998). Differentiation of idiopathic Parkinson's disease from striatonigral degeneration and progressive supranuclear palsy using iodine-123 meta-iodobenzylguanidine myocardial scintigraphy. *Journal of Neurological Sciences,* Vol. 155, pp. 60-67, ISSN 0022-510X

Yoritaka, A., Shimo, Y. & Shimo, Y. (2011). Nonmotor symptoms in patients with PARK2 mutations. *Parkinson's Disease,* Vol. 2011, pp. 1-5, ISSN 2042-0080

Yoshita, M., Taki, J. & Yamada, M. (2001). A clinical role for ^{123}I-MIBG myocardial scintigraphy in the distinction between dementia of the Alzheimer's-type and dementia with Lewy bodies. *Journal of Neurology, Neurosurgery, and Psychiatry,* Vol. 71, pp. 583-588, ISSN 0022-3050